PATHWAYS OF THE PULP

PATHWAYS OF THE PULP

Edited by

Stephen Cohen, M.A., D.D.S., F.I.C.D., F.A.C.D.

Clinical Professor (Adjunct), Department of Endodontics,
University of the Pacific School of Dentistry,
San Francisco, California;
Diplomate, American Board of Endodontics

Richard C. Burns, D.D.S., F.I.C.D., F.A.C.D.

Clinical Professor (Adjunct), Department of Endodontics,
University of the Pacific School of Dentistry,
San Francisco, California;
Diplomate, American Board of Endodontics

Seventh Edition

With 40 contributors, 1703 illustrations, and 34 color plates

Principal illustrator, Richard C. Burns

*Cover image created by Richard C. Burns with
technical assistance of
Eric James Herbranson*

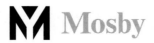

St. Louis Baltimore Boston Carlsbad Chicago Minneapolis New York Philadelphia Portland
London Milan Sydney Tokyo Toronto

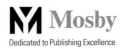
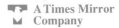

Dedicated to Publishing Excellence

A Times Mirror
Company

Publisher: Don Ladig
Executive Editor: Linda Duncan
Editor: Penny Rudolph
Project Manager: Mark Spann
Production Editor: Steve Hetager
Book Design Manager: Judi Lang
Manufacturing Supervisor: Karen Boehme

SEVENTH EDITION

Composition by The Clarinda Co.
Printing/binding by Maple-Vail Press

Mosby, Inc.
11830 Westline Industrial Drive
St. Louis, Missouri 64146

ISBN 0-8151-8613-4

98 99 00 01 02 / 9 8 7 6 5 4 3 2

Contributors

Robert E. Averbach, D.D.S., F.I.C.D., F.A.C.D.
President's Teaching Scholar,
Dean and Professor of Endodontics,
University of Colorado School of Dentistry,
Denver, Colorado

Scott K. Bentkover, D.D.S.
Clinical Assistant Professor,
Director of Endodontic Microscopy,
Department of Endodontics,
University of Illinois College of Dentistry,
Chicago, Illinois

Cecil E. Brown, Jr., M.S., D.D.S.
Director, Graduate Endodontics,
Associate Professor, Endodontic Section,
Department of Restorative Dentistry,
Indiana University School of Dentistry,
Indianapolis, Indiana

David Clifford Brown, B.D.S., M.D.S., M.S.D.
Assistant Professor,
Department of Endodontics,
University of the Pacific School of Dentistry,
San Francisco, California

Richard C. Burns, D.D.S., F.I.C.D., F.A.C.D.
Clinical Professor (Adjunct),
Department of Endodontics,
University of the Pacific School of Dentistry,
San Francisco, California;
Diplomate, American Board of Endodontics

Joe H. Camp, D.D.S., M.S.D.
Adjunct Associate Professor,
Department of Endodontics,
University of North Carolina School of Dentistry,
Chapel Hill, North Carolina

Gary B. Carr, D.D.S.
Founder and Director,
Pacific Endodontic Research Foundation,
San Diego, California;
Lecturer,
University of California at Los Angeles,
Los Angeles, California;
Consultant in Endodontics,
VA Medical Center Long Beach,
Long Beach, California;
Diplomate, American Board of Endodontics

Noah Chivian, D.D.S., F.A.C.D., F.I.C.D.
Adjunct Associate Professor,
Department of Endodontics,
University of Pennsylvania School of Dentistry,
Philadelphia, Pennsylvania;
Director of Dentistry,
Newark Beth Israel Medical Center,
Newark, New Jersey;
Diplomate, American Board of Endodontics

A. Scott Cohen, D.D.S., B.D.Sc.
Clinical Assistant Professor,
Department of Endodontics,
University of the Pacific School of Dentistry,
San Francisco, California

Stephen Cohen, M.A., D.D.S., F.I.C.D., F.A.C.D.
Clinical Professor (Adjunct),
Department of Endodontics,
University of the Pacific School of Dentistry,
San Francisco, California;
Diplomate, American Board of Endodontics

Samuel O. Dorn, D.D.S.
Director, Postgraduate Endodontics,
Department of Endodontics,
Nova Southeastern University School of Dental Medicine,
Ft. Lauderdale, Florida;
Diplomate, American Board of Endodontics

Lewis R. Eversole, M.A., M.S.D., D.D.S.
Professor of Oral Diagnostic Sciences and Orofacial Pain,
UCLA School of Dentistry,
Los Angeles, California;
Oral and Maxillofacial Pathology,
Pathology Consultants of New Mexico,
Roswell and Santa Fe, New Mexico

Arnold H. Gartner, D.D.S., F.I.C.D.
Clinical Associate Professor,
Department of Endodontics,
University of Detroit Mercy School of Dentistry,
Detroit, Michigan;
Diplomate, American Board of Endodontics

Gerald Neal Glickman, M.S., M.B.A., D.D.S.
Clinical Professor and Director of Endodontics,
Department of Cariology, Restorative Sciences, and
    Endodontics,
Universty of Michigan School of Dentistry,
Ann Arbor, Michigan;
Diplomate, American Board of Endodontics

Alan H. Gluskin, D.D.S., F.I.C.D., F.A.C.D.
Professor and Chairman,
Department of Endodontics,
University of the Pacific School of Dentistry,
San Francisco, California

James L. Gutmann, D.D.S.
Professor and Program Director—Graduate Endodontics,
Department of Restorative Sciences,
The Texas A & M University System—Dallas;
Baylor College of Dentistry,
Dallas, Texas;
Diplomate, American Board of Endodontics

Kenneth M. Hargreaves, D.D.S., Ph.D.
Professor and Chairman,
Department of Endodontics,
Professor, Department of Pharmacology,
University of Texas Health Science Center,
San Antonio, Texas

Eric James Herbranson, M.S., D.D.S.
Assistant Professor (Adjunct)
Department of Endodontics,
University of the Pacific School of Dentistry,
San Francisco, California

William T. Johnson, D.D.S., M.S.
Director, Advanced Education Program in Endodontics,
Department of Endodontics,
University of Iowa College of Dentistry,
Iowa City, Iowa

James D. Kettering, B.A., M.S., Ph.D.
Professor of Microbiology,
Department of Microbiology and Molecular Genetics,
Loma Linda University Schools of Medicine and Dentistry,
Loma Linda, California

Syngcuk Kim, D.D.S., Ph.D.
L.I. Grossman Professor and Chairman,
Department of Endodontics,
School of Dental Medicine,
University of Pennsylvania,
Philadelphia, Pennsylvania

Donald J. Kleier, D.M.D., F.A.C.D., F.I.C.D.
Professor of Endodontics,
President's Teaching Scholar,
Department of Surgical Dentistry,
University of Colorado School of Dentistry,
Denver, Colorado

Stanley F. Malamed, D.D.S.
Professor and Chair,
Section of Anesthesia and Medicine,
University of Southern California School of Dentistry,
Los Angeles, California

Kathy I. Mueller, D.M.D.
Assistant Professor,
Department of Fixed Prosthodontics,
University of the Pacific School of Dentistry,
San Francisco, California;
Diplomate, American Board of Prosthodontics

Carl W. Newton, D.D.S., M.S.D.
Professor,
Department of Restorative Dentistry,
Indiana University School of Dentistry,
Indianapolis, Indiana;
Diplomate, American Board of Endodontics

James B. Roane, B.S., M.S., D.D.S., D.A.B.E., F.A.C.D.
Professor, Department of Endodontics,
University of Oklahoma College of Dentistry,
Oklahoma City, Oklahoma;
Diplomate, American Board of Endodontics

Ilan Rotstein, C.D.
Associate Professor and Acting Chairman,
Department of Endodontics,
Hebrew University—Hadassah Faculty of Dental Medicine,
Jerusalem, Israel

Asgeir Sigurdsson, Cand. Odont., M.S.
Assistant Professor,
Department of Endodontics,
University of North Carolina School of Dentistry,
Chapel Hill, North Carolina

James H.S. Simon, A.B., D.D.S., F.I.C.D., F.A.C.D.
Chief, Endodontic Section,
Veterans Administration Medical Center,
Long Beach, California;
Professor of Endodontics,
Loma Linda University School of Dentistry,
Loma Linda, California;
Clinical Associate Professor of Endodontics,
University of Southern California School of Dentistry,
Los Angeles, California;
Diplomate, American Board of Endodontics

Larz S.W. Spångberg, D.D.S., Ph.D.
Professor and Head,
Department of Restorative Dentistry and Endodontology,
University of Connecticut Health Center,
School of Dental Medicine,
Farmington, Connecticut

Mahmoud Torabinejad, D.M.D., M.S.D., Ph.D.
Professor of Endodontics,
Director of Graduate Endodontics,
Department of Endodontics,
Loma Linda University School of Dentistry,
Loma Linda, California

Martin Trope, D.M.D., F.I.C.D., F.A.C.D.
Professor and Chair,
Department of Endodontics,
University of North Carolina at Chapel Hill,
School of Dentistry,
Chapel Hill, North Carolina

Henry O. Trowbridge, D.D.S., Ph.D.
Emeritus Professor of Pathology,
University of Pennsylvania School of Dental Medicine,
Philadelphia, Pennsylvania

Galen W. Wagnild, D.D.S.
Associate Clinical Professor,
Department of Restorative Dentistry,
University of California, San Francisco,
School of Dentistry,
San Francisco, California;
Diplomate, American Board of Prosthodontics

Richard E. Walton, M.S., D.M.D.
Professor,
Department of Endodontics,
University of Iowa College of Dentistry,
Iowa City, Iowa

John David West, D.D.S., M.S.D.
Clinical Associate Professor,
Department of Endodontics,
University of Washington School of Dentistry,
Seattle, Washington;
Clinical Instructor,
Department of Endodontics,
Boston University,
Goldman School of Graduate Dentistry,
Boston, Massachusetts

Lisa R. Wilcox, M.S., D.D.S.
Associate Professor,
Department of Endodontics,
University of Iowa College of Dentistry,
Iowa City, Iowa

David E. Witherspoon, B.D.S., M.S.
Assistant Professor,
Department of Restorative Sciences,
The Texas A & M University System—Dallas;
Baylor College of Dentistry,
Dallas, Texas

Edwin J. Zinman, D.D.S., J.D.
Former Lecturer, Department of Periodontics,
University of California, San Francisco,
School of Dentistry,
San Francisco, California

This seventh edition is dedicated to
Dr. Nguyen Thanh Nguyen,
selfless teacher, master clinician, and
elegant role model for all who aspire
to heal and to help others.

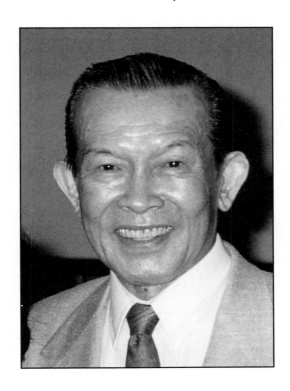

Preface

This, the seventh edition of *Pathways of the Pulp*, has been developed around a major transition occurring in endodontics, the arrival of the digital age. Not only do many of the chapters discuss exciting clinical applications of digital technologies, but, when appropriate, chapter references are linked by Medline to the National Library of Medicine.

It is our belief that clinical excellence today depends upon a commitment to lifelong learning. Every chapter in the book has been either rewritten or substantially revised. The chapters discussing bleaching, retreatment, pharmacology, trauma, obturation, and instruments and materials are new chapters. The latest devices, including digital radiography and rotary filing systems, are fully illustrated, described, and evaluated. New concepts in clinical practice, such as using enlarging files as disposal instruments, are part of the expanded analysis of what will make endodontics even more effective. New nonnarcotic but highly effective pain control medications are evaluated, and new instruments for shaping and sealing root canals are introduced to the reader. As in previous editions, the most current information about the evolving legal definitions of standard of care and ethical guidelines for standard of excellence are included.

Our question sections and the answer section have been replaced by the Challenge at the end of the book, which facilitates broader self-testing. Our emphasis on the uses of microscopy in endodontic therapy reflects our assessment of the primary new directions that the practice of endodontics will take in the next five years. Not only will the microscope and its applications become central to clinical practice by the end of the decade, but the use of enhanced illumination and imaging techniques will become integral to the standard of excellent care.

As in earlier editions, this edition of *Pathways* is built around the belief that accurate diagnosis is the foundation for all effective and successful endodontic treatment. In summary, this seventh edition of *Pathways of the Pulp* is offered to dental students as a comprehensive learning tool, and to practicing clinicians as a support in their continued pursuit of endodontic excellence.

The publication of the seventh edition marks another transition as well, the retirement of our erudite and devoted developmental editor, Ms. Melba Steube. Ms. Steube has organized and overseen with rare skill the development of every edition of *Pathways of the Pulp*. We are deeply grateful for Ms. Steube's support of us, and we will miss her.

We are grateful for the selfless work of all of our excellent authors, whose own deep commitment to learning is reflected in their contributions. Our special thanks to Ms. Katherine Brennan for her wonderful administrative support and to our superb editors, Ms. Linda Duncan and Ms. Penny Rudolph.

Stephen Cohen
Richard C. Burns

Contents

PART ONE

THE ART OF ENDODONTICS

Chapter 1

Diagnostic Procedures

Stephen Cohen

THE ART AND SCIENCE OF DIAGNOSIS

Diagnosis is the "determination of the nature of a diseased condition . . . by careful investigation of its symptoms and history."[7] The sophisticated technology available to clinicians today can support sound diagnostic procedures. However, technology does not alter the fundamental nature of diagnosis as a process of active listening, precise observation, and genuine curiosity about the source of the presenting signs and symptoms. An accurate diagnosis is the result of the synthesis of scientific knowledge, clinical experience, intuition, and common sense. It is both an art and a science.

A good diagnostician is a clinician who has learned the fundamentals of gathering and interpreting clinical information, testing thoroughly, and asking appropriate questions. Systematic recording of the patient's responses to the clinician's tests and inquiries is essential for diagnostic success. The facts about the patient's medical history and dental history, the details of the presenting signs and symptoms, and careful gathering of test results are the analytic core of clinical diagnosis. A chronically inflamed or diseased pulp is a nonurgent condition that will almost always be identified through conscientious application of this protocol.

There are instances, however, when a patient has intense pain, conflicting signs and symptoms, or inconsistent responses to clinical testing. Chapter 2 explores the ways and means to treat these endodontic emergencies, and Chapter 3 explores diagnosis of ostensible "toothache" of nonodontogenic origin.

Medical History

A recent, well-organized record of medical history is a critical part of the picture of the patient that a clinician always needs to create. Although the only systemic contraindications to endodontic therapy are uncontrolled diabetes or a very recent myocardial infarction,[16] only the patient's medical history enables the clinician to determine the need for a medical consultation or premedication of the patient. Completion of a pre-printed, succinct, comprehensive medical history form is mandatory, and it represents the standard of care (Fig. 1-1).

Some patients require antibiotic prophylaxis before clinical examination because of systemic conditions such as heart valve replacement, a history of rheumatic fever, or advanced acquired immunodeficiency syndrome (AIDS).[16] Patients taking daily anticoagulant medications such as warfarin (Coumadin) may need a dosage reduction or suspension of the drug before the periodontal examination, which is integral to a complete endodontic diagnostic workup. Additional barrier protection can be provided to all clinical personnel if the patient's medical history reveals infection with communicable diseases such as hepatitis B or tuberculosis.[8]

An aging population results in an increasing number of patients with continuing disease processes. Before rendering endodontic therapy, the clinician must know what drugs the patient is using to identify possible adverse drug interactions. Such cases mandate consultation with the treating physician. The permanent patient record should include a summary of any conversations with other treating dentists and with treating physicians and an outline of any care recommendations.

Dental History

Although the medical history provides the clinician with the basic health context in which to evaluate the patient's needs, the dental history offers the mechanism for identifying the patient's chief complaint. The patient's completion of the dental history, also an organized, preprinted form, offers the patient the first opportunity to record his or her experiences in a cogent, meaningful way. A report of this kind gives the patient a voice in the process of diagnosis, and it affords the clinician initial information about the patient's signs and symptoms, the duration of the problem, and the patient's own experience of what leads to relief or an increase in symptoms. The dental history form accelerates the clinician's determination of the patient's main concerns (Fig. 1-2).

*LAST NAME*_____ *FIRST NAME*_____

How would you rate your health? Please circle one.　　　　　Excellent　Good　Fair　Poor

*When did you have your last physical exam?*_____

If you are under the care of a physician, please give reason(s) for treatment.

_____

Physician's Name, Address and Telephone Number:

*Name*_____*Address*_____

*City*_____*State*_____*Zip*_____*Telephone*_____

Have you ever had any kind of surgery?　　　　　　　　　Yes___ No___

*If yes, what kind?*_____*Date*_____

_____*Date*_____

Have you ever had any trouble with prolonged bleeding after surgery?　Yes___ No___
Do you wear a pacemaker or any other kind of prosthetic device?　Yes___ No___
Are you taking any kind of medication, or drugs at this time?　　Yes___ No___

If yes, please give name(s) of the medicine(s) and reason(s) for taking them:

*Name*_____*Reason*_____

_____

Have you ever had an unusual reaction to an anesthetic or drug (like penicillin)? Yes___No___

*If yes, please explain:*_____

Please circle any past or present illness you have had:

Alcoholism	Blood Pressure	Epilepsy	Hepatitis	Kidney or Liver	Rheumatic Fever
Allergies	Cancer	Glaucoma	Herpes	Mental	Sinusitis
Anemia	Diabetes	Head/Neck Injuries	Immunodeficiency	Migraine	Ulcers
Asthma	Drug Dependency	Heart Disease	Infectious Diseases	Respiratory	Veneral Disease

Are you allergic to Latex or any other substances or materials?　　Yes___No___

*If so, please explain*_____

If female, are you pregnant?　　　　　　　　　　　Yes___No___

*Is there any other information that should be known about your health?*_____

_____

*Signed: Patient or Parent*_____*Date:*_____

FIG. 1-1 Succinct, comprehensive medical history form designed to gather information that may have relevance to the final diagnosis.

*LAST NAME*_____*FIRST NAME*_____

1. *Are you experiencing any pain at this time? If not , please go to question 6.*　Yes___ No___
2. *If yes, can you locate the tooth that is causing the pain?*　Yes___ No___
3. *When did you first notice the symptoms?*_____
4. *Did your symptoms occur suddenly, or gradually?*_____

Please check the frequency and quality of the discomfort, and the number that most closely reflects the intensity of your pain:

LEVEL OF INTENSITY (On a scale of 1 to 10) 1= Mild 10=Severe	FREQUENCY	QUALITY
1__2__3__4__5__6__7__8__9__10__	___ Constant	__ Sharp
	___Intermittent	__ Dull
	___Momentary	___Throbbing
	___Occasional	

Is there anything you can do to relieve the pain?　　Yes____ No___

*If yes, what?*_____

Is there anything you can do to cause the pain to increase?　Yes____ No___

*If yes, what?*_____

When eating or drinking, is your tooth sensitive to:　Heat____ Cold____ Sweets____

Does your tooth hurt when you bite down, or chew?　　Yes___ No___

Does it hurt if you press the gum tissue around this tooth?　Yes___ No___

Does a change in posture (lying down or bending over) cause your tooth to hurt? Yes___ No___

6. *Do you grind, or clench your teeth?*　　　　　Yes___ No___
7. *If yes, do you wear a night guard?*　　　　　Yes___ No___
8. *Has a restoration (filling or crown) been placed on this tooth recently?*　Yes___ No___
9. *Prior to this appointment, has root canal therapy been initiated on this tooth?*　Yes___ No___
10. *Is there anything else we should know about your teeth, gums or sinuses that would assist us in our diagnosis?*_____

*Signed: Patient or Parent*_____*Date*_____

FIG. 1-2 Dental history form designed to expedite the gathering of information about the patient's symptoms.

The most effective way for the clinician to reconfirm the patient's descriptions of his or her main concern and to evaluate their accuracy is the use of directed relevant questions that build on those that make up the dental history. It is useful to begin with a general question regarding the chief complaint: "Can you tell me about your problem?" This question should be followed by several more specific questions regarding the following:

- inception: "When did you first notice this?"
- provoking factors: "Do heat, cold, biting, or chewing cause pain?"
- attenuating factors: "Does anything relieve the pain? Drinking warm or cold liquids? Lying down or sitting up?"
- frequency: "How often does this pain occur?"
- intensity: "When you have this pain, is it mild, moderate, or severe?"

Careful, sensitive listening to the patient's responses to these queries allows the clinician to develop a narrative description of the patient's chief complaint.

Symptomatic patients, most of whom have obvious problems of pain or swelling, should be led through an additional series of questions that will identify the urgency of the problem. These questions should be phrased to encourage the patient to expand the information already given. These include questions that address the following:

- location: "Could you point to the tooth that hurts or to the area that you feel is swelling?"

- duration: "When heat (or cold) causes pain, is the pain momentary, or does it last longer?"
- postural: "Do you have any pain when you lie down or bend over?"
- stimulated or spontaneous: "Does the pain ever occur without provocation?"
- quality: "What is the nature of the pain? Sharp? Dull? Stabbing? Throbbing?"

The application of the techniques of active listening to the patient's verbal responses to all these questions enables the clinician to sort them into the elements of a preliminary diagnosis. When the clinician uses the dental history form (see Fig. 1-2), many of the questions included in the preceding list may have already been answered by the patient, thereby allowing the clinician to identify the source more quickly. This important dialogue between the patient and the clinician is the first diagnostic step. It is essential to the development of the patient's trust in the openness and receptivity of the clinician, and it guides the selection and sequence of the second diagnostic step, clinical examination.

The most fundamental rule to follow in gathering the dental history is to be appropriate to the presenting clinical situation. If, for example, the clinician observes a grossly decayed tooth or a fractured crown while speaking with the patient, the dental history should be brief and focus on only those questions relevant to the obvious problem. If the patient has severe, acute symptoms at the time of the diagnosis, the gathering of the dental history should be abbreviated to allow prompt action to relieve the patient's pain. If the diagnosis is elusive, even after all the questions regarding the patient's dental history have been asked and answered, additional targeted questions (as described in Chapter 2), should be posed to the patient.

Pain

Frequently dental pain is the result of an inflamed or degenerating pulp. This is the most common symptom offered by patients in need of diagnosis.[3,19] In general, this source of pain is revealed through the dental history, inspection of the tooth, clinical examination, and diagnostic testing. Despite the straightforward nature of this most frequent symptom and its source, the psychobiologic components of pain (i.e., physical, emotional, pain tolerance level) can make the diagnostic process challenging. Pain perception is an area especially susceptible to patient misinterpretation. Fear and other psychologic conditioning can lead to a perception of pain that is out of proportion to the stimulus appplied. Nevertheless, the majority of patients who have a complaint of pain that is determined to be of odontogenic origin will be diagnosed with irreversible pulpitis, with or without partial necrosis.[3,19]

The accuracy and precision of the patient's description of pain depends on whether the inflammatory state is limited to the pulp tissue. If the inflammation has not reached the periodontal ligament, it may be difficult for the patient to localize the pain.[3,9,22] Because the neural portion of the pulp contains sensory fibers that will transmit only pain, the patient may describe the pain with such terms as *sharp, dull, continuous, intermittent, mild,* or *severe.* However, the periodontal ligament also contains proprioceptive sensory fibers. Therefore, when the inflammatory process extends beyond the apical foramen and affects the periodontal ligament, it will be easier for the patient to identify the source of the pain. In this instance percussion and chewing tests can be used to corroborate the patient's perception of the source of the pain.

Pain can also be referred to other areas of the mouth and even to the neck or temple area. It is most common for referred pain to manifest in the adjacent teeth or in the opposing quadrant.[3,9,22] It is rare for odontogenic pain to cross the midline of the head. Referred pain may also be ipsilaterally referred to the preauricular area, down the neck, or up to the temple. In these instances a posterior tooth is almost always the source of the referred pain. Chapter 3 discusses ostensible toothache of nonodontogenic origin (i.e., from neurologic, cardiac, vascular, mental, malignant, or sinus diseases).

Patients may report that their dental pain is exacerbated by lying down or bending over. This change occurs because of the increase in blood pressure to the head, which in turn increases pressure on the inflamed, confined pulp.[9]

In some cases emotional disorders can manifest as dental pain. If no organic cause for the presenting dental pain can be found, the patient should be referred to a pain clinic or to a physician for medical consultation. Patients with atypical facial pain of nonodontogenic origin may begin their long journey through the many specialties of the health sciences in the dentist's office.

If the clinician can reproduce and relieve the patient's pain through clinical testing, it is certain that the pain is of odontogenic origin. Patients with pain will often gain immeasurable psychologic comfort when the clinician provides sincere reassurance that, once the source is discovered, appropriate treatment will be provided immediately to stop the pain.

EXAMINATION AND TESTING

The extraoral visual examination of the patient should begin while the clinician is taking the patient's history. Speaking with the patient affords the clinician the opportunity to observe the patient's facial features. This external observation should be organized as meticulously as all the other portions of the examination. A consistent step-by-step approach helps the clinician develop diagnostic discipline and good examination habits. A careful, methodical approach also minimizes the possibility that significant information will be overlooked.

In observing the patient during this part of the examination, the dentist should look for facial asymmetry (Fig. 1-3, *A*) or distentions that might indicate swelling of odontogenic origin or even a systemic ailment. The patient's eyes should be observed for pupillary dilation or constriction, which may signal systemic disease, premedication, or fear. The patient's skin should be checked for the presence of any lesion(s). If more than one lesion is found, it should be noted whether the lesions appear randomly or follow one of the branches of the trigeminal nerve. Occasionally facial lesions (e.g., a sinus tract draining through the skin) can be traced to a tooth as the source.

After completing a thorough extraoral visual examination of the patient, the clinician should proceed with an oral examination. The necessary tools for a comprehensive oral examination include two mouth mirrors, 2 × 2–inch gauze, cotton rolls, a saliva ejector, a headlamp, and good magnification (Fig. 1-3, *B* and *C*). Abnormalities are easier to see in dry oral issue, so this portion of the examination should begin with drying the first quadrant under examination with 2 × 2–inch gauze. The clinician should look for signs of caries, toothbrush abrasion (Fig. 1-3, *D*), darkened teeth (Fig. 1-3, *E*), observable swelling (Fig. 1-3, *F*), fractured teeth (Fig. 1-3, *G*), and defective restorations. In addition, the clinician should be alert for signs of abrasion, attrition, cervical erosion, or developmental defects (e.g., external tubercles, lingual grooves) (Fig. 1-7, *G* to *I*).

As in the extraoral visual examination, a high index of suspicion will lead the clinician to thorough, patient-sensitive completion of the oral examination. Any unusual changes in the color or contour of the soft tissues should be noted. For example, the clinician should look carefully for lesions of odontogenic origin, such as sinus tracts (fistulas) (Fig. 1-3, *H*) or localized redness or swelling involving the attachment apparatus. Generally, sinus tracts indicate necrosis and periapical suppuration that has burrowed its way from the cancellous bone, through the cortical plate and mucoperiosteum, and finally to the mucosal surface. All sinus tracts should be traced with a gutta-percha cone (Fig. 1-3, *I*) to locate their source no matter how remote[22] (Fig. 1-3, *J* and *K*).

Palpation

Palpation testing is an important element of the oral examination. Palpation is a tactile skill acquired through practice and repetition. Certain clinical situations are primarily evident only during palpation testing. When periapical inflammation develops after pulp necrosis, the inflammatory process may burrow its way through the facial cortical bone and begin to affect the overlying mucoperiosteum. Before incipient swelling becomes

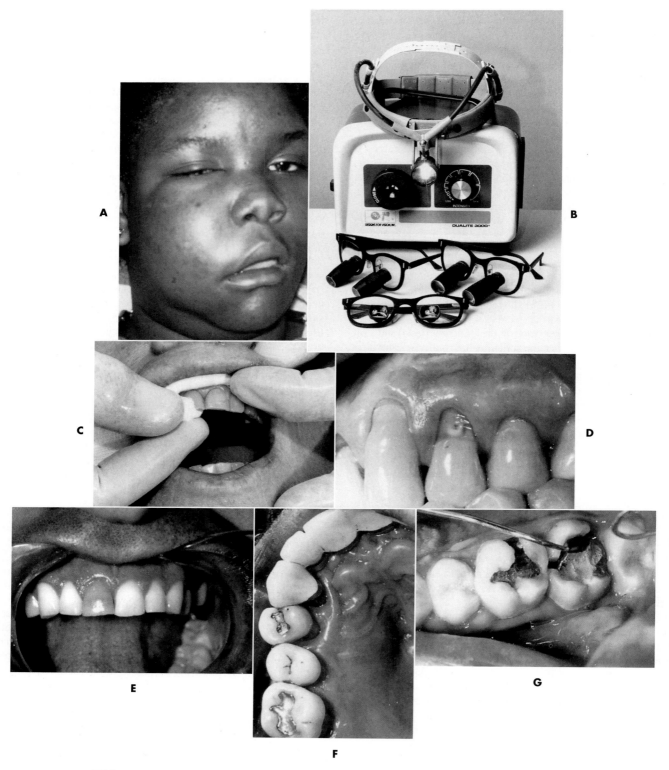

FIG. 1-3 A, While talking with the patient during the gathering of the medical and dental histories, look for facial asymmetry and alertness. When there is evident suffering, the patient appreciates brevity, when it is possible. **B,** Designs for Vision fiberoptic headlamp and 2.5× to 4.5× magnifying telescopes allow the clinician to examine the soft tissues and teeth without shadows. **C,** A thorough clinical examination is facilitated by drying the tissues with gauze and cotton rolls. **D,** Toothbrush abrasion or Class V caries is most likely to be detected during the visual examination. **E,** Tooth discolored after a football injury. Before a diagnosis is made, vitality tests should be conducted, because a discolored tooth may remain vital. **F,** Intraoral swelling is most commonly found on the facial side; however, occasionally it may appear on the lingual side or, as seen here, on the palate. **G,** Careful clinical examination may reveal crown fractures that might not be detected radiographically.

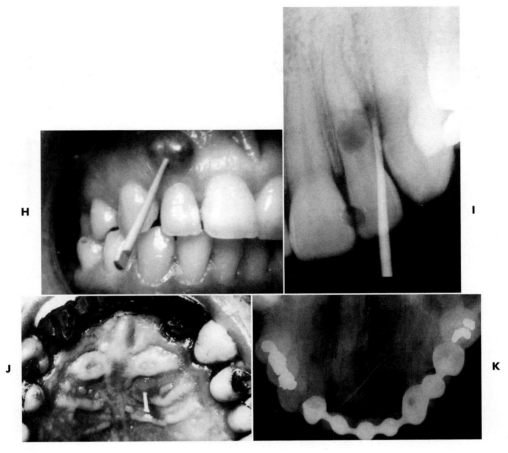

FIG. 1-3, cont'd H, Whenever a sinus tract is found, it should be traced with a gutta-percha cone to its source, **I. J,** Palatal sinus tract traced with a gutta-percha cone. **K,** Occlusal jaw film revealed the remote source as a contralateral cuspid.

clinically evident, it may be detected by gentle palpation with the index finger (Fig. 1-4, *A*). The index finger is rolled while the mucosa is pressed against the underlying cortical bone. If the mucoperiosteum is inflamed, this rolling motion will locate the extent of inflammation.

Occasionally a patient will point to a particular facial area that feels tender during shaving or applying makeup. This information may guide the clinician in locating the source through palpation of the mucofacial fold. If a mandibular tooth is abscessed, for example, it is prudent to palpate the submandibular area bimanually (Fig. 1-4, *B*) to determine whether any submandibular lymph nodes have been affected by the disease process. The patient's responses to this palpation will indicate the extent of the disease process.

Percussion

The percussion test is essential to a comprehensive oral examination. Although the percussion test does *not* indicate the health or integrity of the pulp, it does reveal inflammation in the periapical region, specifically, inflammation of the apical part of the periodontal ligament.

Before testing is performed, the patient should be instructed about the purpose of the test and how to communicate if any tenderness is felt during the test. Most commonly, patients may communicate by either raising a hand or making a soft audible sound. The patient should first be made aware of normal sensation by initial percussion of the teeth on the contralateral side of the mouth. When the patient is familiar with the normal sensation of percussion, the dentist should test the area being examined.

Because digital percussion is less painful than percussion with the handle of the mouth mirror, the first percussion test should be performed with the clinician's finger (Fig. 1-5, *A*). The teeth should be randomly (out of sequence) tapped in all directions so that the patient will be unable to anticipate the percussion of the suspect tooth. If the patient is unable to discern a difference in sensation with digital percussion, then the blunt handle of a mouth mirror should be used. Each tooth should be percussed on the facial, occlusal, and lingual sides (Fig. 1-5, *B*).

Part of the skill acquisition of percussion testing is learning the proper amount of force to be applied. Percussing the tooth too strongly can cause unnecessary pain and anxiety for the patient. The clinician must determine the amount of force to be applied. The force of percussion needs to be strong enough only for the patient to discern a difference between a sound tooth and a tooth with an inflamed periodontal ligament. The sensitivity of the proprioceptive fibers in an inflamed periodontal ligament will aid the clinician in identifying the source of the pain.

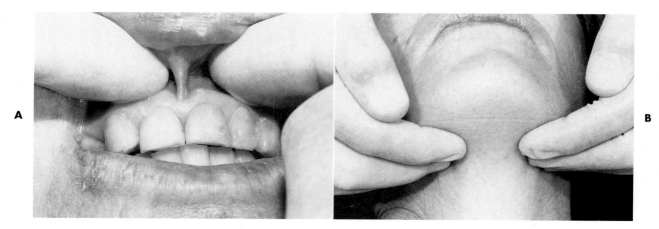

FIG. 1-4 A, Palpation test. With index finger, gently press the mucosa at the mucofacial fold. Search for a spongy or indurated area or a site that elicits tenderness when palpated. If any tenderness is located, the degree of tenderness (+ = mild pain, ++ = moderate pain, +++ = severe pain) should be recorded. Palpating the same area contralaterally helps identify the normal range for each patient. **B,** Bimanual extraoral palpation to tactilely locate swollen submandibular or cervical lymph nodes. A swollen lymph node pressed against the ramus or between two fingers will also feel tender to the patient.

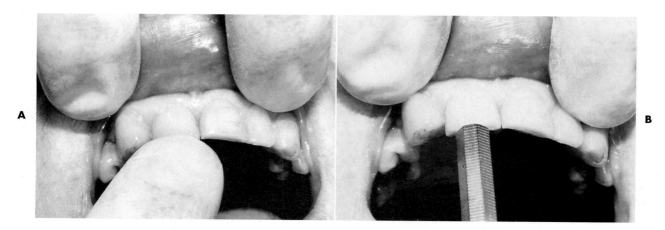

FIG. 1-5 A, Percussion test. If part of the chief complaint is pain with biting or chewing, percussion testing should begin with the index finger tapping the incisal or occlusal surface to avoid unnecessary pain. **B,** If no pain is elicited with digital percussion, a more definitive percussion test can be conducted with the handle of a mouth mirror. If a tooth is found to be tender to percussion, record the degree of pain as described in Fig. 1-4, *A*.

A positive response to percussion indicates not only the presence of inflammation of the periodontal ligament but also the degree of the inflammation. The degree of response is directly proportional to the degree of inflammation. If the pulp inflammation extends beyond the apical foramen, or if the bacterial endotoxins have spilled out beyond the apical foramen, the periodontal ligament will be irritated and an inflammatory response will occur.[2,18,19] Rapid orthodontic movement of teeth, a recently placed restoration in hyperocclusion, or a lateral periodontal abscess may also inflame the periodontal ligament. Where chronic periapical inflammation is present, percussion testing often yields a negative result.

Mobility

Tooth mobility is directly proportional to the integrity of the attachment apparatus (i.e., periodontal disease) or to the extent of inflammation of the periodontal ligament resulting from pulpal inflammation or degeneration. The clinician should use two mouth-mirror handles to apply alternating lateral forces in a facial-lingual direction to observe the degree of mobility of the tooth (Fig. 1-6). The degree of depressibility of the tooth within its alveolus should also be tested by pressing the tooth into its socket and watching for any vertical movement.

First-degree mobility is less than 1 mm of horizontal movement. Second-degree mobility is about 1 mm of horizontal

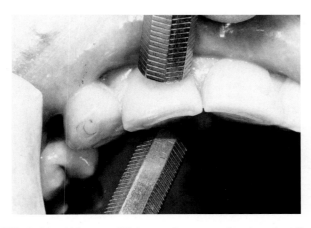

FIG. 1-6 Mobility test. With use of two mouth-mirror handles, apply alternating lateral forces in a facial-lingual direction. Record the degree of any mobility detected.

movement. Third-degree mobility is greater than 1 mm of horizontal movement accompanied by vertical depressibility.

The pressure exerted by the purulent exudate of an acute apical abscess may cause some transient mobility of a tooth.[2,14,22] This mobility is quickly relieved by the establishment of drainage for the exudate. Horizontal root fracture in the coronal half of the tooth, very recent trauma, chronic bruxism, and overzealous orthodontic treatment are also causes of tooth mobility.

Radiographs

Although periapical radiographs cannot be used exclusively for endodontic diagnosis, they are an essential aid to the determination of the source of presenting signs and symptoms. The clinician will need to take any series of films necessary to lead to a full picture of the tooth or teeth involved. These films may include panographs, lateral jaw radiographs, occlusal radiographs, or bite-wing films. Because anatomic aberrations can be misinterpreted, when there is any doubt about the diagnosis, a contralateral exposure of the same type of radiograph is a prudent step. A radiolucency, for example, will not begin to manifest until demineralization extends into the cortical plate of the bone.[4,6,11] A contralateral exposure will reveal this condition. Unfortunately, a few clinicians rely exclusively on radiographs in attempting to arrive at a diagnosis; this naiveté often leads to misdiagnosis and mistreatment.

A high-quality radiograph requires good technique—proper placement, exposure, and processing. High-quality radiographs provide the foundation for accurate interpretation. However, because a radiograph is a two-dimensional image of a three-dimensional tooth, radiographic strategy should involve the exposure of two films at the same vertical angulation but with a 10 to 15-degree change in horizontal angulation. This approach enables the clinician to construct a three-dimensional mental model of the anatomic and possible pathologic features. Examination of the dry films with appropriate magnification and background illumination is critical to accurate radiographic interpretation. Chapters 2 and 5 offer a more extended discussion of the particulars of dental radiology.

The status of the health and integrity of the pulp cannot be determined by radiographic images alone. However, the dis-covery of deep caries, pulp caps, extensive restorations, pulpotomies, pulp stones, extensive canal calcification, resorption, radiolucences at or near the apex, root fractures, a thickened periodontal ligament, and periodontal disease that has caused bone loss should heighten the clinician's suspicion of inflammatory or degenerative pulp changes.

Radiographic interpretation

The interpretation of high-quality pretreatment periapical radiographs must be conducted in a consistent, orderly way. The crown, the root(s), and the root canal system must all be closely studied. The following questions should guide the clinician's examination of the radiographs:

- Is the lamina dura intact, or is there a loss of the lamina dura?
- Is the bony architecture within normal limits, or is there evidence of demineralization?
- Is the root canal system within normal limits, or does it appear to be resorbing or calcifying?
- What anatomic landmarks could be expected in this area?
- Are these films clear, or are additional films needed?

A sound, correct examination protocol includes the process of answering each of these questions thoroughly and carefully.

It is often helpful to prepare bite-wing films in addition to periapical films in the posterior region. Early caries, the depth of existing restorations, pulp caps, and pulpotomies, or dens invaginitus or dens evaginatus can be more easily identified in bite-wing films. Deep caries or extensive restorations increase the likelihood of pulpal involvement. A single root canal should appear tapering from crown to apex; a sudden change in appearance of the canal from dark to light indicates that the canal has bifurcated or trifurcated (Fig. 1-7, *A*). The presence of "extra" roots or canals is much more common than was previously thought.[15,22] The clinician should always carry the suspicion of the presence of "extra" canals. Three-rooted mandibular molars (Fig. 1-7, *B*) and maxillary premolars and two-rooted mandibular canines and incisors (Fig. 1-7, *C*) will be found with greater frequency as the clinician's understanding of anatomy, index of suspicion, and diagnostic sophistication improve.

A necrotic pulp will not cause radiographic changes until the metabolic breakdown products of pulp degeneration or bacterial toxins have begun to demineralize the cortical plate. For this reason significant medullary bone destruction may occur before any radiographic signs start to appear. Toxins and other irritants may exit through a lateral canal, causing periradicular (rather than periapical) demineralization. Conversely, a lateral canal can also be a portal of entry for harmful toxins in teeth affected by periodontal disease (Fig. 1-7, *C* and *D*).

Pulp stones and canal calcifications are not necessarily pathologic; they can also be the result of normal aging of the pulp.[19] Consequently, in the absence of any additional signs or any symptoms, the presence of pulp stones or canal calcification should not be interpreted as pulpal disorders requiring endodontic therapy.

Internal resorption (commonly resulting from trauma) is an indication for endodontic therapy (Fig. 1-7, *E*). The inflamed pulp, asymptomatically expanding at the expense of the surrounding dentin, must be removed as soon as possible to avoid a pathologic perforation of the root. (Chapter 16 discusses this issue in depth.)

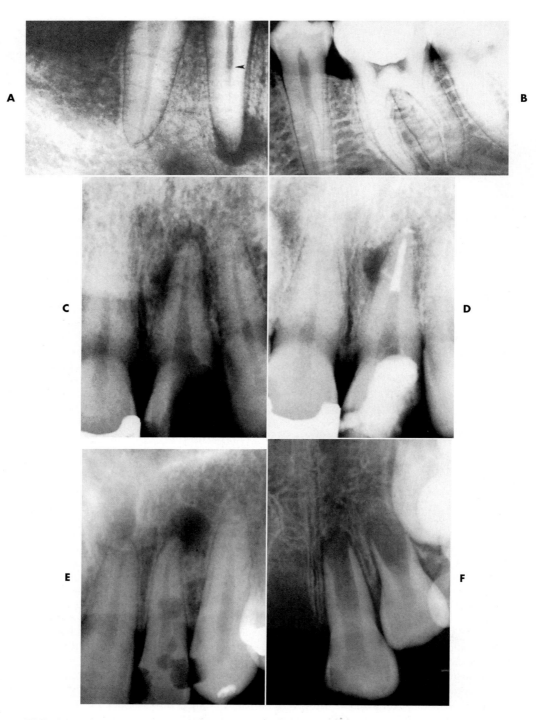

FIG. 1-7 A, Root canal bifurcation. A sudden change from dark to light *(arrow)* indicates that root canal has branched into more than one canal. **B,** Anticipation of "extra" root and canals. The astute clinician will not be surprised to find "extra" canals (premolar) or roots (molar). Anatomic variations will not be overlooked if they are anticipated. **C,** Periapical and periradicular demineralization. Bacteria and their endotoxins may cascade out of lateral canals and apical portals of exit, causing diffuse periradicular demineralization. **D,** When the portals of exit have been sealed well, remineralization will proceed uneventfully. In the presence of periodontal disease, these lateral canals could potentially become infected and ultimately infect the pulp. **E,** Internal resorption, an insidious, asymptomatic inflammatory process, will perforate the root unless endodontic therapy is promptly initiated. **F,** Pulp vitality tests are unreliable when the apices are immature.

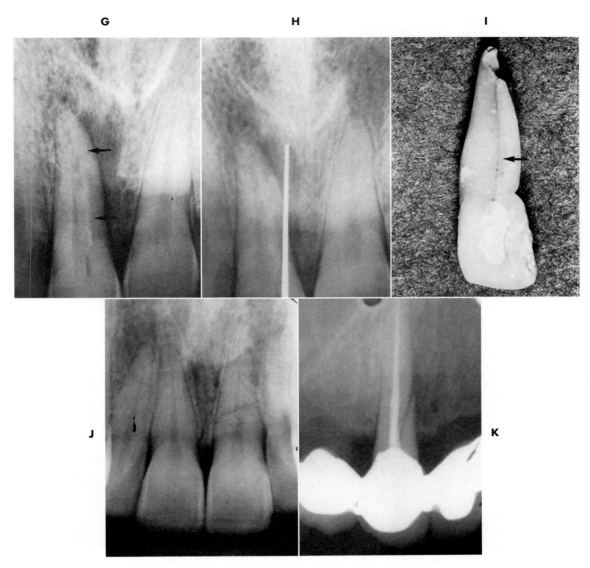

FIG. 1-7, cont'd G, Lingual developmental groove. Note that the canals of the central incisors are distinctly different. Arrows indicate the groove traced along the root. **H,** Silver cone placed in the lingual sulcular defect shows the extent of the associated periodontal breakdown. **I,** The only treatment at this time is extraction. In the future, fusing these grooves by laser surgery may allow these teeth to be retained. **J,** Only horizontal root fractures are readily identifiable shortly after injury. **K,** Oblique and vertical fractures are often not identified until demineralization or root separation makes them evident.

Periapical radiographs also allow the clinician to identify teeth with immature apices (Fig. 1-7, *F*). Knowledge of the presence of immature apices enables the clinician to anticipate erroneous responses to thermal and electric pulp tests.

In addition, lingual developmental grooves would be suspected when the canal appears blurred on the radiograph compared with the contralateral tooth, and there is an irregular demineralized radiolucency surrounding the root (Fig. 1-7, *G* through *I*).

With some exceptions, root fractures may cause pulp degeneration. Only the horizontal root fracture will be identifiable in the early stage (Fig. 1-7, *J*). Vertical and oblique root fractures will eventually cause demineralization (Fig. 1-7, *K*). (Chapters 2 and 16 take the discussion of these issues further.)

Radiographic misinterpretation

Radiographic interpretation, like diagnosis itself, is part science and part art and intuition. For example, in one study[13] three endodontists looking at more than 250 films interpreted the same radiographs 6 to 8 months later; they agreed with their own interpretation only 72% to 88% of the time. In an earlier study six endodontists agreed with each other less than half the time.[12] Certain radiographic phenomena are especially susceptible to multiple interpretations. These include the following:

Radiolucency at the apex (Fig. 1-8, *A*). At first glance a radiolucency at the apex may appear to be a periapical lesion. However, a positive response to thermal or electric pulp testing, an intact lamina dura, the absence of symptoms and prob-

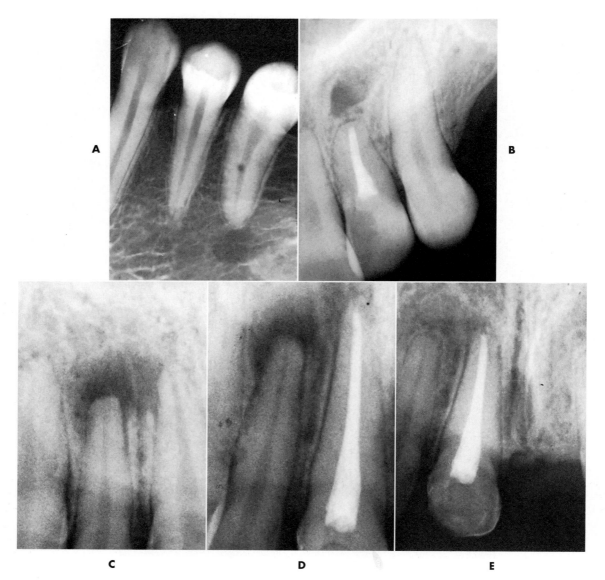

FIG. 1-8 Potential radiographic misinterpretation. **A,** Thermal and electric pulp tests, along with an intact lamina dura, indicate that this asymptomatic radiolucency is the mental foramen. **B,** With a history of prior apical surgery and an intact lamina dura, this asymptomatic radiolucency was identified as an apical scar. **C,** Vitality tests confirmed the nonvital central incisor was source of the radiolucency over the lateral incisor. **D,** Immediately after endodontic therapy. **E,** After 6 months complete remineralization is visible. *(Courtesy Dr. John Sapone.)*

able cause, and the anatomic location of the mass clearly reveal that this is the mental foramen.

Well-circumscribed radiolucency at or near the apex (Fig. 1-8, *B*). At first glance a well-circumscribed radiolucency at or near the apex may also appear to be a periapical lesion. However, the absence of symptoms, the history of apical surgery, and the intact lamina dura make it clear that the correct diagnosis is an apical scar.

Ostensible periapical lesion (Fig. 1-8, *C*). The source of an ostensible periapical lesion can be confirmed only through complete testing, including thermal and electric pulp testing. In this case use of the radiograph alone for diagnosis could

lead to treatment of the wrong tooth. Good differential diagnosis demands the careful consideration of anatomic landmarks in the region being examined.

Thermal Tests

One of the most common symptoms associated with the symptomatic inflamed pulp is pain elicited by thermal stimulation. Thermal tests are especially valuable diagnostic aids because in certain types of inflamed pulps pain may be induced or relieved by applying cold or warm stimuli. Often it is the patient's response to thermal tests that provides the clinician with information about whether the pulp is healthy, inflamed,

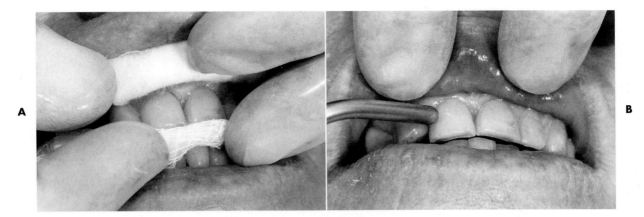

FIG. 1-9 Preparing for vitality testing. **A,** The teeth should be isolated with cotton rolls and dried with gauze to ensure accurate responses. **B,** The teeth should *not* be dried with blasts of air because this may cause thermal shock to a tooth that is sensitive to cold stimuli; additionally, this unsanitary practice may spray saliva on the assistant and the dentist.

or aging and calcifying.[5,15,19] When the patient describes the pain as diffuse, thermal testing involving vital pulps often helps to pinpoint the source.

When the patient's dental history records pain with thermal change (usually cold), the clinician should expect a strong response to thermal testing. In this situation in particular the clinician must explain the necessity of thermal testing to the patient and its value in finding and relieving the source of pain. Before proceeding, the clinician should explain the procedure for thermal testing to the patient and should demonstrate the testing on several teeth on the contralateral side. This approach will be both instructive and reassuring to the patient. In addition, the clinician and the patient must agree on a signal through which the patient can indicate immediately that he or she is feeling pain. The most commonly used signals are a patient's raised hand or a soft, audible sound.

Reliable responses to pulp vitality testing are critical and depend on the teeth being dry. Before initiating testing, the clinician should isolate the teeth to be tested and dry them with a 2 × 2–inch gauze. The area must be kept dry with a saliva ejector (Fig. 1-9, *A*). A blast of air should not be used to dry the teeth because room-temperature air can cause thermal shock if the pulp is inflamed. Additionally, air blasts can spray saliva onto the assistant or the dentist (Fig. 1-9, *B*).

Cold test

Several methods for cold testing teeth yield interpretable results. These are cold-water bath, ethyl chloride, sticks of ice, and carbon dioxide ice sticks (Fig. 1-10, *A* through *E*). Although each of these methods delivers cold to the tooth, ethyl chloride and a cold bath are the most frequently used. Although the ethyl chloride method is the most convenient for the clinician, the cold-water bath, which takes more time, will elicit the most accurate patient response. Sticks of ice are seldom used because they may warm when applied to the tooth and leak onto the gingiva, causing a false-positive response. Carbon dioxide dry ice sticks are extremely cold ($-77.7°$ C, $-108°$ F) and may cause infraction lines in enamel or damage to an otherwise healthy pulp.[1]

In the ethyl chloride method ethyl chloride is sprayed liberally onto a cotton pellet. The cotton pellet is shaken to remove excess liquid, and the chilled pellet is then applied immediately to the middle third of the facial surface of the crown (Fig. 1-10, *C*). The pellet is kept in contact with the crown for 5 seconds or until the patient begins to feel pain.

The cold-water bath method requires isolation of the tooth with a rubber dam. Iced water is sprayed onto the tooth with a plastic syringe for 5 seconds or until the patient begins to feel pain (Fig. 1-10, *D*).

Heat test

Several methods for heat testing teeth yield interpretable results. These include warm sticks of temporary stopping, rotating a dry prophy cup to create frictional heat, and a hot-water bath. Although each method transfers heat to the tooth, the most commonly used methods are the warm sticks of temporary stopping and the hot-water bath. Warm sticks of temporary stopping are the most convenient for the clinician, but the hot-water bath will yield the most accurate patient response.

In the temporary stopping method, a stick of temporary stopping is heated over a flame until it appears glassy (within a few seconds). It is applied immediately to the middle third of the facial surface of the crown (Fig. 1-10, *E* and *F*). The temporary stopping is left on the crown for 5 seconds or until the patient begins to feel pain. Overheating the temporary stopping can damage the pulp and cause unnecessary pain to the patient. The crown should be protected with petroleum jelly to prevent the warm temporary stopping from sticking to the tooth.

Like the cold-water bath, the hot-water bath method requires isolation of the tooth to be tested. Very warm water is sprayed onto the tooth with a plastic syringe for 5 seconds or until the patient begins to feel pain.

Although the cold-water and hot-water bath methods of thermal testing are more time-consuming for the clinician, they are clearly superior in their accuracy. The use of water allows the entire crown to be immersed, not just one section of one surface of the tooth. Even when the tooth has been restored with a full crown (metal and/or porcelain), sufficient contact is made to allow cooling or warming of the pulp. In addition, the cold- and hot-water bath methods prevent excessive temperature-change damage to the tooth.

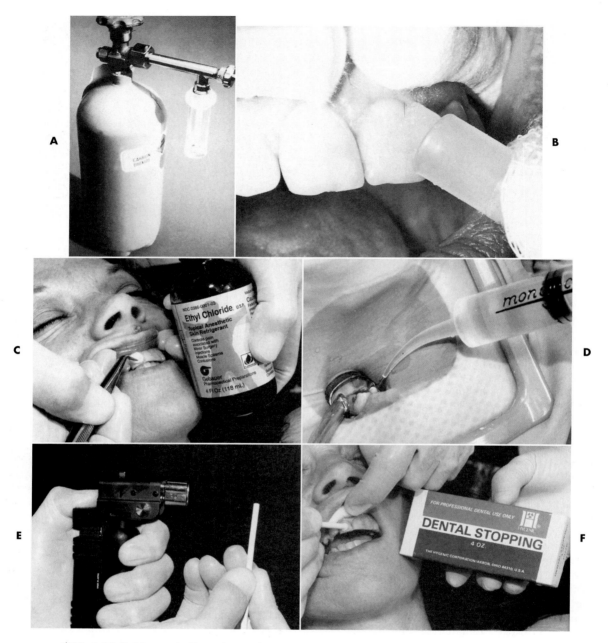

FIG. 1-10 Cold test. **A,** Preparing carbon dioxide dry ice sticks **B,** A carbon dioxide dry ice stick, held in gauze, is applied to the tooth. These cold sticks are so extremely cold that they may cause infraction lines in enamel. **C,** After the excess ethyl chloride is tapped away, a cotton pellet is applied to the tooth for 5 seconds or until the patient begins to feel pain. This is the easiest method for cold testing. **D,** After a tooth has been completely isolated under a rubber dam, a plastic syringe is used to immerse the tooth in ice water. Although this method takes a little more time, the benefit is that *all* surfaces of the tooth are submerged in ice water. Therefore this is the most accurate method for cold testing. When very warm water is used, this is also the most accurate method for heat testing. **E,** Another technique for heat testing is to warm temporary stopping until the surface begins to glisten. Temporary stopping is too warm if it begins to smoke. **F,** After the tooth is moistened with petroleum jelly (Vaseline), the very warm gutta-percha is applied for 5 seconds or until the patient begins to feel pain.

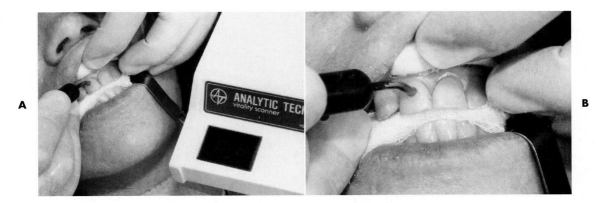

FIG. 1-11 Electric pulp testing. **A,** Before testing, the teeth must be isolated and dried; a lip clip is applied on the side of the mouth. **B,** With a generous amount of conductor between the electrode and the tooth, adjust the rate of current flow to a slow stream. The patient should raise his or her hand as soon as a "tingling" or sensation of warmth is felt within the tooth. Each tooth should be tested at least two to three times to ensure an accurate, reproducible response.

Responses to thermal tests

The sensory fibers of the pulp transmit only pain, whether the pulp has been cooled or heated (see p. 11 for further discussion). There are four possible responses to thermal stimulation:
1. No response
2. Mild to moderate degree of awareness of slight pain that subsides within 1 to 2 seconds after the stimulus has been removed
3. Strong, momentary painful response that subsides within 1 to 2 seconds after the stimulus has been removed
4. Moderate to strong painful response that lingers for several seconds or longer after the stimulus has been removed

If there is no response to thermal testing, a nonvital pulp is indicated. However, no response to thermal testing can also indicate a false-positive response because of excessive calcification, an immature apex, recent trauma, or patient premedication. A momentary mild to moderate response to thermal change is generally considered within normal limits. A painful response that subsides quickly is characteristic of reversible pulpitis. A painful response that lingers after the stimulus is removed is characteristic of irreversible pulpitis.

Electric Pulp Tests

The electric pulp tester is designed to stimulate a response of the sensory fibers within the pulp by electric excitation (Fig. 1-11, *A* and *B*). The patient's response to electric pulp testing does *not* suggest the health or integrity of the pulp; it simply indicates that there are vital sensory fibers present within the pulp.[19] The electric pulp test does *not* provide any information about the vascular supply to the pulp, which is the true determinant of pulp vitality. Several conditions can cause false responses to electric pulp testing. *Therefore it is essential that thermal tests be performed before a final diagnosis is made.*

However, the electric pulp test is necessary when all other clinical testing is inconclusive. In the case of a periapical radiolucency, the electric pulp test can help the clinician determine whether the pulp is vital. When used with thermal and periodontal testing, the electric pulp tester can help differentiate pulpal from periodontal disease or nonodontogenic causes.

Electric pulp testing technique

The teeth to be tested must be isolated and dried with 2 × 2–inch gauze, and the testing area must be kept dry with a saliva ejector if the testing results are to be valid. The clinician must explain to the patient the diagnostic value and the procedure to be followed.

It is also important that the patient be specifically prepared for the tingling or heat sensation that he or she will feel during the testing. The clinician can provide additional reassurance to the patient by first testing several teeth on the contralateral side. The patient should be instructed to raise a hand when any sensation is felt.

The Analytic Technology Pulp Tester is widely used because the digital reading (indicating current flow) always starts at zero and the rate of flow of the current is easily controlled. First the lip clip should be attached, and the electrode of the pulp tester should be generously coated with a viscous conductor (e.g., toothpaste). The electrode should then be applied to the dry enamel on the middle third of the facial surface of the crown of the tooth being tested. The current flow should be adjusted to increase slowly to allow the patient time to respond before the attendant tingling sensation becomes painful. The electrode should not be applied to any restorations because this could lead to a false reading.

Each tooth should be tested at least two or three times. The average of the several readings should be recorded. The patient's response may vary slightly with each test. However, a significant variation in response suggests a false reading. Generally, thicker enamel will lead to a more delayed response. Thinner enamel of anterior teeth will yield a quicker response than the thicker enamel of posterior teeth. *If the patient's medical history reveals that a cardiac pacemaker has been implanted, the use of an electric pulp tester is contraindicated because of potential interference.*[17]

Electric pulp tester false readings

Although the electric pulp tester is generally reliable in determining pulp vitality, false readings can occur in certain circumstances.[10] A *false-positive* reading means that the pulp is necrotic, yet the patient will signal that there is sensation in the tooth. A *false-negative* reading means that the pulp is vital, yet the patient will be unresponsive to electric pulp tests.

Main reasons for a false-positive response

- Electrode or conductor contact with a metal restoration or the gingiva
- Patient anxiety: Without proper instruction about the reasons and methodology for electric pulp testing, and without preparation for the sensations that occur, a frightened or neurotic patient may raise his or her hand immediately when asked: "Do you feel anything?"
- Liquefaction necrosis may conduct current to the attachment apparatus, leading the patient to raise his or her hand slowly near the highest range of current flow
- Failure to isolate and dry the teeth before testing (saliva acts as a conductor)

Main reasons for a false-negative response

- The patient has been heavily premedicated with analgesics, narcotics, alcohol, or tranquilizers
- Inadequate contact between the electrode or conductor and the enamel plate
- A recently traumatized tooth
- Excessive calcification of the canal
- Recently erupted tooth with an immature apex
- Partial necrosis: Although the pulp is vital in the apical half of the root, the absence of a response to the electric pulp test could appear to suggest that there is total necrosis

Periodontal Examination

Testing of the tooth in question is not complete until the integrity of the sulci has been carefully checked through thorough probing. The clinician should use a blunt calibrated probe to explore the integrity of the gingival sulcus around each tooth. The findings should be recorded in the patient's clinical record (Fig. 1-12). It is possible that, in the presence of periodontal disease, the disease through a lateral canal could cause pulp degeneration in an otherwise sound tooth.[20] If a significant pocket is discovered in the *absence* of periodontal disease, it increases the probability of the presence of a vertical root fracture. Occasionally, for diagnostic confirmation (and dental-legal reasons), the depth and direction of a periodontal pocket can be confirmed through placement of a gutta-percha or silver cone in the sulcular defect. To distinguish disease of periodontal origin from disease of pulpal origin, thermal and electric pulp tests along with periodontal probing are essential.[19,20]

Selective Anesthesia Test

The use of intraligamentary anesthesia is an effective diagnostic tool in special clinical situations. This test should be used, for example, when the clinician has determined through prior testing which tooth is the source of pain but the patient reports severe, lingering residual pain, especially from thermal testing. Administration of 0.2 ml of local anesthetic into the distal sulcus will provide welcome relief for the patient (Fig. 1-13). Under these conditions the use of intraligamentary anesthetic effectively breaks the cycle of pain for the patient for several minutes and reconfirms through the elimination of pain what prior testing determined through reproduction of pain.[3,21]

If the patient continues to have vague, diffuse, strong pain and prior testing has been inconclusive, intraligamentary anesthetic may be used to help identify the source of pain. Administration of 0.2 ml of local anesthetic into the distal sulcus of the offending tooth will briefly stop the pain. However, because the diffusion of the local anesthetic is not limited to a single tooth (see Chapter 19), the clinician cannot make a conclusive diagnosis on the basis of pain relief. Nevertheless, the use of anesthetic here can help identify the probable source of the pain.

If the chief complaint is about continuing pain and the pain is not relieved by the administration of intraligamentary anesthesia, the clinician must consider nonodontogenic etiologies. Chapter 3 provides a comprehensive discussion of this kind of pain.

Procedures for Identifying Vertical Crown-Root Fractures

Trauma is the most common cause of vertical root fracture[1] (see Chapter 16). The following paragraphs detail several diagnostic procedures that will aid the clinician in the detection of complete and incomplete vertical crown-root fractures.

A thorough dental history

A thorough dental history may record the patient's memory of a sudden jolt of pain while chewing popcorn or ice or while accidentally biting into a bone or olive pit. Although the tooth appears to be perfectly sound, the patient reports that it has

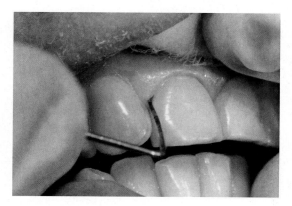

FIG. 1-12 Periodontal examination. A thin, blunt periodontal probe should be used to check the integrity of the gingival sulcus. The findings of the periodontal examination must be recorded.

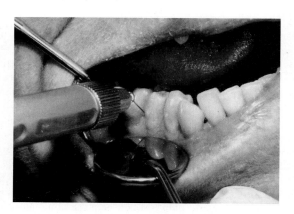

FIG. 1-13 Selective anesthesia test. Intraligamentary anesthesia, where 0.2 ml is injected into the distal sulcus, can be used to confirm the source of pain.

never felt comfortable since the recalled incident. This strongly suggests that a crown-root vertical fracture resulted, and it is the cause of the pain (Fig. 1-14, *A*). Sometimes patients will report that they feel pain in the tooth *after* they release from clenching or moments after chewing.

The dental history may also record that the patient has undergone endodontic therapy more than once on the tooth in question but the tooth remains symptomatic even after both surgical and nonsurgical treatment. This history is commonly associated with the present of an occult root fracture.

When the patient's dental history notes that a properly designed restoration has dislodged several times, a vertical crown fracture should be suspected. Similarly, if the patient reports in the dental history that the tooth hurts only when it is tapped

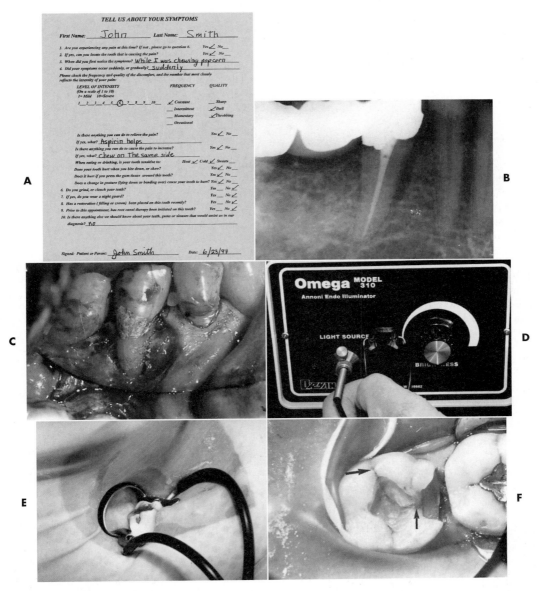

FIG. 1-14 Detecting vertical crown-root fractures. **A,** A careful review of the patient's dental history often provides initial clues regarding the cause of the patient's chief complaint. For example, a sudden onset of moderate pain while chewing popcorn, chewing into a bone unexpectedly, or chewing into a pit in pie are common reports suggesting crown-root fracture. **B,** Periodontal therapy did not resolve this defect. In the absence of periodontal disease, a narrow, vertical loss of bone along one surface of a root strongly suggests vertical root fracture. **C,** A sinus tract draining through the gingival sulcus and a deep pocket on the facial surface raised suspicion of a vertical root fracture. A full-thickness flap confirmed the diagnosis. **D,** Fiberoptic light sources are available with rubber dam clamp attachments. **E,** In a dimly lit room, attaching the fiberoptic rubber clamp to the tooth makes the vertical crown fracture on the mesial surface evident. **F,** If the dental history or associated signs or symptoms suggest vertical crown fracture, removing all restorations from the tooth may reveal an underlying fracture.   *Continued*

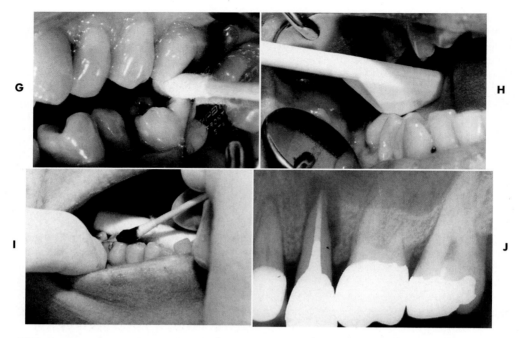

FIG. 1-14, cont'd G, Excursive movements of the jaw while clenching on a cottonwood stick may elicit pain not detected with percussion testing. When there is a vertical crown-root fracture, the patient may also notice an increase in pain when he or she releases the clenching motion. **H,** The Tooth Slooth, an autoclavable plastic device, can be applied to individual cusps while the patient clenches and moves the jaw in reciprocal excursive directions to reproduce the complaint of pain when chewing. This too may help to identify a sheared cusp or a vertical crown fracture. **I,** After the occlusal surface is dried, methylene blue dye can be applied. The patient is directed to clench down on the cottonwood stick and move the jaw in a side-to-side motion. Then gauze moistened in isopropyl alcohol should be used to wipe away the excess dye. Vertical crown fractures will be stained by the dye. **J,** A "halo" radiolucency around a root is a strong sign suggesting vertical root fracture.

on the side of the tooth and the patient can describe and point to the side that produces the pain, an incomplete vertical crown-root fracture must be suspected.

Persistent periodontal defect

Vertical crown-root fracture should be suspected when periodontal therapy has not resolved a recurrent periodontal defect around one and sometimes two surfaces of a root (Fig. 1-14, *B*) and there is no additional evidence periodontal disease. Reflecting a full-thickness mucoperiosteal flap with the aid of strong magnification and illumination, including the endodontic microscope, may reveal the vertical fracture line (Fig. 1-14, *C*).

Fiberoptic examination

Horizontally directing fiberoptic illumination at the gingival sulcus (e.g., from a fiberoptic handpiece) in a dimly lit treatment room may reveal a vertical fracture line or may make a suspected line more visible (Fig. 1-4, *D* and *E*). A preexisting restoration may need to be removed to make the fracture line visible (Fig. 1-14, *F*).

Wedging and staining

A wedging force exerted during mastication may stimulate a patient's complaint of pain with chewing. The two most common techniques for creating wedging force are asking the patient to chew on a cottonwood stick and asking the patient to chew on a Tooth Slooth (Fig. 1-14, *G* and *H*). The patient should be instructed to chew firmly and to move the jaw slightly in excursive directions while pressing firmly on the object between the teeth. This technique aids the clinician in identifying both vertical crown-root fractures and cuspal shear fractures that may not involve the pulp.

The application of methylene blue dye to a cottonwood stick can be a helpful extension of the wedging technique; it can highlight a subtle coronal fracture that might otherwise escape detection. The coronal surface of the tooth should be dried and a cottonwood stick moistened with methylene blue dye placed on the occlusal surface of the tooth. The patient should be instructed to press firmly on the stick and to move the jaw from side to side (Fig. 1-14, *I*). Gauze dampened with 70% isopropyl alcohol should be used to wipe excess dye from the tooth surface. A close inspection of the tooth will then reveal the elusive coronal fracture, darkened with dye.

Periapical radiographs

When the radiograph shows a narrow radiolucency extending from the alveolar crest alongside the root (see Fig. 1-14, *B*) or a "halo" radiolucency that is more periradicular than simply periapical, it is probable that a vertical root fracture is present (Fig. 1-14, *J*).

The accurate diagnosis of vertical crown-root fracture begins with an awareness of the frequency of this finding. Keeping this in mind during the evaluation of the patient's dental history, observation of the presenting signs and symptoms, and active listening to the patient's reporting will aid in an accurate diagnosis.

Probable Cause for Pulpal Disease

Every pulpal disease has a probable cause. Endodontic treatment should not be initiated if the cause for the diagnosis remains unknown. A probable cause for the patient's presenting signs and symptoms must be determined. If careful application of the diagnostic protocols discussed, including diagnostic testing, yields no probable cause for the pulpal-periapical condition, referral for additional diagnostic consultation is mandated.

CLINICAL CLASSIFICATION OF PULPAL AND PERIAPICAL DISEASE

A clinical classification of pulpal and periapical disease cannot list every possible variation of inflammation, ulceration, proliferation, calcification, and degeneration of the pulp and the attachment apparatus and still remain practical. Furthermore, it is unnecessary because the primary purpose of a clinical classification is to provide basic terms and phrases that will be effective within the dental profession in describing the furthest extent of pulpal and periapical disease. In the broadest possible interpretation, the pulp is either healthy or unhealthy, and it must be removed or need not be removed. The extent of the disease processes can affect the method of treatment selected, from a palliative sedative for a reversibly inflamed pulp to pulpectomy.

The terms listed below outline the main clinical signs and symptoms of the degrees of inflammation or degeneration of the pulpal-periapical tissue. The clinical terms applied to periapical disease suggest the nature, duration, and type of exudation found in the disease processes. Current knowledge does not allow an association to be made between these terms and histopathologic findings.[19]

Within Normal Limits

A normal pulp is asymptomatic and produces a mild to moderate transient response to thermal and electrical stimuli. The response subsides almost immediately when the stimulus is removed. The tooth and its attachment apparatus do not cause a painful response when percussed or palpated. Radiographs reveal a clearly delineated canal that tapers smoothly toward the apex. There is no evidence of calcification or root resorption, and the lamina dura is intact.

Reversible Pulpitis

The pulp is inflamed to the extent that thermal stimuli (usually cold) cause a quick, sharp, hypersensitive response that subsides as soon as the stimulus is removed. Otherwise, the pulp remains asymptomatic. Any irritant that can affect the pulp may cause reversible pulpitis, including early caries, periodontal scaling, root planing, and unbased restorations.

Reversible pulpitis is *not* a disease; it is a symptom. If the irritant is removed and the inflamed pulp is palliated, it will revert to an uninflamed state that is asymptomatic. Conversely, if the irritant remains, the symptoms may persist indefinitely or may become more widespread, leading to irreversible pulpitis. Reversible pulpitis can be clinically distinguished from a symptomatic irreversible pulpitis in two ways:

1. Reversible pulpitis causes a momentary painful response to thermal change that subsides as soon as the stimulus (usually cold) is removed. However, symptomatic irreversible pulpitis causes a painful response to thermal change that lingers after the stimulus (usually cold) is removed.
2. Reversible pulpitis does not involve a complaint of spontaneous (unprovoked) pain. Symptomatic irreversible pulpitis commonly includes a complaint of spontaneous pain.

Irreversible Pulpitis

Irreversible pulpitis may be acute, subacute, or chronic; it may be partial or total, infected or sterile. Clinically, the acutely inflamed pulp is symptomatic. The chronically inflamed pulp is usually asymptomatic. Clinically, the furthest extent of irreversible pulpitis cannot be determined until the periodontal ligament is affected by the cascade of inflammatory breakdown products.[1,19] Dynamic changes in the irreversibly inflamed pulp are continual; the pulp may move from quiescent chronicity to acute pain within hours.

Asymptomatic Irreversible Pulpitis

Although uncommon, asymptomatic irreversible pulpitis may be the conversion of symptomatic irreversible pulpitis to a quiescent state. Caries and trauma are the most common causes. This pathologic condition is identified through a synthesis of the information provided in a thorough dental history and a properly exposed radiograph.

Hyperplastic pulpitis

A reddish cauliflower-like growth of pulp tissue through and around a carious exposure is one variation of asymptomatic irreversible pulpitis. The proliferative nature of this type of pulp is attributed to a low-grade chronic irritation of the pulp and the generous vascularity characteristically found in young people.[19] Occasionally this condition may cause mild, transient pain during mastication.

Internal resorption

Internal resorption is the painless expansion of the pulp that results in the destruction of dentin. Internal resorption is most commonly identified during routine radiographic examination (see Fig. 1-7, *E*). If undetected, internal resorption will eventually perforate the root. Before perforation of the crown, the resorption can be detected as a pink spot on the site. Only prompt endodontic therapy will prevent tooth destruction. Chapter 16 contains a further discussion of this issue.

Canal calcification

The physical stress of restorative procedures or periodontal therapy, attrition, abrasion, or trauma all may cause an otherwise healthy pulp to metamorphose into an irreversible pulpitis. This condition appears as excessive deposits of dentin throughout the canal system.[1,19,22] Like internal resorption, canal calcification is most often detected through routine radiographic examination. Sometimes an anterior tooth will reveal coronal discoloration, suggesting chamber calcification.

Symptomatic irreversible pulpitis

Symptomatic irreversible pulpitis is characterized by spontaneous (unprovoked) intermittent or continuous paroxysms of pain. Sudden temperature changes (often with cold) elicit prolonged episodes of pain (i.e., pain that lingers after the thermal stimulus is removed). Occasionally patients may report that a postural change (lying down or bending over) induces pain and results in fitful sleep even with the use of several pillows to stabilize themselves at a comfortable postural level.

Pain from symptomatic irreversible pulpitis is generally moderate to severe, sharp or dull, localized or referred. Chapter 2 offers a comprehensive discussion of referred pain from symptomatic irreversible pulpitis. Radiographs are not generally useful in diagnosing symptomatic irreversible pulpitis. However, radiographs can be helpful in identifying suspect teeth (i.e., teeth with deep caries or extensive restorations). Thickening of the apical portion of the periodontal ligament may become evident on the radiographs in the advanced stage of symptomatic irreversible pulpitis.

Symptomatic irreversible pulpitis can be diagnosed through synthesis of the information provided in a thorough dental history, a complete visual examination, properly exposed radiographs, and carefully conducted thermal tests. If radiating or referred pain is involved, the application of 0.2 ml of intraligamentary anesthesia in the distal sulcus will immediately stop the pain in the correctly identified tooth. The electric pulp test is of little value in the diagnosis of symptomatic irreversible pulpitis.

The inflammatory process of symptomatic irreversible pulpitis may become so severe that it will lead to necrosis of the pulp. In the degenerative transition from pulpitis to necrosis, the usual symptoms of symptomatic irreversible pulpitis may subside as necrosis occurs.

Necrosis

Necrosis, the death of the pulp, results from an untreated irreversible pulpitis, a traumatic injury, or any event that causes long-term interruption of the blood supply to the pulp. Whether the remnants of the pulp are liquefied or coagulated, the pulp is still necrotic.

Pulp necrosis may be partial or total. Partial necrosis may present some of the symptoms associated with irreversible pulpitis. For example, a two-rooted canal could have an inflamed pulp in one canal and a necrotic pulp in the other. Total necrosis before it affects the periodontal ligament is asymptomatic, and there is no response to thermal or electric pulp tests. In anterior teeth some crown discoloration may accompany pulp necrosis.

The protein breakdown products, bacteria and their toxins (primarily endotoxins) that result from necrosis of the pulp, will eventually spread beyond the apical foramen. This will lead to thickening of the periodontal ligament and will manifest as tenderness to percussion and chewing.[1,19,20] As these irritants cascade out of the root canal system, periapical disease will almost always occur.[2]

PERIAPICAL DISEASE

Acute Apical Periodontitis

Acute apical periodontitis means painful inflammation around the apex. This condition can be the result of an extension of pulpal disease into the periapical tissue, an overextension of endodontic instruments or materials, or occlusal trauma such as bruxism. Because acute apical periodontitis may occur around vital and nonvital teeth, *conducting thermal and electric pulp tests is the only way to confirm the need for endodontic treatment.*

Although acute apical periodontitis is present, the apical periodontal ligament may appear within normal limits or only slightly widened on the pretreatment radiograph. However, the tooth may be slightly to extremely painful during percussion and chewing tests. If the tooth is vital, a simple occlusal adjustment will often relieve the pain. If the pulp is necrotic and the resulting acute apical periodontitis remains untreated, additional symptoms may appear as the disease advances to the next stage, acute apical abscess.

Acute Apical Abscess

An acute apical abscess is a painful, purulent exudate around the apex as a result of the exacerbation of acute apical periodontitis from a necrotic tooth. Although this disease can be very serious, the periodontal ligament may appear within normal limits or may be only slightly thickened. The periapical radiograph reveals a relatively normal lamina dura (or slightly thickened) because the fulminating infection has rapidly spread beyond the confines of the cortical plate before demineralization can be detected radiographically.

The presenting signs and symptoms of acute apical abscess include rapid onset of slight to severe swelling, moderate to severe pain, pain with percussion and palpation, and slight increase in tooth mobility; in more advanced cases the patient is febrile. The extent and distribution of the swelling are determined by the location of the apex and the muscle attachments and the thickness of the cortical plate.[2,14] The acute apical abscess can be differentially diagnosed from the lateral periodontal abscess and from the phoenix abscess because of the following:

- The thermal and electric pulp test will confirm that the pulp is vital although the symptoms of the lateral periodontal abscess may mimic those of the acute apical abscess. Additionally, with only rare exceptions, a deep periodontal pocket is found associated with the lateral periodontal abscess.
- The symptoms of the phoenix abscess and the acute apical abscess are identical; when a periapical radiolucency is evident, it is called a *phoenix abscess.*

Chronic Apical Periodontitis

Chronic apical periodontitis is a generally asymptomatic periapical lesion that is manifested radiographically. Bacteria and their endotoxins cascading out into the periapical region from a necrotic pulp causes extensive demineralization of cancellous and cortical bone. The resulting radiographically evident lesions may be large or small, diffuse or circumscribed. Occasionally, there may be slight tenderness to percussion and/or palpation testing. A sinus tract (incorrectly referred to as a "fistula" or "gum boil") represents frank suppuration. As pressure from pus is relieved by drainage through a sinus tract, the sinus tract may close temporarily. When the pressure from pus builds up again (along with slight tenderness to palpation), the sinus tract returns.

The diagnosis of chronic apical periodontitis is confirmed by the general absence of symptoms, the presence of a periapical radiolucency, and the confirmation of pulp necrosis. A totally necrotic pulp provides a safe harbor for the primarily anaerobic microorganisms and their noxious allies; if there is no vascularity, there are no defense cells. For this reason only complete endodontic therapy will create the microenvironment in which these periapical lesions can remineralize.

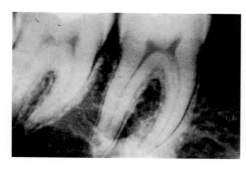

FIG. 1-15 Periapical osteosclerosis, possibly caused by a mild pulp irritant.

Phoenix Abscess

A phoenix abscess is always preceded by chronic apical periodontitis. If chronic apical periodontitis worsens without a sinus tract to relieve the pressure, symptoms identical to those present with an acute apical abscess will appear. Chapter 2 provides a full discussion of the causes and the cures for this pathologic condition.

Periapical Osteosclerosis

Periapical osteosclerosis is excessive bone mineralization around the apex of an asymptomatic, vital tooth (Fig. 1-15). This radiolucency may be caused by low-grade pulp irritation. This condition is asymptomatic and benign, and therefore it does not require endodontic therapy.

ACKNOWLEDGMENT

Special thanks to Ms. Guilana Guerrero for her assistance in preparing the manuscript for this chapter.

REFERENCES

1. Andreasen JO: *Atlas of replantation and transplantation,* Philadelphia, 1992, WB Saunders.
2. Baumgartner JC: Treatment of infections and associated lesions of endodontic origin, *J Endod* 17:418, 1991.
3. Bell WE: *Orofacial pains,* ed 4, Chicago, 1989, Mosby.
4. Bender IB: Factors influencing radiographic appearance of bony lesions, *J Endod* 8:161, 1982.
5. Brannstrom M: The hydrodynamic theory of dentinal pain: sensation in preparations, caries and the dentinal crack syndrome, *J Endod* 12:453, 1986.
6. Cohn SA: *Endodontic radiography: principles and clinical techniques,* Gilberts, Ill, 1988, Dunvale.
7. *The compact Oxford English dictionary,* ed 2, Oxford, 1993, Oxford University Press.
8. Cottone JA, Terezhalmy GT, Molinari JA: *Practical infection control in dentistry,* ed 2, Baltimore, 1996, Williams & Wilkins.
9. Drinnan AL: Differential diagnosis of orofacial pain, *Dent Clin North Am* 31:627, 1987.
10. Gazelius B, Olgart L, Edwall B: Restored vitality in luxated teeth assessed by laser Doppler flowmeter, *Endod Dent Traumat* 4:265, 1988.
11. Goaz PW, White SC: *Oral radiology: principles and interpretation,* ed 3, St Louis, 1994, Mosby.
12. Goldman M, Pearson A, Darzenta N: Endodontic success—who's reading the radiograph? *Oral Surg* 33:432, 1972.
13. Goldman M, Pearson A, Darzenta N: Reliability of radiographic interpretations, *Oral Surg* 32:287, 1974.
14. Hutter JW: Facial space infections of odontogenic origin, *J Endod* 17:422, 1991.
15. Kier DM et al: Thermally induced pulpalgia in endodontically treated teeth, *J Endod* 17:38, 1991.
16. Little JW et al: *Dental management of the medically compromised patient,* ed 5, St Louis, 1997, Mosby.
17. Malamed SF: *Handbook of medical emergencies in the dental office,* ed 4, St Louis, 1993, Mosby.
18. Nissan R et al: Ability of bacterial endotoxin to diffuse through human dentin, *J Endod* 21:62, 1995.
19. Seltzer S: *Endodontology: biologic consideration in endodontic procedures,* ed 2, Philadelphia, 1988, Lea & Febiger.
20. Simon JHS: *Endodontic-periodontal relations.* In Cohen S, Burns RC, editors: *Pathways of the pulp,* ed 6, St Louis, 1994, Mosby.
21. Systematic endodontic diagnosis, Endodontics; Colleagues for excellence, *Am Assoc Endod,* Winter 1996.
22. Walton RE, Torabinejad M: *Principles and practice of endodontics,* ed 2, Philadelphia, 1996, WB Saunders.

Chapter 2

Orofacial Dental Pain Emergencies: Endodontic Diagnosis and Management

Alan H. Gluskin

A. Scott Cohen

David Clifford Brown

PATIENT-DENTIST DYNAMICS

No area of dental practice has more potential for patient fear and discomfort than the emergency visit for acute orofacial pain. A complex interplay between the patient and the dentist has an important effect on the acute pain emergency. Three basic components of this interaction significantly affect the diagnostic approach and treatment:

1. The *patient's perception* of pain, based on a multicomponent model
2. The *professional's assessment* of the patient in pain
3. The *dentist's decision to treat or refer* the patient in pain

The patient presents complaints as a series of descriptions and behavioral patterns. The dentist must then understand and interpret this information. This dialogue is often inadequate to manage the patient, even if the source of the problem is identified. To aid in patient management and to build rapport, pain behavior should be viewed from the following perspectives.

Patient's Perception of Pain

At the most simple and basic level, the patient who seeks care for a "toothache" may be suffering the effects of pain from pulpal and periapical tissue inflammation. However, referred pain, more complex facial pain, temporomandibular disorder (TMD) pain, or nonodontogenic pain in the head and neck demonstrate that the complaint of "toothache" pain is insufficient to diagnose and treat these entities.

When describing their pain, patients will convey a descriptive history of the problem and an interpretive narration, both of which are subjective. The dentist must recognize these personal interpretations and distill all clinically objective terms, such as *acute* ("It came outta nowhere.") or *chronic* ("I knew it would lead to this."). The patient's actual reaction to the pain also can be expressed as body adaptation (e.g., not chewing on one side) and provides valuable behavioral insights, along with the dentist's visual assessment for facial asymmetry, altered constitutional signs (e.g., swelling, flushing, pallor), dysfunctional reflexes, or posturing (e.g., avoiding trigger zones, holding the face).

When the clinician needs to determine an etiologic basis for the pain, there are a multitude of patient presentations that can occur in the interaction with the dentist. The many different ways that individuals respond to pain is a common and dramatic clinical observation. Some patients may show little evidence of clinical disease but may seem to have intolerable pain that is incapacitating. Others with serious pathosis may continue to function at a high level and will not regard themselves to be ill or at risk.[90]

Current models describe pain as a complex event. Pain, by its very nature, is no longer considered a single entity but rather involves many overlapping components: "An unpleasant sensory and emotional experience associated with actual or potential tissue damage defines the physiologic and the psychological components."[70]

Multicomponent model of pain

The pain process involves pain reception (nociception) and its recognition, an emotional-affective component, a cognitive component, and a behavioral component.[90] Current literature and research emphasize the importance of the psychologic components of orofacial pain.[30] Today, accommodating the multidimensional components of pain is crucial in diagnosis and treatment of pain entities. To perform triage for urgent care, this distinction is pivotal.

The receptor system recognizes painful stimuli above a threshold by sending afferent information to the perceptual sensory system. The patient's reaction to the experience in terms of suffering and anxiety involves the emotional-affective component. Emotional factors such as anxiety can decrease the pain threshold and thus heighten the patient's reaction to the pain.

What individuals think about their pain involves the cognitive process. Cognition is implicated in virtually every aspect of the pain experience.[90] What patients understand about their pain is important in modulating how they react to it, and this understanding facilitates pain management. Patients, when told that their palatal swelling is from a pulpal disorder and is not life-threatening, will react more calmly to their condition than uninformed patients will.

Orofacial pain can generate unreasonable anxiety in a fearful patient. Speaking to the patient in a calm, knowledgable manner, in words the patient can readily understand, significantly enhances patient management. Providing information about typical procedures and sensations—sights, sounds, smells, vibrations, and other physical stimuli—is an invaluable management tool[43] that removes much of the patient's uncertainty about the planned treatment.

How patients perceive their control over pain is also important. Increased tolerance for potentially painful procedures is often seen when the dentist affords the patient a means to stop the operation. Patients who have more control over what happens to them feel more comfortable and show higher tolerance for dental procedures.[18]

Patients' experiences with successful or unsuccessful treatments invariably influence their behavior. Reassurance that the dentist can treat and eliminate acute dental pain efficiently helps to modulate anxiety and fear-related behavior. Personality and cultural factors are additional learned behaviors that can modify a patient's responses to pain, and they should be considered in pain management.

Professional's Assessment of the Patient in Pain

In an acute pain emergency both the physical problem and the emotional state of the patient should be considered. The dentist's reactions to the patient are important for management of both pain and patient. The patients' needs, their fears about the immediate problem, and their defenses for coping with the situation must be understood. This assessment and building rapport with the patient are key factors in proper management of the psychodynamic interaction between the dentist and the patient. This psychodynamic exchange involves five key aspects, elucidated by a number of authors:[43,90]

1. Patients are to be treated responsibly. All symptoms and complaints are perceived as real. Patients must see that the dentist is giving their complaints and symptoms serious consideration. Concern and empathy must be shown for the individual. Avoid making negative value judgments. Build patient rapport by stating, "You look like you have been experiencing a great deal of pain; let me begin helping you by asking you some questions." This is far more effective than making an impersonal statement that could have easily come out of a tape recording, such as, "You'll be fine, just relax."

2. A show of support for their complaint is reflected through active listening and expressing empathy, being nonjudgmental, and establishing and maintaining eye contact with patients.[43] Such support does not imply absolute agreement. Be thorough in evaluation of patients' symptoms and complaints. Patients must never feel that the attention is cursory and that less than possible is being done to make the diagnosis and to provide a solution to the problem.

3. Display a calm and confident professionalism. This demeanor can be expressed verbally and nonverbally. Eye contact, supportive touching of the patient's shoulder, or body contact while moving the patient into the treatment chair is reassuring. Providing care without positive statements or gestures is an obstacle to effective patient management. Rapport building requires sensitivity.

4. A positive attitude about patients' problems can make them aware that an efficient and effective treatment or referral can be made to help them. They must never feel that they will be abandoned.

5. Discuss and inform patients about what to expect once a diagnosis is made and treatment determined. Discussing the procedures and the physical sensations patients will feel is very useful. The patients' anxiety should be accepted as common and normal. Do not add guilt to patients' emotional presentation by telling them, "There is nothing to be afraid of." Giving permission to be anxious can help to modulate the emotional responses of an anxious patient in an emergency situation.[43]

Management of the orofacial pain emergency requires a comprehensive understanding of the patient's experience and feelings. The dentist who is perceptive and adaptable and can actively participate in the dynamic interplay will avoid many potential hardships and failures in patient management.

Dentist's Decision to Treat or Refer the Patient in Pain

Accommodating an unexpected patient into a busy schedule can be stressful and difficult for both dentist and staff. To ensure that the emergency patient receives appropriate care, the clinician must decide which dentist is best able to administer the specific treatment and meet the unique needs of a given patient. The dentist must determine what expertise is required to make a difficult diagnosis or render a complicated treatment. The patient's ability to withstand the procedure—emotionally, physically, or medically—and the availability of time for a complex case may be considerations in referring the emergency patient.[20]

INTERPRETATION OF THE LANGUAGE OF OROFACIAL PAIN

Pain Phenomenon[101]

The emergency presentation of orofacial pain may include a series of symptoms in a dental emergency that can be assessed only by the evaluation of each symptom individually. It may be difficult, however, for the patient to objectively describe the painful experience because of modulation and crossover in the central neural pathways. Modulation can intensify or suppress pain, giving it a multidimensional character.

At the neurophysiologic level pain results from noxious stimulation of free nerve endings in orofacial tissues. The peripheral nerve endings, acting as nociceptors or pain receptors, detect and convey the noxious information to the brain, where pain is perceived.

Physiology of Pulpal Pain[51,118]

Odontogenic pain

The sensibility of the dental pulp is controlled by myelinated (A-delta) and unmyelinated (C) afferent nerve fibers (see Fig. 21-1, p. 692). Operating under different pathophysiologic capabilities, both sensory nerve fibers conduct nociceptive input to the brain. Differences between the two sensory fibers enable the patient to discriminate and characterize the quality, intensity, location, and duration of the pain response.

Dentinal pain. The A-delta fibers are large myelinated nerves that enter the root canal and divide into smaller branches, coursing coronally through the pulp. Once beneath the odontoblastic layer, the A-delta fibers lose their myelin sheath and anastomose into a network of nerves referred to as the *plexus of Raschkow*. This circumpulpal layer of nerves sends free nerve endings onto and through the odontoblastic cell layer and into dentinal tubules and in contact with the odontoblastic processes. The intimate association of A-delta fiber with the odontoblastic cell layer and dentin is referred to as the *pulpodentinal complex.*

Disturbances of the pulpodentinal complex in a vital tooth initially affect the low-threshold A-delta fibers. Not all stimuli will reach the excitation threshold and generate a pain response. Irritants such as incipient dental caries and mild periodontal disease are seldom painful but can be sufficient to stimulate the defensive formation of sclerotic or reparative dentin. When the contents of the dentinal tubules (fluid or cellular processes) are disturbed sufficiently to involve the odontoblastic cell layer, A-delta fibers are excited. The vital tooth responds immediately with symptoms of dentinal sensitivity or dentinal pain.

A-delta fiber pain must be provoked. Nociceptive signals, transmitted through fast-conducting myelinated pathways, are immediately perceived as a quick, sharp (bright) momentary pain. The sensation dissipates quickly on removal of the inciting stimulus, such as drinking cold liquids or biting unexpectedly on an unyielding object.

The clinical symptoms of A-delta fiber pain signify that the pulpodentinal complex is intact and capable of responding to an external disturbance. Many dentists have mistakenly interpreted this symptom to indicate reversible pulpitis. However, symptoms are not mutually exclusive, and thus dentinal sensitivity or pain should be distinguished from degenerative pulpal inflammation.

Clinical symptoms correlate poorly with the health or histologic status of the pulp. The dentist should be aware that, for the moment, he or she is dealing with a tooth that is vital. The most appropriate treatment for a vital tooth causing apparent A-delta fiber pain can be determined only by the clinical presentation of the involved tooth. Although pulp preservation procedures can maintain the vitality of the tooth, the clinical circumstances leading to this decision must be reasonable. Nevertheless, A-delta fiber pain (dentinal sensitivity/pain) warrants consideration of pulp preservation measures as a primary treatment option.

Pulpitis pain. An external irritant of significant magnitude or duration injures the pulp. The injury is localized and initiates tissue inflammation. The dynamics of the inflammatory response will determine whether the process can be confined and the tissues can be repaired, restoring pulpal homeostasis. In a low-compliance environment an intense inflammatory vascular response can lead to adverse increases in tissue pressure, outpacing the pulp's compensatory mechanisms to reduce it. The damaged tissue succumbs by degenerating. The inflammatory process spreads circumferentially and incrementally from this site to involve adjacent structures, perpetuating the destructive cycle.[119]

An injured vital tooth with established local inflammation can also emit symptoms of A-delta fiber pain with provocation. In the presence of inflammation, the response is exaggerated and disproportionate to the challenging stimulus, quite often thermal (mostly to cold). The *hyperalgesia* is induced by inflammatory mediators. As the exaggerated A-delta fiber pain subsides, however, pain seemingly remains and is perceived as a dull, throbbing ache. This second pain symptom signifies the inflammatory involvement of nociceptive C nerve fibers.

C fibers are small unmyelinated nerves that innervate the pulp much like the A-delta fibers. They are high-threshold fibers that course centrally in the pulp stroma and run subjacent to the A-delta fibers. Unlike A-delta fibers, C fibers are not directly involved with the pulpodentinal complex and are not easily provoked. C fiber pain surfaces with tissue injury and is modulated by inflammatory mediators, vascular changes in blood volume and blood flow, and increases in tissue pressure. When C fiber pain dominates over A-delta fiber pain, pain is more diffuse and the dentist's ability to identify the diseased tooth becomes more elusive. Just as significant, C fiber pain is an ominous symptom that signifies that irreversible local tissue damage has occurred.

With increasing inflammation of pulp tissues, C fiber pain becomes the only pain feature. Pain that may start as a short, lingering discomfort can escalate to an intense, prolonged episode or a constant, throbbing pain. The pain is diffuse and can be referred to a distant site or to other teeth. Occasionally, the inflamed vasculature is responsive to cold, which vasoconstricts the dilated vessels and reduces tissue pressure. Momentary relief from the intense pain is provided, which explains why some patients bring a container of ice water to the emergency appointment. Relief provided by a cold stimulus is diagnostic and indicates significant pulp necrosis. In the absence of endodontic intervention, the rapidly deteriorating condition will most likely progress to a periapical abscess.[51]

Stressed pulp syndrome. Not all C fiber pain symptoms are associated with a recent injury or acute inflammation of the pulp. In aging persons diffuse pulpal pain is seen increasingly with retained teeth that have been repeatedly or extensively restored. The pathophysiologic process in aging teeth is one of slow deterioration. Under these conditions the pulp of the restored tooth is stressed and is likely undergoing circulatory embarrassment, leading ultimately to ischemic necrosis.

C fiber pain from a stressed pulp is identical to that of degenerative pulpal inflammation. The pain occurs when hot liquids or foods raise intrapulpal pressure to levels that excite C fibers. The process is slow and the delayed response makes the association with heat provocation difficult. At times, coincidental dental treatment or changes in ambient pressure can initiate symptoms in teeth with degenerative pulpal disease. The patient can be confused by the apparently spontaneous appearance of diffuse pain symptoms.

Mediators of pulpal pain[110]

Inflammation of pulp tissue can manifest itself as acute pain, chronic pain, or no pain at all. Biochemical pathways and immunologic mechanisms participate directly or indirectly in initiating and sustaining pulpal inflammation.[49] To set the stage for repair of inflamed tissues, activated pulpal defenses must be able to remove the irritants hemodynamically and moderate the inflammatory process.

Ideally, the inflammatory cycles of vascular stasis, capillary permeability, and chemotactic migration of leukocytes to injured tissues are synchronized with the removal of irritants and drainage of exudate from the area. With moderate to severe injury, an aberrant increase in capillary pressure can lead to excessive permeability and fluid accumulation. A progressive pressure front builds and begins to passively compress and collapse all local venules and lymphatic channels,[119] outpacing the pulp tissue's capacity to drain or shunt the exudate.[49,51] Blood flow to the area ceases, and the injured tissue undergoes necrosis. Leukocytes in the area degenerate and release intracellular lysosomal enzymes, forming a microabscess.

Mediators of vascular inflammation. Metabolites released from specific and nonspecific inflammatory pathways directly and indirectly affect the initiation and control of vascular events, increasing tissue pressure. Pain from pressure heralds the onset of inflammation. Nonspecific biochemical mediators such as histamine, bradykinin, prostaglandins, leukotrienes, and elements of the complement system dilate blood vessels, increase permeability, and thus increase local interstitial pressures. Some mediators are short-lived but are constantly replaced through the newly extravasating plasma.[38] The renewed presence of mediators sustains the inflammatory process beyond the initial traumatic event. Fluid leakage diminishes blood flow and results in vascular stasis and hemoconcentration in the vessel. Platelets aggregated in the vessels release the neurochemical serotonin, which is leaked along with plasma into the interstitial tissues.[38] More detailed information on this phenomenon can be found in Chapter 15.

Mediators of neurogenic inflammation. The neurochemicals serotonin and prostaglandin induce a state of *hyperalgesia* in local nerve fibers.[38,118] In the sensitized state nerve tissues seemingly "overreact" to all low-grade intensity stimulations with acute pain symptoms, which can also occur spontaneously. In addition, neuropeptides such as substance P and calcitonin gene–related peptide are released by the sensitized nerves.[38] At the local level the neuropeptides stimulate the release of histamine, which refuels the vascular inflammatory cycle. The sustained inflammatory cycle is detrimental to pulpal recovery, terminating in tissue necrosis.

Nonodontogenic pain

It is common for orofacial pain from nonodontogenic structures to mimic pulpal-periradicular pain. Pain symptoms are often acute and confusing to the patient, who will interpret the pain as a "toothache." It is up to the dentist, then, to understand the language and symptoms of pain to glean the many subtle clues in the search for a cause. The information that is obtained from the patient is integrated with the dentist's own knowledge of orofacial disorders that can mimic toothache.

With a thorough knowledge of these painful entities, the dentist is able to undertake the task of deliberate and selective elimination of nonessential pain characteristics. Through this process the predominant pathognomonic pain patterns are identified and a definitive diagnosis is achieved.

Of the many entities that mimic endodontic symptoms, seven of the most common nonodontogenic conditions that may be seen for urgent care will be briefly reviewed. The emphasis here is on diagnosis. The discussion contrasts pain features that overlap endodontic symptoms with distinctive clinical features that characterize the entity as nonodontogenic. (A thorough review of the causes and management of orofacial pain entities is found in Chapter 3.)

It is best to put into perspective the overlapping pain features that mimic pulpal-periradicular inflammatory pain. Facial pain typically follows the distribution of blood vessels or neural pathways and can arise from the supplied somatic structures. The area of neural involvement may be greater than, or limited to, the trigeminal nerve distribution. The wide painful region on the face can be confusing to the patient. Pain symptoms are often felt as "diffuse" and, with unilateral confinement, similar to symptoms of irreversible pulpitis. Ultimately, a broadly focused search reveals somatic sensitivity, discloses an area and pattern of cutaneous hypersensitivity, and exposes

a psychologically troubled patient or one whose "textbook" description of pain symptoms cannot always be substantiated with clinical testing.

Disorders associated with acute jaw pain[95]

Although many diseases are marked by pain in the mandible or maxilla, a number of these conditions appear to be more prevalent in elderly populations. People in this age group often exhibit chronic medical problems and take a variety of medications, making differential diagnosis of jaw pain difficult.

Trigeminal neuralgia.[21] The onset of trigeminal neuralgia occurs late in life and is extremely distressing for the patient. Attacks of pain are confined to one side and involve one division of the nerve (although bilateral successive involvements have occurred).[87] The attack produces severe "dental" pain but is described as lancinating, electrical, shocking, shooting, sharp, cutting, or stabbing. When asked, however, the patient will trace a line along the distribution of the nerve on the face. The most prominent feature is the existence of trigger points. These areas are often located in the skin of the lips, cheeks, or gums and when touched provoke a painful response. Nevertheless, the possibility that these symptoms, which resemble trigeminal neuralgia, are being triggered by pulpal disease must be ruled out.[87]

A bout of paroxysmal pain in this degenerative neural condition is characteristically short, lasting several seconds but no longer than 1 minute. There can be secondary pain with a vague burning or aching quality. The patient, usually a woman, tells of rigorously massaging the cutaneous site to deaden the pain.

The attacks come in series and can end abruptly. The period of remission is also free from the thermal and periapical sequelae seen with genuine endodontic disease. The patient quickly learns with each episode of painful attacks to avoid the cutaneous or intraoral site that sets off the attack. Some patients are able to identify and describe a vague prodrome of tingling just before an attack. Characteristically and understandably, the patient is reluctant to have the area examined. The medical community has speculated on the etiologic basis of trigeminal neuralgia; the condition has been proposed to be viral in origin, the result of stroke or cerebral tumor,[25] or caused by dental trauma. A cause-and-effect relationship between advancing age and demyelination of the nerve may prove to be the most promising explanation.[95] Because carbamazepine (Tegretol) provides excellent initial results, it is recommended as a first-line drug in the diagnosis and treatment of the condition.[56]

Myocardial pain.[21] The presence of jaw pain related to cardiac causes underscores the importance of recording each patient's medical history, including relevant symptoms. Reports on the condition of cardiac-induced jaw pain show that approximately 10% of cases involve referred pain to the mandible.[95] In an imminent myocardial infarct, the pain is both sudden and severe and is not induced by oral stimulation. In chronic angina or coronary (ischemic) artery disease, pain may be less intense and may be associated with emotional or physical activity. With cessation of the inducing activity (e.g., by resting in the dental chair), pain from ischemia of heart muscle usually dissipates.

Myocardial pain referred to the jaws has often surfaced on the left side, but bilateral involvement has been documented. It is not unusual to find collateral pain in the shoulder(s), back, neck, and especially down the arms. This important feature is generated as sensory impulses cross through several thoracic and cervical dermatomes to reach the sensory pathways of the jaws. Collateral pain may not be readily apparent or present in every case. Interpretation of body language (e.g., signs and symptoms of shock, nausea, difficulty breathing, sweats, clammy skin, pallor) can give a better sense of the gravity of the patient's situation.

With imminent myocardial infarct, pain symptoms are constant and spread to involve vast areas of the maxilla and mandible, or they travel down into the neck, or up into the temporal and zygomatic regions. During this time the patient becomes anxious and complains of pain that is increasingly unbearable. The cutaneous area over the jaws may be massaged in a desperate attempt to obtund the pain.

Entities associated with acute tooth pain

Maxillary sinusitis. It is not unusual for inflammation of the sinus-lining mucosa to evoke facial pain that involves all of the subjacent maxillary teeth, producing dental discomfort. Maxillary sinusitis can produce a constant dull-to-moderate aching pain in multiple teeth on the involved side.[21,96] To the exclusion of pulpally involved teeth, the teeth adjacent to the sinus are generally healthy but behave identically to each other, being uniformly hypersensitive to thermal stimulation and sensitive on palpation and percussion. Pain may increase with eating, may involve the entire quadrant up to the facial midline, or may be referred to the mandibular teeth on the same side.

Pain from an inflamed sinus membrane and associated nasal mucosa is characteristically felt in the face. Cutaneous pain features share in the clinical description of this condition and include complaints such as a fullness in the face, tenderness of the skin overlying the sinus, pain that increases with lying down or bending over, and pain that spreads to the scalp and toward the nose, often in association with a postnasal drip.

In the differential diagnosis of maxillary sinusitis, the endoantral syndrome and barodontalgia-barosinusitis from chronic pulpal or periapical pathosis must be considered to rule out a coexisting endodontically induced infection of the sinus lining.[98]

Atypical facial pain. Atypical facial pain (AFP) is an affliction that can be manifested as toothache pain.[21] The "toothache" is uncharacteristic and the diagnosis of AFP has become a "wastebasket" for facial pain that does not fit a recognized syndrome. Pain is felt in the teeth and periodontium and is described as steady and pulsating. In a differential diagnosis, however, the involved tooth or teeth are found to have healthy pulps.

The pain is vague and difficult for the patient to localize, suggestive of a chronic onset. It is a constant, aching, burning, and nagging sensation deep in the tissues. The condition is not associated with any identifiable trigger points and crosses over rather than follows known neurologic boundaries. As pain travels, it appears along vascular arborizations into the head region and behind the orbit. Further, the patient often reports that analgesics have no effect.

The intensity of the pain increases with physical exhaustion and general debilitation of the patient, suggesting an underlying psychogenic foundation to this condition. Early recognition of AFP spares the patient unwarranted dental treatment and leads to appropriate referral.

Phantom tooth pain.[65] Phantom tooth pain (PTP) is a syndrome of persistent pain in the teeth and oral structures after pulp extirpation, apicoectomy, or extraction. The incidence of this condition is reported to be 3% of the population undergoing pulp amputation.[6] It is similar to phantom limb pain and is often confused with atypical facial pain. However, although the literature ascribes a psychologic cause or association to AFP, the research pertaining to PTP shows no correlation.[64] *The difficulty of this condition is that it is often misdiagnosed.* The pain is described as a constant, dull, deep ache with occasional spontaneous sharp pains.[63] In chronic cases patients have difficulty localizing the pain to a given tooth. Additionally, the erroneous treatment of neighboring teeth obscures the original condition. Testing and radiographic surveys are negative.

PTP must be differentially diagnosed from two major facial pain disorders and typical odontalgia. Neuralgias, such as recurrent trigeminal neuralgia with sudden, electric stabbing pain, are unlike the dull uninterrupted pain of PTP. Trigeminal neuralgia has a peak onset in the fifth and sixth decades. PTP occurs in both sexes but can be found in any adult age group. Careful differentiation of PTP from AFP requires attention to the lack of boundaries in the somatic distribution of AFP and the patient's psychogenic component.

Herpes zoster (shingles). A recurrence of herpes zoster infection involving the second and third division of the trigeminal nerve can manifest in a rare prodrome of symptomatic pulpitis.[37] The latent virus resides in the gasserian ganglion after a primary chickenpox (varicella virus) infection. Like any trigeminal nerve involvement, pulpal pain is unilaterally confined. Toothache pain can be localized in one or more teeth and is described as sharp, throbbing, and intermittent. *The symptoms are believed to be genuine pulpal pain and not mimicked.*

During the prodrome, which can last for weeks, recognition of a recurrence of herpes zoster is nearly impossible. The symptoms are undeniably those of irreversible pulpitis, and the pulpitic teeth are easily identified by the patient. On examination, the dentist may be baffled to find the teeth intact, noncarious, and free of recent trauma.

The dilemma the dentist faces is whether to believe that the symptoms are genuine and benign to the health of the pulpitic tooth. A recent report suggests that intense symptoms are not benign and can lead to adverse pulpal responses, even necrosis.[37] An early decision to intervene endodontically during the prodrome of a suspected shingles infection can relieve the intense pulpal pain. Understandably, the shingles infection may be followed to its clinical conclusion without intervention. Postshingles infection monitoring for development of pulpal or periapical pathosis is indicated.[102] Patient suffering and the clinical merits of each case should dictate the best course of action.

Neoplastic diseases. Neoplastic diseases are extremely rare but can mimic symptoms of a toothache.[96] The nature of the pain can be severe, escalating with time and involving a developing paresthesia. The pain features are out of character to those typically seen with inflammatory pulpal disease and should prompt the prudent dentist to seek consultation with and a referral to an oral surgeon or a physician.

Fabricated pain

Munchausen's syndrome.[21] This condition is characterized by elaborate description or creation of pain that either is not real or is self-inflicted. The profile of patients with Munchausen's syndrome runs the gamut from the psychotic to the neurotic, the pathologic liar to the chemically dependent addict.

The psychotic or neurotic patient gives a history that is convincingly accurate for orofacial pain but cannot be substantiated by examination and testing. The preoccupied patient may spend countless hours in a health science library to "research" the condition and often boasts of this when questioned. The dentist may be informed that he or she is the most recent of many professionals the patient has seen. The pain is *real* to the patient, who insists on treatment.

The chemically abusive patient occupies the other extreme and gives detailed textbook descriptions of pain. On examination, the dentist may actually find probable cause for the pain. The situation is self-induced or, at the insistence of the patient, "dentistogenic."

The addicted patient purposely shows up unannounced at inconvenient times in the work day, just before a holiday weekend, or even during the holiday with an "emergency" call to the office. This patient conveys convincing stories, such as being from out of town, saying that he or she "forgot or lost my painkillers," alleging dissatisfaction with his or her dentist and seeking someone "new" to take over, or requesting something to "tide me over" until the next work day. The addict may even allow the compassionate dentist to perform treatment. It becomes difficult to deny a prescription to someone who has been rendered urgent care. The patient specifies what type of medication is being sought and may abruptly change demeanor to insist on a strong painkiller.

DIAGNOSIS

As described in Chapter 10, the "standard of care" in dentistry requires that the practitioner provide the quality of care that is expected to be performed by a responsible and prudent dentist in the community. To render care for any orofacial emergency, the dentist must make a prudent and thoughtful diagnosis regarding the etiologic basis and present state of the patient's disease. The dentist's worth as a healer will never be more appreciated than by the patient who has suffered the pain of a throbbing and rapidly degenerating pulpitis that has interfered with eating and sleeping.

The endodontic emergency is a pulpal or periapical pathologic condition that manifests itself through pain, swelling, or both. An urgent endodontic emergency usually interrupts the normal office routine and patient flow. In addition, after-hours accommodations may have to be made to care for the patient.

Triage of the Pain Patient

Emergencies resulting from orofacial pain demand immediate professional attention. The urgency of the situation, however, should not preclude a thorough clinical evaluation of the patient. Orofacial pain can be the clinical manifestation of a variety of diseases involving the head and neck region. The cause must be reliably differentiated, odontogenic from nonodontogenic. The task is made needlessly difficult without a comprehensive knowledge of the pathophysiologic mechanisms of inflammatory pain of the pulp and periradicular tissues.

Triage can expedite the differentiation process by systematically sorting through the signs and symptoms of the presenting pain. Each entity is characterized as having a dental or nondental pain feature. Features that are shared and are not exclusive to either source are also noted. With the signs and symptoms collected in this manner, triage is concluded by noting the preponderance of pain features in either the dental or nondental category. A working differential diagnosis is thus methodically begun and directs the dentist to investigate further.

Triage of odontogenic symptoms should discriminate for sensory and proprioceptive sensations that are produced exclusively by inflammatory pulpal and periradicular diseases. Genuine endodontic pain involves nociceptive transmissions in the maxillary and mandibular branches of the trigeminal nerve.

Identifying orofacial pain definitively to be endodontic pain becomes increasingly difficult as the focus shifts away from a more localized and tooth-specific pain to an ever wider area on the face. Numerous orofacial diseases may mimic endodontic pain and may produce sensory misperception as a result of overlapping between sensory fibers of the trigeminal nerve and adjacent cranial and cervical sensory dermatomes. Convergence of signals in the medulla can cause sensory overload to occur and a perceptual error by the cerebral cortex.

Triage of nonodontogenic symptoms should discriminate for pain patterns that are inconsistent with inflammatory pulpal and periradicular diseases. Organic orofacial pain follows many different peripheral neurologic pathways but can also overlay onto the sensory distribution of the trigeminal nerve. Pain can also follow the vascular arborization of head and neck vessels. The interrelationship between the neural and vascular pathways and the orofacial structures they supply produces symptoms that can be readily distinguished as nondental. Pain features that are episodic with pain-free remissions, that have trigger points, that travel and cross the midline of the face, that surface with increasing mental stress, that are seasonal or cyclic, or that produce paresthesia are characteristics of nondental involvement.[21]

The process of diagnosis of the endodontic emergency, as set forth in this chapter, will concentrate on the acute emergency or the potentially complex orofacial pain emergency. The practitioner must collect the appropriate data—the set of signs, symptoms, and test results that will lead to a diagnosis.

Careful adherence to the basic principles and a systematic approach to procuring an accurate diagnosis cannot be overemphasized. A hasty diagnosis and inappropriate treatment of a suffering patient are pitfalls with the potential for a litigious aftermath. In procuring diagnostic data, the dentist must generate the following:

1. A "subjective" interrogatory examination
2. An "objective" clinical examination
3. A radiographic examination and evaluation

The clinician who reviews and prioritizes patient data in all emergencies in a deliberate and thorough manner can avoid the pitfalls of inaccurate diagnosis and inappropriate treatment.

Developing Data: Medical History

The subjective interrogatory examination of the patient must include a comprehensive evaluation of the patient's medical history. Although numerous authorities agree that there are almost no medical contraindications to endodontic therapy, it is important to understand how an individual's physical condition, medical history, and current medications might affect the treatment course or prognosis.

A medical history informs the evaluator of any "high-risk patient" whose therapy may have to be modified, such as a cardiac patient who might tolerate only short appointments. The medical history would also identify patients who require antibiotic prophylaxis for congenital or rheumatic heart disease. Some patients receiving chemotherapy may require antibiotic coverage because of a compromised immune system.[83] The medical history can identify patients for whom healing and repair of endodontic pathosis could be complicated or delayed, such as those who have uncontrolled diabetes or active acquired immunodeficiency syndrome (AIDS). Knowledge of specific critical blood values, immune status, and medications being used are essential to any therapy provided to a patient with human immunodeficiency virus (HIV).[5]

In situations in which the prognosis is guarded owing to systemic illness, a medical consultation with the patient's treating physician is imperative. The use of antibiotic prophylaxis to prevent infective endocarditis is justified in high-risk patients. It is reasonable to mitigate bacteremia in other selected patients at risk because of implanted prosthetic devices, congenital heart disease, hemodialysis, or impaired host defenses.[62,83]

There are also aspects of a patient's medical background that might have an impact on the chief complaint, the repair potential, or the radiographic appearance of disease. Sickle cell anemia, vitamin D–resistant rickets, and herpes zoster have all been implicated in spontaneous pulpal degeneration.[99] Nutritional disease, stress, and corticosteroid therapy can also decrease the potential for repair.[99]

Forms are available to the dentist that afford quick and efficient evaluation of patient systems to provide a simple means of taking a medical history (see suggested forms in Chapter 1). The dentist should follow up by reviewing what the patient has written and should seek more detailed information that may not impress the patient as important. Some women are reluctant to discuss their use of birth control pills for contraception, yet a number of common antibiotics used to treat endodontic infections significantly decrease the efficacy of oral contraceptives.[17] Possible drug interactions between currently prescribed medications and those prescribed for the emergency must be understood by the dentist and noted on the patient's record.

Against the possibility of nondisclosure of important data by the patient or omission on the medical history form, the diagnostician should ask supplemental questions in the following areas of concern:

1. Current medical condition
2. History of significant illness or serious injury
3. Emotional and psychologic history
4. Prior hospitalizations
5. Current medications, including over-the-counter remedies
6. Habits (alcohol, tobacco, drugs)
7. Any other noticeable sign or symptom that may indicate an undiagnosed health problem (Fig. 2-1)

All significant medical data should be recorded on the patient's record (Fig. 2-2). In the emergency setting, if possible, the dentist should measure and record the patient's vital signs (i.e., pulse rate, blood pressure, respiratory rate, temperature). A hyperventilating patient, one who is febrile, or one who has high blood pressure will require a thoughtful consideration of systemic or emotional complications to treatment. If any question exists regarding the patient's current medical status, the appropriate physician should be consulted.

Dental History

The subjective interrogatory examination continues with the dental history. This is unquestionably the most important aspect of the diagnostic workup and, if carefully done, will build rapport in the dentist-patient relationship. This subjective questioning should attempt to provide a narrative from the patient that addresses the following points:

1. Chief complaint—as expressed in the patient's own words
2. Location—the site(s) where symptoms are perceived

3. Chronology—inception, clinical course, and temporal pattern of the symptoms
4. Quality—how the patient describes the complaint
5. Intensity and severity of symptoms
6. Affecting factors—stimuli that aggravate, relieve, or alter the symptoms
7. Supplemental history—past facts and current symptoms characterizing the difficult diagnosis

The diagnostician should listen carefully to the patient's choice of words, remembering that the patient's descriptions are being filtered through a myriad of complex psychosocial and emotional components that affect not only the account of the pain but also how it is perceived.

Chief complaint

The questions listed in the following sections ensure comprehensive and logical evaluation of the chief complaint. When questioning the patient, the dentist may need to rephrase or completely restate a question to ensure that the patient understands. The dentist should be prepared to paraphrase the patient's responses to verify what was heard.

Location of chief complaint

The patient is asked to indicate the location of the chief complaint by pointing to it directly with one finger. Pointing avoids verbal ambiguity, and the dentist can note if the pain is intraoral or extraoral, precise or vague, localized or diffuse. If the symptoms radiate or if the pain is referred, the direction and extent can also be demonstrated.

The diagnostician should be well aware of referred pain pathways because referred pain is common with advanced pulpitis when the disease has not yet produced signs or symptoms in the attachment apparatus. In posterior molars pain can often be referred to the opposing quadrant or to other teeth in the same quadrant. Maxillary molars often refer pain to the zygomatic, parietal, and occipital regions of the head, whereas lower molars frequently refer pain to the ear, angle of the jaw, or posterior regions of the neck. Corroborating tests and data are necessary to make a definitive diagnosis or to justify invasive therapy whenever referred pain is suspected.

Chronology of symptoms

The dentist must explore the exact nature of the patient's symptoms because of the extreme variability of patients' descriptions of a complaint.

Inception of symptoms

The patient should relate when the symptoms of the chief complaint were initially perceived. He or she may be aware of a history of dental procedures, trauma, or other events such as sinus surgery or tumors in the areas of concern.

Clinical manifestations

Beyond the inception of symptoms, it is extremely important for the dentist to record details of symptoms, emphasizing these features:

1. *Mode:* Is the onset or abatement of symptoms spontaneous or provoked? Is it sudden or gradual? If symptoms can be stimulated, are they immediate or delayed?
2. *Periodicity:* Do the symptoms have a temporal pattern or are they sporadic or occasional? Often, early pulpitis is reported by the patient as recurring symptoms in the

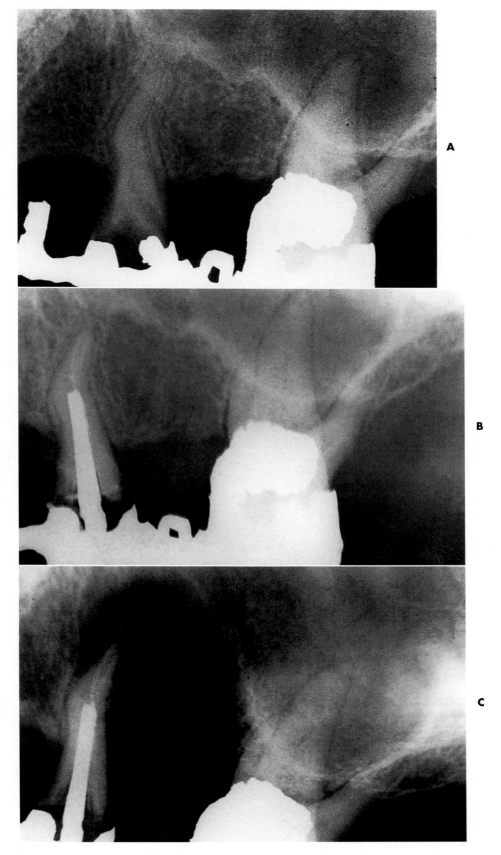

FIG. 2-1 A, Preoperative endodontic involvement of left maxillary first premolar. **B,** Completion of the endodontic treatment. **C,** Reexamination at 6 months. Radiographic evidence of significant bone loss and apical resorption is seen, which is atypical of endodontic failure. Biopsy specimen revealed multiple myeloma, a malignancy of the lymphoreticular system. Discovery of systemic disease on the dental films was confirmed by head and chest films that demonstrated widespread involvement. The patient died 7 months later.

Heart Condition	Anemia / Bleeding	Epilepsy / Fainting	Allergies:	Major Medical Prob:
angina	Diabetes / Kidney	Sinusitis / ENT	penicillin / antibiotics	Females: Pregnant _____ mo
coronary	Hepatitis / Liver	Glaucoma / Visual	aspirin / Tylenol	Recent Hosp. Operation:
surgery	Herpes	Mental / Neural	codeine / narcotics	Current Medical TX:
pacemaker	Thyroid / Hormonal	Tumor / Neoplasms	local anesthetic	Medications:
Rheumatic Fever / Murmur	Asthma / Respiratory	Alcoholism / Addictions	N_2O/O_2	
Hypertension / Circulatory	Ulcers / Digestive	Infectious Diseases	other:	
	Migraine / Headaches	Venereal Disease		Initial:

FIG. 2-2 Chart of a medical systems review common to a comprehensive dental record.

evening or after a meal, giving the inflammation a predictable or reproducible quality.

3. *Frequency:* Have the symptoms persisted since they began, or have they been intermittent?
4. *Duration:* How long do symptoms last when they occur? Are they stated as "momentary" or "lingering"? If they are persistent, the duration should be estimated in seconds, minutes, hours, or longer intervals. If the symptoms can be induced, are they momentary or do they linger? *By this time, the patient may have provided the dentist with enough data to make an endodontic diagnosis.* However, some cases have far more diffuse symptoms and require a more persistent and astute analysis of key descriptions.

Quality of pain

The patient is asked to render a detailed description of each symptom associated with the presenting emergency. This description is important in differential diagnosis of the pain and for selection of objective clinical tests to corroborate symptoms.

Certain adjectives describe pain of bony origin, for example, *dull, drawing,* or *aching.* Other adjectives—*throbbing, pounding,* or *pulsing*—describe the vascular response to tissue inflammation. *Sharp, electric, recurrent,* or *stabbing* pain is usually caused by pathosis of nerve root complexes, sensory ganglia, or peripheral innervation, which is associated with irreversible pulpitis or trigeminal neuralgia. A single episode of sharp, persistent pain can result from acute injury to muscle or ligament, as in temporomandibular joint dislocation or iatrogenic perforation into the periodontal attachment apparatus.

Pulpal and periapical pathosis produce sensations that are described with such terms as *aching, pulsing, throbbing, dull, gnawing, radiating, flashing, stabbing,* or *jolting* pain. Although such descriptions support suspicion of an odontogenic cause, the diagnostician cannot ignore the fact that many of these adjectives can also describe nonodontogenic pathosis.

Intensity of pain

The patient's perception of and reaction to an acute pain emergency, especially one that is odontogenic in origin, is widely variable. For an unremitting toothache, the treating clinician usually makes a diagnosis and renders emergency treatment on the basis of its intensity. The dentist therefore should try to quantify the intensity level of the pain symptoms reported by the patient. There are methods to accomplish this goal:

1. Try to quantify the pain. Assigning to the pain a degree of 0 (none) to 10 (most severe or intolerable pain) helps monitor the patient's perception of the pain throughout the course of treatment.
2. Have the patient classify the pain as mild, moderate, or severe. This classification has implications for the question, *How does the pain affect the patient's lifestyle?* The pain can be classified as severe if it interrupts or significantly alters the patient's daily routine. Generally, pain

that interferes with sleeping, work, or leisure activities is significant. If bedrest or potent analgesics are required, the pain is likewise considered extreme.

Whenever symptoms are clinically reproducible, the intensity of the pain should alert the dentist to which clinical and diagnostic tests are most appropriate. If the clinician can reproduce them, more painful symptoms will help locate the chief complaint and provide corroborative information. Reproducing less intense symptoms, although it "creates data," may not help differentiate the involved tooth from those responses that are within normal limits.

Affecting factors

The objective of the next part of the interrogatory examination is to identify which factors provoke, intensify, alleviate, or otherwise affect the patient's symptoms. Before any corroborative testing is attempted (such as thermal or percussion tests), it is imperative to know the level of intensity of each affecting stimulus and the interval between stimulus and response. The patient who describes a toothache that manifests itself when the patient is about halfway through drinking a cup of coffee is exhibiting a delayed-onset response to heat. This has a significant bearing on how clinical testing should proceed. Unless adequate time between stimulus and response is allowed, coincidence may have the dentist stimulating a second tooth at the same time a previously stimulated tooth is manifesting a delayed response.

The prudent clinician will be cautious and conservative in the use of the percussion test. If by questioning the patient it is learned that percussion may elicit an extreme response, it would be unwise to immediately start percussing teeth and provoke so much discomfort for the patient that the diagnosis is greatly clouded. Symptoms can be more meaningful if the investigator takes the time to hear and understand the circumstances in which they occur.

Local stimuli. The following stimuli are generally associated with odontogenic symptoms: heat, cold, sweets, percussion, biting, chewing, and palpation. The significance of these provoking factors for the diagnosis of endodontic disease is discussed in Chapter 1. In addition, the patient may have spontaneous pain of variable quality, intensity, location, and duration.

Predisposing factors. Just as there are factors that provoke odontogenic pain, there are factors that can precipitate the onset of symptoms, which may indicate a nonodontogenic cause:

Postural Changes: Head or jaw pain accentuated by bending over, blowing the nose, or jarring of the skeleton (e.g., by jogging) may imply involvement of the maxillary sinuses.
Time of Day: Stiffness and pain in the jaws and masticatory muscles on waking may indicate occlusal disharmony or temporomandibular joint dysfunction and possible acute pulpalgia.[125] Pain on strenuous or vigorous activity may indicate pulpal or periapical inflammation.

DENTAL HISTORY:		CHIEF COMPLAINT		SYMPTOMATIC			ASYMPTOMATIC			
SYMPTOMS	Location	Chronology		Quality		Affected By		Prior Tx		Initial:
		Inception	sharp	intensity	hot	palpation	Tx: restorative	Yes No		**TOOTH**
			dull	+ ++ +++	cold	manipulation	emergency	Yes No		
		Clinical Course:		spontaneous			RCT	Yes No		R ——— L
localized	referred		pulsating	provoked	biting	head position	Sx Pre-Tx:	Yes No		
diffuse	radiating	constant momentary	steady	reproducible	chewing	activity				
		intermittent lingering	enlarging	occasional	percussion	time of day	Sx Post-Tx:	Yes No		

FIG. 2-3 Systematic format for charting the dental history.

Pulpal or sinus involvement may also be revealed by changes in barometric pressure, which can occur during scuba diving or flying at high altitudes. Another significant implication would be jaw pain associated with exertion, which may be a warning sign of coronary artery disease.

Hormonal Change: It has been seen that "menstrual toothache" or recurring hypersensitivity may occur when there is an increase in body fluid retention.[10] The teeth may ache and may even become tender to percussion. The symptoms disappear when the cycle ends.

Supplemental history for difficult diagnosis

For many endodontic emergencies there is a cause-and-effect relationship. The dentist restores a fractured filling in a patient's mandibular left first molar, and the patient experiences extreme sensitivity to cold, which lingers several minutes. The diagnosis is uncomplicated: it is irreversible pulpitis, the treatment for which is root canal therapy. However, as biologic variability goes, there will always be cases that perplex and confound even the most astute diagnostician. Every dentist assuredly will be asked to diagnose and treat emergencies whose symptoms are vague and whose cause is far less obvious.

The patient who complains of diffuse, disabling pain presents a challenge. There may be a great deal of pain for the patient but very little evidence that constitutes real information for the dentist. If, in addition, the patient is demanding that something be done, this can compound the stress of the emergency visit. Faced with a dissatisfied, insistent patient, there is a strong temptation to "do something," even before a definitive diagnosis can be made. **This situation is to be avoided at all costs.** Otherwise, the dentist may become vulnerable to claims of misdiagnosis or negligence. Patients who are made aware of the dentist's concern for their problem and empathy for their suffering will be more inclined to accept a cautious approach during the diagnostic process. The clinician must emphasize the scientific nature of the diagnosis and the real possibility that it may take more than one visit to identify the problem.

The dentist does well to tell patients that it might be necessary to wait a while for vague symptoms to localize. This conservative approach is often necessary in pulpal pathosis confined to the root canal space, which can refer pain to other teeth or to nondental sites. It may be necessary for the inflammation to involve the attachment apparatus before it can be localized. Pain generally can be managed with analgesics until a definitive diagnosis can be made.

Pain diary for difficult diagnosis

A daily diary can provide valuable information to aid in the difficult diagnosis. Patients' verbal reports are often vague or overdramatized and can be contradictory. The frequency and severity of symptoms can vary with time, and the patient who is stressed may not report critical information accurately. In these types of cases, especially when the dentist is trying to distinguish between odontogenic and nonodontogenic pain, a pain diary provides an hour-by-hour or day-by-day narrative. The more chronic or diffuse the complaint, the longer the diary should be kept; 2 to 3 weeks is sometimes necessary. Information such as the severity of pain (on a 1 to 10 scale), the duration, the time of day, and the type of provocation or activity associated with the discomfort should be recorded. Patients are often surprised to find out when it hurts or what provokes the pain. Similarly, psychogenic problems triggered by stress may be revealed as the patient begins to correlate his or her pain with certain events. The patterns of discomfort may provide concise information for the dentist and may place the problem in perspective for patients to help modify their behavior toward their pain.

In the final analysis, after they provide descriptive information about their chief complaint, patients should recount any significant incidents in the affected area—trauma, previous symptoms or treatments, and complications. Certain descriptions of pain, such as trigger zones or headaches, and medical conditions such as coronary artery disease or a history of neoplasm are details that should be considered in a differential diagnosis when the cause of pain is sought.

After organizing, analyzing, and assimilating all the pertinent descriptions, facts, and data, the dentist should be ready to proceed with the clinical examination phase of the diagnostic process.

Clinical Examination

Records

If the dentist is to provide a precise and structured appraisal of a patient's chief complaint, an efficient record that quantifies diagnostic data is a necessity. Suggested forms appear in Figs. 2-3 and 2-4. Details of the comprehensive clinical examination and data acquired from diagnostic tests should be recorded.

The clinical examination has three components: (1) physical inspection, (2) diagnostic tests, and (3) radiographic interpretation.

The clinician is to be reminded that even in an area with numerous dental problems, in the true endodontic emergency, it is most likely that only one tooth is responsible for the acute situation. Clinically, it is rare that, on a biologic level, the set of circumstances that could produce the odontogenic emergency would occur in two teeth with the same intensity at the same time.

The physical inspection should include observations of periodontal health; tissue color and texture; tooth discoloration;

CLINICAL FINDINGS

EXAMINATION		RADIOGRAPHIC		CLINICAL		DIAGNOSTIC TESTS						
Tooth		Attachment Apparatus	Tooth	Soft Tissues	Tooth #							
WNL		PDL normal	WNL	WNL	perio							
caries		PDL thickened	discoloration	extra-oral swelling	mobility							
restoration		alveolar bone, WNL	caries	intra-oral swelling	percussion							
calcification		diffuse lucency	pulp exposure	sinus tract	palpation							
resorption		circumscribed lucency	prior access	lymphadenopathy	cold							
fracture		resorption	attrition / abrasion	TMJ	hot							
perforation / deviation		apical	fracture	perio:	EPT							
prior RCTx/RCF		lateral	restoration		transillum							
separated instrument		hypercementosis	amalgam		cavity							
canal obstruction		osteosclerosis	composite		bite / chewing							
post / build-up		perio:	inlay / onlay		date:							
open apex			temporary									
			crown									
			abutment									

FIG. 2-4 Chart for clinical findings and diagnostic data.

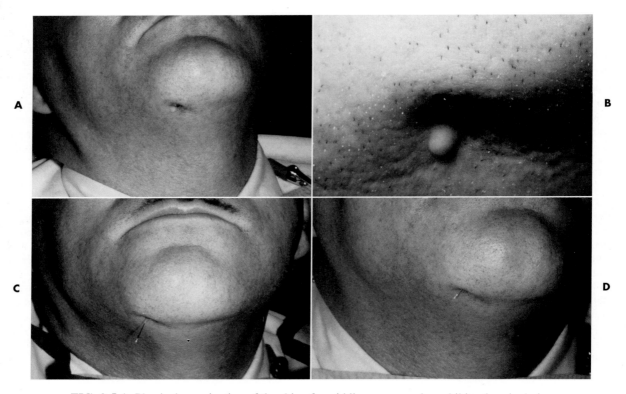

FIG. 2-5 A, Physical examination of the skin of a middle-age man who exhibits chronic drainage in the lower right chin area. The lesion was resistant to dermatologic therapy. **B,** Closer inspection of the area reveals active drainage. **C** and **D,** Presence of an extraoral sinus tract was confirmed by inserting a silver cone to the source, the mandibular first bicuspid. Confirmation was made by dental radiographs and pulp vitality testing.

and presence, condition, and extent of restorations, erosion, fractures, caries, sinus tracts, and swelling (Fig. 2-5). A thorough periodontal assessment, with careful probing of the sulcus and attachment apparatus and notation of mobilities, is a standard and essential element of the physical inspection.

Diagnostic tests (described in Chapter 1) enable the practitioner to do the following:

1. Define the pain by evoking reproducible symptoms that characterize the chief complaint.
2. Provide an assessment of normal responses for comparison with abnormal responses that may be indicative of pathosis.

Obviously, the usefulness of diagnostic testing is a function of the clinician's correct and systematic application of those tests and their proper interpretation. Diagnostic tests may include hot and cold thermal testing, tooth percussion, electric pulp testing, tissue palpation, transillumination and magnification, test cavity preparation, and anesthetic tests to localize pain. All these entities, and the fundamentals of diagnosis, are discussed in Chapter 1. This discussion focuses on those clini-

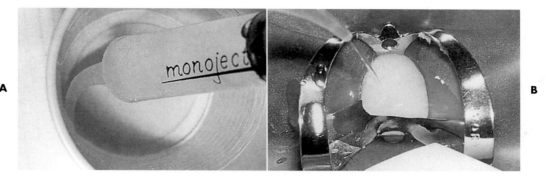

FIG. 2-6 A, Syringe for loading hot water to bathe the suspected tooth. **B,** Rubber dam isolation of a central incisor that is sensitive to heat. The patient should test the water with a finger to identify the affecting temperature.

cal considerations relative to testing that are requisite to identifying and treating the endodontic emergency.

When diagnostic testing is required to evaluate a patient's chief complaint, the success of the analysis depends on the following clinician characteristics:

1. Awareness of the limitations of the various tests and how to administer them
2. Biologic knowledge of the inflammatory process and the pain phenomenon
3. Knowledge of nonodontogenic entities that mimic pulpal and periapical pathosis

Investigators have explained why teeth with radiographically discernible periapical lesions retain pulpal innervation, even when necrosis is anticipated.[60] This fact can confound the interpretation of pulp vitality testing and may engender inaction on the part of the dentist when true pathosis is present. It should reinforce the requirement to provide a thorough evaluation and corroborative data before a definitive diagnosis is made.

The dentist should include adequate controls for any set of applied test procedures. Several adjacent, opposing, and contralateral teeth should be tested before the tooth in question is tested to establish the patient's normal range of response. The dentist should use care not to bias a patient's response by indicating to the patient a suspected culprit tooth before it is evaluated.

Thermal tests

Endodontists remind us that a misdiagnosis can result from misperception of symptoms, misinterpretation of data, and an incomplete diagnostic examination.[96] They have concluded that, in the difficult diagnosis of thermal sensitivity, it is imperative to accurately recreate with the thermal tests the conditions that stimulate the pain. In general, endodontists recommend that each tooth be isolated properly with a rubber dam and bathed in hot water or iced water to reproduce the environment in which the pain is evoked most closely. This method is also very effective in evaluating teeth with full coverage restorations, whether porcelain or metal.

For patients who experience an onset of prolonged moderate or severe pain when taking hot or cold substances into the mouth, rubber dam isolation for thermal testing will reproduce the symptoms more reliably than any other method. Once the complaint is reproduced, the hot or cold fluid should be quickly

aspirated away from the patient's tooth to provide relief. The dentist must use methodical diagnostic technique to avoid producing conflicting and unreliable responses. The sensory response of teeth is refractory to repeated thermal stimulation. To avoid a misinterpretation of a response, the dentist should wait an appropriate time for tested teeth to respond and recover (Fig. 2-6).

Percussion

If the patient's chief complaint involves pain to biting or chewing, an attempt to identify the initiation of the symptoms can be initially assessed with a soft but resistant object. Having the patient chew on a cotton roll, a cotton swab, or the flexible, reverse end of a low-speed suction straw will identify a single tooth more quickly than simple percussion when the pain is elusive (see Chapter 1). Use of the Tooth Slooth for cuspal and dentinal fractures will readily identify cracks hidden under restorations or those newly developed in the crown or root. Finally, selective percussion from various angles will help identify and isolate teeth with early inflammation in the periodontium.

Electric pulp testing

The clinician should be aware of the limitations of electric pulp testing. The potential for erroneous results—either false positive or false negative—is described in Chapter 1. The electric pulp test should be regarded as an aid in detecting pulpal neural response and not a measure of pulpal health or pathosis. Corroborating tests are also mandatory. Basing a diagnosis of necrosis solely on a nonresponsive electric pulp test ignores error of technique or a malfunctioning device. In addition, secondary dentin, trauma, restorations, and dystrophic calcification may all contribute to negative responses on a normal tooth.

Transillumination and magnification

The use of fiberoptic lighting and chairside magnification has become indispensable in the search for cracks, fractures, undetected canals, and obstructions in root canal therapy. The fact that magnification (e.g., Designs for Vision or a surgical microscope) and transillumination might allow the dentist the only means of diagnosing a cracked tooth or managing an obstructed canal requires dentists to practice at new and advancing levels of care.

Radiography

After collecting the details of the chief complaint from the patient's history, physical examination, and clinical or laboratory testing, the dentist should obtain the required radiographic views that will contribute to the location and identification of the patient's stated problem. Occasionally, the contralateral side may need to be viewed, in the event that unusual tooth or alveolar anatomy requires that bilateral symmetry be considered.

Although unnecessary use of radiation is definitely discouraged, the attending dentist is cautioned to use discretion in accepting prior diagnostic radiographs from the patient or another dentist, no matter how recently they were made. Such radiographs may not accurately reflect the present condition of the teeth and surrounding bone. Investigations have shown that for a radiograph to exhibit a periapical radiolucency the lesion must have expanded to the corticomedullary junction and a portion of the bone mineral must be lost.[11] This situation can occur in a short time in the presence of an aggressive infection. New radiographs taken when treatment is actually initiated may corroborate a diagnosis or point to a different, unsuspected tooth. Furthermore, prior iatrogenic mishaps such as ledge formation, perforation, or instrument separation are critical for a newly treating dentist to uncover. The dentist who omits taking a new radiograph assumes legal responsibility for the procedural error because there is no documentation that it occurred before the current treatment of the patient. Good radiographic technique includes proper film placement, exposure, processing, and handling. These principles are the foundation for the attainment of a high-quality diagnostic radiograph and may provide the only legal defense in support of treatment outcomes.

The interpretation of radiographs can be a source of enlightenment and a source of misinformation. A thorough understanding of regional anatomic structures and their variations is critical to proper interpretation. A careful assessment of continuity in the periodontal ligament space, lamina dura, and root canal anatomy will distinguish healthy structures from diseased ones. Changes in the pulp chamber often constitute a record of past pulpal inflammation. Caries, secondary dentin under restorations, very large or narrow pulp chambers compared with adjacent teeth, deep bases, calcifications, and condensing osteitis all can indicate pulpal tissue undergoing chronic inflammation (Fig. 2-7). Use of an optical magnifier and proper illumination will help the examiner discern these subtle and intricate details in the radiographic image. The patient record should provide space to note radiographic changes (see Fig. 2-4). Subtle radiographic changes can often account for the only changes that might potentially identify the tooth causing pain. Proper selection of the appropriate type of radiographs (as discussed in Chapter 5) is paramount to complete differential diagnosis.

Determining the Diagnosis

The final phase of the diagnostic sequence requires a systematic analysis of all pertinent data accumulated from the patient's history, narrative, and clinical and radiographic evaluation. The dentist must be methodical in his or her approach to determine the cause and the diagnosis.

Considerations in treatment planning

The dentist should begin by determining whether the chief complaint is consistent with an endodontic cause. It is impor-

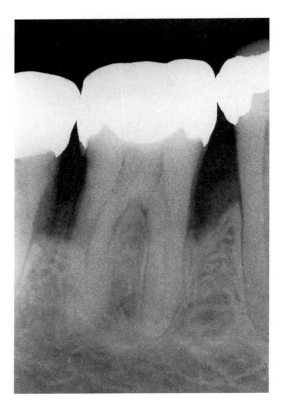

FIG. 2-7 Stressed pulp. A right-angle periapical projection reveals complete cusp coverage, dystrophic calcification of the pulp chamber, and chronic periodontal disease with moderate bone loss. This tooth should be a prime suspect in evaluation of vague pain in the area and is a candidate for endodontics if additional restorative treatment is planned.

tant to go through the mental exercise of narrowing down the possibilities to a specific tooth. Tests should be able to confirm whether pulpal pathosis is confined to the root canal space or has progressed and exhibits periapical extension. Specific etiologic factors such as caries, fracture, trauma, restorations, and other, more subtle, initiators of pulpal inflammation (developmental anomalies, orthodontic tooth movement, viral agents[37]) must also be identified.

Diagnostic determinants

There are specific diagnostic determinants that guide the practitioner into making judgements about diagnosis and treatment. These considerations address whether a given set of symptoms might indicate that treatment should be periodontal, transdentinal, or endodontic.

Periodontal considerations

An acute and painful periodontal abscess can mislead the careful diagnostician into believing a pulp lesion is the actual cause. Prognosis for long-term tooth retention is usually most dependent on the periodontal status, so before the pulpal status is determined, the results of the periodontal examination should be evaluated. If a significant periodontal condition exists, the extent of involvement and the nature of the problem should be elucidated. If extensive bone loss around a tooth has created acute pulpal symptoms, the practitioner must carefully weigh whether endodontic therapy is in the patient's interest, even though it may palliate the acute pain. Extraction of the hopeless tooth may be a better treatment. When endodontic pathosis is diagnosed, the clinician should determine whether periodontal factors are also contributing to the chief complaint. Those causal factors that specifically affect periodontal prognosis, such as inadequate epithelial attachment, lingual developmental grooves, and enamel projections, should be explicitly identified to separate palliative treatment from definitive therapy.

Dentinal considerations

Probably the most common kind of nonurgent odontogenic pain is pain related to exposure of dentinal tubules to outside stimuli. Because the physiologic features of this type of pain have been discussed previously, it is sufficient to describe the pain as very brief and sharp. Causes range from dentin exposure from caries to trauma of the dentin by enamel fracture. The overriding question for the clinician is whether the brief, sharp pain is a "normal" response of a healthy pulp or a sign of pulpal inflammation. Protection and insulation (transdentinal therapy) of exposed dentin in a healthy pulp will normally result in complete resolution of the dentinal symptoms. At this point endodontic therapy is not required unless there is a restorative requirement for such a treatment consideration. The quality of pain described as *dentinal* is usually considered to be normal. Pulp preservation techniques are most commonly indicated in these situations.

Endodontic involvement

Once an endodontic lesion is diagnosed, the dentist must confirm the location and delineate the specific nature of that problem. It is most often seen that irreversible pulpitis without inflammation in the periodontal ligament will exhibit referred pain because of the lack of proprioceptors in the pulp proper. A tooth with a history of deep caries, pulp caps, large and multiple restorations, trauma, or previous painful episodes should be the prime suspect. Once the tooth is identified, endodontic therapy should be instituted as soon as possible. Localization can be achieved by watchful waiting until the inflammation progresses, or it may be delineated by anesthetics or pulpal testing.

Restorative considerations

In considering the future restorability of the tooth in question, the dentist must assess whether he or she has the requisite skills and knowledge to carry out the treatment and serve the patient's best interest. Extraction is sometimes an acceptable and desirable alternative. Extraction has been suggested as a viable choice when no aesthetic, masticatory, or space-maintaining function can be attributed to the tooth in question. In addition, it is indicated if the tooth lacks adequate periodontal support, exhibits severe resorption, is unrestorable, or if the patient refuses endodontic treatment. (See Chapter 4 for a complete discussion of this issue.)

Endodontic treatment planning

An increasing majority of people choose endodontic therapy to alleviate their acute pain and restore their dentition. Providing the most biologic strategies for the management of acute odontogenic pain involves considering which areas of treatment afford the practitioner the greatest potential for a successful endodontic outcome. Pulpal and periapical pathoses that result in endodontic emergencies manifest themselves in a variety of ways.

Local pain, referred pain, spontaneous pain, provoked pain, thermal sensitivity, and swelling are all common features of pulpal and periapical pathosis. During therapy operator judgments and iatrogenic treatment factors, pulpal and periapical irritants, and patient factors (e.g., age, sex, tooth type, allergic history, preoperative pain, periapical lesion size, sinus tracts, and use of analgesics) all have a significant bearing on treatment-related emergencies.[112] Many of these complications also affect the incidence of postobturation pain and swelling and can alter the treatment plan. The remainder of this chapter describes treatment for the odontogenic emergency relative to its clinical presentation. The text focuses on recently investigated areas of emergency management that concentrate on several important themes that are central to efficacious treatment:

1. Pharmacologic control and management of pain and swelling
2. Complete debridement of the pulpal space
3. Treatment and prevention of midtreatment and postobturation flare-ups

MANAGEMENT OF ACUTE DENTAL PAIN

The treatment approaches described next pertain to permanent teeth with mature apices; for a discussion of diagnosis and treatment of primary teeth, immature permanent teeth, and traumatic injuries, see Chapters 16 and 22.

Acute Dental Pain

A number of insults can provoke a quick, sharp, momentary tooth pain that initially causes the patient to seek urgent care and consultation. These symptoms of A-delta pain cue the dentist to look for a vital tooth. Ideally, pulp preservation measures should take priority in the management of pain symptoms.

There are overriding factors that become apparent depending on the individual circumstances. These factors can alter subsequent treatment decisions. Overriding factors may include significant or obvious stained fracture lines, large or deep areas of decay, recurrent decay, or the *chronopathologic status* (age and current health) of the tooth in question. The defensive capabilities of the pulp diminish with successive treatment of the aging tooth, which adversely affects pulp vitality.[108] Chronopathologic factors include history of pulp capping (direct/indirect), history of trauma, orthodontic treatment, periodontal disease, history of extensive restorations (e.g., pins, buildups, crown), and the restorative treatment planned for the tooth (Fig. 2-7).

As the overriding factors are discovered, each must be carefully assessed because of the adverse impact they can have or may have had on current pulpal health. The dentist must then decide on the most appropriate treatment that will conserve the integrity of the pulpal tissue. At times, this may not be practical. The patient must be informed of the situation in an empathetic and compassionate manner. Treatment may shift radically from pulp preservation measures to deliberate removal of the pulp and the sealing of the root canal system in anticipation of a long-term restoration. What is important here is for both dentist and patient to realize that urgent care results in the retention of the tooth as a functioning member of the dentition, regardless of whether the pulp is retained.

Hypersensitive Dentin

Exposed cervical dentin from gingival recession, periodontal surgery, toothbrush abrasion, or erosion may result in root hypersensitivity. Any chemical (osmotic gradient), thermal (contraction/expansion), or mechanical (biting or digital scratching) irritant can disturb the fluid content in the dentinal tubules and excite nociceptive receptors in the pulp.[12]

Treatment of hypersensitive dentin has had limited success. A number of viable treatment modalities focus on the chemical or physical blockage of the patent dentinal tubules to prevent fluid movement from within. *Chemical desensitization* seeks to sedate the cellular processes within the tubules with corticosteroids or to occlude the tubules with a protein precipitate, a crystallized oxalate deposit,[84] or potassium ion formulations.[50] The mechanism of action involves blocking pulpal nociceptor activity by altering the excitability of the sensory nerves. *Physical techniques* attempt to block dentinal tubules with composite resins, varnishes, sealants, soft tissue grafts, and glass ionomer cements. The efficacy of these treatment approaches is often temporary and treatment must be repeated.

With increasing hypersensitivity, treatment can quickly escalate to the use of physical agents and preparation of the tooth surface. Laser techniques may provide the definitive solution for sealing the dentinal tubules permanently.

Recurrent Decay

Patients with large multisurface restorations may feel sharp pain when eating. Often an undetected gap has formed in the interface between dentin and restoration, leading to microleakage and recurrent decay. With sufficient occlusal pressure on the defective restoration, pain is produced as saliva in the gap is compressed against the exposed dentin interface.

Treatment of provoked pain that results from recurrent decay depends on the chronopathologic history of the tooth in question. The tooth may be amenable to pulp conservation measures, provided that A-delta fiber pain is the only symptom present and that it is produced on provocation. Thorough but atraumatic caries removal, placement of indirect pulp capping with calcium hydroxide where indicated, and temporization of the tooth with a sedative filling such as zinc oxide–eugenol material may be beneficial in stabilizing the chronically inflamed pulp. To assess the relative effectiveness of this treatment, the pulp must first be allowed to recover. A more permanent interim restoration is then placed but with the understanding that pulpal degeneration (stressed pulp syndrome) can occur in the future.

Inadvertent exposure of the pulp or emerging pulpal symptoms after careful caries removal are adverse developments for which endodontic treatment takes precedence over pulp preservation.

Recent Restoration

After a restorative procedure a tooth can sense inflammatory pain in both A-delta and C fibers. The common complaint is of pain that is provoked by a thermal stimulus that would normally not evoke a response. This state of hyperalgesia can be produced by inflammatory mediators and warns that significant local injury to the pulp has occurred.

Historically, postrestorative sensitivity, diagnosed as reversible pulpitis, was routinely managed by immediate removal of the restoration and placement of a sedative filling such as zinc

oxide–eugenol; little thought was given to the consequences. Before submitting the tooth to another insult, the dentist must reassess the situation for answers that only he or she knows. This step may prevent the needless removal of the restoration, which increases the likelihood that the pulp will succumb to the inflammatory process. On the other hand, if the sustained injury is significant, there is probably little that can be done to reverse the cascading events that lead eventually to pulpal degeneration.

The rendering of urgent care in this situation requires the differentiation between acts of commission and acts of omission. Acts of commission should seek to rectify poor treatment or faulty techniques. This might entail correction of hyperocclusion in a recent restoration, telltale shiny spot(s) in both centric and excursive occlusion. Inadequate or excessive interproximal contacts, which promote food impaction or excessive stresses along the root, must also be corrected. The tight contact must be reduced. The dentist should allow the tooth several weeks to recover from the restorative episode. The inadequate filling can then be removed and the tooth temporized with a sedative filling such as zinc oxide–eugenol.[118] This approach allows the pulp to recover fully before the final restoration is placed. Ligamental injections to induce operative anesthesia are discouraged in vital teeth that are sensitive on preparation. Anesthetics containing high concentrations of a vasoconstrictor can disrupt the flow of blood to the pulp[52] and can depress efficient hemodynamic clearing of accumulated inflammatory toxins. A vital tooth with pulp that is compromised may never recover.[121] To complete preparation of a tooth that exhibits a chronopathologically stressed pulp, the tooth should be anesthetized through regional and block techniques only.

Acts of omission can be acknowledged only by the provider of the restoration. The detailed technical maneuvers executed in producing the restoration must be honestly assessed for an atraumatic delivery. Use of sharp burs, appropriate preparation depth, ample air/water coolants, application of liners and bases, and avoiding desiccating the dentin are just a few details that, if omitted, can lead to irreversible pulpal damage. If the clinician determines that atraumatic procedures were followed, the tooth should be allowed several weeks to adequately recover before the need for endodontic intervention is assessed.

Cracked Tooth Syndrome

With a cracked tooth, the patient feels a sharp momentary pain on mastication that is surprising. A tooth that is susceptible to cracking is one that is extensively restored but lacks cuspal protection (cuspal crack) or an intact tooth that has an opposing plunger cusp occluding centrically against a marginal ridge (vertical crack).

Pain, generated only on disclusion, drives oral fluids within the crack in the pulpal direction. This phenomenon is unique to a crack, and it has inspired the diagnostic technique of selective closure on the suspected tooth to elicit the pain on release. (See Chapter 1 for tools and techniques used to diagnose the cracked tooth.)

Urgent care of the cracked tooth involves the immediate reduction of its occlusal contacts by selective grinding at the site of the crack or against the cusp(s) of the occluding antagonist.

Definitive treatment of a vertically cracked tooth attempts to preserve pulpal vitality by requiring no less than full occlusal coverage for cusp protection.[96] Cusp coverage may seem drastic, but a vertical crack that is left unprotected will migrate "pulpally" and apically. When the aging defect encroaches on the pulp, emerging endodontic symptoms are indicative of the unavoidable need for root canal treatment. A long-standing defect can be betrayed by heavy staining in a tooth that is asymptomatic. It is possible that slow pulp degeneration explains the absence of symptoms.

Endodontic treatment can alleviate pulpal symptoms in a vertically cracked tooth. Tooth retention, however, remains questionable. The apical extension of and future migration of the defect down onto the root will decide the outcome.[96] Full cuspal coverage from this vantage is the most practical approach to treating a tooth with recent symptoms of disclusion pain.

Treatment of cuspal cracking in an extensively restored tooth depends on the chronopathologic history. Consideration should be given to the planned restorative needs and the possible need to perform elective endodontic treatment first. Tooth retention in cuspal cracking is favorable because the cusp generally separates obliquely in the horizontal plane. The defect usually has no adverse residual effect on the root or periodontal supporting structures.

Acute Degenerative Pulpitis and Associated Periapical Pain and Swelling

Pulpal inflammation is responsible for a variety of the signs and symptoms seen in an endodontic emergency. The symptom constellation of pulpal C fiber pain has already been described. Identifying the affected tooth is most difficult when the disease is still confined entirely within the pulpal space. Nevertheless, the dentist should proceed in a disciplined and orderly manner to gather subjective and objective data, including radiographs.[96]

Selective anesthesia can be the final resort for distinguishing which adjacent teeth are the source for the pain but *only if the pain is determined unequivocally to be odontogenic.* Delaying treatment would be the prudent course in case of any lingering doubt.

An inescapable sequela of pulp inflammation is its eventual spread from the confines of the tooth into the periapical tissue. An inflamed periodontal ligament can be equally painful because of activated A-delta and C nerve fibers in the area. Also activated are proprioceptive mechanoreceptors that enhance the patient's ability to localize the affected tooth. Proprioception is the hallmark of periapical inflammation and signals advanced stages of pulpal disease. As fluid accumulates and pressure increases, the tooth may feel elevated or loose in the socket, and it is increasingly painful on biting or on digital pressure.

Emergency management for the pain of acute degenerative pulpitis involves *initiating root canal treatment* to alleviate pain symptoms and *definitive management* of associated signs and symptoms of soft tissue involvement.

Profound Anesthesia

Attaining profound anesthesia is paramount to rendering emergency treatment. It can be difficult even for an experienced practitioner. Suppression of the nociceptive action potential is hampered by the numerous inflammatory pathways that are operating in the area. As the inflammatory process progresses, local tissue pH falls precipitously. The acidic environment prevents the anesthetic molecule from dissociating into ion form and the cation is unable to migrate through the neural sheath. Further, the inflamed nerve fibers are morphologically and biochemically altered throughout their length by neuropeptides and other neurochemicals. Therefore, in a state of hyperalgesia, nerve block injections at sites distant from the inflamed tooth are rendered less effective.[76]

The clinician must gain the advantage by judiciously selecting alternate and supplementary sites for injecting anesthetic solution. Consideration must be given to the type and amount of anesthetic solution required for the conditions. There may be anatomic limitations such as dense bony plates, aberrant distribution of neural bundles, or accessory innervations, especially in the mandible. The clinician should be skilled in all the various anesthetic techniques that may be required (see Chapter 19).

The nerve block injection of a nerve trunk central to an area or tooth is the standard intraoral approach for achieving initial regional anesthesia. However, conventional local anesthetic techniques are sometimes unsuccessful in obtaining profound anesthesia for endodontic procedures. In difficult cases depositing a greater volume of anesthetic in the region increases the likelihood of achieving pain control. The periodontal ligament injection (intraligamentary injection)[16,121] and intraosseous injection[22] are effective adjuncts to a conventional nerve block. If the pulp chamber is exposed and the pulp remains sensitive, an intrapulpal injection, done expertly into the pulp and with consideration for the patient, will anesthetize the remainder of the pulp tissue. Profound anesthesia is mandatory. Only a complete lack of sensation will allow for effective therapy to ensue.

Endodontic Emergency

No dentist should need reminding that an endodontic emergency has never been an elective visit for the patient in pain. Unscheduled emergency treatment can be reasonably easy, but more often it can be very difficult. The dentist must first make a diagnosis and then achieve pain and infection control within a limited amount of time. The clinician must determine the extent of the disease process (e.g., irreversible pulpitis, partial necrosis, total necrosis, alveolar abscess) or how best to manage a traumatic incident that might involve avulsed dentition. All too often the treatment decision is made not by the urgency of the situation but for expediency, with the least disruption to an already busy schedule. This approach may be a disservice to the patient.

Unless thorough cleaning and debridement is performed, pain symptoms can persist or worsen as the inflammatory process extends into the periradicular area. In most cases, the endodontic treatment can be completed during the next appointment. "Hurried care" may be misinterpreted by the patient and can only reinforce the patient's already distorted perception that root canal treatment is the most painful and least desirable of all dental procedures. A sobering fact is the number of malpractice suits that arise from endodontic complications when patients experience continued pain and suffering, which they attribute to incomplete professional care.[74,97]

Endodontic Swelling

Extension of pulpal disease into the surrounding periapical tissues may result in periapical infection. The infection will spread preferentially along the lines of least resistance, through cancellous bone, until it reaches the cortical plate. Where the plate is thin, the infection will erode through the bone into soft tissues, resulting in swelling. Swelling from a specific tooth will appear in a predictable anatomic location and is determined by two factors: the orientation of the tooth apex and the relationship of the site of perforation to muscle attachments on the maxilla or mandible.[55]

Tissue swelling may be seen at the initial emergency visit, at an interappointment flare-up, or as a postendodontic complication. Swellings may be *localized* or *diffuse*. Localized swellings are confined within the oral cavity. A diffuse swelling or cellulitis is characterized by its spread through adjacent soft tissues, dissecting tissue spaces along fascial planes.

There are three ways to resolve swelling and infection:

1. Establish drainage through the root canal.

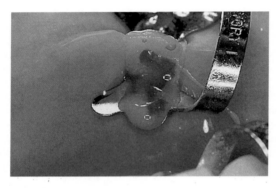

FIG. 2-8 Acute apical abscess relieved by drainage through the access opening. *(Courtesy Dr. Eric Herbranson.)*

2. Establish drainage by incising a fluctuant swelling.
3. Prescribe antibiotics.

The cardinal rule for managing all these infections is to achieve drainage.[39] When a localized swelling is present, it is the consensus among endodontists to thoroughly clean and shape the canal with copious irrigation, allow the drainage to stop, dry the canal, medicate if necessary, and close. Gentle finger pressure to the mucosa overlying the swelling and positive aspiration of the pulp chamber will aid drainage. If pus continues to drain through the canal and cannot be dried within a reasonable period of time, the tooth may be left open. Leaving a tooth open because of persistent drainage is necessary only on rare occasions. When considered a treatment necessity, leaving the pulp chamber open for drainage of pus does not necessarily affect treatment outcomes.[109] If good drainage is achieved by access and instrumentation of the root canal system, often no soft tissue incision and drainage procedure is needed (Figs. 2-8 and 2-9).

The systemic use of antibiotics in treating swelling caused by pulpless teeth should be regarded as an aid to drainage.[31] The objective is to aid the elimination of pus from the tissue spaces. However, if the cause of the infection remains within the root canal system, resolution of the acute condition is compromised.[31,68] Thorough removal of the diseased pulp along with bacteria and their toxins prevents these irritants from overwhelming the periradicular tissues. The use of antibiotics alone, without concurrent attempts to establish drainage and clean the pulpal space, generally is not considered appropriate treatment.[39,45]

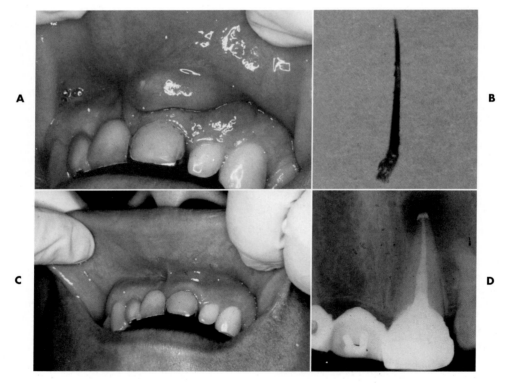

FIG. 2-9 A, Large vestibular swelling associated with failing gutta-percha fill in tooth #9. Tooth #10 tested vital. **B,** After gutta-percha removal, the canal exhibited profuse drainage. Incision and drainage was accomplished. Black discoloration of the gutta-percha is likely pigmentation associated with bacterial growth. **C,** Near complete resolution of the swelling 1 week after cleansing and shaping of the canal. **D,** Postoperative radiograph.

It is difficult to achieve satisfactory levels of antibiotic concentration at a tissue site in the presence of pus. In addition, the localized acute apical abscess may be primarily an inflammatory immunologic phenomenon. Certain immunologic mediators are increased in symptomatic periapical lesions.[57] These endogenous substances can decrease the pain threshold and increase vascular permeability, promoting edema. They may represent a nonbacterial cause for persistent symptoms.

With localized swelling, the clinician is dealing with an abscess that is confined within the oral cavity. The swelling does not have the same potential to spread as a diffuse swelling and is therefore treated less aggressively. A diffuse swelling indicates an advanced infection that is potentially dangerous for the patient. More aggressive treatment is necessary to minimize the possibility of the infection spreading. It is appropriate to use a systemic antibiotic for any diffuse swelling regardless of whether drainage is obtained from the root canal or the soft tissue (Fig. 2-10).

Incision and drainage of localized and diffuse swellings

Management of a localized soft tissue swelling can be facilitated through incision and drainage of the area (Fig. 2-11). Fluctuance, the sensation on palpation that there is fluid move-

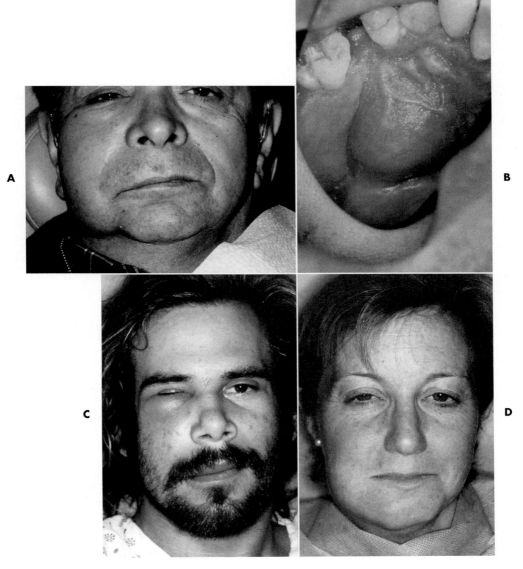

FIG. 2-10 A, Maxillary space infection resulting from phoenix abscess. **B,** Palatal swelling from necrotic lateral incisor. **C,** Canine space abscess spreading into the periorbital spaces. **D,** Submandibular space infection from an endodontically involved mandibular molar. *(B courtesy Dr. Joseph Schulz. C and D courtesy Dr. Alex McDonald.)* Cellulitis and space infections require aggressive therapy for resolution. This would include thorough debridement of the root canal space, intraoral drainage whenever possible, and administration of appropriate antibiotics. Culture and antibiotic sensitivity testing, and possibly referral, are strongly recommended for cases that are refractory to initial conventional therapy.

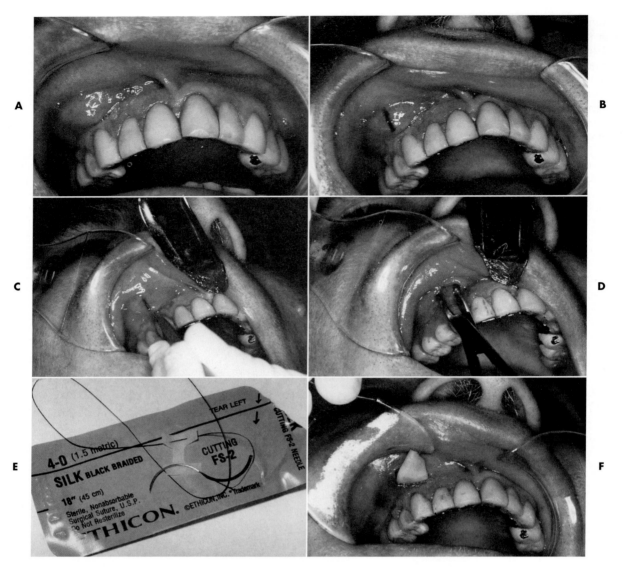

FIG. 2-11 A, Fluctuant intraoral vestibular swelling from a maxillary molar requires incision and drainage. **B,** Vertical placement of incision is marked for location. **C,** Incision is made through the swelling to the base of the alveolar bone. **D,** Surgical hemostat dissects and facilitates drainage. **E,** Suture placement through a rubber dam drain. **F,** Indwelling drain may be sutured into place to maintain drainage. Monitor for resolution of swelling. Drain should be removed in 24 to 48 hours. *(Courtesy Dr. Alex McDonald.)*

ment under the tissue, indicates that pus is present. Profound anesthesia may prove more difficult in the acidic infection site. Soft tissue infiltration of anesthetic around the periphery of the distended tissues may achieve a limited degree of anesthesia that permits tissue manipulation with minimum discomfort. Infiltration into the superficial mucosa overlying the swelling allows anesthesia directly over the site of the infected tissues. The following principles should be observed when incision and drainage therapy is used:

1. Incise at the site of greatest fluctuance down to the level of apical bone.
2. A vertical incision offers improved postoperative healing compared with a horizontal incision.[41]
3. When possible, place the incision in a position to encourage drainage by gravity.

4. Dissect gently through the deeper tissues and explore all parts of the abscess cavity thoroughly so that compartmentalized areas of pus are disrupted and evacuated. Extend the dissection to the roots of the teeth responsible for the infection.
5. The wound should be kept clean with hot salt-water mouthrinses to promote drainage. Intraoral heat application to infected tissues results in a dilation of small vessels, intensifying host defenses through increased vascular flow.[39,45]

Some clinicians recommend suturing an indwelling drain into place to maintain active drainage, whereas others do not place any drains into the incision site. Care must be taken in the region of the mental foramen to prevent damage to the underlying neurovascular bundle. A point of contention is whether to incise an indurated swelling or to wait until the tissues become fluctuant. Some believe that early incision of an indurated swelling can reduce pain from increasing tissue distention, even if only hemorrhagic fluid is obtained;[31] there is no consensus on this issue.

Medical therapy of dentoalveolar abscesses consists mainly of supportive care, hydration, soft diet, analgesics, and oral hygiene.

A diffuse swelling can develop into a medical emergency of potentially life-threatening complications. For this reason most endodontists[31] advise a more aggressive treatment approach. The tooth is opened, and the canal is thoroughly instrumented and irrigated. If no drainage is achieved, the apical foramen is intentionally instrumented through, under anatomic constraints, to encourage drainage from the periapical tissues. In the absence of drainage through the tooth, soft tissue drainage might be established through incision of the diffusely swollen tissues. An indwelling drain is sutured into the incision wound to ensure tissue drainage. Individuals who show signs of toxicity, central nervous system changes, or airway compromise should be considered for immediate hospitalization and aggressive medical and surgical intervention.[73]

Antibiotic therapy

Antibiotic therapy is usually unnecessary for localized swellings if drainage is achieved. Conversely, minor infections in patients with depressed host defenses must be treated with bactericidal drugs as soon as possible. Antibiotics are indicated for a diffuse swelling that drains inadequately or in cases in which it is impossible to gain access to the root canal terminus. Patients with spreading infections or systemic signs of illness (elevated temperature or malaise) also require antibiotic therapy.

Ideally, the choice of antibiotic depends on the definitive laboratory results of culture and antibiotic sensitivity testing. Most dentoalveolar infections and swellings occur in otherwise healthy patients, and cultures are not routinely performed. If the antibiotic choice is based on scientific data and clinical experience, a pragmatic approach to empirical antibiotic selection is acceptable, both ethically and legally. Penicillin and its derivitives have been the empirical antibiotics of choice for dental infections for more than five decades, with a proven record of efficacy.[39,45,73] However, some organisms, such as beta-lactamase–producing *Bacteroides,* are frequently seen to be insensitive to penicillin. Metronidazole is bactericidal against anaerobes. The combination of penicillin and metronidazole in a serious odontogenic infection is recommended. Erythromycin and clindamycin are suitable alternatives for patients who are allergic to penicillin and exhibit mixed anaerobic-aerobic infections.[68,111]

Laboratory Diagnostic Adjuncts

When an infection is severe or if the patient is a medical risk, purulent samples should be collected and sent immediately to a laboratory for culturing and isolation. In these serious situations a clinical diagnosis of any infectious pathogens should be confirmed by laboratory methods before treatment is begun (Fig. 2-12). However, some delay must be expected in awaiting a response from the laboratory because cultures for bacteria require at least 24 hours. Before beginning treatment, the clinician must judge whether rapid initiation of therapy based on clinical criteria will benefit the patient more than an attempt to establish the diagnosis by laboratory confirmation.

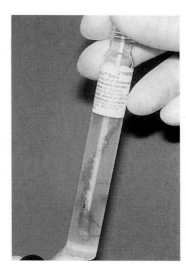

FIG. 2-12 Culture and antibiotic sensitivity testing of pathogenic microorganisms can be conducted with both aerobic and anaerobic techniques. Commercially available sample swabs and transport media are to be used as directed.

As a compromise, antibiotic therapy is often started while waiting for results from the laboratory.

Specimens representative of the site of infection should be collected in an amount sufficient for both direct examination and culture. Specimens can be aspirated with a disposable syringe, recapped, and submitted in toto. This provides a safe method for collection of aerobic and anaerobic bacteria and allows for Gram-staining procedures. Because anaerobic bacteria are always present in dentoalveolar infections,[1] specimens should be submitted in a transport medium that prevents desiccation and oxygen contamination. A variety of commercially prepackaged transport systems are suitable for this purpose. A maximum of 2 hours should be permitted to elapse between collection and microbiologic examination of the specimens.

It should be emphasized to the patient that the dentist may be contacted at any time for additional instructions or an alternative course of action should the situation worsen. Analgesics should be prescribed. The patient must be monitored closely over the next several days until there is improvement.

Progressive deterioration of the patient's condition, as evidenced by increased swelling, a sustained high fever, mental confusion, and difficulty swallowing or breathing, is sufficient reason to hospitalize the patient for more specialized care and around-the-clock monitoring.[73] The laboratory findings may guide the clinician or the subsequent physician in the proper choice of an antibiotic regimen.[7,39,45]

An uneventful resolution of the crisis should be expected. If after 48 hours, improvement is slower than expected, a switch to a broader-spectrum antibiotic may be indicated.

ENDODONTIC FLARE-UPS AND MIDTREATMENT URGENT CARE

Definition

Many researchers and clinicians who write about endodontic flare-ups have differing definitions of this expected treatment complication. Some have defined a flare-up as pain and/or swelling that requires an unscheduled patient visit and active intervention by the dentist.[123] The American Association of

Endodontists defines a flare-up as an acute exacerbation of periradicular pathosis after the initiation or continuation of root canal treatment.[2] As the definition of flare-ups varies, so does the reported incidence, with a range from 1.4% to nearly 45%.[46,71,74,117,123] The great variability in the reported incidence of these exacerbations cautions the critical thinker to be careful in comparing different studies with one another.

Causes

The causes of flare-ups are numerous and often multifactorial. The following discussion of urgent care for midtreatment exacerbations will focus on contributing factors, treatment modalities, and prevention.

Contributing Factors

Inadequate debridement

Persistent pain or onset of acute pain often signals the presence of residual pulp tissue in inadequately instrumented or still undetected canals. In these cases symptoms are usually consistent with irreversible pulpitis. Thorough debridement of the entire root canal system should eliminate the pain. Inadequate debridement of a pulp that has degenerated or is degenerating will allow bacteria and their toxins to remain in the root canal and act as a continuous irritant.[39] Teeth with necrotic pulps, with or without associated periradicular lesions, are more predisposed than vital teeth to develop midtreatment flare-ups.[39] Complete elimination of the irritants from the root canal system is the treatment of choice and usually results in the cessation of the inflammatory response. *Thorough debridement of the entire root canal space is a reasonable goal of initial management of all pulpless teeth.*

Debris extrusion

Despite strict length control of instruments during root canal preparation, pulp tissue fragments, necrotic tissue, microorganisms and their toxins, dentin filings, and other canal irrigants are extruded beyond the apical foramen.[120] This may result in periapical inflammation and midtreatment or posttreatment pain. When flare-ups occur, pulpless teeth are the most problematic. Pulpless teeth with associated periradicular lesions are likely to be infected.[29,107] Inadvertently innoculating the infectious contents of the root canal into the periapical tissues may predispose the pulpless tooth to periapical exacerbation.[29,39]

Debris extrusion is a problem with all instrumentation techniques; however, some techniques cause less extrusion than others. By comparing the mean weights of apically extruded debris, researchers found that sonic instrumentation extruded the least debris, followed by the cervical flaring technique and the ultrasonic technique.[24] Conventional hand instrumentation was shown to extrude the most debris. Shaping the canal in the coronal aspect before apical preparation may reduce the potential for debris extrusion. Crown-down instrumentation techniques[91] and the balanced forces technique[69] have been shown to extrude significantly less debris than step-back filing techniques. Both techniques rely on early coronal flaring and a rotational manipulation of root canal instruments. A recent study reported that the Profile .04 taper Series 29 rotary system forces minimal debris apically even when filing beyond the apical constriction.[9]

Irrigation solutions may also be extruded during instrumentation.[13] Forced irrigation of sodium hypochlorite beyond the apex of the tooth can cause violent tissue reactions and un-

bearable pain. Extruded irrigant in vital cases has been found only in the space created by instrumentation. In necrotic cases the irrigant may go beyond instrumented areas.[94]

The presence of an apical dentinal plug may help prevent extrusion of debris beyond the apical foramen. The plug may reduce the potential for flare-ups, prevent overinstrumentation of the periapical tissues, and often prevent extrusion of the obturating material. However, because the plug could harbor infectious material, the long-term prognosis is compromised. A canal in which patency is maintained allows for more debris extrusion, but the absence of an infected apical plug enhances the long-term prognosis.

Overinstrumentation

The correlation between endodontic overinstrumentation and postoperative pain has been demonstrated.[33] The incidence of moderate to severe pain is reported to be significantly higher if instrumentation occurs beyond the apical foramen. With care and attention, gross overinstrumentation is avoidable. Careful assessment of the preoperative radiographs and the use of an apex locator and corroborating radiographs should allow the instrument to remain within the root canal. Overinstrumentation of vital cases should be avoided because it crushes tissue and produces pain and inflammation.[59] Slight overinstrumentation past the apex in nonvital cases (apical trephination) has long been suggested to increase the likelihood for drainage, allow for release of pressure, and remove any remaining necrotic debris.

Gross overinstrumentation may cause acute apical periodontitis, producing primarily inflammatory pain. Infection is not a factor in vital cases if treatment is rendered using aseptic techniques. In cases of overinstrumentation, a serosanguineous exudate, not pus, is seen when a sterile paper point is placed into the apical extent of the canal(s). In many symptomatic cases involving overinstrumentation, a profuse exudate will continue to be discharged despite repeated and thorough reinstrumentation of the root canals. The problematic exudate can be controlled by placing a calcium hydroxide preparation (e.g., $Ca(OH)_2$ USP plus sterile water, Vitapex, Pulpdent, Hypo-Cal) against or slightly through the perforated foramen. Once the tooth feels comfortable, treatment can be continued by removing the paste and maintaining instrumentation within the canal space.

Overfilling

The extrusion of sealer or gutta-percha into the periapical tissues of teeth with no periapical radiolucent areas is more likely to cause a higher incidence and degree of postobturation pain than in similar teeth filled flush or up to 1 mm short of the radiographic apex.[40,99] This, however, is not a universal finding because clinicians have not found a correlation between the level of obturation, the extrusion of sealer, and the intensity of postobturation pain.[114]

It may be that a small overfill of gutta-percha and/or sealer is not the primary cause of postobturation pain. Rather, some degree of overinstrumentation may have occurred before obturation, and gutta-percha protruding past the apex may be a sign of such an occurrence. Furthermore, it may not be possible to achieve a good apical seal in overinstrumented canals if the foramen has been transported. In such cases residual bacteria from the root canal are not sealed off and percolation of apical tissue fluids into the root canal may provide the nourishment for these bacteria to grow. Symptoms may then ensue because of bacterial proliferation inside the root canal system, which releases toxic substances periapically.

Large overfills are a factor in postobturation pain. Gross overfilling can cause nerve damage resulting from either the chemical toxicity of the extruded material or mechanical nerve damage caused by compressing or crushing forces of the foreign material.[77] Paraformaldehyde pastes are a classic example of neurotoxic substances that can cause extensive irreversible nerve damage when expressed periapically. Surgical intervention is often required to remove such noxious irritants. A slight extrusion of gutta-percha is probably insignificant, affecting neither the long-term prognosis[61] nor the incidence of postoperative pain.[114]

Microbiology and immunology

Seven possible etiologic factors for endodontic flare-ups have been described in the literature:[100]

1. Local adaptation syndrome: the introduction of a new irritant into inflamed tissue exacerbates a chronic problem.
2. Changes in periapical tissue pressure: increased pressure causes pain because of excessive exudate applying pressure to nerve endings; decreased pressure aspirates irritants and microorganisms into the periapical space and exacerbates the inflammatory response.
3. Association between certain microorganisms and clinical signs and symptoms.
4. Chemical mediators of inflammation, such as prostaglandins, leukotrienes, Hageman factor, and the complement cascade.
5. Changes in cyclic nucleotides, such as cyclic adenosine monophosphate (AMP), affect biosynthetic and biodegradative pathways.
6. Immunologic responses: the production of antibodies plays a central role in the inflammatory response.
7. Psychologic factors: fear and anxiety may exacerbate the patient's perception and decrease the tolerance of pain.

Periapical lesion

Some researchers have found apical radiolucencies to be correlated with an increased frequency of flare-ups.[46,74,117,123] The pulps of teeth with large periapical radiolucencies have more bacterial strains and are more infected.[58,74] These bacteria may cause an acute problem if innoculated periapically.

Others found fewer problems when an apical lesion[66,67,71,75,112] or sinus tract[46,112,123] is present because of the potential space for pressure release. In teeth with an intact periodontal ligament, the increased pressure that develops after an inflammatory response has nowhere to vent, so the area becomes more painful.

It is not clear what relationship periapical lesions have to the occurrence of exacerbations because there is evidence supporting both sides of the controversy. It is similarly uncertain what significance pulpal status has on the incidence of flare-ups. Some investigators have found more flare-ups occurring in teeth with necrotic pulps,[71,123] whereas others have not.[35,46,61]

Retreatment

Endodontists have found that retreatment cases have a higher incidence of flare-ups.[46,112,116] In these cases the host response to extruded filling materials and toxic solvents may increase pain.[124] Many retreatment cases have associated periapical pathoses with symptoms, which may also increase the likelihood of flare-ups.[113] Technically these cases are the most

difficult and time consuming, with an increased chance for iatrogenic mishaps.

One-appointment endodontics

Most patients experience little or no spontaneous pain after one-visit root canal therapy; only 2% may have severe pain.[27] In fact, the frequency of pain in single-visit or multivisit root canal therapy does not differ.[4,66,71,75,116,123] Some studies have shown that single-appointment therapy produces postoperative pain *less frequently* than multivisit treatments do.[46,89] The reasons for the variability in studies are many, including the different criteria for completing single visit therapy as described in Chapter 4.

Host factors

The intensity of preoperative pain and amount of patient apprehension are correlated to the degree of postoperative pain.* Patients with dental phobias are difficult to treat because of their low psychophysiologic tolerance. Such patients may be best served by presedation, either oral or intravenous, to make the endodontic experience atraumatic. Other factors that have shown both positive and negative correlations with flare-ups include patient age, gender, tooth position,† and the presence of allergies.[112,123] Race[66,75] and systemic disease[27,74,112] are not associated with increased flare-ups.

Treatment and Prevention of Flare-ups

Studies have shown that postoperative pain will diminish to low levels within 72 hours.[35,40] This is a stressful time for the patient who is consumed by pain and for the practitioner whose job it is to help the patient. During this critical period clinicians must know how to quickly and effectively alleviate patients' pain and prevent its recurrence.

Cleansing and shaping

The single most effective method to reduce flare-ups is thorough and complete cleansing and shaping of the root canal system at the initial treatment visit. *The concepts of crown-down cleansing and shaping and confirming apical patency as described in Chapter 8 are two preeminent factors that are important in the strategic management of teeth most likely to exhibit midtreatment flare-ups.* As stated previously, symptomatic pulpless teeth and retreatment cases may be predisposed to interappointment exacerbations.[112] A crown-down shaping strategy is expeditious for removing the bulk of infected organic debris from the tooth. If the root length can also be determined at the emergency visit, apical patency should be established and maintained throughout crown-down instrumentation.[36]

Incision and drainage for swelling

Treatment of an interappointment or postoperative swelling is similar to the treatment of a preoperative swelling, namely, the establishment of drainage and the prescribing of antibiotics as indicated. If the root canal has not been obturated or is inadequately obturated, reinstrumentation through the root canal should be attempted to achieve drainage (Fig. 2-13). Alveolar trephination may be necessary for teeth with an apical blockage. If the obturation appears adequate, drainage may be achieved through incision and drainage alone. Attempting

---

*References 46, 66, 112-114, 123.
†References 4, 27, 35, 46, 66, 71, 74, 75, 112, 123.

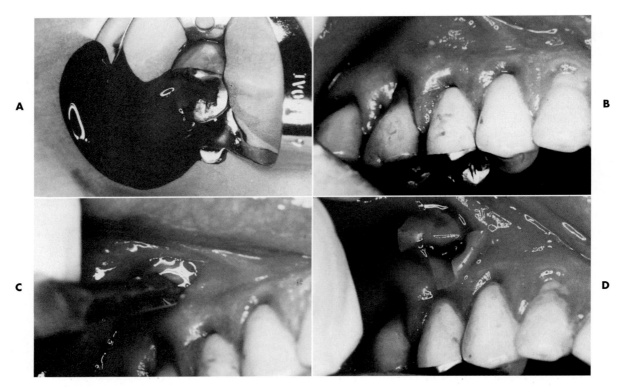

FIG. 2-13 A, Acute flare-up. Inflammatory bleeding through the access opening of a midtreatment emergency 36 hours after initial therapy. **B-D,** After coronal drainage, soft tissue evacuation and placement of a drain are accomplished. Root canal should be thoroughly cleaned, shaped, and closed at this visit. *(Courtesy Dr. Kenneth Tittle.)*

periradicular surgery at the time of an acute infection may be contraindicated because of the difficulty in obtaining profound anesthesia.

Periapical surgery

For most flare-ups nonsurgical root canal therapy is the preferred treatment method because the root canal contents can be thoroughly cleaned in a noninvasive manner. In certain situations, however, periapical surgery may be the treatment of choice. For example, nonsurgical treatment may be impractical because of restorative issues, failing retreatment, gross overfills, or necessary correction of procedural accidents.

Another surgical method for resolving flare-ups is trephination. The American Association of Endodontists defines trephination as the surgical perforation of the mucoperiosteum and alveolar plate to release accumulated tissue exudate.[2] Clinical studies have shown this therapy to provide relief to patients with severe and recalcitrant pain.[15] However, trephination is not routinely recommended because of the additional trauma and invasiveness with a questionably beneficial result.

Leaving teeth open

When a tooth is opened and purulence escapes, the exudate should stop after just a few minutes. Patients are instructed that the tooth will be allowed to drain for up to 20 minutes while the rubber dam is still in place. On the rare occasion when exudate continues to well out of a tooth and prevent closure, the tooth may be left open to the oral environment with a cotton ball or similar barrier to prevent food impaction. The tooth can usually be closed without incident the

next day, after additional cleansing and shaping. It is best to close all teeth immediately after treatment to prevent contamination by the oral cavity[7,31] and to prevent future problems because teeth left open are frequently involved in midtreatment flare-ups.[100]

Although some practitioners recommend routinely leaving teeth open between appointments, this is rarely indicated and is not based on sound scientific research. Researchers have found that teeth left open to the oral environment show higher levels of secretory immunoglobulin A than teeth that are not left open.[115] The significance of this finding is that epithelial growth factor, a polypeptide found in saliva, may stimulate the rests of Malassez, found in periapical lesions, to proliferate.[59,115] The result is that leaving canals open to the oral cavity may increase periapical cyst formation. For this reason all teeth, with rare exception, should be closed aseptically under the rubber dam after treatment.

Occlusal reduction

Teeth with periapical inflammation may be exquisitely sensitive to occlusal forces. Occlusal reduction or selective adjustment of cusps is indicated as a palliative measure.[31,39] Temporary fillings that are overcontoured may cause intense periapical pain because of hyperocclusion and should be adjusted with articulating paper to ensure that the tooth does not hit prematurely.

Intracanal medicaments

For root canals that require more than one visit to complete, there are sufficient remaining bacteria within the system to grow and reinfect the root canal space between appointments.[14]

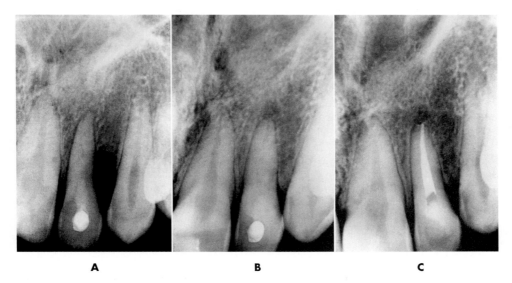

A   **B**   **C**

FIG. 2-14 A, Placement of calcium hydroxide 1 week after blunt trauma has devitalized the upper lateral incisor. After thorough cleaning and shaping, calcium hydroxide was placed to stimulate remineralization of the adjacent bone and to neutralize the acidic intracanal involvement. **B,** One week later. Remarkable remineralization of the alveolar matrix. **C,** Postobturation.

Historically, placement of intracanal medicaments has become a popular method of preventing bacterial regrowth. It may seem that eliminating bacteria would minimize any symptoms associated with reinfection, but numerous studies have found that the use of traditional intracanal medicaments has no effect on flare-ups.[40,112,117]

The decision to use an intracanal medicament should be guided by the antibacterial efficacy, toxicity, and specificity of the drug. For example, despite its superior antibacterial activity against anaerobes,[81] formocresol has been shown to cause periapical irritation and is embryotoxic and teratogenic.[28] Cresatin and phenolic compounds, such as camphorated parachlorophenol, are bactericidal[34,81,82] but they also demonstrate toxicity to human cells.[105] Chlorhexidine gluconate has been shown to have an antimicrobial efficacy comparable to that of sodium hypochlorite,[47] with a similar ability to penetrate dentinal tubules,[82] yet it is less toxic to periradicular tissues.[47] Iodine potassium iodide also has potent antibacterial effects with minimal toxicity.[81,82,93]

Calcium hydroxide and chlorhexidine gluconate are the two primary medicaments to consider if any is to be used. Chlorhexidine is easy to deliver and can be dispensed through a syringe directly into root canals. Furthermore, it has been shown to be as safe and effective as sodium hypochlorite.[47,82] Calcium hydroxide is also a safe and effective intracanal medication that may be potentiated if it is mixed with chlorhexidine gluconate or iodine potassium iodide (Vitapex).

Calcium hydroxide therapy

Calcium hydroxide intracanal dressings may be therapeutic in the treatment of flare-ups. The reasons for flare-ups are numerous, but surely one of the critical factors is viable bacteria still remaining within the root canal system.[14] Application of calcium hydroxide is intended to reduce bacterial colonies and their toxic by-products. It has been shown that the antimicrobial effects of calcium hydroxide are best achieved if the calcium hydroxide remains in root canals for at least 1 week[104]

(Fig. 2-14). Removing the smear layer can facilitate the diffusion of calcium hydroxide through the dentinal tubules.[26] This step may be useful because bacterial lipopolysaccharides, which are involved in numerous inflammatory reactions,[92] can diffuse through dentin.[79]

There are various methods by which calcium hydroxide can be placed in root canals. A Messing gun, vertical condensation, an injectable formulation of calcium hydroxide, a Lentulo spiral, a hand file, and paper points are all acceptable techniques.[103] A study comparing the use of a Lentulo spiral, the injection technique, and a hand file for placement of calcium hydroxide found that use of the Lentulo spiral most consistently delivered calcium hydroxide to working length with density, irrespective of the root canal curvature. In contrast, the injection technique was limited by the root canal curvature and diameter.[103]

The possibility of calcium hydroxide reducing postoperative pain may depend on its ability to kill bacteria and neutralize their by-products. Studies have shown that calcium hydroxide hydrolyzes the lipid moiety of bacterial lipopolysaccharides, rendering it incapable of producing biologic effects such as toxicity, pyrogenicity, macrophage activation, and complement activation.[92] Other investigators suggest that the antibacterial mechanism of calcium hydroxide may be related to its absorption of carbon dioxide, which would nutritionally starve capnophilic bacteria in the root canal system.[53] Additionally, calcium hydroxide may exert its effects by obliterating the root canal space, which minimizes the ingress of tissue exudate, a potential source of nourishment for remaining bacteria.[82] Researchers attribute the soft-tissue–dissolving potential and antibacterial effects of calcium hydroxide to its high pH.[3] The ability of calcium hydroxide to kill *Bacteroides* species may reduce the occurrence of flare-ups.[34]

The exact therapeutic mechanisms of calcium hydroxide have not been clearly elucidated, but certain effects have been well studied. Because calcium hydroxide can dissolve necrotic tissue, the denaturing effect of calcium hydroxide on proteins allows sodium hypochlorite to then more easily dissolve remaining tissue.[42] This tissue-dissolving effect works equally well in aerobic and anaerobic environments.[126]

Placement of calcium hydroxide between appointments is recommended for teeth that have been incompletely cleansed and shaped, are symptomatic, have long interappointment delays, or exhibit periapical infection. For additional uses of calcium hydroxide, refer to traumatic injuries in Chapter 16.

Antibiotics and analgesics

When it is necessary to give an antibiotic to control infection, amoxicillin should be considered the drug of choice; metronidazole can be added to the regimen to enhance the killing of anaerobes. Although erythromycin is frequently administered to patients allergic to penicillin, an alternative might be clindamycin because, unlike erythromycin, it is bactericidal.

For most patients nonsteroidal antiinflammatory drugs (NSAIDs) are appropriate and sufficient to control pain. When this is not the case, opioid analgesics may be used to supplement the NSAIDs.

Although drugs should never be prescribed to satisfy the patient's desire or addiction,[73] a request that is reasonable must be considered, not only for the pharmacologic effect but also for the psychologic value.

Antibiotic prophylaxis

An ongoing controversy exists about whether giving patients antibiotics prophylactically before root canal therapy will reduce the incidence of flare-ups in certain situations. In a double-blind prospective study administration of penicillin prophylactically was unrelated to reducing posttreatment signs and symptoms after root canal preparation.[122] A recent study[123] also supports the conclusion that antibiotic prophylaxis does not reduce the incidence of flare-ups.

However, there is also evidence to support the use of prophylactic antibiotics in preventing flare-ups.[74,113,114] For patients in moderate to severe pain, erythromycin base was the most effective medication for reducing the incidence of postoperative pain after instrumentation.[113] These results suggest that patients in moderate to severe pain may have fewer postoperative sequelae when given erythromycin prophylactically. Penicillin is more slowly absorbed than erythromycin, which may explain observed differences showing penicillin less effective in these circumstances.

Other researchers prefer penicillin because of its bactericidal action and efficacy.[74] They reported flare-up occurrence to decrease from about 20% to 2% in a series of studies.[74] Their rationale is that teeth showing pulpal necrosis with periapical lesions have anaerobic bacteria proliferating inside the root canal system. Penicillin given before root canal therapy is intended to treat an existing infection before it has the opportunity to spread. Penicillin is given to inhibit the synergistic activity between certain microorganisms responsible for flare-ups, such as the gram-positive bacteria that provide vitamin K to *Porphyromonas* species.

Antibiotics also carry inherent risks of morbidity and mortality. Patients may have adverse side effects such as nausea or diarrhea, or an anaphylactic reaction may even develop. Other complications include sensitization to antibiotics, superinfections, and the development of microbial resistance. A dentist who prescribes an antibiotic of questionable benefit places a patient at risk and may be held accountable if the patient has a severe adverse reaction.[122]

The question then remains as to whether antibiotics should be given to patients with pulpal necrosis and periapical lesions. Although there is evidence to support either view, we believe that antibiotics are generally unnecessary for prophylactic use. Careful cleansing and shaping of root canals and the use of crown-down techniques and copious irrigation should result in a flare-up rate that is very low and does not warrant the side effects and risks associated with antibiotic usage.

NSAIDs—oral and injectable

The use of pretreatment and posttreatment analgesics may significantly reduce the incidence of flare-ups,[112,113] especially for patients in moderate to severe pain. Because endodontic pain results from numerous inflammatory and immunologic pathways, most endodontists prefer NSAIDs to narcotics for interfering with this process and reducing pain symptoms.

Studies have evaluated ketorlac tromethamine (Toradol) when given as a local infiltration[86] or as an intramuscular injection.[19,86] Ketorlac is the first NSAID available for intramuscular injection. By blocking cyclooxygenase, ketorlac is a potent inhibitor of prostaglandin synthesis and may be equivalent or superior to morphine sulfate when delivered through the intramuscular route.[19,86] One research group found that nearly all patients in severe pain who were given ketorlac as an intramuscular injection experienced a pain reduction of 67% in 40 minutes, which increased to a 99.5% reduction after 90 minutes.[19] Others found that local infiltration of ketorlac produced a significant analgesic effect, especially in the mandible compared with the maxilla. From these results they concluded that the pharmacokinetics of ketorlac differ significantly from those of local anesthetics, and their ability to provide adjunctive pain relief was promising.

Two NSAIDs, diclofenac and ketoprofen, have been used as intracanal medicaments to control pain.[78] Both medications were superior to a placebo in reducing pain subsequent to instrumentation of root canals.

Corticosteroids—oral and injectable

Corticosteroids inhibit the enzyme phospholipase A_2, which is responsible for conversion of membrane phospholipids into arachidonic acid. Arachidonic acid is the precursor of various inflammatory mediators, including the prostaglandins, thromboxanes, prostacyclin, and leukotrienes. Corticosteroids thus reduce inflammation and pain by blocking the inflammatory cascade.

Researchers have shown that a local infiltration of dexamethasone produces a histologically significant antiinflammatory effect on the periapical tissues of overinstrumented teeth.[80] Studies of dentin and pulp confirm that dexamethasone reduces the immunoreactivity for calcitonin gene-related protein and substance P, and it reduces nerve-sprouting responses to dentin cavity injuries.[44] This inhibition of neural reactions to injury may contribute to steroid effects on clinical dental pain.

Oral methylprednisolone is effective in reducing postoperative symptoms when it is given prophylactically with penicillin to patients in moderate to severe pain.[113] Methylprednisolone also reduces the frequency and intensity of postobturation pain after single-visit treatment.[48] This medication may be easily dispensed as the Medrol Dosepak, a package of 21 tablets taken in decreasing amounts for 6 days.

Researchers evaluating postinstrumentation pain at 8, 24, and 48 hours in patients given either oral dexamethasone or placebo found that those taking placebo experienced significantly more pain at all time periods.[35,54] Other studies evaluating the effect of intramuscular injections of corticosteroids on postoperative pain recorded similar results.[66,67]

Corticosteroids seem to have their greatest impact in the first 24 hours postoperatively. For patients in severe pain it may be beneficial to prescribe or administer some form of corticosteroids. Among the various methods of delivering corticosteroids, intracanal placement may be the least effective because of the difficulty of delivering sufficient quantities periapically.

There is no evidence of dexamethasone injections leading to an increase in infections, such as cellulitis, fever, or lymphadenopathy, regardless of the pulpal or periapical status of teeth to be treated.[66] For this reason antibiotics may be given at the discretion of the practitioner, depending on the other treatment and health variables of the particular patient. However, *it is critical that the practitioner is confident that the recommendation to use corticosteroids is made for the pain of inflammation and injury and not for pain associated with infection and swelling.*

One-appointment endodontics

Endodontists and clinical researchers have found that obturation of root canals is associated with fewer flare-ups and a decrease in pain.[114,123] After obturation, the highest degree of pain occurs in the first 24 hours and diminishes substantially thereafter.[40,114] The popularity of single-visit treatment can be credited to favorable reports that found no difference in treatment complications or success rates compared with teeth treated in multiple visits.[85] The preference of the single-visit approach, however, must be tempered with the understanding that careful case selection and the clinician's expertise factored heavily in achieving the reported outcomes.

Because bacteria are the source of pulpal and periapical infections, eliminating the bacteria will resolve associated symptoms. One author suggests that "the root canal should ideally be completely cleaned at the initial treatment visit when the bacteria are particularly vulnerable to eradication by a disturbance in their sensitive ecology."[106] Between appointments, when the tooth is coronally sealed, "the anaerobiosis is restored and an influx of tissue fluid into the canal can support the regrowth of bacteria."[106] If an intracanal dressing is not placed in the root canal, then resistant bacteria, which have survived the biomechanical treatment, may proliferate and resurrect infections that are difficult to treat.[14,106]

Rather than placing an intracanal dressing to prevent regrowth of resistant bacteria, it would be better to obturate the root canal during the initial treatment visit. Obturation with gutta-percha and sealer is a superior method of obliterating the canal space. In this way any remaining bacteria are entombed within the confines of the tooth and isolated from any source of nutrients. If root canal therapy cannot be completed in a single visit because of time constraints, difficulty of the case, or other limitations, a calcium hydroxide dressing should be applied to keep the root canal system temporarily sealed. (See Chapter 4 for further information about this issue.)

HYPOCHLORITE ACCIDENT

Accidental injection of sodium hypochlorite into the periapical tissues is an experience that neither the patient nor the practitioner will soon forget. The literature contains numerous case reports describing the morbidity associated with such occurrences.[8,23,32,88]

Definition

A hypochlorite accident refers to any event in which sodium hypochlorite is expressed beyond the apex of a tooth and the patient immediately manifests some combination of the following symptoms:

1. Severe pain, even in areas that were previously anesthetized for dental treatment
2. Swelling
3. Profuse bleeding, both interstitially and through the tooth

Causes

Some of the reasons that a hypochlorite accident may occur include forceful injection of the irrigating solution, having an irrigating needle wedged into a root canal, and irrigating a tooth that has a large apical foramen, apical resorption, or an immature apex. Some patients have several days of increasing edema and ecchymosis, accompanied by tissue necrosis, paresthesia, and secondary infection (Fig. 2-15). Although most patients recover within 1 to 2 weeks, long-term paresthesia and scarring have also been reported.[32,88]

Management

1. Recognize that a hypochlorite accident has occurred.
2. Attend to the immediate problem of pain and swelling. Administer a regional block with a long-acting anesthetic solution. With the irrigant spreading rapidly over a wide region, pain management is difficult because symptoms from distant anatomic structures will continue to cause discomfort. This also explains the extreme pain felt during the incident despite establishment of adequate local anesthesia before treatment was begun. A reported incident describes flushing the palatal canal of a maxillary molar with sterile water to dilute the effects of the hypochlorite that was expressed into the sinus through the same route.[23]
3. Reassure and calm the patient. The reaction, although alarmingly fast, is still a localized phenomenon and will resolve with time. If available, nitrous oxide sedation can help the patient cope throughout the remainder of this emergency.
4. Monitor the tooth over the next half hour. A bloody exudate may discharge into the canal. This bleeding is the body's reaction to the irrigant. Remove the fluid with high-volume evacuation to encourage further drainage from the periapical tissues. If drainage is persistent, consider leaving the tooth open over the next 24 hours.
5. Consider antibiotic coverage. If the treated tooth is pulpless and cleansing and shaping procedures have not been completed, consider prescribing amoxicillin, 500 mg, four times a day, over the next 5 days.
6. Consider administering an analgesic. Because of possible bleeding complications with aspirin and other NSAIDs, an acetaminophen-narcotic analgesic combination may be more appropriate. If swelling is extensive, it is best to caution the patient to expect bruising or pooling of blood as it subsides.
7. Consider prescribing a corticosteroid. Steroids will help minimize the ensuing inflammatory process.
8. Give the patient home care instructions. For the first 6 hours

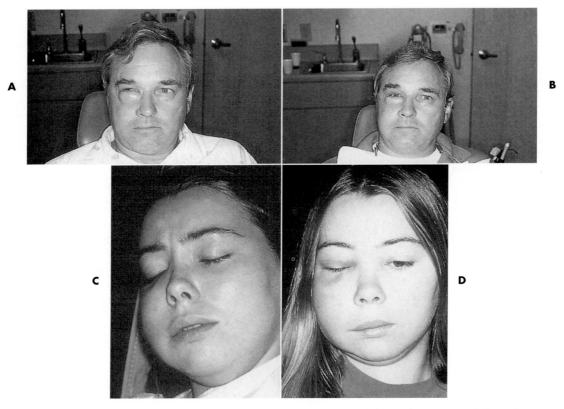

FIG. 2-15 Hypochlorite accident. **A,** Immediate response to a 1.0% solution expressed through the roots of a maxillary premolar. **B,** Presentation 24 hours after the accident. Swelling is evident. *(A and B courtesy Dr. Peter Chalmers.)* **C,** Immediately after mishap through a maxillary canine with 5.25% solution; the swelling had spread to involve the canine and infraorbital spaces. **D,** Twenty-four hours later. Swelling and ecchymosis are evident. *(C and D courtesy Dr. Ronald Borer.)*

the patient should use cold compresses to minimize pain and swelling. Subsequently, warm compresses should be used to encourage a healthy healing response.

9. Consider referring the patient. If the patient continues to be apprehensive or needs additional reassurance or develops complications, referral to the endodontist or oral surgeon is appropriate. Informing the specialist about the patient and the nature of the problem will ensure a smooth transition between offices for the patient.

Prevention

A hypochlorite accident is completely avoidable. As an endodontic irrigant, hypochlorite solution is meant to flush debris from the root canal system. Part of the efficacy of hypochlorite depends on the volume of irrigation and the depth of penetration of the irrigating needle. Even so, the solution must be delivered in a passive manner to avoid apical extrusion. Because root canals are coronally flared during the cleansing and shaping process, the irrigating needle can penetrate deeper into the canal and still not bind against the walls.

The following measures are recommended to prevent a hypochlorite accident:

1. Bend the irrigating needle at the center to confine the tip of the needle to higher levels in the root canal and to facilitate direct access to all teeth regardless of angulation.

2. Never place the needle so deeply into the canal that it binds against the walls.
3. Oscillate the needle in and out of the canal to ensure that the tip is free to express irrigant without resistance.
4. Express the irrigant slowly and gently.
5. Stop irrigating if the needle jams or if there is any detectable resistance when pressing against the plunger of the syringe.
6. Check the hub of the needle for a tight fit to prevent inadvertent separation and accidental exposure of the irrigant to the patient's eyes.

Although a hypochlorite accident requires immediate management, the definitive assessment and accurate identification of any dental emergency must follow the same process as outlined in this chapter.

The art and science of endodontic diagnosis and treatment have undergone a tremendous scientific and technologic evolution over the last half of the twentieth century. As a result, the dental profession is prepared and able to remedy one of the most painful and feared human afflictions with compassion, knowledge, and skill.

REFERENCES

1. Aderhold L, Konthe H, Frenkel G: The bacteriology of dentigerous pyogenic infections, *Oral Surg Oral Med Oral Pathol* 52:583, 1981.

2. American Association of Endodontists: *Glossary, contemporary terminology for endodontics,* ed 5, Chicago, 1994, The Association.
3. Andersen M, Andreasen JO, Andreasen FM: In vitro solubility of human pulp tissue in calcium hydroxide and sodium hypochlorite, *Endod Dent Traumatol* 8:104, 1992.
4. Balaban FS, Skidmore AE, Griffin JA: Acute exacerbations following initial treatment of necrotic pulps, *J Endod* 10:78, 1984.
5. Barr CE: Practical considerations in the treatment of the HIV-infected patient, *Dent Clin North Am* 38:403, 1994.
6. Battrum DE, Guttman JL: Phantom tooth pain: a diagnosis of exclusion, *Int Endod J* 29:190, 1996.
7. Baumgartner JC: Treatment of infections and associated lesions of endodontic origin, *J Endod* 17:418, 1991.
8. Becker GL, Cohen S, Borer R: The sequelae of accidentally injecting sodium hypochlorite beyond the root apex: report of a case, *Oral Surg* 38:633, 1974.
9. Beeson T, Hartwell G: Comparison of debris extruded apically. Conventional filing versus profile .04 taper series 29, *J Endod* 4:212, 1996.
10. Bell WE: *Orofacial pains,* ed 4, Chicago, Year Book Medical Publishers, 1989.
11. Bender IB: Factors influencing radiographic appearance of bony lesions, *J Endod* 8:161, 1982.
12. Brännström M: The hydrodynamic theory of dentinal pain: sensation in preparations, caries, and the dentinal crack syndrome, *J Endod* 12:453, 1986.
13. Brown DC, Moore BK, Brown Jr CE, Newton CW: An in vitro study of apical extrusion of sodium hypochlorite during endodontic canal preparation, *J Endod* 21:587, 1995.
14. Byström A, Sundqvist G: Bacteriologic evaluation of the efficacy of mechanical root canal instrumentation in endodontic therapy, *Scand J Dent Res* 89:321, 1981.
15. Chestner SB, Selman AJ, Friedman J, Heyman RA: Apical fenestration: solution to recalcitrant pain in root canal therapy, *J Am Dent Assoc* 77:846, 1968.
16. Childers M, Reader A, Nist R, Beck M, Meyers WJ: Anesthetic efficacy of the periodontal ligament injection after an inferior alveolar nerve block, *J Endod* 22:317, 1996.
17. Ciancio S: Oral contraceptives, antibiotics and pregnancy, *Dent Manag* 5:54, 1989.
18. Corah NL: Effect of perceived control on stress reduction in pedodontic patients, *J Dent Res* 52:1261, 1973.
19. Curtis P, Gartman LA, Green DB: Utilization of ketorlac tromethamine for control of severe odontogenic pain, *J Endod* 20:457, 1994.
20. Dietz GC Sr, Dietz GC Jr: The endodontist and the general dentist, *Dent Clin North Am* 36:459, 1992.
21. Drinnan AL: Differential diagnosis of orofacial pain, *Dent Clin North Am* 31:627, 1987.
22. Dunbar D, Reader A, Nist R, Beck M, Meyers WJ: Anesthetic efficacy of the intraosseous injection after an inferior alveolar nerve block, *J Endod* 22:481, 1996.
23. Ehrich DG, Brian JD Jr, Walker WA: Sodium hypochlorite accident: inadvertent injection into the maxillary sinus, *J Endod* 19:180, 1993.
24. Fairbourn DR, McWalter GM, Montgomery S: The effect of four preparation techniques on the amount of apically extruded debris, *J Endod* 13:102, 1987.
25. Feinerman DM, Goldberg MH: Acoustic neuroma appearing as trigeminal neuralgia, *J Am Dent Assoc* 125:1122, 1994.
26. Foster KH, Kulild JC, Weller RN: Effect of smear layer removal on the diffusion of calcium hydroxide through radicular dentin, *J Endod* 19:136, 1993.
27. Fox J et al: Incidence of pain following one-visit endodontic treatment, *Oral Surg* 30:123, 1970.
28. Friedberg BH, Gartner LP: Embryotoxicity and teratogenicity of formocresol on developing chick embryos, *J Endod* 16:434, 1990.
29. Fukushima H et al: Localization and identification of root canal bacteria in clinically asymptomatic periapical pathosis, *J Endod* 16:534, 1990.
30. Gatchel RJ: Managing anxiety and pain during dental treatment, *J Am Dent Assoc* 123:37, 1992.
31. Gatewood RS, Himel VT, Dorn SO: Treatment of the endodontic emergency: a decade later, *J Endod* 16:284, 1990.
32. Gatot A, Arbelle J, Leiberman A, Yanai-Inbar I: Effects of sodium hypochlorite on soft tissues after its inadvertent injection beyond the root apex, *J Endod* 17:573, 1991.
33. Georgopoulou M, Anastassiadis P, Sykaras S: Pain after chemicomechanical preparation, *Int Endod J* 19:309, 1986.
34. Georgopoulou M, Kontakiotis E, Nakou M: In vitro evaluation of the effectiveness of calcium hydroxide and paramonochlorophenol on anaerobic bacteria from the root canal, *Endod Dent Traumatol* 9:249, 1993.
35. Glassman G et al: A prospective randomized double-blind trial on efficacy of dexamethasone for endodontic interappointment pain in teeth with asymptomatic inflamed pulps, *Oral Surg* 67:96, 1989.
36. Goerig AC, Michelich RJ, Schulz HH: Instrumentation of root canals in molars using the step-down technique, *J Endod* 8:550, 1982.
37. Goon WWY, Jacobsen PL: Prodromal odontalgia and multiple devitalized teeth caused by a herpes zoster infection of the trigeminal nerve: report of case, *J Am Dent Assoc* 116:500, 1988.
38. Hargreaves KM, Troullos ES, Dionne RA: Pharmacologic rationale for the treatment of acute pain, *Dent Clin North Am* 31:675, 1987.
39. Harrington GW, Natkin E: Midtreatment flare-ups, *Dent Clin North Am* 36:409, 1992.
40. Harrison JW, Baumgartner JC, Svec TA: Incidence of pain associated with clinical factors during and after root canal therapy. 2. Postobturation pain, *J Endod* 9:434, 1983.
41. Harrison JW, Jurosky KA: Wound healing in the tissues of the periodontium following periradicular surgery. 2. The incisional wound, *J Endod* 17:425, 1991.
42. Hasselgren G, Olsson B, Cvek M: Effects of calcium hydroxide and sodium hypochlorite on the dissolution of necrotic porcine muscle tissue, *J Endod* 14:125, 1988.
43. Holmes-Johnson E, Geboy M, Getka EJ: Behavior considerations, *Dent Clin North Am* 30:391, 1986.
44. Hong D, Byers MR, Oswald RJ: Dexamethasone treatment reduces sensory neuropeptides and nerve sprouting reactions in injured teeth, *Pain* 55:171, 1993.
45. Hutter JW: Facial space infections of odontogenic origin, *J Endod* 17:422, 1991.
46. Imura N, Zuolo ML: Factors associated with endodontic flare-ups: a prospective study, *Int Endod J* 28:261, 1995.
47. Jeansonne MJ, White RR: A comparison of 2.0% chlorhexidine gluconate and 5.25% sodium hypochlorite as antimicrobial endodontic irrigants, *J Endod* 20:276, 1994.
48. Kaufman E et al: Intraligamentary injection of slow-release methylprednisolone for the prevention of pain after endodontic treatment, *Oral Surg* 77:651, 1994.
49. Kim S: Microcirculation of the dental pulp in health and disease, *J Endod* 11:465, 1985.
50. Kim S: Hypersensitive teeth: desensitization of pulpal sensory nerves, *J Endod* 12:482, 1986.
51. Kim S: Neurovascular interactions in the dental pulp in health and inflammation, *J Endod* 16:48, 1990.
52. Kim S et al: Effects of local anesthetics on pulp blood flow in dogs, *J Dent Res* 63:650, 1984.
53. Kontakiotis E, Nakou M, Georgopoulou M: In vitro study of the indirect action of calcium hydroxide on the anaerobic flora of the root canal system, *Int Endod J* 28:285, 1995.
54. Krasner P, Jackson E: Management of post-treatment endodontic pain with oral dexamethasone: a double-blind study, *Oral Surg* 62:187, 1986.
55. Laskin DM: Anatomic considerations in diagnosis and treatment of odontogenic infections, *J Am Dent Assoc* 69:38, 1964.
56. Law AS, Lily JP: Trigeminal neuralgia mimicking odontogenic pain, *Oral Surg* 80:96, 1995.
57. Lim G et al: Interleukin 1B in symptomatic and asymptomatic periapical lesions, *J Endod* 20:225, 1994.

58. Lin LM, Shovlin F, Skribner JE, Langeland K: Pulp biopsies from teeth associated with periapical radiolucency, *J Endod* 10:436, 1984.

59. Lin LM, et al: Detection of epidermal growth factor receptor in inflammatory periapical lesions, *Int Endod J* 29:179, 1996.

60. Lin LM, Skribner J: Why teeth associated with periapical lesions can have a vital response, *Clin Prevent Dent* 12:3, 1990.

61. Lin LM, Skribner JE, Gaengler P: Factors associated with endodontic treatment failures, *J Endod* 18:625, 1992.

62. Little JW: Prosthetic implants: risk of infection from transient dental bacteremias, *Compend Contin Educ Dent* 12:160, 1991.

63. Marbach JJ: Is phantom tooth pain a deafferentation (neuropathic) syndrome? I. Evidence derived from pathophysiology and treatment, *Oral Surg Oral Med Oral Pathol Oral Radiol Endod* 75:95, 1993.

64. Marbach JJ: Is phantom tooth pain a deafferentation (neuropathic) syndrome? II. Psychosocial considerations, *Oral Surg Oral Med Oral Path Oral Radiol Endod* 75:225, 1993.

65. Marbach JJ: Orofacial phantom pain: theory and phenomenology, *J Am Dent Assoc* 127:221, 1996.

66. Marshall JG, Walton RE: The effect of intramuscular injection of steroid on posttreatment endodontic pain, *J Endod* 10:584, 1984.

67. Marshall JG, Liesinger AW: Factors associated with endodontic posttreatment pain, *J Endod* 19:573, 1993.

68. Matusow RJ, Goodall LB: Anaerobic isolates in primary pulpal-alveolar cellulitis cases: endodontic resolutions and drug therapy considerations, *J Endod* 9:535, 1983.

69. McKendry DJ: Comparison of balanced forces, endosonic, and step back filing instrumentation techniques: quantification of extruded apical debris, *J Endod* 16:24, 1990.

70. Merskey H et al: Pain terms: a list with definitions and notes on usage, recommended by the IASP sub-committee on taxonomy, *Pain* 6:249, 1979.

71. Mor C, Rotstein I, Friedman S: Incidence of interappointment emergency associated with endodontic therapy, *J Endod* 18:509, 1992.

72. Deleted in proofs.

73. Morse DR: The use of analgesics and antibiotics in endodontics: current concepts, *Alpha Omegan* 83:26, 1990.

74. Morse DR et al: Infectious flare-ups and serious sequelae following endodontic treatment: a prospective randomized trial on efficacy of antibiotic prophylaxis in cases of asymptomatic pulpal-periapical lesions, *Oral Surg* 64:96, 1987.

75. Mulhern JM, Patterson SS, Newton CW, Ringel AM: Incidence of postoperative pain after one-appointment endodontic treatment of asymptomatic pulpal necrosis in single-rooted teeth, *J Endod* 8:370, 1982.

76. Najjar TA: Why can't you achieve adequate regional anesthesia in the presence of infection? *Oral Surg Oral Med Oral Pathol* 44:7, 1977.

77. Neaverth EJ: Disabling complications following inadvertent overextension of a root canal filling material, *J Endod* 15:135, 1989.

78. Negm MM: Effect of intracanal use of nonsteroidal anti-inflammatory agents on posttreatment endodontic pain, *Oral Surg* 77:507, 1994.

79. Nissan R et al: Ability of bacterial endotoxin to diffuse through human dentin, *J Endod* 21:62, 1995.

80. Nobuhara WK, Carnes DL, Gilles JA: Anti-inflammatory effects of dexamethasone on periapical tissues following endodontic overinstrumentation, *J Endod* 19:501, 1993.

81. Ohara P, Torabinejad M, Kettering JD: Antibacterial effects of various endodontic medicaments on selected anaerobic bacteria, *J Endod* 19:498, 1993.

82. Orstavik D, Haapasalo M: Disinfection by endodontic irrigants and dressings of experimentally infected dentinal tubules, *Endod Dent Traumatol* 6:142, 1990.

83. Pallasch TJ: Antibiotic prophylaxis: theory and reality, *Calif Dent Assoc J* 6:27, 1989.

84. Pashley DH: Dentin permeability, dentin sensitivity and treatment through tubule occlusion, *J Endod* 12:465, 1986.

85. Pekruhn RB: The incidence of failure following single-visit endodontic therapy, *J Endod* 12:68, 1986.

86. Penniston SG, Hargreaves KM: Evaluation of periapical injection of ketorlac for management of endodontic pain, *J Endod* 22:55, 1996.

87. Pinsawasdi P, Seltzer S: The induction of trigeminal neuralgia-like symptoms by pulp-periapical pathosis, *J Endod* 12:73, 1986.

88. Reeh ES, Messer HH: Long-term paresthesia following inadvertent forcing of sodium hypochlorite through perforation in maxillary incisor, *Endod Dent Traumatol* 5:200, 1989.

89. Roane JB, Dryden JA, Grimes EW: Incidence of postoperative pain after single- and multiple-visit endodontic procedures, *Oral Surg* 55:68, 1983.

90. Rugh JD: Psychological components of pain, *Dent Clin North Am* 31:579, 1987.

91. Ruiz-Hubbard EE, Guttman JL, Wagner, MJ: A quantitative assessment of canal debris forced periapically during root canal instrumentation using two different techniques, *J Endod* 13:554, 1987.

92. Safavi KE, Nichols FC: Alteration of biological properties of bacterial lipopolysaccharide by calcium hydroxide treatment, *J Endod* 20:127, 1994.

93. Safavi KE, Spangberg LSW, Langeland K: Root canal tubule disinfection, *J Endod* 16:207, 1990.

94. Salzgeber RM, Brilliant JD: An in vivo evaluation of the penetration of an irrigating solution in root canals, *J Endod* 3:394, 1977.

95. Sandler NA, Ziccardi V, Ochs M: Differential diagnosis of jaw pain in the elderly, *J Am Dent Assoc* 126:1263, 1995.

96. Schwartz S, Cohen S: The difficult differential diagnosis, *Dent Clin North Am* 36:279, 1992.

97. Selbst AG: Understanding informed consent and its relationship to the incidence of adverse treatment events in conventional endodontic therapy, *J Endod* 16:387, 1990.

98. Selden HS: The endo-antral syndrome, *J Endod* 3:462, 1977.

99. Seltzer S: *Endodontology: biologic considerations in endodontic procedures*, ed 2, Philadelphia, 1988, Lea & Febiger.

100. Seltzer S, Naidorf IJ: Flare-ups in endodontics. I. Etiological factors, *J Endod* 11:472, 1985.

101. Sessle BJ: Neurophysiology of orofacial pain, *Dent Clin North Am* 31:595, 1987.

102. Sigurdsson A, Jacoway JR: Herpes zoster infection presenting as an acute pulpitis, *Oral Surg Oral Med Oral Pathol Oral Radiol Endod* 80:92, 1995.

103. Sigurdsson A, Stancill R, Madison S: Intracanal placement of Ca(OH)$_2$: a comparison of techniques, *J Endod* 18:367, 1992.

104. Sjögren U, Figdor D, Spångberg L, Sundqvist G: The antimicrobial effect of calcium hydroxide as a short-term intracanal dressing, *Int Endod J* 24:119, 1991.

105. Soekanto A et al: Toxicity of camphorated phenol and camphorated parachlorophenol in dental pulp cell culture, *J Endod* 22:284, 1996.

106. Sundqvist G: Ecology of the root canal flora, *J Endod* 18:427, 1992.

107. Sundqvist G, Johansson E, Sjögren U: Prevalence of black-pigmented *Bacteroides* species in root canal infections, *J Endod* 15:13, 1989.

108. Takahashi K: Changes in the pulp vasculature during inflammation, *J Endod* 16:92, 1990.

109. Tjaderhane LS et al: Leaving the pulp chamber open for drainage has no effect on the complication of root canal therapy, *Int Endod J* 28:82, 1995.

110. Torabinejad M: Mediators of pulpal and periapical pathosis, *Calif Dent Assoc J* 14:21, 1986.

111. Torabinejad M: Management of endodontic emergencies: facts and fallacies, *J Endod* 18:417, 1992.

112. Torabinejad M et al: Factors associated with endodontic interappointment emergencies of teeth with necrotic pulps, *J Endod* 14:261, 1988.

113. Torabinejad M et al: Effectiveness of various medications on postoperative pain following complete instrumentation, *J Endod* 20:345, 1994.

114. Torabinejad M et al: Effectiveness of various medications on postoperative pain following root canal obturation, *J Endod* 20:427, 1994.

115. Torres JOC, Torabinejad M, Matiz RAR, Mantilla EG: Presence of secretory IgA in human periapical lesions, *J Endod* 20:87, 1994.

116. Trope M: Flare-up rate of single-visit endodontics, *Int Endod J* 24:24, 1991.

117. Trope M: Relationship of intracanal medicaments to endodontic flare-ups, *Endod Dent Traumatol* 6:226, 1990.
118. Trowbridge HO: Intradental sensory units: physiological and clinical aspects, *J Endod* 11:489, 1985.
119. Van Hassel HJ: Physiology of the human dental pulp, *Oral Surg* 32:126, 1971.
120. Vande Visse JE, Brilliant JD: Effect of irrigation on the production of extruded material at the root apex during instrumentation, *J Endod* 1:243, 1974.
121. Walton RE: The periodontal ligament injection as a primary technique, *J Endod* 16:62, 1990.
122. Walton RE, Chiappinelli J: Prophylactic penicillin: effect on post-treatment symptoms following root canal treatment of asymptomatic periapical pathosis, *J Endod* 19:466, 1993.
123. Walton RE, Fouad A: Endodontic interappointment flare-ups: a prospective study of incidence and related factors, *J Endod* 18:172, 1992.
124. Wolfson EM, Seltzer S: Reaction of cat connective tissue to some gutta-percha formulations, *J Endod* 1:395, 1975.
125. Wright EF, Gullickson DC: Iden ifying acute pulpalgia as a factor in TMD pain, *J Am Dent Assoc* 127:773, 1996.
126. Yang SF et al: Anaerobic tissue-dissolving abilities of calcium hydroxide and sodium hypochlorite, *J Endod* 21:613, 1995.

Chapter 3

Nonodontogenic Facial Pain and Endodontics: Pain Syndromes of the Jaws That Simulate Odontalgia

Lewis R. Eversole

Pain can be the vilest of human experiences. Sometimes it is merely annoying; at other times it is excruciating to the point where the system can no longer handle the experience and the sufferer loses consciousness. Of all the symptoms that the dentist must confront, pain is the most poignant. Ridding the patient of pain is perhaps the most rewarding aspect of practice. The ultimate purpose of the pain response is to inform the patient of a severe or even life-threatening pathologic process. It is, of course, the intent of our pain pathways to inform us of pathologic processes, and in the practice of endodontics the elimination of pulpal infection is the ultimate goal for odontogenic pain.

To the dismay of the patient, and often the practitioner, this signaling system is occasionally triggered in the absence of noxious stimuli, or it may be exaggerated beyond the severity of the underlying pathologic process. In this regard, the pain experience can be likened to the immune response. Certainly, the intricacies of the immune system were developed to protect the host from foreign agents that have the potential to destroy tissue (i.e., pathogens). In some hosts, however, the immune response is triggered by harmless foreign particles. In the context of a hypersensitivity or allergic reaction, the host immune system is stimulated and the various cellular and biochemical components of this response often result in unpleasant symptoms, including pain. Pain may be analogous to immune hypersensitivity in that symptoms may appear in the absence of a readily identifiable pathologic or detrimental process. Although some pain syndromes are associated with a low-grade inflammatory lesion, others seem not to be associated with an underlying disease process. Many of these pain syndromes are touted as psychogenic problems, but the precise cause and pathogenesis have yet to be deciphered. As more research findings unfold and more is learned about various neurotransmitter peptides, eventually we will solve the puzzles of chronic pain for which we now have no explanations.

NATURE OF PAIN

Normally the pain experience is initiated on a physiologic basis by way of the peripheral nervous system. Recall that nerve fibers have a nucleus, the cell body, that is located either within the central nervous system or in ganglia located in the peripheral tissues. Emanating from the cell body are long processes referred to as *axis cylinders*. A single nerve comprises hundreds of individual axis cylinders that are encased in a fibrous capsule known as the perineurium. Each individual axis cylinder is ensheathed by specialized cells, the Schwann cells. Thus the peripheral nerve can be envisioned as a bundle of electrical cables, all with their own enveloping insulation. Some axis cylinders with their associated Schwann cells have an additional insulating layer known as *myelin,* a specialized lipid synthesized by the Schwann cells. Those fibers capable of transmitting noxious stimuli (i.e., nociceptors) lack a myelin sheath. These nonmyelinated fibers are also referred to as *C fibers* as opposed to certain A or B fibers that transmit nonpainful sensory stimuli. The nerve endings of nociceptor C fibers are found in the skin and mucosa and of course are prevalent throughout the jaws, teeth, and periodontal tissues. In the region of the jaws, the nociceptor fibers are components of the trigeminal nerve. All of these nociceptors in the trigeminal system have their cell bodies located in the gasserian ganglion, and the afferent axis cylinders that feed into these cell bodies exit the ganglion and extend toward the central nervous system through the trigeminal trunk that enters the pons. These fibers then progress from the pons inferiorly into the upper aspects of the cervical region of the spinal cord. It is in this location where the axis cylinders terminate in a region referred to as the *caudate nucleus of V.* Nerves that are transmitting proprioceptive signals and light touch terminate higher in the spinal cord (mesencephalic nucleus). Fibers that terminate in the caudate nucleus are nociceptors that interdigitate with secondary neurons that then pass superiorly into the brain itself. At this synapse in the caudate nucleus neuropeptides are secreted that are capable of transmitting a noxious impulse from the C fiber across the synapse to the secondary nerve fiber. In addition, other fibers have been identified that modulate this neurotransmitter pathway. Interneurons also have fiber endings that contact the incoming nociceptor fiber and are capable of secreting yet other neurotransmitters that are capable of inhibiting propagation of noxious stimuli. Many of these inhibitory neurosecretory molecules fall into a special class of peptides known as *endorphins.*

Some time ago a theory was proposed to explain how noxious stimuli became consciously identifiable in the higher centers of the brain. This *gate theory of pain* was based on observation of a variety of interconnections in the region of the synapse. As noxious stimuli became more accentuated, the so-called gate would open and allow the impulses to be transmitted across the synapse. Indeed, neuroscience researchers have provided evidence that the gatekeeper is, in fact, represented by neurotransmitter molecules. Once noxious stimuli, such as chemical moieties in an acutely inflamed dental pulp, stimulate nociceptor fibers and the impulse is transmitted across the synapse in the caudate nucleus, the signal is further propagated through the secondary neuron to the midbrain. In this region the secondary fibers terminate in the vicinity of the thalamus. This region of the midbrain, the periaqueductal gray matter, is an area under significant neurosecretory molecular influences and is involved in a variety of emotions. It is thus interesting to speculate how some pain syndromes may be modified by the patient's psychologic and emotional status. From this area of the brain tertiary and quaternary neurons synapse and transmit the nerve impulse to the cerebral cortex. It is at this level that the patient actually becomes conscious of the pain symptom.

Nociceptor fibers are stimulated by a variety of physical and chemical stimuli. During an infection or in the face of trauma the tissues release noxious chemicals, including both peptides and lipids. In acute inflammation, the pH often drops below 5, and it is well documented that both acidic and alkaline solutions stimulate firing of nociceptor fibers. Excessive heat, such as that from an electrical burn or thermal injury, stimulates nociceptor fibers as well. In the context of the inflammatory reaction, kinins and prostaglandins, small vasoactive molecules, also have strong nociceptor-stimulating effects. Acute compressive forces on nerve endings may also produce pain, and this compression may be the result of cellular infiltrates into tissues and edema formation. As a rule, the patient is able to localize the specific region of pain where the tissue harbors the pathologic process that has engendered the pain sensation. As clinicians are well aware, severe and acute pain may not always be readily localized. The neuroanatomic basis for the inability to specifically localize severe pain is ill understood. Eventually, sometimes within 2 or 3 hours, sometimes after 2 or 3 days, the pain becomes more precisely localized.

Sharp pains are precipitated by acute pathologic processes. Alternatively, low-grade or chronic inflammatory conditions frequently manifest as dull aches. Acute infectious or traumatic stimuli tend to cause a sudden onset of pain of short duration. *Pain syndromes that fail to show any organic basis commonly present as aching, chronic pains of long duration.* Therefore pain as a symptom must be precisely characterized to arrive at a definitive diagnosis. The clinician is usually confronted with a specific complaint for which more than one entity must be considered. In this chapter we will consider the facial pain syndromes according to the type of pain symptoms that the patient describes, thus constructing differential diagnoses for specific types of complaints.

Pain may be classified as either acute or chronic. Acute pains are of short duration; chronic pains may last weeks, months, or even years. Another characteristic that must be elicited from the patient is the fluctuating nature of the pain. Some pains that are acute appear for a few days and completely disappear, whereas other acute pains are episodic or paroxysmal, appearing once or twice a day and lasting anywhere from seconds to many minutes. With chronic pain the pain experience frequently fluctuates from hour to hour or day to day. Some patients may complain of chronic pain that begins as a mere nuisance in the morning and builds to a more severe ache in the late afternoon. Identification of precipitating factors is diagnostically important. Sometimes gravity influences the severity of the pain; simply by placing the head below the knees the pa-

tient may experience an exacerbation. Exposure of tooth surfaces to hot and cold certainly is a well-recognized precipitating factor for pulpal pain. Patients may relate exacerbation of pain to emotional stress, jaw clenching, turning the head from left to right, or noting an increase in severity during mealtimes. It is therefore important to explore with the patient any factors that could precipitate an exacerbation of symptoms and to evaluate these in the context of the differential diagnosis.

Anatomic considerations are, of course, extremely important in the differential diagnosis of facial pains, although most pain localized to teeth or the jaw bones is odontogenic. From time to time the clinician may encounter nonodontogenic sources for tooth- and jaw-related pain symptoms. The anatomic sites that must be evaluated in the patient who has pain of unknown origin include the teeth, the periodontium, the masticatory musculature, the salivary glands, the sinus linings, the middle ear, and effects within the nerve itself.

In the overall process of patient assessment, particularly when compiling physical findings, it is important to assess the function of cranial nerves. Clinicians are often concerned about the possibility that facial pain is a harbinger of malignancy. In reality, malignant tumors that cause facial pain symptoms are extremely rare.[8] When they do occur, they often invade areas of the skull and cranial base, with resultant neural compression. Therefore motor deficits are common concomitant features. A brief evaluation of cranial nerve function takes only 1 minute and is easy to accomplish. Initially the patient is questioned about subjective complaints. Specifically, questions are directed toward uncovering defects in the special senses. The patient is asked about any changes or differences in the ability to see, smell, hear, or taste and about any numbness or paresthesia in the facial region.

Objective screening of cranial nerves is relatively simple. First, the trigeminal sensory pathways are evaluated by use of a cotton tip to test for light touch sensation of the forehead, the cheek, and the chin for all three divisions. This can also be done intraorally along the lateral border of the tongue and the palate and on the buccal mucosa. The sensory tract of nerve VII can be evaluated by stimulating the skin around the external auditory meatus. This is quickly followed by an assessment of pain sensation, which can be accomplished with a dental explorer. First, the patient is allowed to feel a brief pinprick on their hand from the explorer, to show what sensation they should expect. Then the same areas of the face are stimulated with a light touch of the sharp explorer point to the skin. The patient should feel all stimuli, and if all sensory pathways are intact the sensation should be the same in one site as in the next.

Once sensory pathways have been evaluated, the objective examination turns to motor function. The cranial nerves that innervate the facial musculature are often grouped together. In this regard, those cranial nerves that innervate the extraocular muscles are evaluated together. Nerves III, IV, and VI can be evaluated by having the patient track a moving object with the eyes. The tracking involves vertical upward and downward movements of the object and side-to-side movements. The object is returned to the center of the patient's gaze and moved down and out in both right and left directions. If the patient's eyes are able to follow the up, down, side-to-side, and down-and-out movements, then nerves III, IV, and VI are intact.

The motor function of nerve VII is assessed by asking the patient to wrinkle the forehead, raise the eyebrows, close the eyes, pucker the lips, and smile. Hypoglossal function is evaluated by having the patient protrude the tongue and move it left and right. Finally, spinal accessory innervation is assessed by having the patient shrug the shoulders against the resistance of a hand placed on the top of the shoulder. Among patients with facial pain, should a motor or a sensory deficit be encountered (either paresthesia or hypoesthesia) a serious organic disease should be suspected.

ACUTE PAIN SYNDROMES OF THE JAWS

Acute pain is defined as pain of sudden onset that either lasts only a few days or exhibits short-lived episodic exacerbations. Patients describe these pains as sharp, stabbing, or lancinating. Such comments as, "It feels like a hot poker is jammed into my jaw," or "It feels like a sharp electrical jolt" are commonly related. Once the usual and customary diagnostic approaches have been undertaken to rule out pain of pulpal or periodontal origin, then other disease processes that cause acute pain must be considered. Acute pain syndromes that are episodic or paroxysmal usually represent neuralgias or vasodilatory pain syndromes. Sharp, acute pains that persist for many hours or days are more likely to represent a nociceptor response to organic disease, usually an acute infectious processes. Table 3-1 lists the major pain syndromes subsumed under the rubric of acute pain. For each of these disorders the clinical features, nature, and duration of the pain, and precipitating factors should be considered. Some pain syndromes are diagnosed on the basis of exclusion, although most have unique signs and symptoms that allow a definitive diagnosis.

Trigeminal Neuralgia*

Trigeminal neuralgia, or tic douloureux, is a facial pain disorder that has very specific clinical features. The pain involves one or more of the trigeminal nerve divisions and, although the precise cause is unknown, empiric evidence suggests that the symptoms evolve as a consequence of vascular compression of the gasserian ganglion. The precise neurophysiologic mechanism has not been uncovered, and other theories for this particular disorder include viral infection of either neurons or the Schwann cell sheath.

Two highly characteristic features of tic douloureux allow

---

*References 1, 10, 29, 33, 41, 42, 51, 56, 57.

it to be differentiated from other facial pain syndromes. The character and duration of the symptoms are unique, and a specific anatomic trigger point generally can be identified. The pain tends to involve primarily either the maxillary or the mandibular division, although the ophthalmic division is sometimes involved. The pain is severe and lancinating, shooting into the bone and teeth. Frequently both patient and dentist are convinced that the source of the pain is pulpal. The electrical quality of the pain is unique and is rarely encountered in odontogenic infections. Furthermore, the pain episode lasts only seconds at a time, although paroxysms may occur in rapid succession. Somewhere on the facial skin, or occasionally in the oral cavity, a trigger zone exists. This trigger area may be only 2 mm wide. When it is merely touched with the finger or an instrument the pain paroxysms are triggered. The patient is usually keenly aware of this small anatomic site and will do anything to avoid stimulating the spot.

Treatment modalities are varied and include medical intervention with specific drugs that alleviate the neuralgic pain and various surgical interventions. For the dentist the most salient advice is to establish a diagnosis and avoid any invasive dental procedures. Invariably, patients with trigeminal neuralgia have undergone numerous endodontic procedures and extractions but continue to experience pain because pulpal and periodontal infectious processes have no role in this syndrome. Therefore, despite the insistence by the patient that the symptoms are tooth related, the diagnosis should be established and the patient should be referred to a neurologist for definitive therapy.

Carbamazepine (Tegretol), the standard medical therapy for trigeminal neuralgia, is quite effective. Unfortunately, this particular drug is a bone marrow suppressant and will eventually produce agranulocytosis. This side effect is dose dependent. Therefore many patients may be maintained on Tegretol without untoward effects if the dose can be restricted to a level where agranulocytosis does not occur, yet pain symptoms are alleviated. For patients who do not respond to medical treatment a variety of surgical modalities have been advocated, including peripheral neurectomy, rhizotomy (severance of the nerve trunk at its exit from the ganglion), alcohol injections, and glycerol injections. All these therapies have met with some degree of success. Two surgical procedures are widely accepted among the neurosurgical community for the relief of trigeminal neuralgia. The hypothesis that vascular compression on the

---

Table 3-1. Differentiating acute pains

Condition	Nature	Triggers	Duration
Odontalgia	Stabbing, throbbing, nonepisodic	Hot, cold, tooth percussion	Hours-days
Trigeminal neuralgia	Lancinating, electrical, episodic	1-2 mm locus on skin/mucosa, light touch triggers pain	Seconds
Cluster headache	Severe ache, retroorbital component, episodic	REM sleep, alcohol	30-45 min
Acute otitis media	Severe ache, throbbing, deep to ear, nonepisodic	Lowering head, barometric pressure	Hours-days
Bacterial sinusitis	Severe ache, throbbing in multiple posterior maxillary teeth, nonepisodic	Lowering head, tooth percussion	Hours-days
Cardiogenic	Short-lived ache in left posterior mandible, episodic	Exertion	Minutes
Sialolithiasis	Sharp, drawing, salivary swelling, episodic	Eating, induced salivation	Constant low-level ache, sharp brief episodes when triggered

REM, Rapid eye movement.

ganglion is a causative factor has met with some acceptance, because surgical decompression of the ganglion often results in prolonged reduction of pain symptoms. Another successful approach is transcutaneous ganglionic neurolysis in which a probe is placed into the ganglion and the neurons are ablated by thermal means. Both of these procedures have resulted in 90% success over a 5-year period. Again, it is stressed that dental extraction or endodontic therapy is contraindicated in trigeminal neuralgia.

Cluster Headache*

Cluster headache, also known as *Sluder's neuralgia* or *sphenopalatine ganglion neuralgia,* is an acute paroxysmal pain syndrome of no known cause. The pathogenesis is hypothesized to be a consequence of vasodilatory phenomena that occur on an episodic basis. Presumably nociceptor fibers that encircle vessels are stimulated during acute vasodilatation. If this is the case, cluster headache is a form of migraine.

Cluster headache is generally encountered among males in their 30s through 50s. Although precipitating factors are not always identifiable, many of these patients report onset of pain after consuming alcohol. There is a tendency for the patients who suffer from cluster headaches to have a unique facial appearance: they are often freckled and have a ruddy complexion. Onset and duration of the pain episodes are unique and easily diagnosed. In classic cluster headache the pain is located unilaterally in the maxilla, sinus, and retroorbital area. It is often mistaken for acute pulpitis or apical abscess of a posterior maxillary tooth. The pain frequently occurs just after the patient retires and is entering the early stages of REM (rapid eye movement) sleep. The onset is acute and severe, with patients indicating that it feels like a hot poker has been jammed into the upper jaw and behind the eye. Typically, the pain continues to increase in severity and persists for 30 to 45 minutes. During this period the patient finds it difficult to remain seated and tends to pace the floor. The symptoms occur at approximately the same time, once each evening, though some people suffer two such episodes a day. Interestingly, in the classic form of cluster headache the episodic symptoms persist only 6 to 8 weeks and then spontaneously disappear. Hence the term *cluster headache.* The headache episodes cluster at a certain time of day and during a certain season. They seem to be more prevalent in spring.

Another form of cluster headache is referred to as *chronic cluster.* These headaches are similar to the classic form in that they occur on an episodic basis and typically last 30 to 45 minutes, but they affect the patient year round rather than seasonally.

In the past, because vasodilatation is involved in their pathogenesis, cluster headaches were managed by prescribing ergotamine tartrate. This medication causes significant side effects, including nausea and vomiting, so it is prescribed as a suppository. Because ergot alkaloids induce vasoconstriction, they are contraindicated for patients with hypertension, and many patients with cluster headache are also hypertensive. It was subsequently discovered that oxygen would lessen the headache attacks if administered at the onset of pain. Administration of oxygen is often used as a diagnostic intervention.

The current therapy for cluster headache uses vasoactive

drugs, particularly the calcium channel blockers. Nifedipine or one of its related compounds, when prescribed on a regular basis, prevents the pain paroxysms. This medication is of benefit for both classic and chronic cluster headache. In addition, prednisone in combination with lithium has been shown to be effective in alleviating or preventing pain of cluster headache. Hyperbaric oxygen therapy has been shown to have preventive affects. The vasoactive antimigraine drug sumatriptin, a 5-hydroxytryptamine receptor agonist administered subcutaneously, is effective for treatment of cluster headache, although oral administration is not particularly beneficial.

Acute Otitis Media[16]

Infection of the middle ear is common, particularly in children, and is caused by pyogenic microorganisms, usually streptococci. It is well known that odontogenic infections of posterior teeth may refer pain back to the ear/temporomandibular joint (TMJ) area; similarly, middle ear infections may be confused with odontogenic pain because the symptoms radiate from the ear over the posterior aspects of the maxilla and mandible. It would be unlikely for middle ear infection to be manifested by jaw pain exclusively. The nature of the pain is acute. Patients complain of a severe ache, and throbbing is a frequent accompaniment. Gravitational factors may also come into play. The pain is often exacerbated as the patient lowers the head.

The pathogenesis is straightforward and is, in many ways, similar to that of acute pulp pain. In the dental pulp the noxious components of the inflammatory process and factors secreted by the pathogenic microorganisms accumulate in a confined space. In otitis media the infection occurs within the middle ear, which is confined laterally by the tympanic membrane and posteriorly by the oval window; laterally the eustachian tube serves as an outlet. In the process of acute inflammation, with accumulation of neutrophils, exudate, and associated mucosal edema, the eustachian tube–lining mucosa swells and becomes occluded, thereby confining the noxious components of the infectious process to the middle ear chamber.

The definitive diagnosis is made by using an otoscope to examine the tympanic membrane, which is usually red and bulging. Treatment consists of antibiotic therapy, usually penicillin with β-lactamase inhibitor or clindamycin. Rarely, syringotomy is necessary. Once the diagnosis is established, referral to an otolaryngologist is recommended.

Acute Maxillary Sinusitis[3,26]

Because the roots of the maxillary teeth extend to the sinus floor, it is axiomatic that acute infectious processes involving the sinus mucous membrane will simulate dental pain. Most forms of sinusitis are allergic and are characterized by chronic pain symptoms as manifested by a dull ache in the malar region and maxillary alveolus.

When maxillary sinusitis is the consequence of an acute pyogenic bacterial infection the symptoms are usually acute. The pain may be stabbing, with severe aching pressure and throbbing. Pain is frequently referred upward under the orbit and downward over the maxillary posterior teeth. Importantly, pain is not referred to a single tooth but is perceived in all teeth in the quadrant. Percussion sensitivity of the molar teeth is a common finding. Typically, when the head is placed below the knees, the pain is exacerbated.

The aforementioned signs and symptoms are rather charac-

---

*References 9, 12, 15, 23, 28, 38, 39, 40, 46, 52, 55.

teristic; however, other diagnostic approaches can be used to secure a definitive diagnosis. Transillumination is a diagnostic aid and is easy to perform. A fiberoptic light beam is placed against the palate, and in a darkened room a clear sinus will transilluminate. Antra that are filled with exudate are clouded and will not transilluminate. Radiographic imaging is also of considerable diagnostic utility. Although more advanced imaging such as magnetic resonance imaging (MRI) and computed tomography (CT) may be used, a Waters sinus is usually sufficient.

Because maxillary root apices are separated from the antral floor by a few millimeters of bone, it is understandable that acute periapical infection could spread into the sinus. Therefore, bacterial sinusitis can be a consequence of pulpal infection. It is essential to assess each individual maxillary tooth when a patient presents with acute maxillary sinusitis because treatment of the sinusitis without management of the dental source will only result in recurrence of symptoms.

Although acute bacterial sinusitis is generally readily responsive to antibiotic therapy, induced sinus drainage and lavage may occasionally be necessary when the ostia are closed because of edema. At the time of examination, culture and sensitivity tests should be obtained to select the appropriate antibiotic should preliminary therapy fail to resolve the infection. Referral to an otolaryngologist is recommended.

Cardiogenic Jaw Pain[2,44]

Vascular occlusive disease is one of the most common afflictions of modern society. The accumulation of atherosclerotic plaque in coronary vessels in association with vasospasm will lead to angina pectoris. The most common manifestation of coronary vascular occlusion, particularly in its acute manifestation, is substernal pain with referred pain rotating over the left shoulder and down the arm. This pain is usually precipitated by exertion. Presumably, the pain sensation is transmitted by nociceptor fibers that envelop the coronary vasculature and are stimulated by vasospasm. Of course, angina pectoris is a prelude to acute myocardial infarction. These symptoms are extremely significant and, once diagnosed, the appropriate diagnostic imaging studies are required to ascertain the degree of coronary occlusion. Such symptoms represent a life-threatening event. Occasionally, angina pectoris is manifested as left shoulder and arm pain without a substernal component. Even less frequent is referral of pain up the neck into the left angle of the mandible. In these instances, the referred pain may mimic odontalgia.

When a patient presents with left posterior mandibular pain and there is no obvious odontogenic source of infection, referred cardiogenic pain should be considered. Importantly, the patient should be questioned about the onset of the symptoms. If they occur after exercise or other exertion, then coronary vascular disease should be an important consideration.

Once suspected, specific diagnostic tests can be performed to assess the potential for coronary vascular occlusive disease. Specifically, electrocardiography or stress tests may be in order. If these findings support a diagnosis of coronary ischemia, cardiac catheterization and angiography are indicated. Treatment consists of a variety of interventions including restricted intake of lipids, administration of aspirin to prevent thrombosis, and surgical intervention by coronary angioplasty or bypass surgery should angiography show significant occlusive disease.

Sialolithiasis[32,47]

Unlike kidney and gallbladder stones, sialoliths are unrelated to increased levels of serum calcium or to dietary factors. The cause is unknown, although the pathogenesis is relatively well understood. Desquamated epithelial cells from the major salivary ducts may accumulate and form complexes with salivary mucin to form a nidus for calcification. The salivary stone evolves by sequential concretion of calcium phosphate salts, much like the growth rings of a tree. Once the stone reaches a critical size, the salivary duct becomes occluded and symptoms develop. Sialolithiasis is significantly more frequent in the submandibular duct, and therefore pain associated with submandibular stones is more prone to mimic endodontic pain in the posterior aspect of the mandible. The occluded duct often leads to swelling of the submandibular area and therefore may mimic lymphadenitis associated with an endodontic infection of a posterior mandibular tooth.

With close examination and questioning, the diagnosis is usually made quite easily because the pain has characteristic features. Although a chronic ache may extend into the mandible, the primary location is within the submandibular soft tissues. Typically, the pain is exacerbated by salivation (induced by a lemon drop or at mealtimes). The floor of the mouth can be palpated with a milking motion; when the major duct is occluded, no saliva flows from the duct orifice. The nature of the pain is also revealing in that the patient feels a stringent drawing in the area. When pain of this nature is encountered, salivary occlusion should be investigated before each individual tooth in the vicinity is evaluated. Typically, an occlusal radiograph will disclose the presence of a soft tissue calcification along the course of the duct in the floor of the mouth. It should be noted that panoramic radiographs may reveal an opacity in the mandible. In such instances, the soft tissue calcification is simply superimposed although it may mimic focal sclerosing osteomyelitis.

Although sialolithiasis of the parotid duct is quite rare, its pain can be mistaken for toothache. Again, the symptoms are similar to those of submandibular sialolithiasis in that the pain is exacerbated during meals and with stimulation of salivation. The sialolith is generally demonstrable with a panoramic radiograph.

Treatment consists of physical attempts to remove the stone by manipulating it out the orifice. Larger stones cannot be removed in this fashion and will require a surgical cutdown to the duct. Indeed, stones of large size and long duration usually culminate in ablation of the secretory component of the gland, and the nonfunctional gland then becomes subject to retrograde bacterial infections. In these instances sialoadenectomy, along with removal of the stone, is indicated.

CHRONIC PAIN SYNDROMES OF THE JAWS

Internal Derangement of the Temporomandibular Joint and Facial Myalgia*

Internal derangements of the TMJ include meniscus displacement, formation of intraarticular adhesions, and various forms of arthritis. A variety of etiologic factors have been implicated, but no single hypothesis has been universally accepted. It has been proposed that stress-related jaw clench-

---

*References 14, 17, 21, 22, 24, 30, 36, 43, 54.

ing and bruxism may place stress on the meniscus and cause anterior displacement. Alternatively, traumatic events such as yawning and prolonged jaw opening have been suggested to cause overextension of the ligaments with secondary displacement of the meniscus. Once the meniscus has been anteriorly displaced, adhesions may form, the retrodiscal tissues that are not designed for loading become perforated, and bone-to-bone contact progresses to degenerative joint disease. It is highly unlikely that occlusal discrepancies predispose or even cause these events when one evaluates the literature in a nonbiased fashion (Table 3-2).

Other organic joint diseases may also involve the TMJ and cause pain symptoms in this region. Included here are rheumatoid, gouty, or psoriatic arthritis and arthritis attending collagen diseases. All of these arthritides are quite rare in the TMJ region.

The more common disorders of the TMJ primarily affect young white women[31] and include meniscus displacement with adhesions and progression to degenerative arthritic changes. It is noteworthy that organic lesions of this nature may develop in the absence of any pain symptoms whatsoever. The chief findings are limitation of jaw opening, deviation on opening, clicking or crepitus, and pain directly localized to the joint region in front of the tragus of the ear.

The pain associated with internal derangement is generally a dull, boring ache, but it may be more acute when exacerbated by wide opening of the mandible or chewing. In some patients the chronic symptoms become progressively worse and the degree of pain increases. In such instances the pain symptoms may become more generalized. Odontalgia originating from a pulpally or periodontally infected posterior tooth, either maxillary or mandibular, may refer pain back to the TMJ area. In such instances a joint problem may be perceived by the patient as a dental problem, or conversely a pulp involvement may be mistaken for a TMJ disorder.

Myalgic pains are the consequence of sustained muscle contraction usually associated with tooth clenching. In this context, facial myalgia is generally considered to be equivalent to tension headache, being a stress disorder. The pain is always dull, aching, and diffuse. In general, most patients complain of symptoms over the mandible and temple. Palpitation of the masticatory muscles will often reveal the presence of so-called "trigger points." These trigger zones are painful foci in the masticatory muscles and should not be confused with the trigger zone of trigeminal neuralgia. Myalgia may exist as an isolated entity, or it may be associated with other pain disorders, including TMJ internal derangement or odontalgia. A preexisting pain may predispose to muscle posturing and a tendency for jaw clenching. Thus the pain symptoms become quite variable and confusing to the examiner. In such instances, evaluations of jaw function, auscultation of the TMJ, masticatory muscle palpitation, and endodontic testing must be performed. If an endodontic infection is uncovered, root canal therapy will relieve the primary pain source and secondary myalgia should resolve shortly thereafter.

When odontogenic sources have been ruled out and a diagnosis of internal derangement, myalgia, or internal derangement with myalgia is confirmed, appropriate therapy should be instituted. Psychologic factors have been shown to play a dominant contributing etiologic role in TMJ and myofascial pain disorders. It is generally accepted that a conservative approach to therapy should be initiated and should include behavioral, physical, and medical therapies. Muscle relaxants, nonsteroidal analgesics, physical therapy, stress management therapy, and occlusal splints are all noninvasive procedures. Acupuncture has shown some utility in certain populations but is not universally effective. Extensive tooth grinding and fixed prosthetic reconstruction aimed at curing the disorder should be avoided. When intractable pain persists after conservative therapy, arthroscopic examination may be indicated and either arthroscopic surgery or surgical meniscus replacement may be indicated. Even with surgical intervention, severe pain disorders often recur within months after the procedure. Therefore conservative management is to be encouraged.

Atypical Facial Pain*

Of all the facial pain syndromes, the group that most often simulates endodontic or odontogenic pain is "atypical facial pain." Indeed, patients will insist the pain is of tooth origin and will often plead to have the putatively offending tooth or teeth removed. When diagnosing jaw and endodontic pain, it is imperative that the clinician be well versed in the clinical features of this group of pain disorders because tooth extraction or endodontic therapy will fail to alleviate the symptoms.

Subsumed under the heading of atypical facial pain are a

---

*References 2, 4, 5, 7, 10, 13, 17, 18, 23, 25, 34-37, 45, 48, 50, 51, 58.

Table 3-2. Differentiating chronic aching and burning pains

Condition	Nature	Triggers	Duration
Odontalgia	Dull ache	Hot, cold, tooth percussion	Days-weeks
TMJ internal derangements	Dull ache, sharp episodes	Opening, chewing	Weeks-years
Myalgia	Dull ache, degree varies	Stress, clenching	Weeks-years
Atypical facial pain	Dull ache with severe episodes	Spontaneous	Weeks-years
Phantom tooth pain	Dull ache with severe episodes	Spontaneous	Weeks-years
Neuralgia-inducing cavitational osteonecrosis	Dull ache with severe episodes	Spontaneous	Weeks-years
Allergic sinusitis	Dull ache	Lowering head	Weeks-months
	Malar area, multiple posterior maxillary teeth		Seasonal
Causalgia	Burning	Posttrauma, postsurgical	Weeks-years
Post-herpetic neuralgia	Deep boring ache with burning	Spontaneous after facial shingles	Weeks-years
Cancer-associated facial pain	Variable, motor deficit, paresthesia	Spontaneous	Days-months

variety of disorders (atypical odontalgia, phantom tooth pain, neuralgia-inducing cavitational osteonecrosis) that all share common features. By definition, atypical facial pain represents a pain syndrome that does not conform to a specific organic disease and does not represent another well-defined form of neuralgia. Importantly, there is no identifiable cause. When the pain is localized to the mandible or maxilla without reference to any specific teeth, it is generally termed atypical facial pain. Alternatively, when pain is localized to a given tooth or a group of contiguous teeth in the absence of any pulpal insults or periodontal infection, the condition is termed atypical odontalgia. When pain persists in teeth whose pulp has been extirpated, the condition is referred to as *phantom tooth pain,* a phenomenon akin to phantom limb after amputation. These types of atypical pains are chronic and aching. Patients with atypical facial pain feel it deep within the bones and it is hard to localize. Indeed, many patients with atypical facial pain will report that the symptoms seem to wander from site to site. In addition, many of these patients have pain complaints elsewhere in their bodies. The intensity of these atypical pains varies considerably from one patient to the next. Some complain of a constant nagging ache; others claim that the pain is excruciating at times. The cause of atypical pain has long been a mystery, and many clinicians have emphasized the probability that psychogenic factors play a major role. Some studies have indicated that patients with atypical facial pain also have vascular-type headaches such as migraine and cluster headaches; other studies challenge this relationship.

Phantom tooth pain is estimated to occur in less than 3% of patients undergoing root canal therapy. It has been suggested that surgical extirpation of the pulp results in damage to nerve fibers at the apex of the teeth and should be considered a traumatic neuralgia. Another possible mechanism is formation of a small traumatic neuroma in the apical periodontium. Although psychologic factors have been suggested to be important in phantom tooth pain, there is not a great deal of evidence, on the basis of psychometric testing, that psychopathologic mechanisms are major factors. Deafferentation in experimental animals results in pain behavior and it has therefore, by analogy, been suggested that phantom tooth pain is in fact a form of deafferentation pain. Frequently, although these postendodontic pain foci are subjected to surgical procedures, the pain persists. The organic basis for phantom tooth pain remains an enigma.

Atypical pain localized to edentulous foci can sometimes be alleviated with a subperiosteal injection of local anesthetic. In such instances, it has been proposed that small residual inflammatory foci exist within the endosteum and that focal necrosis occurs with neural damage. These so-called pathologic bone cavities are now referred to as *neuralgia-inducing cavitational osteonecrosis* (NICO). Large series have been reported in which surgical curettage has alleviated pain. Tissue curetted from these cavities often shows minor pathologic changes such as fibrosis and mild inflammation. The validity of this theory of atypical facial pain arising in edentulous regions is not universally accepted and is somewhat controversial. Recent large series studies with long-term follow up have reported favorable outcomes for more than 70% of patients treated for NICO.

Whether atypical facial pains lie in edentulous areas or are poorly localized or centered in teeth, treatment should be approached cautiously. Many patients have submitted to numerous endodontic procedures and extractions for these pains, and subsequent to the invasive procedures the pain has persisted. Many dentists have undertaken such procedures at the insistence of the patient, who firmly believes there is an odontogenic source. When the symptoms are mild, the pain should be managed with analgesics and reassurance. Many patients with atypical facial pain respond favorably to tricyclic antidepressants, particularly amitriptyline. This medication affects neurotransmitter substances and appears to have an analgesic property in addition to its antidepressant effects. In more severe cases, the therapy used for trigeminal neuralgia may be indicated. In particular, microvascular decompression and transcutaneous thermal neurolysis have been found to be effective in treating the more severe atypical facial pain problems in some, but not all, patients.

Allergic Sinusitis[3,26]

As discussed in the differential diagnosis of acute facial pains, inflammatory disease of the antrum is more often chronic and allergic in nature. Allergies tend to be seasonal because most people with upper airway allergic reactions respond to various seeds and pollens. In more northerly climates the prevalence of sinusitis increases in spring and fall. In warmer climates, such as California and Florida, allergies may be encountered year round, and some are actually more common during the winter months.

The contact of an allergen with the sinonasal mucous membranes results in an immediate-type hypersensitivity reaction that is mediated by an antigen that penetrates the respiratory epithelium, enters the submucosa, and is bound to an immunoglobulin E antibody. This antibody is complexed with mast cells and, on binding to the allergen, histamine is released. Vasoactive consequences evolve, with edema formation and transudation of fluids. Involvement of the sinus includes mucosal thickening and the presence of a fluid level within the maxillary sinus cavity. As the ostium becomes occluded, pain symptoms evolve. The pain is preceded by a feeling of pressure within the maxilla for a few hours or days, which then evolves into a dull, chronic ache. Frequently the posterior maxillary teeth seem to "itch," and the patient feels compelled to clench. Percussion sensitivity is evident on all of the molar teeth, and frequently the premolars are percussion sensitive as well. This sensitivity is not acute; rather, it is experienced as a dull discomfort. As with acute sinusitis, the symptoms may be accentuated by having the patient place the head between the knees. The gravitational changes shift the fluid in the sinus and the result is increased pain. Maxillary sinus pain is typically accentuated by changes in barometric pressure, so that traveling to high altitudes or flying may exacerbate the pain. Without treatment these symptoms persist throughout the period when allergens circulate in the air.

The diagnosis is supplemented by antral transillumination in which light will not illuminate an affected maxilla in a darkened room. Waters sinus radiographs will disclose either soft tissue membrane thickening of the antral walls or an air-fluid level will be discernable. Mucosal changes are also evident on MRI and CT scans.

Because chronic sinusitis is generally allergic in nature, the treatment differs from that of acute bacterial sinusitis. Decongestants and nasal sprays, along with antihistamines, are the treatment of choice. Identification of the allergen and desensitization may offer relief for some of these patients, and referral to either an otolaryngologist or an allergist should be considered.

CHRONIC BURNING PAIN

Causalgia[18,19,25]

Causalgia is a pain syndrome that is rarely encountered in the head and neck. When present, it is unlikely to be confused with odontalgia. Causalgic pain occurs as a consequence of trauma, jaw fracture, or laceration or may evolve after surgery.

It has been hypothesized that nociceptor fibers become retracted in association with sympathetic fibers in causalgia. The skin overlying the painful area often becomes erythematous during pain episodes. Patients have a tendency to rub and scratch the involved area, producing what are known as *trophic foci*. The skin becomes encrusted and keratotic with scaling. The pain is characteristically paroxysmal and burning and may be both superficial and deep. When a deep component is the predominant complaint, it may be confused with toothache.

Thus, to arrive at a definitive diagnosis of causalgia, the events and clinical features must be identified and administration of an ipsilateral stellate ganglion block will alleviate pain. In these cases, sympathectomy has been advocated.

Postherpetic Neuralgia[5,11,27,49]

Primary infection with varicella zoster virus causes chickenpox, a disease that affects over 95% of the population during early childhood. In its secondary or recurrent form, the disease is referred to as *herpes zoster* or *shingles*. This disease represents a recrudescence of a latent virus that is located in sensory ganglia. In the head and neck area it is the trigeminal ganglion that harbors latent virus. The factors that activate the virus and allow it to exit from the ganglion and enter the axis cylinder are unknown. Importantly, once the virus is liberated from the nerve endings, it enters epithelial cells and induces a rather characteristic vesicular eruption. Unlike herpes simplex, recrudescence of varicella zoster results in a vesicular eruption that outlines the entire distribution of the sensory pathways. Therefore the vesicles terminate at the midline and involve only one division of the trigeminal nerve, although sometimes more than one division may be involved. Bilateral involvement is extremely rare. The painful lesions of shingles cause a deep boring ache that involves not only the superficial mucosal and cutaneous tissues but also the maxillary or mandibular bones. Before the onset of the vesicular eruption it is common for the patient to experience prodromal pain, and when that happens the diagnosis may be obscured. These prodromal symptoms frequently simulate trigeminal neuralgia in that they last only seconds and have an electrical quality. Once vesicles appear, the diagnosis is straightforward. If any doubts persist, samples of the vesicular fluid collected within the first 3 days can be cultured for virus or subjected to cytologic smear examination with immunoperoxidase staining to identify the specific viral capsid antigen.

In fewer than 5% of varicella zoster infections patients show clearing of vesicles though pain persists. Postherpetic neuralgia may persist weeks, months, or years. Although the prodromal pain is acute and electrical and pain associated with vesicular eruption is a deep boring ache, the pain symptoms of postherpetic neuralgia differ yet again. Once the vesicles clear,

the residual pain has a burning quality and is chronic. Deeper aching pains occasionally may be associated with this burning element and may suggest pain of odontogenic origin. Nevertheless, the classic sequence of events with an antecedent vesicular eruption is sufficient to make the diagnosis.

The management of postherpetic neuralgia is problematic, and there is no way of knowing when the symptoms may resolve of their own accord. A variety of techniques have been used to manage the pain, including transcutaneous electrical nerve stimulation (TENS), antiseizure drugs, analgesics, and topical preparations. Referral to a neurologist is recommended.

FACIAL PAIN RESULTING FROM MALIGNANT NEOPLASIA[20]

Although cancer involving the maxilla and mandible rarely manifests itself with pain, there is a published case report regarding prodromal facial pain from a glioblastoma.[8] Typically, paresthesia or hypoesthesia is the complaint. Carcinoma arising in the maxillary sinus may proliferate and begin to erode the bony margins of the sinus walls. Encroachment on the infraorbital nerve as the tumor extends into the floor of the orbit induces paresthesia over the malar region and in the maxillary teeth. Similarly, a malignant tumor in the mandible such as metastatic carcinoma from a distant site such as lung, breast, or colon can invade the nerve. Therefore numbness is the ominous symptom of cancer in the jaws, although occasionally such tumors produce pain symptoms. In particular, multiple myeloma (malignant neoplasia of B lymphocytes) is notorious for causing intense bone pain. Therefore in the jaws such lesions could easily mimic toothache. Rarely does myeloma manifest itself only in the jaws because it is a disseminated disease and pain would be experienced in other bones. The tumor induces "punched-out" radiolucencies that are poorly marginated. Such lesions should be investigated by obtaining a biopsy specimen.

A variety of cancer-associated pain syndromes of the face have been reported in the literature. These are rare conditions and are designated by a host of eponyms. In general, they represent metastatic tumors that have metastasized to the base of the skull, where they encroach on exiting cranial nerves. Most such tumors will invade not only sensory nerves but motor nerves as well. Therefore muscular weakness or paralysis in conjunction with pain are the usual accompaniments. When tumors affect the upper aspects of the nasopharynx and skull base, upper facial pain is experienced and the cranial nerves III, IV, and VI become involved, leading to ophthalmoplegia. Tumors that arise around the exit of the trigeminal nerve generally affect the motor fibers of nerve V and masticatory muscle weakness is identifiable. A combination of atypical facial pain with ocular, facial, or masticatory muscle paresis should alert the clinician that a malignant disease may be present. At this point, more sophisticated imaging studies should be undertaken, such as MRI and CT scans. The tumor will then be localized on such images, and referral to an oncologist is recommended.

A variety of pain syndromes involving the head and neck have the potential to refer pain to the jaw areas. In evaluating pulpal and periapical pain, these specific syndromes must be considered in the differential diagnosis, particularly when the usual physical findings fail to implicate a particular tooth. It must always be remembered that individual patients may suffer from more than one disorder. In this context it is certainly possible for a patient who has one of these pain disorders also to harbor a dental pulp infection. For this reason the importance of conducting a thorough history with comprehensive physical examination procedures to evaluate the dentition and other anatomic sites cannot be overemphasized.

REFERENCES

1. Barker FG II et al: The long-term outcome of microvascular decompression for trigeminal neuropathy, *N Engl J Med* 334:1077-1083, 1996.
2. Batchelder BJ, Krutchkoff DJ, Amara J: Mandibular pain as the initial and sole clinical manifestation of coronary insufficiency: report of case, *J Am Dent Assoc* 115:710, 1987.
3. Berg O, Lejdeborn L: Experience of a permanent ventilation and drainage system in the management of purulent maxillary sinusitis, *Ann Otol Rhinol Laryngol* 99:192, 1990.
4. Bouquot JE, Christian J: Long-term effects of jawbone curettage on the pain of facial neuralgia, *J Oral Maxillofac Surg* 53:387-399, 1995.
5. Bernstein JE et al: Topical capsaidcin treatment of chronic postherpetic neuralgia, *J Am Acad Dermatol* 21:265, 1989.
6. Bouquot JE et al: Neuralgia-inducing cavitational osteonecrosis (NICO), *Oral Surg Oral Med Oral Pathol* 73:307, 1992.
7. Brooke RI: Atypical odontalgia, *Oral Surg Oral Med Oral Pathol* 49:196, 1980.
8. Cohen S et al: Oral prodromal signs of a central nervous system malignant neoplasm-glioblastoma multiforme, *J Am Dent Assoc* 121:643, 1986.
9. Connors MJ: Cluster headache: a review, *J Am Osteopathic Assoc* 95:533-539, 1995.
10. Dalessio DJ: Management of the cranial neuralgias and atypical facial pain. A review. *Clin J Pain* 5:55, 1989.
11. De Benedittia G, Besana F, Lorenzetti A: A new topical treatment for acute herpetic neuralgia and post-herpetic neuralgia: the aspirin/diethyl ether mixture. An open-label study plus a double blind controlled clinical trial.
12. Dechant KL, Clissold SP: Sumatriptan. A review of its pharmacodynamic and pharmacokinetic properties, and therapeutic efficacy in the acute treatment of migraine and cluster headache.
13. Donlon WC: Neuralgia-inducing cavitational osteonecrosis. *Oral Surg Oral Med Oral Pathol* 73:319, 1992.
14. Dworkin SF et al: Brief group cognitive-behavioral intervention for temporomandibular disorders, *Pain* 59:175-187, 1994.
15. Ekbom K et al: Cluster headache attacks treated for up to three months with subcutaneous sumatriptan (6 mg). Sumatriptan Cluster Headache Long-Term Study Group, *Cephalalgia* 15:230-236, 1995.
16. Froom J et al: Diagnosis and antibiotic treatment of acute otitis media: report from International Primary Care network, *BMJ* 300:582, 1990.
17. Gallagher RM et al: Myofascial face pain: seasonal variability in pain intensity and demoralization, *Pain* 61:113-120, 1995.
18. Graff-Radford SB, Solberg WK: Atypical odontalgia, *J Craniomand Dis* 6:260-265, 1992.
19. Graff-Radford SB et al: Thermographic assessment of neuropathic facial pain, *J Orofacial Pain* 9:138-146, 1995.
20. Greenberg HS: Metastasis to the base of the skull: clinical findings in 43 patients, *Neurology* 31:530, 1981.
21. Hapak L et al: Differentiation between musculoligamentous, dentoalveolar, and neurologically based craniofacial pain with a diagnostic questionnaire, *J Orofacial Pain* 8:357-368, 1994.
22. Harness DM, Donlon WC, Eversole LR: Comparison of clinical characteristics in myogenic TMJ internal derangement and atypical facial pain patients, *Clin J Pain* 8:4, 1990.
23. Harness DM, Rome HP: Psychological and behavioral aspects of chronic facial pain, *Otolaryngol Clin North Am* 22:1073, 1989.
24. Helms CA et al: Staging of internal derangements of the TMJ with magnetic resonance imaging: preliminary observations, *J Craniomandib Dis* 3:93, 1989.
25. Hoffman KD, Matthews MA: Comparison of sympathetic neurons in orofacial and upper extremity nerves: implications for causalgia, *J Oral Maxillofac Surg* 48:720, 1990.
26. Kennedy DW, Loury MC: Nasal and sinus pain: current diagnosis and treatment, *Semin Neurol* 8:303, 1988.
27. Kishore-Kumar R, et al: Desipramine relieves postherpetic neuralgia, *Clin Pharmacol Ther* 47:305, 1990.
28. Kudrow L: Cluster headache. A review, *Clin J Pain* 6:29, 1989.
29. Lichtor T, Mullan JR: A 10-year follow-up review of percutaneous microcompression of the trigeminal ganglion, *J Neurosurg* 72:49, 1990.
30. Linde A, Isacsson G, Jonsson BG: Outcome of 6-week treatment with transcutaneous electric nerve stimulation compared with splint on symptomatic temporomandibular joint disk displacement without reduction, *Acta Odont Scand* 53:92-98, 1995.
31. Lipton JA, Ship JA, Larach-Robinson D: Estimated prevalence and distribution of reported orofacial pain in the United States, *J Am Dent Assoc* 124:115, 1993.
32. Lustmann J, Regev E, Melamed Y: Sialolithiasis. A survey on 245 patients and a review of the literature, *Int J Oral Maxillofac Surg* 19:135, 1990.
33. Main JH, Jordan RC, Barewal R: Facial neuralgias: a clinical review of 34 cases, *J Can Dent Assoc* 58:752-755, 1992.
34. Marbach JJ: Is phantom tooth pain a deafferentation (neuropathic) syndrome? Part I: Evidence derived from pathophysiology and treatment, *Oral Surg Oral Med Oral Pathol* 75:95-105, 1993.
35. Marbach JJ: Is phantom tooth pain a deafferentiation (neuropathic) syndrome? II. Psychosocial considerations, *Oral Surg Oral Med Oral Pathol* 75:225-232, 1993.
36. Marbach JJ, Raphael KG, Dohrenwend BP: Do premenstrual pain and edema exhibit seasonal variability? *Psychosom Med* 57:536-540, 1995.
37. Marbach JJ et al: Incidence of phantom tooth pain: an atypical facial neuralgia, *Oral Surg Oral Med Oral Pathol* 53:190, 1982.
38. Mathew NT: Advances in cluster headache, *Neurol Clin North Am* 8:867, 1990.
39. Mauskop A, Altura BT, Cracco RQ, Altura BM: Intravenous magnesium sulfate relieves cluster headaches in patients with low serum ionized magnesium levels, *Headache* 35:597-600, 1995.
40. Medina JL, Diamond S, Fareed J: The nature of cluster headache, *Headache* 19:309, 1979.
41. Moller AR: The cranial nerve vascular compression syndrome: I. A review of treatment, *Acta Neurochirurgica* 113:18, 1991.
42. Moraci M et al: Trigeminal neuralgia treated by percutaneous thermocoagulation: comparative analysis of percutaneous thermocoagulation and other surgical procedures, *Neurochirurgia* 35:48, 1992.
43. Murakami K et al: Four-year follow-up study of temporomandibular joint arthroscopic surgery for advanced stage internal derangements, *J Oral Maxillofac Surg* 54:285-291, 1996.
44. Natkin E, Harrington GW, Mandel MA: Anginal pain referred to the teeth, *Oral Surg Oral Med Oral Pathol* 40:678, 1975.
45. Nicolodi M, Sicuteri F: Phantom tooth diagnosis and an anamnestic focus on headache, *New York State Dent J* 59:35-37, 1993.
46. Pascual J, Peralta G, Sanchez U: Preventive effects of hyperbaric oxygen in cluster headache, *Headache* 35:260-261, 1995.
47. Pollack CV Jr, Severance HW Jr: Sialolithiasis: case studies and review, *J Emerg Med* 8:561, 1990.
48. Pollmann L: Determining factors of the phantom tooth, *N Y State Dent J* 59:42-45, 1993.
49. Robertson DR, George DP: Treatment of post-herpetic neuralgia in the elderly, *Br Med Bull* 48:113, 1990.
50. Schnurr RR, Brooke RI: Atypical odontalgia: update and comment on long-term follow-up, *Oral Surg Oral Med Oral Pathol* 73:445, 1992.
51. Sicuteri R et al: Idiopathic headache as a possible risk factor for phantom tooth pain, *Headache* 31:577, 1991.
52. Stovner LJ, Sjaastad O: Treatment of cluster headache and its variants, *Curr Opin Neurol* 8:243-247, 1995.

53. Taarhj P: Decompression of the posterior trigeminal root in trigeminal neuralgia: a 30-year follow-up review, *J Neurosurg* 57:14, 1982.

54. Truelove EL: The chemotherapeutic management of chronic and persistent orofacial pain, *Dent Clin North Am* 38:669-688, 1994.

55. Wilkinson M et al: Migraine and cluster headache—their management with sumatriptan: a critical review of the current clinical experience, *Cephalalgia* 15:337-357, 1995.

56. Zakrewska JM: Medical management of trigeminal neuralgia, *Br Dent J* 168:399, 1990.

57. Ziccardi VB et al: Trigeminal neuralgia: review of etiologies and treatments, *Compendium* 14:1256-1264, 1993.

58. Ziccardi VB et al: Peripheral trigeminal nerve surgery for patients with atypical facial pain, *J Cran Maxillo Fac Surg* 22:355-360, 1994.

Chapter 4

Case Selection and Treatment Planning

Samuel O. Dorn
Arnold H. Gartner

Once a thorough examination and diagnosis have determined that an endodontic problem exists, the process of case selection begins. The dentist must use the factors discussed in this chapter to determine whether treatment is indicated, what treatment will best serve this patient, and whether this patient will be best served by being referred to a specialist or treated by the examining clinician. Rating systems have been devised to aid the dentist in determining which cases to treat and which to refer.[39]

EVALUATION OF THE PATIENT

Each patient must be evaluated both physically and mentally. Even the simplest endodontic case can turn into an extremely difficult one when the patient's physical or mental health is seriously compromised. The clinician must use all available knowledge and experience in assessing all aspects of the patient as well as the dental problem.

Physical Evaluation

Most medical conditions do not contraindicate endodontic therapy. However, the patient's medical condition should be thoroughly evaluated to properly manage the case. If the treating dentist does not feel comfortable treating medically compromised patients, that patient should be referred to an endodontist who may be able to provide more expeditious treatment.

The following considerations are not meant to be a thorough treatise on the subject, but decisions that the dentist should consider when planning treatment. For a thorough review of the management of the medically compromised patient, the reader is referred to textbooks on the subject.[27,28]

Cardiovascular disease

A history of a myocardial infarction within the past 6 months is a contraindication of elective dental treatment.[27] Emergency relief, however, should be provided with consultation with the patient's cardiologist. These patients should be treated with a stress reduction protocol that includes short appointments, psychosedation, and pain and anxiety control. Patients with prosthetic cardiac valves or with a heart murmur with regurgitation should be premedicated with amoxicillin or clindamycin according to current American Heart Association guidelines.[9]

Bleeding disorders

Laboratory screening tests and physician consultation are necessary for any patient with a bleeding disorder. The dentist should be aware that dialysis patients, alcohol abusers, and patients taking aspirin may have severe bleeding problems. Although endodontic therapy is preferable to extraction in these patients, the dentist should be prepared to handle in consultation with the patient's physician any bleeding resulting from impingement of the rubber dam clamp, vital pulp extirpation, or surgical procedures.

Diabetes

An acute endodontic infection can compromise even a well-controlled diabetic patient; therefore all diabetic patients must be carefully monitored. Prophylactic antibiotics may be necessary even when there are no signs of periradicular infection. Patients with uncontrolled or brittle diabetes should be monitored carefully for signs of insulin shock or diabetic coma. Appointments should be scheduled so as not to interfere with the patient's normal insulin and meal schedule. A stress reduction protocol should be followed.[27]

Cancer

A thorough history will reveal what type of cancer the patient has and what type of treatment is being rendered. Because some cancers can mimic an endodontic lesion (Fig. 4-1), the dentist should perform a biopsy of any suspicious lesions. Because chemotherapy and radiation to the head and neck region can severely compromise the healing process, endodontic treatment should be done in close consultation with the patient's oncologist.[27]

AIDS

Human immunodeficiency virus (HIV) infection, including acquired immunodeficiency syndrome (AIDS), is not a contraindication to endodontic therapy. In most instances the patient is at less risk with endodontic therapy than with extraction. Consultation with the patient's physician, antibiotic coverage, and strict adherence to universal precautions are necessary.[27]

Pregnancy

Pregnancy is not a contraindication to endodontic therapy. Pain and infection should be controlled for the health and well-being of the fetus and the mother. The patient's obstetrician should be consulted when any medications are to be prescribed.[27] The use of electronic apex locators can reduce the already minimal radiation risk.

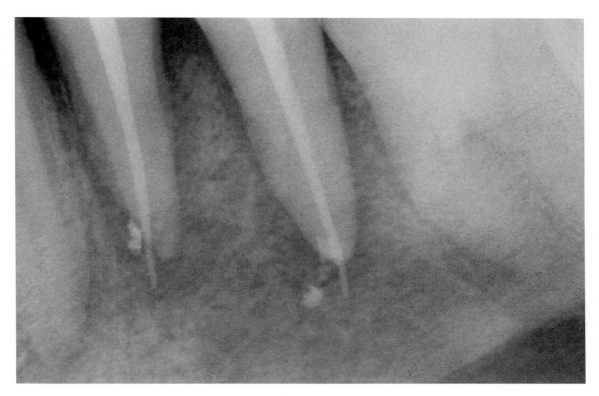

FIG. 4-1 Malignancy. This patient was referred to the endodontist because of continued mobility of the mandibular premolars after the generalist endodontically treated and retreated these teeth. Biopsy specimen showed this diffuse lesion to be metastatic cancer from the prostate.

Allergies

A thorough medical history should be taken to determine any possible allergies. Brand and generic names of medications should be checked against those being prescribed. Possible cross-allergencity should also be considered (e.g., 10% of patients who are allergic to penicillin are also allergic to cephalosporins).[27]

If the patient is allergic to latex, a nonlatex dental dam should be used, along with vinyl gloves. A highly allergic patient may be more prone to interappointment flare-ups, which may be preventable by antihistamine premedication.[42,48]

Steroid therapy

Adrenal suppression should be suspected when a patient is taking 20 mg of hydrocortisone per day or its equivalent. It may be necessary to increase the steroid dose for treatment. Any patient receiving steroid therapy has an increased susceptibility to infection and, in consultation with his or her physician, should be appropriately protected with antibiotics.[27]

Infectious diseases

The strict adherence to universal infection control precautions will prevent the spread of infectious diseases between patients and dental personnel. All dental office personnel should be inoculated for the hepatitis B virus. There is now increasing concern of airborne diseases, especially multiple-drug-resistant tuberculosis. Barrier protection is mandatory. See Chapter 5 for more information about this issue.

Physical disabilities

Because patients with physical disabilities such as Parkinson's disease, spinal cord injury, or stroke may not be able to hold radiographic film in position because of impairment, the electronic apex locator is recommended. If a patient has a limited mouth opening or cannot lie on his or her back, a routine case can become a difficult one.

Organ transplants

Organ transplant patients are usually taking high doses of immunosuppressive drugs. Antibiotic coverage is mandatory in these patients. The treating physician should be consulted to determine the proper level of antibiotic coverage.[27]

Dialysis

The physical condition of the kidney dialysis patient changes during the time between dialysis sessions. The physician should be consulted regarding the best day and time for the patient to be treated. The patient should be premedicated to protect the integrity of the arteriovenous shunt.[27]

Orthopedic implants

There is much controversy regarding whether to premedicate patients with orthopedic implants. There are no studies that have proved any relationship between orthopedic implants and bacteria of endodontic origin.[26,43] Most implant infections occur within 6 months of implant surgery and are caused by staphylococci, which are uncommon in endo-

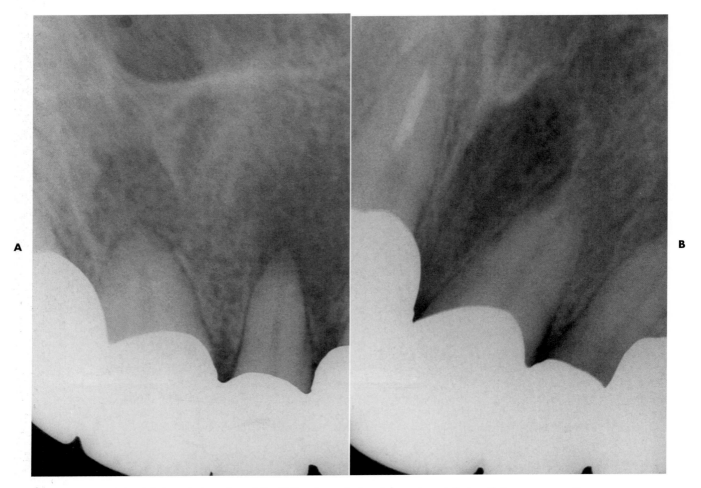

FIG. 4-2 Angulation. **A** and **B,** Shift of angulation demonstrated that radiolucency over the maxillary central incisor is the incisive canal. Note that in **A** the lamina dura appears intact.

dontic infections. Premedication is recommended only when the patient is immunocompromised, has rheumatoid arthritis, is an insulin-dependent diabetic, has had previous prosthetic joint infections, or has had the joint replaced within the past 2 years.[5a]

Psychologic Evaluation

Motivation

Before the patient can be motivated, the dentist needs to be motivated. The dentist must believe in the value of keeping a tooth compared with a denture or placing an implant. The best and most predictable implants are still our own teeth.

A patient who shows no effort to maintain good oral hygiene or one who constantly misses appointments may not be a good candidate for endodontic therapy unless the dentist can motivate this patient to change his or her neglectful ways.

Difficult patients

Even the most routine central incisor can become a problem to treat when the patient exhibits a difficult personality. Claustrophobia or fear of ionizing radiation, pain, or needles can impair a patient's ability to behave well in the dental of-

fice. Many of these psychologic problems can be overcome by a gentle, caring, honest chairside manner.

Economic Evaluation

Endodontic therapy provides good value for treatment rendered.[4] Although 46% of the respondents in a recent survey falsely perceived endodontic therapy to be more expensive than extraction and replacement by a fixed prosthesis,[5] another survey placed the market value of a tooth at over $300,000.[4] Accordingly, the patient should understand that, in concert with endodontic therapy, orthodontic, periodontic, or surgical procedures may also be necessary.

EVALUATION OF TOOTH

A number of factors should be considered to determine whether a tooth should be endodontically treated and, if so, whether by a general dentist or an endodontist.

One of the most important aids we have to assess the tooth during case selection and treatment planning is the radiograph. It is important to have properly exposed and processed radiographs taken from at least two different horizontal angles (Fig. 4-2). At least one of the radiographs should be taken with a paralleling device.

Morphologic Features

Unusual length

Teeth that are either unusually long (greater than 25 mm) or unusually short (less than 15 mm) are difficult to treat. By measuring the approximate length of the tooth on a radiograph exposed with the paralleling technique, the general dentist can determine whether he or she has the necessary skill or whether an endodontist would better serve the patient.

Unusual canal shapes

Unusual canal shapes (Fig. 4-3) require special techniques. An open apex ("blunderbuss") canal will need either apexification or apexogenesis. C-shaped canals, dens-in-dente, taurodontism, and roots with bulbous ends are more difficult to treat and will often require more specialized techniques that are more likely to be acquired by the advanced general dentist or an endodontist.

Canal curvature

Extreme curvature of the root canal (Fig. 4-4) can be challenging for even an experienced clinician. The use of anticurvature filing and nickel-titanium files can help avoid strip perforations and ledging. Radiographs exposed at a 15-degree horizontal angle can help visualize canal curvatures in the buccolingual plane.

Number of canals

Always look for and expect extra canals (Fig. 4-5). All molars should be considered to have four canals unless proved otherwise. When a large canal stops abruptly, look for a branching into two or more smaller canals.

Resorptions

Internal resorption can be differentiated from external resorption by the radiographic appearance[20] (Fig. 4-6). External resorption appears to be superimposed on the canal, whereas internal resorption appears continuous with the canal. When the resorptive process causes a perforation from the outside of the tooth to the canal, the prognosis remains questionable.

Calcifications

Calcification in the root canal, whether isolated or continuous, can make treatment difficult even for the most skilled clinician. The use of chelating agents, magnification, fiberoptic transillumination, and path-finding files can aid the dentist in finding and treating calcified canals. The use of the endodontic microscope adds extraordinary visibility for searching for the elusive canal spaces.

Previous Treatment

Canal blockage

Previously treated teeth may need to be retreated because of persistent pathologic conditions resulting from incomplete root canal debridement or obturation (Fig. 4-7). Any material blocking access to the apical extent of the canal must be removed. Ultrasonic instruments have made it much easier to remove posts, silver points, broken instruments, and paste fillings. Gutta-percha can be carefully removed with mechanical instruments, Hedstrom files, and solvents (such as chloroform, rectified turpentine, eucalyptol, or xylene). Care must be taken not to ledge or block these canals. A dentist not familiar with retreatment techniques should refer these cases to an endodontist.

Ledging

A previously treated tooth that has a ledge in the canal can be difficult to treat, even for the most experienced clinician. Using a file where the apical 2 mm has been bent at a 30-degree angle can aid in bypassing the ledge and eventually eliminating it.

Perforations

If a previously treated tooth has a perforation that is not properly sealed, there may be a very poor prognosis. When the perforation is in the apical two thirds of the root it may be treated surgically. If the perforation is in the furcation area, it may be possible to pack a matrix of hydroxyapatite and seal the perforation with a glass ionomer cement (Fig. 4-8). If bone loss has already occurred, microsurgery hemisection, root amputation, or extraction may be indicated.

Location of the Tooth

Accessibility

Location in the arch is directly related to accessibility. The further posterior the dentist goes, the less ability there is to see and treat all the canals. The compromised range of motion, especially in cases of limited opening from trismus, scarring from burns or surgical procedures, or systemic diseases such as scleroderma can create problems. If the clinician does not think that he or she has the dexterity and speed necessary to best serve the patient, referral should be considered. Angulation of the tooth can also present problems with accessibility. Molars that are tipped to the mesial or teeth that are in lingual or labial version can also present problems for the inexperienced dentist.

Proximity to other structures

Certain anatomic structures in close proximity to the apex of the tooth to be treated may cause case selection concerns. Paresthesia can be caused by overinstrumentation, overfilling, or endodontic pathologic conditions in close approximation to the mental foramen or mandibular canal (Fig. 4-9, *A*). Periradicular infections can cause concomitant infections of the maxillary sinus (Fig. 4-9, *B*), nasal cavities, or endosseous implants.

The malar process, impacted teeth (Fig. 4-9, *C*), tori, or overlapping roots can make radiographic visualization of the apex and periradicular region difficult for both diagnosis and treatment. In these situations the use of electronic apex locators is recommended.

Restorability

The restorability of the tooth in question should be carefully evaluated (Fig. 4-10). All caries should first be removed so that the extent of remaining tooth structure may be evaluated. If caries has progressed subgingivally or into the furcation area, the feasibility of restoring the tooth after root amputation or periodontal procedures should be evaluated before proceeding with endodontic therapy.

Periodontal Status

The prognosis for all endodontically involved tooth should be evaluated in relation to its periodontal status. A tooth with

Text continued on p. 71

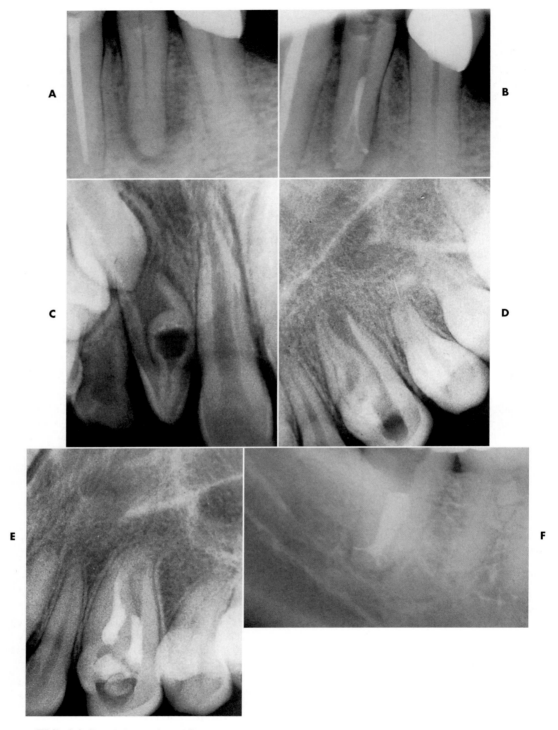

FIG. 4-3 Canal shape. **A** and **B,** Multiple portals of exit require thermoplastic obturation techniques. **C,** Dens-in-dente. **D** and **E,** Fusion. (**D,** preoperative; **E,** difficult obturation). **F,** Taurodont teeth have large pulp chambers and short roots that are often difficult to locate and treat.

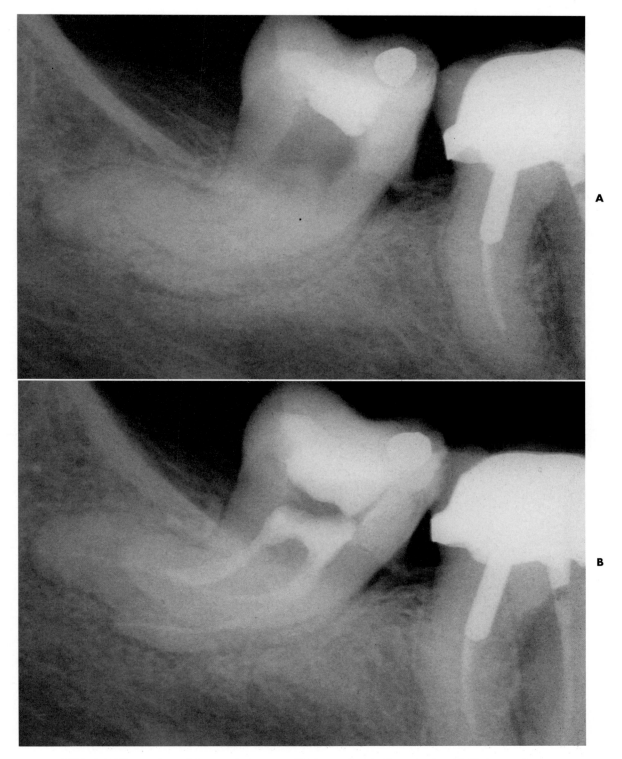

FIG. 4-4 Dilaceration of the canals in a mandibular molar. **A,** Preoperative. **B,** Postoperative.

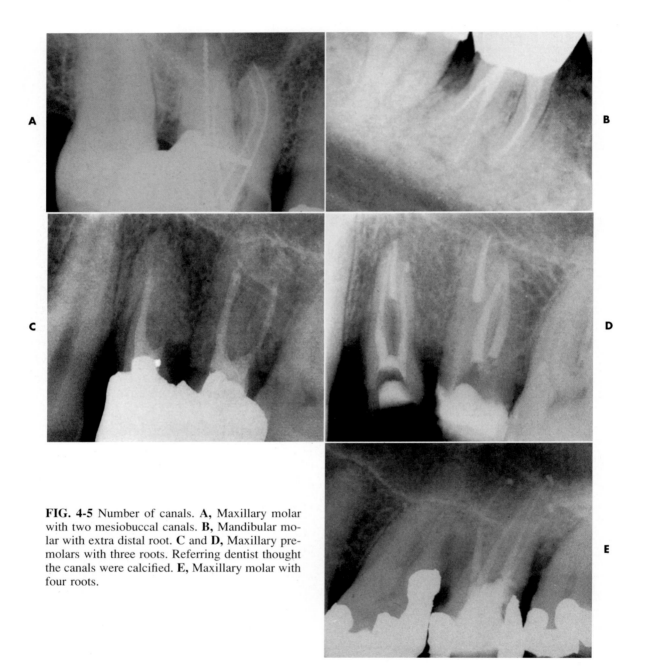

FIG. 4-5 Number of canals. **A,** Maxillary molar with two mesiobuccal canals. **B,** Mandibular molar with extra distal root. **C** and **D,** Maxillary premolars with three roots. Referring dentist thought the canals were calcified. **E,** Maxillary molar with four roots.

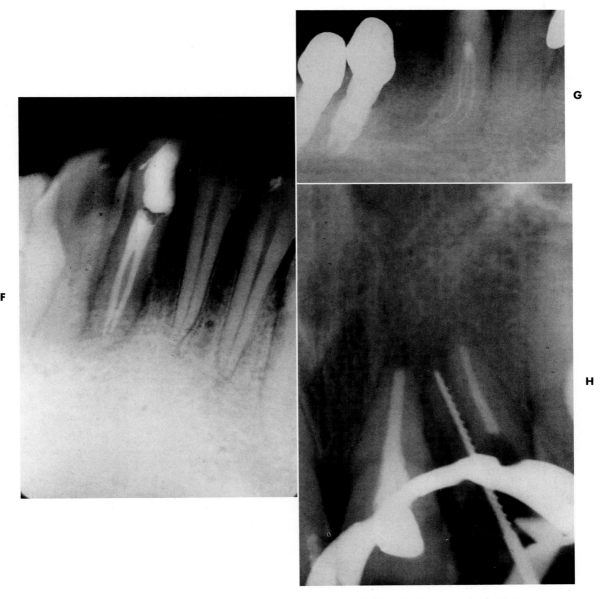

FIG. 4-5, cont'd F, Mandibular incisor with two canals. **G,** Mandibular premolar with three canals. **H,** Maxillary lateral incisor with two roots. Always suspect extra canals until proved otherwise.

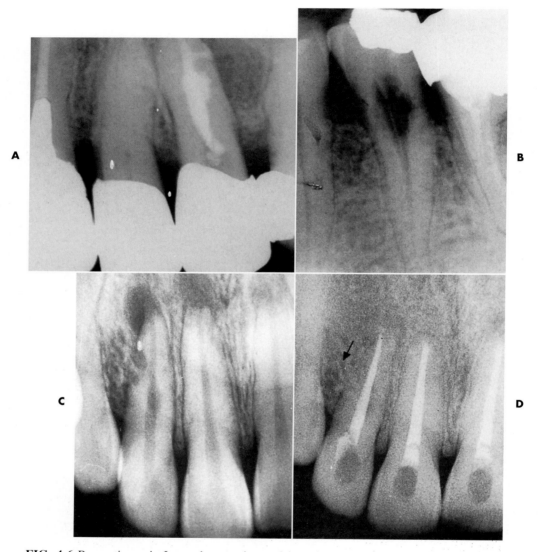

FIG. 4-6 Resorptions. **A,** Internal resorption and lateral canal were obturated with thermoplasticized gutta-percha. **B,** External resorption. Note outline of root canal in the resorptive area. **C** and **D,** Replacement (external) resorption caused by trauma on the maxillary lateral incisor. This was arrested with calcium hydroxide treatment before gutta-percha obturation. Arrow in **D** shows bone.

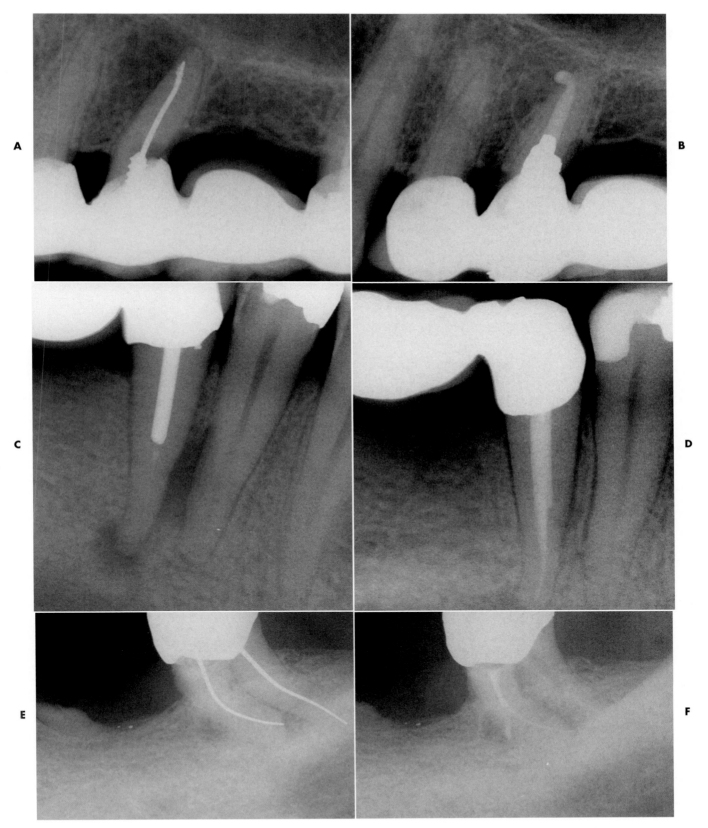

FIG. 4-7 Retreatment. **A** and **B,** Retreatment of a silver point case. **C** and **D,** Retreatment of paste filling after removal of post. Note healing of lateral area after 6 months. **E** and **F,** Retreatment of silver point case. Gutta-percha now fills lateral canal.

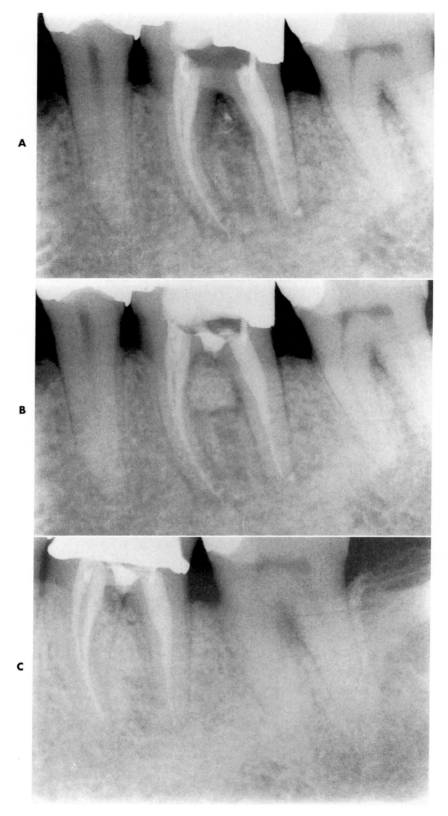

FIG. 4-8 Perforation repair. **A,** Perforation into the furcation area occurred during endodontic treatment 2 years earlier and was repaired with Intermediate Restorative Material (IRM). The patient had a sinus tract to the furcation but with no periodontal communication. **B,** Defect is packed tightly with hydroxyapatite through the perforation and covered with Ketac-Silver. **C,** Two years postoperatively the patient is asymptomatic with no reappearance of the sinus tract.

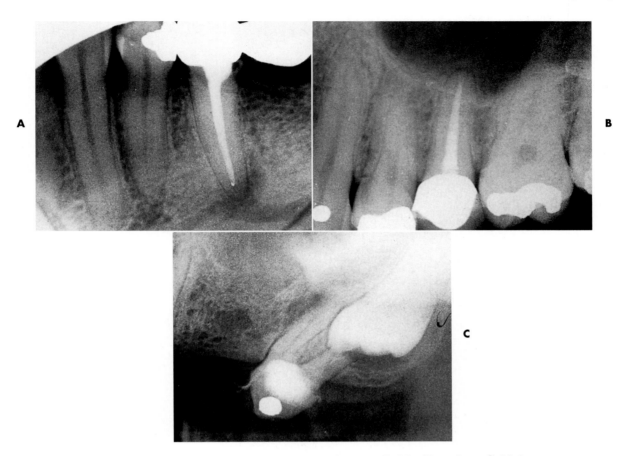

FIG. 4-9 Proximity to other structures. **A,** Mental foramen. **B,** Maxillary sinus. **C,** Malar process and impacted tooth.

very little bone support and class III mobility will have a poor endodontic prognosis. Some advanced endodontic-periodontal combined lesions may never heal. If the endodontic problem is caused by a vertical fracture, periodontal healing is most unlikely; the tooth will most likely require extraction. The need for hemisection or root amputation should be determined before proceeding with endodontic treatment.

Evaluation of the Clinician

Self-evaluation by the clinician should include the following questions:

1. *Do I have the experience to effectively manage this problem?* Complicated treatment procedures should not be attempted until the clinician has had advanced training or experience with more situations of the same type.

2. *Do I have the skill to treat this endodontic case?* Not every clinician has the ability or patience to carefully clean and shape and fill curved, narrow canals or to do surgical procedures if necessary. The clinician should be honest in evaluating his or her abilities to treat complicated cases. The internal question must always be, who can best serve this patient's needs?[10]

Patients with medical problems or disabilities might need special or rapid care beyond the ability of this clinician.

3. *Do I have the appropriate equipment?* Are unusually long or flexible files needed? Does this case call for the use of a microscope (Fig. 4-11), ultrasonic device, or electronic apex locator? Will special obturation techniques be necessary because of the canal anatomy? Will other special techniques and materials be advantageous, such as guided tissue regeneration, bone grafting, or endodontic stabilizers?

These questions should be asked by the clinician of himself or herself and answered truthfully. It is much easier to refer a patient to a specialist before a problem occurs than it is after the problem creates stress for everyone.

TREATMENT PLANNING

As described in Chapter 1, a proper diagnosis must be made before endodontic therapy is initiated.

To determine the correct treatment and avoid misdiagnosis, it is essential to follow a thorough and systematic approach.

1. Determine the patient's chief complaint.
2. Take an accurate medical and dental history.
3. Perform a methodical and thorough examination of the patient, including all necessary tests.
4. Carefully evaluate all necessary radiographs.
5. Analyze and synthesize the results to arrive at the proper diagnosis.
6. Evaluate the difficulty of the case and the ability of the clinician.
7. Establish an appropriate treatment plan.

Any shortcuts to this systematic approach may result in misdiagnosis and incorrect treatment.

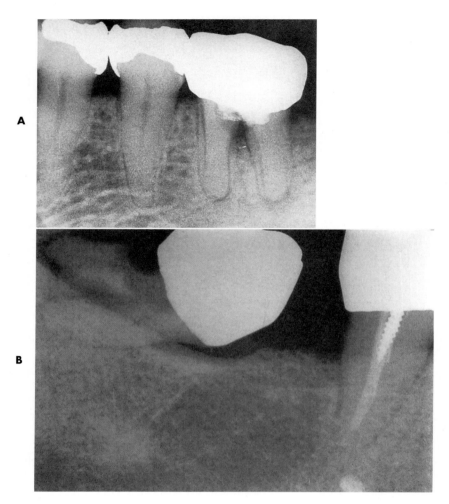

FIG. 4-10 Restorability. **A,** Caries into the furcation may render a tooth untreatable or unrestorable. **B,** Angulation, caries, and lack of bone support render this tooth hopeless.

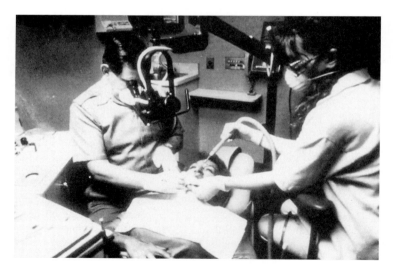

FIG. 4-11 Operating microscope may be necessary to find calcified or additional canals.

Emergency Treatment

The first goal of endodontic therapy is to relieve acute pain and provide drainage of infection. Initiating root canal therapy by itself may alleviate the patient's acute symptoms. Often emergency treatment, such as establishing drainage by opening the tooth or performing an incision and drainage procedure, may be needed before the root canal can be initiated.[12,13]

Once the patient's acute symptoms have been alleviated, the completion of the root canal therapy can be set aside while the clinician conducts a comprehensive examination of the patient and develops a customized treatment plan. This written sequenced document will provide the patient information on planned therapy. Complete patient awareness will help prevent embarrassment and patient dissatisfaction. The following sequence is recommended[55]:

1. Management of acute pulpal or periodontal pain
2. Oral surgery for the extraction of nonsalvageable teeth
3. Caries control of deep lesions
4. Periodontal procedures to manage soft tissue
5. Endodontic therapy for asymptomatic teeth with irreversibly inflamed or necrotic pulp and retreatment of failing root canals
6. Restorative procedures

One-Appointment Root Canal Therapy

History

In recent years one-appointment endodontics has gained increased acceptance as the best treatment for most cases. Some endodontists even feel there are few cases that cannot be treated successfully in one appointment. Recent studies (see Tables 4-1 and 4-2) have shown little or no difference in the quality of treatment, incidence of posttreatment complications, or success rates between single-visit and multiple-visit root canal treatment. Not all studies agree,[37] however, about the efficacy of this technique for every case.

Completing endodontic treatment in a single visit is a concept that can be traced through the literature for at least 100 years. Dodge[11] described varying techniques that included root canal sterilization by hydrogen dioxide and sodium dioxide, hot platinum wire sterilization, potassium permanganate sterilization, or sulfuric acid irrigation. The canals were filled with chloropercha, formopercha, sectional gutta-percha, or zinc oxide and eugenol paste.

Single-visit endodontics enjoyed a resurgence during and after World War II; however, it was generally performed in conjunction with resection of the root apex immediately after the canals were filled. Trephination, or artificial fistulation, was also used in conjunction with single-visit endodontics to prevent or alleviate postoperative pain and swelling.[34] Many of these early reports involved opinions based on limited clinical observation and inadequate scientific studies. In 1959 Ferranti[18] reported that there was little difference in postoperative sequelae between single-visit and two-visit root canals. However, relatively few comprehensive studies of one-visit endodontics were published until the 1970s.

In more recent years studies have been published attempting to answer two basic questions: (1) Is endodontic therapy performed in a single visit any more or less painful postoperatively than when it is performed in multiple visits? (2) Is single-visit endodontic therapy more or less successful than endodontic therapy performed in multiple visits?

Postoperative pain and flare-ups

The reported incidence of postoperative pain after single- versus multiple-visit endodontic treatment varies considerably. However, most studies show that one-visit root canal procedures produce no more pain than multiple-visit cases do (Table 4-1).

In 1970 Fox et al[19] treated 291 teeth in single visits and reported severe pain within 24 hours in only 7% of those cases. He found that 90% of the teeth were free of spontaneous pain after 24 hours, whereas 82% had little or no pain on percussion. Wolch[54] in 1970 also reported on more than 5000 nonvital cases treated in one visit. He found severe pain in only 5% of these cases. In 1978 Soltanoff[45] found that 64% of the single-visit and 38% of the multiple-visit cases experienced postoperative pain, although his figures seem high compared with those of the many studies that followed (see Table 4-1). These all confirmed the earlier studies that suggest that one-visit procedures produce no more pain and *in some cases less pain* than multiple-visit root canals. Most studies showed that when pain occurred it was invariably the most intense during the first 24 to 48 hours and declined after the first week. In a recent series of studies Fava[14-17] found no difference in the incidence of postoperative pain between single-visit and multiple-visit endodontic therapy despite use of a variety of instrumentation and filling techniques and materials.

Recently the term *flare-up* has become popular in describing posttreatment symptoms, although there is little agreement at which point pain and swelling become a bona fide flare-up.[23] Morse et al.[31] define a flare-up as swelling and pain combined or swelling alone that necessitates unscheduled emergency appointments. Pain by itself is not considered a flare-up. Walton's definition of a flare-up is this:

> Within a few hours to a few days after a root canal treatment procedure a patient has either pain or swelling or a combination of both. The problem must be of sufficient severity that there is a disruption of the patient's lifestyle such that the patient initiates contact with the dentist. Required then are both: (a) an unscheduled visit and (b) active treatment (incision and drainage, canal debridement, opening for drainage, etc.).[53]

Morse and co-workers, in an exhaustive series of clinical studies covering a period of 24 years,[1,29-32] investigated factors that could reduce the incidence of flare-ups and non-flare-up–associated pain and swelling. They concluded that one-appointment endodontics combined with prophylactic administration of antibiotics (penicillin V or erythromycin) and intentional overinstrumentation of the root canal into the approximate center of the bony lesion reduced flare-ups from about 20% to 1.5%. Their strict definition of a flare-up, excluding many cases of non-flare-up–associated pain and swelling, may account for the unusually low incidence of flare-ups in these cases.

These findings are somewhat controversial because avoiding overinstrumentation has long been a standard of endodontic treatment, and the prophylactic use of antibiotics, other than for premedication for medical reasons, has long been frowned on because of its questionable value and the possibility of allergic reactions.[41] If Morse's work is correct, however, then these techniques should be considered for all one-appointment nonvital cases without sinus tracts. Moderate overinstrumentation past the apex in nonvital cases has long been taught to increase the likelihood of drainage and relief of pressure. How-

Table 4-1. One-visit endodontics—comparative studies on incidence of postoperative pain and flare-ups

| Investigator | Year | No. of Cases | Pulp Status | One-Visit Postoperative Pain (%) | | Multiple-Visit Postoperative Pain (%) | |
				None or Slight	Moderate to Severe	None or Slight	Moderate to Severe
Ferranti[18]	1959	340	N	91.0	9.0	96.2	3.8
Fox et al.[19]	1970	270	V-N	90.0	10.0	Not studied	
O'Keefe[35]	1976	55	V-N	98.0	2.0	91.0	7.0
Soltanoff[45]	1978	282	V-N	81.0	19.0	86.0	14.0
Ashkenaz[7]	1979	359	V	96.0	4.0	Not studied	
Rudner & Oliet[40]	1981	98	V-N	88.5	11.5	88.5	11.5
Mulhern et al.[33]	1982	30	N	76.5	23.5	73.3	26.7
Oliet[34]	1983	382	V-N	89.0	11.0	93.4	6.5
Roane et al.[38]	1983	359	V-N	85.0	15.0	68.8	31.2
Alacam[3]	1985	212	V	86.0	14.0	Not studied	
Mata et al.[29]*	1985	150	N	Not studied		98.0	2.0
Morse et al.[31]*	1986	200	N	98.5	1.5	Not studied	
Morse et al.[32]*	1987	106	N	93.4	6.6	Not studied	
Abbott et al.[1]*	1988	195	N	97.4	2.6	Not studied	
Fava[14-17]	1989	60	V	97.0	3.0	100.0	0.0
	1991	120	N	95.0	5.0	Not studied	
	1994	90	V	94.0	6.0	Not studied	
	1995	60	N	94.0	6.0	Not studied	
Trope[49,50]*	1990	474	V-N	—	—	97.4	2.6
	1991	226		98.2	1.8	—	
Walton & Fouad[53]*	1992	935	V-N	97.4	2.6	96.3	3.3
Abbott[2]	1994	100	V-N	95.0	5.0	Not studied	

V, Vital; *N,* nonvital.
*Used strict definition for flare-ups.

Table 4-2. One-visit endodontics—comparative success-failure studies

| Investigator | Year | Pulp Status | Total Cases | Recall Period | One-Visit (%) | | Multiple-Visit (%) | |
					Success	Failure	Success	Failure
Soltanoff[45]	1978	V-N	266	6 mo-2 yr	85	15	88	12
Ashkenaz[7]	1979	V	101	1 yr	97	3	Not studied	
			44	2 yr	97.7	1.3		
Rudner & Oliet[40]	1981	V-N	41	6-12 mo	90.2	9.8	85.7	14.3
			27	12-14 mo	88.8	11.2	90.0	10.0
			30	>24 mo	90	10.0	91.8	8.2
Oliet[34]	1983	V-N	153	Min 18 mo	88.8	11.2	88.6	11.4
Pekruhn[37]	1986	V-N	925	1 yr	94.8	5.2	Not studied	
Jurcak et al.[24]	1993	V-N	167	NA	89.0	11.0	Not studied	

V, Vital; *N,* nonvital; *NA,* not available.

ever, the literature is clear that overinstrumentation of vital cases is to be avoided because it crushes tissue and produces pain and inflammation.[41]

Trope[50] reported that the flare-up rate for one-appointment retreatment cases with apical periodontitis was unacceptably high and should be avoided. Walton[53] indicated that the over-riding factor as to predicting a flare-up was the presence of pain or other symptoms before treatment. If these symptoms exist, it would be reasonable to administer antibiotics in an attempt to control a possible flare-up. It also should be noted that single-visit endodontic treatment of posterior teeth seems to produce more postoperative discomfort.[38]

Success rates

The number of prognosis studies of one-appointment root canal treatment is less than the number of pain studies, but most studies indicate that there is no substantial difference in the success rate of one- and two-visit cases (Table 4-2). Despite Soltanoff's[45] report of considerably more pain in multiple-visit endodontic treatment, he found that both techniques provided success rates exceeding 85%. Ashkenaz[7] claimed that one-appointment root canals succeeded 97% of the time, but he did not evaluate multiple visits. Rudner and Oliet[40] compared one-visit with multiple-visit treatments and found that both healed with a frequency approximating 88%

to 90%. Southard[46] described total healing of all recalled cases when one-appointment endodontics was combined with incision and drainage and antibiotic therapy. Pekruhn,[36] in a study of 1140 single-visit cases, found a failure rate of only 5.2%. He noted that teeth not previously opened showed three times the number of failures as those that had been previously opened. This was especially true of teeth with periapical extension of pulpal disease. There was also a higher incidence of failure in teeth being retreated. Stamos et al[47] described two cases in which total healing occurred after one-visit treatments in which combined hand instrumentation and ultrasonic technique was used. Recently Jurcak et al.[24] performed one-visit endodontics on 167 patients who were rapidly deployed during the initial stages of Operation Desert Shield. This study is unique because the short time frame in which the treatments were performed did not allow for the screening for pretreatment symptoms. All cases were performed in one visit regardless of the presence of pain, swelling, sinus tracts, or radiographic lesions. All patients were prescribed an antibiotic and a nonsteroidal antiinflammatory agent. The results revealed a success rate of 89% despite the uncontrolled conditions of the study.

Survey results

The exact extent of the practice of one-appointment endodontics is not known. In 1980 Landers and Calhoun[25] questioned the directors of postgraduate endodontic programs concerning one-appointment endodontic therapy. Most of the directors saw little difference between one- and multiple-appointment endodontic therapy with respect to flare-ups, successful healing, and patient acceptance. One-visit endodontics was taught in 85.7% of the programs, and 91.4% of the directors, faculty, and residents treated some types of cases in one visit. Calhoun and Landers[8] polled 429 endodontists randomly in 1982 and found that 67% would treat vital case whereas only 12.8% would treat necrotic cases in one visit. The majority of endodontists thought that there would be more pain if treatment was completed on one appointment.

In a 1985 survey of 35 directors of endodontic programs by Trope and Grossman,[51] 54% indicated that they completed vital cases in one appointment. Only 9% said they would fill teeth with necrotic pulps in one visit. When a periapical lesion was present, 70% of the respondents preferred multiple treatments with an intracanal medicament.

Gatewood et al.,[21] in a 1990 survey of 568 diplomates, reported that 35% would complete cases in one visit for teeth with a normal periapex, whereas only 16% would do so if apical periodontitis were present. Fewer than 10% of the diplomates would complete a nonvital case in one visit despite the previously cited evidence that there is little difference in pain or healing between multiple- and single-visit root canals. Despite strong evidence to the contrary, there has existed within the endodontic community a resistance to one-appointment root canal treatment. However, anecdotal evidence seems to indicate that this resistance may be lessening. Recently educators have begun to strongly recommend one-visit endodontics for most cases in conjunction with use of the endodontic surgical operating microscope. Further surveys need to be undertaken to evaluate the extent of these changing attitudes.

Advantages and disadvantages

There are many advantages to one-visit endodontic therapy.[6,30,31,34,39]
1. It reduces the number of patient appointments while still maintaining predictably high levels of success and patient comfort.
2. It eliminates the chance for interappointment microbial contamination and flare-ups caused by leakage or loss of the temporary seal.
3. It allows for the immediate use of the canal space for retention of a post and construction of an aesthetic temporary crown, when required by restorative needs.
4. It is the most efficient way of performing endodontic treatment because it allows the practitioner to prepare and fill the canals at the same appointment without the need for refamiliarization with the canal anatomy at the next visit.
5. It minimizes fear and anxiety in the apprehensive patient. Few patients ever request to have the root canal treatment completed in several appointments!
6. It eliminates the problem of the patient who does not return to have the case completed.

There are a few disadvantages to one-appointment endodontic therapy[6,30]:
1. The longer appointment required may be tiring and uncomfortable for the patient. Some patients, especially those with temporomandibular dysfunction or other physical or mental conditions, may not be able to keep the mouth opened long enough for a one-appointment procedure.
2. Flare-ups cannot be easily treated by opening the tooth for drainage.
3. If hemorrhage or exudation occurs, it may be difficult to control it and still complete the case at the same visit.
4. Difficult cases with extremely fine, calcified, multiple canals may not be treatable in one appointment without causing undue stress to both the patient and the clinician.
5. The clinician may lack the expertise to properly treat a case in one visit. This could result in failures, flare-ups, and legal repercussions.

Guidelines for one-appointment endodontics

One-appointment endodontics should not be undertaken by inexperienced clinicians. The dentist must possess a full understanding of endodontic principles and the ability to exercise these principles fully and efficiently. There can be no shortcuts to success. The endodontic competence of the practicing dentist should be the overriding factor in undertaking one-visit treatment. *As a guideline, the case should be able to be completed in approximately 60 minutes.* Treatments taking considerably longer should be done in multiple visits.

Oliet's criteria[34] for case selection include (1) positive patient acceptance, (2) sufficient treatment time available to complete the procedure properly, (3) absence of acute symptoms requiring drainage through the canal and absence of persistent continuous flow of exudate or blood, and (4) absence of anatomic obstacles (calcified canals, fine tortuous canals, bifurcated or accessory canals), and procedural difficulties (ledge formation, blockage, perforations, inadequate fills).

Within the confines of the clinician's ability, one-appointment root canal therapy should be considered in the following circumstances:
1. Uncomplicated vital teeth
2. Fractured anterior or bicuspid teeth where aesthetics is a concern and a temporary post and crown are required
3. Patients who are physically unable to return for the completion

4. Medically impaired patients who require repeated regimens of prophylactic antibiotics
5. Necrotic uncomplicated teeth with draining sinus tracts
6. Patients requiring sedation or operating room treatment

One-appointment root canal therapy should be avoided in the following instances:

1. Most painful, necrotic teeth with no sinus tract for drainage
2. Teeth with severe anatomic anomalies or cases fraught with procedural difficulties
3. Most asymptomatic nonvital molars with periapical radiolucencies and no sinus tract
4. Patients who have acute apical periodontitis with severe pain to percussion
5. Most retreatments

Careful case selection and proper and thorough adherence to standard endodontic principles, with no short cuts, should result in successful one-appointment endodontics.

Premedication

The need for premedication may affect the treatment plan. Patients requiring the American Heart Association regimen of prophylactic antibiotics for protection of damaged or prosthetic heart valves must take the first dose 1 hour before the initiation of treatment (see Chapter 2). Administration of the proper antibiotics in the office may be necessary in the case of an emergency or when the patient has forgotten medication.

Some orthopedists may request premedication for patients who have undergone prosthetic surgery, such as a hip replacement. [5a,26,52]

Patients undergoing corticosteroid replacement therapy may need to adjust their dosage before each endodontic appointment. Also, patients receiving anticoagulant therapy require close attention to blood test results and may require adjustments in anticoagulant dosage. These and other medical conditions may require consultation with the patient's physician before initiation of treatment. It also may be advisable to perform one-appointment endodontics on such patients to avoid the need for repeated premedication.

Retreatment Versus Periradicular Surgery

Retreatment is required when previous endodontic therapy is failing. The retreatment should not be attempted until the cause of the patient's symptoms is ascertained. Often a patient is certain that the symptoms are originating in a previously treated tooth, when, instead, an adjacent or nearby tooth is the source. Complaints of hot or cold sensitivity in an existing root canal should be followed up with the appropriate tests. Occasionally a tooth remains sensitive to thermal change after endodontic therapy because all the canals were not initially located and treated.

If the failure is obviously caused by poor or incomplete debridement or obturation of all the canals, conventional retreatment should be instituted (see Fig. 4-7). Although the success rate of retreatments is high, it may be lower than that for initial endodontic therapy.[44] Removal of failing silver points can be easy if the points are small and can be easily grasped. However, large, well-fitted silver points may be difficult to remove, and the treatment plan may require additional appointments in these cases. Old gutta-percha can be easily removed with Hedstrom files and rectified turpentine as a solvent.

When molars are retreated, it is essential to look for additional canals. Despite poor obturation of the major canals, the cause of such failures is often a missed fourth or fifth canal, which must be located, debrided, and obturated to achieve success. The use of the surgical operating microscope greatly facilitates successful resolution of such cases.

Nonsurgical retreatment is always preferable and should be attempted before resorting to surgery. The presence of a crown is not in itself an indication for choosing surgery over nonsurgical treatment. In certain cases treatment may be impossible because of obstructions, calcifications, and prosthetic considerations. The presence of a post is not always an impediment to retreatment. Often the post can be removed with ultrasonics and the surgical operating microscope to allow retreatment of all canals (See Chapter 24.) If only one canal was not previously treated, the access opening can be made beside the post to locate and treat only the failing canal.

When material that can be harmful to the periradicular tissues, such as nitrogen, is extruded past the apex, it is necessary to immediately enter the area surgically to remove the material (Fig. 4-12). However, if an inert material, such as gutta-percha or a tip of a file, is expelled past the apex, it is not necessary to remove it surgically provided that the canal system is adequately debrided and sealed.

Surgery should be planned only when the practitioner is certain that the failing case was initially treated properly and cannot be improved on, when retreatment is impossible for prosthetic or other reasons, or when the lesion is large and biopsy is prudent. In planning surgeries, the first visit is generally for examination, consultation, and informed consent. Most surgeries are not done as emergencies; they must be carefully scheduled to allow enough time. Often the profound anesthesia required for periradicular surgery cannot be obtained in the presence of severe inflammation and infection. Acute symptoms should be alleviated by incision and drainage or trephination before periradicular surgery is performed. The surgery can be performed once the patient is comfortable. Many surgical cases are asymptomatic or have a draining sinus tract and can be scheduled at a time convenient to everyone.

Coordination With Other Dental Specialists

In some instances cases must be evaluated by other dentists or specialists before endodontic treatment is instituted. The first concern is the restorability of the tooth. Root canal therapy should not be initiated until it is certain that the tooth is restorable. Severe furcation caries or caries below the bony crest may contraindicate endodontic therapy (see Fig. 4-10, *A*) or may necessitate root extrusion. Inadequate root structure may not allow for placement of a post after endodontic therapy. It is imperative that coordination with all dentists treating the case be done before definitive endodontic therapy is initiated.

Second, the integrity of the attachment apparatus must be ascertained before endodontic therapy is undertaken (Fig. 4-13), and a periodontist or endodontist should be consulted when the status is in question. A *periodontal explorer should always be included on the examination tray and should be used on all cases.* Although endodontic therapy is usually done before periodontal therapy, it is nonetheless essential to be sure that the tooth is periodontally sound. Occasionally a combination of root canal therapy and resection of periodontally diseased roots is necessary. This should be determined as part of the original treatment plan after necessary consultations.

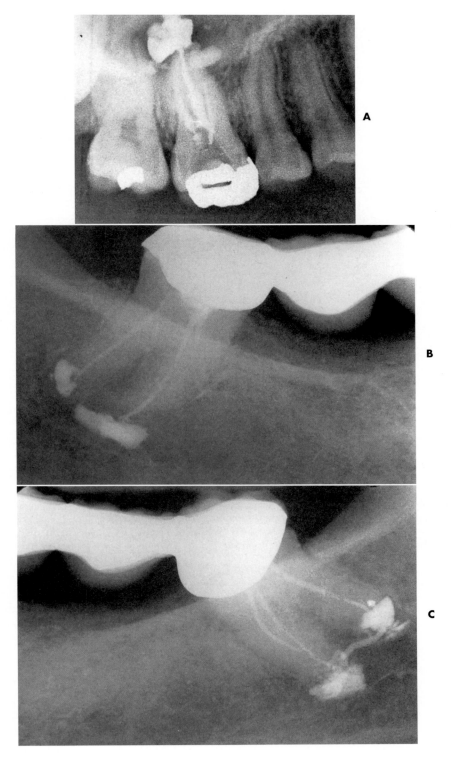

FIG. 4-12 A, Immediate surgery is required to remove extruded paraformaldehyde-ZOE paste from the sinus. **B** and **C,** Extruded paraformaldehyde-ZOE paste from both distal abutments in proximity to the mandibular canal caused bilateral paresthesia. *(Courtesy Dr. Ed Ruiz-Hubard.)*

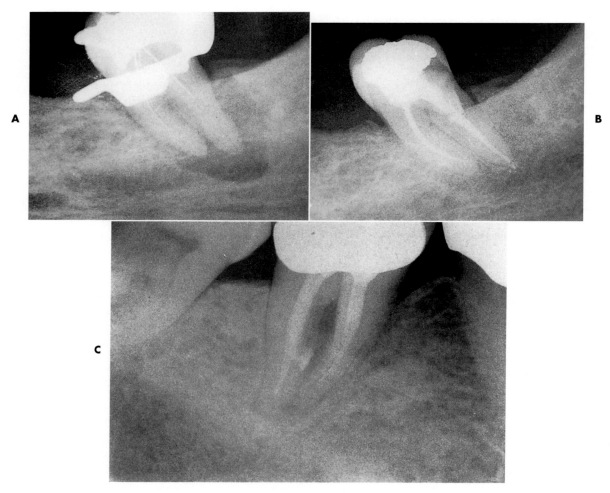

FIG. 4-13 Often lesions that appear to be of periodontal origin are primarily endodontic. **A** and **B,** Successful resolution of an apparent periodontal lesion in a 79-year-old woman with a significant history of cardiovascular disease and diabetes. **C,** Furcation involvement often heals after proper endodontic treatment.

Pain that is difficult to diagnose may be of nonendodontic origin. When careful examination does not reveal the cause of symptoms, referral is in order. *Endodontic treatment must never be instituted unless the cause of the distress is known with certainty.* It is always wise to refer patients to other specialists rather than to guess and risk making an improper diagnosis. In cases of difficult diagnosis, referral to an endodontist is recommended.[22] When pain of nondental origin is suspected, referral to a neurologist, an otolaryngologist, or an orofacial pain clinic is also recommended

REFERENCES

1. Abbott AA et al: A prospective randomized trial on efficacy of antibiotic prophylaxis in asymptomatic teeth with pulpal necrosis and associated periapical pathosis, *Oral Surg* 66:722, 1988.
2. Abbott PV: Factors associated with continuing pain in endodontics, *Australian Dent J* 39:157, 1994.
3. Alacam T: Incidence of postoperative pain following the use of different sealer in immediate root canal filling, *J Endod* 11:135, 1985.
4. American Association of Endodontists: *Public knowledge and opinion about endodontics,* Opinion Research Corp, Princeton NJ, 1987, The Association.
5. American Association of Endodontists: *Market value of tooth,* Princeton NJ, 1989, Opinion Research Corp.
5a. American Dental Association, American Academy of Orthopaedic Surgeons: Antibiotic prophylaxis for dental patients with total joint replacements, *J Am Dent Assoc* 128:1004, 1997.
6. Ashkenaz PJ: One-visit endodontics, *Dent Clin North Am* 28:853, 1984.
7. Ashkenaz PJ: One-visit endodontics: a preliminary report, *Dent Surv* 55:62, 1979.
8. Calhoun RL, Landers RR: One-appointment endodontic therapy: a nationwide survey of endodontists, *J Endod* 8:35, 1982.
9. Council on Dental Therapeutics and American Heart Association: Preventing bacterial endocarditis: a statement for the dental professional, *J Am Med Assoc* 277:1794, 1997.
10. Dietz GC, Dietz GC: The endodontist and the general dentist, *Dent Clin North Am* 36:459, 1992.
11. Dodge JS: Immediate root-filling in the late 1800's, *J Endod* 4:165, 1978.
12. Dorn SO et al: Treatment of the endodontic emergency: a report based on a questionnaire, Part I, *J Endod* 3:94, 1977.
13. Dorn SO et al: Treatment of the endodontic emergency: a report based on a questionnaire, Part II, *J Endod* 3:153, 1977.
14. Fava LRG: A comparison of one versus two appointment endodontic therapy in teeth with non-vital pulps, *Int Endod J* 22:179, 1989.

15. Fava LRG: One-appointment root canal treatment: incidence of post-operative pain using a modified double flared technique, *Int Endod J* 24:258, 1991.

16. Fava LRG: A clinical evaluation of one and two-appointment root canal therapy using calcium hydroxide, *Int Endod J* 27:47, 1994.

17. Fava LRG: Single visit root canal treatment: incidence of post-operative pain using three different instrumentation techniques, *Int Endod J* 28:103, 1995.

18. Ferranti P: Treatment of the root canal of an infected tooth in one appointment: a report of 340 cases, *Dent Dig* 65:490, 1959.

19. Fox J et al: Incidence of pain following one visit endodontic treatment, *Oral Surg* 30:123, 1970.

20. Gartner AH, Mack T, Somerlott RG, Walsh LC: Differential diagnosis of internal and external root resorption, *J Endod* 2:329, 1976.

21. Gatewood RS, Himel VT, Dorn SO: Treatment of the endodontic emergency: a decade later, *J Endod* 16:284, 1990.

22. Goerig AC, Neaverth EJ: Case selection and treatment planning. In Cohen S, Burns RC, editors: *Pathways of the pulp*, ed 5, St Louis, 1991, Mosby.

23. Goldman M et al: Immunological implications and clinical management of the endodontic flare-up, *Compend Contin Educ Dent* 10:126, 1987.

24. Jurcak JJ et al: Successful single-visit endodontics during Operation Desert Shield, *J Endod* 19:412, 1993.

25. Landers RR, Calhoun RL: One-appointment endodontic therapy: an opinion survey, *J Endod* 6:799, 1980.

26. Little JW: Antibiotic prophylaxis for prevention of bacterial endocarditis and infectious major joint prostheses, *Curr Opin Dent* 2:93, 1992.

27. Little JW, Falace DA, Miller CS, Rhodus NL: *Dental management of the medically compromised patient*, ed 5, St Louis, 1997, Mosby.

28. Malamed SF: *Handbook of medical emergencies in the dental office*, ed 4, St Louis, 1993, Mosby.

29. Mata et al: Prophylactic use of penicillin V in teeth with necrotic pulps and asymptomatic periapical radiolucencies, *Oral Surg* 60:201, 1985.

30. Morse DR: One-visit endodontics, *Hawaii Dent J* 12:14, Dec 1987.

31. Morse DR et al: Clinical study: infectious flare-ups: induction and prevention, Parts 1-5, *Int J Psychosom* 33:5, 1986.

32. Morse DR et al: A prospective randomized trial comparing periapical instrumentation to intracanal instrumentation in cases of asymptomatic pulpal-periapical lesions, *Oral Surg* 64:734, 1987.

33. Mulhern JM et al: Incidence of postoperative pain after one-appointment endodontic treatment of asymptomatic pulpal necrosis in single rooted teeth, *J Endod* 8:370, 1982.

34. Oliet S: Single visit endodontics: a clinical study, *J Endod* 9:147, 1983.

35. O'Keefe EM: Pain in endodontic therapy: preliminary study, *J Endod* 2:315, 1975.

36. Pekruhn RB: Single-visit endodontic therapy: a preliminary clinical study, *J Am Dent Assoc* 103:875, 1981.

37. Pekruhn RB: The incidence of failure following single visit endodontic therapy, *J Endod* 12:68, 1986.

38. Roane JB, Dryden JA, Grimes EW: Incidence of post-operative pain after single- and multiple-visit endodontic procedures, *Oral Surg* 55:68, 1983.

39. Rosenberg RJ, Goodis HE: Endodontic case selection: to treat or to refer, *J Am Dent Assoc* 123:57, 1992.

40. Rudner W, Oliet S: Single-visit endodontic: a concept and clinical study, *Compend Contin Educ* 2:63, 1981.

41. Seltzer S: Endodontology: biologic consideration in endodontic procedures, ed 2, Philadelphia, 1988, Lea & Febiger.

42. Seltzer S, Naidorf IJ: Flare-ups in endodontics. II. Therapeutic measures, *J Endod* 11:559, 1985.

43. Simmons NA et al: Case against antibiotic prophylaxis for dental treatment of patients with joint prostheses, *Lancet* 339:301, 1992.

44. Sjogren U et al: Factors affecting the long-term results of endodontic treatment, *J Endod* 16:498, 1990.

45. Soltanoff W: A comparative study of single-visit and multiple visit endodontic procedures, *J Endod* 9:278, 1978.

46. Southard DW: Effective one-visit therapy for the acute periapical abscess, *J Endod* 10:580, 1984.

47. Stamos DE et al: The use of ultrasonics in single-visit endodontic therapy, *J Endod* 13:246, 1987.

48. Torabinejad M et al: Factors associated with endodontic interappointment emergencies of teeth with necrotic pulps, *J Endod* 14:261, 1988.

49. Trope M: Relationship of intracanal medicaments to endodontic flare-ups, *Endod Dent Traumatol* 6:226, 1990.

50. Trope M: Flare-up rate of single visit endodontics, *Int Endod J* 24:24, 1991.

51. Trope M, Grossman LI: Root canal culturing survey: Single-visit endodontics, *J Endod* 11:511, 1985.

52. Wahl MJ: Myths of dental-induced endocarditis, *Arch Int Med* 154:137, 1994.

53. Walton R, Fouad A: Endodontic interappointment flare-ups: a prospective study of incidence and related factors, *J Endod* 18:172, 1992.

54. Wolch I: One appointment endodontic treatment, *J Can Dent Assoc* 41:24, 1970.

55. Wood NK: Treatment planning: a pragmatic approach, St Louis, 1978, Mosby.

Chapter 5

Preparation for Treatment

Gerald Neal Glickman

Before initiation of nonsurgical root canal treatment, a number of treatment, clinician, and patient needs must be addressed. These include proper infection control and occupational safety procedures for the entire health care team and treatment environment; appropriate communication with the patient, including case presentation and informed consent; premedication, if necessary, followed by effective administration of local anesthesia; a quality radiographic survey; and thorough isolation of the treatment site.

PREPARATION OF THE OPERATORY

Infection Control

Because all dental personnel risk exposure to a host of infectious organisms that may cause a number of infections, including influenza, upper respiratory disease, tuberculosis, herpes, hepatitis (B, C, D, and G), or acquired immunodeficiency syndrome (AIDS), it is essential that effective infection control procedures be used to minimize the risk of cross-contamination in the work environment.[17,18,42,54] These infection control programs must not only protect patients and the dental team from contracting infections during dental procedures but also must reduce the number of microorganisms in the immediate dental environment to the lowest level possible.

As the AIDS epidemic continues to expand, it has been established that the potential for occupational transmission of human immunodeficiency virus (HIV) and other fluid-borne pathogens can be minimized by enforcing infection control policies specifically designed to reduce exposure to blood and other infected body fluids.[8-10,42,54] Since HIV has been shown to be fragile and easily destroyed by heat or chemical disinfectants, the highly resistant nature of the hepatitis B virus, along with its high blood titers, makes it a good model for infection control practices to prevent transmission of a large number of other pathogens via blood or saliva. Because all infected patients are not readily identifiable through the routine medical history and many are asymptomatic, the American Dental Association (ADA) recommends that each patient be considered potentially infectious; this means that the same strict infection control policies or "universal precautions" apply to all patients.[18,54] In addition, the Occupational Safety and Health Administration (OSHA) of the U.S. Department of Labor, in conjunction with both the ADA and Centers for Disease Control and Prevention (CDC), has issued detailed guidelines on hazard and safety control in the dental setting.[2,8-10,35,54] In 1992 laws specifically regulating exposure to blood-borne disease became effective through OSHA's "Occupational Exposure to Bloodborne Pathogens, Final Rule."[20] Primarily designed to protect any employee who could be "reasonably anticipated" to have con-

tact with blood or any other potentially infectious materials, the standard encompasses a combination of engineering and work practice controls, personal protective clothing and equipment, training, signs and labels, and hepatitis B vaccination and authorizes OSHA to conduct inspections and impose financial penalties for failure to comply with specific regulations.[20]

In 1993 the ADA, CDC, and OSHA recommended or mandated that infection control guidelines include the following measures*:

I. The ADA and CDC recommend that all dentists and their staff members who have patient contact be vaccinated against hepatitis B. The OSHA standard requires that employers make the hepatitis B vaccine available to occupationally exposed employees, at the employer's expense, within 10 working days of assignment to tasks that may result in exposure. A declination form, using specific language requested by OSHA, must be signed by an employee who refuses the vaccine. In addition, postexposure follow-up and evaluation must be made available to all employees who have had an exposure incident.

II. A thorough patient medical history, which includes specific questions about hepatitis, AIDS, current illnesses, unintentional weight loss, lymphadenopathy, oral soft tissue lesions, and so on, must be taken and updated at subsequent appointments.

III. Dental personnel must wear protective attire and use proper barrier techniques. The standard requires the employer to ensure that employees use personal protective equipment and that such protection is provided at no cost to the employee.

  A. Disposable latex or vinyl gloves must be worn when contact with body fluids or mucous membranes is anticipated or when touching potentially contaminated surfaces; the gloves may not be washed for reuse. OSHA requires that gloves be replaced after each patient contact and when torn or punctured. Sturdy unlined utility gloves for cleaning instruments and surfaces may be decontaminated for reuse if their integrity is not compromised. Polyethylene gloves may be worn over treatment gloves to prevent contamination of objects such as drawers, light handles, or charts.

  B. Hands, wrists, and lower forearms must be washed with soap at the beginning of the day, before and after gloving, at the end of the day, and after removal

---

*References 2, 3, 8-10, 17, 18, 20, 35, 42, 54.

of any personal protective equipment or clothing; for surgical procedures, an antimicrobial surgical hand scrub should be used. The standard requires that any body area that has contact with any potentially infectious materials (including saliva) must be washed immediately after contact. Sinks should have electronic or elbow-, foot-, or knee-action faucet controls for asepsis and ease of function. Employers must provide washing facilities (including an eyewash) that are readily accessible to employees.

C. Masks and protective eyewear with solid side shields or chin-length face shields are required when splashes or sprays of potentially infectious materials are anticipated and during all instrument and environmental cleanup activities. When a face mask is removed, it should be handled by the elastic or cloth strings, not by the mask itself. It is further suggested that protective eyewear be worn by the patient.

D. Protective clothing, either reusable or disposable, must be worn when clothing or skin is likely to be exposed to body fluids and should be changed when visibly soiled or penetrated by fluids. OSHA's requirements for protective clothing (i.e., gowns, aprons, laboratory coats, clinic jackets) are difficult to interpret, since the "type and characteristics [thereof] will depend upon the task and degree of exposure anticipated." The ADA and CDC recommend long-sleeved uniforms; but according to OSHA, long sleeves are required only if significant splashing of blood or body fluids to the arms or forearms is expected. Thus endodontic surgery would likely warrant long-sleeved garments. OSHA requires that the protective garments not be worn outside the work area. The standard prohibits employees from taking home contaminated laundry to be washed; it must be washed at the office or by an outside laundry service. Contaminated laundry must be placed in an impervious laundry bag that is colored red or labeled BIO-HAZARD. Although OSHA does not regulate nonprotective clothing such as scrubs, such clothing should be handled like protective clothing once fluids have penetrated it.

E. Patients' clothing should be protected from splatter and caustic materials, such as sodium hypochlorite, with waist-length plastic coverings overlaid with disposable patient bibs.

F. High-volume evacuation greatly reduces the number of bacteria in dental aerosols and should be employed when using the high-speed handpiece, water spray, or ultrasonics.

G. Use of the rubber dam as a protective barrier is mandatory for nonsurgical root canal treatment, and failure to use such is considered to be below standard care.[12,13,23]

IV. OSHA regulates only contaminated sharps. Contaminated *disposable* sharps such as syringes, needles, and scalpel blades and contaminated *reusable* sharps such as endodontic files must be placed into separate, leakproof, closable, puncture-resistant containers, which must be colored red or labeled BIOHAZARD and marked with the biohazard symbol. The standard states that before decontamination (i.e., sterilization) contaminated reusable sharps must not be stored or processed in such a manner that employees are required to reach by hand into the containers to retrieve the instruments. The OSHA ruling allows picking up sharp instruments by hand only after they are decontaminated.[17,35,42]

A. A suggested format for handling contaminated endodontic files is this: With tweezers, place used files in glass beaker containing a nonphenolic disinfectant–detergent holding solution; at the end of the day, discard the solution and rinse with tap water; add ultrasonic cleaning solution; place the beaker in an ultrasonic bath for 5 to 15 minutes (use time adequate for thorough cleaning); discard ultrasonic solution and rinse with tap water; pour contents of the beaker onto a clean towel; use tweezers to place clean files into the metal box for sterilization. Files with any visible debris should be separately sterilized; once sterilized, these files can be picked up by hand and debrided using 2×2 sponges; once cleaned, files are returned to the metal box for sterilization.

B. The standard generally prohibits bending or recapping of anesthesia needles; however, during endodontic treatment, reinjection of the same patient is often necessary, so recapping is essential. Recapping with a one-handed method or using a mechanical device is the only permissible technique. Shearing or breaking of contaminated needles should never be permitted.

V. Countertops and operatory surfaces such as light handles, x-ray unit heads, chair switches, and any other surface likely to become contaminated with potentially infectious materials can be either covered or disinfected. Protective coverings such as clear plastic wrap, special plastic sleeves, or aluminum foil can be used and should be changed between patients and when contaminated. OSHA mandates, however, that work surfaces must be decontaminated or recovered at the end of each work shift and immediately after overt contamination. The coverings should be removed by gloved personnel, discarded, and then replaced with clean coverings after gloves are removed. Alternatively, countertops and operatory surfaces can be wiped with absorbent toweling to remove extraneous organic material and then sprayed with an Environmental Protection Agency (EPA)-registered and ADA-accepted tuberculocidal disinfectant such as a 1:10 dilution of sodium hypochlorite, an iodophor, or a synthetic phenol. With the advent of endodontic microscopy, appropriate barriers should be placed on the handles and controls of the microscope or the entire unit can be draped to prevent cross-contamination. Disinfection should be performed according to the microscope manufacturer's recommended guidelines if the system becomes contaminated.

VI. Contaminated radiographic film packets must be handled in a manner to prevent cross-contamination. Contamination of the film when it is removed from the packet and subsequent contamination of the processing equipment can be prevented either by properly handling the film as it is removed from the contaminated packet or by preventing the contamination of the packet during use.[26] After exposure, "overgloves" should be placed over contaminated gloves to prevent cross-contamination of processing equipment or darkroom surfaces.[34] For darkroom procedures, films should be carefully manipulated out of their holders and dropped onto a disinfected surface or into a clean cup without touching them. Once the film has been removed, the gloves are removed and discarded and the film can be processed. All contaminated film envelopes must be accumulated, after film removal, in a strategically positioned impervious bag and disposed of properly. For daylight loaders, exposed film packets are placed into a paper cup; gloves are discarded and hands are washed; a new pair of gloves is donned; the paper cup with the films and an empty cup are placed into the chamber; the chamber is entered with gloved hands; packets are carefully opened, allowing the film to drop onto a clean surface in the chamber; empty film packets are placed into the empty cup; gloves are removed and also discarded in the cup; the films can then be processed.[35] Plastic envelopes such as the ClinAsept Barriers (Eastman Kodak, Rochester, N.Y.) have simplified the handling of contaminated, exposed films by protecting films from contact with saliva and blood during exposure. Once a film is exposed, the barrier envelope is easily opened and the film can be dropped into a paper cup or onto a clean area before processing. The barrier-protected film, however, should be wiped with an EPA-approved disinfectant as an added precaution against contamination during opening.[26]

VII. In conjunction with the above guidelines for infection control, it has been advocated that before treatment patients rinse with a 0.12% chlorhexidine gluconate mouth rinse such as Peridex (Procter & Gamble, Cincinnati, Ohio) to minimize the number of microbes in the mouth and consequently in any splatter or aerosols generated during treatment.[17,42,54]

VIII. Following treatment, all instruments and burs must be cleaned and sterilized by sterilizers monitored with biological indicators. Cassettes, packs, or trays should be rewrapped in original wrap, and individually packaged instruments should be placed in a covered container. Air or water syringes must be flushed, cleaned, and sterilized. Antiretraction valves (one-way flow check valves) should be installed to prevent fluid aspiration and to reduce the risk of transfer of potentially infective material. Heavy-duty rubber gloves must be worn during cleanup. The ADA and CDC recommend that all dental handpieces and "prophy" angles be heat sterilized between patients.[2,17,35,42] Before sterilization, all handpieces should be wiped with an EPA-registered disinfectant and high-speed handpieces should be run to discharge water and air for a minimum of 30 seconds, with spray directed into a high-volume evacuation system. Dental unit water lines should be periodically flushed with water or a 1 : 10 dilution of 5.25% sodium hypochlorite (NaOCl) to reduce biofilm formation. All regulated infectious waste must be immediately disposed of in containers that meet specific criteria. Disposal must be in accordance with applicable federal, state, and local regulations.

In 1987 the infection control decision-making process was transferred to the U.S. Government through OSHA.[54] The ongoing goal of OSHA is to establish a routine and practical program of enforcing infection control standards based on published CDC guidelines to ensure the health and safety of all members of the dental health team. According to OSHA,[35,42,54] dentists must classify personnel and tasks in the dental practice according to levels of risk of exposure and must establish "standard operating procedures" to protect the patient and staff from infection transmission. OSHA requires the dentist to provide infection control training for all employees and maintain records of such training; properly label all hazardous substances that employees are exposed to on the job; and have a written hazard communications program with manufacturers' Material Safety Data Sheets (MSDS) for all hazardous substances. With the enactment of OSHA's bloodborne pathogens standard in 1991, employers must make exposure determinations and develop an exposure control plan. As mentioned above, the rule encompasses a number of critical areas: universal precautions, engineering and work practice controls, employee training, specific record keeping, and many others, all ultimately designed to protect employees from exposure to blood-borne pathogens, particularly the HIV and the hepatitis B virus. Although the OSHA standard was written principally to protect employees, it does not encompass all the infection control practices recommended by the ADA and CDC to protect dentists and patients. In 1994 the CDC issued its position on the prevention of transmission of tuberculosis in dental settings by allowing for the deferral of elective dental treatment until the patient is confirmed to not have tuberculosis and further stating that emergency care for a patient with tuberculosis should only be provided in facilities with appropriate respirators, negative pressure treatment areas, and other respiratory engineering controls.[11] Compliance with OSHA regulations and with evolving infection control policies of the ADA and CDC will help provide a safer workplace for the entire dental treatment team.[17,35,42,54]

PATIENT PREPARATION

Treatment Planning

Aside from emergency situations that require immediate attention, endodontic treatment usually occurs early in the total treatment plan for the patient so that any asymptomatic but irreversible pulpal and periradicular problems are managed before they become symptomatic and more difficult to handle. The most important rationale for the high priority of endodontics is to ensure that a sound, healthy foundation exists before any further treatment is attempted. A stable root system within sound periradicular and periodontal tissues is paramount to the placement of any definitive restorations.

Regardless of the specifics of the case, it is the responsibility of the clinician to explain effectively the nature of the treatment and inform the patient of any risks, prognosis, and other pertinent facts. As a result of bad publicity some believe root canal treatment to be a horrifying experience. Consequently, some patients may be reluctant, anxious, or fearful of undergoing root canal treatment. Thus it is imperative that the dentist educate the patient before treatment (i.e., informing before performing)[13] to allay concerns and minimize misconceptions about it.

Good dentist-patient relationships are built on effective communication. There is sufficient evidence to suggest that dentists who establish warm, caring relationships with their patients through effective case presentation are perceived more favorably and have a more positive impact on the patient's anxiety, knowledge, and compliance than those who maintain impersonal, noncommunicative relationships.[16] Most patients

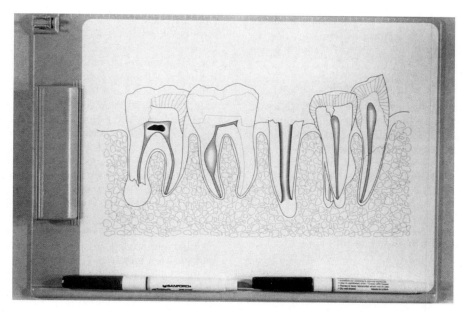

FIG. 5-1 The Endoboard is a handy erasable board for educating patients needing endodontic therapy. *(Courtesy Kilgore International, Coldwater, Mich.)*

also experience an increase in anxiety while in the dental chair; a simple but informative case presentation that leaves no questions unanswered not only reduces patient anxiety but also solidifies the patient's trust in the dentist.

Case Presentation

The ADA and the American Association of Endodontists (AAE) publish brochures such as *Endodontics: Your Guide To Endodontic Treatment*[1] to help patients understand root canal treatment. Valuable educational aids of this nature should be available to the patient, either before or immediately after the case presentation. This supportive information addresses the most frequently asked questions concerning endodontic treatment. These questions are reviewed. Accompanying each question is an example of an explanation that patients should be able to understand. In addition, the dentist will find it useful to have a set of illustrations or drawings to help explain the procedure. An excellent case presentation aid is the Endoboard (Fig. 5-1), a plastic-coated erasable drawing board, allowing for visualization of various types of endodontic problems and treatment options.

What is endodontic (root canal) treatment?

Endodontics is the specialty in dentistry that is concerned with the prevention, diagnosis, and treatment of diseases or injuries to the dental pulp. The pulp, which some people call "the nerve," is the soft tissue inside the tooth that contains the nerves and blood vessels and is responsible for tooth development. Root canal treatment is a safe and effective means of saving teeth that otherwise would be lost.

What causes the pulp to die or become diseased?

When a pulp is injured, diseased, and unable to repair itself, it becomes inflamed and eventually dies. The most frequent causes of pulp death are extensive decay, deep fillings, trauma such as a severe blow to a tooth, cracks in teeth, and periodontal or gum disease. When a pulp is exposed to bacteria from decay or saliva that has leaked into the pulp system, infection can occur inside the tooth and, if left untreated, can cause infection to build up at the tip of the root, forming an abscess. Eventually the bone supporting the tooth will be destroyed, and pain and swelling will often accompany the infection. Without endodontic treatment, the tooth will eventually have to be removed.

What are the symptoms of a diseased pulp?

Symptoms may range from momentary to prolonged, mild to severe pain on exposure to hot or cold or on chewing or biting; or the condition may produce no symptoms at all.

The patient should be informed that the radiographic examination may or may not demonstrate abnormal conditions of the tooth and that sometimes there is radiographic evidence of pulpal or periradicular disease in the absence of pain.

What is the success rate of root canal treatment?

Endodontics is one of the few procedures in dentistry that has a predictable prognosis if treatment is performed properly. Studies indicate that root canal treatment is usually 90% to 95% successful. Those in the failure group may still be amenable to retreatment or surgical treatment to save the tooth, although no treatment's success can be guaranteed. In addition, patients must understand that the prognosis may vary depending on the specifics of each case and that, without good oral hygiene and a sound restoration following endodontics, there may be an increased chance for failure. The need for periodic follow-up must be addressed to assess the long-term status of the tooth and periradicular tissues.

Will the endodontically treated tooth discolor following treatment?

If the treatment is done correctly, discoloration seldom occurs. Bleaching with heat or chemicals can be used to treat discolored teeth. Some endodontically treated teeth appear discolored because they have been restored with tooth-colored fillings that have become stained or with amalgam restorations that leach silver ions. In these instances the fillings may be replaced, but often the placement of crowns ("caps") or veneers is indicated.

What are the alternatives to root canal treatment?

The only alternative to root canal treatment is to extract the tooth, which often leads to shifting and crowding of surrounding teeth and subsequent loss of chewing efficiency. The patient should understand that often extraction is the easy way out and, depending on the case, may prove to be more costly for the patient in the long run. Part of patient autonomy includes the right to do nothing about the problem, provided the associated risks of this decision have been explained by the dentist.

Will the tooth need a crown or cap following the treatment?

If there is no previously existing crown, the necessity of a crown or cap depends on the amount of remaining sound tooth structure following endodontic treatment, the type of tooth, and the amount of chewing force to which the tooth will be subjected. Loss of tooth structure significantly weakens the tooth and renders it more susceptible to fracture; as a result, it may be necessary to protect what is left with a restoration such as a crown. Significant loss of tooth structure with a concomitant loss of retentive areas for coronal buildups may necessitate the placement of a metallic post in a canal to retain the buildup material (Fig. 5-2, *I* and *J*). For further information on these issues, the reader is referred to Chapter 21.

What does root canal treatment involve?

Treatment generally requires only one appointment, but more appointments may be necessary depending on the diagnosis, the number of roots, and the complexity of the case. During this appointment the clinician removes the injured or diseased pulp tissue. The root canals are cleaned, enlarged, and sealed to prevent recontamination of the root canal system. The following steps (Fig. 5-2) describe the technical aspects of the treatment (illustrations, diagrams, and radiographs should be used as aids to the presentation):

1. Local anesthesia is usually administered.
2. The tooth is isolated with a rubber dam to prevent contamination from saliva and to protect the patient. This procedure is followed at each subsequent visit.
3. An opening is made through the top of the tooth to gain entrance to the root canal system.
4. The pulp tissue is painlessly removed with special instruments called *files.*
5. Periodic images or radiographs must be taken to ensure that these instruments correspond to the exact length of the root so that the entire tissue can be removed.
6. The root canal is cleaned, enlarged, and shaped so that it can be filled or sealed properly.
7. Sometimes medications and a temporary filling are placed in the opening to prevent infection if an additional appointment is necessary.
8. Finally, the canal is sealed to safeguard it from further contamination.
9. A final restoration should be placed within 30 days after completion of the root canal treatment.

Some additional points should be conveyed to the patient after treatment. The patient should not be given the impression that there will be no pain following the treatment.[52] In most cases, whatever mild discomfort the patient experiences is transitory and can usually be treated with an over-the-counter antiinflammatory or analgesic agent such as aspirin or an ibuprofen-containing compound. In fact, prophylactic administration of these drugs before the patient leaves the office helps reduce postoperative discomfort by achieving therapeutic blood levels of analgesic before the local anesthetic wears off[30] (see Chapter 19). In certain cases, simply handing the patient a written prescription for a stronger analgesic, "just in case," conveys a feeling of empathy and caring toward the patient and strengthens the doctor-patient relationship.

If the dentist wishes to refer the patient to an endodontist for treatment, skillful words of encouragement and explanation convey the caring and concern behind this recommendation. Many patients already feel comfortable with their dentists and thus are fearful of "seeing someone new." In addition, they may not understand why a general dentist chooses not to do the root canal treatment. The referring dentist can only help his or her cause by carefully explaining the complex nature of the case and why it would be in the patient's best interests to visit the endodontist, who is specially trained to handle complex cases.[52]

Informed Consent

With today's continuous rise in dental litigation, a good rule to follow is to realize that "no amount of documentation is too much and no amount of detail is too little."[45] For further information on this subject, the reader is referred to Chapter 10.

Radiation Safety

A critical portion of the endodontic case presentation and informed consent is educating the patient about the requirement for radiographs as part of the treatment. The dentist must communicate to the patient that the benefits of radiographs in endodontics far outweigh the risks of receiving the small doses of ionizing radiation, as long as techniques and necessary precautions are properly executed.[25] Although levels of radiation in endodontic radiography range from only 1/100 to 1/1000 of the levels needed to sustain injury,[41,50] it is still best to keep ionizing radiation to a minimum, for the protection of both the patient and dental delivery team. Two simple analogies can be used to help the patient conceptualize the minimal risk levels with dental radiographs. A patient would have to receive 25 complete full-mouth series (450 exposures) within a very short time frame to significantly increase the risk of skin cancer.[41] One full-mouth survey (i.e., 20 E-speed films with rectangular collimation) has been found to deliver one third the amount of radiation of a single chest film and less than 1% the amount of a barium study of the intestines.[26] Nevertheless, the principles of ALARA (**a**s **l**ow **a**s **r**easonably **a**chievable), which are essentially ways to reduce radiation exposure, should be followed as closely as possible to minimize the amount of radiation that both patient and treatment team receive. ALARA also implies the possibility that no matter how small the radiation dose, there still may be some deleterious effects.[26,41]

Principles of ALARA

In endodontic radiography, one should select fast (sensitive)-speed film, either D (Ultraspeed) or E (Ektaspeed).[40] Although E-speed film allows for a reduction of approximately 50% of the radiation exposure required for D-speed film,[21] findings in observer preference studies have been mixed with regards to

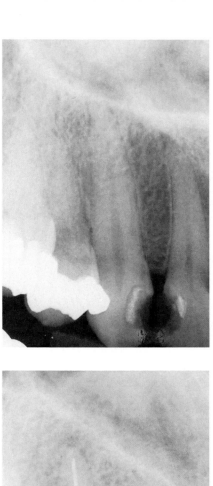

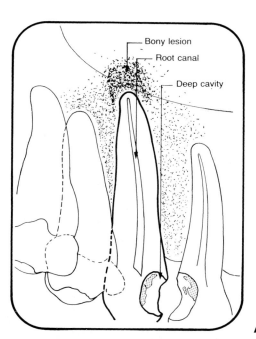

Bony lesion
Root canal
Deep cavity

A, B

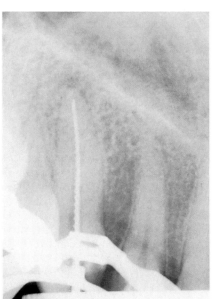

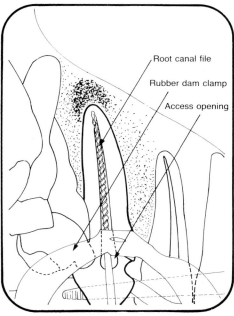

Root canal file
Rubber dam clamp
Access opening

FIG. 5-2 Series of radiographs and illustrations demonstrating root canal treatment and restoration of a maxillary canine. **A** and **B,** Maxillary canine with periradicular lesion of endodontic origin. **C** and **D,** Endodontic file corresponding to length of canal; isolation with rubber dam throughout procedure. **E** and **F,** Endodontic filling material placed after cleaning and shaping of canal.

Continued

C, D

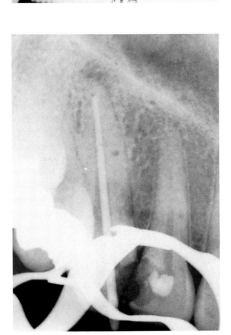

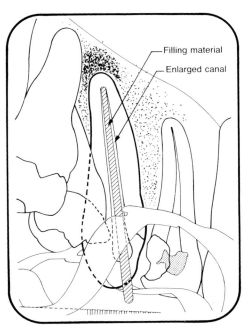

Filling material
Enlarged canal

E, F

G, H

I, J

FIG. 5-2, cont'd **G** and **H,** Canal system filled and post space made. **I** and **J,** One-year follow-up shows completed restoration and healed periradicular bone.

the quality, clarity, and diagnostic capability of E-speed film compared to D. Processing of the E-speed film is also more sensitive.[21,22,33] Specialized radiographic systems[26,44] such as Computed Dental Radiography and radiovisiography involve the digitization of ionizing radiation and use considerably smaller amounts of radiation to produce an image that is available immediately after exposure (see Digitization of Ionizing Radiation later in this chapter).

Meticulous radiographic technique helps reduce the number of retakes and obviates further exposure. Film-holding devices, discussed later in the chapter, along with correct film and tube head positioning, are essential for maintaining film stability and producing radiographs of diagnostic quality.[26,41] A quality assurance program for film processing should also be set up to ensure that films are properly processed.[26,41]

Dental units should be operated using at least 70 kVp. The lower the kilovoltage, the higher the patient's skin dose. Optimally, 90 kVp should be used. Units operating at 70 kVp or higher must have a filtration equivalent of 2.5 mm of aluminum to remove the extraneous low-energy x-rays before they are absorbed by the patient.[26,41]

Collimation also reduces exposure level. Collimation, essentially, is the restriction of the x-ray beam size by means of a lead diaphragm so that the beam does not exceed 2.75 inches (7 cm) at the patient's skin surface. Open-ended, circular or rectangular lead-lined cylinders, known as position-indicating devices (PIDs), help direct the beam to the target (Fig. 5-3); however, the rectangular cylinder additionally collimates the x-ray beam by decreasing beam size even more, subsequently reducing the area of skin surface exposed to x-radiation (Fig.

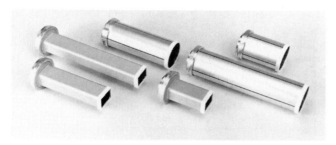

FIG. 5-3 Rectangular and round, collimating, lead-lined position-indicating devices (PIDs). The rectangular PID reduces as much as half the tissue area exposed to radiation. *(Courtesy Rinn Corp., Elgin, Ill.)*

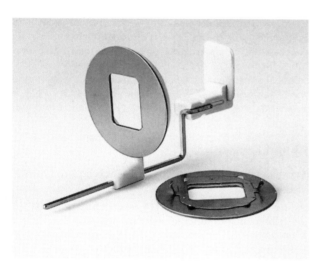

FIG. 5-4 Ring collimator snaps on aiming ring to extend the extra protection of a rectangular collimator to round, open-ended cones. *(Courtesy Rinn Corp., Elgin, Ill.)*

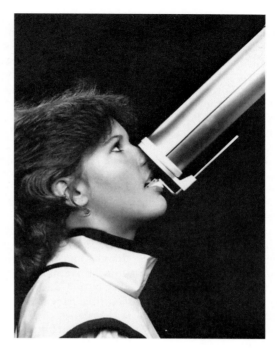

FIG. 5-5 Film-holding and aiming device (XCP instrument) with PID on a patient protected with a lead apron and thyroid collar. *(Courtesy Rinn Corp., Elgin, Ill.)*

5-4). These PIDs or cones should be at least 12 to 16 inches long because the shorter (8-inch) cones, which provide shorter source-to-film distances, cause more divergence of the beam and more exposure to the patient.[26,41] Pointed cones, illegal in some states, should not be used because of the increased amount of scatter radiation they produce.

The patient should be protected with a lead apron and a thyroid collar for each exposure (Fig. 5-5). When exposing films, the clinician should stand behind a barrier. Plaster, cinderblock, and at least 2.5 inches of drywall provide the necessary protection from the radiation produced by dental units. If there is no barrier, the clinician should stand in an area of minimal scatter radiation: at least 6 feet away from the patient and in an area that lies between 90 degrees and 135 degrees to the beam.[26,41] Film badges for recording occupational exposure should be worn by all dental personnel who might be exposed to occupational x-radiation. If the concept of ALARA is strictly adhered to, no member of the dental team should receive doses close to their MPD, or maximum permissible dose (i.e., 0.02 Sv or 2 rem per year per whole body).[26] For "declared" pregnant workers, the Nuclear Regulatory Commission limits the radiation dose to the fetus to 0.005 Sv during the gestation period. It is important to note that the MPD is specified as occupational exposure and thus should not be confused with expo-

sure that patients receive as a result of radiographic procedures. Although there are no state recommended maximum patient exposures, it is the responsibility of anyone who administers ionizing radiation to consult the respective state's bureau of radiation control to obtain information on current laws. Nonetheless, every effort should be made to keep the radiation dose to all individuals as low as practicable and to avoid any unnecessary radiation exposure.

Premedication with Antibiotics

Prophylactic coverage with antibiotics or antiinfectives is indicated for patients who are susceptible to systemic disease following bacteremia. Although it has been documented that the incidence of bacteremia associated with nonsurgical root canal treatment is essentially negligible as long as endodontic instruments are confined to the root system,[5,6] the American Heart Association (AHA) recommends prophylactic antibiotic coverage for patients who have prostheses, shunts, or certain diseases to prevent any blood-borne microorganisms from lodging on shunts and prostheses or from multiplying within a depressed system and potentially causing infection and a life-threatening situation.[19,36,43,46]

With respect to premedication for dental patients with total joint replacements, there has been considerable controversy as to whether such patients require routine prophylaxis. Recently, the ADA and AAOS (American Academy of Orthopedic Surgeons) published an advisory statement on antimicrobial premedication for dental patients with total joint replacements.* The joint organizations recognized that there was no agreed upon scientific evidence to support the contention that antibi-

---

*Advisory statement: antibiotic prophylaxis for dental patients with total joint replacements, *J Am Dent Assoc* 128:1004, 1997.

otic prophylaxis is necessary to prevent hematogenous infection in patients with total joint prostheses. The risk/benefit and cost/effectiveness ratios fail to justify the administration of routine antibiotic prophylaxis. They agreed that the analogy between late prosthetic joint infections with infective endocarditis was invalid because the anatomy, blood supply, types of microorganisms involved, and mechanisms of infection are all different. Both the ADA and AAOS concluded that antibiotic prophylaxis is not indicated for dental patients with pins, plates, and screws, nor is it routinely indicated for most dental patients with total joint replacements. However, since there is limited evidence that some dental procedures are high-risk procedures (e.g., extractions, periodontal probing, intraligamentary local anesthesia, endodontic surgery, replantation of avulsed teeth, endodontic filing beyond the apical foramen and that some medically compromised patients with total joint replacements (e.g., insulin-dependent diabetes, inflammatory arthropathies such as rheumatoid arthritis, immunosuppression, hemophilia, history of infections in the arthroplasty, first 2 years following joint placement) may be at higher risk for hematogenous infections, an antibiotic regimen may be employed. The antibiotic regimen is cephalexin, cephradine, or amoxicillin, 2 g PO, 1 hour before procedure; for those allergic to penicillin, the recommended antibiotic is clindamycin, 600 mg PO, 1 hour before procedure; for patients not allergic to penicillin but unable to take oral medications, the recommended antibiotic is cefazolin 1 g or ampicillin 2 g IM or IV, 1 hour before procedure; and for patients allergic to penicillin and unable to take oral medications, the recommended antibiotic is clindamycin, 600 mg IV, 1 hour before procedure. Similar to the new AHA guidelines (see below) for prevention of bacterial endocarditis, follow-up doses are not recommended. The advisory statement only represents recommended guidelines and is not intended as a standard of care, since it is impossible to make recommendations for all clinical situations in which late infection might occur in total joint prostheses. Practitioners must exercise their own clinical judgment in determining whether to premedicate.

Patients with certain cardiac conditions are candidates for antibiotic coverage in order to prevent subacute bacterial endocarditis (SBE.).[46] In 1997, the AHA revised its recommendations for the prevention of bacterial endocarditis that may be the result of an invasive procedure.[19] The major modifications include the recognition and emphasis that most cases of endocarditis are not the result of an invasive procedure, that predisposing cardiac conditions are stratified into high, moderate, and negligible risk categories based upon the potential outcome if endocarditis were to develop, and modification of the drugs and dosages necessary for prophylaxis.

Based upon the new guidelines, prophylaxis is recommended for individuals in high-risk and moderate-risk categories. Individuals at highest risk are those who have prosthetic heart valves, previous history of endocarditis, complex cyanotic congenital heart disease, and surgically constructed systemic pulmonary shunts. Those conditions in the moderate-risk category include most other congenital cardiac malformations, rheumatic heart disease, hypertrophic cardiomyopathy, and mitral valve prolapse with valvular regurgitation and/or thickened leaflets. Conditions that are in a negligible-risk category (no greater risk than the general population) and for which prophylaxis is not recommended include previous coronary artery bypass graft surgery, mitral valve prolapse without valvular regurgitation, previous rheumatic fever without valvular dys-

function, and cardiac pacemakers (both intravascular and epicardial).

The AHA has developed a standard prophylactic antibiotic regimen for patients at risk and a set of alternative regimens for those unable to take oral medications, for those who are allergic to the standard antibiotics, and for those who are not candidates for the standard regimen.[19] The recommended standard prophylactic regimen for all dental, oral, and upper respiratory tract procedures is currently amoxicillin because it is better absorbed by the gastrointestinal tract and provides higher and more sustained serum levels than does penicillin. The major modification in the new regimen is that the postoperative dose has been eliminated; the rationale for this is that amoxicillin has a sufficiently high plasma level for an adequate period of time to prevent endocarditis. Erythromycin has also been eliminated as a recommended drug in the penicillin-allergic patient because of the high incidence of gastrointestinal upset and the variability of the pharmacokinetics of the various erythromycin preparations. The official AHA recommendations for prophylactic antibiotic regimens do not specify all clinical situations for which patients may be at risk; thus, it is the responsibility of the clinician to exercise his or her own judgment or consult with the patinet's physician before giving treatment.

The current AHA guidelines for prophylactic antibiotic coverage are as follows[19]:

Standard regimen for patients at high and moderate risk

Adults. Amoxicillin, 2 g PO, 1 hour before procedure. For amoxicillin/penicillin-allergic patients, clindamycin 600 mg PO, or cephalexin or cefadroxil 2 g PO, or azithromycin or clarithromycin 500 mg PO, 1 hour before procedure.

Children. Amoxicillin, 50 mg/kg PO 1 hour before procedure. For amoxicillin/penicillin-allergic patients, clindamycin, 20 mg/kg PO 1 hour before procedure; or cephalexin or cefadroxil, 50 mg/kg PO 1 hour before procedure; or azithromycin or clarithromycin, 15 mg/kg PO 1 hour before procedure.

Alternative regimens for patients at high and moderate risk

Patients unable to take oral medications

Adults. Ampicillin, 2 g IV or IM, within 30 minutes before procedure.

Children. Ampicillin, 50 mg/kg IV or IM, within 30 minutes before procedure.

Ampicillin/amoxicillin/penicillin-allergic patients unable to take oral medications

Adults. Clindamycin, 600 mg IV, within 30 minutes before procedure, or cefazolin, 1 g IV or IM, within 30 minutes before procedure.

Children. Clindamycin, 20 mg/kg IV, within 30 minutes before procedure, or cefazolin, 25 mg/kg IV or IM, within 30 minutes before procedure.

Chlorhexidine mouth rinses before treatment are recommended for all patients requiring prophylactic antibiotic coverage.

Antianxiety Regimens

Because patients very often have been misinformed about root canal treatment, it is understandable that some may experience an increased anxiety. Fortunately, however, the vast majority of patients are able to tolerate their anxiety, control their behavior, and allow treatment to proceed with few problems. Appropriate behavioral approaches can be used to manage most anxious dental patients. Retrospective studies[16] concerning dental anxiety have clearly demonstrated that patients' anxiety states can be effectively reduced by explaining procedures before starting, giving specific information during treatment, warning about the possibility of mild discomfort that can be controlled, verbal support and reassurance, and showing personal warmth. Many of these measures can be taken during the case presentation.

Although the clinician's hope and desire may not cure a patient's fear of root canal treatment, each clinician should realize that anxious patients are not all alike and each patient should be managed individually. If behavioral solutions are not feasible or effective in a particular case, pharmacologic approaches to managing the patient may be exercised. Selection of such pharmacotherapeutic techniques must involve a careful assessment of the relative risks and benefits of the alternative approaches. All pharmacologic treatment regimens include the need for good local anesthetic technique, and range from nitrous oxide plus oxygen sedation, oral sedation, or intravenous or conscious sedation for the management of mild to moderate anxiety states. For further information on these issues, the reader is referred to Chapter 19.

Pain Control with Preoperative Administration of NSAIDs

The reader is referred to Chapter 17 for a complete discussion about this issue.

PREPARATION OF RADIOGRAPHS

Radiographs are essential to all phases of endodontic therapy. They inform the diagnosis and the various treatment phases and help evaluate the success or failure of treatment. Because root canal treatment relies on accurate radiographs, it is necessary to master radiographic techniques to achieve films of maximum diagnostic quality. Such mastery minimizes retaking of films and avoids additional exposure of patients. Expertise in radiographic interpretation is essential for recognizing deviations from the norm and for understanding the limitations associated with endodontic radiography.

Functions, Requirements, and Limitations of the Radiograph in Endodontics

The primary radiograph used in endodontics is the periapical radiograph. In diagnosis this film is used to identify abnormal conditions in the pulp and periradicular tissues and to determine the number of roots and canals, location of canals, and root curvatures. Because the radiograph is a two-dimensional image, which is a major limitation, it is often advantageous to take additional radiographs at different horizontal or vertical angulations when treating multicanaled or multirooted teeth and those with severe root curvature. These supplemental radiographs enhance visualization and evaluation of the three-dimensional structure of the tooth.

Technically, for endodontic purposes a radiograph should depict the tooth in the center of film. Consistent film placement in this manner will minimize errors in interpretation, as this is the area of the film where distortion is least. In addition, at least 3 mm of bone must be visible beyond the apex of the tooth. Failure to capture this bony area may result in misdiagnosis, improper interpretation of the apical extent of a root, or incorrect determination of file lengths for canal cleaning and shaping. Finally, the image on the film must be as anatomically correct as possible. Image shape distortion caused by elongation or foreshortening may lead to interpretative errors during diagnosis and treatment.[24,26]

The bite-wing radiograph may be useful as a supplemental film. This film normally has less image distortion because of its parallel placement, and it provides critical information on the anatomic crown of the tooth. This includes the anatomic extent of the pulp chamber, the existence of pulp stones or calcifications, recurrent decay, the depth of existing restorations, and any evidence of previous pulp therapy.[25,52] The bite-wing also indicates the relationship of remaining tooth structure relative to the crestal height of bone and thus can aid in determining the restorability of the tooth.

In addition to their diagnostic value, high-quality radiographs are mandatory during the treatment phase. Technique is even more critical, however, since working radiographs must be taken while the rubber dam system is in place. Visibility is reduced and the bows of the clamp often restrict precise film positioning. During treatment periradicular radiographs are used to determine canal working lengths; the location of superimposed objects, canals, and anatomic landmarks (by altering cone angulations); biomechanical instrumentation; and master cone adaptation (Fig. 5-2, C to F). Following completion of the root canal procedure, a radiograph is taken to determine the quality of the root canal filling or obturation. Recall radiographs taken at similar angulations enhance assessment of the success or failure of treatment (Fig. 5-2, I and J).

The astute clinician can perceive that precise radiographic interpretation is undoubtedly one of the most valuable sources of information for endodontic diagnosis and treatment, but the radiograph is only an adjunctive tool and can be misinterpreted. Information gleaned from proper inspection of the radiograph is not always absolute and must always be integrated with information gathered from a thorough medical and dental history, clinical examination, and various pulp-testing procedures as described in Chapter 1.

Use of the radiograph depends on an understanding of its limitations *and* its advantages. The advantages are obvious: the radiograph allows a privileged look inside the jaw. The information it furnishes is essential and cannot be obtained from any other source, yet its value is not diminished by a critical appraisal of its limitations.

One of the major limitations of radiographs is their inability to detect bone destruction or pathosis when it is limited to the cancellous bone. Studies[48] have proven that radiolucencies usually do not appear unless there is external or internal erosion of the cortical plate (Fig. 5-6). This factor must be considered in evaluating teeth that become symptomatic but show no radiographic changes. In most cases root structure anatomically approaches cortical bone, and if the plate is especially thin, radiolucent lesions may be visible before there is significant destruction of the cortical plate. Nevertheless, inflammation and resorption affecting the cortical plates must still be sufficiently extensive before a lesion is present radiographically.

Principles of Endodontic Radiography

Film placement and cone angulation

For endodontic purposes the paralleling technique produces the most accurate periradicular radiograph. Also known as the *long cone* or *right-angle technique*, it produces improved im-

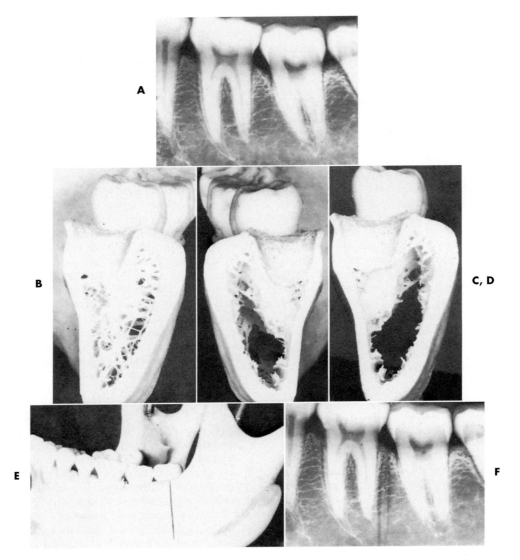

FIG. 5-6 A, Radiograph before any bone removal. **B,** Buccolingual section demonstrating cortical and cancellous bone. **C,** Removal of cancellous bone *without* infringement on the junctional trabeculae or cortical bone. **D,** Block section removed, demonstrating extent of destruction. **E,** Block section rearticulated to mandible with acrylic splint. **F,** Radiograph after removal of cancellous bone. Note there is no radiographic evidence of periradicular bone destruction. *(Courtesy Dr. Stephen F. Schwartz.)*

ages; the film is placed parallel to the long axis of the teeth, and the central beam is directed at right angles to the film and aligned through the root apex (Fig. 5-7, *A* and *B*). To achieve this parallel orientation it is often necessary to position the film away from the tooth, toward the middle of the oral cavity, especially when the rubber dam clamp is in position.[26] The long cone (16 to 20 inches) aiming device is used in the paralleling technique to increase the focal spot-to-object distance. This has the effect of directing only the most central and parallel rays of the beam to the film and teeth, thus reducing size distortion.[26,40,41] This technique permits more accurate reproduction of the tooth's dimensions, thus enhancing a determination of the tooth's length and relationship to surrounding anatomic structures.[24] In addition, the paralleling technique reduces the possibility of superimposing the zygomatic processes over the apexes of maxillary molars, which often occurs with more an-

gulated films, such as those produced by means of the bisecting-angle technique (Fig. 5-7, *C* and *D*). Thus if properly used, the paralleling technique provides the clinician with films with the least distortion, minimal superimposition, and utmost clarity.

Variations in size and shape of the oral structures (e.g., a shallow palatal vault, tori, and extremely long roots) or a patient's gagging often render absolutely true parallel placement of the film highly unlikely. To compensate for difficult placement, the film can be positioned so that it diverges as much as 20 degrees from the long axis of the tooth, with minimal longitudinal distortion. With maxillary molars, any increase in vertical angulation increases the chances of superimposing the zygomatic process over the buccal roots. A vertical angle of not more than 15 degrees should usually project the zygomatic process superiorly and away from the molar roots. To help achieve

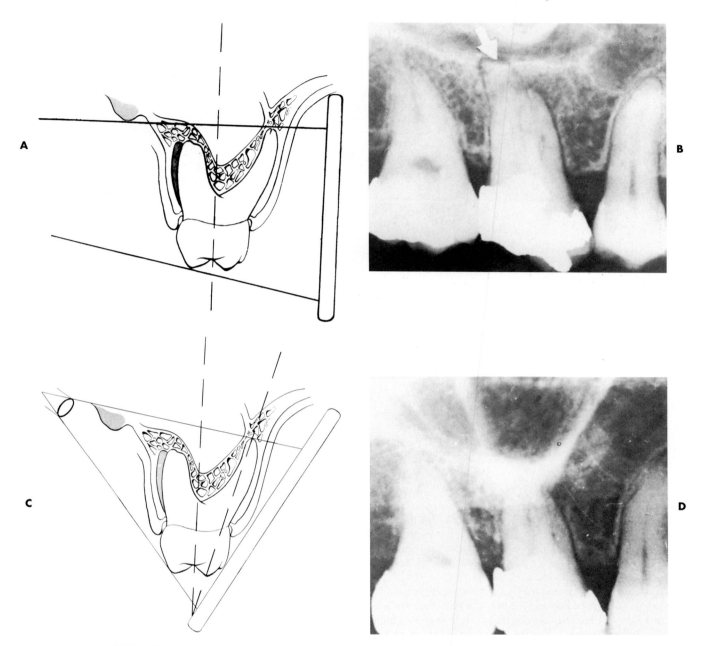

FIG. 5-7 A, Paralleling or right-angle technique. **B,** Projection of the zygomatic process above the root apexes with the right-angle technique allowing visualization of the periradicular pathosis *(arrow)*. **C,** Bisecting-angle technique. **D,** Superimposition of the zygomatic process over the root apexes of the maxillary first molar with the bisecting-angle technique.

this, a modified paralleling technique[15] that increases vertical angulation by 10 to 20 degrees can be used. Though this orientation introduces a small degree of foreshortening, it increases periradicular definition in this troublesome maxillary posterior region. The Dunvale Snapex system (Dunvale Corp., Gilberts, Ill.), a film holder and aiming device originally designed for the bisecting-angle technique, has been altered for the modified paralleling technique.[15] In conjunction with this technique, a distal angulated radiograph (i.e., a 10- to 20-degree horizontal shift of the cone from the distal [beam is directed toward the mesial]) tends to project buccal roots and the zygomatic process to the mesial, thus enhancing anatomic clarity.[15]

The bisecting-angle technique is not recommended for endodontic radiography; however, when a modified paralleling technique cannot be used, there may be no choice because of difficult anatomic configurations or patient management problems.[15,26,40,41] The basis of this technique is to place the film directly against the teeth without deforming the film (Fig. 5-7, *C* and *D*). The structure of the teeth, however, is such that with the film in this position there is an obvious angle between the plane of the film and the long axis of the teeth. This causes distortion because the tooth is not parallel to the film. If the x-ray beam is directed at a right angle to the film, the image on the film is shorter than its actual tooth, or foreshortened; if

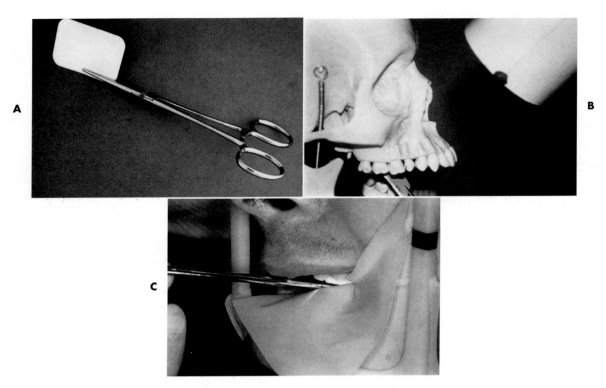

FIG. 5-8 A, Hemostat aids in film placement and in cone alignment. **B,** With the paralleling technique, the tube head is positioned at a 90-degree angle to the film. Note the hemostat is resting on the mandibular anterior teeth so that the film is parallel with the long axis of the maxillary central incisors. *(Courtesy Dr. Eddy Tidwell.)* **C,** Releasing a corner of the rubber dam aids in hemostat placement so that the film can be properly aligned. *(Courtesy Dr. Michelle Speier.)*

the beam is directed perpendicularly to the long axis of the teeth, the image is much longer than the tooth, or elongated. Thus by directing the central beam perpendicular to an imaginary line that bisects the angle between tooth and film, the length of the tooth's image on the film should be the same as the actual length of the tooth.

Even though the projected length of the tooth is correct, the image shows distortion because the film and object are not parallel and the x-ray beam is not directed at right angles to both. This distortion increases along the image toward its apical extent. The technique produces additional error potential, as the clinician must imagine the line bisecting the angle, an angle that in itself is difficult to assess. Beside producing more frequent superimposition of the zygomatic arch over apexes of maxillary molars, the bisecting-angle technique causes greater image distortion than the paralleling technique and makes it difficult for the operator to reproduce radiographs at similar angulations to assess healing following root canal treatment[26] (Fig. 5-7, *C* and *D*).

Film holders and aiming devices

Film holders and aiming devices are required for the paralleling technique because they reduce geometric distortion caused by misorientation of the film, central beam, and tooth.* They also minimize cone cutting, improve diagnostic quality,

and allow for similarly angulated radiographs to be taken during treatment and at recall. By eliminating the patient's finger from the x-ray field and thus the potential for displacing the film, these devices help minimize retakes and make it easier for the patient and clinician to properly position the film.

A number of commercial devices are available that position the film parallel and at various distances from the teeth, but one of the most versatile film-holding devices is the hemostat (Fig. 5-8, *A*). A hemostat-held film is positioned by the operator, and the handle is used to align the cone vertically and horizontally. The patient then holds the hemostat in the same position, and the cone is positioned at a 90-degree angle to the film (Fig. 5-8, *B*). When taking working radiographs, a radiolucent plastic rubber dam frame, such as an Ostby or Young frame, should be used and not removed. To position the hemostat or other film-holding device, a corner of the rubber dam is released for visibility and to allow the subsequent placement of the device-held film (Fig. 5-8, *C*). Another film-holding device, ideal for taking preoperative and postoperative films, is the Greene Stabe disposable film holder (Rinn Corp., Elgin, Ill.) (Fig. 5-9).

Beside the Dunvale Snapex system that was mentioned earlier, the major commercial film-holding and aiming devices include the extension cone paralleling (XCP) instruments, the EndoRay endodontic film holder, the Uni-Bite film holder, the EZ-Grip film holder, the EZ-Grip IIe film holder with aiming device, and the Crawford film holder system (Figs. 5-10 to 5-13). Variations in the use of the XCP system, for example, can prevent displacement of the rubber dam clamp and increase

---

*References 15, 25, 26, 40, 41, 52.

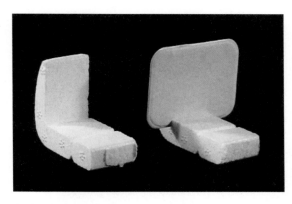

FIG. 5-9 The Greene Stabe disposable film holder.

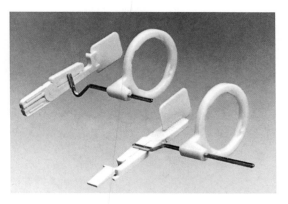

FIG. 5-12 EZ-Grip IIe film holder and aiming ring. The biting portion of the instrument is reduced to make it easier to place the instrument around the rubber dam. *(Courtesy Rinn Corp., Elgin, Ill.)*

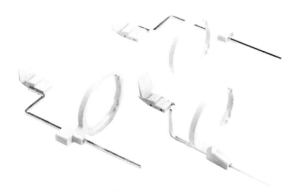

FIG. 5-10 Extension cone paralleling (XCP) instruments hold the x-ray film packets and aid in cone alignment. Cone cutting is prevented, and consistent angulation can be achieved. *(Courtesy Rinn Corp., Elgin, Ill.)*

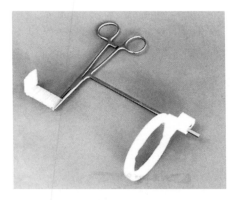

FIG. 5-13 Crawford film holder system. Components include Kelly hemostat with aiming rod attached, aiming ring, and bite block. *(Courtesy Dr. Frank Crawford, Palm Desert, Calif.)*

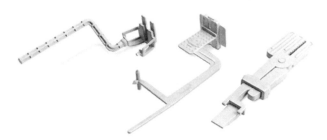

FIG. 5-11 Film-holding devices *(from left):* EndoRay, Uni-Bite, and EZ-Grip. *(Courtesy Rinn Corp., Elgin, Ill.)*

periradicular coverage during endodontic procedures. The film is placed off center in the bite block, and the cone is similarly placed off center with respect to the aiming ring. This allows for placement of the bite block adjacent to the rubber dam clamp without altering the parallel relation of the cone to the film (Fig. 5-14). A customized hemostat with rubber bite block attached can also be made to assist film placement during the taking of working radiographs. Other specialized film holders such as the EndoRay and the Crawford film holder system have been designed to help the dentist to secure parallel working

films with the rubber dam clamp in place. These holders generally have in common an x-ray beam–guiding device, for proper beam-film relationship, and a modified bite block and film holder, for proper positioning over or around the rubber dam clamp (Figs. 5-15 and 5-16).

Exposure and film qualities

The intricacies of proper kilovoltage, milliamperage, and time selection serve as examples of how the diagnostic quality of a film may be altered by changes in the film's density and contrast.[26,41] Density is the degree of darkening of the film, whereas contrast is the difference between densities. The amount of darkening depends on the quantity and quality of radiation delivered to the film, the subject thickness, and the developing or processing conditions. Milliamperage controls the electron flow from cathode to anode; the greater the electron flow per unit of time, the greater is the quantity of radiation produced. Proper density is primarily a function of milliamperage and time. Kilovoltage also affects film density by controlling the quality and penetrability of the rays. Higher kilovoltage settings produce shorter wavelengths that are more penetrating than the longer wavelengths produced at lower settings.[26,41] The ability to control the penetrability of the rays

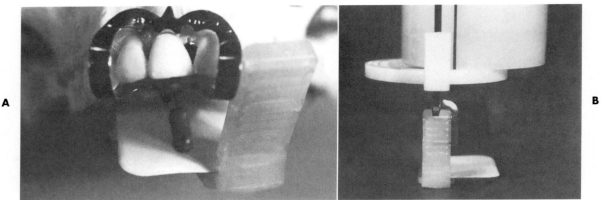

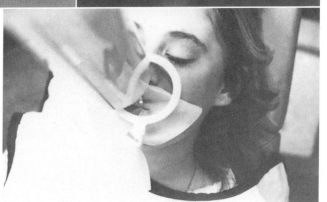

FIG. 5-14 A, Placement of a bite block on the tooth adjacent to the rubber dam clamp. **B,** Placement of the film off center in the bite block. **C,** Alignment of the x-ray cone. *(Courtesy Dr. Stephen F. Schwartz.)*

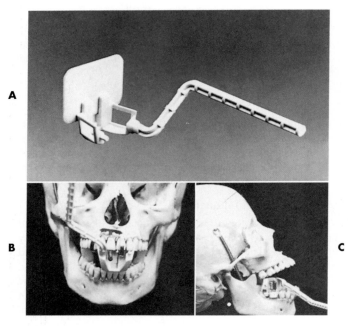

FIG. 5-15 A, EndoRay (posterior) film holder has a positioning arm to guide the cone to the center of the film. *(Courtesy Rinn Corp., Elgin, Ill.)* **B** and **C,** Anterior and posterior EndoRay film holders in place over the rubber dam clamp. Handle aids in determining cone position and angulation.

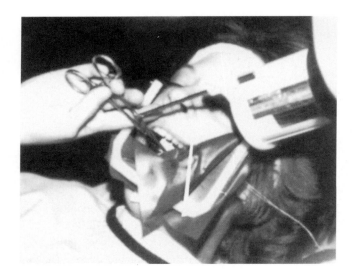

FIG. 5-16 Patient maintains position of film by holding handle of the hemostat of the Crawford film holder system. Note the bite block is not used when rubber dam is in place.

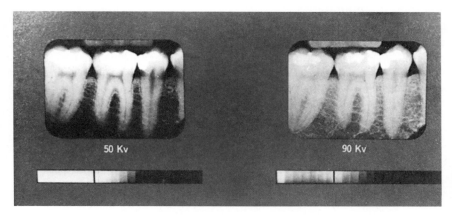

FIG. 5-17 Comparison of short-scale and long-scale contrast produced by altering the kilo-voltage. Note the increased shades of gray in the film produced at 90 kVp. *(Courtesy Rinn Corp., Elgin, Ill.)*

by alterations in kilovoltage affects the amount of radiation reaching the film and the degree of darkening or density. Variations in density can be controlled by altering exposure time or milliamperage for each respective unit.[26,41]

Contrast is defined as the difference between shades of gray or the difference between densities. Most of the variation observed in endodontic radiography is due to subject contrast, which depends on the thickness and density of the subject and the kilovoltage used. Thus kilovoltage is really the only exposure parameter under the clinician's control that directly affects subject contrast.[25,26,41] Exposure time and milliamperage control the number of x-ray beams only and therefore have most of their impact on the density of the film image. A radiographic film may exhibit a long scale of contrast (low contrast) (i.e., more shades of gray or more useful densities); high-kilovoltage techniques (90 kVp) produce this long scale of contrast as a result of the increased penetrating power of the rays. This results in images with many more shades of gray and less distinct differences (Fig. 5-17). Films exposed at low-kilovoltage settings (60 kVp) exhibit short-scale contrast (high contrast) with sharp differences between a few shades of gray, black, and white.[25,26,41] Although perhaps more difficult to read, films exposed at higher kilovoltage settings (90 kVp) make possible a greater degree of discrimination between images, often enhancing their diagnostic quality; films exposed at a lower kilovoltage (70 kVp) have better clarity and contrast between radiopaque and radiolucent structures, such as endodontic instruments near the root apex. Nevertheless, the optimal kilovoltage and exposure time should be individualized for each x-ray unit and exposure requirement.

Processing

Proper darkroom organization, film handling, and adherence to the time-temperature method of film processing play important roles in producing films of high quality.[41] For the sake of expediency in the production of working films in endodontics, rapid-processing methods are used to produce relatively good films in less than 1 to 2 minutes (Fig. 5-18).[25,26,41] Although the contrast in using rapid-processing chemicals is lower than that achieved by means of conventional techniques, the radiographs have sufficient diagnostic quality to be used for treat-

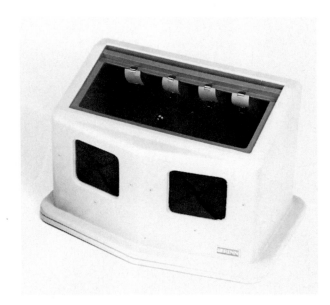

FIG. 5-18 Chairside darkroom allows rapid processing of endodontic working films. *(Courtesy Rinn Corp., Elgin, Ill.)*

ment films and are obtained in less time and with less patient discomfort. Rapid-processing solutions are available commercially but tend to vary in shelf life and tank life and in the production of films of permanent quality. To maintain the radiographic image for documentation, it is recommended that after it has been evaluated it be returned to the fixer for 10 minutes more and then washed for 20 minutes and dried. An alternative is to reprocess the film by means of the conventional technique. Double film packets can also be used for working films: one can be processed rapidly and the other conventionally. Regardless of what method is used for working films, a controlled time-temperature method should be used for the diagnostic qualities desired in pretreatment, posttreatment, and recall radiographs. All radiographs taken during the course of endodontic treatment should be preserved as a part of the patient's permanent record.

Radiographic Interpretation in Endodontics

Examination and differential interpretation

Radiographic interpretation is not strictly the identification of a problem and the establishment of a diagnosis. The dentist must read the film carefully, with an eye toward diagnosis and treatment. Frequently overlooked are the small areas of resorption, invaginated enamel, minute fracture lines, extra canals or roots, calcified canals, and, in turn, the potential problems they may create during treatment (Fig. 5-19). Problems during treatment, additional time, and extra expense can be avoided or at least anticipated if a thorough radiographic examination is conducted. As mentioned earlier, additional exposures at various angulations may be necessary to gain a better insight into the three-dimensional structure of a tooth.

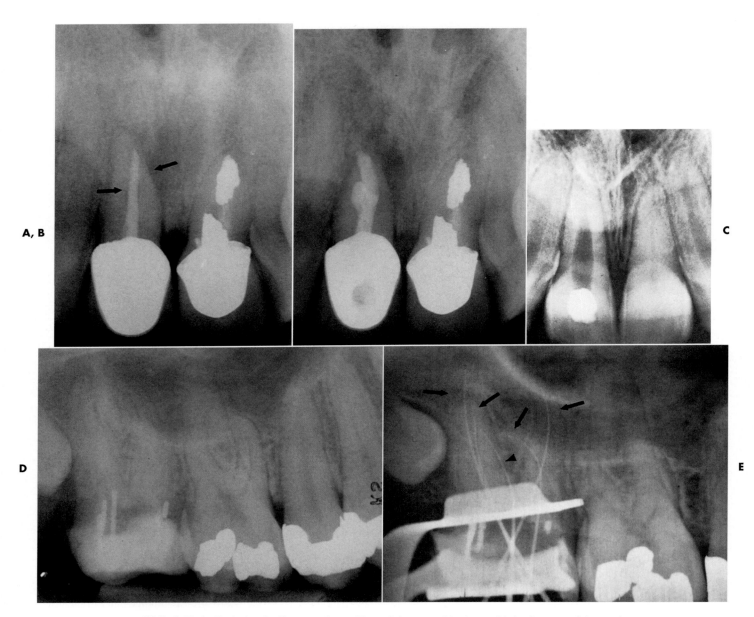

FIG. 5-19 A, Endodontically treated maxillary right central incisor with both external *(arrow)* and internal *(arrow)* root resorption. **B,** Nonsurgical retreatment on tooth in **A** and obturation with thermoplasticized gutta-percha were necessary to correct the internal resorptive defect; surgery was later performed to arrest the external resorption. **C,** Opposite reactions to traumatic injury to the maxillary central incisors. The maxillary right central incisor exhibits an excessively large canal as a result of internal resorption in the coronal two thirds, whereas the left one exhibits almost complete calcification of the canal. **D,** Maxillary second molar with complex root anatomy requiring endodontic treatment. **E,** Working length radiograph of tooth in **D** demonstrates five separate roots *(arrows):* two mesiobuccal roots, two palatal roots, and one distobuccal root.

Many anatomic structures and osteolytic lesions can be mistaken for pulpoperiradicular lesions. Among the more commonly misinterpreted anatomic structures are the mental foramen (Fig. 5-20) and the incisive foramen. These radiolucencies can be differentiated from pathologic conditions by exposures at different angulations and by pulp-testing procedures. Radiolucencies not associated with the root apex move or are projected away from the apex by varying the angulation. Radio-

lucent areas resulting from sparse trabeculation can also simulate radiolucent lesions and in such cases must be differentiated from the lamina dura and periodontal ligament space.

A commonly misinterpreted osteolytic lesion is periapical cemental dysplasia or cementoma (Fig. 5-21). The use of pulp-testing procedures and follow-up radiographic examinations prevents the mistake of diagnosing this as a pulpoperiradicular lesion. The development of this lesion can be followed ra-

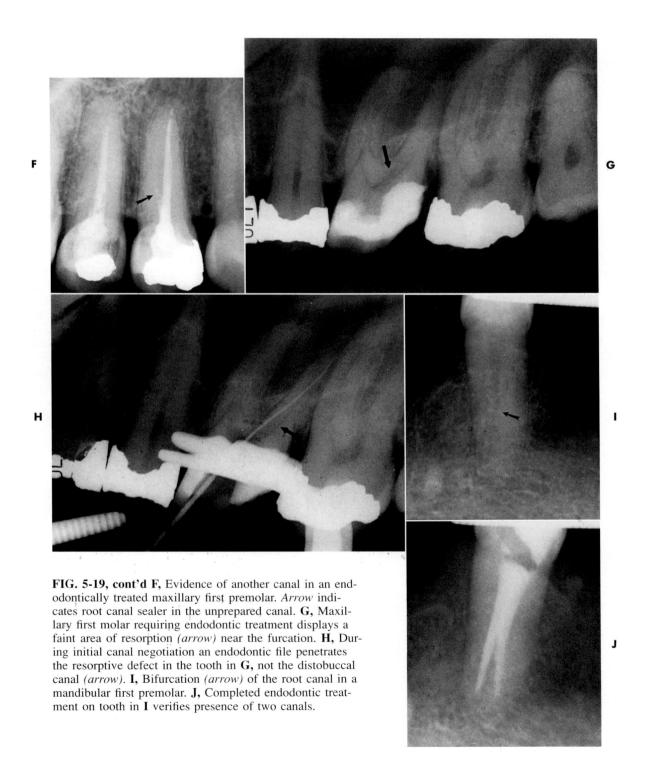

FIG. 5-19, cont'd F, Evidence of another canal in an endodontically treated maxillary first premolar. *Arrow* indicates root canal sealer in the unprepared canal. **G,** Maxillary first molar requiring endodontic treatment displays a faint area of resorption *(arrow)* near the furcation. **H,** During initial canal negotiation an endodontic file penetrates the resorptive defect in the tooth in **G,** not the distobuccal canal *(arrow)*. **I,** Bifurcation *(arrow)* of the root canal in a mandibular first premolar. **J,** Completed endodontic treatment on tooth in **I** verifies presence of two canals.

diographically from its osteolytic stage through its osteogenic stage.

Other anatomic radiolucencies that must be differentiated from pulpoperiradicular lesions are maxillary sinus, nutrient canals, nasal fossa, and the lateral or submandibular fossa. Many systemic conditions can mimic or affect the radiographic appearance of the alveolar process. A discussion of these conditions is beyond the scope of this chapter, but the reader is referred to Chapters 1 and 2 for further discussion.

Lamina dura: a question of integrity

One of the key challenges in endodontic radiographic interpretation is understanding the integrity, or lack of integrity, of the lamina dura, especially in its relationship to the health of

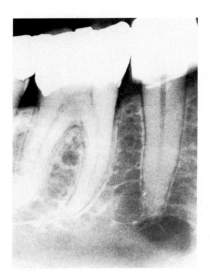

FIG. 5-20 A mandibular second premolar with an apparent periradicular radiolucency. Pulp-testing procedures indicated a normal response; the radiolucency is the mental foramen.

the pulp. Anatomically the lamina dura[25,26] is a layer of compact bone (the cribriform plate or alveolar bone proper) that lines the tooth socket; noxious products emanating from the root canal system can effect a change in this structure that is visible radiographically. X-ray beams passing tangentially through the socket must pass through many times the width of the adjacent alveolus and are attenuated by this greater thickness of bone, producing the characteristic "white line" (Fig. 5-22). If, for example, the beam is directed more obliquely so that it is not as attenuated, the lamina dura appears more diffuse or may not be discernible at all. Therefore the presence or absence and integrity of the lamina dura are determined largely by the shape and position of the root, and, in turn, by its bony crypt, in relation to the x-ray beam. This explanation is consistent with the radiographic and clinical findings of teeth with normal pulps and no distinct lamina dura.[48]

Changes in the integrity of the periodontal ligament space, the lamina dura, and the surrounding periradicular bone certainly have diagnostic value, especially when recent radiographs are compared to previous ones. However, the significance of such changes must be tempered by a thorough understanding of the features that give rise to these images.

Buccal object rule (cone shift)

In endodontic therapy it is imperative that the clinician know the spatial or buccolingual relation of an object within the tooth or alveolus. The technique used to identify the spatial relation of an object is called the cone or *tube shift technique*. Other names for this procedure are the *buccal object rule, Clark's rule*, and the *SLOB* (same lingual, opposite buccal) *rule*.[26,27,41,47] Proper application of the technique allows the dentist to locate additional canals or roots, to distinguish between objects that have been superimposed and between various types of resorption, to determine the buccolingual position of fractures and perforative defects, locate foreign bodies, and to locate anatomic landmarks in relation to the root apex, such as the mandibular canal.[25,52]

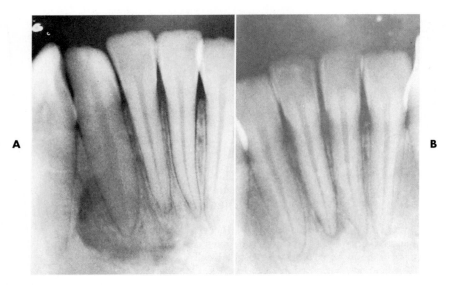

FIG. 5-21 Variations in appearance of periapical cemental dysplasia (cementoma). **A,** Osteolytic stage at apex of the mandibular lateral incisor. **B,** One year later: regeneration of bone around the apex of the lateral incisor and appearance of a radiolucency around the central incisor.

The buccal object rule relates to the manner in which the relative position of radiographic images of two separate objects changes when the projection angle at which the images were made is changed. The principle states that the object closest to the buccal surface appears to move in the direction opposite the movement of the cone or tube head when compared to a second film. Objects closest to the lingual surface appear on a film to move in the same direction that the cone moved, thus "same lingual, opposite buccal" rule. Fig. 5-23 shows three simulated radiographs of a buccal object (circle) and a lingual object (triangle) exposed at different horizontal angles. The position of the objects on each radiograph is compared with the reference structure (i.e., the mesial root apex of the mandibular first molar). The first radiograph (Fig. 5-23, *A* and *B*) shows superimposition of the two objects; in this case the tube head was positioned for a straight-on view. In the first radiograph (Fig. 5-23, *C* and *D*) the tube head shifted mesially, and the beam was directed at the reference object from a more mesial angulation. In this case the lingual object (triangle) moved mesially with respect to the reference object, and the buccal object (circle) moved distally with respect to the reference object. In the third radiograph (Fig. 5-23, *E* and *F*) the tube head shifted distally, and the beam was directed at the reference object from a more distal angulation; here the triangle moved distally with respect to the mesial root of the mandibular first molar, and the circle moved mesially. These radiographic relations confirm that the lingual object (triangle) moves in the same direction with respect to reference structures as the x-ray tube and that the buccal object (circle) moves in the opposite direction of the x-ray tube. Thus according to the rule, the object farthest (most buccal) from the film moves farthest on the film with respect to a change in horizontal angulation of the x-ray cone. In an endodontically treated mandibular molar with four canals (Fig. 5-24), a straight-on view results in superimposition of the root-filled canals on the radiograph. If the cone is angled from mesial to distal, the mesiolingual and distolingual canals move mesially and the mesiobuccal and distobuccal canals move distally on the radiograph when compared with the straight-on view.

The examples cited above involve application of the buccal object rule using changes in horizontal angulation. The clinician should be aware that this rule applies to changes in vertical angulation as well (Fig. 5-25). To locate the position of the mandibular canal relative to mandibular molar root apexes, one must take radiographs at different vertical angulations. If the canal moves with or in the same direction as the cone head, the canal is lingual to the root apexes; if the mandibular canal moves opposite the direction of the cone head, the canal is buccal to the root apexes. The clinician should recognize the wide range of applicability of the buccal object rule in determining the buccolingual relationship of structures not visible in a two-dimensional image.

Digitization of ionizing radiation

The evolution of computer technology to radiography has allowed for instantaneous image acquisition, image enhancement, storage, retrieval, and even transmission of images to remote sites in a digital format. Major advantages of digital radiography in endodontics are that radiographic images are obtained immediately, eliminating developing time and film processing, and radiation exposure is reduced from 50% to 90% compared to conventional film-based radiography.[26,44] The primary disadvantages of all the currently available systems are their high costs and potential reduction in image quality when compared to conventional radiography.

Digital imaging systems require an electronic sensor or detector, an analog to digital converter, a computer, and a monitor or printer for image display.[26] The computer is in charge of the components of the imaging system. It instructs the x-ray generator when to begin and end the exposure, controls the digitizer, constructs the image by mathematical algorithm, determines the method of image display, and provides for storage and transmission of the acquired data. The most common sensor is the CCD or charged-coupled device. When a conventional x-ray unit is used to project the x-ray beam onto the sensor, an electrical charge is created, an analog output signal is generated, and the digital converter converts the analog output signal from the CCD to a numeric representation that is recognizable by the computer. The radiographic image then appears on the monitor and can be manipulated electronically to alter contrast, resolution, orientation, and even size. Working lengths of root canals can even be electronically measured.

Digitization of ionizing radiation first became a reality in the late 1980s with the development of the original RVG, or

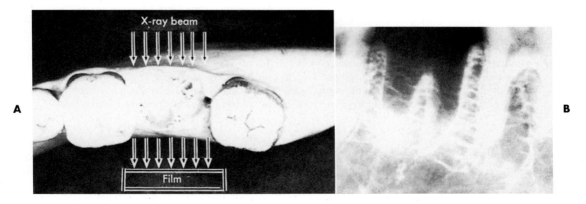

FIG. 5-22 A, Attenuation of x-ray beams passing tangentially through the socket by the greater thickness of bone on the periphery of the socket. This results in a greater radiopacity of the periphery as compared with the adjacent alveolar bone. **B,** White lines (lamina dura) produced by these attenuated rays.

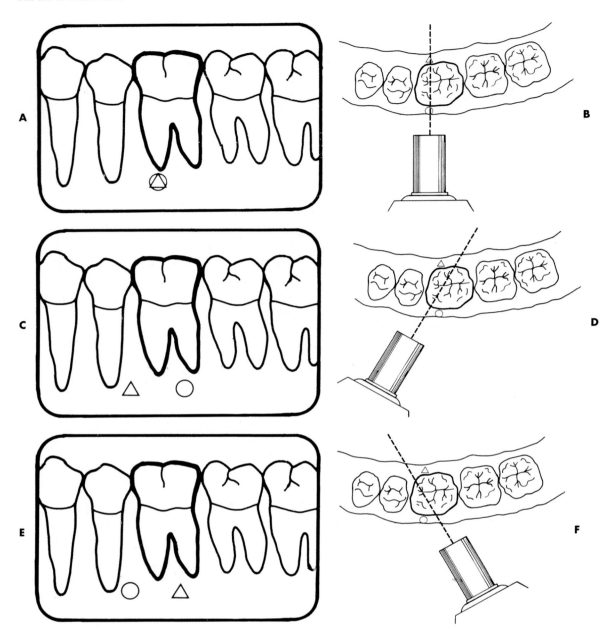

FIG. 5-23 Objects may be localized with respect to reference structures by using the buccal object rule (tube shift technique). **A** and **B,** A straight-on view causes superimposition of the buccal object *(circle)* with the lingual object *(triangle)*. **C** and **D,** Using the tube shift technique, the lingual object *(triangle)* appears more mesial with respect to the mesial root of the mandibular first molar, and the buccal object *(circle)* appears more distal on a second view projected from the mesial aspect. **E** and **F,** The object *(triangle)* on the lingual surface appears more distal with respect to the mesial root of the mandibular first molar, and the object *(circle)* on the buccal surface appears more mesial on a view projected from the distal aspect.

radiovisiography, system by Dr. Francis Mouyen[44]; it has since technologically evolved and is now known as the Everest RVG (Fig. 5-26, *A*). Another system that is currently available is computed dental radiography, or CDR (Fig. 5-26, *B*). Both are approved by the Food and Drug Administration (FDA).

As the name suggests, the Everest RVG has three components. The "radio" component consists of a high-resolution sensor, 40 mm × 24 mm × 6.95 mm, and has an active area of 30 mm × 20 mm (Fig. 5-26, *C*). The sensor is protected from

x-ray degradation by a fiberoptic shield and can be cold sterilized. For infection control, disposable latex sheaths are used to cover the sensor when it is in use. The second component, the "visio" portion, consists of a video monitor and display-processing unit. As the image is transmitted to the processing unit, it is digitized and memorized by the computer. The unit magnifies the image four times for immediate display on the video monitor and has the additional capability of producing colored images. It can also display multiple images simulta-

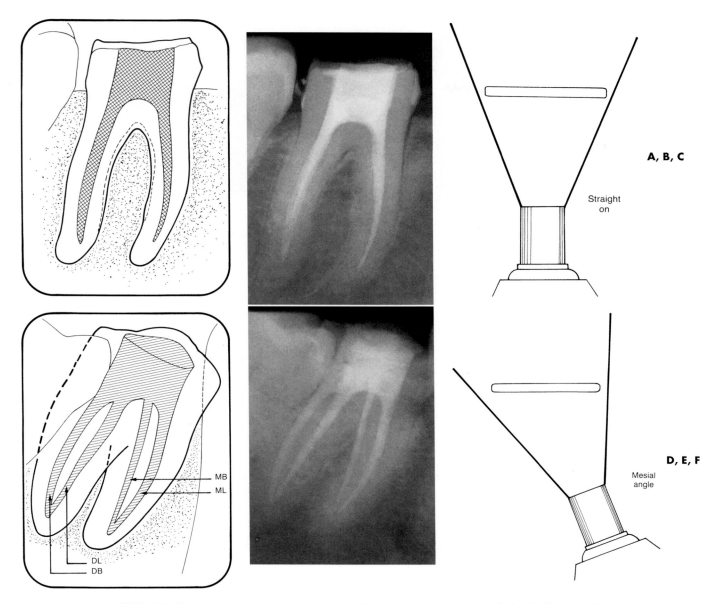

FIG. 5-24 Comparison of straight-on and mesial-angled views of an endodontically treated mandibular molar with four canals. **A, B,** and **C,** Straight-on view of the mandibular molar shows superimposition of the root canal fillings. **D, E,** and **F,** Mesial-to-distal angulation produces separation of the canals. The mesiolingual and distolingual root-filled canals move mesially (toward the cone), and the mesiobuccal and distobuccal root-filled canals move distally (away from the cone) on the radiograph.

neously, including a full-mouth series on one screen. Because the image is digitized, further manipulation of the image is possible; this includes enhancement, contrast stretching, and reversing. A zoom feature is also available to enlarge a portion of the image up to full-screen size. The third component is the "graphy," a high-resolution videoprinter that instantly provides a hard copy of the screen image, using the same video signal. In addition, a digital intraoral camera can now be integrated with the Everest system.

CDR essentially operates similarly and provides the same basic functions as the Everest RVG. One of the advantages of CDR, however, is that multiple sensors are available, corresponding to film sizes 0, 1, and 2 (Fig. 5-26, *D*). The CDR

sensor that is similar in size to the Everest sensor is also slightly thinner, being 41 mm × 23 mm × 5 mm, and has a slightly larger active area, 35 mm × 19 mm. The CDR also has specially designed multiple types of sensor holders available.

The advantages of digital imaging seem numerous, but the primary ones include the elimination of x-ray film, a significant reduction in exposure time (80% to 90% reduction when compared to D-speed film), and instantaneous image display. An exposure time in the range of hundredths of a second is all that is needed to generate an image.[26] A recent study showed that RVG resolution was slightly lower than that produced with silver halide film emulsions, but radiographic information can be increased with the electronic image treatment capabilities

FIG. 5-25 Examples of the buccal object rule using shifts in vertical and horizontal angulations. **A,** Bite-wing radiograph (straight-on view with minimal horizontal and vertical angulation) depicts amalgam particle superimposed over the mesial root of the mandibular first molar. To determine the buccolingual location of the object, the tube shift technique (buccal object rule) must be applied. **B,** The periapical radiograph was taken by shifting the vertical angulation of the cone (i.e., the x-ray beam was projected more steeply upward). Since the amalgam particle moved in the opposite direction to that of the cone compared with the bite-wing radiograph, the amalgam particle lies on the buccal aspect of the tooth. **C,** The periapical radiograph was taken by shifting the horizontal angulation of the cone (the x-ray image was taken from a distal angle). Compared to both **A** and **B,** each taken straight-on with minimal horizontal angulation, the amalgam particle moved opposite the direction of movement of the cone or tube head, confirming that the amalgam particle lies on the buccal aspect of the tooth.

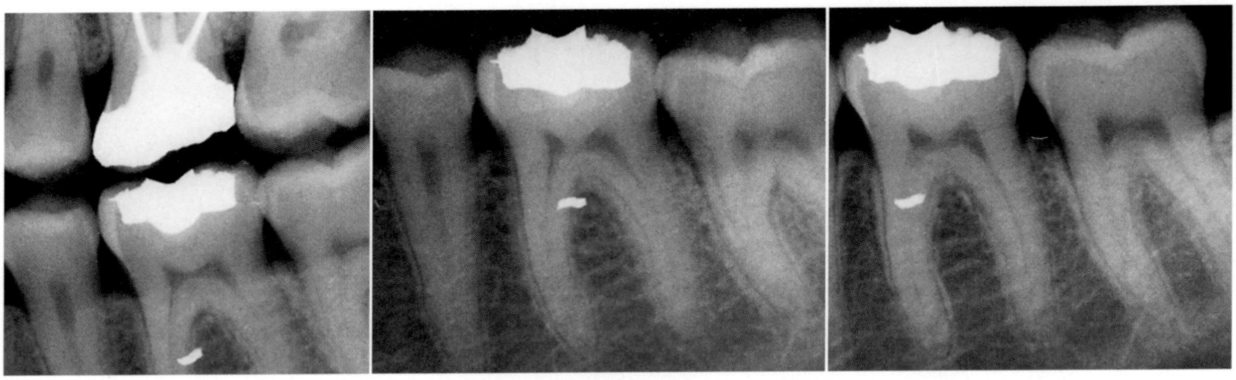

of the system.[44] These systems appear to be very promising for endodontics and general dentistry.

PREPARATION FOR ACCESS: TOOTH ISOLATION

Principles and Rationale

The use of the rubber dam is mandatory in root canal treatment.[13,14] Developed in the nineteenth century by S. C. Barnum, the rubber dam has evolved over the years from a system that was designed to isolate teeth for placement of gold foil to one of sophistication for the ultimate protection of both patient and clinician.[52] The advantages[10,12,28] and absolute necessity of the rubber dam must always take precedence over convenience and expediency, a rationale often cited by clinicians who condemn its use. Properly placed, the rubber dam facilitates treatment by isolating the tooth from obstacles such as saliva and the tongue, which can disrupt any procedure. Proper rubber dam placement can be done quickly and enhances the entire procedure.

The rationale for use of the rubber dam in endodontics is that it ensures the following[12,23,31,52]:

1. Patient protection from aspiration or the swallowing of instruments, tooth debris, medicaments, and irrigating solutions

2. Clinician protection: Today's litigious society certainly focuses on the negligent clinician who fails to use a rubber dam on a patient who subsequently swallows or aspirates an endodontic file. *Routine placement of the rubber dam is mandatory; i.e., it represents the minimum standard of care.*[13,14] The reader is referred to Chapter 10 for further discussion about this issue.

3. A surgically clean operating field isolated from saliva, hemorrhage, and other tissue fluids: The dam reduces the risk of cross-contamination of the root canal system and provides an excellent barrier to the potential spread of

infectious agents.[12,23] *It is a required component of any infection control program.**

4. Retraction and protection of the soft tissues.

5. Improved visibility: The rubber dam provides a dry field and reduces mirror fogging.

6. Increased efficiency: The rubber dam minimizes patient conversation during treatment and the need for frequent rinsing. It relaxes the patient and saves time.

The dentist should be aware that in some situations, especially in teeth with crowns, access into the pulp system may be difficult without first orienting root structure to the adjacent teeth and periodontal tissues. Radiographically the coronal pulp system is often obscured by the restoration, and as a result the dentist may misdirect the bur during access. In these cases it may be necessary to locate the pulp chamber first, before the dam is placed. In doing so, the dentist can visualize root topography, making it easier to orient the bur toward the long axis of the roots and prevent perforation. Once the root canal system is located, however, the rubber dam is immediately placed.

Armamentarium

The mainstay of the rubber dam system is the dam itself. These autoclavable sheets of thin, flat, latex rubber come in various thicknesses (thin, medium, heavy, extra heavy, and special heavy) and in two different sizes (5×5 inches and 6×6 inches). For endodontic purposes, the medium thickness is probably best because it tends to tear less easily, retracts soft tissues better than the thin type, and is easier to place than the heavier types. However, a thinner gauge may be desirable to decrease tension if retainer placement is questionable or if the

---

*References 2, 10, 11, 17, 20, 42.

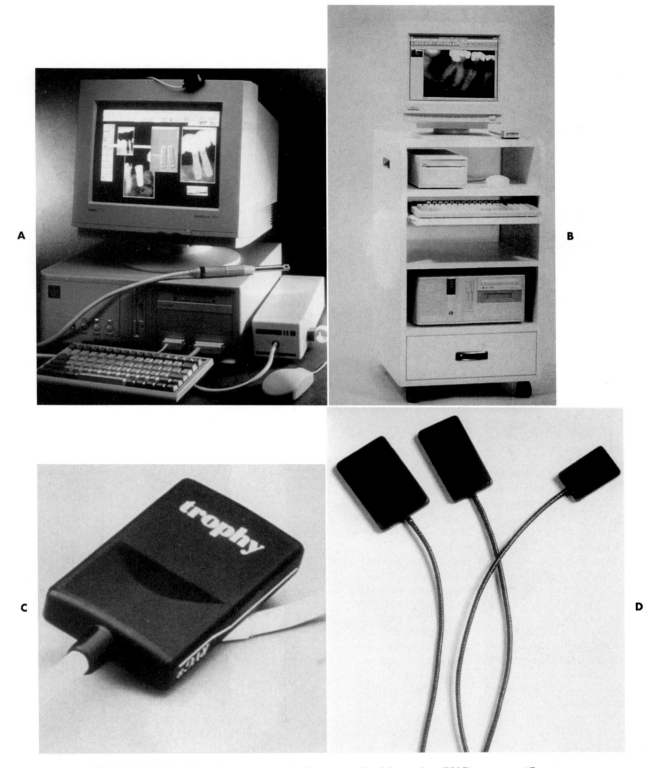

FIG. 5-26 Digital imaging systems. **A,** Everest radiovisiography (RVG) system. *(Courtesy Trophy Radiology, Marietta, Ga.)* **B,** Computed dental radiography (CDR) system. *(Courtesy Schick Technologies, Long Island City, N.Y.)* **C,** Everest RVG's high-resolution intraoral sensor replaces film. *(Courtesy Trophy Radiology, Marietta, Ga.)* **D,** CDR offers three different sizes of high resolution intraoral sensors. *(Courtesy Schick Technologies, Long Island City, N.Y.)*

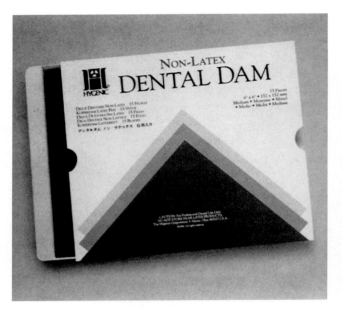

FIG. 5-27 Nonlatex rubber dam is ideal for patients with known latex allergies. *(Courtesy Coltene/Whaledent (Hygenic), Manwah, N.J.)*

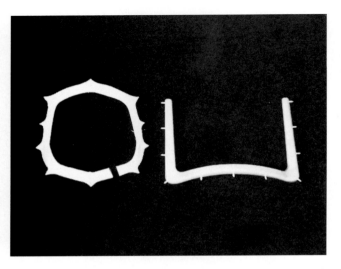

FIG. 5-28 Plastic radiolucent rubber dam frames. *Left,* Nygaard-Ostby (N-O) frame. *Right,* Young's frame.

retainer is resting on a band. The dam is also manufactured in a variety of colors ranging from light yellow to blue, green, or gray. The darker colored dams may afford better visual contrast, thus reducing eyestrain, but the lighter colored ones, because of their translucency, have the advantage of naturally illuminating the operating field and allowing easier film placement underneath the dam. Depending on individual preference and specific conditions associated with a tooth, the dentist may find it necessary to vary the color or thickness of the rubber dam used. Glare and eyestrain can be reduced and contrast enhanced by routinely placing the dull side of the dam toward the operator.

For patients with latex allergies, a nonlatex rubber dam is available from Coltène/Whaledent (Hygenic) (Fig. 5-27). This powder-free teal-green synthetic dam comes in one size (6 × 6 inches) and in one thickness, medium gauge. It has a shelf life of 3 years but only one third the tensile strength of latex dam.

Another component of the rubber dam system is the rubber dam frame, which is designed to retract and stabilize the dam. Both metal and plastic frames are available, but plastic ones are recommended for endodontic procedures. They appear radiolucent, do not mask key areas on working films, and do not have to be removed before film placement. The Young's rubber dam frame (plastic type), the Star Visi frame, and the Nygaard-Ostby (N-O) frame are examples of radiolucent frames used in endodontics (Fig. 5-28). The disposable Handidam rubber dam system also provides a radiolucent plastic frame (Fig. 5-29). The Quickdam is another disposable single isolation device with a flexible outer ring, eliminating the need for an additional frame (Fig. 5-30). Metal frames are seldom used today; because of their radiopacity, they tend to block out the radiograph and, if removed, may result in destabilization of the dam and salivary contamination of the canal system, thus negating the disinfected environment that was previously attained.

Rubber dam clamps or retainers anchor the dam to the tooth

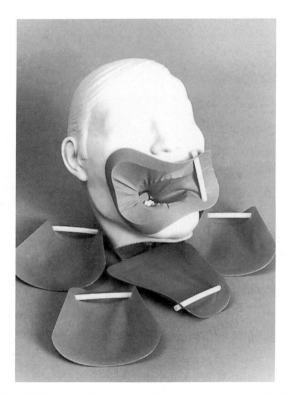

FIG. 5-29 The Handidam is a rubber dam system with built-in plastic frame. The disposable frame bends easily for film placement. *(Courtesy Aseptico, Woodinville, Wash.)*

requiring treatment or, in cases of multiple tooth isolation, to the most posterior tooth. They also aid in soft tissue retraction. The clamps are made of shiny or dull stainless steel, and each consists of a bow and two jaws. Regardless of the type of jaw configuration, the prongs of the jaws should engage at

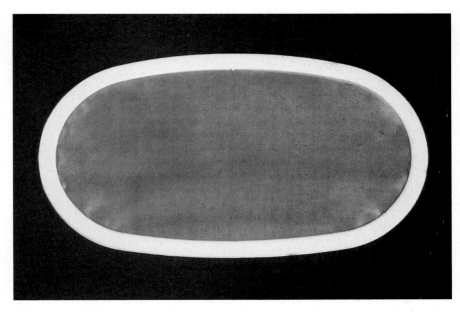

FIG. 5-30 The Quickdam is a disposable isolation system with a pliable outer ring. *(Courtesy Ivoclar/Vivadent, Amherst, N.Y.)*

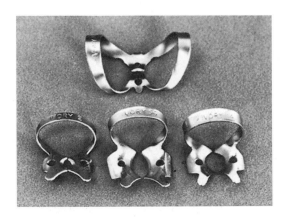

FIG. 5-31 Basic set of ivory winged rubber dam clamps: on top, no. 9 butterfly clamp for anterior teeth; on bottom, from left, No. 2 premolar clamp, No. 56 mandibular molar clamp, and No. 14 maxillary molar clamp. *(Courtesy Columbus Dental, Division of Miles Inc., St. Louis, Mo.)*

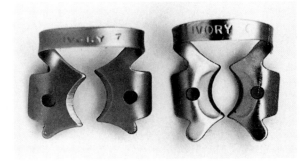

FIG. 5-32 Mandibular molar clamps. Clamp on right has jaws inclined apically to engage tooth with minimal tooth structure remaining. *(Courtesy Columbus Dental, Division of Miles Inc., St. Louis, Mo.)*

least four points on the tooth. This clamp-to-tooth relationship stabilizes the retainer and prevents any rocking which, in itself, can be injurious to both hard and soft tissues.[32,39]

Clamps are available from a variety of manufacturers and are specifically designed for all classes of teeth with a variety of anatomic configurations. For most uncomplicated endodontic isolations, the dentist's basic armamentarium should consist of winged clamps; a butterfly-type clamp for anterior teeth; a universal premolar clamp; a mandibular molar clamp; and a maxillary molar clamp (Fig. 5-31). The wings, which are extensions of the jaws, not only provide for additional soft tissue retraction but also facilitate placement of the rubber dam, frame, and retainer as a single unit (see Methods of Rubber Dam Placement, which follows). Other retainers are designed for specific clinical situations in which clamp placement may be difficult. For example, when minimal coronal tooth structure remains, a clamp with apically inclined jaws may be used to engage tooth

structure at or below the level of the free gingival margin (Fig. 5-32). Retainers with serrated jaws, known as tiger clamps, also may increase stabilization of broken-down teeth. Another type of retainer, the Silker-Glickman (S-G) clamp should also be included in the dentist's armamentarium (Fig. 5-33). Its anterior extension allows for retraction of the dam around a severely broken-down tooth while the clamp itself is placed on a tooth proximal to the one being treated (Fig. 5-34).

The Annoni Endo-Illuminator (Analytic Technology, Redmond, Wash.) system is new to the specialty of endodontics (Fig. 5-35). Through its fiber-optic attachment to specially designed autoclavable retainers, the high-intensity light generated by the Endo-Illuminator transilluminates pulp chambers and canal orifices so that pulp systems are easier to identify and locate.

The remaining components of the rubber dam system include the rubber dam punch and the rubber dam forceps. The punch has a series of holes on a rotating disc from which the

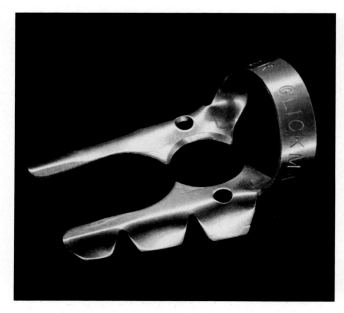

FIG. 5-33 The Silker-Glickman (S-G) clamp for isolation of severely broken-down teeth. *(Courtesy The Smile Center, Deerwood, Minn.)*

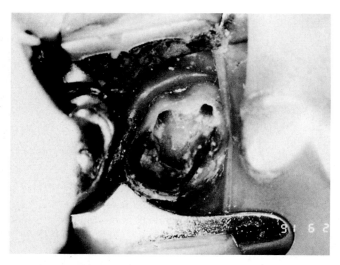

FIG. 5-34 The S-G clamp is placed on the maxillary second molar to isolate a severely broken-down maxillary first molar.

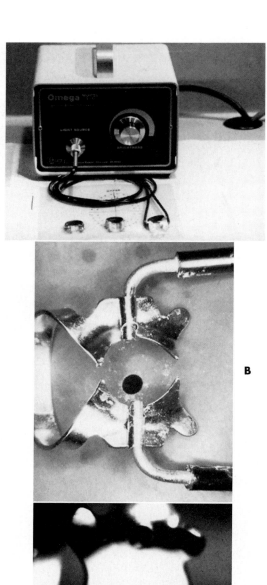

dentist can select according to the size of tooth or teeth to be isolated. The forceps hold and carry the retainer during placement and removal.

Methods of Rubber Dam Placement

As mentioned earlier, an expedient method of dam placement is to position the bow of the clamp through the hole in the dam and place the rubber over the wings of the clamp (a winged clamp is required).[25,52] The clamp is stretched by the forceps to maintain the position of the clamp in the dam, and the dam is attached to the plastic frame, allowing for the placement of the dam, clamp, and frame in one motion (Fig. 5-36). Once the clamp is secured on the tooth, the dam is teased under the wings of the clamp with a plastic instrument.

Another method is to place the clamp, usually wingless,

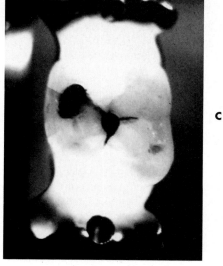

FIG. 5-35 The Annoni Endo-Illuminator system. **A,** Fiberoptic unit with attachments to clamp. **B,** Clamp specially designed for fiberoptic attachments. **C,** Maxillary molar "illuminated" via fiberoptics. *(Courtesy Analytic Technology, Redmond, Wash.)*

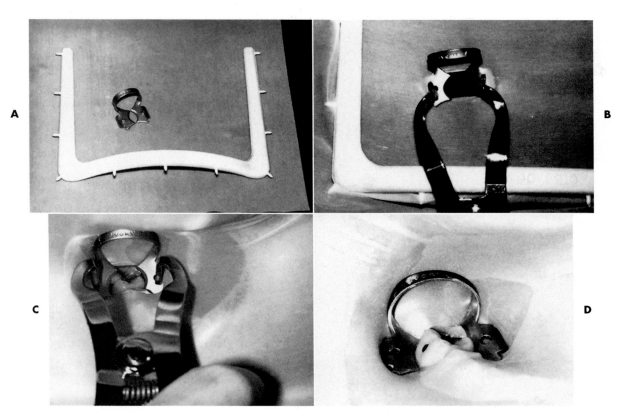

FIG. 5-36 **A,** Rubber dam, clamp, and frame. **B,** Clamp positioned in the dam with frame attached and held in position with rubber dam forceps. **C,** Dam, clamp, and frame carried to mouth as one unit and placed over the tooth. **D,** Clamp in place with four-point contact with rubber tucked under the wings.

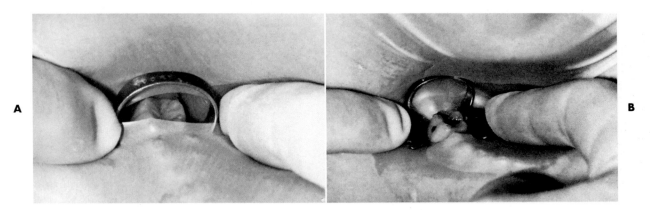

FIG. 5-37 **A,** After the clamp is placed, the dam is attached to the frame and gently stretched over the clamped tooth with the index finger of each hand. **B,** Clamp is tested for a secure fit with gentle finger pressure alternately on the buccal and lingual aspects of the clamp apron.

on the tooth and then stretch the dam over the clamped tooth (Fig. 5-37).[25,52] This method offers the advantage of enabling the clinician to see exactly where the jaws of the clamp engage the tooth, thus avoiding possible impingement on the gingival tissues. Gentle finger pressure on the buccal and lingual apron of the clamp before the dam is placed can be used to test how securely the clamp fits. Variations of this method include placing the clamp and dam first, followed by the frame, or placing the rubber dam first, followed by the clamp and then the frame.[52]

A third method, the split-dam technique,[25] may be used to isolate anterior teeth without using a rubber dam clamp. Not only is this technique useful when there is insufficient crown structure, as in the case of horizontal fractures, but it also prevents the possibility of the jaws of the clamp chipping the margins of teeth restored with porcelain crowns or laminates. Studies[32,39] on the effects of retainers on porcelain-fused-to-metal restorations and tooth structure itself have demonstrated that there can be significant damage to cervical porcelain, as well as to dentin and cementum, even when the clamp is properly sta-

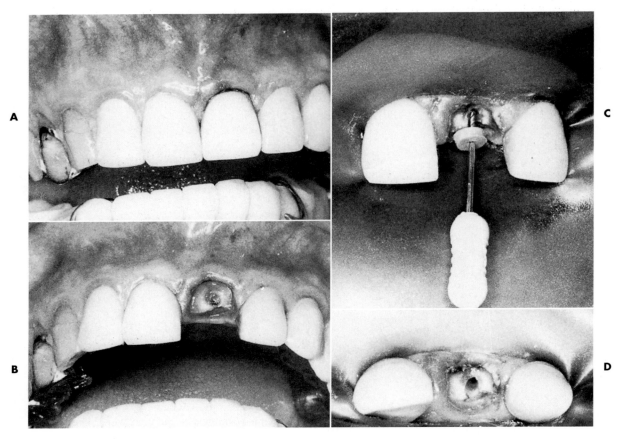

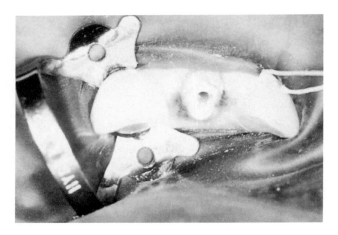

FIG. 5-38 Split-dam technique. **A,** Maxillary central incisor with a horizontal fracture at the cervical area. **B,** Appearance after removal of the coronal fragment. **C,** Cotton roll in place in the mucobuccal fold and rubber dam stretched over the two adjacent teeth. **D,** Appearance after pulp extirpation.

bilized. Thus for teeth with porcelain restorations, ligation with dental floss is recommended as an alternate method to retract the dam and tissues, or the adjacent tooth can be clamped.

In the split-dam method, two overlapping holes are punched in the dam. A cotton roll is placed under the lip in the mucobuccal fold over the tooth to be treated. The rubber dam is stretched over the tooth to be treated and over one adjacent tooth on each side. The edge of the dam is carefully teased through the contacts on the distal sides of the two adjacent teeth. Dental floss helps carry the dam down around the gingiva. The tension produced by the stretched dam, aided by the rubber dam frame, secures the dam in place. The tight fit and the cotton roll should help provide a dry field (Fig. 5-38). If saliva leakage remains a problem, pressing the puttylike OraSeal caulking around the margins of the overlapping holes will assure a dry field. If the dam has a tendency to slip, a premolar clamp may be used on a tooth distal to the three isolated teeth or even on an adjacent tooth (Fig. 5-39). The clamp is placed over the rubber dam, which then acts as a cushion against the jaws of the clamp.

Aids in Rubber Dam Placement

Punching and positioning of holes

The rubber dam may be divided into four equal quadrants, and the proper place for the hole is estimated according to which tooth is undergoing treatment. The more distal the tooth,

FIG. 5-39 Split-dam technique. Premolar clamp on maxillary central incisor along with ligation on the maxillary canine prevents dam slippage and aids in dam retraction during endodontic treatment on broken-down maxillary lateral incisor. *(Courtesy Dr. James L. Gutmann.)*

the closer to the center is the placement of the hole.[25] This method becomes easier as the clinician gains experience. The hole must be punched cleanly, without tags or tears. If the dam is torn, it may leak or permit continued tearing when stretched over the clamp and tooth.

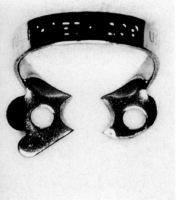

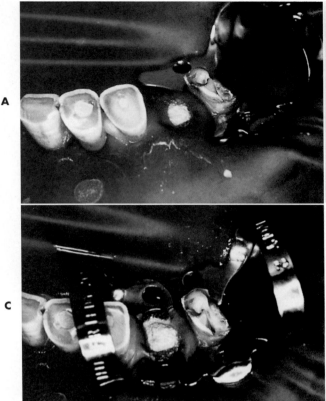

FIG. 5-40 A, Isolation rendered difficult by multiple, severely broken-down mandibular premolars. **B,** Modified premolar rubber dam clamp. **C,** Modified clamp in place on first premolar to accommodate wings of distal clamp. *(Courtesy Dr. Robert Roda.)*

Orientation of the dam and bunching

The rubber dam must be attached to the frame with enough tension to retract soft tissues and prevent bunching, without tearing the dam or displacing the clamp. The rubber dam should completely cover the patient's mouth without infringing on the patient's nose or eyes. To prevent bunching of the dam in the occlusal embrasure, only the edge of the interseptal portion of the dam is teased between the teeth. Dental floss is then used to carry the dam through the contacts. These contacts should always be tested with dental floss before the dam is placed. A plastic instrument is used to invert the edge of the dam around the tooth to provide a seal.

Problem-Solving in Tooth Isolation

Leakage

The best way to prevent seepage through the rubber dam is meticulous placement of the entire system. Proper selection and placement of the clamp, sharply punched, correctly positioned holes, use of a dam of adequate thickness, and inversion of the dam around the tooth help reduce leakage through the dam and into the root canal system.[4,31,38,52] Nevertheless, there are clinical situations in which small tears, holes, or continuous minor leaks may occur. These often can be patched or blocked with Cavit, OraSeal Caulking, rubber base adhesive,[7] "liquid" rubber dam, or periodontal packing. If leakage continues, the dam should be replaced with a new one.

Because salivary secretions can seep through even a well-placed rubber dam, persons who salivate excessively may require premedication to reduce saliva flow to a manageable level. Failure to control salivation may result in salivary contamination of the canal system and pooling of saliva beneath the dam, as well as drooling and possible choking. Such occurrences can disrupt treatment and should be prevented. Excessive saliva flow can be reduced through the use of an anticholinergic drug such as atropine sulfate, propantheline bromide (Pro-Banthine), methantheline (Banthine), or the new drug, glycopyrrolate (Robinul).[29] Therapeutic doses of atropine sulfate for adults range from 0.3 to 1 mg PO, 1 to 2 hours before the procedure. The synthetic anticholinergic drug propantheline bromide (Pro-Banthine) reportedly has fewer side effects than Banthine.[29] The usual adult dose of Pro-Banthine for an adult is 7.5 to 15 mg taken orally 30 to 45 minutes before the appointment. Because they can cause undesirable autonomic effects, especially through various drug interactions, the anticholinergics should be used only in specific cases and only as a last resort.

Unusual tooth shapes or positions that cause inadequate clamp placement

Some teeth do not conform to the variety of clamps available. These include partially erupted teeth, teeth prepared for crowns, and teeth fractured or broken down to the extent that their margins are subgingival. To handle these cases, rubber dam retainers may be customized by modifying the jaws to adapt to a particular tooth (Fig. 5-40).[53] In partially erupted teeth or cone-shaped teeth such as those prepared for full coverage, one technique[51] is to place spots of self-curing resin on the cervical surface of the tooth. These resin beads act as a scaffold for the retainer during treatment. Another method[28] is to place small acid-etched composite lips on the teeth; these resin lips serve as artificial undercuts and remain on the teeth between appoint-

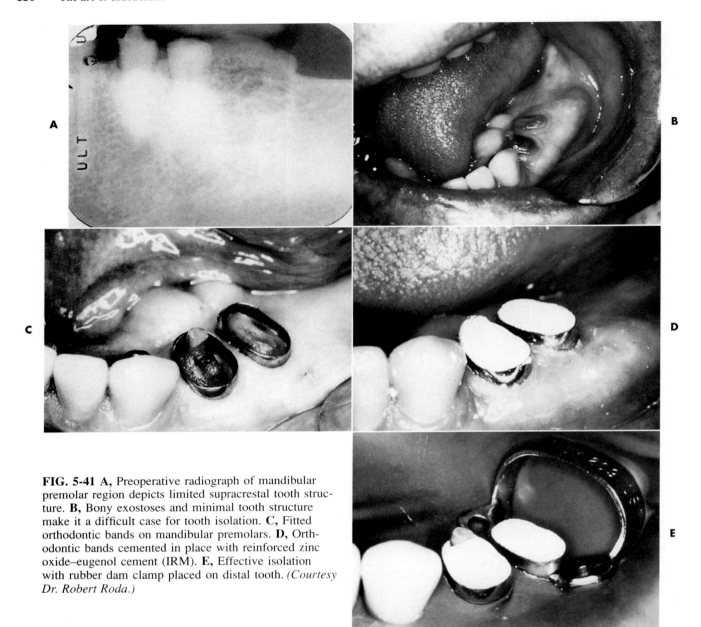

FIG. 5-41 A, Preoperative radiograph of mandibular premolar region depicts limited supracrestal tooth structure. **B,** Bony exostoses and minimal tooth structure make it a difficult case for tooth isolation. **C,** Fitted orthodontic bands on mandibular premolars. **D,** Orthodontic bands cemented in place with reinforced zinc oxide–eugenol cement (IRM). **E,** Effective isolation with rubber dam clamp placed on distal tooth. *(Courtesy Dr. Robert Roda.)*

ments. When the root canal treatment is complete, the resin beads are easily removed. In multiple-treatment cases involving misshapen teeth, a customized acrylic retainer[49] can be used in conjunction with a dam to isolate the operating field.

Loss of tooth structure

If insufficient tooth structure prevents the placement of a clamp, the clinician must first determine whether the tooth is periodontally sound and restorable. Meticulous and thorough treatment planning often can prevent embarrassing situations for both the dentist and patient. One example is the case in which the endodontic treatment is completed before restorability was determined; later it is then discovered that the tooth cannot be restored.

Once a tooth is deemed restorable but the margin of sound tooth structure is subgingival, a number of methods should be considered. As mentioned earlier, less invasive methods, such as using a clamp with prongs inclined apically or using an S-G clamp, should be attempted first (see Fig. 5-34). If neither of these techniques effectively isolates the tooth, the dentist may consider the clamping of the attached gingiva and alveolar process. In this situation, it is imperative that profound soft tissue anesthesia exists before clamp placement. Although the procedure may cause some minor postoperative discomfort, the periodontal tissues recover quickly with minimal postoperative care.

Restorative procedures

If none of the techniques mentioned above is desirable, a variety of restorative methods may be considered to build up the tooth so that a retainer can be placed properly.[37,38,52] A preformed copper band, a temporary crown, or an orthodontic band (Figs. 5-41 and 5-42) may be cemented over the remaining natural crown. This band or crown not only enables the

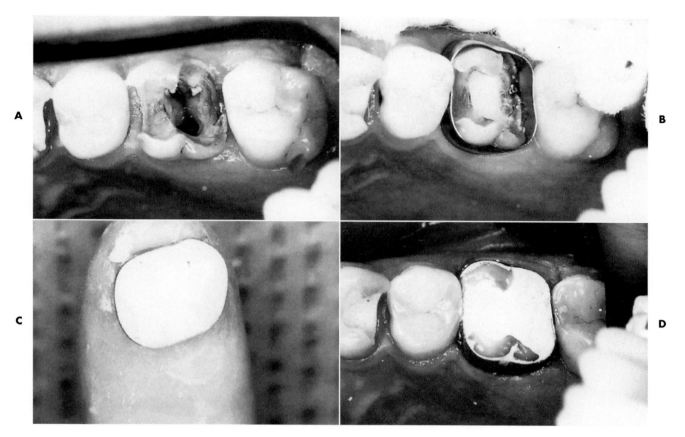

FIG. 5-42 A, Broken-down maxillary molar following removal of restoration, post, and caries. **B,** Fitted orthodontic band; cotton in access opening to protect orifices. **C,** IRM loaded into band before cementation. **D,** Completed temporary restoration before rubber dam placement. *(Courtesy Dr. Robert Roda.)*

clamp to be retained successfully, it also serves as a seal for the retention of intracanal medicaments and the temporary filling between appointments. These temporary bands or crowns have several disadvantages. One of their main problems is their inability to provide a superior seal. Another concern is that particles of these soft metals or cement can block canal systems during access opening and instrumentation. Third, these temporary crowns and bands, if they become displaced or are not properly contoured, can cause periodontal inflammation.

Occasionally so little tooth structure remains that even band or crown placement is not possible. In these cases it becomes necessary to replace the missing tooth structure to facilitate placement of the rubber dam clamp and prevent leakage into the pulp cavity during the course of treatment.[37,38,52] Replacement of missing tooth structure can be accomplished by means of pin-retained amalgam buildups, composites, glass ionomer cements such as Ketac-Silver, Fuji II (Fig. 5-43), or Photac-Fil, or dentin-bonding systems such as Scotchbond 2, Tenure Bond, Gluma, Optibond, PermaQuik (Fig. 5-44), or C&B Metabond.[52] Although these newer dentin-bonding systems form a very strong immediate bond and are generally simple to use, any restorative method for building up a broken-down tooth is time consuming, can impede endodontic procedures, and may duplicate restorative treatment. Many restorations that have been hollowed out by access cavities are weakened and require redoing.

Canal Projection

Canal projection technique using the Projector Endodontic Instrument Guidance System (Moyco Union Broach, York, Pa.) allows for preendodontic buildup of teeth with severe coronal breakdown (Fig. 5-45, *A*) while preserving individualized access to the canals. The technique is as follows. After gaining access, all orifices are dimpled to the depth of a No. 2 slow-speed round bur. The chamber is then etched with 37% phosphoric acid, and a moist-field primer is applied. Projectors (tapered plastic sleeves) are placed onto endodontic files, the files are inserted into the canals, and the projectors are slid apically until they are precisely seated into the dimples (Fig. 5-45, *B*). Bonding agent is then applied to the primed surfaces and a composite buildup material is injected from the chamber floor to the occlusal surface. Following polymerization, the files are removed, the projector tops are cleared of resin with a diamond bur, and the projectors are removed by inserting a No. 60 Hedstrom file, engaging the flutes in the walls of the lumen, and withdrawing. The external surfaces of the projectors are treated with a releasing agent, enabling easy removal from the buildup material. The occlusal surface is then flattened with a diamond bur to provide ideal reference points (Fig. 5-45, *C*). Once the canals have been cleaned, shaped, and obturated, the projected portion of the canals (from the level of the chamber floor to the cavosurface) is filled by injecting a resin-based material, either composite or glass ionomer (Fig. 5-45, *D*).

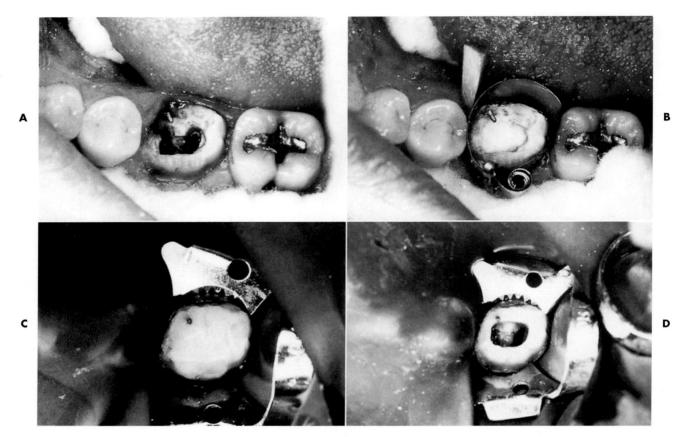

FIG. 5-43 A, Broken-down mandibular molar following crown and caries removal; preexisting pin aids retention of restorative material. **B,** Isolation with wedged Automatrix. **C,** Completed temporary restoration using glass ionomer cement (Fuji II). **D,** Access through completed restoration following rubber dam placement. *(Courtesy Dr. Robert Roda.)*

Periodontal procedures

As a result of excessive crown destruction or incomplete eruption, the presence of gingival tissue may preclude the use of a clamp without severe gingival impingement. Various techniques of gingivectomy (Fig. 5-46) or electrosurgery have been suggested for cases in which the remaining tooth structure still lies above the crestal bone. With an inadequate zone of attached gingiva, osseous defects, or a poor anatomic form, an apically positioned flap with a reverse bevel incision is the technique of choice to "lengthen" the crown.[37,38]

Electrosurgery and the conventional gingivectomy are crown-lengthening procedures for teeth that have sufficient attached gingiva and no infrabony involvement.[37,38] The electrosurgery method offers the advantage of leaving a virtually bloodless site for immediate rubber dam placement. Electrosurgery units have become highly sophisticated and are capable of providing both cutting and coagulating currents that, when used properly, will not cause cellular coagulation. The wide variety of sizes and shapes of surgical electrodes enables the clinician to reach areas inaccessible to the scalpel. Furthermore, electrosurgery facilitates the removal of unwanted tissue in such a manner as to recreate normal gingival architecture. This feature, combined with controlled hemostasis, makes the instrument extremely useful in the preparation of some teeth for placement of the rubber dam clamp. The main drawback of electrosurgery is the potential for damage to the adjacent tissues; if the electrode contacts bone, significant destruction of bone can occur. As a result, this technique is not recommended when the distance between the crestal level of bone and the remaining tooth structure is minimal. Compared to electrosurgery, conventional gingivectomy presents the major problem of hemorrhage following the procedure; this forces delay of endodontic treatment until tissues have healed.

The apically positioned flap[37,38] is a crown-lengthening technique for teeth with inadequate attached gingiva, infrabony pockets, or remaining tooth structure below the level of crestal bone. With this technique as well, endodontic treatment should be delayed until sufficient healing has taken place.

Orthodontic procedures

The most common indication for orthodontic extrusion is a fracture of the anterior tooth margin below the crestal bone.[37,38] The clinician should be aware that, because bone and soft tissue attachments follow the tooth during extrusion, crown-lengthening procedures after extrusion are often necessary to achieve the desired clinical crown length and restore the biologic and aesthetic tissue relationships. Ultimately, the purpose of orthodontic extrusion is to erupt the tooth to provide 2 to 3 mm of root length above crestal bone level.

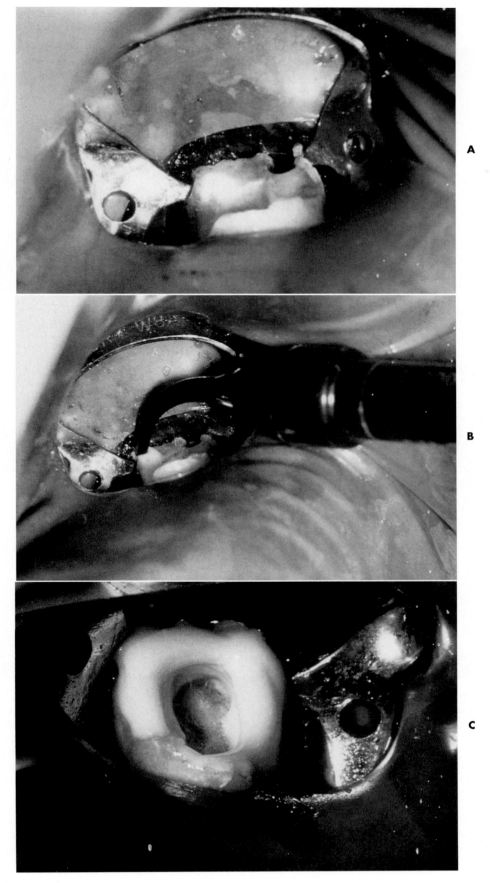

FIG. 5-44 A, Poor isolation because of a severely broken-down tooth. Jaws of the retainer are barely engaging the tooth. **B,** The dentin is etched and bonded using PermaQuik Primer and Bonding Resin. "Donut"-shaped layers of Ultrablend, a light-activated glass ionomer, are added to the bonded resin and incrementally cured. **C,** "Donut" buildup can be accessed for endodontic treatment and can later serve as a matrix for a resin core once the endodontic treatment is completed. *(Courtesy Ultradent Products, South Jordan, Utah.)*

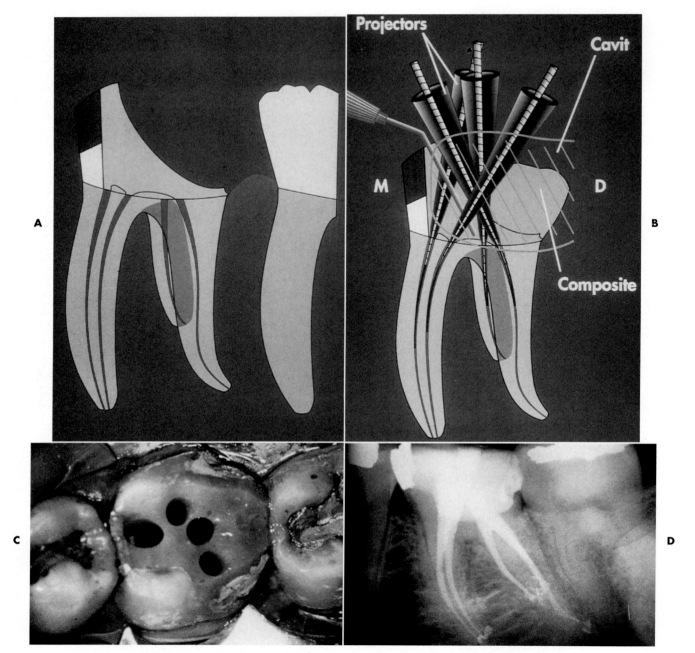

FIG. 5-45 A, Buccal view of severely broken-down mandibular molar with unusual second distal root following caries removal; isolation problems lead to severe leakage. The coronal structures may now be etched and primed before bonding composite projection material into the chamber. Files are selected. **B,** Projectors are placed, files are inserted, and the projectors are slid to the chamber floor using cotton pliers. Since the canals are now occluded, bonding agent is applied to the etched surfaces. A composite core material is injected to the cavosurface using a small-tipped delivery system such as the Centrix syringe. **C,** Occlusal view after removal of files and projectors following composite polymerization. Note the projectors emerged from the chamber floor in their natural orientations: the distobuccal orifice was projected toward the mesial marginal ridge, the distolingual to the center of the occlusal surface, and the mesial canals to either side of the projected distolingual orifice. The risk of contamination has been eliminated, and treatment can now proceed. **D,** Cleaning, shaping, and obturation are completed. An alloy-impregnated resin such as Ketac Silver may be injected directly over the root filling to fill the "created" portion of the projected canal. This creates a unique radiographic appearance in which the root filling flares from the end of the canal to the occlusal surface. *(Courtesy Dr. C. John Munce, Moyco Union Broach Co., York, Pa.)*

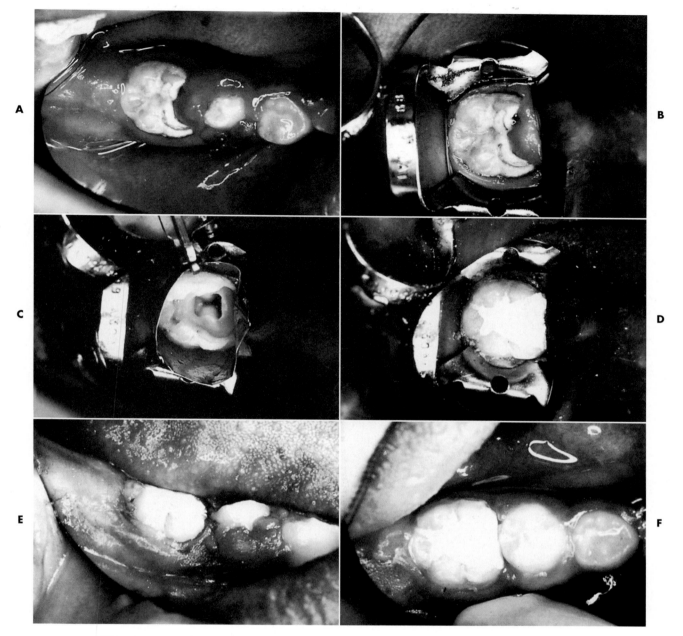

FIG. 5-46 A, Gingival hypertrophy on mandibular molar and erupting premolar of young patient; mandibular molar requires root canal treatment. **B,** Rubber dam clamp impinging on gingival tissues; tissue removed with scalpel. **C,** Automatrix placed immediately following tissue removal; bleeding was minimal. **D,** Placement of Intermediate Restorative Material (IRM) temporary restoration following pulpectomy. **E,** Postoperative facial view immediately following gingivectomy; note hemostasis. **F,** Six-week postoperative occlusal view exhibits fully exposed mandibular molar and recently erupted premolar. *(Courtesy Dr. Robert Roda.)*

REFERENCES

1. American Association of Endodontists: *Endodontics: your guide to endodontic treatment,* Chicago, 1996, The Association.
2. American Dental Association: *OSHA: what you must know,* Chicago, 1992, The Association.
3. American Dental Association: *Statement regarding dental handpieces,* Chicago, 1992, The Association.
4. Antrim DD: Endodontics and the rubber dam: a review of techniques, *J Acad Gen Dent* 31:294, 1983.
5. Baumgartner JC, Heggers JP, Harrison JW: The incidence of bacteremias related to endodontic procedures. I. Nonsurgical endodontics, *J Endod* 2:135, 1976.
6. Bender IB, Seltzer S, Yermish M: The incidence of bacteremia in patients with rheumatic heart disease, *Oral Surg* 13:353, 1960.
7. Bramwell JD, Hicks ML: Solving isolation problems with rubber base adhesive, *J Endod* 12:363, 1986.
8. Centers for Disease Control: Recommended infection control practices for dentistry, *MMWR* 35:237, 1986.

9. Centers for Disease Control: Recommendations for prevention of HIV transmission in health care settings, *MMWR* 36(suppl 2S):1, 1987.

10. Centers for Disease Control: Recommendations for preventing transmission of human immunodeficiency virus and hepatitis B virus to patients during exposure-prone invasive procedures, *MMWR* 40:1, 1991.

11. Centers for Disease Control and Prevention: Guidelines for preventing the transmission of *Mycobacterium tuberculosis* in health care facilities, *Federal Register* 59:54242-54303, 1994.

12. Cochran MA, Miller CH, Sheldrake MA: The efficacy of the rubber dam as a barrier to the spread of microorganisms during dental treatment, *J Am Dent Assoc* 119:141, 1989.

13. Cohen S: Endodontics and litigation: an American perspective, *Int Dent J* 39:13, 1989.

14. Cohen S, Schwartz SF: Endodontic complications and the law, *J Endod* 13:191, 1987.

15. Cohn SA: *Endodontic radiography: principles and clinical techniques,* Gilberts, Ill, 1988, Dunvale Corp.

16. Corah NL, Gale EN, Illig SJ: Assessment of a dental anxiety scale, *J Am Dent Assoc* 97:816, 1978.

17. Cottone JA, Terezhalmy GT, Molinari JA: *Practical infection control in dentistry,* ed 2, Baltimore, 1996, Williams & Wilkins.

18. Council on Dental Materials, Instruments, and Equipment, Council on Dental Practice, Council on Dental Therapeutics: Infection control recommendations for the dental office and the dental laboratory, *J Am Dent Assoc* 116:241, 1988.

19. Dajani AS et al: Prevention of bacterial endocarditis, recommendations by the American Heart Association, *JAMA* 277:1794, 1997.

20. Department of Labor, Occupational Safety and Health Administration, 29 CFR Part 1910.1030: Occupational exposure to bloodborne pathogens, final rule, *Federal Register* 56(235):64004, 1991.

21. Donnelly JC, Hartwell GR, Johnson WB: Clinical evaluation of Ektaspeed x-ray film for use in endodontics, *J Endod* 11:90, 1985.

22. Farman AG, Mendel RW, von Fraunhofer JA: Ultraspeed versus Ektaspeed x-ray film: endodontists' perceptions, *J Endod* 14:615, 1988.

23. Forrest W, Perez RS: The rubber dam as a surgical drape: protection against AIDS and hepatitis, *J Acad Gen Dent* 37:236, 1989.

24. Forsberg J: Radiographic reproduction of endodontic "working length" comparing the paralleling and bisecting-angle techniques, *Oral Surg* 64:353, 1987.

25. Glickman GN: Preparation for treatment. In Cohen S, Burns RC, editors: *Pathways of the pulp,* ed 6, St Louis, 1994, Mosby.

26. Goaz PW, White SC: *Oral radiology: principles and interpretation,* ed 3, St Louis, 1994, Mosby.

27. Goerig AC, Neaverth EJ: A simplified look at the buccal object rule in endodontics, *J Endod* 13:570, 1987.

28. Greene RR, Sikora FA, House JE: Rubber dam application to crownless and cone-shaped teeth, *J Endod* 10:82, 1984.

29. Holroyd SV, Wynn RL, Requa-Clark B: *Clinical pharmacology in the dental practice,* ed 4, St Louis, 1988, Mosby.

30. Jackson DJ, Moore PA, Hargreaves KM: Preoperative nonsteroidal anti-inflammatory medication for the prevention of postoperative dental pain, *J Am Dent Assoc* 119:641, 1989.

31. Janus CE: The rubber dam reviewed, *Compend Contin Dent Ed* 5:155, 1984.

32. Jeffrey IWM, Woolford MJ: An investigation of possible iatrogenic damage caused by metal rubber dam clamps, *Int Endod J* 22:85, 1989.

33. Kantor ML et al: Efficacy of dental radiographic practices: options for image receptors, examination selection, and patient selection, *J Am Dent Assoc* 119:259, 1989.

34. Kelly WH: Radiographic asepsis in endodontic practice, *J Acad Gen Dent* 37:302, 1989.

35. Kolstad RA: *Biohazard control in dentistry,* Dallas, Tex, 1993, Baylor College of Dentistry Press.

36. Little JW et al: *Dental management of the medically compromised patient,* ed 5, St Louis, 1997, Mosby.

37. Lovdahl PE, Gutmann JL: Periodontal and restorative considerations prior to endodontic therapy, *J Acad Gen Dent* 28:38, 1980.

38. Lovdahl PE, Wade CK: Problems in tooth isolation and postendodontic restoration. In Gutmann JL et al, editors: *Problem solving in endodontics: prevention, identification, and management,* ed 3, St Louis, 1997, Mosby.

39. Madison S, Jordan RD, Krell KV: The effects of rubber dam retainers on porcelain-fused-to-metal restorations, *J Endod* 12:183, 1986.

40. Messing JJ, Stock CJR: *Color atlas of endodontics,* St Louis, 1988, Mosby.

41. Miles DA et al: *Radiographic imaging for dental auxiliaries,* Philadelphia, 1989, WB Saunders.

42. Miller CH: Infection control, *Dent Clin North Am* 40:437, 1996.

43. Montgomery EH, Kroeger DC: Principles of anti-infective therapy, *Dent Clin North Am* 28:423, 1984.

44. Mouyen F et al: Presentation and physical evaluation of radiovisiography, *Oral Surg* 68:238, 1989.

45. Pollack BR, editor: *Handbook of dental jurisprudence and risk management,* Littleton, Mass, 1987, PSG Publishing.

46. Requa-Clark B, Holroyd SV: Antiinfective agents. In Holroyd SV, Wynn RL, Requa-Clark B, editors: *Clinical pharmacology in dental practice,* ed 4, St Louis, 1988, Mosby.

47. Richards AG: The buccal object rule, *Dent Radiogr Photogr* 53:37, 1980.

48. Schwartz SF, Foster JK: Roentgenographic interpretation of experimentally produced bony lesions, part I, *Oral Surg* 32:606, 1971.

49. Teplitsky PE: Custom acrylic retainer for endodontic isolation, *J Endod* 14:150, 1988.

50. Torabinejad M et al: Absorbed radiation by various tissues during simulated endodontic radiography, *J Endod* 15:249, 1989.

51. Wakabayashi H et al: A clinical technique for the retention of a rubber dam clamp, *J Endod* 12:422, 1986.

52. Walton RE, Torabinejad M: *Principles and practice of endodontics,* ed 2, Philadelphia, 1996, WB Saunders.

53. Weisman M: A modification of the no. 3 rubber dam clamp, *J Endod* 9:30, 1983.

54. Wood PR: *Cross-infection control in dentistry: a practical illustrated guide,* St Louis, 1992, Mosby.

Chapter 6

Armamentarium and Sterilization

Robert E. Averbach
Donald J. Kleier

Armamentarium

Robert E. Averbach

Endodontic treatment has become a routine facet of comprehensive patient care in many dental practices. General dentists graduating in 1987 or later spend approximately 10% of their workweek providing endodontic care for their patients.[1] The rapidly expanding market for new endodontic products and techniques has produced an extensive array of contemporary approaches to root canal treatment. Although this chapter highlights many of these new trends, it is vitally important to maintain a sound scientific perspective based on biologic principles in navigating this constantly changing sea of ideas. Critical thinking by the clinician, based on independent long-term scientific studies, remains the bedrock of making thoughtful, sound choices while embracing change.

RADIOGRAPHS

Obtaining a high-quality preoperative radiograph is essential before initiating endodontic treatment. As described in Chapter 5, the paralleling technique, using special film holders, produces radiographs with minimal image distortion. Tooth length measurements and diagnostic information from the radiograph tend to be more accurate when the paralleling technique is used.

The radiographs obtained during endodontic treatment pose a different set of problems. These views include root length determination, verification of filling cone placement, and other procedures in which the rubber dam is in place. The rubber dam may make the positioning of these "working" radiographs more difficult. A variety of film holders are available to overcome radiograph distortion problems (Figs. 5-4, 5-12, and 5-15). All these devices are specifically designed to aid in the placement of the film and tube head in proper relationship to the tooth undergoing endodontic treatment. These devices are of considerable value in obtaining an accurate and distortion-free "working film" with files or filling materials placed within the tooth and with the rubber dam in place.

The choice of dental x-ray film for endodontic radiographs is shifting from Ultraspeed* to Ektaspeed,* since Ektaspeed is twice as fast and consequently requires one-half the x-ray exposure. Although it may be more grainy and demonstrate less contrast compared to Ultraspeed film, careful attention to exposure and processing variables produces an image of good

*Eastman Kodak Company, Rochester, N.Y.

diagnostic quality. The use of a rapid, automated film processor is helpful in producing high-quality films. Daylight loading, manual quick-processing boxes are also useful for "working" radiographs (Fig. 6-1).

Radiovisiography uses a conventional dental x-ray unit and a microprocessor. An intraoral radiation detector, more sensitive than conventional silver halide films, is used in place of radiographic film. The combination of the highly sensitive intraoral sensor (charged-coupling device) and the precision microprocessor results in a dramatic reduction in radiation. In addition, the displayed image may be altered by the computer control, enhancing and enlarging details and converting negative to positive images. Illustrations and a more complete explanation of these new high-technology digital radiography systems are found in Chapter 5.

DIAGNOSIS

The armamentarium for diagnosis has been detailed in Chapter 1. The technology of pulp testing continues to become more sophisticated and reliable. Examination techniques for disclosing tooth fractures with a fiberoptic light source have been shown in Chapter 1. This transillumination technique is also of value in determining the extent of a pulpal "blush" following extensive tooth preparation. The operatory lights are dimmed, and the transilluminator is placed on the lingual surface of the preparation (Fig. 6-2).

The technique of detecting a cracked tooth by wedging cusps with a cotton roll, cotton-wood stick, or the equivalent has been described in Chapter 1. An additional wedging modality for the diagnosis of fractured teeth is the "Tooth Slooth" pictured in Fig. 6-3, *A*. This plastic device is used as a selective wedge on or between the cusps as the patient bites. Yet another technique for fracture diagnosis is the use of a rubber wheel to simulate chewing on a bolus of food (Fig. 6-3, *B*). Sharp pain on *release* of biting pressure often indicates a cracked tooth.

LIGHT AND MAGNIFICATION

The use of high-quality magnification while practicing dentistry is growing rapidly, and users are convinced that magnification improves both the quality and speed of treatment.[6] Adding a headlight to the system of surgical telescopes significantly enhances both depth of field and magnified resolution, greatly increasing visual acuity. The headlight provides line of sight illumination, which is shadowless and also avoids multiple adjustments to the traditional overhead dental operating light. The combination of light and magnification is especially useful in endodontics, as the clinician often operates in inaccessible areas

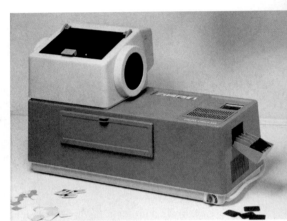

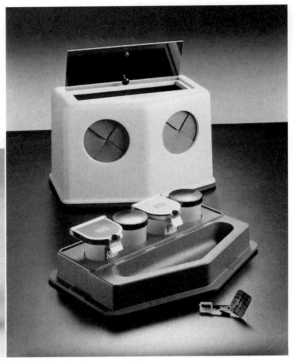

FIG. 6-1 A, Peri-Pro III film processor. *(Courtesy Air Techniques Inc., Hicksville, N.Y.)*
B, Rapid-processing box. *(Courtesy ASI Medical, Englewood, Colo.)*

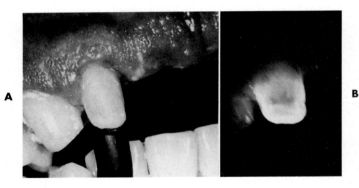

FIG. 6-2 Transillumination of pulpal "blush." **A,** Transillumination of lingual of full crown preparation. **B,** Operatory lights out—demonstration of "blush."

searching for elusive targets such as calcified root canals, following the completion of endodontic access. It is not uncommon to hear clinicians remark, once they have tried working with additional light and magnification, "How did I ever practice dentistry without these?" Although operating using magnification requires a brief learning period, most clinicians comment that returning to unaided vision is a distinct handicap. The most popular surgical telescopes provide magnification in the 2.0× to 3.5× range, with average working distances of 14 to 16 inches. They retain a very adequate clinical depth of field. Examples of some of the more popular light and magnification systems can be found in Fig. 6-4.

The use of the surgical operating microscope in endodontics has become the next logical extension of the operating theory of enhanced light and magnification. Although initially introduced to aid a variety of endodontic surgical procedures, the operating microscope is finding more and more utilization for problematic nonsurgical endodontic approaches such as removal of posts, fracture diagnosis, and endodontic retreatment. Surgical operating microscopes offer a wide range of magnification, usually from 4× to 25×. More detailed information about surgical operating microscopes is found in Chapter 18.

ORGANIZATION SYSTEMS

The trend toward preset trays and cassettes in endodontics has simplified and streamlined the organization, storage, and delivery of endodontic instruments. Particular instruments and tray setups are the choice of the individual clinician, but certain basic principles are common to all systems. A standard cassette contains the most used long-handled instruments, such as mouth mirror, endodontic explorer, long spoon excavator, plastic instrument, and locking forceps. These are often supplemented by items such as irrigating syringe and needles, ruler, sterile paper points, burs, and rubber dam clamps. A sample cassette setup is shown in Fig. 6-5. A wide variety of file stands and file boxes are now available, facilitating organizational simplicity and sterility (Fig. 6-6). Whatever system is chosen, the emphasis is on keeping the setup easy for the staff to restock and sterilize and convenient for the clinician, whether he or she is working alone or with a chairside assistant.

RUBBER DAM

Rubber dam isolation is the standard of care in endodontics, yet a recent national survey revealed that only 59% of general dentists always use the rubber dam for endodontics, compared with more than 92% of practicing endodontists.[30]

Text continued on p. 123

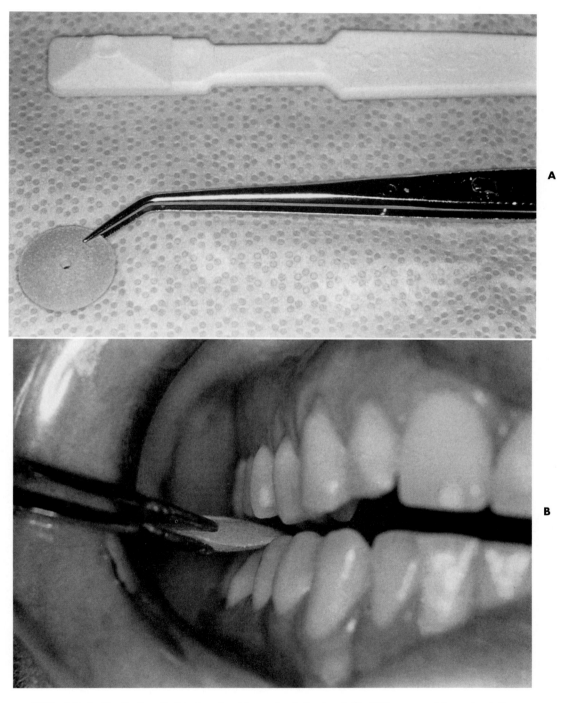

FIG. 6-3 A, Tooth Slooth *(top)* and rubber wheel *(bottom).* **B,** Biting on rubber wheel for cracked tooth diagnosis.

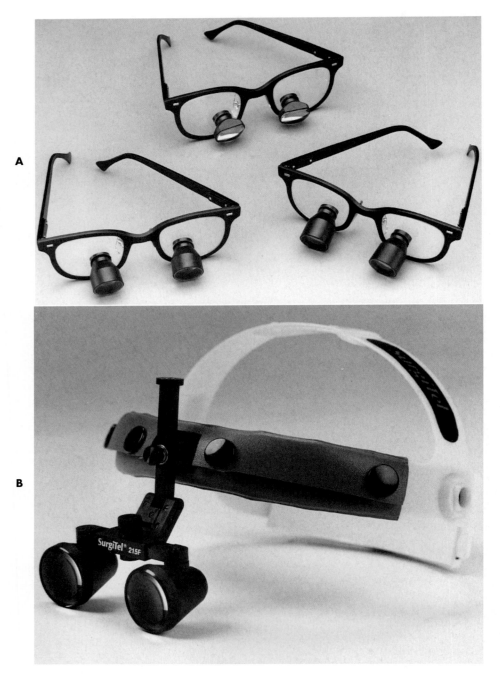

FIG. 6-4 A, Surgical telescopes. *(Courtesy Designs for Vision, Ronkonkoma, N.Y.)* **B,** Surgical telescopes on headband. *(Courtesy SurgiTel, Ann Arbor, Mich.)*

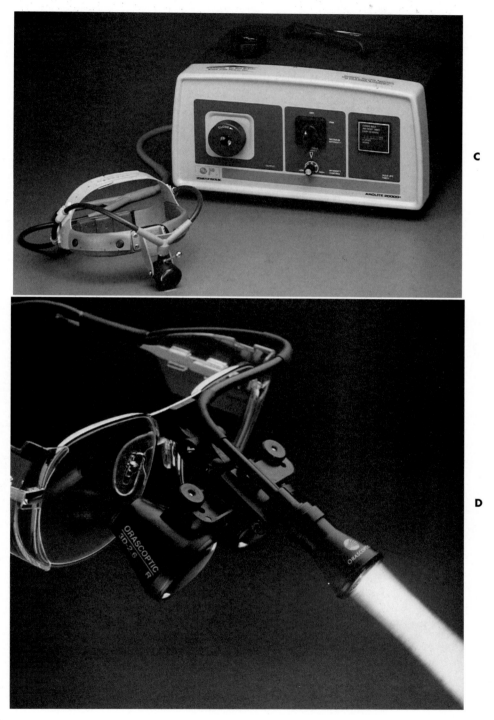

FIG. 6-4, cont'd C, Headlight system. *(Courtesy Designs for Vision, Ronkonkoma, N.Y.)*
D, Surgical telescopes plus headlight. *(Courtesy Orascoptic, Madison, Wis.)*

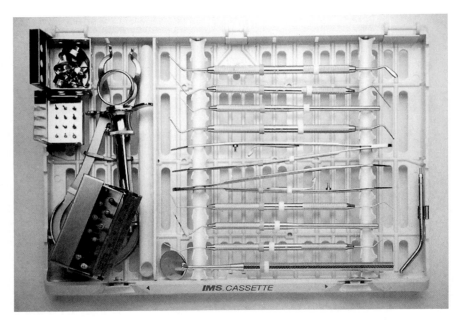

FIG. 6-5 IMS instrument cassette. *(Courtesy Hu-Friedy Co., Chicago, Ill.)*

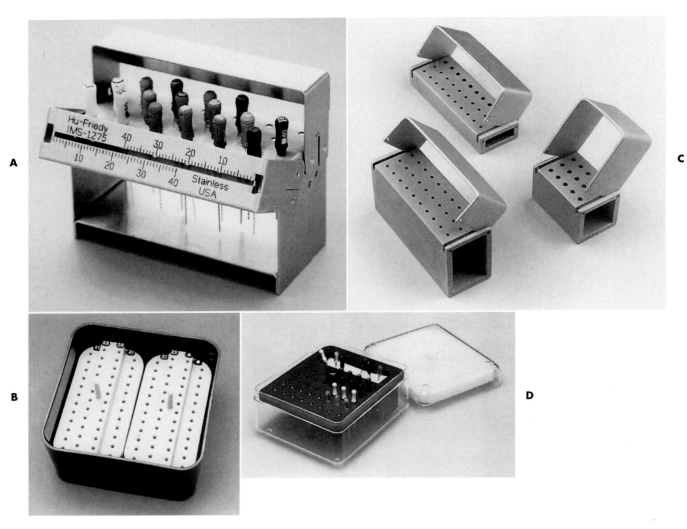

FIG. 6-6 A, File stand. *(Courtesy Hu-Friedy Co., Chicago, Ill.)* **B,** File stand. *(Courtesy Premier Dental Products, Norristown, Pa.)* **C,** File stand. *(Courtesy Brasseler USA, Savannah, Ga.)* **D,** File stand. *(Courtesy Caulk/Dentsply, Milford, Del.)*

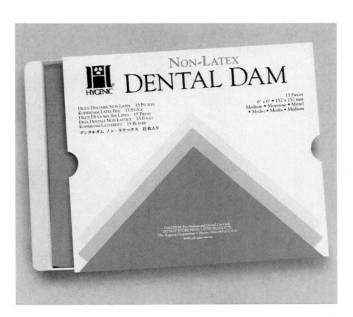

FIG. 6-7 Nonlatex dam. *(Courtesy Hygenic Corp., Akron, Ohio.)*

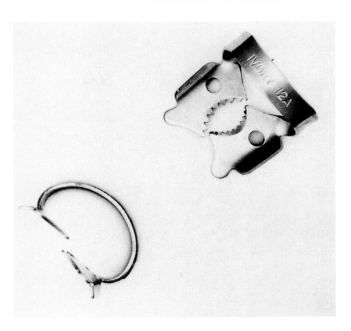

FIG. 6-8 Ivory "tiger-jaw" serrated rubber dam clamp. *(Courtesy Miles Dental Products, South Bend, Ind.)*

This important point must be reemphasized: teeth undergoing endodontic treatment should always be isolated with a rubber dam unless the clinical situation makes this approach physically impossible.

Rubber dam material for endodontic treatment is currently available in a variety of colors, thicknesses, scents, and materials. With the increased recognition of latex allergies, the traditional latex rubber dam has been supplemented by the availability of nonlatex dam material.[27] This nonlatex product is a synthetic elastomeric material that is 100% latex free and powder free (Fig. 6-7). The tear resistance is reportedly similar to latex, and the new product has a minimum 3-year shelf life.

When using a traditional latex rubber dam, many clinicians prefer the medium or lightweight dam material, citing its increased resilience and ease of application. Color is also a matter of personal preference. Dark-colored dam material provides sharp contrast between the tooth and dam, while the light-colored dam permits visualization of the x-ray film holder's position when a working radiograph is being exposed. Options include green dam scented with wintergreen and royal blue, which yields good visual contrast plus "eye appeal." Regardless of which color or thickness is chosen, all dam material should be stored away from strong heat and light to prevent the latex from drying and becoming less flexible. Tearing of the dam on application usually indicates the material is dried out and should be discarded. Refrigeration of dam material seems to extend its shelf life.

An almost endless array of rubber dam clamps are available to isolate special problem situations. The "tiger-jaw" clamps (Fig. 6-8) are especially useful for retaining the dam on broken-down posterior teeth. The winged style of clamp is preferred, since it provides better tissue retraction and allows the use of the "unit" placement technique described in Chapter 5.

Any good-quality rubber dam punch will accomplish the goal of creating a clean hole for the tooth. Care must be taken to punch a hole without "nicks" in the rim to prevent acciden-

tal tearing and leakage. Small leaks can be conveniently patched using OraSeal, a flexible, puttylike product packaged in a plastic syringe (Fig. 6-9). A radiolucent plastic rubber dam frame eliminates the need for removing the frame while exposing "working" radiographs.

ACCESS PREPARATION THROUGH A CROWN

Gaining access through a porcelain-fused-to-metal crown is more difficult than gaining access through natural tooth structure or other restorative materials. One approach is to use a small round diamond with copious water spray to create the outline form in the porcelain. The metal substructure is then penetrated with either a tungsten-tipped or new carbide end-cutting bur (Fig. 6-10). This two-stage technique reduces the possibility of porcelain fracture or chipping.

Uncovering receded or calcified root canal orifices is often a challenge. A useful adjunct for these types of problems is the use of low-speed Mueller burs. These burs have an extra long, flexible shaft that allows visualization by the operator as the bur advances into the deeper portions of the access preparation. A clinical case illustrating their use can be found in Fig. 6-11.

HAND INSTRUMENTS

A sample cassette for endodontics is shown in Fig. 6-5. The long, double-ended spoon excavator is specifically designed for endodontic therapy. It allows the clinician to remove coronal pulp tissue, caries, or cotton pellets that may be deep in the tooth's crown (Fig. 6-12). The double-ended endodontic explorer is used to locate and probe the orifice of the root canal as it joins the pulp chamber (Fig. 6-13). Locking endodontic forceps facilitate the transfer of paper points and gutta-percha cones from assistant to dentist (Fig. 6-14). Plastic filling instruments are designed to place and condense temporary restorations (Fig. 6-15). A periodontal probe completes the basic setup.

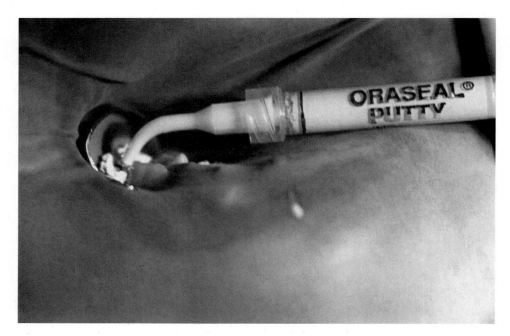

FIG. 6-9 OraSeal may be placed around leaking rubber dam.

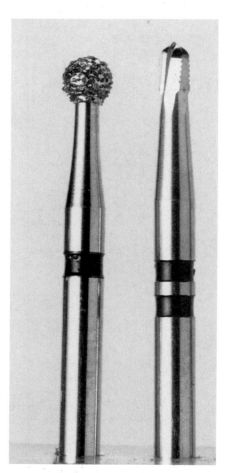

FIG. 6-10 Round diamond and carbide bur for porcelain-fused-to-metal crown access. *(Courtesy Brasseler USA, Savannah, Ga.)*

CANAL PREPARATION

Techniques for determining the "working length" of the root canal before instrumentation are detailed in Chapter 8. Measuring blocks and special millimeter thumb rulers are useful to manually set silicone stops (Fig. 6-16). The use of electronic apex locators as an adjunct to radiographic length determination is becoming more accepted (Fig. 6-17). As they improve, the accuracy of these devices is becoming more predictable.[9,15]

Cleaning, shaping, and sealing of the root canal, as described in Chapters 8 and 9, are primary components of clinical success. The barbed broach is used primarily for the gross removal of pulp tissue from large canals (Fig. 6-18). The disposable broach is inserted into the canal and rotated to engage the tissue. Because these instruments are fragile and prone to breakage, great care must be exercised in their use. The most commonly used hand instruments in canal preparation are endodontic files. Introduction of new file designs and metals has increased dramatically during the past few years. Triangular, square, and rhomboid blanks are usually used in the manufacturing of these hand instruments. Variations in metallurgy, taper, cutting blade angle, degree of twist, flute spacing, and cutting or noncutting tip have complicated the clinician's choice of instruments (Fig. 6-19). In addition, there is recent evidence to suggest that flexible nickel-titanium files, when compared to files of stainless steel, may produce more consistent root canal preparations.[12,13,26] A detailed description of these file variations is found in Chapter 14.

The use of automated handpiece systems for canal preparation is accelerating with the introduction of nickel-titanium, engine-driven files. One of the more popular mechanized systems is illustrated in Fig. 6-20. Other contemporary nickel-titanium rotary instruments include the LightSpeed system and the Quantec Series 2000. Although the engine-driven systems differ in file design, taper, and flute angle, certain characteristics are common to all these devices. Conceptually, they all use nickel-titanium's unique ability to follow canal curvature, a very low-speed high-torque handpiece system, and full 360-

Text continued on p. 133

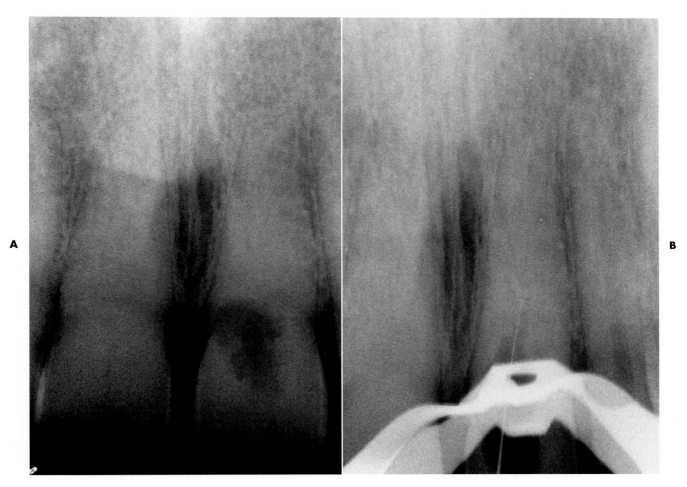

FIG. 6-11 Mueller burs. **A,** Preoperative radiograph—calcified canal. **B,** Initial file penetration following access.

Continued

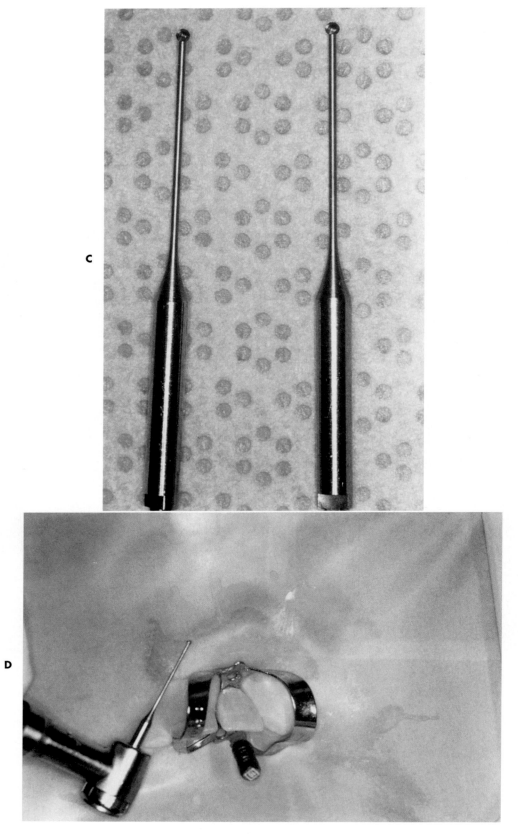

FIG. 6-11, cont'd C, Mueller burs. **D,** File penetration after use of Mueller bur.

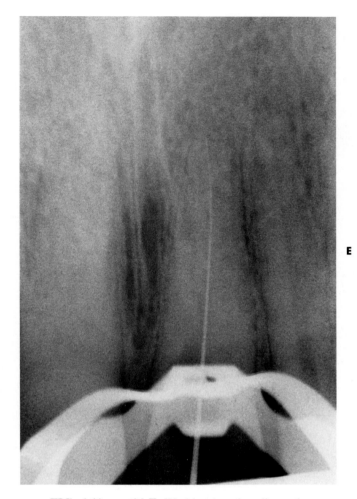

E

FIG. 6-11, cont'd E, Working length radiograph.

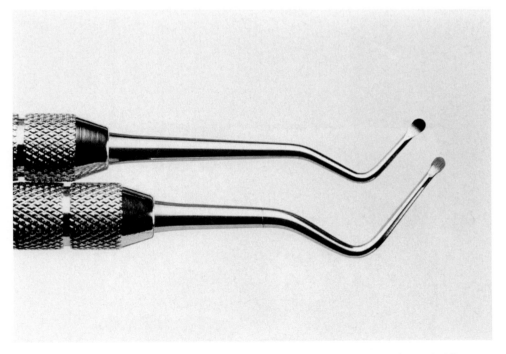

FIG. 6-12 Operative spoon excavator *(top)* and Endo Spoon excavator *(bottom). (Courtesy Brasseler USA, Savannah, Ga.)*

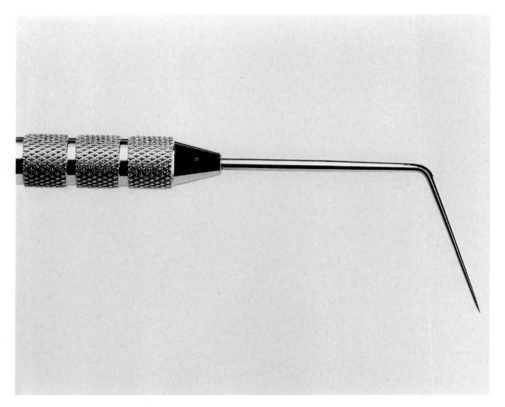

FIG. 6-13 Endodontic explorer. *(Courtesy Brasseler USA, Savannah, Ga.)*

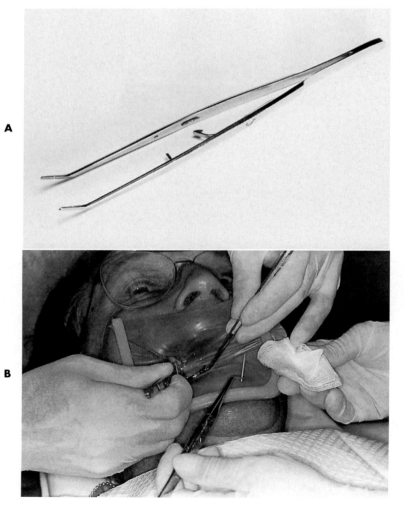

FIG. 6-14 A, Locking forceps. *(Courtesy Brasseler USA, Savannah, Ga.)* **B,** Locking forceps transfer of paper points.

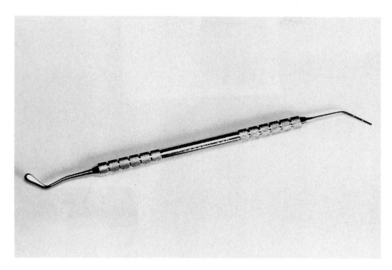

FIG. 6-15 Instrument for placement of temporary seal. *(Courtesy Brasseler USA, Savannah, Ga.)*

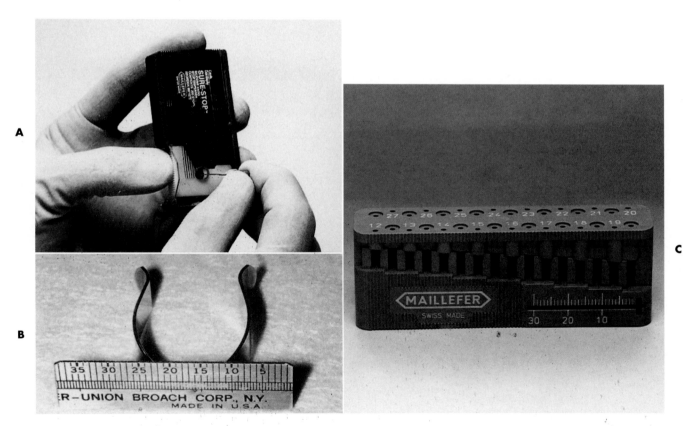

FIG. 6-16 **A,** Silicone stop dispenser. *(Courtesy Caulk/Dentsply, Milford, Del.)* **B,** Millimeter thumb ruler. **C,** Measuring block. *(Courtesy Caulk/Dentsply, Milford, Del.)*

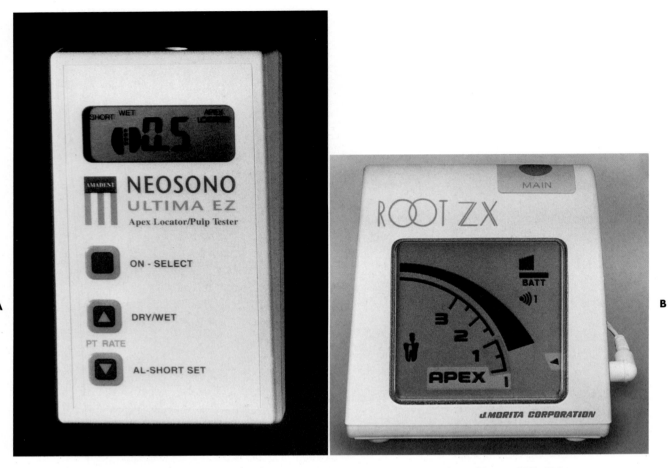

FIG. 6-17 Electronic apex locators. **A,** Neosono. *(Courtesy Amadent, Cherry Hill, N.J.)*
B, Root ZX. *(Courtesy J. Morita USA, Tustin, Calif.)*

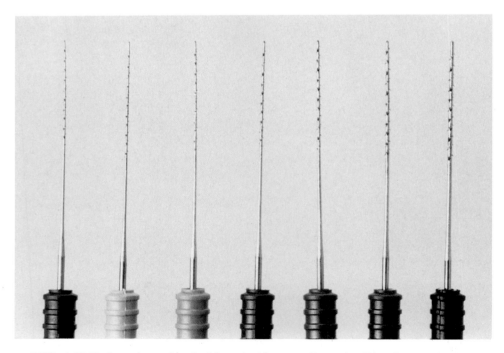

FIG. 6-18 Various sizes of barbed broach. *(Courtesy Brasseler USA, Savannah, Ga.)*

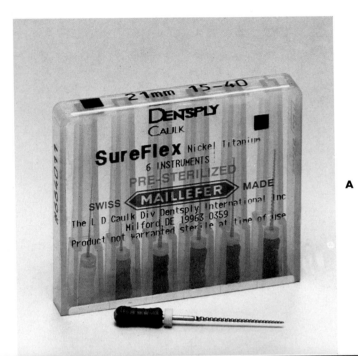

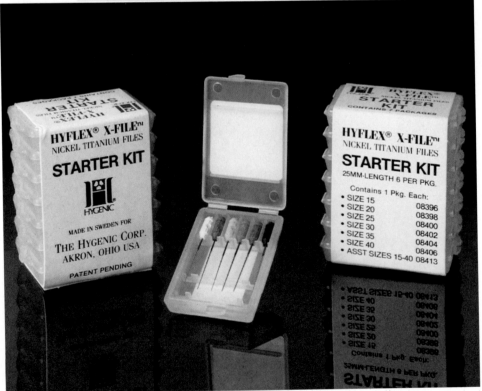

FIG. 6-19 Various endodontic files. **A,** SureFlex. *(Courtesy Caulk/Dentsply, Milford, Del.)*
B, Hyflex. *(Courtesy Hygenic Corp., Akron, Ohio.)*

Continued

FIG. 6-19 cont'd C, Files of Greater Taper. *(Courtesy Tulsa Dental Products, Tulsa, Okla.)*

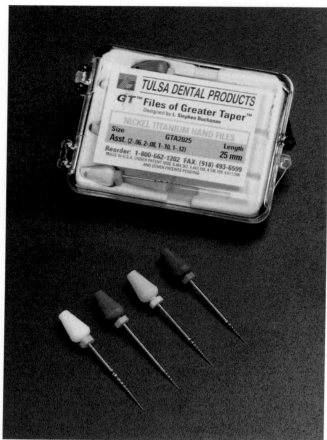

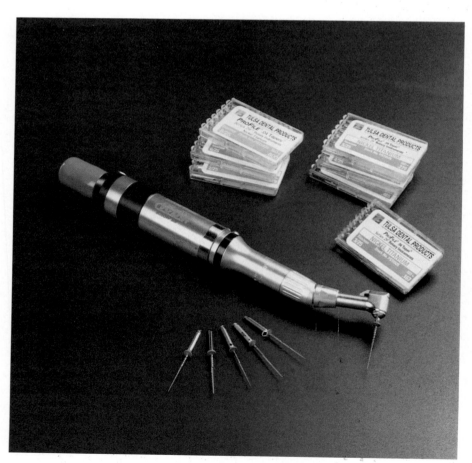

FIG. 6-20 ProFile 0.04 taper system. *(Courtesy Tulsa Dental Products, Tulsa, Okla.)*

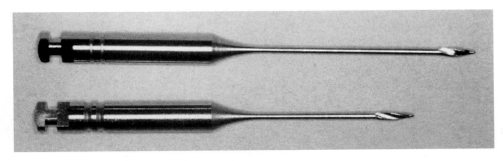

FIG. 6-21 Regular and short Gates-Glidden drills.

degree file rotation, as opposed to an oscillatory movement. All systems should be used with a light touch (the same pressure as applied to writing with a sharp-tipped lead pencil) and minimal apical pressure to avoid instrument breakage. The emphasis is on preflaring of the upper portion of the root canal to allow more control in the preparation of the apical third. Clinical studies on these various systems are demonstrating the ability of this new technology to provide smooth, clean canal walls while maintaining natural anatomic curvatures.[14,25]

The use of sonic and ultrasonic systems as adjuncts in refining canal preparations seems to be increasing. All these devices more or less share certain basic principles that allow the instrument to flush and clean the canal while maintaining much of the natural root curvature (see Chapter 8). The devices oscillate or vibrate at various frequencies when energized. The energy is then transferred to the intracanal instruments used to flare and smooth canal walls. No actual rotation of the instrument is used, thus theoretically preserving the canal shape and natural anatomic apical constriction. In addition, all the sonic and ultrasonic devices deliver copious streams of irrigant into the canal space during use, providing enhanced flushing action and debris removal.[20]

Conventional rotary instruments are used primarily as flaring devices for the coronal portion of the canal. The most commonly used is the Gates-Glidden drill, now available in a short version to facilitate use in posterior teeth (Fig. 6-21). Sized in increasing diameters from No. 1 through No. 6, the Gates-Glidden drill should be used in a passive manner to enlarge the canal orifice and flare the root canal. The use of excessive force may either perforate the canal or fracture the instrument. The Gates-Glidden drill is designed to break high on the shaft if excessive resistance is encountered, allowing the clinician to easily remove the fragment. Other types of rotary orifice openers are pictured in Fig. 6-22.

IRRIGATION

Irrigation of the canal during instrumentation is described in Chapter 8. Systems for the delivery of irrigating solution into the root canal range from simple disposable syringes to complex devices capable of irrigating and aspirating simultaneously. The choice for the clinician is one of convenience and cost. The smaller syringe barrels (less than 10 ml) require frequent refilling during the instrumentation phase of therapy. Plastic syringes in the 10- to 20-ml range may offer the best combination of sufficient solution volume and ease of handling. "Backfilling" of the syringe from a 500-ml laboratory plastic wash bottle filled with the irrigant of choice, saves time and effort over aspirating the solution into the barrel from a container (Fig. 6-23). The barrel tip should be a Luer-Lok de-

sign rather than friction fit, to prevent accidental needle dislodgment during irrigation.

A new design of irrigating needle tip is shown in Fig. 6-24. This design helps prevent the accidental forcing of irrigating solution into the periapical tissues should the needle bind in the canal and has been reported to provide superior apical third irrigation compared to other styles.[20]

Various sizes of paper points are available to dry the canal following irrigation. Paper points are used sequentially in the locking forceps until no moisture is evident on the paper point. Presterilized "cell" packaging is preferred over bulk packaging to maintain asepsis (Fig. 6-25).

OBTURATION

Most root canal filling methods employ root canal sealer as an integral part of the obturation technique. The most popular class of sealer cements used in endodontics are based on zinc oxide–eugenol formulations. These products require a glass slab and cement spatula for mixing to the desired consistency. Sealers containing calcium hydroxide are also available. Root canal obturation techniques are discussed in Chapter 9. Gutta-percha is the best and the most commonly used canal filling material in contemporary endodontics. Gutta-percha is available as standardized cones corresponding to the approximate size of root canal instruments (Nos. 15 to 140). Nonstandardized cones are more tapered and are designated in size from extra fine through extra large. The two styles are compared in Fig. 6-26.

Specialized hand instruments used in obturating the root canal with gutta-percha include spreaders and pluggers. Spreaders are available in a wide variety of lengths and tapers and are used primarily in the lateral condensation technique to compact gutta-percha filling material. Nickel-titanium spreaders offer increased flexibility compared with stainless steel (Fig. 6-27). Pluggers, also called condensers, are flat ended rather than pointed and are used primarily to compact filling materials in a vertical fashion. A nickel-titanium rotary instrument for the removal of compacted gutta-percha is available (Fig. 6-28). This device breaks up and removes gutta-percha from the canal, facilitating retreatment procedures.

On the "high-technology" front, devices for the heating, delivery, and compaction of gutta-percha into the prepared root canal are now available. A detailed description of these systems is found in Chapter 9. Examples of these warm gutta-percha systems are shown in Fig. 6-29. Controversy abounds concerning the purported superiority of one system versus another.[10,18]

Temporary restorative materials used in endodontics must provide a high-quality seal of the access preparation to prevent microbial contamination of the root canal. Premixed products such as Cavit and TERM have become popular for

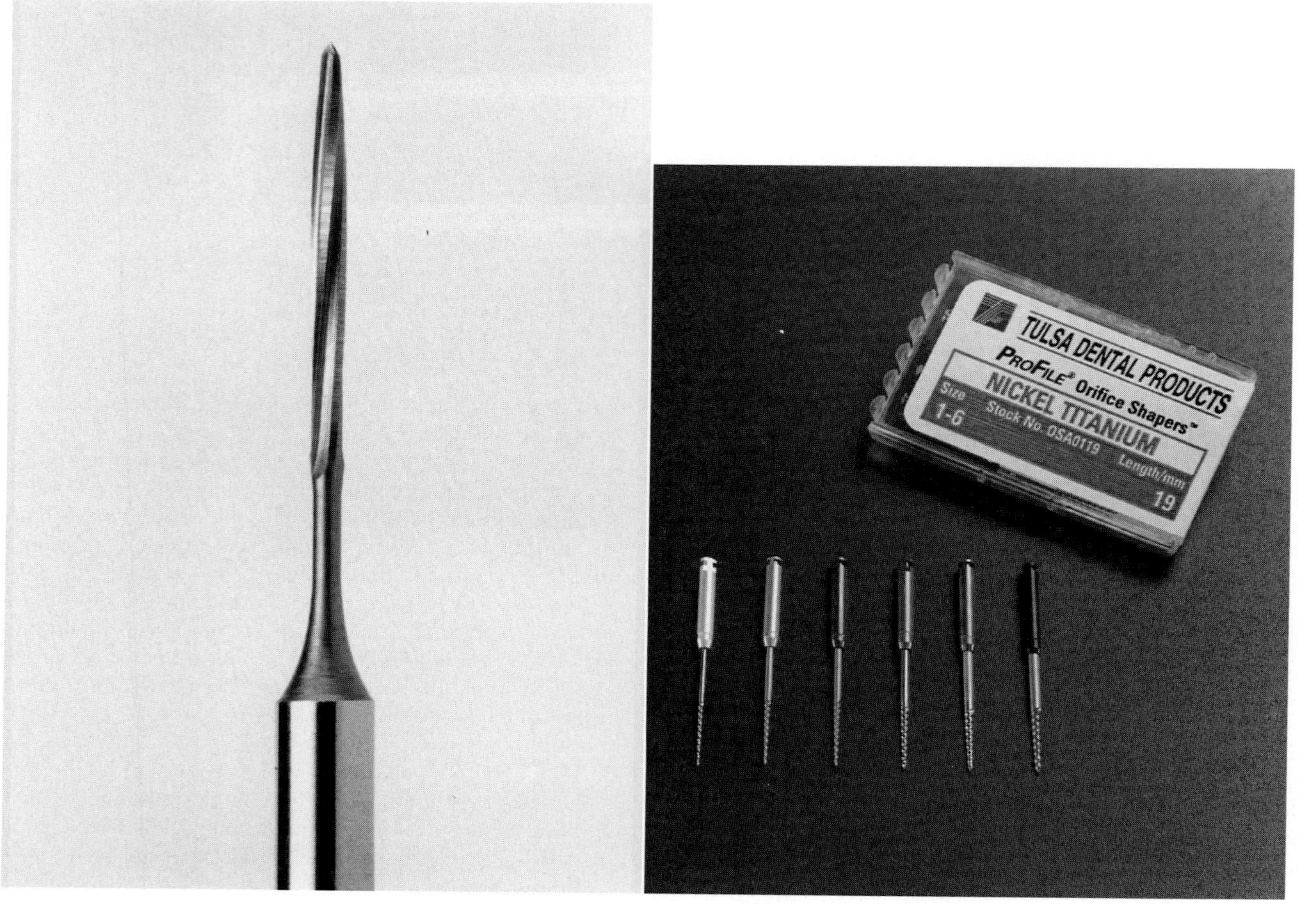

FIG. 6-22 A, Orifice opener bur. *(Courtesy Brasseler USA, Savannah, Ga.)* **B,** ProFile orifice shapers. *(Courtesy Tulsa Dental Products, Tulsa, Okla.)*

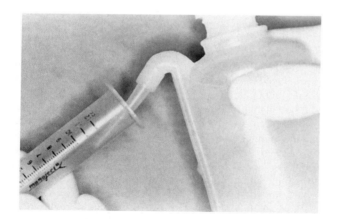

FIG. 6-23 Backfilling of irrigation syringe from wash bottle.

temporary access cavity sealing. Cavit (Fig. 6-30) is a moisture-initiated, autopolymerized, premixed calcium sulfate–polyvinyl chloride acetate, whereas TERM is a visible light-initiated, composite-like product whose main component is urethane dimethacrylate polymer. A recent study comparing the sealing ability of Cavit, TERM, and IRM reported that under the experimental conditions, Cavit provided superior resistance to bacterial leakage.[4]

Sterilization

Donald J. Kleier

As the science of infection control has advanced, permanent changes have occurred in the dental office. This is also true in dental offices where endodontic therapy is practiced. The dentist has a significant responsibility for the health of patients, employees, and co-workers. In addition to infection control changes in the office, dentists must modify their health history procedures to reflect a changed attitude about infectious disease. Questioning patients about infectious diseases and health history responses is an essential part of understanding the patient's health status.[16]

The concept of universal precautions has been adopted by health care facilities because of the inability to distinguish between contagious and noncontagious patients. Furthermore, some patients decide to not disclose their infectious disease status.[21] This section of the chapter examines some of the basics of infection control as it relates to the theory and practice of universal precautions.

VACCINATION

Although acquired immunodeficiency syndrome (AIDS) is of concern to dental health care workers, the risk of contracting hepatitis B is far greater. A recent study conducted by the Centers for Disease Control and Prevention reported that

Text continued on p. 140

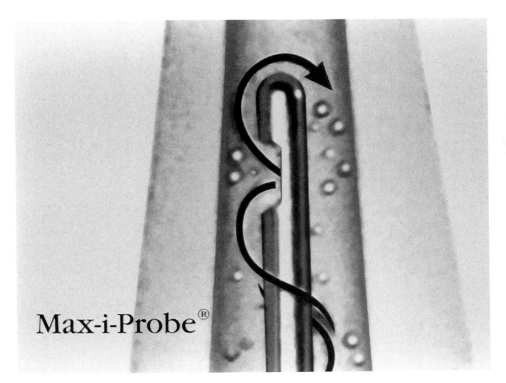

FIG. 6-24 Max-I-Probe irrigating needle. *(Courtesy MPL Technologies, Franklin Park, Ill.)*

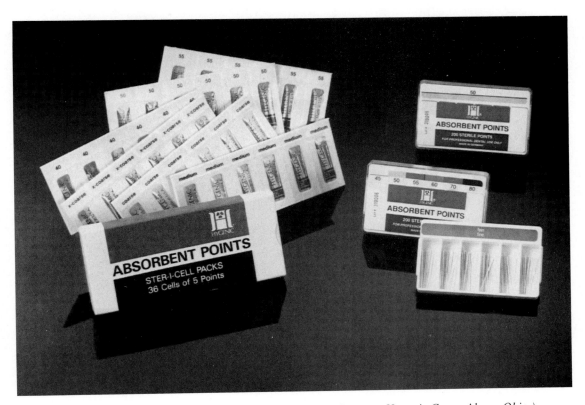

FIG. 6-25 Paper point—bulk versus "cell" packaging. *(Courtesy Hygenic Corp., Akron, Ohio.)*

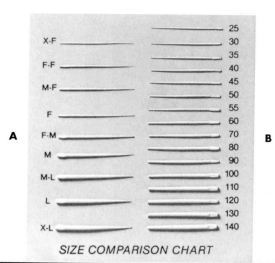

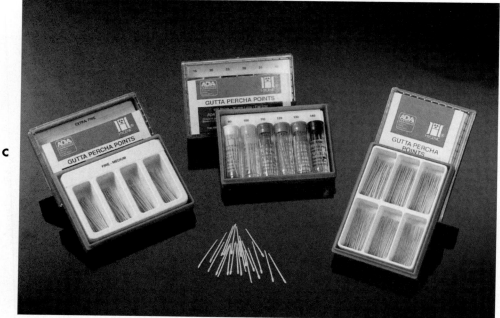

FIG. 6-26 Nonstandardized **(A)** versus standardized **(B)** gutta-percha cones. *(Courtesy Hygenic Corp., Akron, Ohio.)* **C,** Packaging of gutta-percha cones.

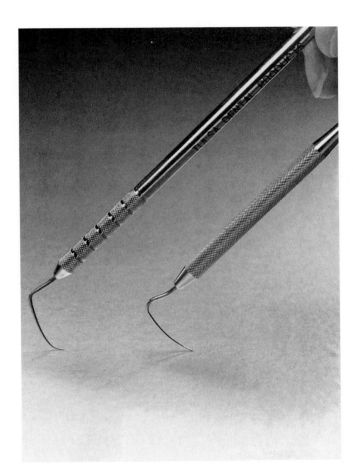

FIG. 6-27 Nickel-titanium spreader *(top)* versus stainless steel spreader *(bottom)* showing different tip flexibility. *(Courtesy Tulsa Dental Products, Tulsa, Okla.)*

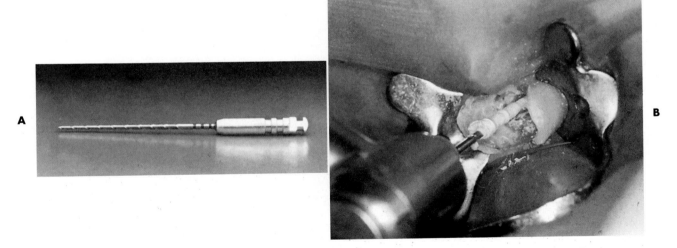

FIG. 6-28 A, GPX gutta-percha remover. *(Courtesy Brasseler USA, Savannah, Ga.)* **B,** Gutta-percha being removed by GPX.

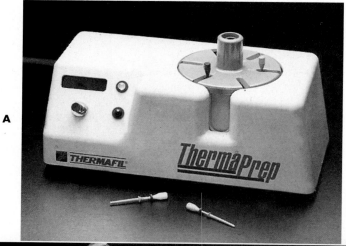

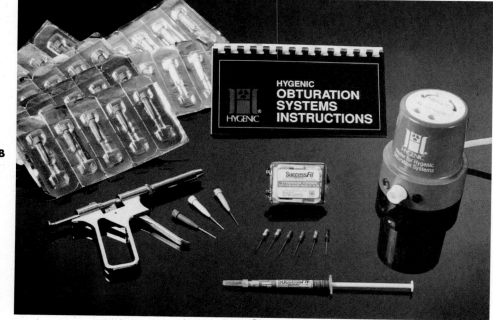

FIG. 6-29 Warm gutta-percha systems. **A,** ThermaPrep oven for heating Thermafil obturators. *(Courtesy Tulsa Dental Products, Tulsa, Okla.)* **B,** UltraFil and SuccessFil systems. *(Courtesy Hygenic Corp., Akron, Ohio.)*

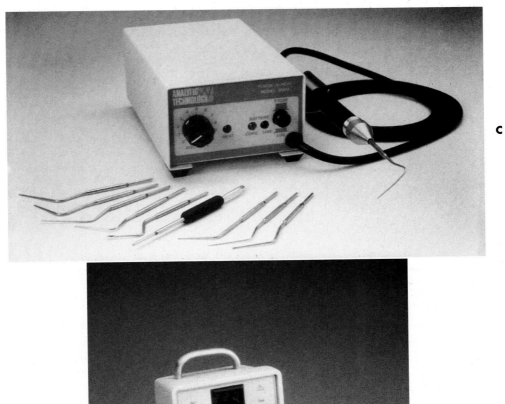

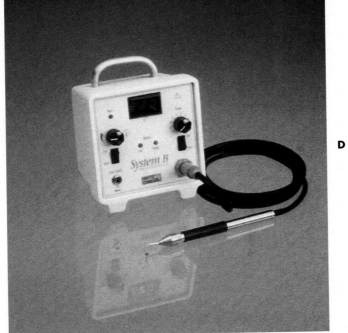

FIG. 6-29, cont'd C, Touch 'N Heat. *(Courtesy EIE/Analytic Technology, San Diego, Calif.)*
D, System B. *(Courtesy EIE/Analytic Technology, San Diego, Calif.)*

hepatitis B vaccination among dentists increased substantially from 1983 to 1992 and that serologic evidence of hepatitis B virus (HBV) infection decreased. These findings support continued emphasis on early vaccination of dental health care workers.[7]

BARRIER TECHNIQUES

The Occupational Safety and Health Administration (OSHA) requires that dentists follow infection control guidelines established by the Centers for Disease Control and Prevention.[11] These guidelines define the use of universal precautions to prevent cross-contamination while treating patients. The most effective method of preventing cross-contamination is the use of personal and environmental barrier techniques (Fig. 6-31). Dentists are increasing their use of gloves, masks, eyewear, and protective clothing.[16] While performing endodontic therapy, however, some general dentists fail to take advantage of protection from sodium hypochlorite irrigating solution afforded by using the rubber dam.[30]

DEFINITION OF TERMS

The purpose of this section is to help clarify certain terms that are used in reference to office infection control.

Aerosols: Fine moisture droplets and debris generated by high-speed dental equipment. This material is usually 5 μm or less in size, can remain suspended in air, and penetrate deep into the lungs. Pathogenic bacteria have been found associated with aerosol droplets.
Bacterial Spore Form (Endospore): A more complex structure than the vegetative cell from which it forms. Spores form in response to environmental conditions and are more highly resistant to sterilization methods than vegetative forms.
Bacterial Vegetative Form: Active, multiplying microorganisms.
Biofilm: The colonization and proliferation of microorganisms at a surface-solution interface. Especially problematic in the small-bore water lines of dental units.
Biologic Indicator: A preparation of microorganisms, usually bacterial spores, that serves as a challenge to the efficiency of a given sterilization process or cycle. Negative bacterial growth from a biologic indicator verifies sterilization.
Cross-Infection: Transmission of infectious material from one person to another.

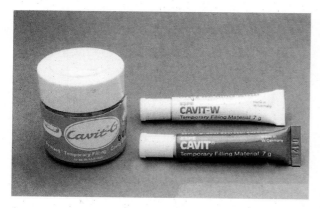

FIG. 6-30 Cavit-G and Cavit temporary filling materials. *(Courtesy Premier Dental Products Co., Norristown, Pa.)*

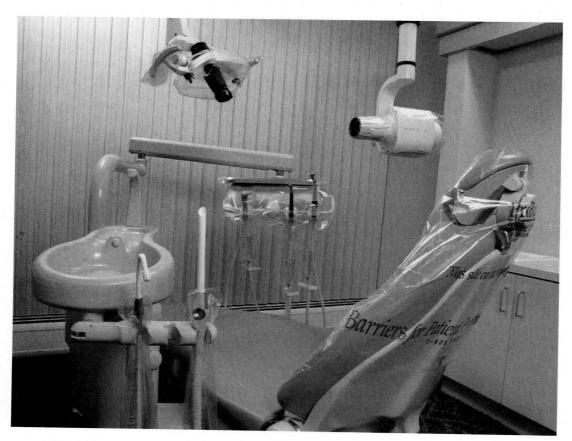

FIG. 6-31 Operatory plastic film barriers in place. *(Courtesy Cottrell Ltd., Englewood, Colo.)*

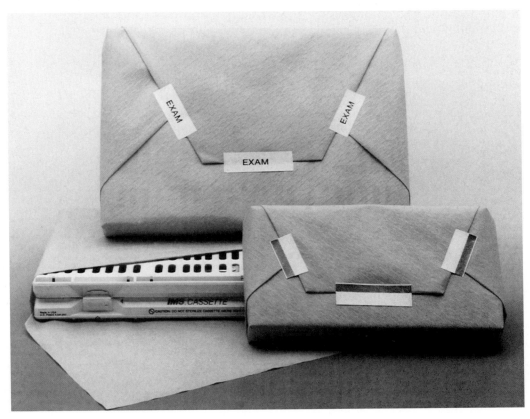

FIG. 6-32 Cassette wrapped in porous autoclave paper in preparation for sterilization. *(Courtesy Hu-Friedy Co., Chicago, Ill.)*

Disinfection: A less lethal process than sterilization. It eliminates virtually all pathogenic vegetative microorganisms but not necessarily all microbial forms (spores). This process usually is reserved for large environmental surfaces that cannot be sterilized (e.g., a dental chair). Disinfection lacks the margin of safety achieved by sterilization procedures. Disinfection is nonverifiable.

Pathogenic Microorganism: A microorganism that causes or is associated with disease.

Process Indicator: Strip, tape, or tab applied to or packaged in a sterilizer load. Special inks or chemicals within the indicator change color when subjected to heat, steam, or chemical vapor and indicate that the indicator has been cycled through the sterilizer. Process indicators do *not* verify sterilization.

Sterilization: The use of a physical or chemical procedure to destroy all microbial life, including highly resistant bacterial endospores. Sterilization is a verifiable procedure.

Universal Precautions: The same infection control procedures are used for all patients regardless of medical history.

Virus: An extremely small agent that grows and reproduces only in living host cells. The virus particle consists of a central core of nucleic acid and an outer coat of protein. It is generally agreed that virus particles are much *less* resistant to thermal inactivation than bacterial spores.[5]

INSTRUMENT PREPARATION

The preoperative handling, cleaning, and packaging of contaminated instruments are frequently sources of injury and possible infection. Dental staff performing such procedures should wear reusable heavy rubber work gloves similar to household cleaning gloves. Contaminated instruments that will not be cleaned immediately should be placed in a holding solution so that blood, saliva, and tissue do not dry on the instrument surfaces. Ultrasonic cleaner detergent, iodophor solution, or an enzyme presoak, placed in a basin, is an effective holding solution.

Use of an ultrasonic cleaner, which is many times more effective and safer than hand scrubbing, should be the choice for definitive instrument cleaning. Instruments cleaned in an ultrasonic device should be suspended in a perforated basket. When an ultrasonic cleaner is on, nothing should come into contact with the tank's bottom, and its lid should be in place. The cleaner should be run for at least 5 minutes per load. Once the cycle is complete, the clean instruments are rinsed under a high volume of cool water, placed on a clean dry towel, rolled or patted, and then air dried. The ultrasonic solution should be discarded daily, and the tub of the ultrasonic machine disinfected. The contaminated instruments are now very clean but not sterile. With the introduction of cassette systems, large-volume ultrasonic and dental thermal disinfectors are being introduced to the dental market. With cassettes, the contaminated instruments are placed back in the cassette holder and circulated through an ultrasonic cleaner or disinfector, resulting in minimal hand contact by staff during instrument preparation. Instruments packaged in a cassette may require additional time in an ultrasonic cleaner or thermal disinfector. The manufacturer recommendations should be strictly followed. Continued precautions are necessary until the instruments have been sterilized.

Clean instruments or cassettes ready for sterilization should be packaged in materials designed for the specific sterilization process to be employed (Fig. 6-32). The sterilizing agent must be able to penetrate the wrapping material and come into inti-

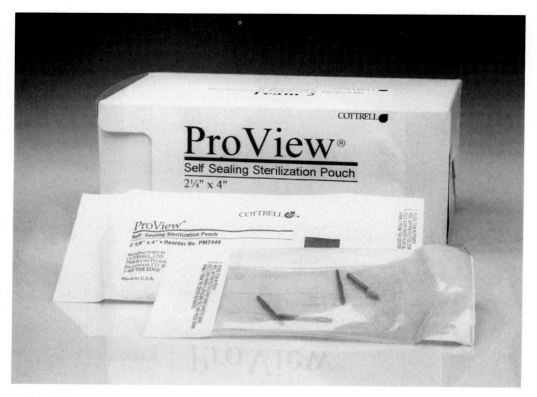

FIG. 6-33 Self-sealing sterilization pouches. *(Courtesy Cottrell Ltd., Englewood, Colo.)*

mate contact with microorganisms (Fig. 6-33). Contaminated endodontic hand files must be cleaned in an ultrasonic bath and autoclaved to completely eliminate microorganisms and measurable endotoxin.[29]

METHODS OF STERILIZATION

The most reliable agent for destroying microorganisms is heat. Methods of sterilization in endodontic practice include steam under pressure, unsaturated chemical vapor, prolonged dry heat, rapid dry heat, intense dry heat, ethylene oxide gas, and glutaraldehyde solutions.

Steam Under Pressure

The autoclave is the most common means of sterilization, except when penetration of steam is limited or heat and moisture damage is a problem. Moist heat kills microorganisms through protein coagulation, RNA and DNA breakdown, and release of low-molecular-weight intracellular constituents.[5] The autoclave sterilizes in 15 to 40 minutes at 249.8° F (121° C), at a pressure of 15 psi. The time required depends on the type of load placed in the autoclave and its permeability. Once the entire load has reached temperature 249.8° F (121° C), it will be rendered sterile in 15 minutes. An adequate margin of safety for load warm-up and steam penetration requires an autoclave time of at least 30 minutes. The clinician should always allow more time for load warm-up if there is any doubt. Existing chamber air is the most detrimental factor to efficient steam sterilization. Modern autoclaves use a gravity displacement method to evacuate this air, thus providing a fully saturated chamber with no cold or hot spots. Instruments and packages placed in an autoclave must be properly arranged so that the pressurized steam may circulate freely around and through the

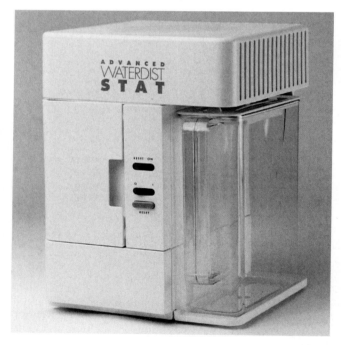

FIG. 6-34 Countertop water distiller. *(Courtesy SciCan, Pittsburgh, Pa.)*

load. Since recirculation of water tends to concentrate contaminants in an autoclave, only fresh deionized (distilled) water should be used for each cycle. Several manufacturers now provide countertop water distillers, which simplifies autoclave operation (Fig. 6-34). Caution must be exercised to never allow

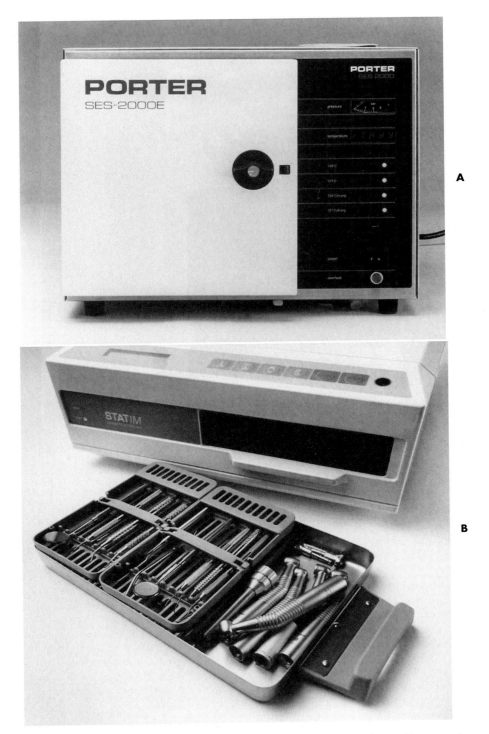

FIG. 6-35 Rapid-cycle autoclaves. **A,** Automatic programmable autoclave. *(Courtesy Porter Instrument Co. Inc., Hatfield, Pa.)* **B,** Statim cassette autoclave. *(Courtesy SciCan, Pittsburgh, Pa.)*

amalgam from teeth or instruments to be sterilized in an autoclave. Mercury vapor is released during the heat of sterilization and could pose a health risk or contaminate the autoclave.[24] When instruments are heated in a steam autoclave, rust and corrosion can occur. Commercially available chemical corrosion inhibitors protect sharp instruments.

Several rapid-speed autoclaves have been developed primar-ily for use in dentistry. Some of these devices may limit the chamber load size but have a sterilization cycle much shorter than the traditional steam autoclave (Fig. 6-35).

Advantages

1. Steam under pressure has a relatively quick turnaround time for instruments.

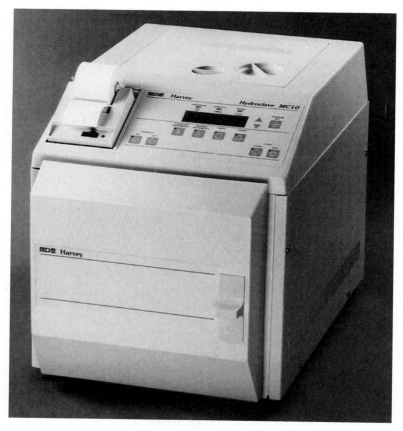

FIG. 6-36 Chemical vapor sterilizer. *(Courtesy MDT Co., Gardena, Calif.)*

2. Steam under pressure offers excellent penetration of packages.
3. Steam under pressure will not destroy cotton or cloth products.
4. Sterilization is verifiable.

Disadvantages

1. Materials must be air dried at completion of the cycle.
2. Because certain metals may corrode or dull, antirust pretreatment may be required. Most stainless steel instruments are resistant to autoclave damage.
3. Steam under pressure can destroy heat-sensitive materials.

Unsaturated Chemical Vapor

The 1928 patent of Dr. George Hollenback and the work of Hollenback and Harvey in the 1940s culminated in the development of an unsaturated chemical vapor sterilization system. This system, using a device that is similar to an autoclave, is named a Harvey chemiclave or chemical vapor sterilizer (Fig. 6-36). The principle of chemiclave sterilization is that although some water is necessary to catalyze the destruction of all microorganisms in a relatively short period of time, water saturation is not necessary. Like autoclave sterilization, chemical vapor sterilization kills microorganisms by destroying vital protein systems. Unsaturated chemical vapor sterilization uses a solution containing specific amounts of various alcohols, acetone, ketone, and formaldehyde and a water content well below the 15% level where rust and corrosion occurs. When the chemiclave is heated to 270° F (132° C) and pressurized to at least 20 psi, sterilization occurs in 20 minutes. As in the autoclave, sterilization in the chemiclave requires careful arrangement of the load to be sterilized. The vapor must be allowed to circulate freely within the chemiclave and penetrate instrument wrapping material. The chemiclave solution is not recirculated; a fresh mixture of the solution is used for each cycle. The chemiclave loses over half its solution to ambient air as vapor. Although it has been shown that this vapor does not contain formaldehyde and is environmentally safe, the vapor has a definite characteristic odor. Adequate ventilation is a necessity when a chemical vapor sterilizer is being used. New models have built in filters or vacuum manifolds that remove the odor of the residual vapors.

Advantages

1. Unsaturated chemical vapor will not corrode metals.
2. Unsaturated chemical vapor has a relatively quick turnaround time for instruments.
3. Load comes out dry.
4. Sterilization is verifiable.

Disadvantages

1. Vapor odor may be offensive, requiring increased ventilation.
2. Special chemicals must be purchased and inventoried.
3. Unsaturated chemical vapor can destroy heat sensitive materials.

Prolonged Dry Heat

There are complicating factors associated with sterilization by dry heat. The time and temperature factors may vary considerably according to heat diffusion, amount of heat available from the heating medium, amount of available moisture present, and heat loss through the heating container's walls. Dry heat kills microorganisms primarily through an oxidation process. Protein coagulation also takes place depending on the water content of the protein and the temperature of sterilization. Dry heat sterilization, like chemical vapor and autoclave sterilization, is verifiable. Dry heat is very slow to penetrate instrument loads. Dry heat sterilizes at 320° F (160° C) in 30 minutes, but instrument loads may take 30 to 90 minutes to reach that temperature. A margin of safety requires instruments to be sterilized at 320° F (160° C) for 2 hours. An internal means of determining and calibrating temperature is an essential component of any dry heat sterilizer. If the sterilizer has multiple heating elements on different surfaces, together with an internal fan to circulate air, heat transfer becomes much more efficient. It is important that loads be positioned within the dry heat sterilizer so that they do not touch each other. Instrument cases must not be stacked one on the other. The hot air must be allowed to circulate freely within the sterilizer.

Mercury vapor in high concentrations can develop in a dry heat sterilizer that has been used to sterilize amalgam instruments. Great care must be exercised to keep scrap amalgam out of any sterilizing device. Once contaminated with mercury or amalgam, a sterilizer continues to produce mercury vapor for many cycles.

Advantages

1. Prolonged dry heat has large load capability.
2. Prolonged dry heat offers complete corrosion protection for dry instruments.
3. Equipment is of low initial cost.
4. Sterilization is verifiable.

Disadvantages

1. Prolonged dry heat provides slow instrument turnaround because of poor heat exchange.
2. Sterilization cycles are not as exact as in moist heat sterilization.
3. Dry heat sterilizer must be calibrated and monitored.
4. If sterilizer temperature is too high, instruments may be damaged.

Rapid Dry Heat

Small chamber, high-speed dry heat sterilizers have been developed primarily for use in dentistry. Load limitations exist, but these devices are much faster than prolonged dry heat. This type of sterilizer has the advantages of prolonged dry heat described above without many of the disadvantages (Fig. 6-37).

Intense Dry Heat

In the past one method of sterilizing endodontic files was the use of a glass bead or salt sterilizer. These sterilizers often need extensive warm-up times and periodic calibration and produce a wide range of temperature gradients within the transfer medium. The salt sterilizer does not predictably sterilize contaminated hand files, is not verifiable, and should not be depended on for sterilization of endodontic hand files between use on different patients.[17]

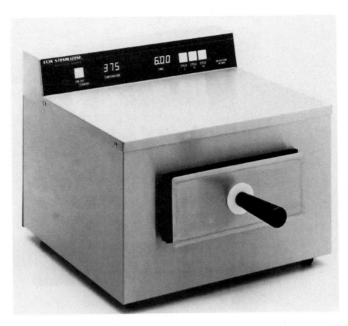

FIG. 6-37 Rapid heat transfer sterilizer. *(Courtesy Cox Sterile Products Inc., Dallas, Tex.)*

Ethylene Oxide Gas

The extreme penetrability of the ethylene oxide (ETO) molecule and ETO's effectiveness at low temperatures (70° to 140° F; 21° to 60° C) make ETO ideal for sterilizing heat-sensitive materials. Even though ETO seems ideal for some dental instruments, such as handpieces, it is best used in a hospital or strictly controlled environment. ETO is thought to be potentially mutagenic and carcinogenic, and its use must be weighed against its possible benefits.

Glutaraldehyde Solutions

Whenever possible, reusable dental instruments should be heat sterilized by a method that can be biologically monitored. However, some dental and medical instruments are destroyed or damaged by the heat of sterilization. In these cases the use of aqueous glutaraldehyde preparations for high-level disinfection or sterilization can be employed. The glutaraldehyde molecule has two active carbonyl groups, which react with proteins through cross-linking reactions. Most activated glutaraldehyde preparations have a shelf life of 14 to 28 days. These products are 2.4% or 3.4% glutaraldehyde and must be discarded once their minimum effective concentration (MEC) of 1.5% is reached or their recommended shelf life has expired. Dipstick or test kit products are available to measure the MEC of glutaraldehyde solutions.

The biocidal activity of glutaraldehyde may be adversely affected by substandard preparation of "activated" glutaraldehyde, contamination of the solution by protein debris, failure to change the solution at the proper time intervals, water dilution of residual glutaraldehyde by washed instruments that have not been dried, and the slow but continuous polymerization of the glutaraldehyde molecule. Instruments contaminated with blood or saliva must remain submerged in glutaraldehyde long enough for spore forms to be killed. Sterilization may require 6 to 10 hours, depending on the product used.

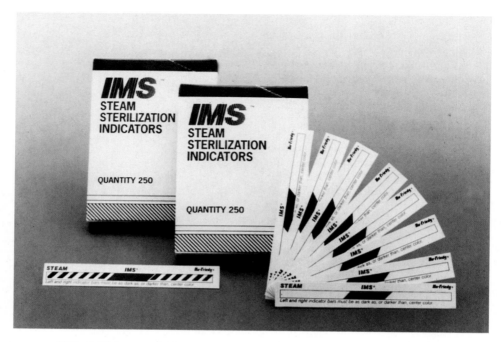

FIG. 6-38 Process indicator strips. *(Courtesy Hu-Friedy Co., Chicago, Ill.)*

Advantages

1. Glutaraldehyde solutions can sterilize heat-sensitive equipment.
2. Glutaraldehyde solutions are relatively noncorrosive and nontoxic.

Disadvantages

1. Glutaraldehyde solutions require long immersion time.
2. Glutaraldehyde solutions have some odor, which may be objectionable, especially if the solutions are heated.
3. Sterilization is nonverifiable.
4. Glutaraldehyde solutions are irritating to mucous membranes (e.g., eyes)

Handpiece Sterilization

Dental handpieces and related instruments should be sterilized between each patient to help prevent cross-infection. Continued improvement in handpiece design has made repeated sterilization of dental handpieces possible. To reduce problems related to sterilization such as loss of torque, turbine wear, and fiber-optic degradation, the manufacturers' instructions should be strictly followed. Although all handpieces can be sterilized, the use of steam under pressure, unsaturated chemical vapor, prolonged dry heat, or rapid dry heat can affect various handpieces differently. Continued product development is necessary to extend handpiece durability and reduce clinical problems.

MONITORING STERILIZATION

There are two methods commonly used to monitor in-office sterilization: process indicators and biologic indicators. Both types of indicators are necessary parts of infection control.

Process indicators are usually strips, tape, or paper products marked with special ink that changes color with exposure to heat, steam, or chemical vapor (Fig. 6-38). The ink changes color when the items being processed have been subjected to sterilizing conditions, but a process indicator usually does not monitor the length of time that such conditions were present. There are specific process indicators for different methods of sterilization. The process indicator's main role in infection control is to prevent accidental use of materials that have not been circulated through the sterilizer. A color change in a process indicator does not ensure proper function of the equipment or that sterilization has been achieved.

Biologic indicators are usually preparations of nonpathogenic bacterial spores that serve as a challenge to a specific method of sterilization. If a sterilization method destroys spore forms that are highly resistant to that method, it is logical to assume that all other life forms, including viruses, have also been destroyed. The bacterial spores are usually attached to a paper strip within a biologically protected packet. The spore packet is placed between instrument packages or within an instrument package itself. After the sterilizer has cycled, the spore strip is cultured for a specific time. Lack of culture growth indicates sterility.

Every sterilizer load should contain at least one process indicator. A safer method is to attach a process indicator to each item sterilized. Each sterilizer should be checked weekly with a biologic indicator to ensure proper functioning of sterilizer equipment and proper loading technique.[8] Records should be maintained, especially of the biologic indicator results. Without periodic biologic monitoring, the clinician cannot be positive that sterilization failures are not occurring. An increasing number of universities and private companies provide mail-in biologic monitoring services (Fig. 6-39).

Causes of sterilization failure

1. Improper instrument preparation
2. Improper packaging of instruments
3. Improper loading of the sterilizer chamber
4. Improper temperature in the sterilization chamber
5. Improper timing of the sterilization cycle
6. Equipment malfunction

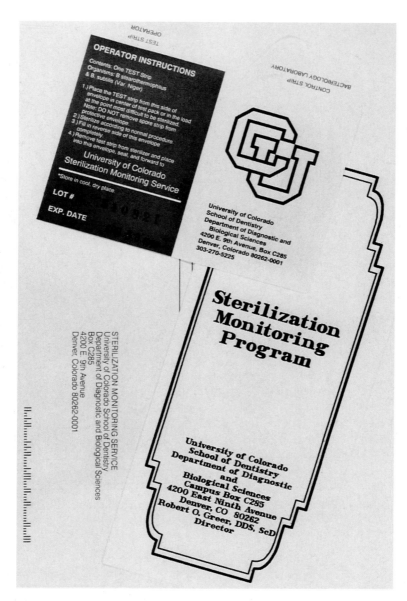

FIG. 6-39 Sterilization monitoring program: instructions, spore test strips, and microbiology report. *(Courtesy University of Colorado School of Dentistry, Denver.)*

METHODS OF DISINFECTION

Disinfection, which does not kill spore forms, should be reserved for the cleaning and decontamination of large surfaces such as countertops and dental chairs. Environmental Protection Agency (EPA)-approved surface disinfectants include iodophors, synthetic phenolics, and chlorine solutions. Surface disinfectants should have an EPA registration number and should be capable of killing *Mycobacterium tuberculosis* in 10 minutes.

Sodium hypochlorite or household bleach in a dilute solution (¼ cup bleach to 1 gallon tap water) can be used to wipe down environmental surfaces. The surfaces to be disinfected should be kept moist for a minimum of 10 minutes, with 30 minutes an ideal. The free chlorine in solution is thought to inactivate sulfhydryl enzymes and nucleic acids and to denature proteins. Sodium hypochlorite is very biocidal against bacterial vegetative forms, viruses, and some spore forms. It is, however, corrosive to metals and irritating to skin and eyes.

Iodophors are combinations of iodine and a solubilizing agent. The manufacturer's recommendations for dilution must be strictly followed to achieve the optimal amount of free iodine in the disinfecting solution. Iodophors have a built-in color indicator that changes when the free iodine molecules have been exhausted. This method of disinfecting offers an effective, practical approach without the problems associated with other disinfectants.

Dental Water Line Contamination

Dental handpieces, water syringes, and sonic and ultrasonic handpieces can be contaminated after sterilization but before patient use by biofilm-contaminated dental unit water lines. The usual source of this contamination is the commercial water

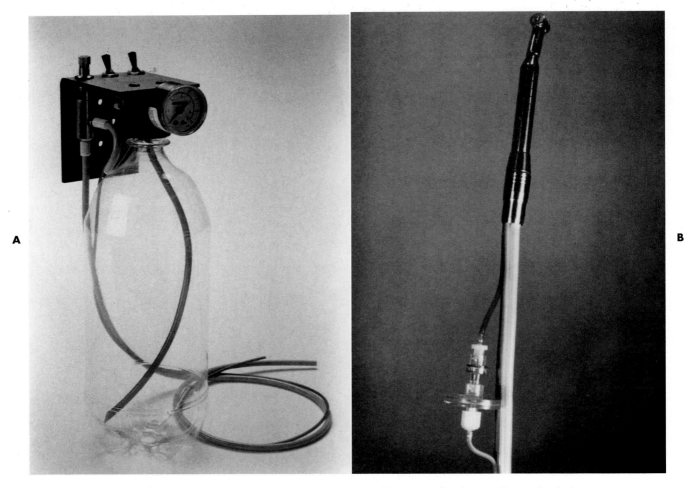

FIG. 6-40 Devices for dealing with dental unit water line contamination. **A,** External solution container. *(Courtesy EIE/Analytic Technology, San Diego, Calif.)* **B,** Clearline microfiltration system. *(Courtesy Sci Tech Dental, Seattle, Wash.)*

supply entering the dental office. The result of biofilm contamination is that the water emitted from handpieces, syringes, and ultrasonic devices may contain elevated concentrations of microorganisms.[2] This is of particular concern, since *Pseudomonas, Mycobacterium,* and *Legionella* species have been isolated from biofilm-contaminated water lines. The following interim recommendations for improving dental unit water quality have been proposed by the American Dental Association (ADA)[3]:

1. Discharge water lines without handpieces attached for several minutes at the beginning of each clinic day.
2. High-speed handpieces should be run to discharge water and air for a minimum of 20 to 30 seconds after use on each patient.
3. Follow the manufacturer's instructions for maintenance of water lines.
4. Possible use of commercial options for water filters or independent water supplies (Fig. 6-40).
5. Use of sterile saline or sterile water for use as a coolant or irrigant when surgical procedures involving the cutting of bone are performed.

The use of disinfectants such as povidone-iodine 10% coupled with sterile water reservoirs appears to reduce dental

unit contamination.[22] Further product development and clinical research are needed in this area.

STERILIZATION OF GUTTA-PERCHA AND ENDODONTIC INSTRUMENTS

The sterilization of gutta-percha cones is of importance in endodontic practice because gutta-percha is the material of choice for root canal obturation. Since this material may come into intimate contact with periapical tissue during obturation, it should not be allowed to serve as a vehicle for pathogenic microorganisms. Immersing gutta-percha cones in 5.25% sodium hypochlorite (full-strength household bleach) for 1 minute is very effective in killing vegetative microorganisms and spore forms.[28]

EFFECT OF REPEATED STERILIZATION ON INSTRUMENTS

The effect of repeated sterilization on the physical characteristics of endodontic files has been studied.[19,23] Repeated sterilization of stainless steel endodontic files, using any heat method described in this chapter, does not cause corrosion, weakness, or an increased rate of rotational failure.

REFERENCES

1. American Dental Association: *Survey of dental practice,* Chicago, 1994, The Association, p 46.

2. American Dental Association Council on Scientific Affairs: ADA statement on dental unit waterlines, *J Am Dent Assoc* 127:185, 1996.

3. American Dental Association Council on Scientific Affairs: Interim recommendations for improving water quality, *J Am Dent Assoc* 127:188, 1996.

4. Beach C et al: Clinical evaluation of bacterial leakage of endodontic temporary filling materials, *J Endod* 22:459, 1996.

5. Block S et al: *Disinfection, sterilization and preservation,* ed 4, Philadelphia, 1991, Lea & Febiger.

6. Christensen G: Magnification, *Clinical Research Associates Newsletter* 19:8, 1995.

7. Cleveland J: Hepatitis B vaccination and infection among U.S. dentists, 1983-1992, *J Am Dent Assoc* 127:1385, 1996.

8. Cottone J et al: *Practical infection control in dentistry,* Philadelphia, 1991, Lea & Febiger.

9. Czerw R et al: In vitro evaluation of the accuracy of several electronic apex locators, *J Endod* 21:572, 1995.

10. Dalet D, Spångberg L: Comparison of apical leakage in root canals obturated with various gutta-percha techniques using a dye vacuum tracing method, *J Endod* 20:315, 1994.

11. Department of Labor, Occupational Safety and Health Administration 29 CFR Part 1910.1030: Occupational exposure to bloodborne pathogens, final rule, *Federal Register* 56(235):64004-64182, 1991.

12. Esposito P, Cunningham C: A comparison of canal preparation with nickel-titanium and stainless steel instruments, *J Endod* 21:173, 1995.

13. Gambill J, Alder M, del Rio C: Comparison of nickel-titanium and stainless steel hand-file instrumentation using computed tomography, *J Endod* 22:369, 1996.

14. Glossen C et al: A comparison of root canal preparations using Ni-Ti hand, Ni-Ti engine-driven, and K-Flex endodontic instruments, *J Endod* 21:146, 1995.

15. Gutmann J, Leonard J: Problem solving in endodontic working length determination, *Compendium* 16:288, 1995.

16. Hazelkorn H, Bloom B, Jovanovic B: Infection control in the dental office: has anything changed? *J Am Dent Assoc* 127:786, 1996.

17. Hurtt C, Rossman L: The sterilization of endodontic hand files, *J Endod* 22:321, 1996.

18. Ingle J: A new paradigm for filling and sealing root canals, *Compendium* 16:306, 1995.

19. Iverson G et al: The effects of various sterilization methods on the torsional strength of endodontic files, *J Endod* 11:266, 1985.

20. Kahn F, Rosenberg P, Gliksberg J: An in vitro evaluation of the irrigating characteristics of ultrasonic and subsonic handpieces and irrigating needles and probes, *J Endod* 21:277, 1995.

21. McCarthy G et al: Rates of nondisclosure and rejection of dental treatment among HIV patients, *Oral Surg Oral Med Oral Pathol* 80:655, 1995.

22. Mills S, Lauderdale P, Mayhew R: Reduction of microbial contamination in dental units with povidone-iodine 10%, *J Am Dent Assoc* 113:280, 1986.

23. Morrison S et al: The effects of steam sterilization and usage on cutting efficiency of endodontic instruments, *J Endod* 15:427, 1989.

24. Parsell D et al: Mercury release during autoclave sterilization of amalgam, *J Dent Ed* 60:453, 1996.

25. Poulson WB, Dove SB, del Rio C: Effect of nickel-titanium engine-driven instrument rotation speed on root canal morphology, *J Endod* 21:609, 1995.

26. Royal J, Donnelly J: A comparison of maintenance of canal curvature using balanced-force instrumentation with three different file types, *J Endod* 21:300, 1995.

27. Safadi G et al: Latex hypersensitivity, *J Am Dent Assoc* 127:83, 1996.

28. Senia S et al: Rapid sterilization of gutta-percha cones with 5.25% sodium hypochlorite, *J Endod* 1:136, 1975.

29. Tittle K, Kettering J, Torabinejad M: Research abstract #50: residual endotoxin on endodontic files after routine infection control procedures, *J Endod* 21:227, 1995.

30. Whitten B et al: Current trends in endodontic treatment: report of a national survey, *J Am Dent Assoc* 127:1333, 1996.

Chapter **7**

Tooth Morphology and Cavity Preparation

Richard C. Burns
Eric James Herbranson

The hard tissue repository of the human dental pulp takes on many configurations that must be understood before treatment begins. This chapter examines anatomic structure and its relationship to the initial clinical goal of endodontics, which is the preparation of an ideal access to the pulp chambers. Only with the successful completion of this first step can thorough cleaning and shaping procedures take place.

COMPLEX ANATOMY

From the early work of Hess and Zurcher[13] to the most recent studies demonstrating anatomic complexities of the root canal system, it has been established that the root with a graceful tapering canal and a single apical foramen is the exception rather than the rule. Investigators have shown multiple foramina, fins, deltas, loops, furcation accessory canals, and more in most teeth. Kasahara et al.[15] studied transparent specimens of 510 extracted maxillary central incisors for anatomic detail and found that 60% of the specimens showed accessory canals that were impossible to clean mechanically. Apical foramina located away from the apex were observed in 45% of the teeth. The student and the clinician must approach the tooth to be treated assuming that the "aberrations" occur so often that they must be considered normal anatomy.

A sagittal section of the mandibular first premolar (Fig. 7-1) reveals one of the truly difficult situations facing the clinician. Instead of distinct individual canals, this tooth presents a fine ribbon-shaped canal system that is almost impossible to clean, shape, and seal thoroughly. The section shown in Fig. 7-2 was located 8 mm apical to the cementum-enamel junction; the root was 14 mm long.[9] This example of anatomic complexity illustrates that internal morphology is far from predictable. The teeth shown in Fig. 7-3 may be the longest on record. The maxillary cuspid (Fig. 7-3, *A*) measures 41 mm from incisal edge to apex. The central incisor (Fig. 7-3, *B*) is 30 mm long. These teeth, removed before placement of immediate dentures by Dr. Gary Wilkie of Korumburra, Victoria, Australia, belonged to a 31-year-old, 5-foot 2-inch tall European female.[3] The decision to remove the teeth was made jointly by patient and dentist.[30] Average tooth lengths are shown in Table 7-1.

It is humbling to be aware of the complexity of the spaces we are expected to access, clean, and fill. We can take comfort, however, in knowing that even under the difficult circumstances of unusual morphology our current methods of root canal therapy result in an astoundingly high rate of success.

ENTERING THE PULP CHAMBER

Access preparations can be divided into the visual, or what you can see, and the visualized, or what you cannot. The coronal anatomy in whatever state it exists, is the first indication of the visualized and is the first key to the root position and root canal system.

A thorough investigation of the sulcus, coronal clefts, restorations, tooth angulation, cusp position, occlusion, and contacts is mandatory before access is begun. Palpation of buccal or labial soft tissue helps determine root position (see Fig. 7-10). In the case of a malaligned tooth some clinicians advocate access cavity preparation before rubber dam placement as a visual aid to prevent disorientation.

Before entry, the clinician must attempt to visualize the expected location of the coronal pulp chamber and canal orifice position. Unnecessary removal of enamel and dentin may compromise final restoration of the tooth. It is important at this time to call on one's knowledge of tooth morphology.

Initial entry into the pulp chamber through enamel or restorative materials is best made with a fissure bur or inverted cone bur (see Fig. 7-9). A true-running high-speed turbine handpiece is mandatory for gaining access into the endodontically involved tooth. The addition of fiberoptics to the handpiece improves visibility during examination of the deeper reaches of the interior of the tooth.

Ideal outline form is illustrated for each tooth in Plates I through XVI (see pp. 157-189). If doubt exists as to the location of the pulp chamber and canal orifice(s), the outline form may be made conservatively until the chamber is unroofed (Fig. 7-4, *A*). The next step is performed with a No. 2, 4, or 6 round bur. When the bur has dropped through the roof of the chamber (Fig. 7-4, *B*), no further cutting in an apical direction should be attempted. All action must be in a "sweeping-out" motion until clear access is gained to the canal orifice(s) for all future instrumentation (Fig. 7-4, *C*). Occasionally it is necessary to remove occlusal tooth structure to achieve straight line access (Fig. 7-5). Any pulp stones, loose calcifications, restorative materials, and other debris must be removed at this time.

USE OF THE PATHFINDER FOR LOCATING ORIFICES

After the pulp chamber is opened, the canal orifices are located with the endodontic pathfinder (Fig. 7-6). This instrument is to the endodontist what a probe is to the periodontist.

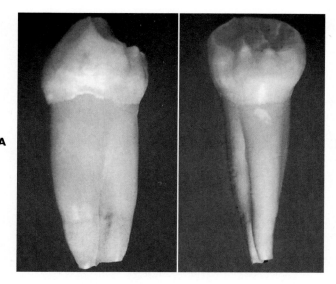

FIG. 7-1 Mandibular first premolar. **A,** Distal view. **B,** Lingual view.

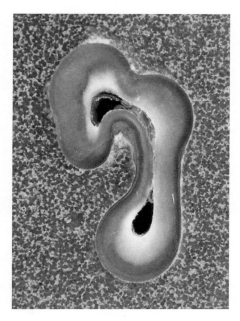

FIG. 7-2 Root section of the premolar shown in Fig. 7-1.

Table 7-1. Tooth length determination

Maxillary	Length (mm)	Mandibular	Length (mm)
Central incisor		Central incisor	
Average	22.5	Average	20.7
Greatest	27.0	Greatest	24.0
Least	18.0	Least	16.0
Lateral incisor		Lateral incisor	
Average	22.0	Average	21.1
Greatest	26.0	Greatest	27.0
Least	17.0	Least	18.0
Canine		Canine	
Average	26.5	Average	25.6
Greatest	32.0	Greatest	32.5
Least	20.0	Least	18.0
First premolar		First premolar	
Average	20.6	Average	21.6
Greatest	22.5	Greatest	26.0
Least	17.0	Least	18.0
Second premolar		Second premolar	
Average	21.5	Average	22.3
Greatest	27.0	Greatest	26.0
Least	16.0	Least	18.0
First molar		First molar	
Average	20.8	Average	21.0
Greatest	24.0	Greatest	24.0
Least	17.0	Least	18.0
Second molar		Second molar	
Average	20.0	Average	19.8
Greatest	24.0	Greatest	22.0
Least	16.0	Least	18.0
Third molar		Third molar	
Average	17.1	Average	18.5
Greatest	22.0	Greatest	20.0
Least	14.0	Least	16.0

Modified from Black GV: *Descriptive anatomy of the human teeth,* ed 4, Philadelphia, 1897, SS White Dental Manufacturing Co.

Reaching, feeling, often digging at the hard tissue, it is the extension of the clinician's fingers. Natural anatomy dictates the usual places for orifices, but restorations, dentinal protrusions, and dystrophic calcifications can alter the actual configuration encountered. While probing the chamber floor, the pathfinder often penetrates or dislodges calcific deposits blocking an orifice.

Positioning the instrument in the orifice enables the clinician to check the shaft for clearance of the orifice walls. Additionally, the pathfinder is used to determine the angle at which the canals depart the main chamber (see Fig. 7-8, *B*).

The endodontic pathfinder is preferred over the rotating bur as the instrument for locating canal orifices (Fig. 7-6). The double-ended design offers two angles of approach.

ACCESS CAVITY PREPARATION IN INCISORS
(Fig. 7-7)

Incisors, particularly mandibular incisors, are often weakened coronally by excessive removal of tooth structure. The mesiodistal width of the pulp chamber is often narrower than the bur used to make the initial access. Because of the ease of visibility and clear definition of external anatomy, lateral perforations (toward the cervical or root surface) are rare.

Labial perforations (cervical or root surface) are common, however, especially with calcifications. To prevent this occurrence, the clinician must consider the relationship between the incisal edge and the location of the pulp chamber. If the incisal edge is intact, it is almost impossible to perforate lingually. Therefore in calcified cases when the bur does not drop easily into the chamber, the clinician should change to smaller diameter burs and, keeping the long axis in mind, direct the cutting action in apicolingual version. If the canal orifice still does not materialize after cutting in an apical direction, the clinician should remove the bur, place it in the access

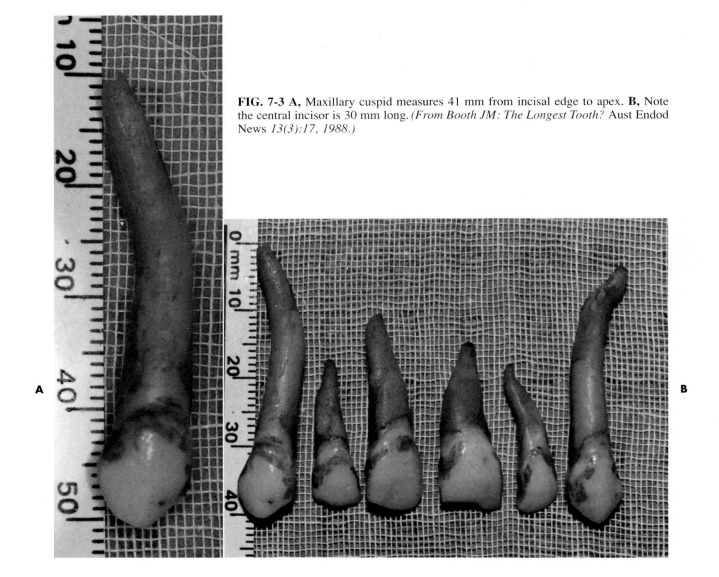

FIG. 7-3 A, Maxillary cuspid measures 41 mm from incisal edge to apex. **B,** Note the central incisor is 30 mm long. *(From Booth JM: The Longest Tooth? Aust Endod News 13(3):17, 1988.)*

cavity, and expose a radiograph to reveal the depth of cutting and the angulation of cutting from within the dentin.

ACCESS THROUGH FULL VENEER CROWNS

Properly made crowns are constructed with the occlusal relationship of the opposing tooth as a primary consideration. A cast crown may be made in any shape, diameter, height, or angle; this cast crown alteration can destroy the visual relationship to the true long axis. Careful study of the preoperative radiograph identifies most of these situations.

Achieving access through crowns should be done with coolants, even when the rubber dam is used. Friction-generated heat can damage adjacent soft tissue, including the periodontal ligament; and with an anesthetized or nonvital tooth the patient is not aware of pain. Once penetration of the metal is accomplished, the clinician can change to a sharp round bur and move toward the central pulp chamber. Metal filings and debris from the access cavity should be removed frequently because small slivers can cause large obstructions in the fine canal system.

When sufficient access has been gained, the clinician should search margins and internal spaces for caries and leaks and the pulpal floor for signs of fracture or perforation. Occasionally caries can be removed through the occlusal access cavity, and the tooth can be properly restored. The interior of a crown can be a surprise package, containing everything from extensive caries to intact dentin (as seen in periodontally induced necrosis).

METHODS OF DETERMINING ANATOMIC DETAIL

The root canal system is often complex. The clinician must use every available means to determine the anatomic configuration before commencing instrumentation. Fig. 7-8 illustrates several techniques and methods:

1. A radiograph reveals many clues to anatomic "aberrations": lateral radiolucencies indicating the presence of lateral or accessory canals (Fig. 7-8, *A, 1*); an abrupt ending of a large canal signifying a bifurcation, where it is assumed that it has bifurcated (or trifurcated) into much finer diameters. To confirm this division, a second radiograph is exposed from a mesial angulation of 10 to 30 degrees. The resultant film shows either more roots or multiple vertical lines indicating the peripheries of addi-

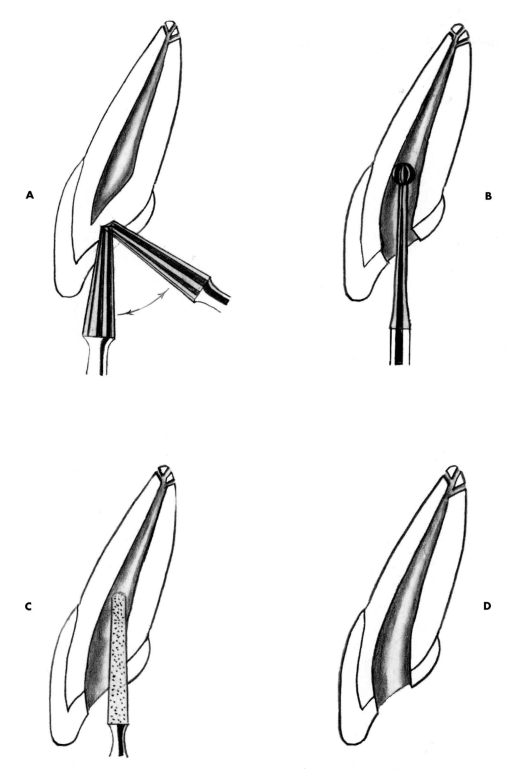

FIG. 7-4 A, Fissure bur in a high-speed handpiece. Moving from a right angle to the long axis facilitates entrance to the chamber. **B,** After "dropping through" the roof of the chamber, the clinician switches to a long-shanked No. 2, 4, or 6 round bur and with a "sweeping-out" motion cleans and shapes the wall of the chamber. **C,** A tapered diamond instrument is used to smooth the entry in the coronal access. **D,** Completed shaping of the upper pulp chamber.

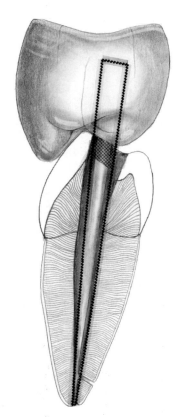

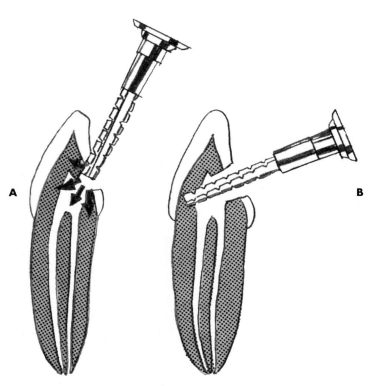

FIG. 7-5 Straight-line access to canals. In some circumstances, coronal tooth structure must be sacrificed to obtain direct access to pulp chambers. Most posterior endodontically treated teeth require full coronal coverage. Ultraconservative access preparation is usually contraindicated. The *hatched area* represents the removal of cuspal hard tissue necessary for ideal access.

FIG. 7-7 A, A sweeping motion in a slightly downward lingual-to-labial direction *(arrows),* until the chamber in engaged, to obtain the best access to the lingual canal. **B,** Incorrect approach: directing the end-cutting bur in a straight lingual-to-labial direction. Mutilation of tooth structure and perforation are the results in this small and narrow incisor.

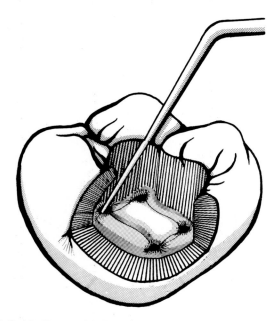

FIG. 7-6 Indispensable in endodontic treatment, the endodontic pathfinder serves as an explorer to locate orifices, as an indicator of canal angulation, and often as a chipping tool to remove calcification.

tional root surfaces (Fig. 7-8, *A, 2* and *A, 4*); a knoblike image indicating an apex that curves toward or away from the beam of the x-ray machine (Fig. 7-8, *A, 3*); multiple vertical lines, as shown in this curved mesial root (Fig. 7-8, *A, 4*), indicating the possibility of a thin root, which may be hourglass-shaped in cross section and susceptible to perforation.

2. The endodontic pathfinder inserted into the orifice openings reveals the direction that the canals take in leaving the main chamber (Fig. 7-8, *B*).
3. Digital perception with a hand instrument can identify curvatures, obstruction, root division, and additional canal orifices (Fig. 7-8, *C*).
4. Fiber-optic illumination can reveal calcifications, orifice location, and fractures (Fig. 7-19).
5. Further knowledge of root formation can save the clinician difficulties with instrumentation, for example, in what appears radiographically to be a normal palatal root of a maxillary first permanent molar (Fig. 7-8, *E, 1*) but is actually a root with a sharp apical curvature toward the buccal (Fig. 7-8, *E, 2*).
6. Ethnic characteristics and other physical differences can be manifested in tooth morphology, for example, the common occurrence of four canals in Asian people (Fig. 7-8, *F*).

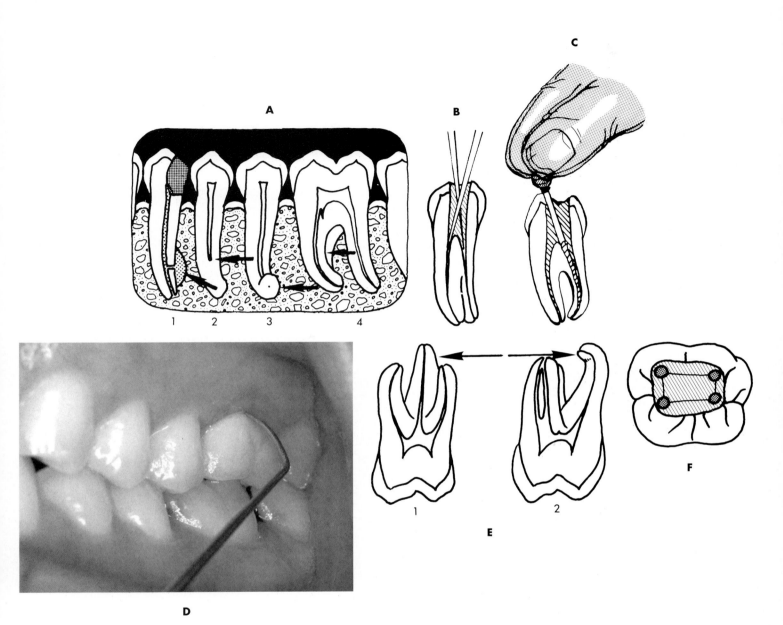

FIG. 7-8 A, A radiograph also reveals many clues to anatomic "aberrations": lateral radiolucencies indicating the presence of lateral or accessory canals *(1);* an abrupt ending of a large canal signifying a bifurcation *(1* and *2);* a knoblike image indicating an apex that curves toward or away from the beam of the x-ray machine *(3);* multiple vertical lines, as shown in this curved mesial root *(4),* indicating the possibility of a thin root, which may be hourglass shaped in cross section and susceptible to perforation. **B,** The endodontic pathfinder inserted into the orifice openings reveals the direction the canals take in leaving the main chamber. **C,** Digital perception with a hand instrument can identify curvatures, obstruction, root division, and additional canal orifices. **D,** Using a tactile sense, cervical anatomy can be tactilely identified with a pathfinder. **E,** Further knowledge of root formation can save the clinician difficulties with instrumentation, for example, in what appears radiographically to be an average palatal root of a maxillary first permanent molar *(1)* but is actually a root with a sharp apical curvature toward the buccal aspect *(2).* **F,** Ethnic characteristics and other physical differences can be manifested in tooth morphology (e.g., the common occurrence of four canals in Asian people).

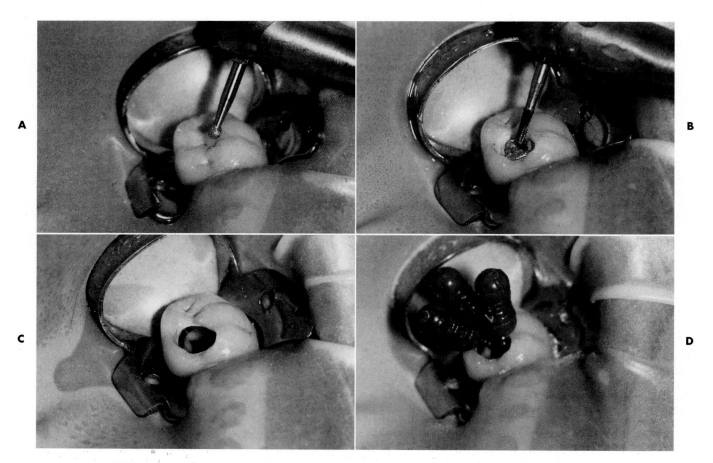

FIG. 7-9 Access cavity preparation through a ceramometal crown. **A,** Diamond-impregnated round instrument. **B,** Following access outline made with the round diamond, an end-cutting or round carbide bur cuts through the metal. **C,** Access cavity prepared allowing direct approach to the canals. **D,** Test files placed without impingement on the access cavity walls.

INTRODUCTION TO PLATES I THROUGH XVI

The anatomy presented in the following plates is a combination of examples of human teeth, illustrations representing ideal morphology,* and radiographs of completed endodontic procedures demonstrating usual pulpal configuration.† The average time of eruption and average time of calcification data are from *Anatomy of Orofacial Structures* by Brand and Isselhard.[5] The narrow strip illustrating anatomic variations for each tooth is from the work of the late Quintiliano de Deus of Brazil.‡

---

*Contained in this series are many classic illustrations from Zeisz and Nuckolls.[31] These extremely accurate and excellent drawings are reproductions of the work of these authors, aided by the artistic talents of Mr. Walter B. Schwarz.
†Also included are photographs and radiographs provided by Dr. L. Stephen Buchanan.
‡de Deus QD: *Endodontia,* ed 4, Rio de Janeiro, 1986, Medsi Editôra Médica e Científica, Ltda.

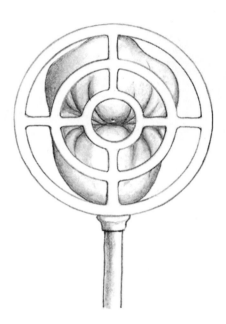

PLATE I
Maxillary Central Incisor

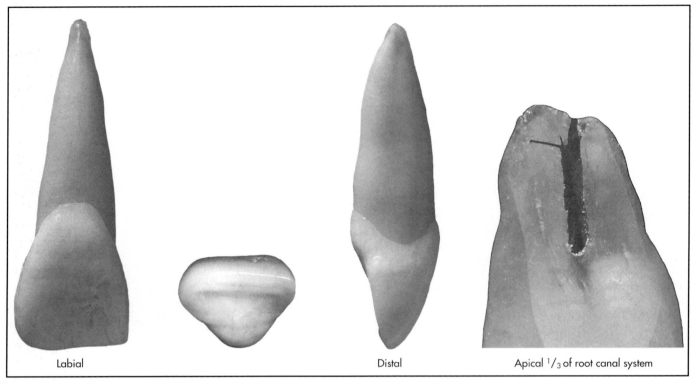

Labial   Distal   Apical ¹/₃ of root canal system

Average time of eruption: 7 to 8 years
Average age of calcification: 10 years
Average length: 22.5 mm

Somewhat rectangular from the labial aspect and shovel shaped from the proximal aspect, the crown of the maxillary central incisor is more than adequate for endodontic access and is positioned ideally for direct mirror viewing. This tooth is especially suitable for a first clinical experience because more than a third of its canal is directly visible. Viewing of the canal proper may be enhanced with fiber-optic illumination.

The first entry point, with the end-cutting fissure bur, is made just above the cingulum (see Fig. 7-4, A). The direction should be in the long axis of the root. A roughly triangular opening is made in anticipation of the final shape of the access cavity. Often penetration of the shallow pulp chamber occurs during initial entry. When the sensation of "dropping through the roof" of the pulp chamber has been felt, the long-shanked No. 4 or 6 round bur replaces the fissure bur (see Fig. 7-4, B).

The round bur is used to sweep out toward the incisal edge; one must be certain to expose the entire chamber completely (see Fig. 7-4, B). It may be necessary to return to the fissure bur to extend and refine the final shape of the access cavity. All caries, grossly discolored dentin, and pulp calcifications are removed at this time. Leaking restorations or proximal caries should be removed and an adequate temporary restoration placed.

Conical and rapidly tapering toward the apex, the root morphology is quite distinctive. Cross-sectionally the radicular canal is slightly triangular at the cervical aspect, gradually becoming round as it approaches the apical foramen.

Multiple canals are rare, but accessory and lateral canals are common. Kasahara et al.[15] studied 510 maxillary central incisors to determine thickness and curvature of the root canal, the condition of any accessory canals, and locations of the apical foramen. Data revealed that the thickness and curvature of canals showed adequate preparation at approximately a size 60 instrument at the apical constriction, that over 60% of the specimens showed accessory canals, and that the apical foramen was located apart from the apex in 45% of the teeth.

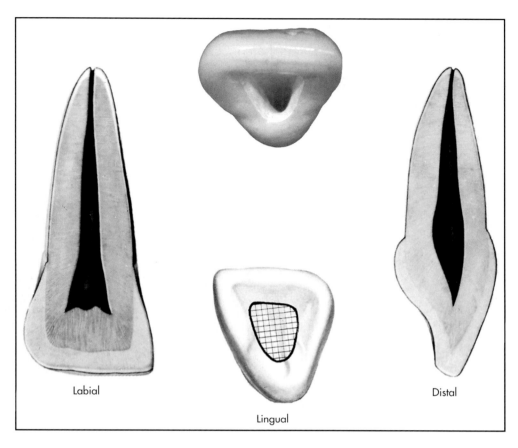

Labial

Lingual

Distal

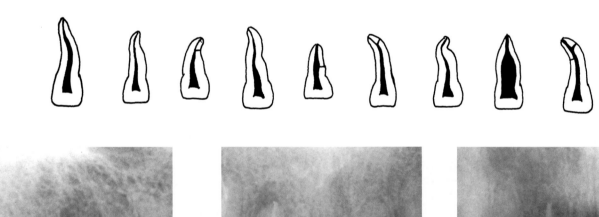

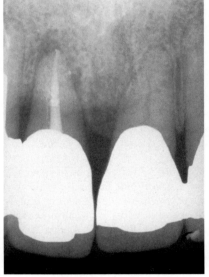

PLATE 7-I-5 Curved accessory canal with straight lateral canal intersecting.

PLATE 7-I-6 Parallel accessory canal to main canal with simple lateral canal.

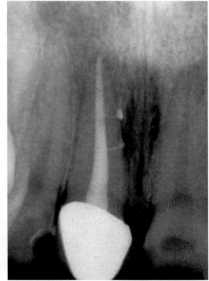

PLATE 7-I-7 Double lateral canals.

PLATE II
Maxillary Lateral Incisor

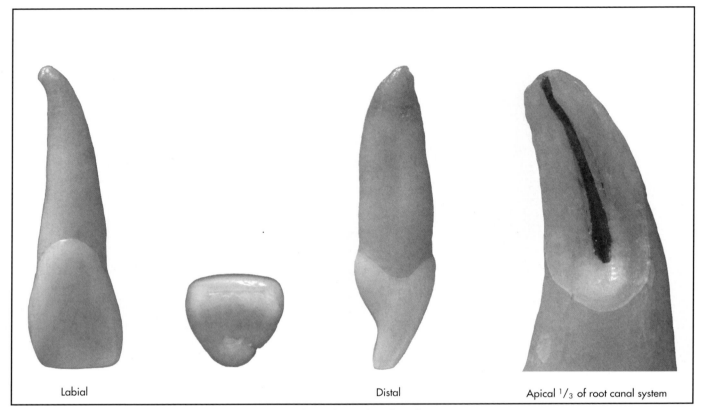

Labial   Distal   Apical $1/3$ of root canal system

Average time of eruption: 8 to 9 years
Average age of calcification: 11 years
Average length: 22.0 mm

Tending toward an oval shape, the crown of the maxillary lateral incisor is as near to ideal for endodontic access as that of the central incisor. Fiberoptic illumination is always helpful during access to this tooth.

The initial entry, with the end-cutting fissure bur, is made just above the cingulum. The access cavity is ovoid. Often the fissure bur engages the shallow pulp chamber while making the initial opening. When the chamber roof is removed, a No. 4 or 6 round bur is used to sweep out all remaining caries, discoloration, and pulp calcifications.

It may be necessary to return to the fissure bur in refining the ovoid access cavity. Adequate flaring is then accomplished with round burs. Care must be exercised that explorers, endodontic cutting instruments, and packing instruments do not contact the access cavity walls.

There are a number of rare morphology oddities that occur in the lateral incisor. Occasionally the crown is "pegged" and assumes the shape of a blunt-ended pencil. Access would still be on the lingual surface, but significant tooth structure will be removed. Some lateral incisors have a groove on the lingual, starting at the cingulum, that on rare occasions extends deep into the root structure, creating an untreatable periodontal defect.

To ensure the canals remain clean and tightly sealed, all car-ies and leaking restorations must be removed and replaced with temporary sealing materials.

The radicular cross-sectional pulp chamber varies from ovoid at the cervical foramen to round at the apical foramen. The root is slightly conical and tends toward curvature, usually toward the distal surface, in its apical portion. The apical foramen is generally closer to the anatomic apex than in the maxillary central incisor but may be found on the lateral aspect within 1 or 2 mm of the apex.

On rare occasions, access is complicated by a dens in dente, an invagination of part of the lingual surface of the tooth into the crown. This creates a space within the tooth that is lined by enamel and communicates with the mouth. Dens in dente most often occurs in maxillary lateral incisors, but it can occur in other teeth. These teeth are predisposed to decay because of the anatomic malformation, and the pulp may die before the root apex is completely developed.[14] Estimates of occurrence range from 0.04% to 10%. Although the pulp often becomes nonvital, cases have been reported of teeth whose pulps maintain their vitality.[14]

Goon et al.[10] reported the first case of complex involvement of the entire facial aspect of a tooth root. An alveolar crest to apex facial root defect led to early pulpal necrosis and periapical rarefaction.[10]

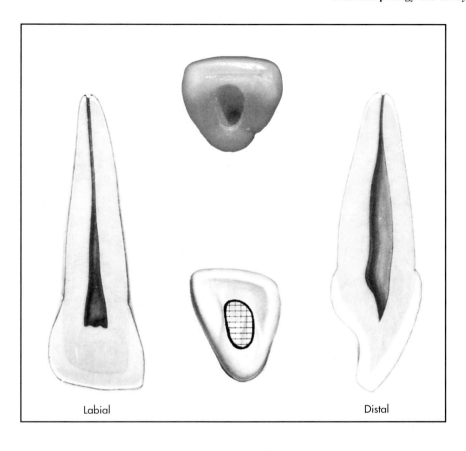

Labial   Distal

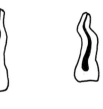

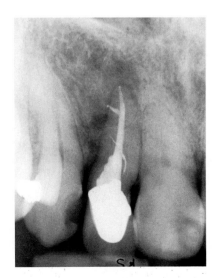

PLATE 7-II-5 Lateral incisor with a canal loop and multiple canals with associated lesions.

PLATE 7-II-6 Multiple portals of exit.

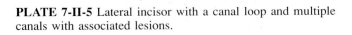

PLATE III
Maxillary Canine

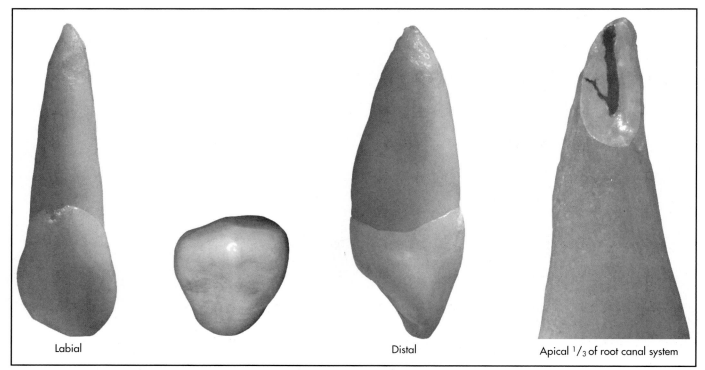

Labial   Distal   Apical $1/3$ of root canal system

Average time of eruption: 10 to 12 years
Average age of calcification: 13 to 15 years
Average length: 26.5 mm

The longest tooth in the dental arch, the canine has a formidable shape designed to withstand heavy occlusal stress. Its long, thickly enameled crown sustains heavy incisal wear but often displays deep cervical erosion with aging.

The access cavity corresponds to the lingual crown shape and is ovoid. To achieve straight-line access, one often must extend the cavity incisally but not so far as to weaken the heavily functioning cusp. Initial access is made slightly below midcrown on the palatal side. If the pulp chamber is located deeper, a No. 4 or 6 long-shanked round bur may be required. The sweeping-out motion of this bur reveals an ovoid pulp chamber. The chamber remains ovoid as it continues apically through the cervical region and below. Attention must be given to circumferential filing so that this ovoid chamber is thoroughly cleaned.

The radicular canal is reasonably straight and quite long. Most canines require instruments that are 25 mm or longer. The apex often curves, in any direction, in the last 2 or 3 mm.

The thin buccal bone over the eminence often disintegrates, and fenestration is a common finding. The apical foramen is usually close to the anatomic apex but may be laterally positioned, especially when apical curvature is present.

Canine morphology seldom varies radically, and lateral and accessory canals occur less frequently than in the maxillary incisors.

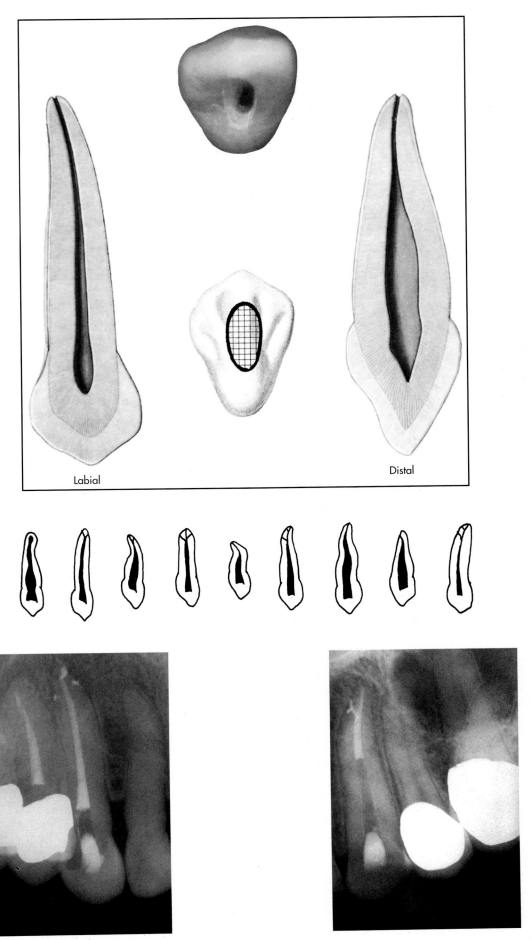

Labial

Distal

PLATE 7-III-5 Canine with multiple accessory foramina.

PLATE 7-III-6 Maxillary canine with lateral canal dividing into two additional canals.

PLATE IV
Maxillary First Premolar

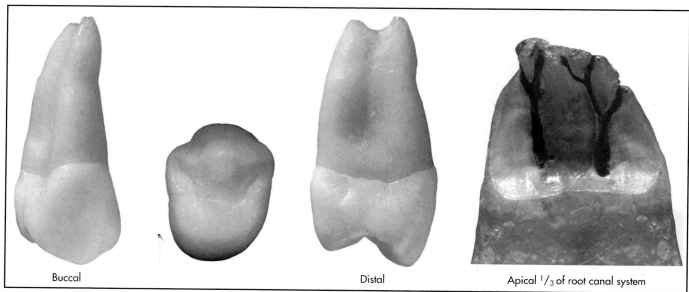

Buccal   Distal   Apical ¹/₃ of root canal system

Average time of eruption: 10 to 11 years
Average age of calcification: 12 to 13 years
Average length: 20.6 mm

Most commonly birooted, the maxillary first premolar is a transitional tooth between incisor and molar. Loss of the posterior molars subjects the premolars to heavy occlusal loads. Removable appliances increase torque on these frequently clasped teeth, and the additional forces, in concert with deep carious lesions, can induce heavy calcification of the pulp chambers. Early posterior tooth loss often causes rotation, which can complicate the locating of pulp chambers.

The canal orifices lie below and slightly central to the cusp tips. The initial opening is in the central fossa and is ovoid in the buccopalatal dimension. When one orifice has been located, the clinician should look carefully for a developmental groove leading to the opening of another canal. The angulation of the roots may be determined by the positioning of the endodontic pathfinder (see Fig. 7-8, *B*). Radiographic division of the roots on a routine periapical film often indicates tooth rotation (see Fig. 7-8, *A, 4*). Divergent roots require less occlusal access extension. Conversely, parallel roots may require removal of tooth structure toward the cusp tips. All caries and leaking restorations must be removed and a suitable temporary restoration placed.

Radicular irregularities consist of fused roots with separate canals, fused roots with interconnections or "webbing," fused roots with a common apical foramen, and the unusual three-rooted tooth. In the last situation the buccal orifices are not clearly visible with a mouth mirror. Directional positioning of the endodontic pathfinder or a small file will identify the anatomy. Carns and Skidmore[6] reported that the incidence of maxillary first premolars with three roots, three canals, and three foramina was 6% of the cases studied. The root is considerably shorter than in the canine, and distal curvature is not uncommon. The apical foramen is usually close to the anatomic apex. Root lengths, if the cusps are intact and used as reference points, are usually the same. The apical portion of the roots often tapers rapidly, ending in extremely narrow and curved root tips.

The prevalence of mesiodistal vertical crown or root fracture of the first premolar requires that the clinician remove all restorations at the inception of endodontic therapy and carefully inspect the coronal anatomy with a fiberoptic light and if necessary with an operating microscope.

After endodontic treatment, full occlusal coverage is mandatory to ensure against cuspal or crown-root fracture.

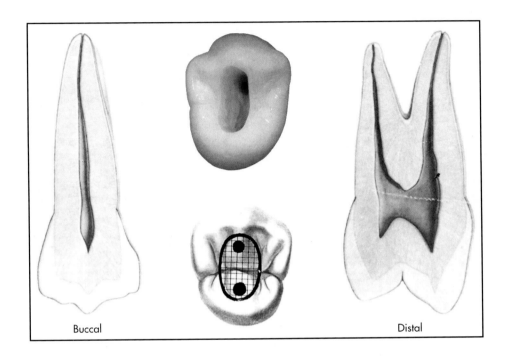

Buccal

Distal

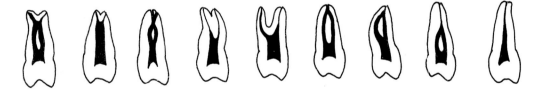

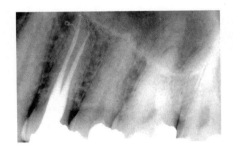

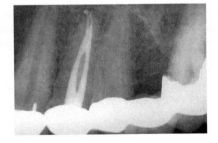

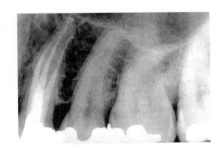

PLATE 7-IV-5 Lateral bony lesion associated with filled lateral canal.

PLATE 7-IV-6 Two canals fusing and redividing.

PLATE 7-IV-7 Three canals in a maxillary first bicuspid.

PLATE V
Maxillary Second Premolar

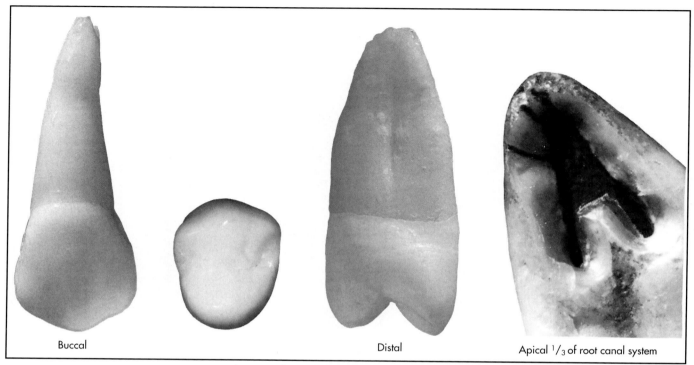

Buccal   Distal   Apical ¹/₃ of root canal system

Average time of eruption: 10 to 12 years
Average age of calcification: 12 to 14 years
Average length: 21.5 mm

Similar to the first premolar in coronal morphology, the second premolar varies mainly in root form. Its crown is narrower in the buccopalatal dimension and slightly wider in the mesiodistal dimension. The basic outline of the tooth is slightly ovoid, but wider from mesial to distal than the outline of the first premolar. The canal orifice is centrally located but often appears more as a slot than as a single ovoid opening. When the slot-shaped opening appears, the clinician must assume that the tooth has two canals until proved otherwise.

Radicular morphology may present two separate canals, two canals anastomosing to a single canal, or two canals with interconnections or "webbing." Accessory and lateral canals may be present but less often than in incisors. Vertucci et al.[27] stated that 75% of maxillary second premolars in their study had one canal at the apex, 24% had two foramina, and 1% had three foramina. Of the teeth studied, 59.9% had accessory canals.

These clinicians also reported that when two canals join into one, the *palatal* canal frequently exhibits a straight-line access to the apex. They further pointed out that "if, on the direct periapical exposure, a root canal shows a sudden narrowing, or even disappears, it means that at this point the canal divides into two parts, which either remain separate (type V) or merge (type II) before reaching the apex."[27]

The root length of the maxillary second premolar is much like that of the first premolar, and apical curvature is not uncommon, particularly with large sinus cavities.

Like the upper first premolar, the upper second premolar is susceptible to vertical crown and root fractures. All caries and leading restorations must be removed and replaced with a suitable temporary restoration. After endodontic treatment, full occlusal coverage is mandatory to ensure against final cuspal or crown-root fracture.

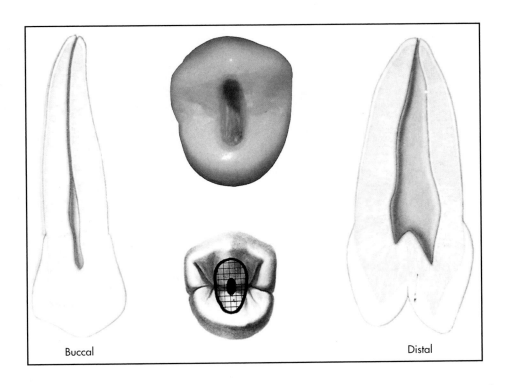

Buccal

Distal

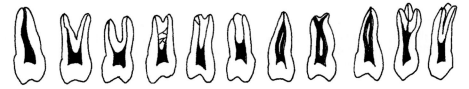

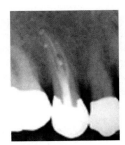

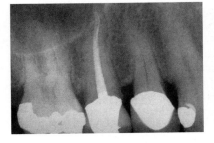

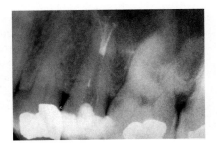

PLATE 7-V-5 An unusual three-canaled second bicuspid with a large lateral canal.

PLATE 7-V-6 Single canal dividing into two canals.

PLATE 7-V-7 Single canal splitting into three canals.

PLATE VI
Maxillary First Molar

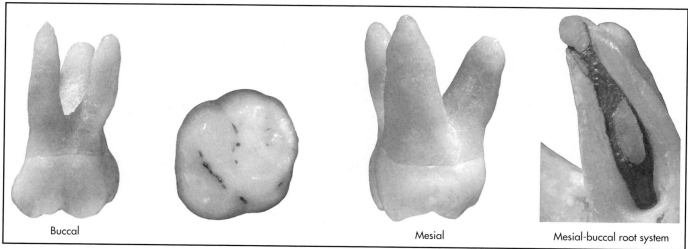

Buccal   Mesial   Mesial-buccal root system

Average time of eruption: 6 to 7 years
Average age of calcification: 9 to 10 years
Average length: 20.8 mm

The tooth largest in volume and most complex in root and root canal anatomy, the "6-year molar" is possibly the most treated, least understood, posterior tooth. It is the posterior tooth with the highest endodontic failure rate and unquestionably one of the most important teeth.

Three individual roots of the maxillary first molar provide a tripod: the palatal root, which is the longest, and the distobuccal and mesiobuccal roots, which are about the same length. The palatal root is often curved buccally in its apical third. Of the three canals, it offers the easiest access and has the largest diameter. Its orifice lies well toward the palatal surface, and the root is sharply angulated away from the midline. Cross-sectionally it is flat and ribbonlike, requiring close attention to debridement and instrumentation; fortunately there is rarely more than one apical foramen. The distobuccal root is conical and usually straight. It usually has a single canal but occasionally has two canals that fuse into one toward the apex.

The mesiobuccal root of the first molar has generated more research, clinical investigation, and pure frustration than has probably any other root in the mouth. Green[11] stated that two foramina were present in 14% of mesiobuccal roots of the maxillary first molars studied, and two orifices were noted in 36%. Pineda[21] reported that 42% of these roots manifested two canals and two apical foramina. Slowey[23] supported Pineda's conclusions within a few percentage points. Kulild and Peters[17] indicated that a second mesiolingual canal was contained in the coronal half of 95.2% of the mesiobuccal roots examined. The canals were located with hand instruments (54.2%), bur (31.3%), and microscope (9.6%). Each tooth was sectioned in 1-mm increments; although not all canals reached the apex, this study revealed that 71.1% had two patent canals at the apex. The fact that almost half these roots bear two canals is enough reason to *always assume that two canals exist* until careful examination proves otherwise. The extra orifice lies somewhere between the mesiobuccal and lingual canals. It may at times lie quite mesial to a line between these two canals, appearing to be almost under the marginal ridge. A rhomboid-shaped access preparation helps locate these mesially located canals. Very rarely this root has three canals.

Kulild and Peters[17] also reported that the mesiolingual canal orifice averaged 1.82 mm lingual to the mesiobuccal orifice. Searching for the extra orifice is aided by using fiber-optic transillumination to locate the developmental line between the mesiobuccal and palatal orifices. Magnification using loupes or a surgical operating microscope is often necessary to locate these extra canals.

All caries, leaking restorations, and pulpal calcifications must be removed before endodontic treatment is initiated. After treatment it is mandatory to institute full coverage to ensure against vertical cuspal or crown-root fracture. It is also advisable to place internal metal reinforcement whenever there is a significant loss of coronal tooth structure.

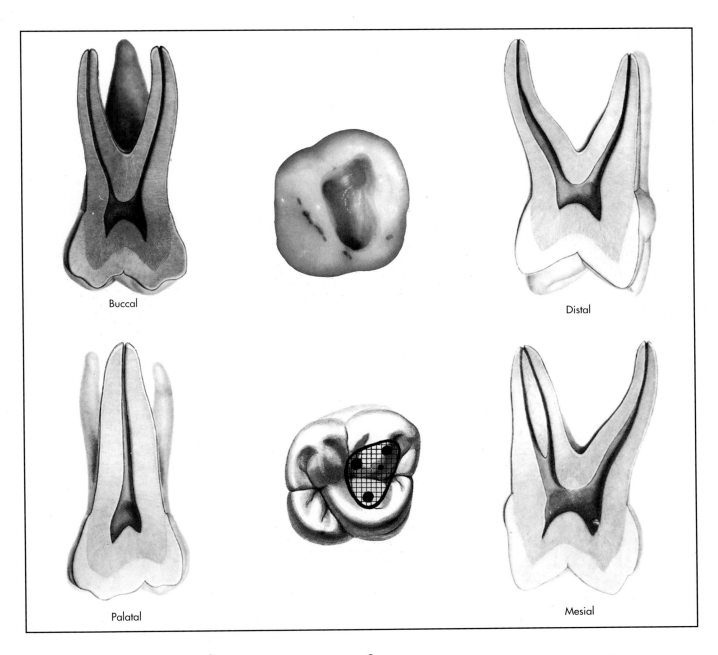

Buccal

Distal

Palatal

Mesial

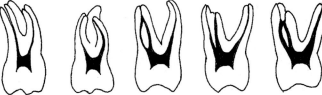

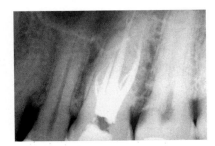

PLATE 7-VI-7 Fourth canal in mesiobuccal root; loops and accessory canals.

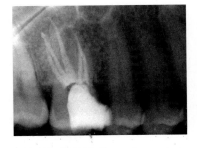

PLATE 7-VI-8 Second canals in both the mesiobuccal and distobuccal roots, both with common foramen.

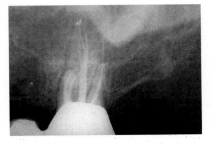

PLATE 7-VI-9 Second canals in both mesiobuccal and lingual canals.

PLATE VII
Maxillary Second Molar

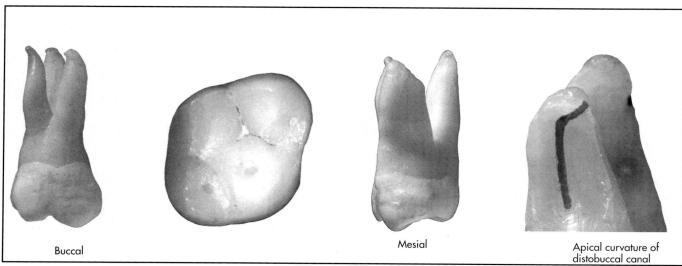

Buccal   Mesial   Apical curvature of
                                                    distobuccal canal

Average time of eruption: 11 to 13 years
Average age of calcification: 14 to 16 years
Average length: 20.0 mm

Coronally, the maxillary second molar closely resembles the maxillary first molar, although it is not as large. Access in both teeth can usually be adequately prepared without disturbing the transverse ridge. The second molar is often easier to prepare because of the straight-line access to the orifice.

The distinguishing morphologic feature of the maxillary second molar is that its three roots are grouped close together and sometimes fused. These fused roots occasionally have only two canals and rarely only one canal. Two-canaled teeth have a buccal and lingual canal of equal length and diameter. The parallel root canals are frequently superimposed radiographically. They are usually shorter than the roots of the first molar and not as curved. The three orifices may form a flat triangle, sometimes almost a straight line. The floor of the chamber is markedly convex, giving a slightly funnel shape to the canal orifices. Occasionally the canals curve into the chamber at a sharp angle to the floor, making it necessary to remove a lip of den-

tin so the canal can be entered more in a direct line with the canal axis (see Fig. 7-5).

Complications in access occur when the molar is tipped in distal version. Initial opening with an end-cutting fissure bur is followed by a short-shanked round bur, which is best suited to uncover the pulp chamber and shape the access cavity. Then small hand instruments are used to establish canal continuity and working length. The bulk of the cleaning and shaping may now be accomplished with engine-driven files.

To enhance radiographic visibility, especially when there is interference with the malar process, a more perpendicular and distoangular radiograph may be exposed.

All caries, leaking restorations, and pulpal calcifications must be removed before endodontic treatment is initiated. Full occlusal coverage is mandatory to ensure against cuspal or crown-root fracture. Internal reinforcement, when indicated, should be incorporated immediately after endodontic treatment.

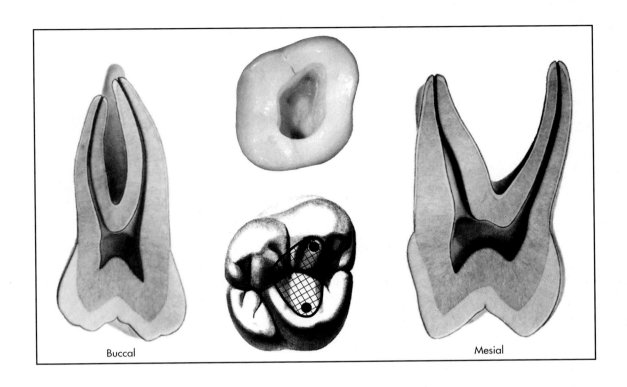

Buccal   Mesial

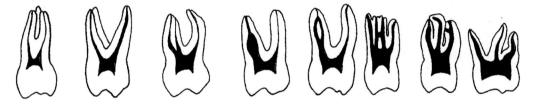

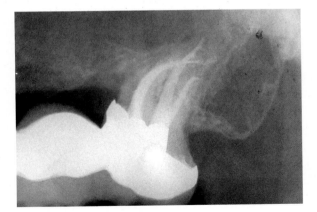

PLATE 7-VII-5 Severely curved mesiobuccal root with right angle curve in distobuccal root.

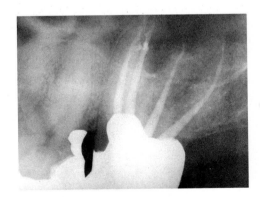

PLATE 7-VII-6 Four-rooted maxillary second molar.

PLATE VIII
Maxillary Third Molar

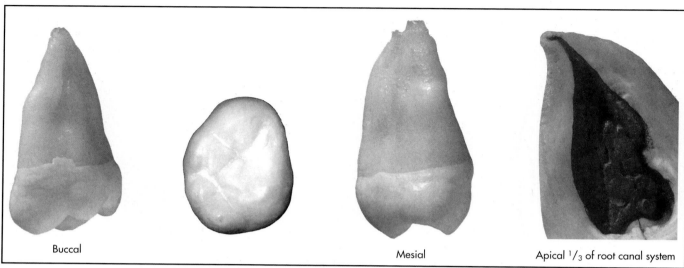

Buccal   Mesial   Apical ¹/₃ of root canal system

Average time of eruption: 17 to 22 years
Average age of calcification: 18 to 25 years
Average length: 17.0 mm

Loss of the maxillary first and second molars is often the reason for considering the third molar as a strategic abutment. The other indication for endodontic treatment and full coverage is a fully functioning mandibular third molar.

Careful examination of root morphology is important before recommending treatment. The radicular anatomy of the third molar is completely unpredictable, and it may be advisable to explore the root canal morphology before promising success. Many third molars present adequate root formation, however, and given reasonable accessibility, there is no reason why they cannot remain as functioning dentition after endodontic therapy.

Some third molars have only a single canal, some two, and most three. The orifice openings may be made in either a triangular arrangement or a nearly straight line.

For visual and mechanical convenience the access may be overextended slightly with the knowledge that full coverage is mandatory. All caries, leaking restorations, and pulpal calcifications must be removed before endodontic treatment is initiated. Precurving the instruments helps guide them through tortuous canals.

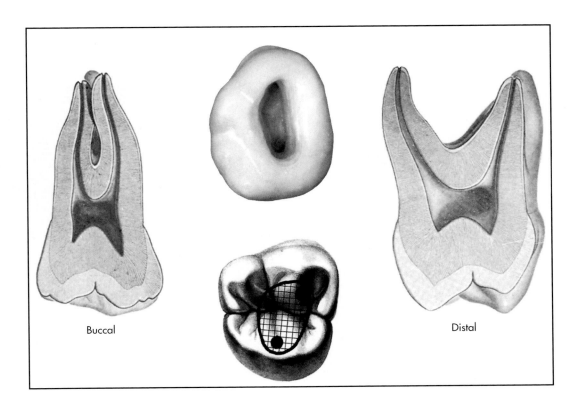

Buccal

Distal

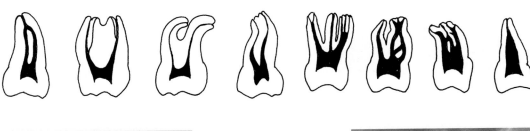

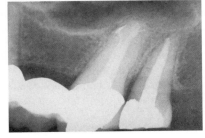

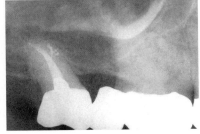

PLATE 7-VIII-5 Showing canals fuses into single canal. (Note multiple accessories in second molar).

PLATE 7-VIII-6 Distal bridge abutment with major accessory canal.

PLATE IX
Mandibular Central and Lateral Incisors

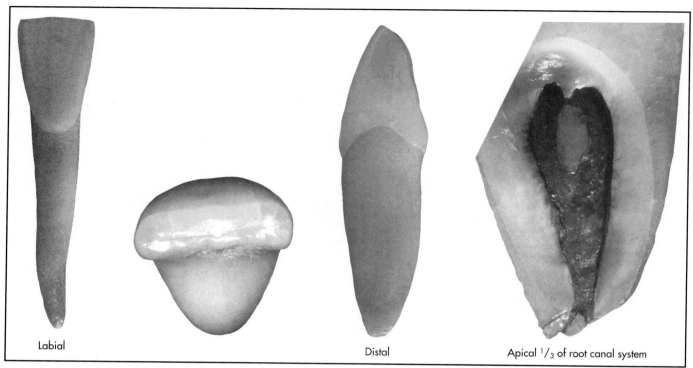

Labial   Distal   Apical $^{1}/_{3}$ of root canal system

Average time of eruption: 6 to 8 years
Average age of calcification: 9 to 10 years
Average length: 20.7 mm

Narrow and flat in the labiolingual dimension, the mandibular incisors are the smallest human adult teeth. Visible radiographically from only two planes, they often appear more accessible than they really are. The narrow lingual crown offers a limited area for access. Smaller fissure burs and No. 2 round burs cause less mutilation of coronal dentition. The access cavity should be ovoid, with attention given to a lingual approach, as seen in Fig. 7-4.

Frequently the mandibular incisors have two canals. One study[2] reported 41.4% of mandibular incisors studied had two separate canals; of these, only 1.3% had two separate foramina. The clinician should search for the second canal immediately on completing the access cavity. Endodontic failures in mandibular incisors usually arise from uncleaned canals, most commonly toward the lingual pulp chamber. Access may be ex-

tended incisally when indicated to permit maximal labiolingual freedom. Two rooted lower incisors are common (Fig. 7-7).

Although labial perforations are common, they may be avoided if the clinician remembers it is nearly impossible to perforate in a lingual direction because of the bur shank's contacting the incisal edge. The ribbon-shaped canal (see Fig. 7-2) is common enough to be considered normal and demands special attention in cleaning and shaping.

Ribbon-shaped canals in narrow hourglass cross-sectioned anatomy invite lateral perforation by endodontic files and Peeso or Gates-Glidden drills. Minimal flaring and dowel space preparation are indicated to ensure against ripping through proximal root walls.

Apical curvatures and accessory canals are common in mandibular incisors.

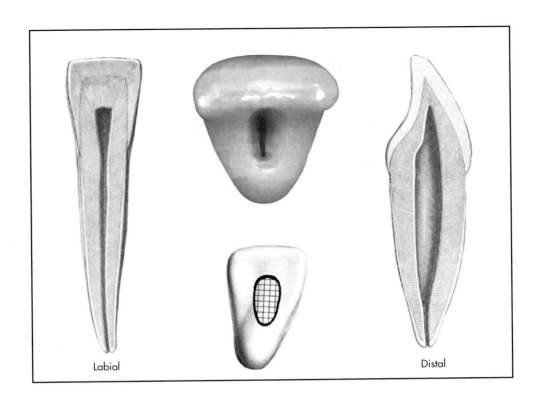

Labial   Distal

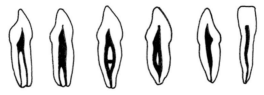

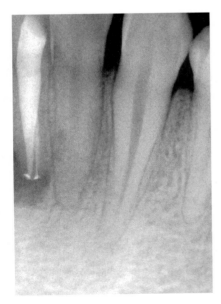

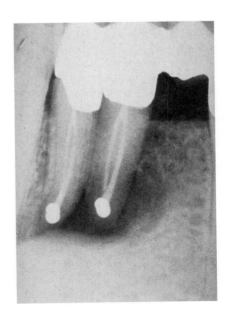

PLATE 7-IX-5 Two rooted mandibular lateral incisor.

PLATE 7-IX-6 Mandibular lateral and central, both with two canals.

PLATE X
Mandibular Canine

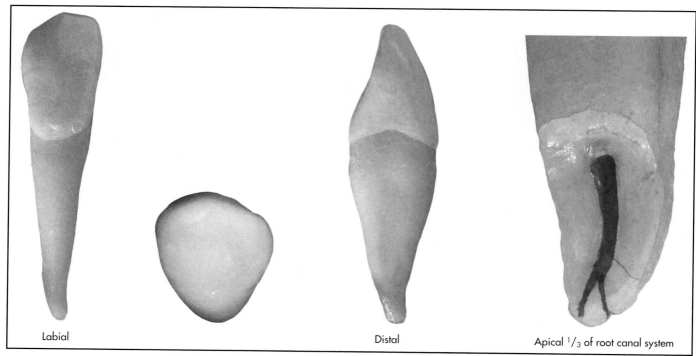

Labial   Distal   Apical ⅓ of root canal system

Average time of eruption: 9 to 10 years
Average age of calcification: 13 years
Average length: 25.6 mm

Sturdy and considerably wider mesiodistally than the incisors, the mandibular canines seldom present endodontic problems. They occasionally have two canals and sometimes two roots, which can create difficulty, but this is rare.

The access cavity is ovoid and may be extended incisally for labiolingual accessibility. The canal is somewhat ovoid at the cervical, becoming round at midroot. Directional instrumentation is necessary to debride the canal walls completely.

If there are two roots, one is always easier to instrument. The other must be opened and funneled in concert with the first to prevent packing of dentin debris and loss of access (see Fig. 7-30). Precurving of instruments at initial access enables the clinician to trace down the buccal or lingual root wall until the tip engages the orifice. When the difficult canal is located, every effort should be made to shape and funnel the opening to maintain continued access.

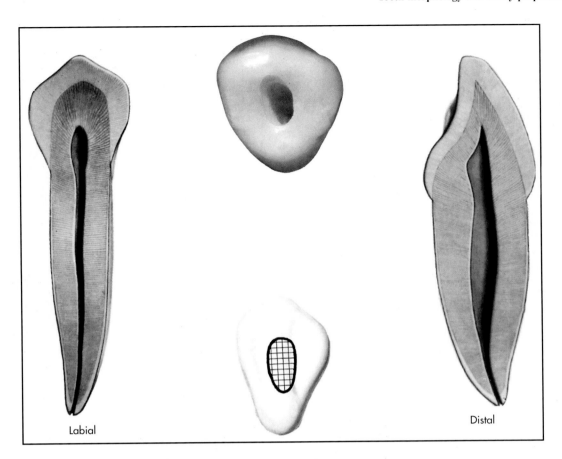

Labial

Distal

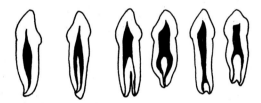

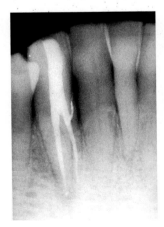

PLATE 7-X-5 Two-rooted mandibular canine.

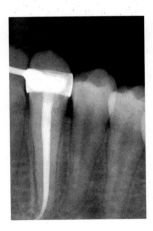

PLATE 7-X-6 Sharp distal curvature at apex.

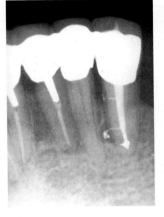

PLATE 7-X-7 Two lateral canals. The incisal canal is above the crest of bone and was probably responsible for pocket depth.

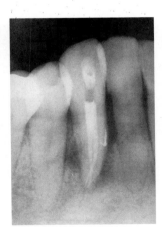

PLATE 7-X-8 Twin-canaled mandibular canine with significant lateral canals feeding a periodontal defect.

PLATE XI
Mandibular First Premolar

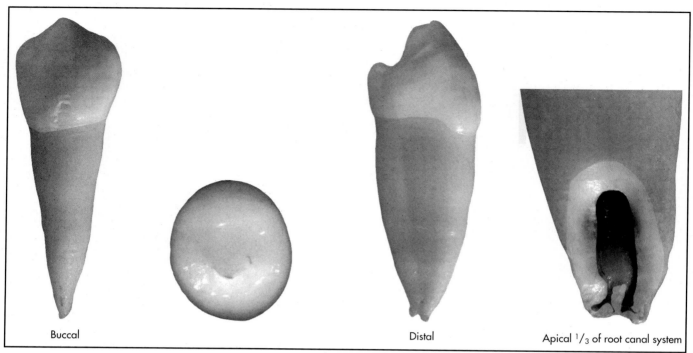

Buccal   Distal   Apical ¹/₃ of root canal system

Average time of eruption: 10 to 12 years
Average age of calcification: 12 to 13 years
Average length: 21.6 mm

Often considered an enigma to the endodontist, the mandibular first premolar with dual canals dividing at various levels of the root can generate complex mechanical problems.

The coronal anatomy consists of a well-developed buccal cusp and a small or almost nonexistent lingual outgrowth of enamel. Access is made slightly buccal to the central groove and is directed in the long axis of the root toward the central cervical area. The ovoid pulp chamber is reached with end-cutting fussure burs and long-shanked No. 4 or 6 round burs. The cross section of the cervical pulp chamber is almost round in a single canal tooth and is ovoid in two canal teeth.

One investigation[32] reported that "a second or third canal exists in at least 23% of first mandibular premolars." The canals may divide almost anywhere down the root. Because of the absence of direct access, cleaning, shaping, and filling of these teeth can be extremely difficult.

A study by Vertucci et al.[27] revealed that the mandibular first premolar had one canal at the apex in 74% of the teeth studied, two canals at the apex in 25.5%, and three canals at the apex in the remaining 0.5% (Fig. 7-2). Baisden et al.[1] reported the existence of C-shaped canals in 14% of the roots of mandibular first premolars that had one root canal and two apical foramina.

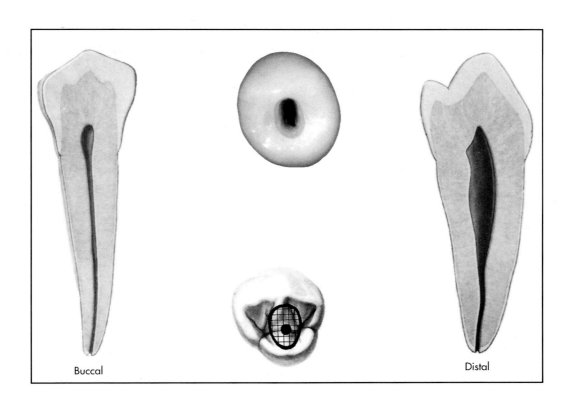

Buccal   Distal

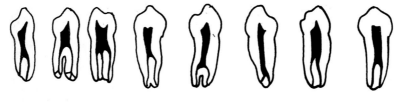

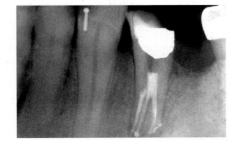

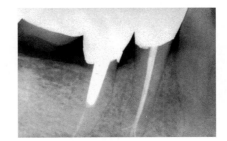

PLATE 7-XI-5 Three-rooted mandibular first bicuspid.   **PLATE 7-XI-6** Single canal dividing at apex.

PLATE XII
Mandibular Second Premolar

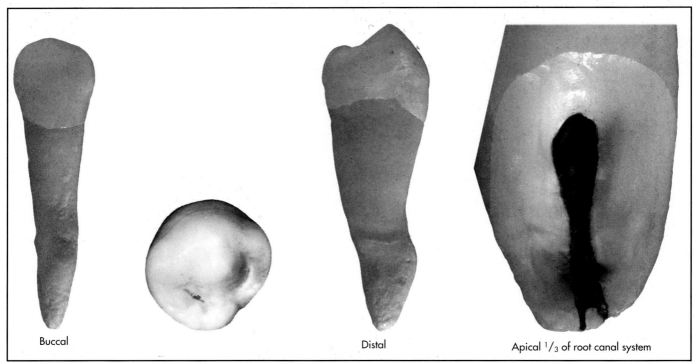

Buccal   Distal   Apical ¹/₃ of root canal system

Average time of eruption: 11 to 12 years
Average age of calcification: 13 to 14 years
Average length: 22.3 mm

Very similar coronally to the first premolar, the mandibular second premolar presents less of a radicular problem. Its crown has a well-developed buccal cusp and a more well-formed lingual cusp than the first premolar. Access is made slightly ovoid, wider in the mesiodistal dimension. The first opening, with the end-cutting fissure bur, is made approximately in the central groove and is extended and refined with Nos. 4 and 6 round burs.

Investigators[29] reported that only 12% of mandibular second molars studied had a second or third canal. Vertucci et al.[27] showed that the second premolar had one canal at the apex in 97.5% and two canals at the apex in only 2.5% of the teeth stud-

ied. In 1991 Bram and Fleisher[4] reported a case of four distinct canals.

An important consideration that must not be overlooked is the anatomic position of the mental foramen and the neurovascular structures that pass through it. The proximity of these nerves and blood vessels can result in temporary paresthesia from the fulminating inflammatory process when acute exacerbation of the mandibular premolars occurs. Exacerbations in this region seem to be intense and more resistant to nonsurgical therapy than in other parts of the mouth.

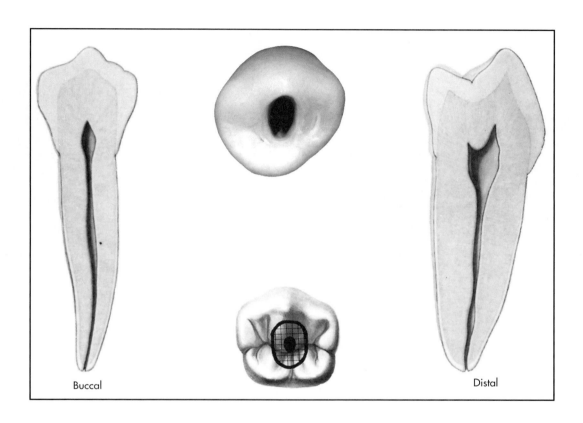

Buccal

Distal

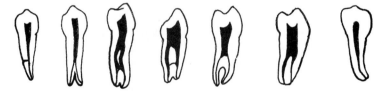

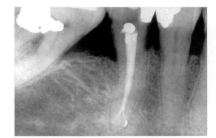

PLATE 7-XII-5 Single canal dividing at apex.

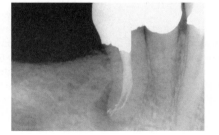

PLATE 7-XII-6 Single canal dividing and crossing over at apex.

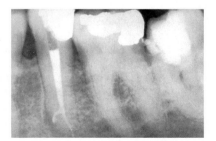

PLATE 7-XII-7 Single canal with lateral accessory canal.

PLATE XIII
Mandibular First Molar

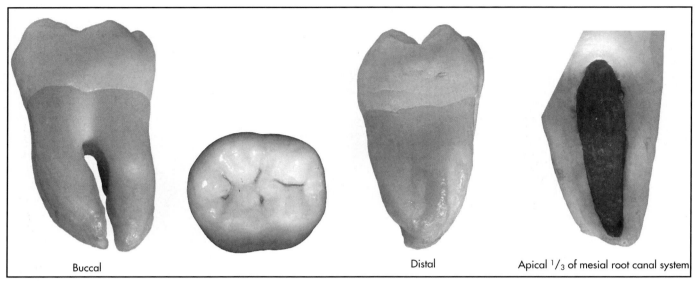

Buccal   Distal   Apical $^1/_3$ of mesial root canal system

Average time of eruption: 6 years
Average age of calcification: 9 to 10 years
Average length: 21.0 mm

The earliest permanent posterior tooth to erupt, the mandibular first molar seems to be the most frequently in need of endodontic treatment. It usually has two roots but occasionally three, with two canals in the mesial and one or two canals in the distal root.

The distal root is readily accessible to endodontic cavity preparation and mechanical instrumentation, and the clinician can frequently see directly into the orifice(s). The canals of the distal root are larger than those of the mesial root. Occasionally the orifice is wide from buccal surface to lingual. This anatomy indicates the possibility of a second canal or a ribbonlike canal with a complex webbing that can complicate cleaning and shaping.

The mesial roots are usually curved, with the greatest curvature in the mesiobuccal canal. The orifices are usually well separated within the main pulp chamber and occur in the buccal, and lingual aspects under the cusp tips.

This tooth is often extensively restored. It is almost always under heavy occlusal stress; thus the coronal pulp chambers are frequently calcified. The distal canals are easiest to locate; once these locations are positively identified, the mesial canals are found in the aforementioned locations in the same horizontal plane.

Because the mesial canal openings lie under the mesial cusps, they may be impossible to locate with conventional cavity preparations. It is then necessary to remove cuspal hard tissue or restoration to locate the orifice. As part of the access preparation, the unsupported cusps of posterior teeth must be reduced.[29] The mandibular first molar, like all posterior teeth, should always receive full occlusal coverage after endodontic therapy (see Chapter 22). Therefore a wider access cavity to locate landmarks and orifices is better than ignoring one or more canals for the sake of a conservative preparation, which may lead to failure.

Skidmore and Bjorndal[22] stated that approximately one third of the mandibular first molars studied had four root canals. When a tooth contained two canals, "they either remained two distinct canals with separate apical foramina, united and formed a common apical foramen, or communicated with each other partially or completely by transverse anastomoses . . . If the traditional triangular outline were changed to a more rectangular one, it would permit better visualization and exploration of a possible fourth canal in the distal root."

On rare occasions, a smaller and shorter third root is present. It is usually found on the distolingual aspect and may possess a sharp apical hook toward the buccal. Orifice locations of the two distally located canals may be found in extreme buccal and lingual positions.

Multiple accessory foramina are located in the furcation areas of mandibular molars.[16] These foramina are usually impossible to clean and shape directly and are rarely seen, except occasionally on a posteroperative radiograph if they have been filled with root canal sealer or warmed gutta-percha. Because sodium hypochlorite solutions have the property of dissolving protein degeneration products, the furcation area of the pulp chamber should be thoroughly exposed (calcific adhesions removed, etc.) to allow the solutions to reach the tiny openings.

All caries, leaking restoration, and pulpal calcifications must be removed before endodontic treatment is initiated, and full cuspal protection and internal reinforcement are recommended.

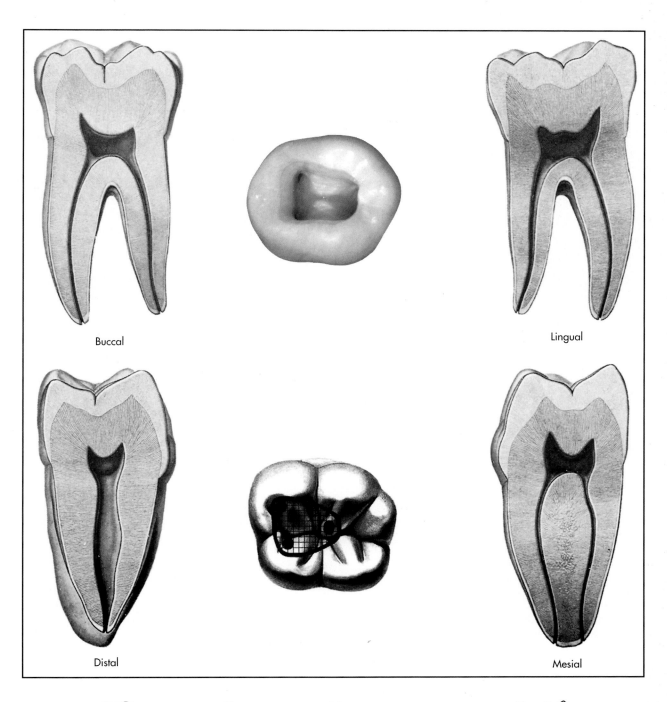

Buccal

Lingual

Distal

Mesial

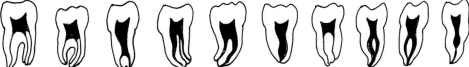

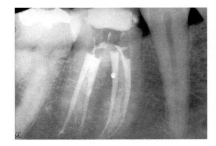

PLATE 7-XIII-7 Mandibular first molar with four roots.

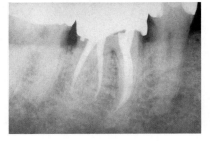

PLATE 7-XIII-8 Mandibular first molar with four roots with wide division of the distal roots.

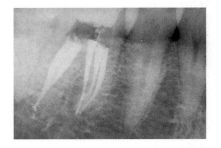

PLATE 7-XIII-9 Mandibular first molar with three mesial canals.

PLATE XIV
Mandibular Second Molar

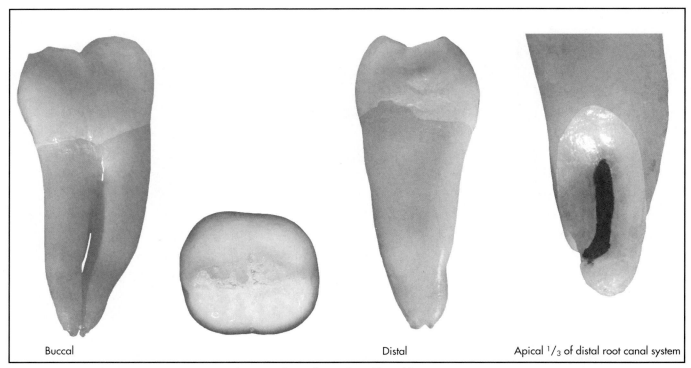

Buccal   Distal   Apical ¹/₃ of distal root canal system

Average time of eruption: 11 to 13 years
Average age of calcification: 14 to 15 years
Average length: 19.8 mm

Somewhat smaller coronally than the mandibular first molar and tending toward more symmetry, the mandibular second molar is identified by the proximity of its roots. The roots often sweep distally in a gradual curve with the apexes close together. The degree and configuration of canal curvature were studied in the mesial roots of 100 randomly selected mandibular first and second molars. One hundred percent of the specimens demonstrated curvature in both buccolingual and mesiodistal views.[7] Weine et al.[29] reported that 4% of mandibular second molars had one root with a **C**-shaped canal, or less often, only one canal. They also reported that 4% had two roots with two canals, most had two roots with three canals, and two-canaled distal roots were less common than in the lower first molar.

Access is made in the mesial aspect of the crown, with the opening extending only slightly distal to the central groove. After penetration with the end-cutting fissure bur, the long-shanked round bur is used to sweep outwardly until unobstructed access is achieved. The distal angulation of the roots often permits less extension of the opening than in the mandibular first molar.

Close attention should be given to the shape of the distal orifice. A narrow, ovoid opening indicates a ribbon-shaped distal canal, requiring more directional type filing. All caries, leaking fillings, and pulpal calcifications must be removed and replaced with a suitable temporary restoration before endodontic therapy is initiated.

The mandibular second molar is the most susceptible to vertical fracture. After access preparation the clinician should use the fiber-optic light to search the floor of the chamber before endodontic treatment is initiated.

Full occlusal coverage after endodontic therapy is mandatory to ensure against future problems with vertical fractures.

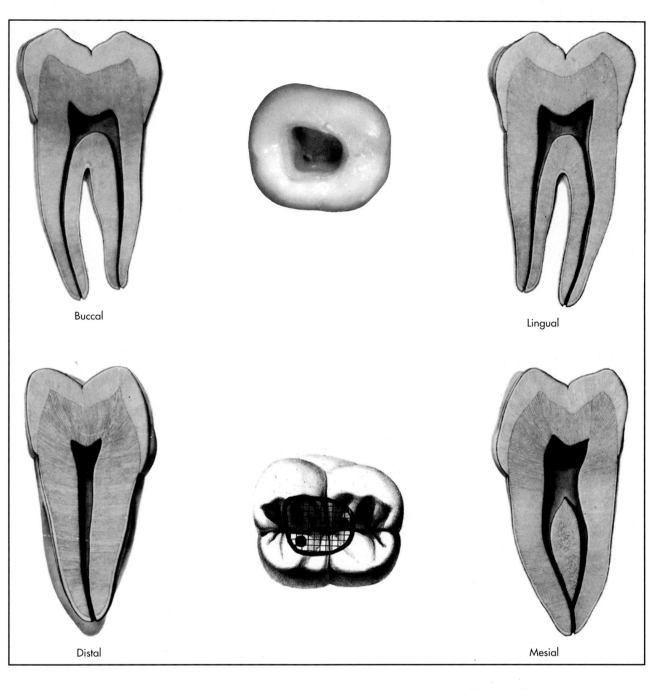

Buccal

Lingual

Distal

Mesial

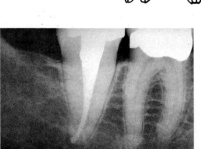

PLATE 7-XIV-8 Mandibular second molar with anastamosis of all canals into one.

PLATE 7-XIV-9 Accessory canal at distal root apex.

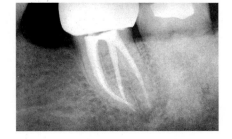

PLATE 7-XIV-10 Fusion of mesial canals at mesial root apex.

PLATE XV
Mandibular Third Molar

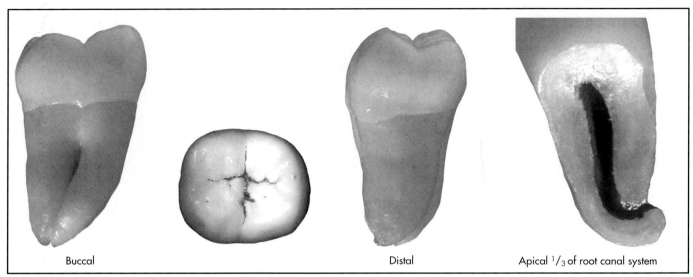

Buccal   Distal   Apical $^1/_3$ of root canal system

Average time of eruption: 17 to 21 years
Average age of calcification: 18 to 25 years
Average length: 18.5 mm

Anatomically unpredictable, the mandibular third molar must be evaluated on the basis of its root formation. Well-formed crowns are often supported by fused, short, severely curved, or malformed roots. Most teeth can be successfully treated endodontically, regardless of anatomic irregularities, but root surface volume in contact with bone is what determines long-term prognosis.

The clinician may find a single canal that is wide at the neck and tapers to a single apical foramen. Access is gained through the mesial aspect of the crown. Distally angulated roots often permit less extension of the access cavity.

All caries, leaking restorations, and pulpal calcifications should be removed and replaced with adequate temporary restoration. If the tooth is in heavy occlusal function, full cuspal protection is indicated postendodontically.

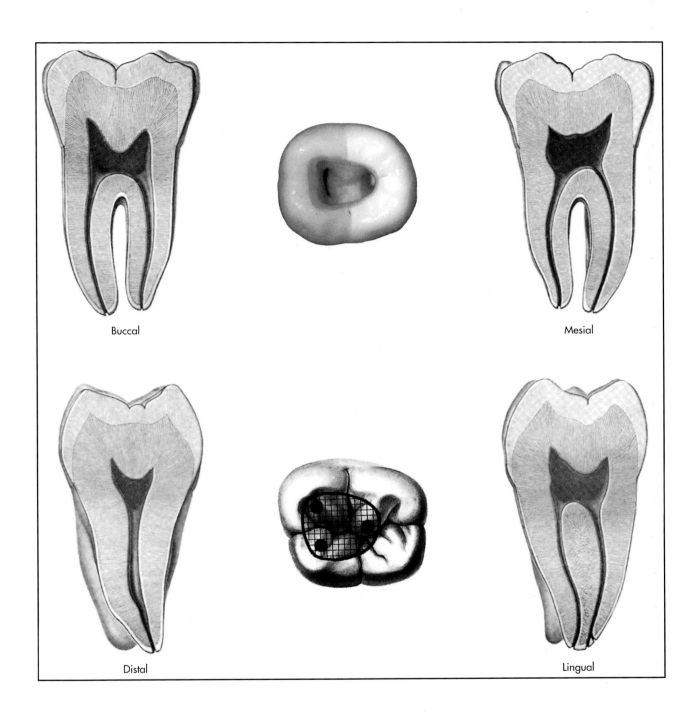

Buccal

Mesial

Distal

Lingual

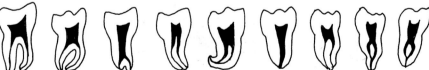

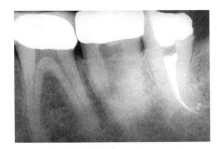

PLATE 7-XV-7 Third molar with accessory foramina at apex.

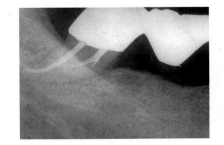

PLATE 7-XV-8 Complex curved root anatomy.

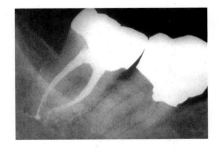

PLATE 7-XV-9 Complex apical anatomy.

PLATE XVI
The C-Shaped Mandibular Molar

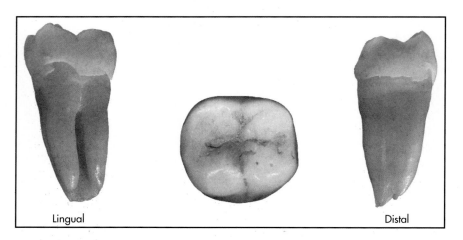

Lingual   Distal

The C-shaped molar is so named for the cross-sectional morphology of the root and root canal. Instead of having several discrete orifices, the pulp chamber of the C-shaped molar has a single ribbon-shaped orifice with a 180-degree arc, starting at the mesiolingual line angle, sweeping around the buccal to end at the distal aspect of the pulp chamber (Plate 7-XVI-2).

Below the orifice level, the root structure of C-shaped molars can harbor a wide range of anatomic variations. These can be classified into two basic groups: (1) those with a single ribbonlike C-shaped canal from orifice to apex and (2) those with three distinct canals below the usual C-shaped orifice.

Fortunately C-shaped molars with a single swath of canal are the exception rather than the rule. Melton et al.[19] found that the C-shaped canals can vary in number and shape along the length of the root, with the result that debridement, obturation, and restoration in this group may be unusually difficult (Plates 7-XVI-6 and 7-XVI-7). More common is the second type of C-shaped molar, with its discrete canals having an unusual form. The mesiolingual canal is separate and distinct from the apex, although it may be significantly shorter than mesiobuccal and distal canals (Plate 7-XVI-4). These canals are easily over-instrumented in C-shaped molars with a single apex (Plate 7-XVI-5) as they may end 2 to 4 mm short of the apex.

In these molars the mesiobuccal canal swings back and merges with the distal canal, and these exit onto the root surface through a single foramen. A few of these molars with C-shaped orifices have mesiobuccal and distal canals that do not merge but have separate portals of exit.

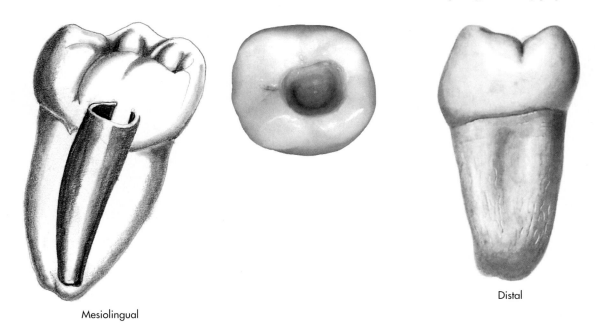

Mesiolingual

Distal

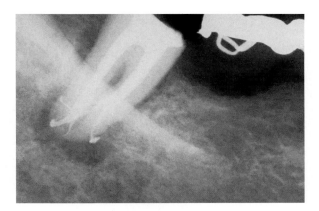

PLATE 7-XVI-4 Mandibular second molar with multiple foramina.

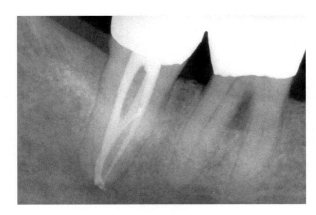

PLATE 7-XVI-5 Mandibular second molar with interconnecting canal anatomy.

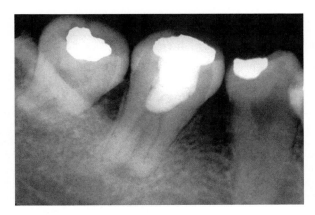

PLATE 7-XVI-6 Preop of mandibular first molar with C-shaped canal.

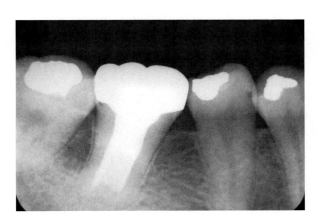

PLATE 7-XVI-7 Finished endodontics showing complete obturation of the ribbon-like canal spaces.

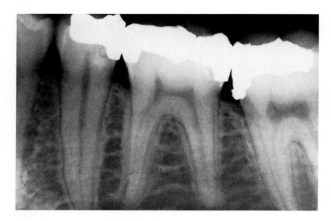

FIG. 7-10 Radiograph of actual case taken in 1976 at the time of first symptoms. The tooth was not treated endodontically because tests showed it to be vital. Caries was removed from under the mesial amalgam, calcium hydroxide was placed.

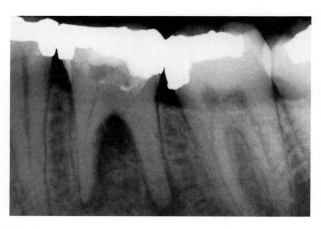

FIG. 7-11 Radiograph of tooth in Fig. 7-11 taken in 1989 reveals severe calcification of the pulp chambers and periapical and furcal radiolucencies.

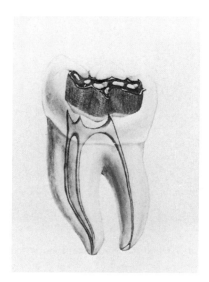

FIG. 7-12 Mandibular first molar with class I amalgam restoration and average pulp chambers.

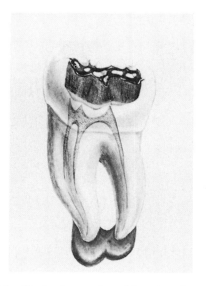

FIG. 7-13 Mandibular first molar with a class I amalgam, calcified canals, and periapical radiolucency. The assumption is that a pulpal exposure has occurred, causing calcification and, ultimately, necrosis of the pulp tissue.

METHODS OF LOCATING CALCIFIED CANALS

Preoperative radiographs (Fig. 7-11) often appear to reveal total or nearly total calcification of the main pulp chamber and radicular canal spaces. Unfortunately the spaces have adequate room to allow passage of millions of microorganisms. The narrowing of these pulpal pathways is often caused by chronic inflammatory processes such as caries, medications, occlusal trauma, and aging.

Despite severe coronal calcification the clinician must assume that all canals exist and must be cleaned, shaped, and filled to the canal terminus. Canals become less calcified as they approach the root apex. There are many methods of lo-

cating these spaces (Figs. 7-11 through 7-24). It is recommended that the illustrated sequences be followed to achieve the most successful result.

In the event of inability to locate either canal orifice, the prudent clinician will stop excavating dentin or the tooth structure will be weakened. Serious errors can occur when overzealous or inappropriate attempts are made to locate canals (Figs. 7-26, 7-28, and 7-32). Root wall or furcal perforations can occur even with the most careful search for canals. Immediate attention must be given to repair communication with the ligament space and surrounding bone (Fig. 7-29). Retrograde procedures become conservative when compared with perfo-

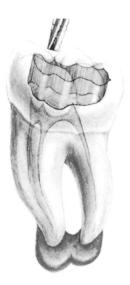

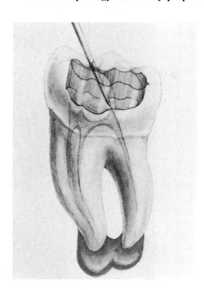

FIG. 7-14 Illustration showing excavation of amalgam and base material. The cavity preparation should be extended toward the assumed location of the pulp chamber. At this phase of treatment the clinician must attempt to provide maximum visibility of the roof of the main chamber. All caries, cements, and discolored dentin should be removed.

FIG. 7-16 The endodontic explorer, DG 16 (Hu-Friedy Co., Chicago, Ill.), is used to explore the region of the pulpal floor. It is as important to the clinician doing endodontic therapy as the periodontal probe is to the dentist performing a periodontal examination. It is both an examining instrument and a chipping tool, often being called on to "flake away" calcified dentin. Reparative dentin is slightly softer than normal dentin. A slight "tugback" in the area of the canal orifice often signals the presence of a canal.

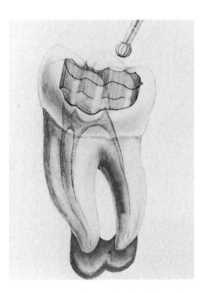

FIG. 7-15 Using a long-shanked No. 4 or 6 round bur, the clinician explores the assumed location of the main pulp chamber.

rations or root fractures. There is no rapid technique for dealing with calcified cases. Painstaking removal of small amounts of dentin has proven to be the safest approach.

ACHIEVING ACCESS THROUGH COMPLEX RESTORATIONS

Most teeth in need of endodontics have or have had major caries. Extensive coronal tooth loss requires multiple restorations of many types. Subgingival caries requires amalgam re-

storative procedures, which often result in the recession of coronal and radicular canals. Because of this, achieving access in these teeth requires major excavation of filling materials, caries, and calcified tooth structure. Coronal access most often is made through multiple layers of materials placed over long periods of time. Straight-line access can be difficult (Fig. 7-30), particularly in teeth with calcified canals (see Fig. 7-12) or malpositioned teeth (see Fig. 7-26, *F*). Inclined teeth that have been crowned can create difficult access situations if the dentist uses only the anatomy of the cast crown as a guide. The orifices to the canals can be hidden (Fig. 7-27).

Ideal access can only be achieved by total removal of all materials. In the case of gold crowns and porcelain-fused-to-metal crowns, economic factors may influence the choice for gaining access. Under these circumstances, one is well advised that the patient must be thoroughly informed of the potential risks (e.g., perforation, fracture). If the patient accepts these risks, the clinician should make one careful attempt at access through the existing restoration, with the understanding that if the access opening is unsatisfactory, the restoration will have to be completely removed and a new restoration prepared following endodontic treatment (Fig. 7-25, *A* through *D*).

PERIODONTAL-ENDODONTIC SITUATION

Complications of aging alone make locating canal orifices difficult. The problems of bone loss, chronic inflammation of the periodontal ligament, mobility, and leakage into the root canal system are a combined periodontal-endodontic situation. The gradual closure of the internal spaces may be observed as the protective bone enclosure melts away from the root surfaces. The height of the pulp space now moves apically, making occlusal access difficult. Perforations of root walls and furcations are most common as the clinician reaches deeper and

Text continued on p. 201

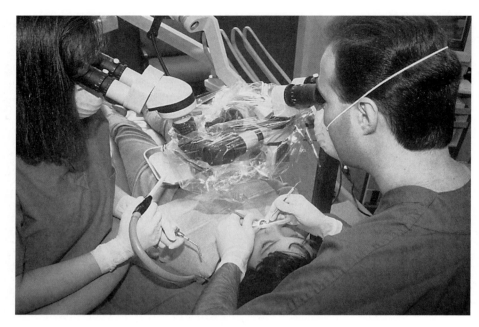

FIG. 7-17 The widespread adaptation of the operating microscope has provided exceptional advances in locating canal anatomy.

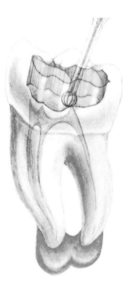

FIG. 7-18 Deeper excavation with Nos. 2 and 4 round burs, following landmarks (without a rubber dam), usually produces a small orifice.

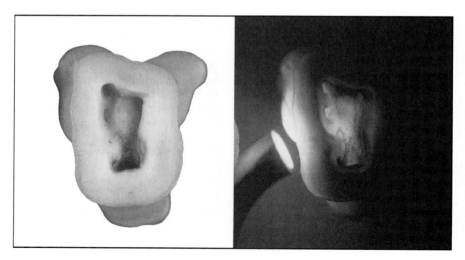

FIG. 7-19 As an adjunct to maximal visibility with magnification, the fiber-optic light can be applied to the cervical aspect of the crown. Transillumination often reveals landmarks otherwise invisible to the unaided eye.

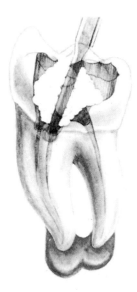

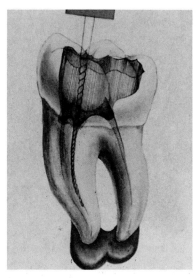

FIG. 7-20 If access does not occur at this point in the search, the clinician should begin to feel concern about the loss of important tooth structure, which could lead to vertical root fracture. The bur may be removed from the handpiece and placed in the excavation site. Packing cotton pellets around the shaft maintains the position and angulation of the bur. The radiograph exposed at right angles through the tooth reveals the depth and the angulation of the search.

FIG. 7-21 At the first indication of a space the smallest instrument (a No. .06 or .08 file) should be introduced. Gentle passive movement, both apical and rotational, often produces some penetration. A slight pull, signaling resistance, is usually an indication that one has located the canal. Careful file manipulation, frequent recapitulation, and canal lubricants (e.g., Calcinase, Glyoxide, R-C Prep) assist in gaining access to the apical terminus. It is suggested that the access to the canal orifice be widened using Gates-Glidden drills until the clinician can readily relocate the orifice.

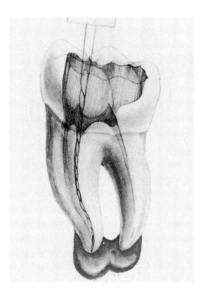

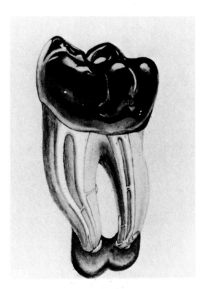

FIG. 7-22 A larger instrument is shown passing two curvatures to the apex by locating one canal in a multicanal tooth. It is usually possible to locate the second, third, or fourth canal once the first one has been located.

FIG. 7-23 Final canal obturation and restoration revealing anatomic complexities. This drawing appeared on the cover of the fifth edition of *Pathways of the Pulp. (The simulations of the prepared and filled canals are courtesy Dr. Clifford Ruddle, Santa Barbara, Calif.)*

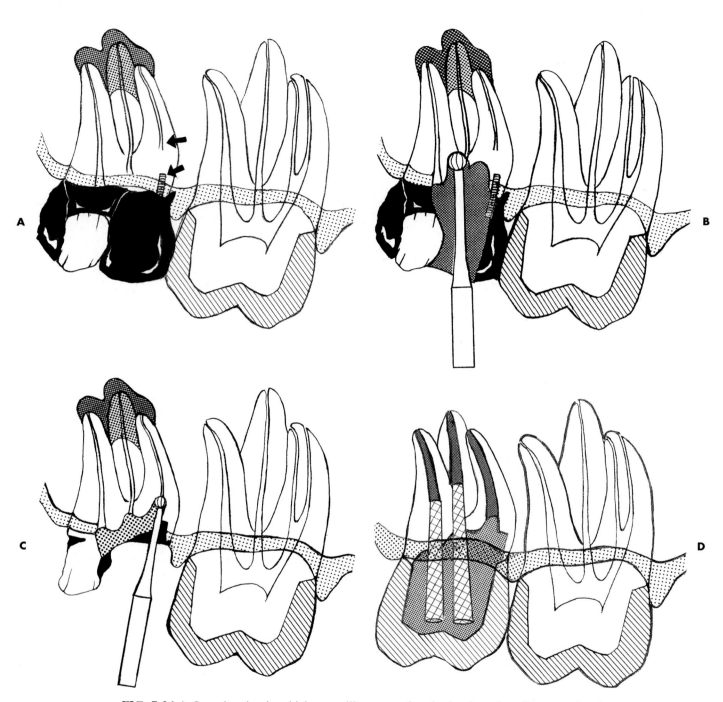

FIG. 7-24 A, In a situation in which a maxillary second molar has been heavily restored and is in need of endodontics, the clinician may elect to attempt access to the canals. The restoration itself presents some clues: (1) a reinforcing pin is visible *(arrow);* (2) at least two thirds of the coronal portion is restorative material; and (3) the mesiobuccal canal appears calcified *(arrow).* These factors alone suggest complete excavation. **B,** On occasion, however, a patient requests a clinician to attempt an unexcavated search for the canals, which might result in a furcal perforation, thereby compromising the prognosis. At this point the patient should be engaged in the decision to continue treatment, which most certainly involves removal of the existing restoration. **C,** A safer and more conservative approach is to remove the amalgam, the pin, and any old cements. **D,** Careful excavation, using enhanced vision, results in access to the pulp chambers and gives the clinician the opportunity to perform routine endodontic therapy followed by internal reinforcement and full coverage.

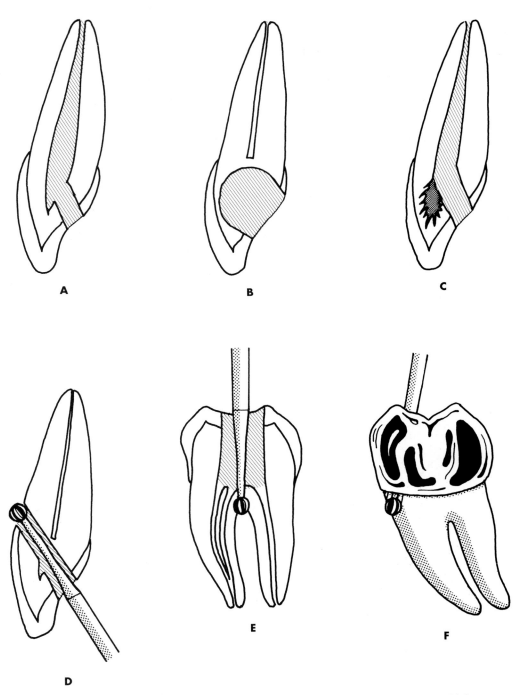

FIG. 7-25 Difficulties created by poor access preparation. **A,** Inadequate opening, which compromises instrumentation, invites coronal discoloration and prevents optimal obturation. **B,** Overzealous tooth removal, resulting in weakening and mutilation of coronal tooth structure, leading to coronal fracture. **C,** Inadequate caries removal, resulting in future carious destruction and discoloration. **D,** Labial perforation (lingual perforation with intact crowns is all but impossible in incisors). Surgical repair is possible, but permanent disfiguration and periodontal destruction will result. **E,** Furcal perforation of any size, which is difficult to repair, causes periodontal destruction and weakens tooth structure, thus inviting fracture. **F,** Misinterpretation of angulation (particularly common with full crowns) and subsequent root perforation. Even when repaired correctly, because it occurs in a difficult maintenance area, the result becomes a permanent periodontal problem.

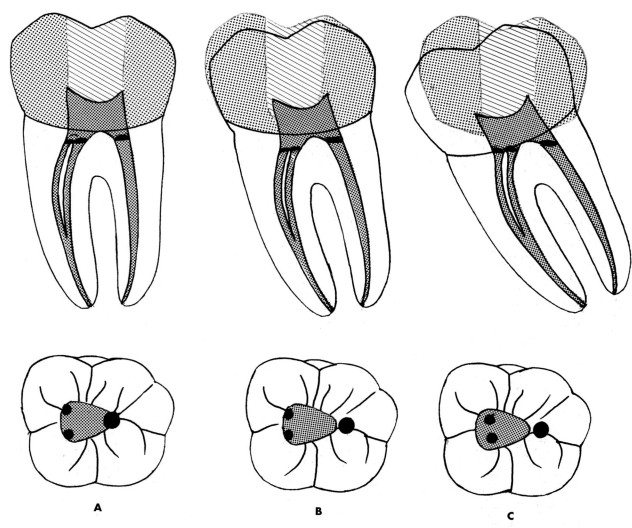

FIG. 7-26 Orifice positions in inclined molars. Inclined posterior teeth occur frequently following tooth loss. Often full veneer crowns are placed with biting surfaces prepared to engage the opposing tooth. The appearance of the occlusal surface can be misleading to the clinician. Even an 11-degree incline can move subcervical orifices dramatically. Careful excavation is required especially with teeth with 18-degree angulations or even more. Severely tipped molars have a high incidence of root perforations (see Fig. 7-25). **A,** Conservative access made in full veneer crown of a mandibular molar in a normal vertical position. **B,** Same access in an occlusal surface made to occlude with maxillary molar in a tooth with an 11-degree angle. **C,** A crown made on an 18-degree angle (see Fig. 7-26, *F*).

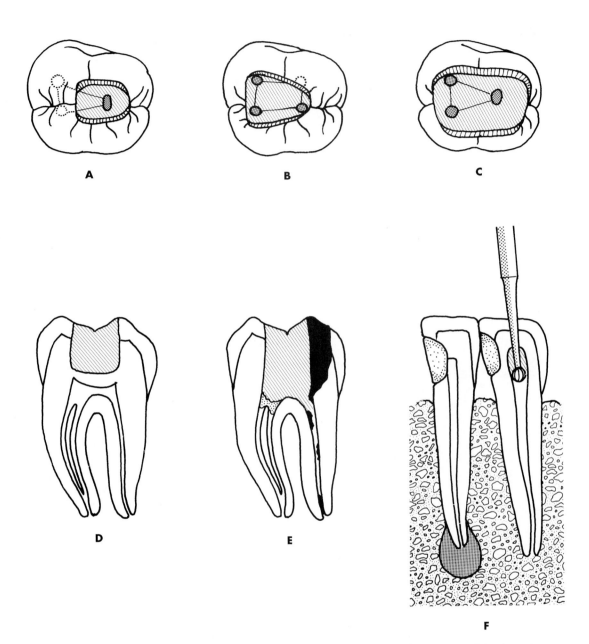

FIG. 7-27 Common errors in access preparation. **A,** Poor access placement and inadequate extension, leaving orifices unexposed. **B,** Better extension but not including the fourth canal orifice. **C,** Overextension, which weakens coronal tooth structure and compromises the final restoration. **D,** Failure to reach the main pulp chamber is a serious error unless the space is heavily calcified. Bite-wing radiographs are excellent aids in determining vertical depth. **E,** Allowing debris to fall into the orifice(s) becomes an iatrogenic problem. Amalgam filings and dentin debris can block access and result in endodontic failure. **F,** The most embarrassing error, and the one with the most damaging medicolegal potential, is entering the wrong tooth. A common site of this mishap is with teeth that appear identical coronally; the simple mistake is placing the rubber dam on the wrong tooth. Beginning the access cavity *before* placement of the rubber dam helps avoid this problem.

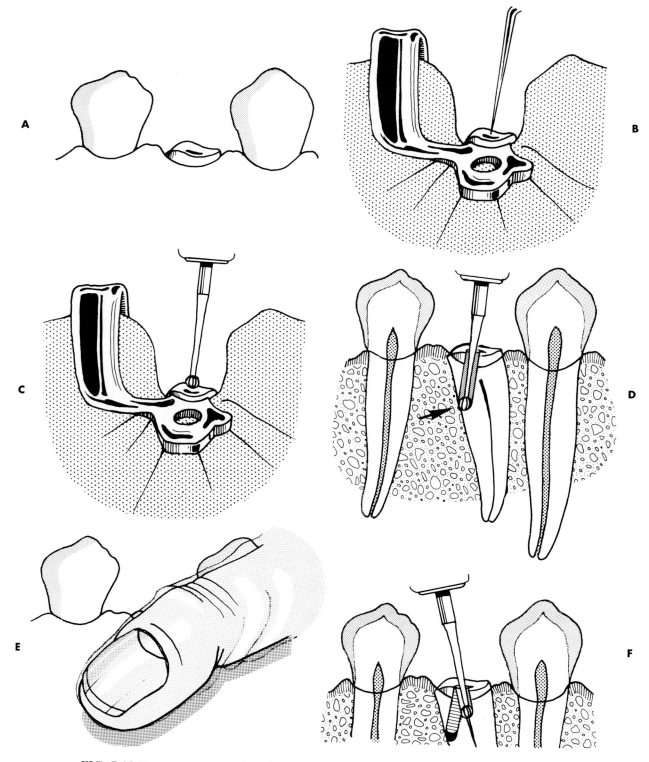

FIG. 7-28 Errors in access cavity when the anatomic crown is missing. **A,** Mandibular first premolar with the crown missing. **B,** An endodontic explorer fails to penetrate the calcified pulp chamber. **C,** Long-shanked round bur directed in the assumed long axis of the root. **D,** Perforation of the root wall *(arrow)* because of the clinician's failure to consider root angulation. **E,** Palpation of the buccal root anatomy to determine root angulation. **F,** Correct bur angulation following repair of the perforation.

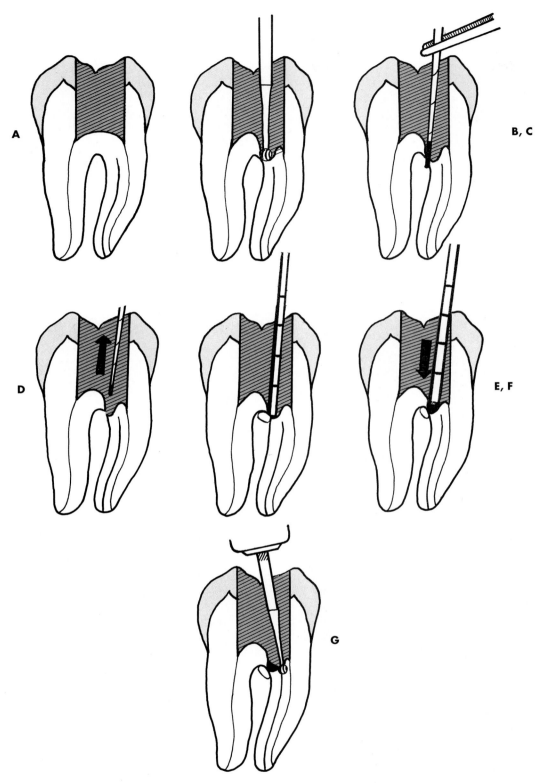

FIG. 7-29 Perforation repair. **A,** Access achieved in two canals but not in the calcified third canal. **B,** Minute furcal perforation during search for the elusive canal. **C,** Using absorbent point for hemorrhage control. **D,** Removing absorbent point immediately before placing matrix. **E,** Introducing Collacote[8] to provide a base for repair material. **F,** Introducing mineral trioxide aggregate (MTF).[25] **G,** On a subsequent appointment, attempt to locate missed canal. (Magnified vision, including the endodontic microscope, is recommended.)

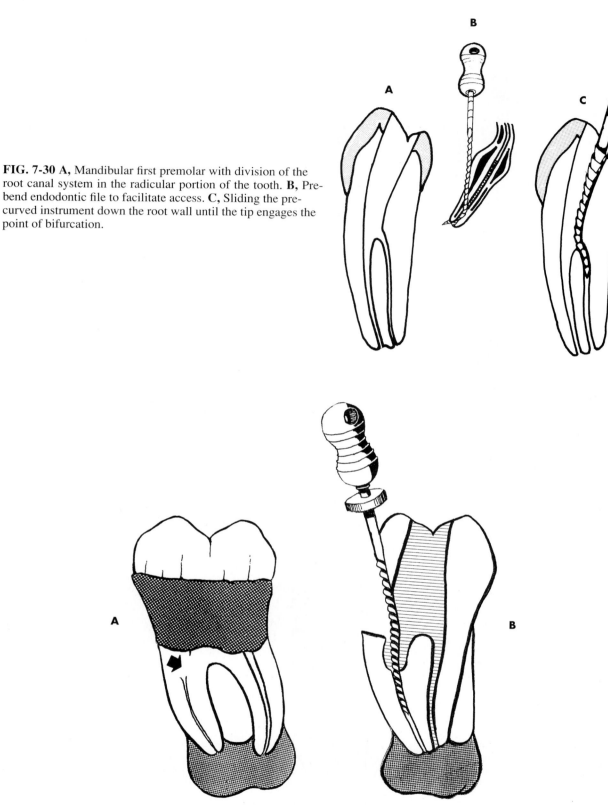

FIG. 7-30 A, Mandibular first premolar with division of the root canal system in the radicular portion of the tooth. **B,** Pre-bend endodontic file to facilitate access. **C,** Sliding the pre-curved instrument down the root wall until the tip engages the point of bifurcation.

FIG. 7-31 A, Extensive class V restoration necessitated by root caries and periodontal disease leading to canal calcification *(arrow).* **B,** Gaining access to these canals occluded by calcification may require removing the facial restoration and obtaining access from the buccal surface.

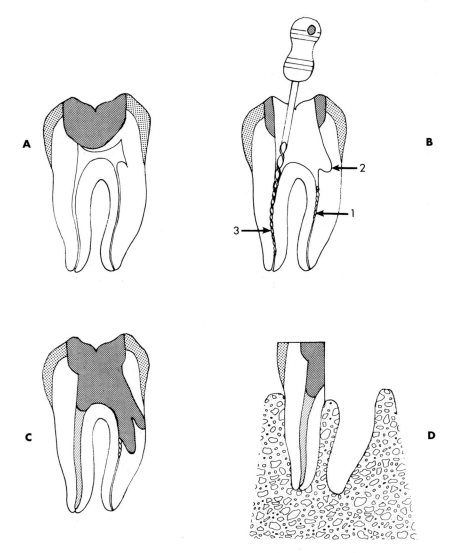

FIG. 7-32 Hemisection as an alternative when mutilation occurs during access preparation. **A,** Calcification after advanced caries and the application of calcium hydroxide can result in serious difficulties in making access. **B,** (1) An instrument has fractured in the mesial canal; (2) a second mesial canal seems totally calcified; and (3) the third canal in the distal root is navigable. **C,** Searching for canals and instrument fragments can result in mutilation of tooth structure. **D,** Obturation of one root and placement of amalgam in access areas restore the intracanal spaces (**C**) in preparation for routine hemisection. Reinforcement with a dowel and core may be performed before final restoration.

deeper with long-shanked burs. One means of locating the position of the bur tip and proper angle of approach is to stop, remove the bur from the handpiece, replace it in the cavity, pack the cavity around the bur with cotton (see Fig. 7-21), and expose a periapical film.

Periodontal patients may have caries on exposed root surfaces and thus require extensive class V restorations. These restorations and the calcification often accompanying them can make gaining occlusal access to some canals impossible. It may become necessary in unusual cases to remove the restorative material and then locate, clean, and shape the canals from the buccal aspect (Fig. 7-31).

REFERENCES

1. Baisden MD, Kulild JC, Weller RN: Root canal configuration of the mandibular first premolar, *J Endod* 18:505, 1992.
2. Benjamin KA, Dowson J: Incidence of two root canals in human mandibular incisor teeth, *Oral Surg* 38:122, 1974.
3. Booth JM: The longest tooth? *Aust Endod News* 13:17, 1988.
4. Bram SM, Fleisher R: Endodontic therapy in a mandibular second bicuspid with four canals, *J Endod* 17:513, 1991.
5. Brand RW, Isselhard DE: *Anatomy of orofacial structures,* ed 5, St Louis, 1994, Mosby.
6. Carns EJ, Skidmore AE: Configurations and deviations of root canals of maxillary first premolars, *Oral Surg* 36:880, 1973.
7. Cunningham CJ, Senia ES: A three dimensional study of canal curvatures in the mesial roots of mandibular molars, *J Endod* 18:294, 1992.

8. Carr GB: Surgical endodontics. In Cohen S, Burns RC, editors: *Pathways of the pulp,* ed 6, St Louis, 1994, Mosby, pp 531-567.

9. Gher ME, Vernino AR: Root anatomy: a local factor in inflammatory periodontal disease, *Int J Periodont Restor Dent* 1:53, 1981.

10. Goon WW et al: Complex facial radicular groove in a maxillary lateral incisor, *J Endod* 17:244, 1991.

11. Green D: Double canals in single roots, *Oral Surg* 35:689, 1973.

12. Grossman LI: *Endodontic practice,* ed 10, Philadelphia, 1981, Lea & Febiger.

13. Hess W, Zurcher E: The anatomy of the root canals of the teeth of the permanent and deciduous dentitions, New York, 1925, William Wood & Co.

14. Hovland EJ, Block RM: Nonrecognition and subsequent endodontic treatment of dens invaginatus, *J Endod* 3:360, 1977.

15. Kasahara E et al: Root canal system of the maxillary central incisor, *J Endod* 16(4):158, 1990.

16. Koenigs JF, Brilliant JD, Foreman DW Jr: Preliminary scanning electron microscope investigation of accessory foramina in the furcation areas of human molar teeth, *Oral Surg* 38:773, 1974.

17. Kulild JC, Peters DD: Incidence and configuration of canal systems in the mesiobuccal root of maxillary first and second molars, *J Endod* 16:311, 1990.

18. Loushine RJ, Jurak JJ, Jeffalone DM: A two rooted mandibular incisor, *J Endod* 19:250, 1991.

19. Melton DC, Krall KV, Fuller MW: Anatomical and histological features of C-shaped canals in mandibular second molars, *J Endod,* vol 17, no. 8, August 1991.

20. Meyer VWE: Die anatomie der Wurzelkanale, dargestellt and mikroskopischen, Rekonstruktionsmodellen, *Dtsch Azhnarztl Z* 25:1064, 1970.

21. Pineda F: Roentgenographic investigations of the mesiobuccal root of the maxillary first molar, *Oral Surg* 36:253, 1973.

22. Skidmore AE, Bjorndal AM: Root canal morphology of the human mandibular first molar, *Oral Surg* 32:778, 1971.

23. Slowey RR: Radiographic aids in the detection of extra root canals, *Oral Surg* 37:762, 1974.

24. Szajkis S, Kaufman A: Root invagination: a conservative approach in endodontics, *J Endod* 11:576, 1993.

25. Torabinejad M: Sealing ability of a mineral trioxide aggregate for repair of lateral root perforations, *J Endod* 11:541, 1993.

26. Vertucci FJ: Root canal morphology of mandibular premolars, *J Am Dent Assoc* 97:47, 1978.

27. Vertucci F, Seelig A, Gillis R: Root canal morphology of the human maxillary second premolar, *Oral Surg* 38:456, 1974.

28. Weine FS et al: Canal configuration in the mesiobucal root of the maxillary first molar and its endodontic significance, *Oral Surg* 28:419, 1969.

29. Weine FS, Pasiewicz RA, Rice RT: Canal configuration in the mandibular second molar using a clinically oriented in vitro method, *J Endod* 14:207, 1988.

30. Wilkie G: Personal communication, Melbourne, Australia, 1993.

31. Zeisz RC, Nuckolls J: *Dental anatomy,* St Louis, 1949, Mosby.

32. Zillich R, Dowson J: Root canal morphology of mandibular first and second premolars, *Oral Surg* 36:738, 1973.

Chapter **8**

Cleaning and Shaping the Root Canal System

John David West
James B. Roane

Techniques for cleaning and shaping root canals differ as a result of extensive clinical observations and research, new products and techniques, and conventional wisdom. For example, there is universal agreement that one should irrigate, yet the type and strength of irrigant is debatable. All agree that the canal system should be cleaned and shaped; however, debate continues over the best method. There are differing views concerning the apical terminus location for cleaning, shaping, and obturating the root canal system. The clinical value of chelating agents used during the cleaning and shaping process has not been proven. These examples illustrate a simple truth: The best procedure for all conditions has not been described. Methods, materials, and techniques change while each clinician faces a different mix of patients. Therefore the astute clinician must be proficient in a variety of cleaning and shaping techniques to provide the best care possible. In this chapter the authors provide the concepts and applications of the most widely used cleaning and shaping techniques supported by the most current research.

ANATOMICALLY GENERATED ENDODONTICS

There is now general consensus about what makes endodontic therapy work so predictably. Every portal of exit is important, because every portal of exit is *potentially* significant.[76] Lesions of endodontic origin may exist anywhere along the surface of the root, including bifurcations, trifurcations, and the base of infrabony pockets.[74] With this awareness, dentists began to think of endodontics in a different manner. The rationale of endodontic treatment is based on simple biologic principles. The connective tissue of dental pulp is similar to other connective tissues of the body. Because the pulp is surrounded by unyielding dentin it cannot swell during the body's natural inflammatory response. Dentists must remain mindful of three facts: (1) the microcirculatory system of the pulp lacks a significant collateral circulation; (2) the pulp consists of a relatively *large* volume of tissue with a relatively small blood supply; and (3) the pulp of the root canal system is *locked* into the unyielding walls of surrounding dentin and cannot expand to accommodate inflammatory fluids. As a result of caries, restorative procedures, or trauma, a vascular pulp may degenerate into avascular necrosis. Products of this degeneration seep out of the root canal system through portals of exit and into the supporting attachment apparatus, where their presence generates lesions of endodontic origin (Fig. 8-1). Therefore when the root canal system is cleaned, shaped, and sealed in three

dimensions, resolution will result. The longevity of a tooth is based, not on the pulp, but on a healthy attachment apparatus. The attachment apparatus is truly the *vital organ of a tooth.* Therefore treatment must be based on thoroughly cleaning, shaping, and obturating the root canal system with a permanent, biologically inert root canal filling.

ROOT CANAL SYSTEM

The root canal system is the clinician's road map to success (Fig. 8-2, *J*). We understand now that the critical issue is three-dimensionality. Root canal systems are not cylinders but ribbons, sheets, and banners. They can be more than six times wider in a buccolingual direction than in a mesiodistal direction. Eccentricity and irregularity are common. Maxillary first and second molars have four canal systems more than 90% of the time.[52] A quarter or more of mandibular molars have two distal canals.

PURPOSE

Cleaning and Shaping: The Master Skill

About 30 years ago, Schilder introduced the concept of "cleaning and shaping,"[75] which is the foundation of successful endodontic therapy. In fact, most obturation problems are really the result of improper cleaning and shaping. The two concepts, cleaning and shaping *and* three-dimensional obturation, are *inseparable.*

What is the modern meaning of cleaning and shaping?

Cleaning is the removal of *all* contents of the root canal system before and during shaping: infected material, antigenic material, organic substrates, microflora, bacterial by-products, food, caries, tissue remnants, denticles, pulp stones, collagen, inflammatory chemicals, contaminated canal filling materials, and dentinal debris created during canal shaping procedures (Figs. 8-2 and 8-3). Cleaning entails both the mechanical removal of canal contents and the chemical dissolution, detoxification, and flushing away of inflammatory and potentially inflammatory substances. Successful cleaning entails the use of instruments to physically remove substances, irrigating systems to flush loosened materials away, and chemicals to dissolve contents from inaccessible regions.

Shaping is the establishment of a specific cavity form with five mechanical objectives. The shape or radicular preparation permits pluggers, spreaders, and other obturation instruments to fit freely within the root canal system and to generate the

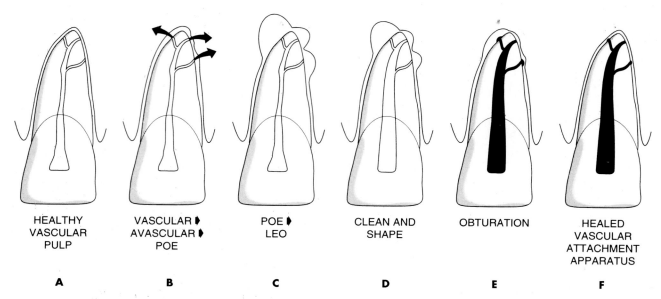

HEALTHY VASCULAR PULP   VASCULAR ▶ AVASCULAR ▶ POE   POE ▶ LEO   CLEAN AND SHAPE   OBTURATION   HEALED VASCULAR ATTACHMENT APPARATUS

A   B   C   D   E   F

FIG. 8-1 Rationale of endodontics. **A,** Healthy, vascular pulp, having the disadvantage of lack of significant collateral circulation, a large volume of tissue to a relatively small blood supply, and locked into unyielding walls of dentin. **B,** When the pulp becomes necrotic, irritants spill through the portals of exit *(POE)* into the attachment apparatus. **C,** Lesions of endodontic origin *(LEO)* are produced. **D,** Healing commences with cleaning and shaping. **E,** Three-dimensional obturation eliminates the source of the LEO. The attachment apparatus is cured. **F,** The LEO has healed.

pressures needed to transform and capture a maximal obturation cushion, forcing gutta-percha and a microfilm of sealer into all foramina. Equally important, shaping facilitates three-dimensional cleaning by providing easy direct access for files, reamers, rotary instruments, and irrigants during the treatment process. Inadequate shaping leads to inadequate obturation. In a poorly shaped canal safe harbors remain open in the avascular pulp canal space and provide room for formation, accumulation, and persistence of noxious irritants. Slow dissemination of these biologically active substances through unsealed portals of exit is reported to be the most common cause of long-term endodontic failures.[45] Shaping is a mechanical process accomplished with files, reamers, Gates-Glidden drills, slow-speed burs, high-speed diamonds-tipped drills, and sonic, ultrasonic, and nickel-titanium instruments of variable taper and other unique designs.

Cleaning and shaping have two special distinctions. The first is that endodontic therapy is the *only* dental procedure that relies almost entirely on "feel." Our tactile sense is extremely important in endodontic treatment. A light touch and delicate manipulation of instruments, will produce better results. In endodontics: *treatment is perfected by the touch.*

The second distinction of cleaning and shaping is accountability. Our ability and willingness to thoroughly clean and shape the anatomic complexities of the root canal system is the primary determinant of endodontic success.

PRINCIPLES

Access

The first step toward successful cleaning and shaping is an appropriate custom design access cavity as described in Chapter 7.

Apical Shape

The ideal apical shape is to leave nature's apical foramen alone, clean it so that it is patent, and obturate it in three dimensions. Both the shape and position of the apical foramen should remain the same to fulfill the requirements of the rationale of endodontics. Since the cementum is fragile in this region, tearing can easily reduce the opportunity for complete obturation. The last few millimeters of canal that approach the apical foramen are critical in that the shape developed there must be a tapering funnel form that allows distortion of obturation materials by compacting into the asymmetric perimeter of the foramen.

Body Shape

Although a continuously tapering cone is the ideal shape for obturating the root canal system, this shape must be appropriate for the external root structure. Overshaping risks weakening the tooth structure or perforating the root. Undershaping leaves tissue, substrate, and contamination and reduces compaction pressures, thus it increases the likelihood of a cemented, undistorted gutta-percha cone with a wider sealer interface.

Taper Convergence Toward the Apex

The five mechanical objectives added together describe the tapered preparation and how it enables total foraminal obturation. Regardless of the obturation technique, this shape is the most conducive preparation for a successful seal.

Foraminal Patency

To successfully complete the rationale of endodontics, foraminal patency is essential. Too often, portals of exit are transported internally or externally. Diligently and carefully con-

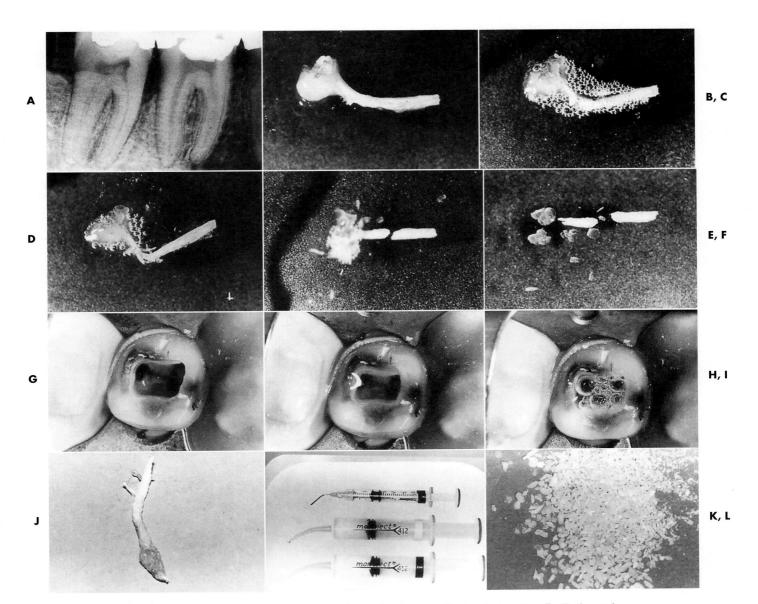

FIG. 8-2 Irrigation. **A,** Pretreatment radiograph of a mandibular first molar. **B,** Extirpated pulp. **C,** A drop of 3% sodium hypochlorite is placed on the pulp and photographed. **D,** Ten minutes later, dissolution of the organic matrix is evident. **E,** At 30 minutes, organic material is essentially in solution. **F,** After 45 minutes, all organic material is dissolved, leaving denticles and calcifications remaining. Remember these potential calcifications in all cleaning and shaping. **G,** Mandibular molar with sodium hypochlorite only at the base of the access cavity. **H,** Mandibular molar with sodium hypochlorite properly filled to the top of the access cavity. **I,** Combination of 3% hydrogen peroxide with sodium hypochlorite creates effervescence and elevates dentin mud away from the apical third and toward the chamber for aspiration. **J,** Extirpated pulp with foraminal appendages, revealing the true three-dimensional nature of the root canal system. **K,** Irrigating syringes for 3% sodium hypochlorite and hydrogen peroxide. Larger syringes for chamber irrigation, and sodium hypochlorite is in a smaller syringe for delicate irrigation slightly deeper into the cervical third of the canal. **L,** Dissolved pulp collection of 50 pulps showing numerous denticles, calcifications, and small pulp stones. Their presence is a major reason that endodontics requires such a light touch.

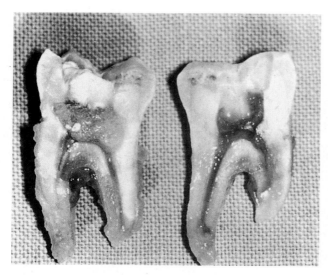

FIG. 8-3 Fractured mandibular molar reveals the canal contents of an endodontically involved tooth. Note the gross discoloration, debris, and contaminated appearance of the canal passages. Treatment must shape and cleanse these passages before predictable clinical response can occur.

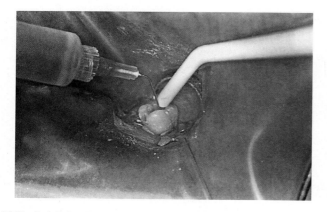

FIG. 8-4 Irrigation is easily accomplished with a 25- to 28-gauge needle and a disposable Luer-Lok syringe. Needle should be bent near the hub to facilitate access into the canals. Suction must accompany irrigation to accidental leakage.

firming patency throughout the cleaning and shaping process ensures preservation of the apical anatomy and produces a cleaned, patent foramen ready to be obturated.

IRRIGATION

Irrigation should always precede probing and length determination. The simple act of irrigation in itself flushes away loose, necrotic, contaminated materials before they are inadvertently pushed deeper into the canal and apical tissues (Fig. 8-4).[17] Using a chemically active irrigant is important. The use of sodium hypochlorite for irrigation provides (1) gross debridement, (2) lubrication, (3) destruction of microbes, and (4) dissolution of tissues.[37] Including a chelating agent or a dilute acid adds a fifth effect: (5) removal of the smeared layer.

Irrigation Solutions

Isotonic saline

Isotonic saline solution has been advocated by a few investigators as an irrigation fluid to minimize tissue irritation and inflammation. In isotonic concentration, saline produces no recognized tissue damage and has been demonstrated to flush debris from the canals as thoroughly as sodium hypochlorite.[8] Saline provides gross debridement and lubrication. Sterile isotonic saline is available in 1-L intravenous containers for parceling out and use in individual treatments. Caution should be used in storage, loading, and handling. This solution can be contaminated with foreign biologic materials by improper handling before, during, and between use. Irrigation with saline alone sacrifices chemical destruction of microbiologic matter and dissolution of mechanically inaccessible tissues (e.g., tissues in accessory canals and intercanal bridges). Isotonic saline is too mild to thoroughly clean canals.

Sodium hypochlorite

Sodium hypochlorite is by far the most commonly used irrigant in endodontic therapy. It can fulfill the first four actions listed previously. Such products as Chlorox and Purex bleach are common sources of concentrated sodium hypochlorite (5.25%). Many clinicians prefer diluted concentrations to reduce the irritation potential of sodium hypochlorite.[10] A 2.5% solution is commonly recommended, although full-strength and 1.25% solutions may also be used. One should be aware that dilution reduces the dissolution power. Sodium hypochlorite is an inorganic solution that is consumed in the dissolution process.[12] The rate and extent of dissolution are related to the concentration of the irrigating solution.[40]

Hydrogen peroxide

Hydrogen peroxide is used as an irrigation fluid in conjunction with sodium hypochlorite. When irrigated into a canal flooded with sodium hypochlorite, an effervescent action takes place, wherein the two chemicals actively release nascent oxygen and cause a strong agitation of the canal contents. Bubbling oxygen rising to the access opening tends to carry loose debris along. Both chemicals produce some tissue dissolution and bacterial destruction. The combined irrigation is mechanically effective; the last irrigant should always be sodium hypochlorite.

Chelating agents

Disodium ethylenediaminetetraacetic acid (EDTA) and a disodium ethylenediaminetetraacetate, sodium hydroxide, cetyltrimethylammonium bromide, and water mixture (REDTA) are chelating agents that may be used as a supplement to sodium hypochlorite to irrigate the canal.[65] They remove the smear layer, soften dentin, and facilitate the removal of calcific obstructions. These agents are not used in all situations, and a specific indication should exist when they are employed. They can soften the dentin throughout the canal system if they are sealed into the canal between visits or if they are used for an extended period during cleaning and shaping.[28]

Lubricants

RC-Prep, Glyoxide, and surgical jelly may be useful during initial canal negotiation procedures (Fig. 8-5). These agents have lubricating properties and facilitate instrument movement

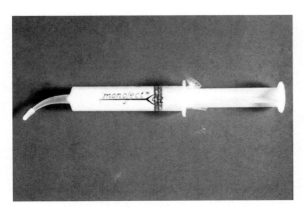

FIG. 8-5 RC-Prep loaded into a large disposable syringe to allow filling of the access cavity during initial preparation. Files carry this lubricant into the canal, thereby decreasing the chance of fibrous apical blockage early in treatment.

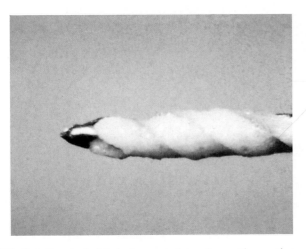

FIG. 8-6 Dentinal debris is created by the cutting action of files and other shaping instruments. Portion of that debris may be packed against the blades and removed with the file, some debris is compacted into the dentin surface forming a smear layer, and the remainder is removed by irrigation.

within the canal. They are recommended only for use during the early stages of preparation to eliminate soft tissue blockage.[12]

Benefits of Irrigation

Gross debridement

Infected root canal systems are filled with materials that have an inflammatory potential. The act of shaping generates debris, which also can elicit an inflammatory response (Fig. 8-6). Irrigation can simply wash away these materials and minimize or eliminate their effect. This gross debridement is analogous to the simple washing of an open and contaminated wound. This is a most important process of treatment.

Frequency of irrigation and volume of irrigant used are important factors in the removal of debris.[10,17,68] The frequency of irrigation should increase as instrumentation approaches the apical constriction.[12] An appropriate volume of irrigant is at least 1 to 2 ml each time the canal is flushed.[11,76] A key to improving the apical efficacy of irrigants is to use a patency file before each irrigation.[11] This small procedural refinement, patency confirmation before irrigation, works significantly better than irrigating without recapitulation. The reason is easy to appreciate. The patency file loosens debris, compacted into the apex, and helps suspend the debris in the canal fluids; thus, apical debris is more likely to be flushed out of the canal by irrigation. When the preparation diameter is small, placing a file into the apical third is the best way to move an irrigant to the apical region. The instrument displaces canal contents; when it is removed, irrigant flows into the vacated space. However, this action alone is not sufficient to remove tissues from small-caliber canal preparations.[81]

Elimination of microbes

Sodium hypochlorite has proven to be a most effective antimicrobial agent.[20,37,42] It can kill all microbes in root canals, including spore-forming bacteria and viruses. This microbicidal effect can be accomplished even with diluted concentrations of sodium hypochlorite.[20,42]

Dissolution of pulp remnants

Using sodium hypochlorite in a low concentration (below 2.5%) predictably eliminates infection but does not consistently dissolve pulpal remnants[40,43] unless extensive time is used during treatment. Baumgartner and Mader[8] have demonstrated that sodium hypochlorite 2.5% is extremely effective in removal of vital pulp tissue from dentinal walls.[11] They also disclosed that walls untouched by files (Fig. 8-7) were cleaned when an adequate concentration of sodium hypochlorite was used. Cunningham and Balekjion[19] and Cunningham and Joseph[20] investigated the relationship between temperature and activity of sodium hypochlorite. Their finding indicated that warming the solution produced more rapid tissue dissolution.

The dissolving efficacy of sodium hypochlorite is influenced by the structural integrity of the connective tissue components of the pulp.[2] If the pulp is already decomposed, it quickly dissolves the soft tissue remnants. If the pulp is vital and little structural degradation has occurred, it takes longer for sodium hypochlorite to dissolve the remnants. In this respect vital pulp removal is greatly dependent on shaping, and time should be allowed for dissolution of tissues located within accessory canals and intercanal connections.

Removal of the smear layer

The smear layer is composed of debris compacted into the surface of dentinal tubules by the action of instruments (i.e., it is burnished into the surfaces as the edges of instruments slide by). It is composed of fractured bits of dentin and soft tissue from the canal. These materials are released into the flute space of preparation instruments (see Fig. 8-6) and smeared over the canal surface by passage of trailing cutting edges (see Fig. 8-7). Since the smear layer is primarily calcific, it is most effectively removed by the action of mild acids and chelating agents (e.g., EDTA and REDTA).

Exceptional removal capability has been demonstrated for a combination of sodium hypochlorite and REDTA solutions.[30] This combination removes soft tissue remnants and the organic-inorganic smear layers. Baumgartner and Mader[8] demonstrated that all canal walls that are planed with cutting in-

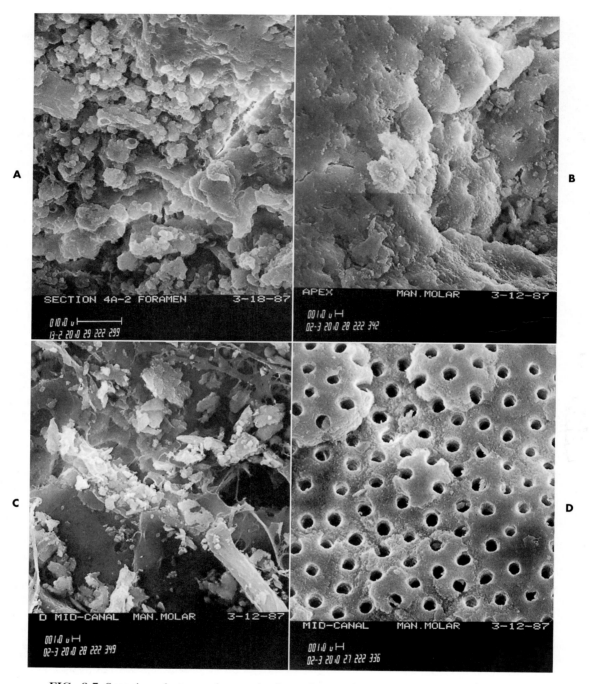

FIG. 8-7 Scanning electron micrographs from the canal system of a mandibular molar. **A,** Near the apical foramen. It has an irregular surface and may retain cellular debris. **B,** The control zone displaying tubules filled with a smear layer. **C,** Narrow crevice region in the midcanal area. Cellular fragments and a small vessel-like structure remain. **D,** Another open but still uninstrumented region in the midcanal area. All cellular debris has been removed by the action of 5.25% sodium hypochlorite. The tubules are clean and open. No smear was formed.

struments develop smear layers. Therefore if one desires to re-move the smear layer and reopen the tubules, all cleaned and shaped regions must be washed with a chelating agent. Canal walls not touched by files do not develop a smear layer and therefore are cleaned by the action of sodium hypochlorite alone (see Fig. 8-7).[3]

There is no clinical consensus as to whether the smear layer should be removed. Those in favor of leaving the smear argue that it could be a clinical condition that actually enhances end-odontic success. It appears to plug the dentinal tubules, mi-crobes and tissue included. This plugging may help prevent bacterial egress from the tubules after treatment. One study[96]

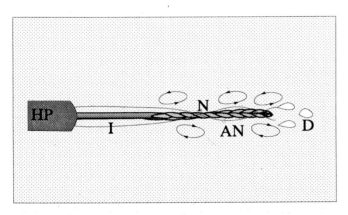

FIG. 8-8 Fluid flow about an instrument activated by ultrasonic energy waves. *HP,* Ultrasonic handpiece; *I,* fluid flow; *N,* nodal region. Little or no movement occurs in these areas. *AN,* Antinode. Oscillating file displacement occurs in this region. Maximal displacement occurs at the instrument tip. Elliptic flow patterns are eddies of acoustic streaming. *D,* Droplets of water that are sprayed from the end of a free instrument.

demonstrated that the smear layer slows bacterial movement, but it does not prevent eventual egress. Others[49,88] have demonstrated that teeth obturated with gutta-percha are more completely sealed when the smear layer is removed. It appears prudent to create the cleanest dentinal surface possible.

Ultrasonic irrigation

Ultrasonic handpieces have not performed as well as expected in apical shaping efficiency;[57,66,97] however, ultrasonic vibration is unparalleled in its ability to enhance cleaning with irrigants.[3,4,12,51,56] Used with a small file fit loosely into the canal, ultrasonic energy warms the irrigating solution, and the resonant vibrations cause movement of the irrigants: *acoustic streaming* (Fig. 8-8). Used as irrigating instruments, ultrasonic handpieces must be handled with care to avoid transporting the apical portion of the canal and to avoid the risk of producing a ledge in the apical third.[13-16] Because the cleaning effects of ultrasonic energy are most ideal when the energized instrument is loose in the canal, it is probably best to use ultrasonic irrigation after shaping is completed.[33,51]

Ultrasonic irrigation adds significantly to the cost and complexity of the clinical irrigation system. These factors must be weighed against its' potential value,[33,38] considering that mixtures of chemicals placed with inexpensive syringes are also effective in removing tissues and smear layer from the canal wall.[8,29] Exposure is a limiting factor to all cleaning, including ultrasonic irrigation. Exposure is significantly influenced by the shaping[48] because space must be created and contents removed before any irrigation fluids can enter an area.[16,89] Acoustic streaming causes flow along the outside of an instrument, and a small instrument of 0.15 mm diameter can be used to deliver the irrigant. This would be an ideal solution; however, acoustic streaming is limited by the amplitude of the sonic vibration, and requires a minimal canal diameter of about 0.25 mm for the No. 15 file.[3,5,90] If the canal is narrower, the instrument suffers a dampening effect and no flow occurs. Curvature may also dampen the oscillations and stop acoustic streaming, especially when the file is not precurved properly.

Syringes, on the other hand, are limited by the diameter of their delivery needle, both the internal bore and external diameter. The smallest practical irrigation needle size is 27 gauge. Its external diameter is 0.39 mm. When a needle is used, the canal area must be greater than the needle diameter plus its lumen area. This relationship provides sufficient canal dimension to enable fluids to escape freely past the needle and return into the access cavity.[17,68] The canal must be enlarged to the diameter of at least a No. 45 file to provide enough space for irrigation fluid return to the access chamber.

LENGTH DETERMINATION

Every part of endodontic treatment is controlled by a measurement of the instrument's penetration depth into the canal. This length is typically determined in millimeters. It is measured from a reference point on the tooth's cavosurface that is within the clinician's field of view. It varies from the complete canal length to some arbitrarily determined point near the termination of the canal space (Fig. 8-9).

Biologic Rationale for Working Length

Working length determines the extent of canal cleaning and shaping that will be accomplished. This measurement limits the penetration depth of subsequent instruments and determines the ultimate form of the shaping process. Cleaning and shaping can have no greater precision than the working length. It is extremely important to make an accurate determination. The most clinically relevant working length landmark is the apical constricture, regardless of whether it is in dentin or cementum.[22] The constricture is the narrowest point within the canal[53] and therefore the narrowest diameter of the blood supply. Beyond the constricture the canal widens and develops a broad vascular supply. Therefore from a biologic perspective the constricture is the most rational point to end the canal preparation, since the existence of a functional blood supply controls the inflammatory process. Intraradicular termination of the cleansing process leaves a canal content interface equal in area to the total inflammatory capable vital tissue surface (1:1). Termination beyond the constricture provides a greater area of vital tissue than irritant interface. Extraradicular termination can theoretically provide a hemisphere of vascular support to the inflammatory process. Such a condition alone gives the inflammatory process a volume, area, and numerically superior relationship. The surrounding vital tissues should have more capacity to destroy irritants and return the area to a biologically functional and repaired state. Thus cleaning and shaping through the apical constricture completely eliminates pathogenic canal contents and allows the inflammatory healing mechanism to progress.

Optimal Length

Procedurally, it is advantageous to treat to the constricture because it is a morphologic landmark[34-36] that can be identified and sometimes felt by the experienced clinician. As the canal is shaped, coronal to the apical constricture, it becomes progressively easier to locate the constricture with a small patency file and tactile sense. The experienced hand can detect an abrupt increase in resistance followed by a rapid decline as the instrument tip passes beyond the constricture.

Using the apical constricture as the working length landmark is recommended because it means that the terminus of the preparation will be located at the narrowest canal diameter.

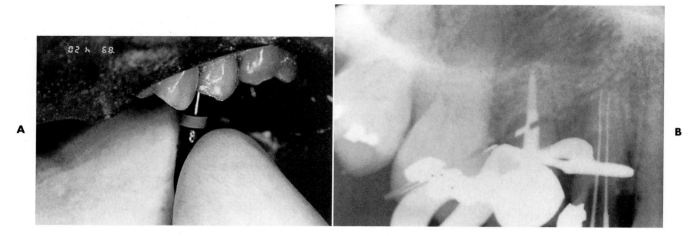

FIG. 8-9 A, File is being oscillated right and left to place it to the estimated radiographic length. When it stops or the marker reaches the cusp tip, a working length radiograph is exposed. **B,** Desired file position has been achieved in both canals. These lengths are carefully measured and recorded.

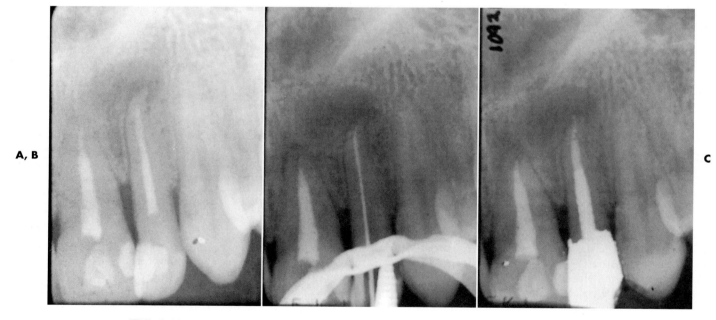

FIG. 8-10 A, Endodontic failure resulting from treatment completed short of the apex. Tooth has an associated apical radiolucent area, and clinical symptoms have returned. **B,** Canal was blocked at the obturation point; however, this was bypassed and the canal successfully negotiated to the apex. **C,** Posttreatment film revealing a three-dimensional fill to the apex; healing response is expected.

This preparation shape helps to optimize the apical seal when the canal is subsequently filled.[6,26,76]

Clinicians are urged to treat root canals to this apical end point because lateral and accessory canals are more common near the apex. Considering the possibility of an accessory canal, treating just 1 to 2 mm short of the apical constricture can leave 2 to 4 mm of untreated canal system. Such a length could significantly increase the chances for persistent periapical infection or inflammation. A region of canal 0.25 mm in diameter and 1 mm long can contain approximately 80,000 streptococci. This is surely a sufficient number to produce an inflammatory reaction (Fig. 8-10).

Methods of Canal Length Determination

Because we cannot directly visualize the ends of root canals in vivo, length determination requires careful clinical assessment. Only by correlating many confirming pieces of evidence can clinicians visualize the true terminus of root canals.

Radiographic

The most commonly used method of determining the length of a canal is radiographic. The clinician starts by placing a file to an estimated length and then exposes a film. The location of the instrument tip is read from this film, and any necessary changes in length to reach the apical constricture are made. Changes greater than 0.5 mm should be verified by an additional radiograph. The exact canal preparation depth depends on the technique and philosophy of the clinician. The periodontal ligament typically is used to identify the apical termination of the canal. This point includes the expanding portion of the canal beyond the constricture; consequently, techniques routinely make an allowance. The preparation length is shortened from the full length to the periodontal ligament by at least 0.5 mm initially. Greater adjustments are recommended in some techniques.

Electronic

Apex locators may be used to determine the canal length (see Fig. 6-17).[44,46,47] The unit leads are connected to a file that is inserted into the canal and to a lip clip that contacts the oral mucosa. The pulp is extirpated, the canal is irrigated and dried, and the attached file is inserted to the terminus. A dry canal and chamber eliminates ionic conduction, which can cause a premature indication that the apex has been reached. This is always necessary when the apex locator works on a resistance principle. Most inexpensive units use this principle. Impedance and frequency type models are not sensitive to ionic solutions like the resistance-based units; however, only the canal should contain fluid, and the chamber should be dry to prevent conduction through metal restorations to gingival tissues.[59,60]

Apex locators are most helpful in placement of the first length-determining file. Without a locator, the working length must be estimated from a preoperative radiograph or other data. This estimation requires considerable clinical experience before it may be used dependably; therefore controlling the initial penetration depth with an apex locator removes the guesswork. An apex locator guides the clinician as he or she develops tactile awareness and gains clinical experience that can further develop the clinician's clinical judgment skills.

One must be careful to avoid contaminating the file while connecting the electrical lead and inserting the measurement instrument. It is usually better to place the measurement file into the canal before the lead is attached. This action reduces the chance of accidental contamination. Once attached, the file is carefully oscillated back and forth and gently guided toward the canal terminus. As it approaches the foramen, the electrical resistance or impedance changes and an indication of the apex is displayed when the file tip first makes contact to apical tissues. This determination is verified by repeated withdrawal and reinsertion. The indicator must be observed during this action to assure the same apical indication is given each time the instrument passes through the foramen. When the point repeats several times, it should be a reliable measurement. To confirm its accuracy, leave the file at the indicated position and expose a radiograph. Used in conjunction with a radiograph, the locator is a most effective adjunct.[25] Without a radiograph mistakes are possible. For example, accidental passage through an accessory canal would indicate contact with the periodontal ligament; however, this length would be inappropriate (Fig. 8-11). A radiograph can disclose the need for

an additional adjustment. Electronic apex locators are especially useful when treating teeth with calcified pulp chambers. They test potential canal openings and detect a perforation before it is enlarged as a canal. The apex locator is superior to a radiograph in such situations.

Tactile

The experienced clinician develops a keen tactile sense and gains considerable information from the passage of an instrument through a canal. This ability must be developed, and for clinicians beginning a career additional bits of information may speed the development of such ability. Once radicular access has removed dentinal interference from the coronal third of a canal, the observant clinician can detect a sudden rise of resistance as a file approaches the apex.[12] Careful study of the apical anatomy discloses two facts that make tactile identification possible: (1) the unresorbed canal commonly constricts just before exiting the root, and (2) it frequently changes course in the last 2 to 3 mm.[53] Both situations apply pressure to the file. A narrowing presses more tightly against the instrument, whereas curvature deflects the instrument and resists its passage. Both consume energy, and the sensitive hand can detect a sudden change in the pressure needed to maintain movement. The awareness of an apex can be enhanced by use of a file diameter that is equal or slightly larger than the constricture.[69]

When a canal is constricted in its coronal two thirds, clinicians cannot discern apical anatomy with accuracy. This inability results from contacts in the cervical regions that interfere with and often mask contacts in the apical area. After preparation develops space in the coronal two thirds (i.e., radicular access), the quality of tactile information improves. With the canal enlarged coronally, files bind only in the apical area; therefore any resistance must lie in the apical region. When only the tip of a file binds in the canal, it becomes a sensitive instrument with which the clinician can accurately determine passage through the foramen. With the canal properly accessed a curved instrumented may access and pass through apical accessory canals (Fig. 8-11, *B*).

Paper point evaluation

Once the preparation is complete, a paper point may yield more than a dry canal.[12] After the canal is rendered dry, an additional paper point may be used to seek out apical moisture or bleeding. A bloody or moist tip suggests an overextended preparation or seepage of fluids into the canal. Further assessment of the apical preparation and working length should be made in this event. The point of wetness gives an approximate location to the actual canal end point. A wet or bloody point may also indicate that the foramen has been zipped or the apex perforated during preparation. These conditions call for additional canal shaping once an appropriate length has been determined.

Radiographs, electronic apex locators, tactile sense, and paper point evaluation used in harmony ensure that the final shaping and obturation will extend the full length of a canal.

MOTIONS OF INSTRUMENTATION

Several methods of manipulation are useful for generating or controlling the cutting activity of an endodontic file. These may be referred to as *envelopes of motion* and are more specifically defined as (1) file, (2) ream, (3) watch-winding, (4) serial shaping, and (5) balanced force motions.

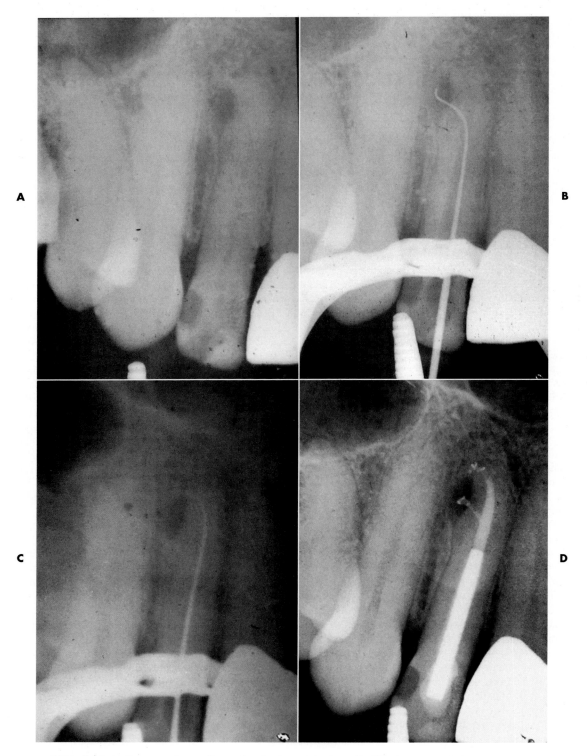

FIG. 8-11 A, Preoperative radiograph of a lateral incisor. **B,** File has passed through an accessory canal. Radiograph identifies this condition, whereas an apex locator would have adjusted the length and resulted in a short preparation. **C,** Additional working film disclosing the primary canal and its radiographic terminus. **D,** Final radiograph demonstrating that both portals of exit have been obturated.

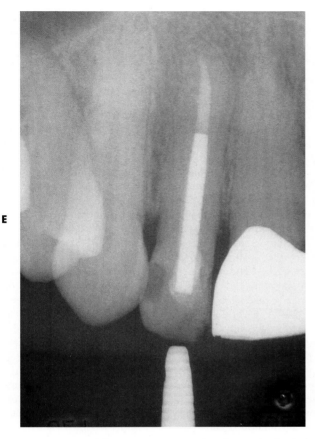

E

FIG. 8-11, cont'd E, Nine-year recall radiograph disclosing complete osseous repair and a reestablished periodontal ligament. Crown has not yet been placed.

File

The term *file* indicates a push-pull action with the instrument (Fig. 8-12). These two motions are the most limited of all motions used for preparation. The inward passage of a K-type file under working loads is capable of damaging the canal wall very quickly even when the slightest curvature is encountered. During the inward stroke, the cutting load is composed of both the instrument's resistance to bending and the inward hand pressure (Fig. 8-13). These two combine at the junctional angle of the instrument tip and gouge the curving canal wall very quickly. The gouge imparts a shape into the canal wall that does not allow even a small instrument to pass beyond that location. This procedural error can occur anywhere apical to a canal curvature, no matter how slight that curvature. The error does not occur in the straight regions because there is no deflection of the file in that circumstance. Without deflection there is no force that can hold the instrument tip consistently against the canal wall. Canal ledging is responsible for more short, underfilled, canal obturations than any other procedural error. The withdrawal or pull portion of a filing motion produces very little potential for canal wall damage. Most techniques use a minimal insertion force or a one-quarter turn clockwise to position an instrument, and follow that with a pull-driven cut as the instrument is withdrawn from the canal. Such techniques can enlarge canals to accepted diameters.

Filing is an effective technique to use with Hedström-type

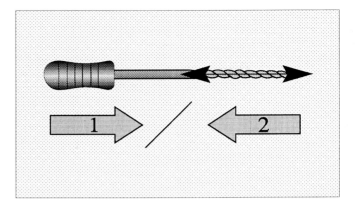

FIG. 8-12 Motion of filing. Arrow indicates pushing into (1) and pulling straight back (2) from the canal. Inward motion is powered by the hand and the rigidity of the file. Canal walls can be damaged very quickly by this motion. Damage can occur with very small diameter files.

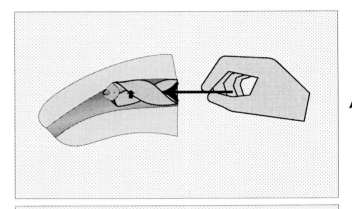

A

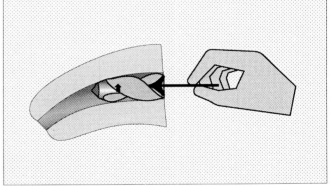

B

FIG. 8-13 A, If a standard K-type file is pushed into a curved canal, the junctional angles gouge the wall rather than reorient to the curvature. This action can form a ledge very rapidly (i.e., within five or six strokes). B, Same motion with a modified tip Flex-R file produces little alteration of the canal wall, since most of the cutting capacity of its tip has been removed. This is not a desirable motion in most canals. It is used only to smooth a previously roughened area.

instruments. Hedström instruments do not engage during the insertion action and cut efficiently during the withdrawal motion. A major limitation of filing with a conventional Hedström is that it can easily cut through the middle of a curvature and cause a strip perforation of the root. Precurving the file and anticurvature directing of the stroke must be used to avoid a mishap. The Unifile and S-file designs are less efficient with filing motions than a conventional Hedström file. The blades of these instruments spiral around the file with a steeper inclination, more like a file of the K-type design. This blade configuration allows the cutting edges to slip more during the withdrawal stroke.

Ream

The term *ream* indicates clockwise or right-hand rotation of an instrument (Fig. 8-14). Rotating any endodontic hand instrument to the right is risky, although the risk is subtle and goes unnoticed until an instrument fractures. The cutting edges of nearly all endodontic files and reamers spiral clockwise about the shaft. This configuration pulls the instrument into the canal as it rotates to the right and causes more of the instrument to engage into the canal substance. That action, in turn, increases the strain and working loads that act on the instrument. Loads continue to increase as the instrument turns clockwise until it ceases to move and is bent by the rotation. Continuing rotation after distortion has occurred eventually fractures the instrument; therefore clinicians must be sensitive to load changes and cease rotation when unusual sensations are present. When a sensation of unwinding is felt during filing, there is considerable risk of instrument fracture while attempting to remove the file.

Reamers manage the complexity and consequences of clockwise rotation by using a different helical spiral than a file. Reamers use a more axial orientation of their cutting edges and therefore feed themselves into the canal less than K- or H-type files. This altered design decreases a reamer's potential to aggressively thread into the canal. Reamers can be used in a

counterclockwise balanced force motion, just as other K-type instruments. Reamers are relatively ineffective shapers when a withdrawal motion is employed, consequently they are normally intermixed with files when used.

Combined Ream and File Motions

Turn-and-pull

The turn-and-pull cutting motion is a combination of the reaming and filing motions previously described (Fig. 8-15). The file is inserted with a one-quarter turn clockwise rotation and inwardly directed hand pressure (i.e., reaming). Positioned into the canal by this action the file is subsequently withdrawn as a cutting action (i.e., filing). The rotation during placement sets the cutting edges of the file into dentin, and the nonrotating withdrawal breaks loose the dentin that has been engaged. The resulting shaping is a spiraling groove in the canal wall, a groove that duplicates the spiraling axis of the instruments' cutting edges. Repeated placement with additional one-quarter turn and straight withdrawal, gradually enlarges the canal diameter to match that of the file. In this process the instrument is allowed to cut actively without guidance, and a ledge can be generated with rather small diameter files. Weine et al.[93] demonstrated a tendency toward "hourglass" canal shapes when one-quarter turn-and-pull techniques were used to create apical stop preparations. It may be concluded that a one-quarter turn-and-pull cutting motion is detrimental when used to create an apical stop preparation. On the other hand, clinical experience has demonstrated it is relatively safe when step-back instrumentation is employed.[62]

Schilder[76] recommends clockwise rotation of one-half revolution followed by withdrawal. Unlike the preceding description he does not encourage insertion toward the apex but rather gradually allows the preparation to progress out of the canal. Each time a file is withdrawn, it is followed by the next in the series. Each is inserted once and withdrawn. After the instrumentation series the canal is recapitulated with a patency file,

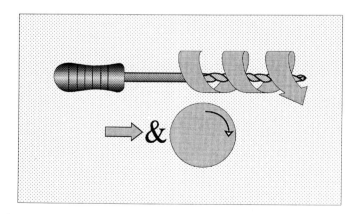

FIG. 8-14 Motion of reaming. This is a simple clockwise or right-hand rotation of the preparation instrument. Instrument must be restrained from insertion to generate a cutting effect. Instrument fracture is increased when this motion is employed.

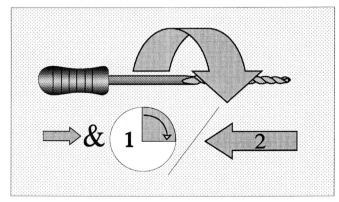

FIG. 8-15 A turn-and-pull motion is illustrated. One-quarter turn to the right is followed by a straight outward pull. Small arrow indicates a light inward force that engages the file before rotation. Pull motion *(arrow 2)* strips out treads started by the one-quarter turn clockwise motion. This can be an effective motion if the instrument is not forcefully pushed toward the apex and subsequent instruments are stepped-back from the apical terminus.

and the process is repeated. Each time the instrumentation series is repeated, each file penetrates deeper into the canal. The process is continued until the canal is shaped adequately to ensure complete cleansing. Accomplished in this manner the turn-and-pull motion can be used very effectively and produce excellent clinical results; however, the process requires careful thoughtful mechanics.

Watch-winding

The watch-winding motion is the back and forth oscillation of a file (30 to 60 degrees) right and (30 to 60 degrees) left as the instrument is pushed forward into the canal (Fig. 8-16). It is a definite advancement in file motion, and is very effective. The back-and-forth movement of K-type files and reamers causes them to plane dentinal walls rather efficiently. This motion is very useful during many shaping procedures. It is less aggressive than one-quarter turn-and-pull motions. The instrument tip is not pushed aggressively into the canal with each motion, and therefore the chance of ledging is somewhat reduced. In a way the watch-winding motion is a predecessor to the balanced force technique (discussed later in this chapter), as the 30 to 60 degrees of clockwise rotation pushes the file tip and working edges into the canal, and the 30 to 60 degrees of counterclockwise turn partially cuts away the engaged dentin. Each cut opens space and frees the instrument for deeper insertion with the next clockwise motion. The watch-winding technique is effective with all K-type files, and the oscillating movement easily inserts small instruments through canals.

Watch-winding-and-pull

When used with Hedström files, the watch-winding motion cannot cut dentin with the backstroke. It can only wiggle and wedge the nearly horizontal unidirectional cutting edges tightly into opposing canal walls. Properly positioned, the instrument removes dentin with a pull stroke. Hence, with Hedström files the watch-winding technique must become a watch-winding-and-pull technique (Fig. 8-17). With each clockwise rotation the instrument is moved apically and meets resistance. It is freed by a pull stroke. When apical placement becomes slug-

gish or very difficult, it is time to change to a smaller file size. When the working length is reached without resistance, one progresses to the next larger instrument.

Serial Shaping Motions

Cleaning and shaping are dynamically delicate motions, flowing, rhythmic, and energetic. To use files and reamers efficiently, the movements require distinction. There are six unique motions of files and reamers used in serial shaping, they are *follow, follow-withdraw, cart, carve, smooth, and patency.*

Follow

Follow (Fig. 8-18, *A* through *F*) is usually performed with files. Files are used initially during cleaning and shaping or any time an obstruction blocks the foramen. Irrigating, precurving, different kinds of curves, curving all the way to the tip of the instrument, and multiple curves in multiple directions of the instrument are all part of follow.

Follow-withdraw

For follow-withdraw (Fig. 8-18, *G* and *H*) the file is the instrument of choice. The motion is used when the foramen is reached, and the next step is to create the path to the foramen. The motion is follow and then withdraw, or "follow and pull," or "follow and remove." It is, simply, an in-and-out, passive motion that makes no attempt to shape the canal.

Cart

Carting (Fig. 8-18, *I*), which actually means transporting, refers to the extension of a reamer to or near the radiographic terminus. The precurved reamer should gently and randomly touch the dentinal walls at the radiographic constriction and "cart" away dentinal debris and pulp remnants.

Carve

Carving (Fig. 8-18, *J* through *L*) is for shaping. It is the most difficult motion to teach and to learn. Reamers are the best instruments for carving, sculpting, forming, and fashioning a continuously tapering cone preparation. The key is not to press

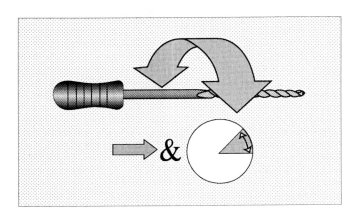

FIG. 8-16 Watch-winding motion. Arched arrow indicates a gentle right and left rocking motion, which causes the instrument to cut while a light inward pressure *(straight arrow)* keeps the file engaged and progressing toward the apex. Arc of rotation is indicated by the shaded region in the circle.

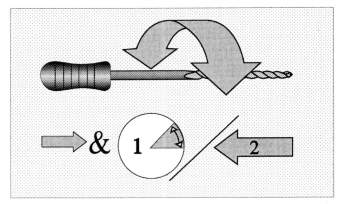

FIG. 8-17 Watch-winding-and-pull motion. This is used primarily with Hedström files. *1,* Inward pressure is maintained *(straight arrow),* while the file is gently rocked right and left, through the arc indicated by the shaded region of the circle; *2,* when insertion stops, all rotation is ceased and the instrument is withdrawn.

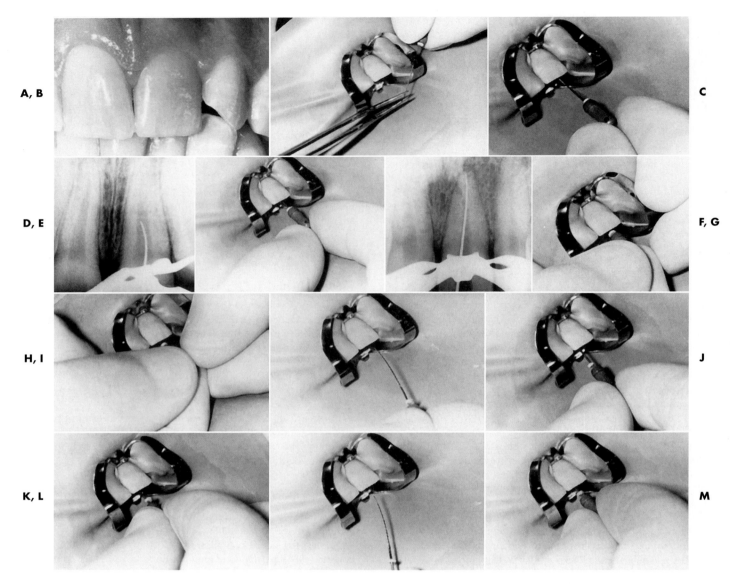

FIG. 8-18 Motions of serial cleaning and shaping. **A,** Pretreatment view of the central incisor. **B,** Careful curving of the apical portion of the file with appropriate cotton pliers. **C,** Follows the No. 10 file into the root canal system. **D,** Radiograph of advancing file. **E,** Continue to follow the instrument with almost no finger contact until the radiograph terminus is reached. **F,** Radiograph, verifying first instrument. **G** and **H,** Demonstrate the follow-withdraw reproduction of the path to the portal of exit. Notice small amplitude. Unlike following, this motion requires stable finger rest positions. **I,** File is followed by the same size reamer to cart away any dentin mud. **J** to **L,** Carving using the envelop of motion of the precurved reamer, randomly shaving the dentinal walls. **M,** Similar motion is needed to smooth the walls and also to confirm patency. All six motions are not static, but rhythmic and in combination. However, their distinctions allow the clinician greater mastery in producing proper shape.

the instrument apically but simply snuggle into the dentin with a precurved reamer and shape on withdrawal, thinking *gentleness*. The clinician never forces an instrument by penetrating to the maximal physical depth.

Smooth

Smoothing (Fig. 8-18, *M*), which is circumferential filing, is usually accomplished with files. If the previous four motions are followed, smoothing is rarely required.

Patency

Patency (Fig. 8-18, *M*) is achieved with files or reamers. It means simply that the portal of exit has been cleared of any debris in its path. If the clinician has been diligent with the other motions, confirming patency is simplified.

Balanced Force Motions

The balanced force technique[69,70] is a most efficient way to cut dentin. This technique calls for the oscillation of the prepa-

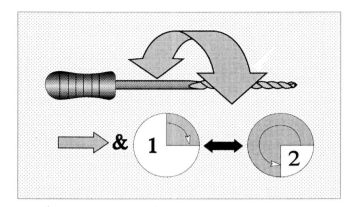

FIG. 8-19 Balanced force motions. Small straight arrow indicates a sustained light inward pressure. *1*, Initiating one-quarter turn to the right; *2*, larger arc used when the file is rotated to the left to drill the canal open. Black arrow indicates one should alternate these two directions until the working depth is reached. Inward pressure and the rotating force should always be very light.

ration instruments right and left with a different arc in each direction (Fig. 8-19). To insert an instrument it is rotated to the right (clockwise) a quarter turn or less as gentle inward pressure is exerted by the clinician's hand. This action pulls the instrument into the canal and positions the cutting edges "equally" into the surrounding walls. Next, the instrument is rotated left (counterclockwise) at least one third of a revolution. Rotation of one or two full turns is preferred but may be used only when little curvature or a generalized curvature is present. Left-hand rotation attempts to unthread the instrument and drives it from the canal, so the clinician must press inwardly to prevent outward movement and to obtain a cutting action. File fracture is unlikely unless pressures that exceed the torque resistance of the instrument are applied.

As described in the preceding section on reaming, right-hand rotation must be applied cautiously. The insertion forces press an instrument into the tooth structure; if excessive insertion occurs, the file may lock and become distorted. When so placed, the file may not be able to move when counterclockwise rotation begins. If it does not rotate to the left, the file can fracture very quickly in that direction of rotation (i.e., usually less than one revolution). *Very light pressure* should be used with balanced force instrumentation. The instruments should feed into the canal in very shallow increments, and the canal should be drilled open to the file diameter at each depth before further insertion is attempted. Gentle, patient oscillation of the instruments gradually carries them to the working depth. Once at that depth, they must undergo one final motion. Positioned at this deepest point of insertion, the instrument should be rotated to the right for about half to one entire revolution while the clinician gradually pulls it from the canal. This action sweeps the walls and loads debris from the canal space against the coronal side of the cutting edges. Loaded in this manner, the file removes most of the dentinal debris and other contents from the canal as it is withdrawn (see Fig. 8-6). Balanced force instrumentation has been demonstrated to extrude less debris through the apex than other techniques of canal preparation.[23,61] *Balanced force instrumentation is specifically designed to operate K-type endodontic instruments* and should not be used with

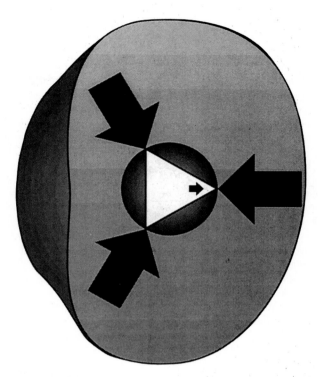

FIG. 8-20 White triangle represents the cross section of a file. Small black arrow, within the triangle, indicates the direction and magnitude of its restoring force. Three large dark arrows shown on the root surface represent forces derived from dentin as it resists the insertion of the edges of the file. Similar magnitude forces (not illustrated) arise from the structure of the file and interact at the points of the triangle. Since the restoring force is the smallest, it is unnoticed when rotation of the instrument keeps the larger forces in constant application. This relationship is the secret of balanced forces; keeping larger forces interacting such that a smaller detrimental force (i.e., restoring force) can be controlled.

broach-type or Hedström-type instruments, as neither possesses left-hand cutting capacity.

Simultaneous apical pressure and counterclockwise rotation of the file sustains a balance between tooth structure and instrument elastic memory (Fig. 8-20). This balance locates the instrument very near the canal axis even in severely curved canals. This technique avoids recognizable transportation of the original canal path,[7,9,55,67,70-73,82] when used with files that have a modified tip configuration (Flex-R, Moyco/Union Broach, York, Pa.). The technique has been shown to work effectively without precurving;[85] however, a tip bend may be required before a file can pass through a sharply deviated apical foramen. The more the canal curves, the less balanced force follows its true central axis. An instrument that has a triangular cross section is preferred, since that cross section contains the least metal mass of any current K-type cross section; the smaller the mass, the more flexible is the instrument. This means less force is required to bend the instrument into the shape of the canal, and the preparation result is less canal transportation during cleaning and shaping. Triangular instruments *must* be used with light working loads because they are not as strong as diamond-shaped or square configurations.[69]

Clinicians should be aware when using this technique that files can be broken.[71] When a rotational cutting technique is used, one must constantly monitor file integrity and discard files that show overwinding or unwinding of the blade spirals. Additionally, files should be replaced following each curved case, as many of the characteristics of instrument fatigue and impending file breakage are invisible to the human eye.[84] To minimize the risk of instrument fracture, all files up through No. 30 should be used only once and then discarded.

CURVATURE: THE ENGINE OF COMPLICATIONS

An engine is a power source for an action. Any instrument action requires an engine. An endodontic file has two: the operators hand and the instrument shaft. The hand force engine is obvious, but the instrument engine is not. As an instrument is curved, elastic forces develop internally. These forces attempt to return the instrument to its original shape and are responsible for straightening of the final canal shape (Fig. 8-21). If it were not for these forces, the final shaping would have the same central axis as the original canal. These internal elastic forces (i.e., restoring forces) act on the canal wall during preparation and influence the amount of dentin removed. They are particularly influential at the junction of the instrument tip and its cutting edges. This junctional point is the most efficient cutting surface along an instrument;[63] when activated by the restoring forces, it removes more tissue than can any other region of the file. This phenomenon is responsible for apical transportation and its consequences. Restoring forces are what power the changes in canal shape as they act through the sharp surfaces of an instrument. The strength of the engine is directly related to the metal composition of the instrument, the cross-sectional area of the instrument, and the angle of deflection. The greater the angle of deflection, the greater is the power developed. The larger the instrument, the larger is the cross section and the greater is the power. The more rigid the material the instrument is manufactured from, the greater is the power. Evaluation of these relationships gives guidance in the following ways:

1. Radicular access minimizes the deflection of all subsequent instruments.
2. A triangular cross section is preferred, especially as apical preparation diameter increases beyond a No. 25 file.
3. Less rigid metals are advantageous, provided they do not introduce undesirable characteristic like unpredictable fracture.

Nickel-titanium instruments are presently being investigated and offer improved preparation accuracy as a result of reduced engine force;[41] however, they suffer from unpredictable fracture. Specialized designs, like Light Speed (Light Speed Inc., San Antonio, Tex.),[94] also reduce the power of the instrument engine. These instruments do not cut over most of the canal length and have a small-diameter shaft that reduces its total cross-sectional area.[95]

Precurved Instruments

A precured file is a valuable tool, useful to search for canal passages and for moving around calcification and ledges and through foramina. When properly shaped, a file is curved smoothly to its tip. Its shape should accurately replicate the expected canal curvature. Sharp kinks should be avoided, as they predispose the instrument to fracture (Fig. 8-22).[12]

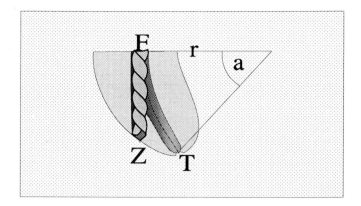

FIG. 8-21 Interaction between an instrument and a curved canal. *a,* Angle of canal curvature; *r,* radius of that arc; *FT* curvature; *FZ,* passive position of the instrument. As the canal curves the file to FT, a restoring force is developed within the file. That force attempts to return the file to FZ. The greater the angle a, the shorter the radius r; and the larger the file, the more likely it is that the preparation will progress to the path FZ. This is one of the forces that activate the junctional angles of K-type files.

Investigators[85] discovered that an S-shaped curvature is present in many of the molar canals. Their work disclosed that this curvature is not revealed in the clinical radiograph in about 20% of their sample. An example of this situation is provided in (Fig. 8-23). When compound curvature is present, precurvature of an instrument to match the canal is not feasible. However, when an S-shaped curvature is present, a tip curvature would be helpful in exploring the remaining apical curvature once a radicular access preparation is complete.

The primary difficulty of precurving is limited by canal shape and size coronal to the curvature. To insert a precurved instrument and maintain the shape, there must be adequate width in the coronal region to allow undisturbed passage of the curved file. If the canal is not curved the same as the file or is not as wide as the file curvature, the canal reshapes the file and straightens its curvature. Early radicular access solves much of this dilemma in that it widens the coronal regions and establishes clearance to pass the precurved instrument into the canal without altering its shape. If the canal is arched through its entire length, precurving may be accomplished very easily. Precurving is not required by the balanced force technique, but it is common in others.

Anticurvature Filing

Anticurvature is a method of applying instrument pressure such that shaping occurs away from the inside of the root curvature in the coronal and middle third of a canal (Fig. 8-24). Abou-Rass et al.[1] described the anticurvature filing concept for curved canals, emphasizing that during shaping procedures files should be pulled from canals as pressure is applied to the outside wall (i.e., away from the danger zones of furcations and midcurvatures). This directionally applied load, they suggest, prevents dangerous midcurvature straightening in curved canals and associated laceration of the furcal area during preparation. Anticurvature pressure application is effective until the

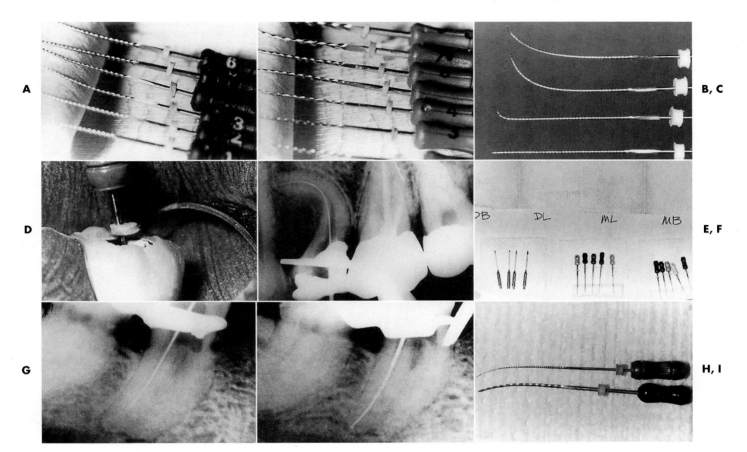

FIG. 8-22 A and **B,** Eventual rubber stop position of the final shaping. Note the instruments are progressively set short of the full length of the root canal system. Cleaning and shaping is achieved through serial reaming, filing, and recapitulation. **C,** Lower straight instrument can be transformed into multiple curves, including abrupt apical turns, gentle curvatures, and finally curves in multiple planes to randomize the directional possibilities of instruments as they advance apically. **D,** Rubber stop reference is essential to successful cleaning and shaping. **E,** Radiographic terminus is the only reproducible guideline for successful cleaning and shaping. **F,** Anticipate four canals in all molars by identifying them with their own 2 × 2 gauze. At completion of cleaning and shaping, each gauze square will store the first and last instrument to the radiographic terminus, as well as the gutta-percha cone. **G,** First instrument to the radiograph terminus. **H,** Last instrument to the radiographic terminus. **I,** Notice the length difference between the first and last instrument of this molar, demonstrating the shortening of canal length after several recapitulations. It is important to expose a treatment film after several recapitulations to prevent external transportation.

canal bends or deflects the file. *Then canal curvature determines the cutting pressures.*

RADICULAR ACCESS

Radicular access creates space in the coronal regions of the canal, which facilitates placing and manipulating subsequent files and increases the depth and effectiveness of irrigation (Fig. 8-25). Radicular access may be accomplished with rotary instruments or by shaping using an instrument's envelope of motion.[54]

Generous enlargement of the coronal half of the canal developed with radicular access provides important advantages in irrigation efficacy,[68] apical control,[27] cone fit, and compaction procedures, regardless of the obturation technique used.[24,76]

Apical preparation is easier and more consistent. Apical blocking, ledging, ripping, and perforation are less likely.[11,54,75]

Engine-Driven Radicular Access

The preferred method of developing a radicular access is to use Gates-Glidden drills[27,69,77] mounted in the right-angle low-speed handpiece. Different sequences may be employed. One approach is to begin after the canal length has been determined and the canal space has been increased in diameter with a No. 25 or larger file (Fig. 8-26). The access cavity is flooded with sodium hypochlorite, and the radicular access is initiated by passing a rotating No. 2 Gates-Glidden drill into the canal. This drill pulls inwardly as a result of rotation. The drill should be backed out of the canal after penetrating 1 to 2 mm and cleared

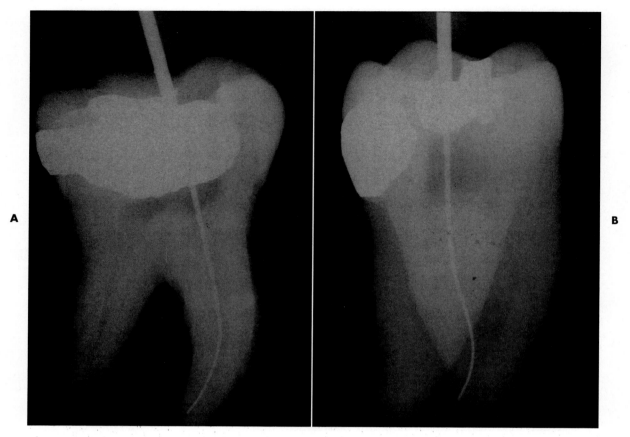

FIG. 8-23 A, Radiograph discloses a J-shaped curvature of the mesial root of this molar. File could be precurved to fit only after the coronal two thirds are enlarged enough to provide passage without the canal restraightening the instrument. **B,** Mesiodistal view of the same file discloses an unidentified S-shaped curvature, which the clinician would not be able to adjust for because it is invisible in the clinical view. Occurrence of this S-shaped curvature is somewhat common in the molar teeth. *(Radiographs courtesy Dr. Denny Southard.)*

of debris before moving it closer to the apex. Irrigating fluids within the chamber area are used to wash debris from the rotating instrument as it is withdrawn from the canal. The drill is then returned to the previous depth, clean and ready to continue shaping. In-and-out movements are repeated until the No. 2 Gates-Glidden drill reaches its intended depth or until the clinician determines that a curvature is preventing further penetration. Gates-Glidden drills are not intended for use around curvatures, and any attempt to do so can cause a serious procedural error. Situations range from a canal blocked by a broken Gates-Glidden drill (Fig. 8-27) to a root perforated by an excessively large diameter preparation (Fig. 8-28).

After using the No. 2 Gates-Glidden drill, the clinician thoroughly irrigates the canal. Next, a No. 3 Gates-Glidden drill is introduced into the canal. The clinician must be alert and ready to stop rapid apical movement of this and any subsequent drill. The preceding drill has enlarged the canal enough that it now offers little resistance against inward movement. Also the length of cutting surface has increased, and the present drill generates a greater inward force. Together these changes mean each subsequent Gates-Glidden drill passes more freely and rapidly into the canal than did its predecessor. A progression of drill diameters and shorter working depths is continued un-

til the coronal portions of the canal are well cleaned and shaped. Generally, only the smaller Gates-Glidden drills are used in molars because of the risk of furcal perforation.

The crown-down technique recommends initiating the radicular access with the larger instruments (Fig. 8-29).[58,64] Each instrument is used to penetrate approximately 2 mm into the canal. In this method each drill is pressing against approximately the same canal resistance, and there is no tendency for large instruments to insert rapidly. Small Gates-Glidden drills may penetrate quickly and possibly reach beyond their intended depth. Generally, a crown-down sequence achieves more depth with the smaller drills and less with the larger, and it produces a better taper within the radicular access preparation. Drill fracture at the head is rare to nonexistent when crown-down methods are used properly.

While preparing a radicular access, the clinician must be guided by the shape of each canal. If the canal is oval or oblong, the shape must be developed by preparation from both ends of the oval (Fig. 8-30). The drills are inserted to an appropriate depth, and the walls are planed with an outward stroke. An exception is made for the inward side of curved and concave roots (i.e., the mesial roots of molars), wherein the preparation is always directed away from the curvature (i.e.,

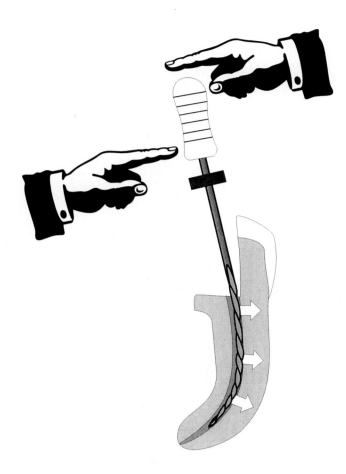

FIG. 8-24 File used in an anticurvature fashion. Hands represent the direction of pressure applied to the file handle. Top of the handle is pulled into the curvature while the base of the handle is pushed away (anticurvature) from the inside of the curve. This action presses the cutting flutes more heavily against the thicker outer regions of the root and away from the furcation.

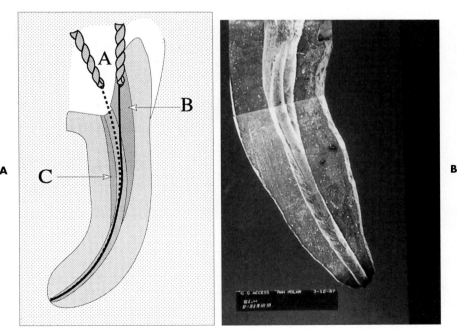

FIG. 8-25 A, Changes of instrument passage resulting from a radicular access. Dashed line represents the initial path of the file. Solid line represents the resultant path of the file. *A,* Angle of reduction in curvature; *B,* dentin intentionally removed to facilitate the angle change; *C,* dentin lost as a result of canal enlarging. Reduction in the region C must be kept to a minimum. **B,** Scanning electron micrograph reconstructs the mesial root of a mandibular molar. Wide coronal space is that of the radicular access. Original canal channel can be seen in the coronal and middle thirds, and the angular change is obvious. Apical half of this canal exhibits completely planed walls. File can pass through this canal in a nearly straight condition, thereby allowing for a larger diameter preparation. Apical preparation was completed with a No. 45 file.

FIG. 8-26 Canal when a typical radicular access is made with Gates-Glidden drills. **A,** Canal is enlarged apically with files through No. 35. **B,** File is removed and the canal flooded with sodium hypochlorite. **C,** No. 2 G-G drill is worked in and out of the canal, making small penetrations each pass, until it reaches a depth 3 to 5 mm short of the apex.

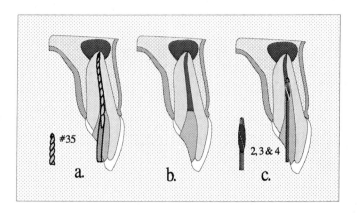

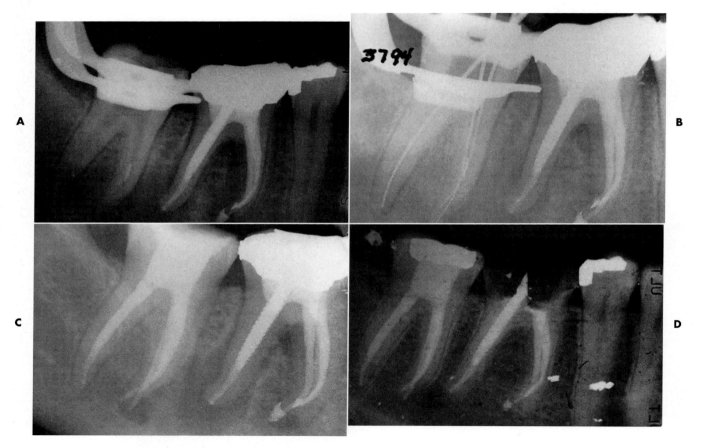

FIG. 8-27 **A,** Mesial canal of this molar is blocked by the cutting head of a No. 2 Gates-Glidden drill. **B,** Careful manipulation of a small file reestablishes a passage through the flute space of the drill head. **C,** Following the bypass instrumentation the canal system was successfully obturated. **D,** Twelve-year recall radiograph indicates complete remineralization has occurred.

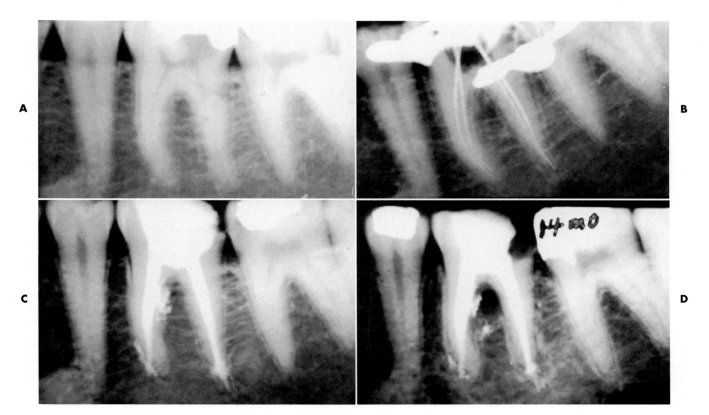

FIG. 8-28 **A,** Preoperative. The mesial root is curved throughout its entire length. **B,** Working files placed to the apex in four canals. **C,** Obturation film discloses a mesial furcal perforation from excessive Gates-Glidden drill depths, a mesial apical perforation, and a short mesial fill. The distal foramen has been zipped and the fill overextended. **D,** Fourteen-month recall discloses the osseous damage which resulted. This tooth was lost.

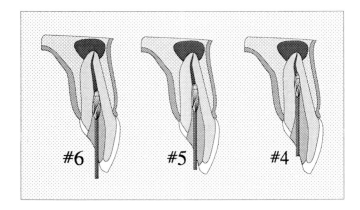

FIG. 8-29 Crown-down technique begins with the larger Gates-Glidden drill first. In the maxillary incisor the No. 6 Gates-Glidden drill starts the procedure and is passed into the canal a depth of 2 to 3 mm from the point it first engaged the canal. No. 5 Gates-Glidden drill extends the preparation an additional 2 mm and the No. 4 Gates-Glidden drill another 2 mm. Nos. 3 and 2 Gates-Glidden drills complete the penetration depth and should leave 3 mm or more of canal remaining before the foramen is encountered.

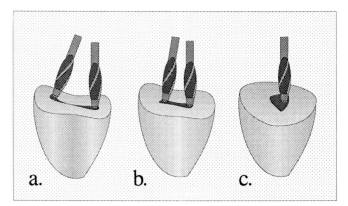

FIG. 8-30 Illustration of Gates-Glidden drill positioning for radicular access preparations in different shapes of canals. **A,** Figure-eight canal typical of mesial roots of molars and some single-rooted premolars. Each canal receives a single pass with pressure applied away from the curvature. **B,** Oval-shaped canal typical of the larger roots of molars and single-rooted premolars. Anastomosing area can be cleaned with a small Gates-Glidden drill. Passage is made down both ends of the oval shape as if two canal existed. **C,** Irregular round canal typical of maxillary incisors, two-rooted premolars, and distal-facial roots of maxillary molars. Single pass is usually sufficient.

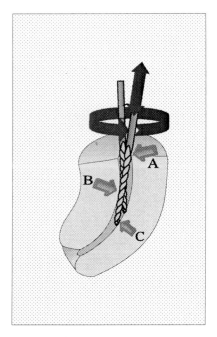

FIG. 8-31 Circumferential filing used to establish a radicular access. This may be accomplished effectively provided the files are not pushed too deeply into the canal to cause bending of the instruments (i.e., past point C).

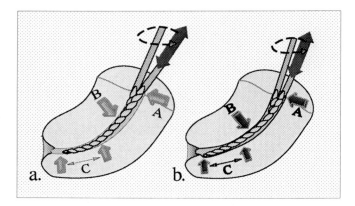

FIG. 8-32 Reaction of an instrument after it passes into a curve (i.e., past point C). **A,** The instrument remains in the same apical location regardless of how the clinician moves the upper shaft and handle. **B,** Continued filing beyond the coronal-most arrow C causes transportation of the canal in regions A, B, and C. Changes are most apparent in region C, since the instrument tip functions in that area.

anticurvature). Round canals should finish round and larger, oval canals should finish oval, and separate figure-eight canals should end as two separate round to oval spaces. Figure-eight canals are flared away from the interconnecting groove. Each drill is withdrawn outwardly in an active manner so as to slightly flare the opening and increase its coronal diameter to near that of the next drill. This flaring prevents the creation of parallel walls, a condition that adversely affects the distribution of compaction pressures during obturation.

Manual Radicular Access

Techniques to manually shape the coronal two thirds of the canal with a circumferential filing action are well established.[91] The body of the canal is repeatedly filed about its diameter in an effort to grossly flare that portion of the canal and create space to better reach the apical regions (Fig. 8-31). This process works best when there is no curvature in the portion of the canal being flared. If a curvature is present, the portion of the file that passes beyond the curve consistently presses against the same wall regardless of the direction the clinician moves his or her hand (Fig. 8-32). Circumferential filing is slow with K-type files but may be accomplished more rapidly with H-type files.

IATROGENIC COMPLICATIONS ARISING FROM CLEANING AND SHAPING

Procedural errors in the canal wall occur rapidly and subtly. The majority of cleaning and shaping complications are a result of improper control of the enlarging instruments, resulting in damage to the canal system. Blockage, laceration, and foraminal damage are the most common errors. Each compromises the reliability of the procedure and *must* be prevented.

Blockage

The canal may suddenly lose patency during a cleaning and shaping process. This can be a result of tissue compression, debris accumulation, wall perforation, or instrument separation. Any of these conditions block access into the deeper regions of the canal. Early detection and proper corrective action can prevent further exacerbating damage. Correcting canal blockage requires considerable experience; therefore an inexperienced clinician should refer to an endodontist when a blockage persists.

Soft Tissues

When the pulp tissue is intact, it can be packed into the apical region by insertion of instruments that are too large. Extirpation of the entire pulp is an important factor in reducing this potential problem. Generally, placing a sharp file down to the apical foramen and carefully rotating it cuts the pulp cleanly and facilitates its removal.

Clinical experience suggests that lubricants such as RC-Prep or Glyoxide help to emulsify the pulp stump and prevent cohesion of collagenous debris. These solutions are recommended for use only during the initial phase of cleaning and shaping (i.e., until enough coronal enlargement is created to allow the effective use of sodium hypochlorite irrigation).[8]

Hard Tissues

Dentin chips (dentin mud) generated by the cutting action of files and drills settle into the apical regions; if not removed by recapitulation and irrigation, they can obstruct that region. Filing near the canal terminus exaggerates apical blockage by packing debris into the smaller apical regions (Figs. 8-33). Once the canal is blocked by chips, continued generation extends the depth of blockage and causes obturation to fall short of the canal terminus. Accumulation of debris also contributes to the formation of ledges.

As the pulp ages, natural calcifications may have accumulated along the vascular channels and on canal walls (see Fig. 8-2). Pulp stones and secondary calcifications (denticles) that

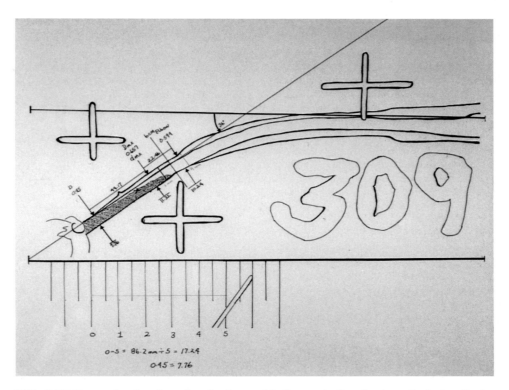

FIG. 8-33 Composite drawing of a plastic canal before and after shaping, disclosing the influence of debris on shaping. Inner lines indicate the original canal shape, and outer dark lines the final canal shape. Note the inner and outer outlines merge along the inside in the apical region, beyond the radicular access. Speckled region indicates accumulated chips that have aided the restoring forces in moving the final canal shape to the outer side. If this debris were completely removed during shaping, there would be a more equal shaping of the apex (inside wall versus outside wall).

project from the canal wall may be moved down the canal and become lodged by the insertion of a file. These can occasionally be bypassed by precurving the tip of the file. Loose pulp stones that are wedged apically into the small diameter of deep canal spaces are very difficult to remove or to file beyond. Once bypassed, the calcification is often reoriented to again obstruct the canal. Frequent, generous irrigation and early radicular access help reduce the risk of accidental blockage with calcifications. Teeth with a diminished pulp chamber, narrowed canals, long-standing periodontal involvement, or multiple previous restorations are more likely to contain calcifications and manifest hard tissue blockage.

Broken Instruments

During the cleaning and shaping process, excessive stress on an instrument can cause it to break in the canal. The fragment blocks the canal system and prevents routine cleaning and shaping (see Fig. 8-27). Clinical recall evaluation indicates that broken instruments with a tip that rests in the apical constriction are not as likely to fail as those with a tip that lies more coronally. In all situations a broken instrument compromises cleaning, shaping, and sealing. This type of blockage is preventable and requires focused attention on the force used to manipulate instruments. Frequent and close instrument examination and instrument disposal are the best preventives. Keen awareness of the minute stress that each instrument can withstand without suffering irreversible structural damage is essen-

tial. Minimal torque resistance and angle to fracture for standardized instruments provide a valuable relative measure of the strength of instruments in relationship to their cutting diameter. Filing forces should not exceed the pressure required to write with a sharp lead pencil.

Furcal Perforations

A furcal perforation is a midcurvature root perforation into the periodontal ligament and is the worst possible outcome of any cleaning and shaping procedure. Furcal perforations are difficult to repair. Their location is close to the clinical crown, and consequently they are very likely to continue microleakage from the coronal restorations into the furcal tissues, thereby compromising the long-term prognosis (see Fig. 8-28, *C* and *D*).

Furcal perforations result from improper file manipulation or oversized radicular access preparations. The risk of occurrence can be minimized by incorporating anticurvature pressure when cutting instruments are pushed or pulled in a curved canal system. Anticurvature pressure is extremely effective when used with Gates-Glidden drills in early radicular access preparations. Anticurvature technique is commonly advocated by clinicians who employ conventional Hedström files for the preparation of curved canals. Too much Hedström filing risks furcal perforation.

Another way to prevent furcal perforations is to *never* take large Gates-Glidden or Peeso drills deep into root canals (see Fig. 8-28). Deep insertion generally is not the clinician's intention but rather a result of self-propelled inward motion of the drill. New drills of the larger sizes (No. 3 to 6) often grab the canal walls and pull themselves deeply into the canal before the clinician can stop the handpiece. *A helpful technique to prevent this is to run the handpiece in reverse direction with new drills.* The drills tend to back out of the canal when rotated counterclockwise. By the application of more apical pressure the drill can be moved into the canal and made to cut dentin. It will only go to the intended depth, since it does not self-propel when rotated counterclockwise, and the propelling pressure can be terminated as the desired depth is obtained. A reverse order of drill sizes is also very reliable in reducing furcal lacerations. This technique is described as the crown-down technique in the engine-driven shaping discussion (see Fig. 8-29).

Apical Perforations

When the apical third of a canal is curved (almost all canals are curved), there is a risk of carving out a new portal of exit. This portal of exit is, most often, a result of uncontrolled transportation and ledge formation. Attempts to reestablish the length past a ledge result in the file tip cutting straight through the root structure and into the periodontal ligament (Fig. 8-34). This error leaves a debris-clogged apical canal space, which severely compromises the prognosis for apical repair.

Altered Foramina: Rip or Zip

When files are passed through the apical foramen they can change its shape very rapidly and irreversibly. A file concentrates its internal forces against the structure of the foramen. This delicate foramen must provide resistance to the abrasive effects of instrument movements. A few in-and-out movements can convert a round apical foramen into a delta-shape (zipped) (Fig. 8-35).

When the foramen is zipped, it cannot be thoroughly cleansed of tissue. This apical transportation may severely compromise apical repair; therefore it is recognized with special terminology (i.e., teardrop transportation, rip, or zip). Opening of the foramen should be kept relatively small; few passes should be made through it. If enlargement of the foraminal diameter is preferred, it should be the last step of canal shaping and it should be performed with a rotary motion with a piloted (safe tip) file.

Delicate apical foramina are situated at the interface between a canal system and the attachment apparatus. Foramina must be maintained in their original position. Files that pass through apical foramina are routinely kept small (i.e., No. 10 or 15) and are precurved. For obturation the foramen must be smaller than the apical shaping diameter, free of tissues, and contoured so that a gutta-percha cone adapts tightly into the patent space (round is optimal) (Fig. 8-36).

CLEANING AND SHAPING TECHNIQUES

The principles common to most endodontic preparation methods have been discussed; we can now focus on the specific mechanics of techniques. The following descriptions provide greater detail about the sequencing for each technique. After completing this section the reader should be able to clean and shape a routine endodontic case.

Serial Shaping Technique

Schilder taught endodontists to think and operate in the third dimension[75,76] by stressing five mechanical objectives for successful cleaning and shaping. Since their introduction, the de-

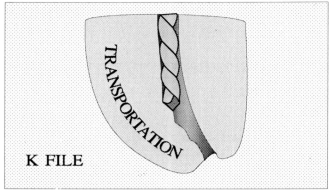

A

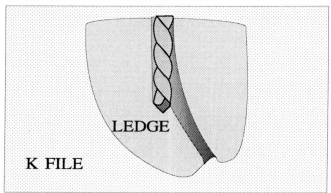

B

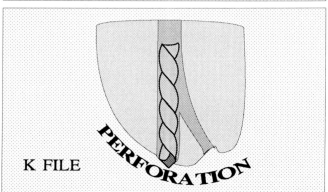

C

FIG. 8-34 Apical perforation. **A,** This event is always preceded by transportation, which is disproportional shaping that creates shallow tip-shaped recesses along the outer wall. **B,** Allowing a file to continually reach the same depth forms a ledge that prevents deeper passage. **C,** Perforation is made when attempts to forcefully bypass a ledge cause an instrument to penetrate from the ledge to the periodontal ligament.

sign objectives have become widely accepted. The use of each instrument has a specific purpose in achieving the optimal canal form.

Mechanical objectives

1. *Develop a continuously tapering conical form in the root canal preparation.* This shape mimics the natural shape of canals before they undergo calcification and formation of secondary dentin. The goal is to create a conical form from access cavity to foramen (Fig. 8-37, *A* through *F*). When this vision is imprinted in the clinician's mind during cleaning and shaping procedures, instrument selection is simplified. In addition, the preparation should be smooth and ap-

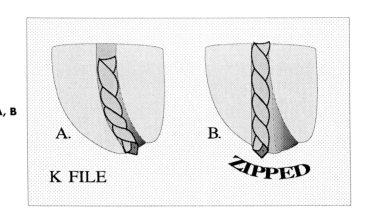

A, B

A. **K FILE**   B. **ZIPPED**

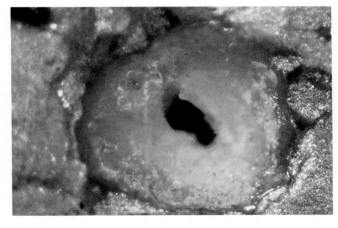

C

FIG. 8-35 **A,** When a small file is placed through a curved foramen, it presses against the outer side of that curvature. **B,** Pushing the instrument in and out (filing) of the foramen transports the contacted area and zips the foramen rapidly. The shaded area, to the inside of the curvature, retains tissues, dentin debris, and other canal contents. Obturation cannot eliminate this debris or seal the resulting shape; this invites failure. **C,** Micrograph of an apex reveals an irregular oval-shaped zip that has resulted from overextended instrumentation. When this occurs clinically, debris accumulates in the original canal space and obturation cannot successfully close the area; this too invites failure.

propriate for the length, shape, and size of the root that surrounds it. There must be a funnel shape beginning from the access cavity so that instruments will slide into the canal. The access cavity and the root canal preparation are continuous. The narrowest part of the continuously tapering cone is located apically, and the widest is found coronally. Irrigation and instruments can now clean and shape all the walls of the root canal preparation. The continuously tapering cone allows hydraulic principles to operate by the restricted flow principle. As flow is restricted during the compaction procedures, it causes the gutta-percha and sealer to take the path of least resistance; namely the apical and lateral foramina.

Watch Words: *Carve, shave, natural form*
Major Benefit: *Obturation, hydraulics, and cleaning*

2. *Make the canal narrower apically, with the narrowest cross-sectional diameter at its terminus.* The second objective is a corollary of the first. The diameter becomes narrower as

the preparation extends apically (Fig. 8-37, *G* and *H*). The only exception is a tooth with internal resorption or an unusual bulge in the natural shape of the root canal. This objective creates control and compaction at *every* level of the preparation. The second objective focuses on harmonizing cavity form with the thermomechanical properties of gutta-percha to achieve a hermetic seal.[31,32,79,80] To seal all foramina the preparation must be shaped serially in a decreasing taper. To preserve apical patency the dentin mud must be suspended in sodium hypochlorite and the radiographic terminus used as the reference (see Fig. 8-22, *E*). The cementodentinal junction is not clinically meaningful and its location may vary histologically up to several millimeters; therefore to use it as *the guide* could jeopardize mechanical objectives 3, 4, and 5. The clinician may clean to the apex, the anatomic apex, the radiographic apex, the apical constriction, the apical foramen, the cementodentinal junction, or the radiographic terminus (see Fig. 8-22, *E*). Clinically the only landmark that can be identified consistently is the radiographic terminus.

Watch Words: *Patency, radiographic terminus*
Major Benefit: *Facilitates the achievement of mechanical objective 1*

3. *Make the preparation in multiple planes.* It is often valuable for learning to analyze the root canals of extracted teeth. The root canals *within* curved roots are similarly curved. The third objective preserves this natural curve of "flow" (Fig. 8-38).

Watch Words: *Delicate, precurve, restraint*
Major Benefit: *Three-dimensional portal of exit seal*

4. *Never transport the foramen.* If the root canals of extracted teeth are examined, few of the exit foramina are located at the apex of the root. They usually are located to the side of the apex.[52] In addition, many root tips have several foramina with root tips that curve significantly at the apical third or occasionally in the middle third. Delicate foramina can be lost during root canal preparation by improper sequencing of instruments, insufficient irrigation, inadequate tactile finesse, or inadequate delicacy. This objective facilitates the achievement of mechanical objective 3, "flow." Maintaining patency to the radiographic terminus and carefully shaping, sculpting, and shaving the inside of the canal are essential to mastering shaping.

Often the angle of access and angle of incidence differ. The angle of access refers to the orientation of the instrument as it slides down the body of the root canal. The angle of incidence refers to the turn required to *follow* the path of the root canal (see Fig. 8-22, *E*).

Foramina may be transported externally or internally (Fig. 8-39). *External transportation* is caused by failing to precurve files, using large instruments, or being too heavy handed. The original apical foramen is torn. Instruments should be used only a few seconds at a time. When an instrument is overused, the elastic memory of the instrument may create the teardrop and tearing of the apical foramen. This "hourglass" shape makes it more difficult to properly obturate the foramen. Many endodontic failures result from external transportation.

The second form of external transportation is direct perforation. This egregious error usually begins with a ledge or apical blockage. The deflected instrument continues its misdirection until it perforates the root surface (see Fig.

Text continued on p. 232

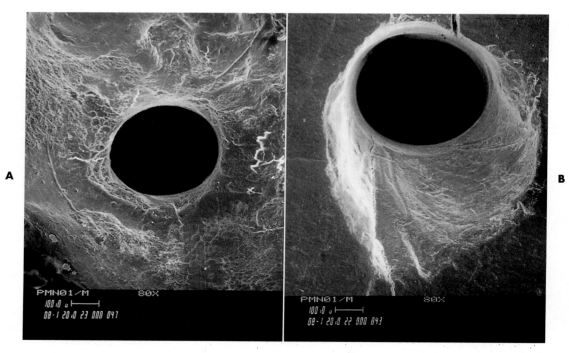

FIG. 8-36 Scanning electron micrograph of a prepared mesial apex from a mandibular molar. The canals were prepared using balanced force technique and Flex-R files. **A,** External view of the foramen discloses a round and clear status; patency was made with a No. 25 file. **B,** Internal view of the control zone region reveals the clean machined and tapering form developed. Outer white elliptical diameter is that created by a No. 45 file, and the black opening is the patency of a No. 25 file.

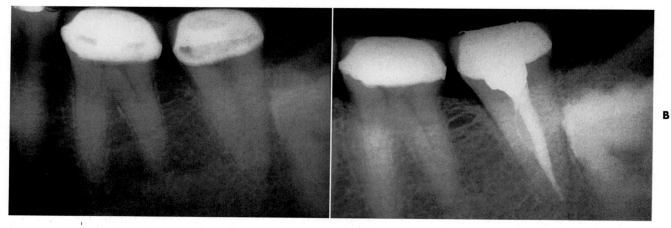

FIG. 8-37 Mechanical objectives 1 and 2: *Develop a continuously tapering conical form in the root canal preparation and make the canal narrower apically, with the narrowest cross-sectional diameter at its terminus.* **A,** Pretreatment radiograph of a maxillary second molar. **B,** Continuously tapering conical form allowed for internal hydraulics to obturate an internal loop toward the mesial side. Although this particular loop had no communication with the attachment apparatus, significant internal hydraulic pressures are always considered a benefit toward achieving the rationale of endodontics.

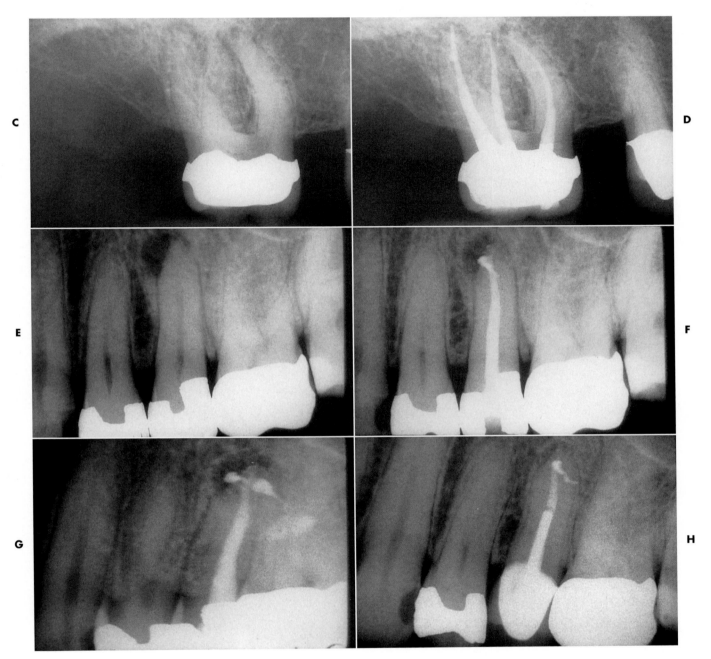

FIG. 8-37, cont'd C, Pretreatment radiograph of a maxillary molar. **D,** Appropriate shapes provide restrictive flow so that the gutta-percha–dentin interface is minimal. **E,** Pretreatment radiograph of a maxillary second premolar. **F,** Perpendicular radiographic final record. **G,** Oblique film better demonstrates the three-dimensionality of the multiple apically obturated portals of exit. **H,** Six-month recall radiograph shows excellent healing of the attachment apparatus around all obturated foramina.

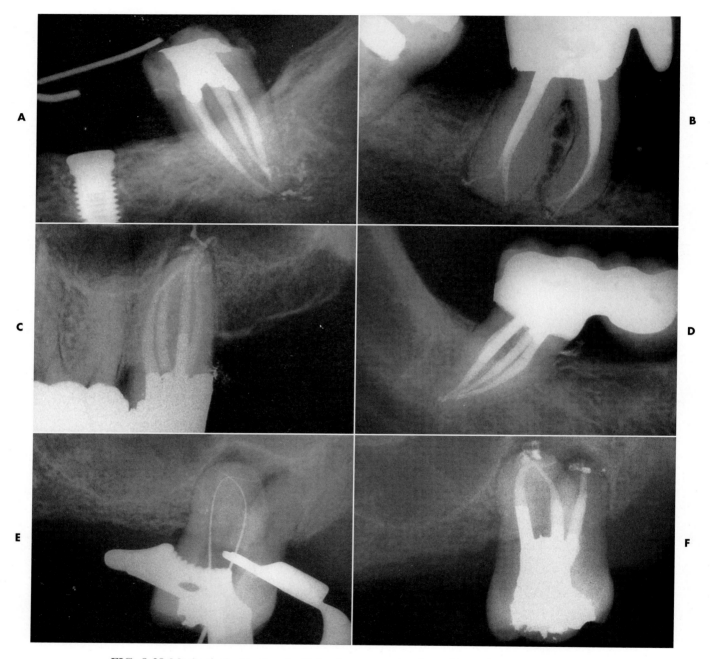

FIG. 8-38 Mechanical objective 3: *Make the preparation in multiple planes.* **A** through **D,** Final pack records of obturated molar root canal systems demonstrating the concept of "flow." Even the radiographs give a sense of three-dimensionality, whereby the anatomy appears to flow in and out of the flat plane of the film. **E,** Two 0.06 files in place to assess the relationship of the two buccal systems. **F,** Obturation shows preservation of the "flow" of the buccal system in the obturation.

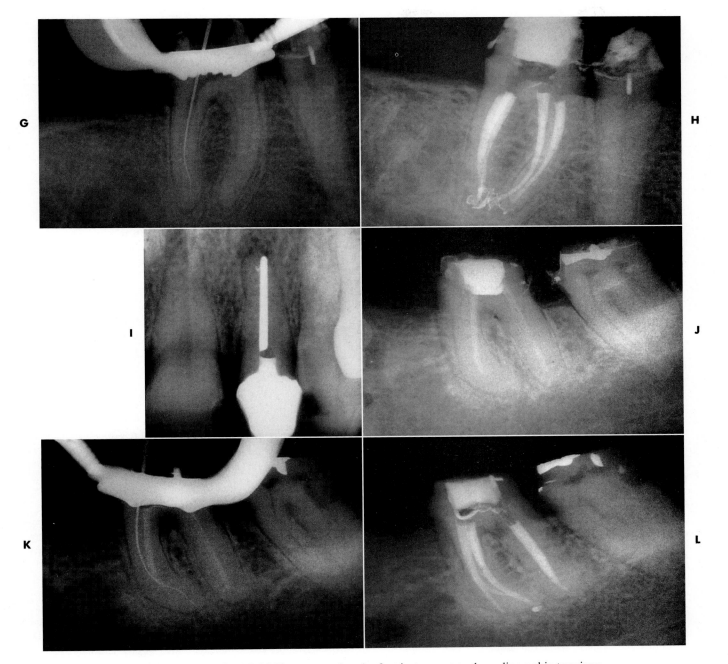

FIG. 8-38, cont'd G, A 0.06 file representing the first instrument to the radiographic terminus. **H,** Again, obturation of this four-canal molar reveals the natural flow of the root canal system is preserved. **I,** Failure to achieve mechanical objective 3 resulted in an unfilled portal of exit and a resulting lesion of endodontic origin. **J,** Patient was referred with a mandibular first molar that was failing endodontically with the symptom of percussion sensitivity. **K,** Rediscovery of the flow of the root canal system within 0.06 file to the radiographic terminus. **L,** Obturation of the original root canal system with subsequent asymptomatic molar abutment.

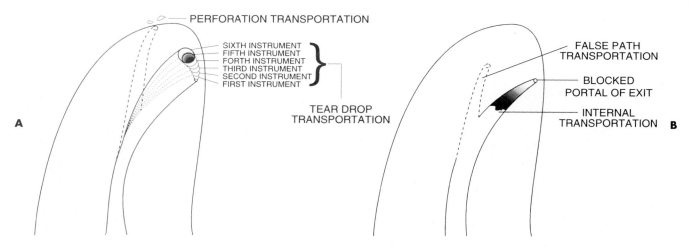

FIG. 8-39 Portal of exit transportation. **A,** External transportation occurs when the same instrument or progressively larger instruments tear the portal of exit into a teardrop shape on the external root surface. External transportation can occur in two forms: a teardrop shape or a direct perforation, which can become a tangential tear. **B,** Internal transportation occurs when the portal of exit is moved internal to its external position by blocking the canal with dentin mud. A new false path will begin.

8-39). This external perforation also can become an external teardrop tear.

Internal transportation occurs when the foramen becomes clogged with dentin mud or denticles. These particles may irritate the attachment apparatus after root canal filling or the particles may prevent obturation of other apical foramina that branch off the main canal. Finally, this internally transported foramen may perforate the external root surface through a false path.

Watch Words: *Save, retain, sanctuary, foraminal patency, loose suspension of dentin mud, prevention*
Major Benefit: *Facilitates the achievement of mechanical objective 3*

5. *Keep the apical foramen as small as is practical.* The final foramen size varies depending on the canal (Fig. 8-40). Some foramina are small and some are large; some are round, some are oval, and some have unusual shapes. The goal of mechanical objective 4 is to preserve foraminal size and shape at the apical constricture. This can be achieved only by carefully maintaining patency to the radiographic terminus by constantly reconfirming patency *through* the foramen with a loose-fitting instrument. Since patency is so important to success, the clinician discovers a sense of security. The clinician cleans the foramen but does not enlarge or distort it. After careful probing to the radiographic terminus, the canal is shaped inside.

To clean and predictably seal the foramen, the size of the file used at the *end* of the cleaning and shaping should be at least a No. 20 or 25 in the ISO sizing, or in the newer series 29 sizing, the foramen size is often a No. 3. Correct shaping and observance of mechanical objectives 1 through 4 produces an apical constriction of minimal diameter. By creating a continuously tapering cone, precurving instruments, and maximizing irrigation, the flow of the root canal preparation is preserved. There is no advantage to creating a wider foramen unless the canal is too small to predictably compact gutta-percha and sealer (ISO No. 10 or 15).

The goal is to clean but not enlarge the foramen. If the diameter of a foramen is increased from an ISO No. 20 to an ISO No. 40 instrument, the *area* of the foramen has increased four times. Not only does this increase the risk of tearing, but it increases the potential of microleakage (Fig. 8-41) around the obturation margin.

Watch Words: *Keep safe, shelter, foster*
Major Benefit: *Predictable corkage*

In summary, the goal is to produce a three-dimensional, continuously tapering, multiplaned cone from access cavity to radiographic terminus while preserving foraminal position and size (Fig. 8-42).

The "look"

The "look" refers to the radiographic appearance of three-dimensional obturation when all five mechanical objectives have been achieved. The mechanical objectives are in harmony with the natural root canal anatomy. The "look" is unmistakable (Fig. 8-43).

Clinical description of the serial shaping technique

The following description is a simulation of the serial shaping technique for a "generic" tooth (Fig. 8-44, *A*). Just as an artist would never use the exact order of brush strokes to paint, this sequence of dental maneuvers should not be memorized; rather it serves as a guide to understanding the concept of cleaning and shaping. The reader should get a sense of the dynamics and sequence of root canal cleaning and of how the sculpted form develops during the *shaping.* In this example, four recapitulations are necessary to achieve the proper shape for the *cone fit,* which is the *last* step of successful cleaning and shaping.

With a good access cavity copiously irrigated with sodium hypochlorite, the precurved No. 10 file is guided gently into the access cavity. The position of the rubber stop and the length of the tooth are not significant at this time. The clinician must

Text continued on p. 237

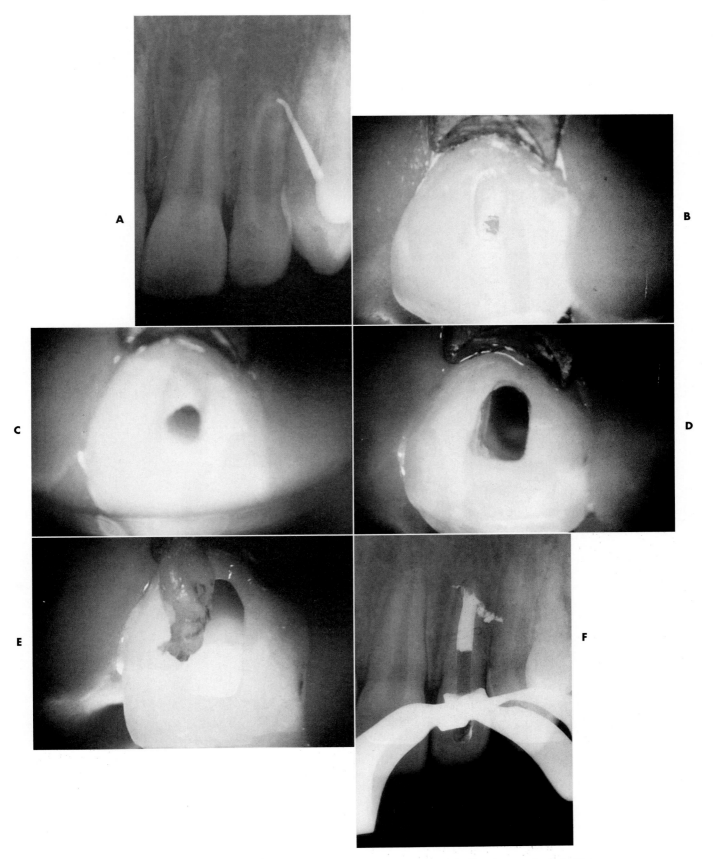

FIG. 8-40 Mechanical objective 5: *Keep the apical foramen as small as is practical.* **A,** Pretreatment radiograph showing the sinus tract being traced by a gutta-percha cone. **B,** Access cavity showing both triangle 1 and 2 still present. **C,** Triangle 1, essentially in enamel, has been removed, but triangle 2, essentially in dentin, is still present. **D,** Completion of triangle 2 removal. **E,** Extirpation of pulp remnants. **F,** Down pack film.

Continued

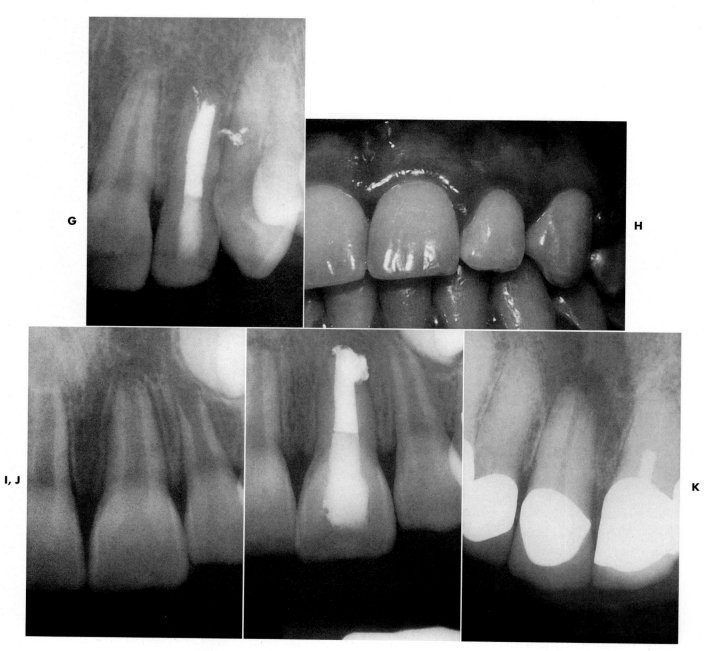

FIG. 8-40, cont'd G, Final obturation. **H,** Two-month recall radiograph shows closure of the sinus tract. **I,** Maxillary central incisor with an underformed apex. **J,** Preservation of apical size and obturation. **K,** Maxillary central incisor. Note that in the obturation the diameter of the apical opening has been preserved.

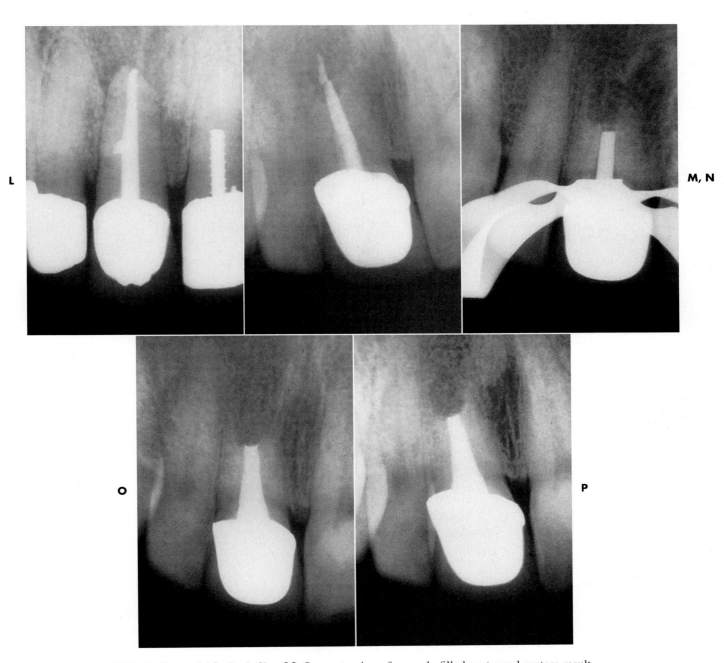

FIG. 8-40, cont'd L, Pack film. **M,** Overextension of an underfilled root canal system resulting in the continued lesion of endodontic origin. **N,** Cone fit. **O,** Obturation demonstrating proper internal shaping and again preservation of the apical foramen and therefore achieving mechanical objective 5. **P,** Oblique radiographic confirmation of obturation at the foraminal constriction.

Continued

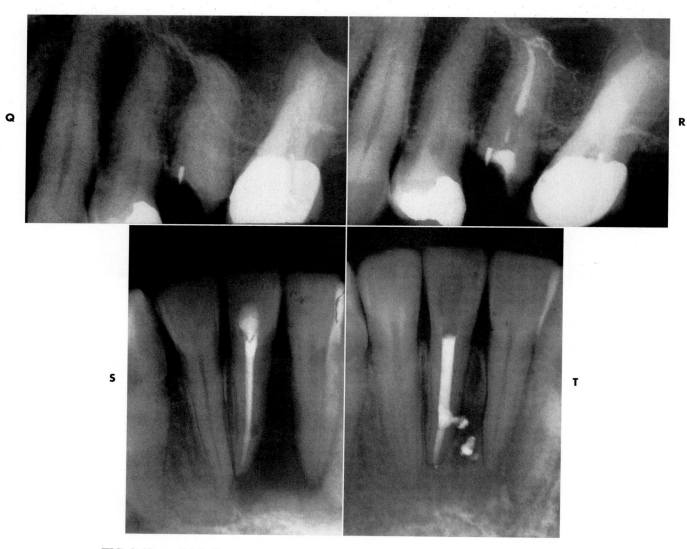

FIG. 8-40, cont'd Q, Pretreatment radiograph where the clinician may suspect the apical portal of exit to be relatively small as an ISO No. 20 file. **R,** Obturation shows good apical constriction and proper shaping internally without enlarging the apical foramen. **S,** Developing lesion of endodontic origin and resorbed apical foramen. **T,** Obturation and subsequent healing after keeping the foramen as small as is practical.

AREA OF CIRCLE = πr^2

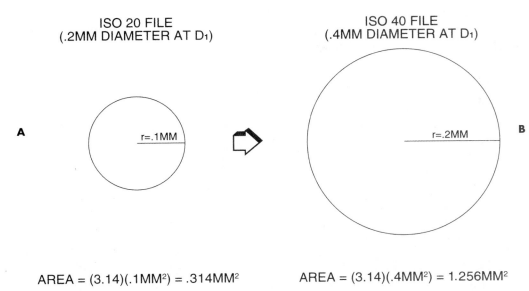

ISO 20 FILE
(.2MM DIAMETER AT D_1)

A

r=.1MM

ISO 40 FILE
(.4MM DIAMETER AT D_1)

r=.2MM

B

AREA = (3.14)(.1MM²) = .314MM²   AREA = (3.14)(.4MM²) = 1.256MM²

FIG. 8-41 Enlarging the foramen results in a significant increase in surface area and circumference, increasing the potential for microleakage. **A,** Radius of 0.1 mm. **B,** When this radius is increased to 0.2 mm, the area of the circle is increased four times and the circumference doubles.

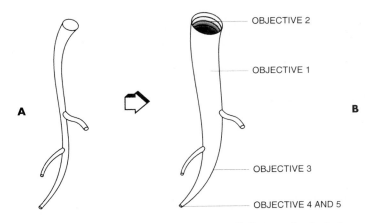

A

OBJECTIVE 2

OBJECTIVE 1

B

OBJECTIVE 3

OBJECTIVE 4 AND 5

FIG. 8-42 Line drawing demonstrates all five mechanical objectives. **A,** Example of a root canal network consisting of an orifice and three foramina. **B,** Cleaning and shaping is a concept that produces a three-dimensional, continuously tapering, multiplaned cone from access cavity to radiographic terminus while preserving foraminal position and size.

tactilely feel and "see" with the instrument tip. Specific knowledge of the individual root canal system anatomy and any potential problems are identified at this time. If the instrument easily glides down the canal, the next step is to follow the paths through the radiographic terminus. The path is always present, but occasionally the instrument suddenly stops. However, with a gentle turn of the precurved No. 10 file, the instrument usually progresses apically through or around the necrotic debris, dense collagen, or small pulp stones and denticles. If the in-

strument does not bypass the obstacle or is confined by restrictive dentin, the file is withdrawn (Fig. 8-45). Again the file is precurved with a slightly different curvature and the chamber is gently irrigated. This sequence is repeated until the radiographic terminus is reached; however, after several unsuccessful attempts, the clinician must consider restrictive dentin as the culprit. Therefore serial coronal shaping with the Nos. 2 and 3 reamers usually allows freedom to the No. 10 file to advance further apically.

Why are we spending so much time on the first instrument? Because the first instrument is the key. Once the radiographic terminus has been reached, success depends solely on the cleaning and shaping mechanics. The fundamental techniques are *patency confirmation* and *serial carving,* which were previously described as *serial filing, reaming,* and *recapitulation.*[18,76,78]

Recapitulation is sequential reentry and reuse of each previous instrument. Recapitulation does not merely confirm patency; it involves careful, rhythmic sequencing of the series of files and reamers to create the shape that achieves the five mechanical objectives. Successful cleaning and shaping depends on the first instrument that reaches the radiographic terminus. At some point, we have weaved and threaded our way to the radiographic terminus. This must be verified by an accurate radiograph and confirmed with an electronic apex locator. The clinician must not manipulate the instrument while waiting for the radiograph. There are two reasons for this. If the foramen has been passed, it could be inadvertently torn. If the instrument is positioned coronal to the foramen, dentin mud could be packed into the foraminal opening. *There is one chance in three that the instrument is in the correct position.* Patience is paramount. Sodium hypochlorite is used to irrigate. If the radiograph indicates that the file is long, the dentist must pull back, adjust the rubber stop to the reference, and expose an-

Text continued on p. 242

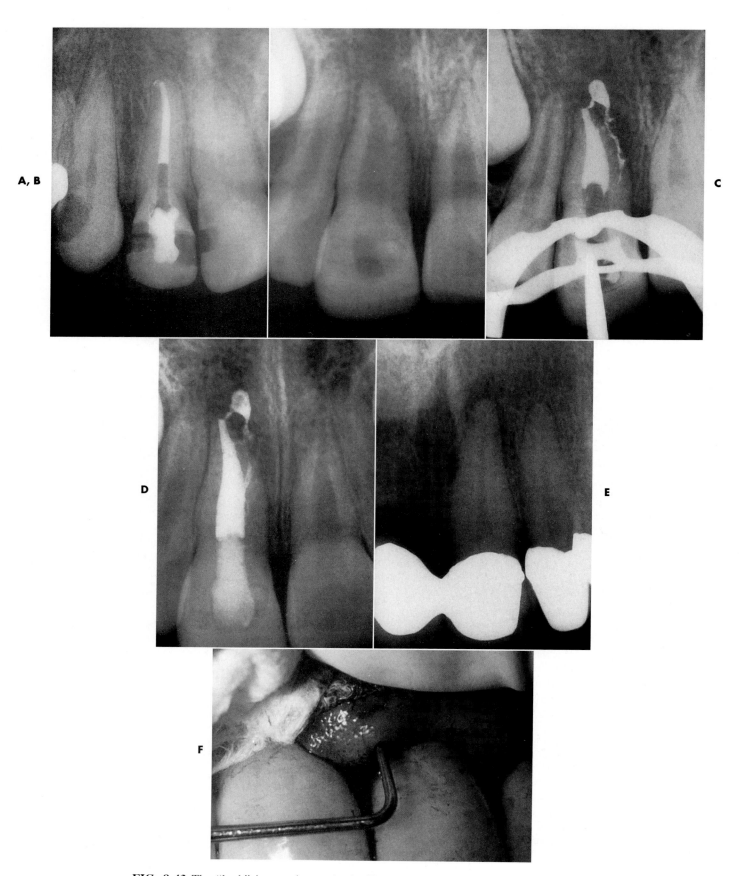

FIG. 8-43 The "look" in anterior teeth. **A,** Simple and appropriate shaping of a maxillary lateral incisor. **B,** Pretreatment radiograph of maxillary incisor. **C,** All mechanical objectives have been met in the down pack. **D,** Completed packing where all five mechanical objectives have been met. **E,** Pretreatment radiograph of maxillary central incisor. **F,** Severe draining through the gingival crevice as evidenced by deep probing.

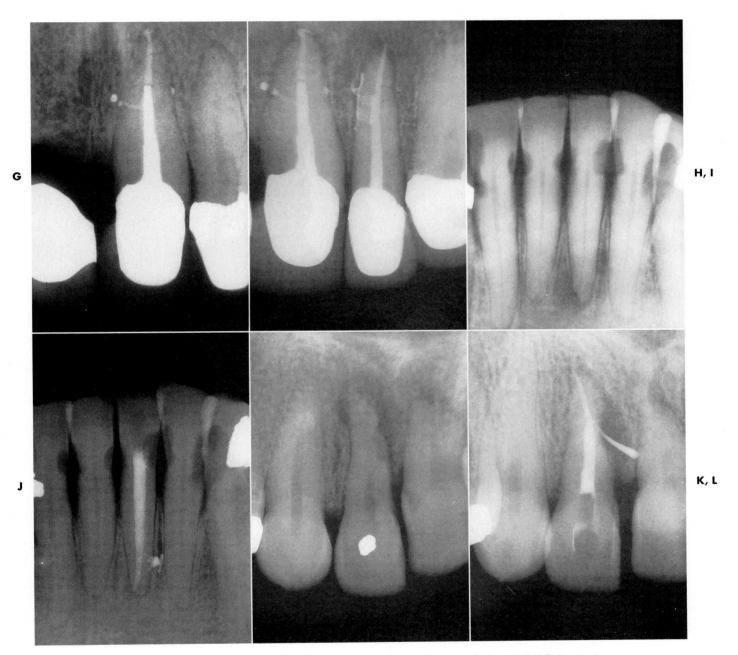

FIG. 8-43, cont'd G, Finished obturation. **H,** Maxillary incisors with the "look." **I,** Pretreatment radiograph of a mandibular central incisor. **J,** Obturation and healing. **K,** Pretreatment radiograph of a maxillary lateral incisor. **L,** Previous attempt resulted in continued sinus tract drainage as evidenced by the gutta-percha cone tracer.   *Continued*

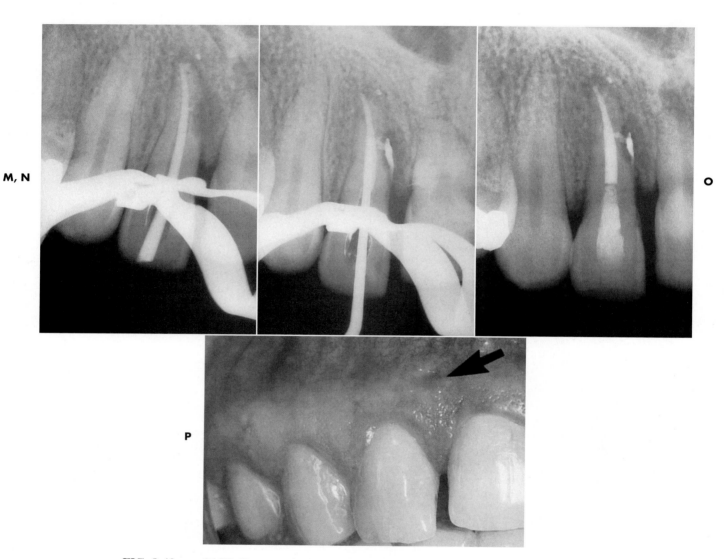

M, N

O

P

FIG. 8-43, cont'd M, Gutta-percha has been removed. Appropriate shape is now created, and the cone fits. **N,** Deepest point of compaction showing a plugger to the depth of 5 to 7 mm from the radiographic terminus. *Note:* Two apical foramina and one major lateral canal has been obturated in this second attempt now that the mechanical objectives have been achieved. **O,** Three-month follow-up radiograph shows good healing. **P,** Sinus tract has closed *(arrow).*

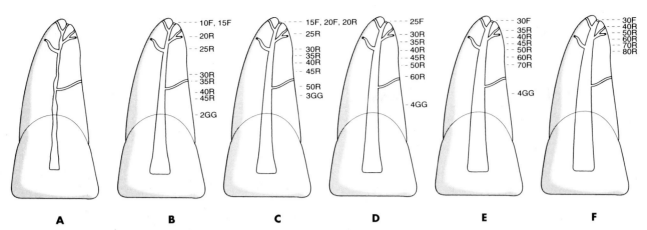

FIG. 8-44 Proper root canal preparation through serial shaping and recapitulation. **A,** Canal requiring cleaning and shaping. **B,** Developing shape after the first series of files and reamers. Notice that the larger reamers are never placed to their maximal physical depth but rather short of the radiographic terminus. **C,** Position of instrument depth after the first recapitulation. No. 20 file now falls to the radiographic terminus where previously it did not extend. Nos. 25, 30, 35, 40, and 45 reamers are now easily advanced apically. Gates-Glidden drills are used only in the cervical third. **D,** After the second recapitulation the root canal begins to take on the correct shape. Position of the instruments is dictated by the developing shape of the canal. Notice how the apical and middle thirds of the shape begin to blend now with the access cavity. **E,** After the third recapitulation the shaping is almost complete with larger instruments progressing apically. **F,** After the final recapitulation it is discovered that the foramen minimal size is a No. 30 file, and the continuously tapering cone shape of the last few millimeters is verified by each subsequent-sized instrument sliding short of the radiographic terminus. Each subsequent instrument should fall easily to its position and then meet resistance from the remaining tapering cone. Cone fit is then the final evidence that all five mechanical objectives have been achieved.

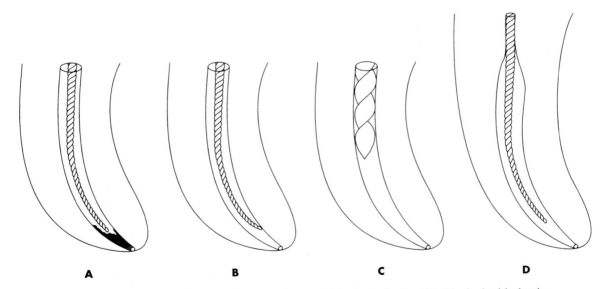

FIG. 8-45 There are four possible causes for canal blockage. **A,** Canal is blocked with dentin mud. Irrigate with sodium hypochlorite, place a significant apical curve on the file or reamer as shown in Fig. 8-22, *C,* and slide the instrument back into the root canal system. Before the instrument reaches maximal resistance, remove it from the root canal and irrigate again. Do this enough times that the dentin mud is disrupted and each instrument moves apically toward the radiographic terminus until finally patency is again achieved. **B,** Angle of access is divergent from the angle of incidence. Solution is to remove the instrument, recurve it, and replace it. As soon as the curvature matches the original curvature of the root canal, the instrument extends to the radiographic terminus, and cleaning and shaping can continue. **C,** Tip of the instrument is too wide for the existing shape. Remove the instrument and return to a narrower one. Do not proceed until that instrument fits loosely. **D,** Instrument experiences restriction somewhere short of the apical third. Correction is to lightly and serially shape the restrictive area so that the file easily falls to the radiographic terminus.

other radiograph, or advance immediately to the No. 15 file and repeat the same steps. If the file is coronal to the radiographic terminus, the clinician carefully slides it apically by continuing to follow the curvature of the canal; the adjusted length is confirmed with a new radiograph. If the file does not advance, it is removed, the canal is irrigated, and the file is recurved before another try is made (see Fig. 8-45). Once the first file easily reaches the radiographic terminus, the rubber stop is set against the closest access reference and the file is moved in vertical strokes of a 0.5-mm to a 1- or 2-mm amplitude; the tighter the canal, the less the amplitude (see Fig. 8-22, D). Sometimes when the first file is snug, flexing the fingers produces enough movement of the instrument (see Fig. 8-18, H). At some point the file begins to release as the dentin is worn away and the instrument is freed. It is essential to recognize that these are vertical strokes and no attempt is made to circumferentially create shape with the small instrument. The purpose is to navigate and establish the path to the foramen using the long axis of the precurved file with a short in-and-out motion. The file is loosening dense collagen, dentin mud, and dentinal filings from the canal walls. When this material surrounds the file, the file is withdrawn and the root canal is irrigated with sodium hypochlorite.

Now the pace quickens, but the light touch is maintained. The rubber stop of a No. 15 file is set the same length as the No. 10 file. The clinician follows the No. 15 file in the same fashion as the No. 10 file, and the sequence is repeated. Once the No. 15 file is loose through gentle vertical strokes, the canal is irrigated and the precurved No. 20 reamer slides short of the radiographic terminus. Random sculpting occurs on withdrawal of the reamer. Any dentin shavings or debris that have accumulated are drawn away. The rubber stops are set by comparing the length of the two instruments. A ruler is an unnecessary step, a step that can add error to the measurement.

In the past, files were for filing, reamers were for reaming, and Gates-Glidden drills were for drilling (see Fig. 8-22). The distinction now is that files are for following and maintaining patency while finding a pathway to the foramen. Reamers are for carrying away dentinal debris and for carving. The envelope of motion of the precurved reamer randomly shaves the dentinal walls,[78] sculpting on *withdrawal*. This is how to avoid ledges. Reamers are for carving in relatively straight canals and the relatively straight portion of curved canals. It is difficult to carve delicately with files without forcing dentin into apical foramina (see Fig. 8-18). The Gates-Glidden drill is used simply as a brush to shape the coronal third (sometimes half) of the root canal so that it blends smoothly with the access cavity. The clinician always shapes away from the furcation with the Gates-Glidden drill. Nickel-titanium files also facilitate the recapitulation process (see new technology). The precurved No. 25 reamer shaves the dentinal walls *coronal* to the point of maximal resistance and is withdrawn in a light carving fashion. The Nos. 30, 35, 40, and 45 reamers are used in the same way (see Fig. 8-44, B). If the No. 50 reamer barely fits into the orifice, it is removed. The access cavity flows to the coronal third of the root canal with the No. 2 Gates-Glidden drill. This essential step removes restrictive dentin and allows larger reamers to fall freely and deeper into the evolving shape. Confirm patency with a No. 15 file, and the *first recapitulation* begins by reintroducing the initial series of files and reamers (see Fig. 8-44, C).

In the first recapitulation, the No. 20 file should advance to the apical foramen. The No. 20 precurved reamer carries away dentin debris. At least 2 ml of sodium hypochlorite is used to irrigate between *every* instrument use. Now that the No. 25 reamer is not restricted, it should advance deeper into the root canal. The clinician should use the envelope of motion to gently carve the walls of the root canal. The precurved Nos. 30 and 35 reamers are gently advanced into the root canal but not to the maximal physical depth. The technique is to slip in and allow the withdrawing envelope of motion of the precurved reamer to carve the internal shape.

Now the Nos. 40 and 45 reamers should easily advance deeper into the root canal. For the first time, the No. 50 reamer should fit into the middle region of the root canal, and a slight amount of sculpting and carving can be accomplished. The No. 50 reamer is followed by a No. 3 Gates-Glidden drill, which is shimmied against the walls in the coronal third of the root canal. The canal is irrigated with 2 ml of sodium hypochlorite after each instrument. In a mandibular tooth, RC-Prep or hydrogen peroxide is alternated with sodium hypochlorite to create effervescence and elevate the dentin mud into the chamber. Then sodium hypochlorite irrigating solution can be aspirated easily, and new irrigation is introduced. Confirm patency with a small file and begin a *second recapitulation* (see Fig. 8-44, D). It is unlikely that the canal could be blocked at this point if this step-by-step procedure is followed. However, it is still possible that some dentin mud has accumulated (Fig. 8-46). After irrigating, the smallest instrument that reached the apical foramen is retrieved and an abrupt apical curve is created (not a bend) so the last half millimeter is not straight (see Fig. 8-22, C). This instrument dislodges the dentin mud (see Fig. 8-46). The technique should be careful and light; sliding and irrigating, sliding and irrigating. The canal is still there (see Fig. 8-44, A through D), and with time the foramen *will* be reached.

Now the No. 25 file should reach to the apical foramen and suddenly and *gently* hug the dentinal walls (see Fig. 8-44, D). The instruments are loose until the canal narrows to their diameter; then they fit loosely against the dentinal walls. The No. 30 reamer should be 1 to 2 mm from the apical foramen when it is advanced into the canal. The Nos. 35, 40, 45, and 50 reamers provide further shaping after the second recapitulation. The No. 60 reamer should now extend into the middle third of the root. One or two carvings with the No. 60 reamer selectively enlarges the midportion of the root canal. The No. 5 Gates-Glidden drill is used to brush the walls in the cervical third and to continue to blend the shape of the apical third with the

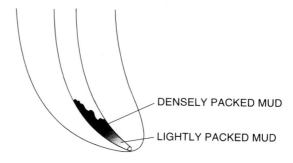

FIG. 8-46 Densest dentin mud is usually most coronal. Disrupt the dentin mud in this area, and the instruments easily move to the radiographic terminus.

coronal third. Again rotary nickel-titanium instruments of greater than 0.02 standard ISO taper can contribute to successful serial shaping.

Patency is confirmed before the *third recapitulation*. If recapitulation is done properly, no instrument goes to the same place twice. Files automatically extend deeper into the canal. In our example, the No. 30 file nearly reaches the foramen, while the Nos. 35, 40, 45, 50, 60, and 70 reamers are subsequently used in sequential order for shaping and sculpting (see Fig. 8-44, *E*). A progress radiograph (see Fig. 8-22, *G* through *I*) is exposed. The No. 4 Gates-Glidden drill is used for final blending of the coronal third and the access cavity. After irrigation and confirmation of patency, the *fourth* and final *recapitulation* begins. If the desired shape has not been achieved, another recapitulation is necessary (see Fig. 8-22, *A* and *B*). At times one or two additional recapitulations make the difference between an adequate and an excellent result.

When are cleaning and shaping complete? They are complete when the cone fits. If the conventional gutta-percha cone fits to the radiographic terminus, the shape is conducive to compaction of gutta-percha and sealer into the canal system.

Balanced Force and Predesigned Preparations

Commitment to a single visit endodontic concept and a desire to establish reliable and reproducible quality controls led to the endodontic cleaning and shaping technique that is discussed in this section.

Preparation design

Canal systems are three-dimensional spaces seen in two dimensions with clinical radiographs. Generally, the visual dimensions are the lesser, not the greater, diameter of the canal system. Also two-dimensional images do not disclose curvatures that course in or out with the radiographic beam (see Fig. 8-23).[85] As a solution to these variances between the seen and the actual canal shapes, predesigned preparations set criteria that assume average canal diameters and call for complete shaping based on prior successful cases.[69,72] The preparation sizes recommended match closely the morphometric sizes de-

termined by Kerekes and Tronstad in their 1977 papers.[50] Predesigned preparations result in a well-controlled and complete cleaning and shaping of the canal system (Fig. 8-47). The specified dimensions of preparation are selected to assure tooth-guided preparation sufficient to fill the greatest width of the canal.[69,70] The required shaping is not altered downward even around a curve, since curvature does not directly influence the canal diameter but rather only the difficulty experienced in accomplishing complete cleaning and shaping. The minimal dimensions of a predesigned preparation are at least one half the greater canal diameter when the canal is straight, and preparation may proceed from both ends of an oval-shaped space. The dimensions must equal the greatest canal diameter whenever cleaning and shaping goes beyond a curvature. This change is necessary because the curvature drives all instruments to a single wall as they pass through the curvature (Fig. 8-48 and see Fig. 8-32). As a result, one wall controls the file position and the final canal shape. Consequently, the preparation dimension must at least equal the greater diameter of the canal when curvature is present. This assumes, of course, that one expects to remove the pulpal tissues, debris, and microbial contents by mechanical means.

A specific final shape is defined for each canal by using a combination of three preparation designs: Nos. 45, 60, and 80. No. 45 for small roots (Fig. 8-49), No. 60 for medium roots (Fig. 8-50), and No. 80 for large roots (Fig. 8-51). These three preparation designs can be employed independently and in combinations to fit the anatomic makeup of any tooth. Hence, a maxillary central incisor would receive a large diameter design, whereas a maxillary first premolar with two roots would dictate two small No. 45 preparations. A maxillary molar would require small preparations for its facial roots and a medium one for its palatal root.

Predesigned preparations impart a specific rate of taper to the canal. The radicular access tapers at a rate of 0.1 mm per millimeter of canal length. The apical preparation tapers at 0.02 mm per millimeter of canal length. The control zones taper at a rate that varies from 0.1 to 0.2 mm per millimeter of canal length. This greater rate of taper is needed in a control zone to

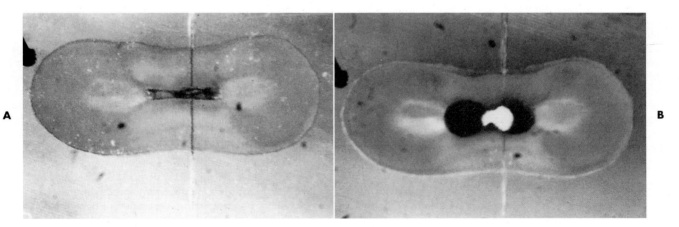

FIG. 8-47 A, Cross section made about 5 mm coronal to the foramen in a maxillary premolar. Note how the canal space is oval and narrow in the mesial to distal plane. Treatment must clear this space of all debris and shape the walls. **B,** Posttreatment view of the same section reveals that instrumentation has cleaned the canal completely and shaped the entire perimeter. There is a confluence of two preparations, each proceeding from opposite ends of the oval space.

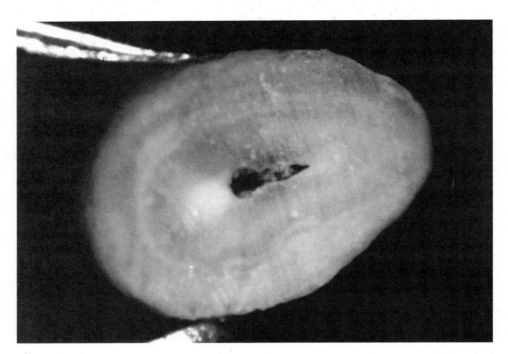

FIG. 8-48 Cross section of the mesial facial root of a maxillary molar is at a point 3 mm coronal to the apex. Round opening is that of a No. 25 file. Note that it lies completely to one end of the narrow oval space. This preparation gives the sensation of tightness, and white filings would certainly be generated. Curvature positioned the file against this wall, and only diameter of the preparation can move it to the other. Required diameter is approximately that of a No. 70 file or No. 2 Gates-Glidden drill.

provide resistance against the condensation pressures of obturation. At least a 50% reduction of canal diameter is defined for each control zone. This taper provides a resistance of at least four times that of the canal shape itself and allows the use of an apical patency with minimal risk for extrusion of obturation materials.

An apical control zone establishes an apical constriction by forming a rapid canal taper at a clinician-defined location. This location is near the location of the natural constriction but is mechanically defined relative to the canal exit itself. Three or more 0.5-mm step-backs establish this terminating taper before the canal exits to the periodontal ligament. This procedural nuance eliminates extensive searching for the natural constriction (Fig. 8-49, *A* and *C*). Preparing to the natural constriction, although desirable, is fraught with difficulty because of the great variability in the location of the constriction. An apical control zone demands strict attention to preparation length, knowledge of cutting dynamics, and awareness of file design. Properly done, a control zone dependably and easily establishes a round and clean apical foramen for obturation.

Apical foraminal patency

Confirming apical foraminal patency is the last step of any cleaning and shaping. It is a feature of the control zone and is important to provide a complete severance of the pulp from the periodontal ligament. Endodontic files lack sufficient sharpness to cut fibrous connective tissues unless those tissues are trapped between the cutting edges and the canal wall. To assure that a severance occurs very near the periodontal ligament, the clinician must slightly enlarge the diameter of the foramen. *This should not be done early in any cleaning procedure,* as to

do so invites an overextended preparation and subsequently an overextended obturation. The patency opening should be completed with the first file that fits tightly in the foraminal passage. Pulpal severance is accomplished by extending the file just through the apical foramen and with a very light pressure rotating it one revolution to cause the cutting edges to engage, trap, and sever the remaining tissues. Be very careful. Inspect each instrument for damage before placing it into the preparation and do not force the rotation to avoid a separated instrument.

Clinical description of the balanced force preparation

The access cavity is aligned to provide straight unimpeded entry into the canal orifice. The chamber and canal are irrigated with sodium hypochlorite, removing debris and microbial matter. The orifice of each canal is identified with a DG 16 explorer, then a No. 15 Flex-R file is marked with a rubber stop to identify the approximate length of the canal as it appears in the pretreatment radiograph. This file is moved to the estimated length using a one-quarter clockwise then a one-half to one-revolution counterclockwise rotation. This action is repeated to gradually move the file into a depth equal that marked on the file. With an apex locator attached, an indication of the apex should correspond to a sensation of tightening and to the approximation of the mark to the occlusal reference point. A radiograph, exposed with this file in place, gives visual confirmation of the correctness of its position (Fig. 8-53, *A*). The canal length is measured and recorded for continued use. The Nos. 20 and 25 files are marked 0.5 mm short of the full canal length; the Nos. 30 and 35 files are marked 1 mm short of the full canal length; and the Nos. 40 and 45 files are marked

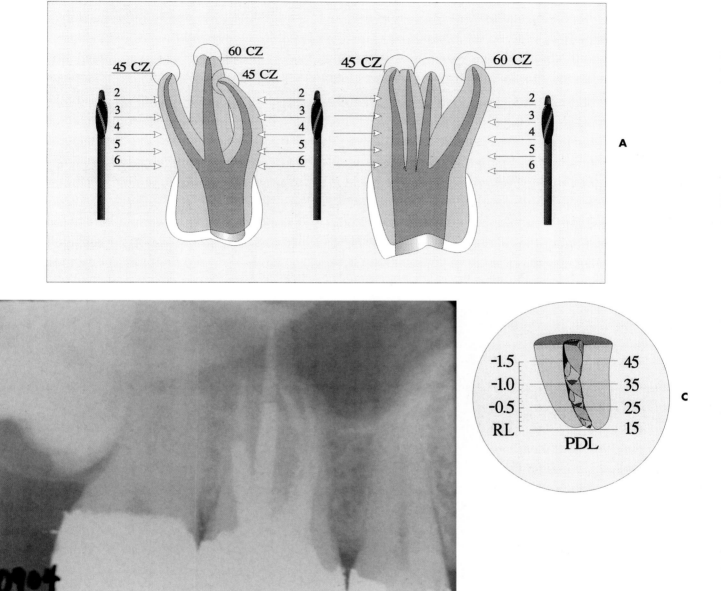

FIG. 8-49 A, No. 45 preparation defines the look for a small curved root such as the facial roots of a maxillary molar. Gates-Glidden drill depths are defined with 2 mm separations. Larger Gates-Glidden drills are used to open the orifice. **B,** Maxillary molar cleaned and shaped using the No. 45 preparation. **C,** Step-backs (0.5 mm each) used to establish a control zone and mechanically determine the minor diameter at the apex. Largest size file used in each step is given.

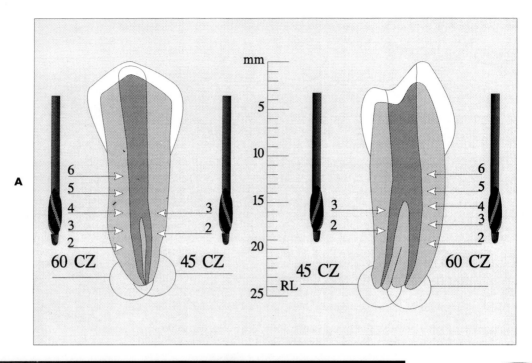

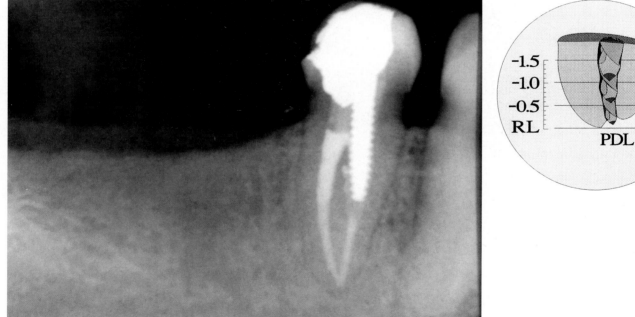

FIG. 8-50 A, No. 60 preparation defines the look for a medium-sized root such as this mandibular premolar with a medium-sized F and smaller (No. 45) L canal. Gates-Glidden drill depths are defined with 2 mm separations. **B,** Mandibular premolar with two canals cleaned and shaped using the 60 F and 45 L preparation. **C,** Step-backs (0.5 mm each) used to establish a No. 60 control zone and mechanically determine the minor diameter at the apex. Largest size file used in each step is given.

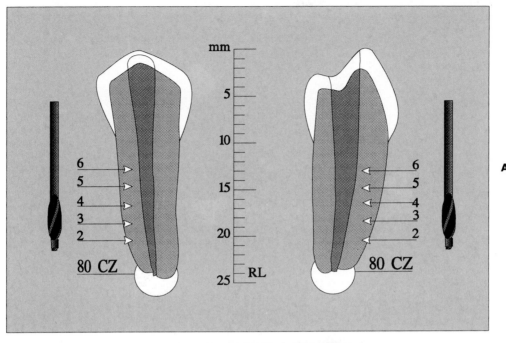

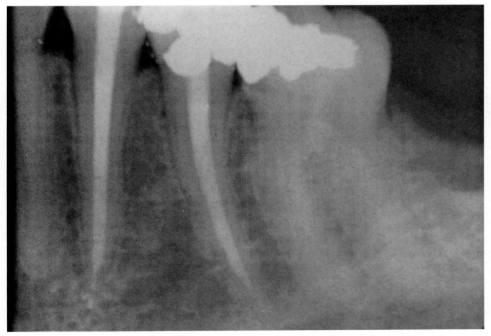

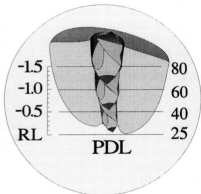

FIG. 8-51 A, No. 80 preparation defines the look for large bulky roots such as the mandibular premolar. Gates-Glidden drill depths are defined with 2 mm separations. **B,** Straight and curved mandibular premolar cleaned and shaped using the No. 80 preparation. **C,** Step-backs (0.5 mm each) used to establish a No. 80 control zone and mechanically determine the minor diameter at the apex. Largest size file used in each step is given.

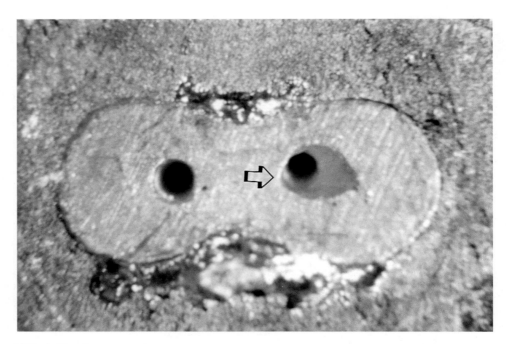

FIG. 8-52 Micrograph of the mesial apex of a mandibular molar. Both canals have a No. 45 control zone. Larger light opening is a curving canal space cut somewhat obliquely. Small black hole, seen in both canals, is the patent foramen. Note how the foraminal shape is clean and round. Both control zones were prepared with Flex-R files.

1.5 mm short of the full canal length. Shaping progresses through the Nos. 20 and 25 files using irrigation between each instrument. The rotational cutting motions described previously in the balanced force section are used for all files. No in-and-out strokes are employed. Before completing the hand enlargement further (beyond file size No. 25), the body of the canal is shaped with Gates-Glidden drills. A radicular access quickly shapes the coronal two thirds of the canal. The best sequence is to begin with the No. 6 Gates-Glidden drill and cut into the canal opening a distance no more than 2 mm (Fig. 8-53, *B*). Flush the canal and chamber with sodium hypochlorite. Then proceed with the No. 5 Gates-Glidden drill and extend the depth an additional 2 mm (Fig. 8-53, *C*). Repeat the irrigation and move to the No. 4 Gates-Glidden drill, moving the preparation an additional 2 mm into the canal (Fig. 8-53, *D*). Continue this process until the No. 2 Gates-Glidden drill has either entered the canal to a completion depth of 10 mm or a curvature prevents its penetration (Fig. 8-53, *E* and *F*). *Do not force a Gates-Glidden drill through a curvature; breakage or a ledge will result!* Irrigate the canal and return to the No. 25 file. Debris will most likely block the canal and a one-quarter turn push, hold then pull motion will be needed to regain the full canal length. Repeat until length is regained, irrigate the canal and move to the No. 30 file. Use balanced force motions and continue the hand shaping through file size No. 45. Be sure to irrigate the canal between each instrument and to accurately maintain the shaping length changes. Having increased the apical diameter to 0.45 mm 1.5 mm short of the canal termination, it is now time to complete the cleaning and shaping by redefining the control zone and establishing apical patency (Fig. 8-53, *H*). Return to the No. 15 file and pass it to the full canal length. Irrigate the canal, fit the No. 25 file to its length (0.5 mm

short), and rotate it at that level. Irrigate the canal. Place the No. 35 file to depth (1 mm short) (Fig. 8-53, *I*) and rotate, then remove it. Irrigate the canal and do the same with the No. 45 file (1.5 mm short) (Fig. 8-53, *J*). Irrigate the canal and now pass a No. 20 file to the full canal length and carefully rotate it through the foramen. Irrigate and then dry the canal. Inspect it for cleanliness (Fig. 8-53, *K*) and fit of a gutta-percha point. When the point fits to the full canal length, preparation is complete (Fig. 8-53, *L*).

Crown-Down Technique

The fundamental importance of cleaning, shaping, debris removal, irrigation, tactile sense, and common sense have been described and the authors are in complete accord concerning the goals for cleaning and shaping the root canal system. The techniques already described have considerable merit and enjoy wide support. However, the crown-down technique for cleaning and shaping is gaining more acclaim. The crown-down technique follows medical principles of cleaning before probing into a wound. To accomplish that goal, the crown-down technique begins with a thorough cleaning and shaping of the coronal regions of the canal and gradually progresses toward the apical region (Fig. 8-54). The apical foraminal area is cleaned and shaped as a final step after the coronal regions of the canal system have been completely cleaned, shaped, and disinfected.

The benefits of the crown-down technique are as follows:
1. It eliminates constrictions in the coronal regions of the canal, reduces the effect of canal curvatures, and gives the clinician better tactile awareness during the apical cleaning and shaping.
2. It allows irrigation to be effective to the complete depth that the cleaning and shaping instruments reach. It cleans

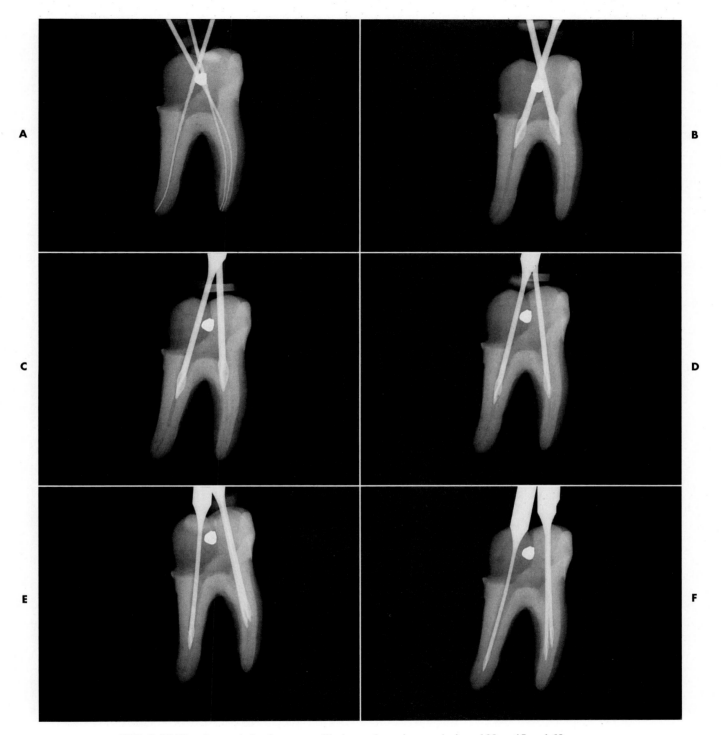

FIG. 8-53 Cleaning and shaping a mandibular molar using predesigned Nos. 45 and 60 preparations. **A,** Complete canal length has been established and verified radiographically. **B,** After increasing the canal diameter to that of a No. 25 file or more, a No. 6 Gates-Glidden drill is used to enlarged the orifice of each canal. **C,** After irrigation, the canals are enlarged 2 mm deeper with a No. 5 Gates-Glidden drill. **D,** Again following irrigation, the radicular access is extended 2 mm further with a No. 4 Gates-Glidden drill. **E,** No. 3 Gates-Glidden drill extends the shaping an additional 2 mm beyond the initial curvature. **F,** No. 2 Gates-Glidden drill completes mechanical shaping by extending the shaping a final 2 mm.

Continued

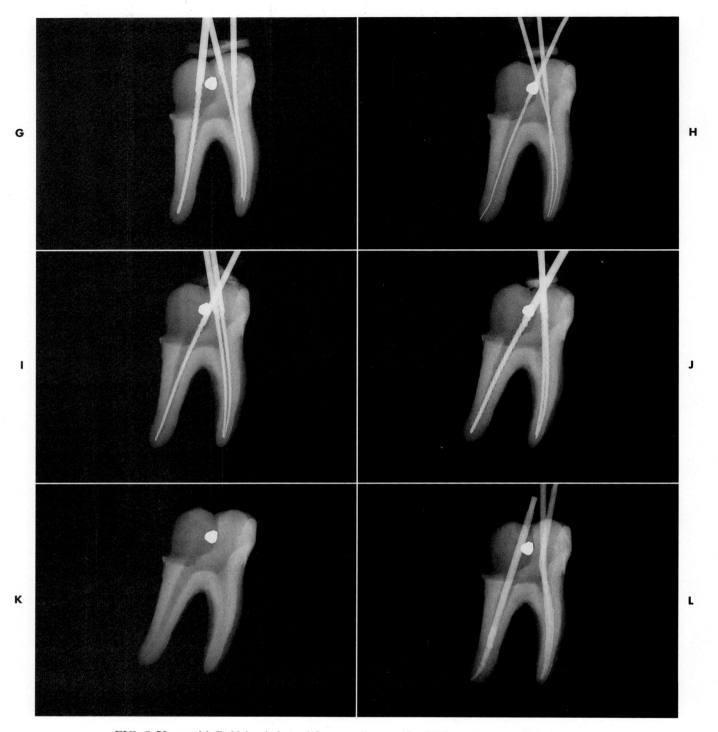

FIG. 8-53, cont'd G, Using balanced force motions, a No. 45 file shapes to within 2 mm of the mesial apex and a No. 60 to 1.5 mm of the distal apex following the Gates-Glidden drill radicular access. **H,** No. 20 file is passed to full length in the mesial and a No. 25 in the distal canal. **I,** No. 35 file is passed to within 1 mm of the mesial length and a No. 45 in the distal canal. **J,** Final shaping of a control zone is made as a No. 45 cleans 1.5 mm short of the mesial canal terminus and a No. 60 file 1.5 mm short of the distal terminus. **K,** After recapitulation of the foramen the dry canal is inspected, and the smooth gradual taper is evident. **L,** Gutta-percha has been adapted to the full-canal lengths in the mesial and distal roots. Apical impression can be examined to determine the control zone shape.

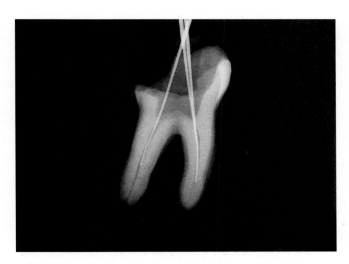

FIG. 8-54 Initial working length radiograph of a crown-down treatment reveals that instruments, inserted 17 mm into the canal system, reside several millimeters short of the apex. This short position assures the apex remains undisturbed until the coronal portions are completely cleaned and shaped.

and disinfects the coronal two thirds of the canal before the apical third is entered.

3. It removes the majority of the pulp and infecting microbes before the apical third is approached, thereby it minimizes the risk of pushing pulpal and microbial irritants into the periapical regions.

4. The working length is less likely to change during apical instrumentation because canal curvature has been reduced before working length is actually established.

Procedures to assure apical patency, as described earlier in this chapter, are not used while the coronal two thirds of the canal system are cleaned and shaped. However, after the coronal two thirds are prepared, light pressure instrumentation, recapitulation, and apical patency are used to clean and shape the apical third of the canal. Either of the previously described techniques or another reliable technique may be used to clean and shape the apical portion. Some type of step-back procedure is needed at the apical foramen with a safe-ended file like Flex-R.

Once the access opening is correctly established, the chamber and accessible coronal reaches of the canal(s) are irrigated with sodium hypochlorite and an approximate length of the canal is established radiographically or electronically. One must determine that greater than 18 mm of canal length is present between the occlusal reference and the periodontal ligament. All initial instrumentation should remain several millimeters short of the apex. To establish a path for Gates-Glidden drills, K-type files No. 15 to 25 are used to sequentially enlarge the canal through its coronal two thirds (i.e., 18 mm more or less). A Flex-R file is recommended because a conventional K-type file can damage the canal wall during a crown-down approach. Balanced force motions are most efficient and reliable for this portion of the cleaning and shaping effort. Each instrument is followed by copious irrigation of the canal with sodium hypochlorite (at least 2 ml after each file). The Gates-Glidden drills are used in a large to small sequence. The first Gates-Glidden drill is used to open into the canal space only 2 or 3 mm. This Gates-Glidden drill is withdrawn from the canal several times using an anticurvature stroke to taper its path outwardly from curvature and root concavities. The canal is irrigated to wash away debris; then the next smaller Gates-Glidden drill is passed into the opened canal space and used to extend the shaping 2 or 3 mm further apically. This progression is continued through Gates-Glidden drill No. 2. A series of three Gates-Glidden drills (Nos. 4 to 2) can shape 6 to 9 mm into the canal depending on the penetration depth achieved per drill size. In large single roots, a complete series of No. 6 to 2 Gates-Glidden drills may be used to rapidly clean and shape the coronal 10 mm or so of the canal. A 2-mm penetration depth is used with each Gates-Glidden drill when the complete series is used. This coronal flaring may also be completed with other rotary instruments.

After the coronal two thirds of the canal are sculpted by Gates-Glidden drills, the apical portion is cleaned and shaped and disinfected as described earlier in the chapter. When a predesigned preparation is employed, the apical preparation may continue from the large final diameter file to smaller instruments. Recapitulation of the instrument series will gradually bring them into the appropriate apical position. Length is established when the first small instrument can pass out the apical foramen. An apex locator and a radiograph precisely determine the full canal length. Tactile sensation is enhanced by coronal shaping thereby allowing only the tip of the files to bind. This technique deserves practice in extracted teeth before clinical use. It is the clinically superior technique for managing acute infections, retreatments, and symptomatic necrotic conditions because of its emphasis on cleaning; this reduces the risk of inoculating the periapical tissue.

Good judgment and common sense must prevail with this technique. If the canal is large, cleaning and shaping go rapidly. If the canal is excessively curved and calcified, a serial shaping technique, held several millimeters short of the apex, would be a the more prudent option for early shaping followed by a crown-down radicular access and finally completing the apical with a step-back technique to open and clean the foramen.

Engine-driven shaping for the crown-down technique

Shaping of the canal in the coronal two thirds may be accomplished with a watch-winding handpiece: M4 (Kerr Manufacturing, Romulus, Mich.) or Endogripper (Moyco/Union Broach, York, Pa.). Both are effective and efficient in the molar regions. They accept hand files and cut as the clinician pushes them into the canal. They will cut 8 to 10 mm of canal length with a stainless steel file but less with a nickel-titanium file. A Flex-R file does not ledge the canal but may not have enough action to reach the apex of a long canal in one preparation pass. Engine-driven shaping easily prepares the approximate 18 mm needed for crown-down procedures. Incorporation of these handpieces in a crown-down preparation is a wise decision for posterior teeth.

Rotary Nickel-Titanium Techniques

Instrument design and materials are finally catching up with concepts, which make today's cleaning and shaping procedures so successful. One material, nickel-titanium, has brought new blade designs, greater instruments tapers, alternative sizing systems, and the introduction of full rotary motion for cleaning and shaping canals. This does not change the protocols for every clinician to adhere to the timeless principles of cleaning and shaping (see the checklist for finishing (p. 226).

Profile Variable Taper Series No. 29 rotary instrumentation

Nickel-titanium endodontic instruments were developed by Quality Dental Products, a subsidiary of Tulsa Dental Products. Nickel-titanium instruments include a variety of rotary instruments including Orifice Shapers, Profile 0.04 tapers, and Profile 0.06 tapers. The principal value of these instruments is their ability to repeatedly recover from gentle distortions. Nickel-titanium instruments have a unique ability to rapidly alter their crystalline state; they possess remarkable flexibility that can withstand the rapid, repeated distortions of rotation in curved canals. A radial land separates their bidirectional cutting edges, a U-shaped flute receives debris, and a rounded guiding tip directs these instruments allowing them to clean and shape canals when they are operated at low rpm and a constant velocity. The radial lands keep the instrument centered in the body of the canal while the guiding tip seeks out the canal and prevents apical transportation.

Two different tapers are available (Profile 0.04 and 0.06) and are used similarly during cleaning and shaping. Their greater taper is assumed to provide a crown-down preparation. The tip guides the instrument into and down the canal while the blade regions contact the dentinal wall and begin shaping. As the instrument progresses apically, the contact with the dentinal wall moves closer to the tip of the instrument. The clinician notices an increased resistance as the instrument moves apically, since there is an increasing surface area of the radial lands contacting dentinal walls. A change of instrument is made when the instrument no longer advances apically.

Smear layer production (Fig. 8-55, E and F) is a consideration when using nickel-titanium rotary instruments. Smear layer is produced when the instrument contacts and begins to plane the dentinal walls. Production of a smear layer is actually accentuated with nickel-titanium rotary instruments. Alternate irrigation with sodium hypochlorite and EDTA can be used throughout the procedure to continually remove the smear layer.

Clinical description of the Profile rotary technique

All rotary instruments should be used in high-torque constant-speed handpieces capable of maintaining speeds of between 150 to 350 rpm (see Fig. 8-55). Begin each case by estimating the canal length from a well-angulated preoperative periapical radiograph. Select a standard ISO taper hand instrument that is estimated to bind one half to two thirds down the length of the canal. Confirm this positioning is correct by inserting with a balanced force motion or a watch-winding motion and following the instrument into the canal. After advancing the hand instrument to midcanal, select a Profile 0.04 taper of the same size, place it into the handpiece, and proceed to slowly advance it into the canal. Continue until it reaches the same depth as the hand instrument or until increased resistance is encountered. Remove this instrument, irrigate the canal, select the next larger Profile 0.04 taper, and repeat the preparation process inserting to approximately the same depth. This concludes the first shaping wedge of the coronal portion of the canal. Irrigate the canal system and select a Profile 0.4 taper one size smaller than the first instrument used. Place it into the handpiece, start rotation (150 to 300 rpm), and begin progressing slowly into the canal approximately three quarters of the estimated working length. Remove this instrument using several outward strokes of the canal wall, and repeat irrigation. Now determine working length using a combination tac-

tile sense, radiograph, and apex locator. Coronal interferences have been eliminated, and a working length is much easier to determine. Proceed to the working length using a Profile 0.04 taper or ISO standard hand instrument one size smaller than the last instrument. After the full canal length has been determined, continue to use increasingly larger rotary 0.04 tapers until adequate apical enlargement has been accomplished. Use a Profile 0.06 taper with the same tip size as the current Profile 0.04 taper each time additional coronal shaping is needed. Continue cleaning and shaping until the canals meet the five objectives shown on p 226. Once the clinician has experience, the Profile rotary 0.04 tapers can be used closer to the radiographic terminus; however, this should not be attempted with difficult cases.

Quantec Series 2000 Graduating Tapers

The Quantec Series 2000 are nickel-titanium instruments manufactured in a graduate series of taper ranging from the conventional 0.02 to a 0.06 taper (see Fig. 8-55). These instruments, like the Profile 0.04 taper above, require a high-torque handpiece that can provide a constant velocity at a rotational speed of approximately 340 rpm (see Fig. 8-55).

First, several general recommendations. Pressure applied to each instrument must be light. The amount of pressure required will vary, dependent on the narrowness of the canal. Once the necessary pressure for instrument advancement has been established, it must not be increased. Never attempt to bypass an obstruction by increasing the force. Use a slight pecking or pumping motion and progress through the canal in 1-mm increments; this motion enhances the removal of debris toward the coronal and frees the cutting edges, allowing them to work under lighter loads. Always have the rotating instrument gently pumping into the canal. Holding the instrument in one position, while it continues to rotate, increases the possibility of ledging. Routinely examine every instrument for distortion and discard the questionable ones. Abrupt changes in applied load can and must be avoided by using a handpiece that has sufficient torque that it can maintain a constant speed. The Quantec E electric handpiece and Quantec Air handpiece accomplish this well (see Fig. 8-55).

Clinical description of the Quantec Series technique

Cleaning and shaping is initiated with a Quantec No. 1 instrument. This is a 17 mm long, size 25 instrument with a 0.06 taper that is used as an orifice opener. Next the canal system is irrigated with sodium hypochlorite. Rotation of 340 rpm is commenced and the No. 1 instrument carefully advanced into the canal employing a very light inward pressure. The No. 1 instrument removes coronal canal interferences because of its rapid taper; subsequent instruments therefore operate with less stress. Before proceeding further, a working length is estimated from the preoperative radiograph(s). A Quantec No. 2 instrument (size 15, ISO taper) is marked with the estimated working length and introduced to that depth. The position is confirmed by radiograph or apex locator. If an obstruction is still present, irrigate and recapitulate with the Quantec No. 1 instrument; then renegotiate with the No. 2 instrument. Repeat until the working length is reached. Select a Quantec No. 3 (size 20, ISO taper) and prepare the canal to full working length with this instrument. Irrigate. Repeat the process with a Quantec No. 4 (size 25, ISO taper). Irrigate. Now select a Quantec No. 5 instrument (size 25, 0.03 taper) to merge the coronal and apical preparations. It is gradually taken to the full

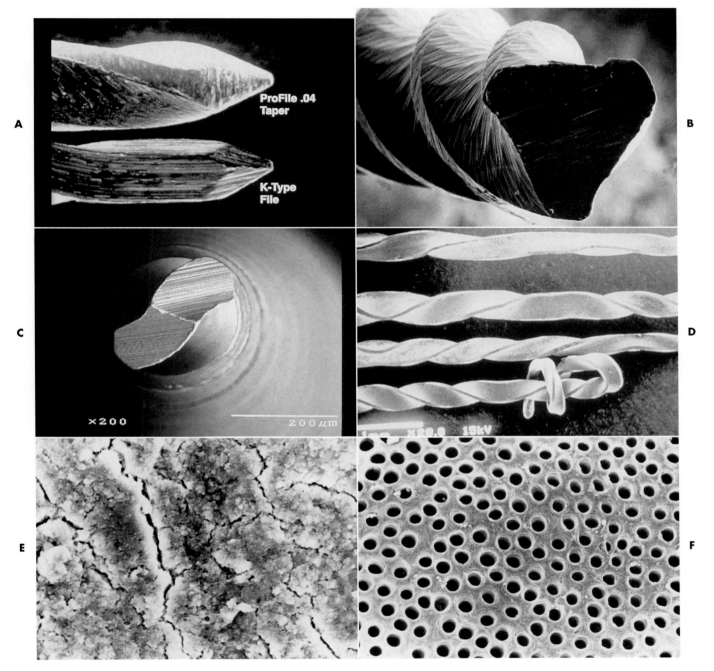

FIG. 8-55 New generation for cleaning and shaping instrumentation. **A,** Comparing a 0.04 taper instrument next to a conventional K-type file. Note the difference in tips. The 0.04 taper has a bullet-nose tip. Sixty-degree tip joins the flat radial lands. Instead of a sharp transition angle, there is a smooth radius from the shank of the instrument to the end of the tip. **B,** Scanning electron micrograph of a U-file cross section. Scanning electron micrograph looking at the cross section near the tip of a Profile 0.04 taper clearly demonstrates the radial lands that prevent rotary nickel-titanium instruments from self-threading into the dentinal walls. **C,** Scanning electron micrograph of a Quantec design instrument shows a more desirable approach for preparing small curved, calcified canals by using an instrument tip that eliminates burnishing action. Configuration is known as a faceted tip. **D,** Scanning electron micrograph of a deformed 0.04 taper instrument shows that as the instruments become overstressed, they tend to unwind and wind in reverse. **E,** Scanning electron micrograph of a smear layer after instrumentation. Smooth preparations obtained with rotary nickel-titanium instruments result in a packed smear layer when sodium hypochlorite is the only irrigant used. *(Courtesy Dr. Guiseppe Caniatori.)* **F,** Scanning electron micrograph of a smear layer after alternating sodium hypochlorite with EDTA as irrigants, whereas instrumenting with rotary nickel-titanium instruments results in smooth, clean, dentinal walls. *(Courtesy Dr. Guiseppe Caniatori.)*

Continued

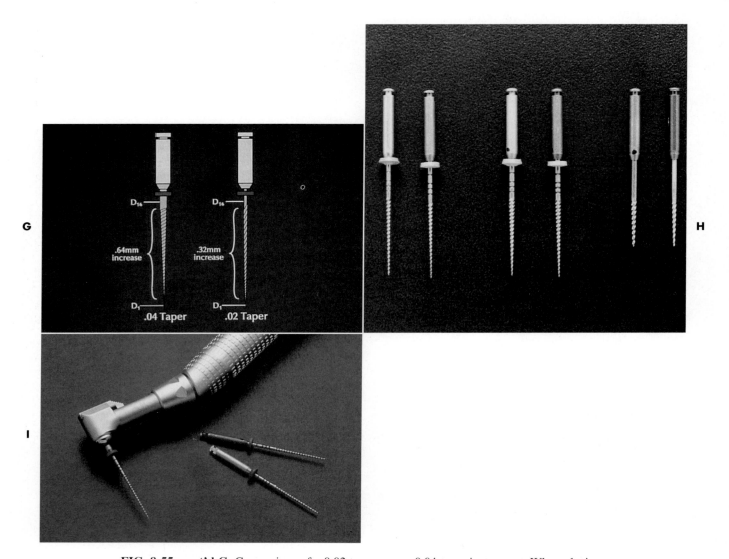

FIG. 8-55, cont'd G, Comparison of a 0.02 taper versus 0.04 taper instrument. When placing a 0.04 taper next to a normal ISO 0.02 taper instrument, the difference in taper is clearly visible. Nonstandard 0.04 taper accelerates flaring and develops a smoothly tapered canal shape. **H,** From left to right: 0.02 taper, 0.04 taper, and Orifice Shapers. **I,** Micromega 324 handpiece for delivering preferred speed ranges of 150 to 325 rpm.

working length; however, the shaping is concentrated in the midportion of the canal. Remember, the coronal portion was previously flared with a 0.06 taper and the apex was shaped with a size 25. Irrigate and continue with the Quantec No. 6 instrument (size 25, 0.04 taper) and the Quantec No. 7 instrument (size 25, 0.05 taper). These instruments continue the preparation in the midportion of the canal, which requires that they are used to the full working length. The Quantec No. 8 instrument (size 25, 0.06 taper) is also used to full working length and completes the flaring of the canal midportion. The Quantec No. 9 instrument (size 40, ISO taper), working the flutes in the apical portion, is used to complete the apical preparation. The Quantec No. 10 instrument (size 45, ISO taper) is used to circumferentially file while being rotated by the 340 rpm handpiece. This final shaping step should incorporate fins or anastomoses into the canal preparation. The canal is given a final irrigation, dried, and prepared for obturation.

These new rotary shaping systems have been in clinical use for only a short period of time. Due to limited experience, no one knows the limits of application, extent of risk, or true advantages they offer. These systems, like all other new techniques, should be experimented with in extracted teeth before attempting to use them clinically. Instrument separation is easily experienced if an instrument tip becomes lodged and handpiece rotation continues. Instrument guidance has only begun to be tested, and *the canal may be quickly and effortlessly ledged, stripped and perforated with these rotating instruments.* Nickel-titanium has given a means to advance cleaning and shaping, yet at the same time has presented a new challenge in defining the safest and most efficient means for using this new technology.

Guidelines for new instrument technologies

1. Integrate all cleaning and shaping techniques with what you already know. Endodontics has too little room for error to go too far out of your "comfort zone." Cautiously integrate these new technologies with the "tried and true" conventional methods for cleaning and shaping.
2. Keep the principles and mechanical objectives of successful cleaning and shaping in mind at all times. Always ask the question of whether new instruments or techniques are enhancing the five mechanical objectives.
3. Start slowly.
4. Seek expert training.
5. Practice first at benchtop with extracted teeth and plastic blocks.
6. Know how to create ideal canal preparations by hand before using nickel-titanium rotary instruments.
7. Using rotary instrumentation to the working length requires practice. Until comfortable with the procedure, the apical control zone should be prepared with hand instruments.
8. All rotary instruments should be used in a high-torque, controlled-speed handpiece.
9. Remember, 0.04 tapers above size No. 6 and 0.06 tapers above size No. 5 have a tendency to "self-thread," pulling themselves into the canal. This tendency can be minimized with additional coronal flaring or with lesser tapered instruments.
10. Nickel-titanium is much more flexible than stainless steel. Therefore nickel-titanium instruments have a tendency to bend on themselves and break during rotation in certain clinical situations, including broad canals with abrupt apical curvature, when two canals join, or double S-shaped curvatures. In these situations the nickel-titanium rotary instruments should be preceded with files to avoid buckling and instrument separation.
11. Gentle apical pressure must be applied at all times.
12. The instrument should be promptly withdrawn after the desired depth has been reached.
13. Straight-line access from the chamber must be maintained.
14. Use continuous apical-coronal movement of the instrument.
15. Allow the instrument to progress slowly.
16. Irrigate the canal frequently and copiously with sodium hypochlorite throughout the procedure.
17. Maintain apical patency to the radiographic terminus after rotary instrumentation.
18. Be aware that instructions that accompany products may be inappropriate, incomplete, inaccurate, or clinically insufficient due to lack of scientific studies or the test of time.
19. Do not hurry.
20. Always maintain a constant speed.
21. Check files often for stress or deformation and discard them frequently.
22. Knowledge of and visualization of root canal systems anatomy helps minimize procedural mishaps.
23. In calcified, narrow, or curved canals the files are subjected to much more stress and more likely to break. Tests have shown that nickel-titanium files break when rotating in a curved canal after 400 to 800 rotations.
24. When two canals unite at a sharp angle into one small canal, create a smoother, more gradual transition from two canals to one by using sharp hand instruments that can be precurved or by using nickel-titanium hand files.
25. Canals with sharp or abrupt curves in the apical regions should be cleaned with new precurved hand instruments.
26. When large canals suddenly become small canals (such as the distal root canal system of mandibular molars), create a smoother, more gradual transition from the larger or wide canal to the smaller and narrower canal by using new hand instruments that can be precurved or by using nickel-titanium hand files.

CONCLUSION

Let this wisdom guide the cleaning and shaping endodontic clinicians perform.

1. *Establish a vision* of cleaning, shaping, and three-dimensional obturation as inseparable accomplishments. Our result is also not merely mechanical but a reflection of a striving for excellence.
2. *Take responsibility* for the outcome. The greatest variable is the clinician. Dedicate your effort to perfecting your skill. Aspire to make every case better than the one before.
3. *Clear the mind* by concentrating on each canal separately. Complete coronal shaping early and focus on the apex separately.
4. *Train the team.* When the assistants know how to provide timely and appropriate support, the clinician can focus on the details of the canal system and perfect the cleaning and shaping results.

5. *Practice delicacy.* The light touch is the most sensitive and the best eye for visualizing the deep canal anatomy and producing a proper shape.

6. *Time is our ally.* Slow down, practice patience, and find the reward in quicker results. Time spent in obtaining the correct result is saved when retreatment and surgery are avoided. If there is not time to do it right, when will there be time to fix it?

7. *Customize the access* and insist on straight-line entry to all canals.

8. *Keep dentin chips (mud) in suspension.* Use sodium hypochlorite freely and frequently and keep the chamber full at all times.

9. *Visualize the shape.* Shaping is the secret of an exceptional obturation. Imagine the obturation and establish the appropriate shape.

10. *Practice efficiency.* Use each instrument to its maximal benefit, not to its maximal possible time or strength. Do not use instruments forcefully. Use a light touch and frequent sequencing.

11. *Use new instruments.* It is more profitable to throw away instruments than to lose time with a bent one or try to bypass a separated one.

12. *Remember pulpal anatomy.* Ribbons, sheets, laterals, accessories, culs-de-sac, and bends form a complex system that challenges the best. Always expect four canals in molars, two canals in mandibular incisors, and acute apical bends in most canals.

13. *Produce detailed radiographs.* Demand exact angulation to obtain maximal detail. Visualize the relationship between the chamber, canal, and furcations. Obtain extra detail and information with multiple preoperative and operative radiographs. Insist on great detail and accuracy in the length determination film. Use the radiographic terminus only for patency.

14. *Do it once and do it well!*

REFERENCES

1. Abou-Rass M, Frank AL, Glick DH: The anticurvature method to prepare the curved root canal, *J Am Dent Assoc* 101:792, 1980.
2. Abou-Rass M, Oglesby SW: Effects of temperature, concentration and tissue type on the solvent ability of sodium hypochlorite, *J Endod* 7:376-377, 1981.
3. Ahmad M, Pit Ford TR, Crum LA: Ultrasonic debridement of root canals: an insight into the mechanisms involved, *J Endod* 13:93, 1987.
4. Ahmad M, Pit Ford TR, Crum LA: Acoustic cavitation and its implications an ultrasonic root canal debridement, *J Endod* 13:131, 1987 (abstract 14).
5. Ahmad M, Pitt Ford TR, Crum LA: Ultrasonic debridement of root canals: acoustic streaming and its possible role, *J Endod* 13:490, 1987.
6. Allison CA, Weber CR, Walton RE: The influence of the method of canal preparation on the quality of apical and coronal seal, *J Endod* 5:298, 1979.
7. Backman CA, Oswald RJ, Pitts DL: A radiographic comparison of two root canal instrumentation techniques, *J Endod* 18:19, 1992.
8. Baumgartner JC, Mader CL: A scanning electron microscopic evaluation of four root canal irrigation regimens, *J Endod* 13:147, 1987.
9. Baumgartner JC et al: Histomorphometric comparison of canals prepared by four techniques, *J Endod* 18:530, 1992.
10. Becker GL, Cohen S, Borer R: The sequelae of accidentally injecting sodium hypochlorite beyond the root apex, *Oral Surg* 38:633, 1974.
11. Buchanan LS: Management of the curved root canal: predictably treating the most common endodontic complexity, *J Calif Dent Assoc* 17:40, 1989.
12. Buchanan LS: Paradigm shifts in cleaning and shaping, *J Calif Dent Assoc* 23:24-34, 1991.
13. Cameron JA: The use of ultrasound in the cleaning of root canals: a clinical report, *J Endod* 8:472, 1982.
14. Cameron JA: The use of ultrasonics in the removal of smear layer: a scanning electron microscope study, *J Endod* 9:289, 1983.
15. Chenail BL, Teplitsky PE: Endosonics in curved root canals, *J Endod* 11:369, 1985.
16. Chenail BL, Teplitsky PE: Endosonics in curved root canals. II, *J Endod* 14:214, 1988.
17. Chow TW: Mechanical effectiveness of root canal irrigation, *J Endod* 9:475, 1983.
18. Cohen S, Burns RC, Schilder H: canal debridement and disinfection: *Pathways of the pulp*, ed 2, St Louis, 1980, Mosby, p 111.
19. Cunningham W, Balekjion A: Effect of temperature on collagen-dissolving ability of sodium hypochlorite irrigating solution, *Oral Surg* 49:175, 1980.
20. Cunningham W, Joseph S: Effect of temperature on the bacteriocidal action of sodium hypochlorite endodontic irrigant, *Oral Surg* 50:569, 1980.
21. Cunningham W et al: A comparison of antibacterial effectiveness of endosonic and hand root canal therapy, *Oral Surg* 54:238, 1982.
22. Dummer PMH, McGinn JH, Rees DG: The position and topography of the apical canal constriction and apical foramen, *Int Endod J* 17:192, 1984.
23. Fairbourn DR, McWalter GM, Montgomery S: The effect of four preparation techniques on the amount of apically extruded debris, *J Endod* 13:102, 1987.
24. Fava LRG: The double-flared technique: an alternative for biomechanical preparation, *J Endod* 9:76, 1983.
25. Fouad AF et al: A clinical evaluation of five electronic root canal measuring instruments, *J Endod* 16:446, 1990.
26. George JW, Michanowicz AE, Michanowicz JP: A method of canal preparation to control apical extrusion of low-temperature thermoplasticized gutta-percha, *J Endod* 13:18, 1987.
27. Goerig AC, Michelich RJ, Schultz HH: Instrumentation of root canals in molars using the step-down technique, *J Endod* 8:550, 1982.
28. Goldberg F, Speilberg C: The effect of EDTAC and the variations of its working time analyzed with scanning electron microscopy, *Oral Surg* 53:74, 1982.
29. Goldman LB et al: Scanning electron microscope study of a new irrigation method in endodontic treatment, *Oral Surg* 48:79, 1979.
30. Goldman M et al: The efficacy of several endodontic irrigating solutions: a scanning electron microscope study, *J Endod* 8:487, 1982.
31. Goodman A, Schilder H, Aldrich W: The thermomechanical properties of gutta-percha. II. The history of molecular chemistry of gutta-percha, *Oral Surg* 37:954, 1974.
32. Goodman A, Schilder H, Aldrich W: The thermomechanical properties of gutta-percha. IV. A thermal profile of the warm gutta-percha packing procedure, *Oral Surg* 51:544, 1981.
33. Goodman A et al: An in vitro comparison of the efficacy of the step-back technique versus the step-back/ultrasonic technique in human mandibular molars, *J Endod* 11:249, 1985.
34. Green D: A stereomicroscopic study of the root apices of 400 maxillary and mandibular anterior teeth, *Oral Surg* 9:249, 1956.
35. Green D: Stereomicroscopic study of 700 root apices of maxillary and mandibular posterior teeth, *Oral Surg* 13:728, 1960.
36. Green EN: Microscopic investigation of root canal diameters, *J Am Dent Assoc* 57:636, 1958.
37. Grossman LI, Melman B: Solution of pulp tissue by chemical agents, *J Am Dent Assoc* 28:223, 1941.
38. Haidet J et al: An in vivo comparison of the step-back technique versus a step-back/ultrasonic technique in human mandibular molars, *J Endod* 15:195, 1989.
39. Haller R, Glosson C, Dove S, Del Rio C: Nickel-titanium hand and engine-driven root canal preparations: a comparison study, *J Endod* 21:220, 1995 (abstract 21).

40. Hand RE, Smith ML, Harrison JW: Analysis of the effect of dilution on the necrotic tissue dissolution property of sodium hypochlorite, *J Endod* 4:60, 1978.

41. Harlan AL, Nichols JI, Steiner JC: A comparison of curved canal instrumentation using nickel-titanium or stainless steel files with the balanced force technique, *J Endod* 22:410-413, 1996.

42. Harrison JW, Hand RE: The effect of dilution and organic matter on the antibacterial property of 5.25% sodium hypochlorite, *J Endod* 7:128, 1981.

43. Huang L: The principle of electronic root canal measurement, *Bull 4th Milit Med Coll* 8:32, 1959.

44. Huang L: An experimental study of the principle of electronic root canal measurement, *J Endod* 13:60, 1987.

45. Ingle JI, Bakland LK: *Endodontics,* ed 4, Philadelphia, 1994, Lea & Febiger.

46. Inoue N: A study of audiometric devices for determining root length, *Shikwa-Gakuo* 76:1121, 1976.

47. Inoue N: A clinico-anatomical study for the determining of root canal length by use of a novelty low frequency oscillation device, *Bull Tokyo Dent Coll* 18:71, 1977.

48. Jackson FJ, Nyborg WL: Small scale acoustic streaming near a locally excited membrane, *J Acoust Soc Am* 30:614, 1958.

49. Kennedy WA, Walker WA III, Gough RW: Smear layer removal effects on apical leakage, *J Endod* 12:21, 1986.

50. Kerekes K, Tronstad L: Morphometric observations on root canals of human teeth, *J Endod* 3:24, 74, 114, 1977.

51. Krell KV, Johnson RJ, Madison S: Irrigation patterns during ultrasonic canal instrumentation. I. K-type files, *J Endod* 14:65, 1988.

52. Kulilid JC, Peters DD: Incidence and configuration of canal systems in the mesiobuccal root of maxillary first and second molars, *J Endod* 7:311, 1990.

53. Kuttler Y: Microscopic investigation of root apexes, *J Am Dent Assoc* 50:544, 1955.

54. Leeb J: Canal orifice enlargement as related to biomechanical preparation, *J Endod* 9:463, 1983.

55. Leseberg DA, Montgomery S: The effects of Canal Master, Flex-R, and K-flex instruments on root canal configuration, *J Endod* 17:59, 1991.

56. Lev R et al: An in vitro comparison of the step-back technique versus a step-back/ultrasonic technique for 1 and 3 minutes, *J Endod* 13:523, 1987.

57. Loushine RJ, Weller RN, Hartwell GR: Stereomicroscopic evaluation of canal shape following hand, sonic and ultrasonic instrumentation, *J Endod* 15:417, 1989.

58. Marshall FJ, Pappin J: *A crown-down pressureless preparation root canal enlargement technique: technique manual,* Portland, Ore, 1980, Oregon Health Sciences University.

59. McDonald NJ: The electronic determination of working length, *Dent Clin North Am* 36:293, 1992.

60. McDonald NJ, Hovland EJ: An evaluation of the apex locator Endocater, *J Endod* 16:5, 1990.

61. McKendry DJ: Comparison of balanced forces, endosonic, and step-back filing instrumentation techniques: quantification of extruded apical debris, *J Endod* 16:24, 1990.

62. Mullaney TP: Instrumentation of finely curved canals, *Dent Clin North Am* 23:575, 1979.

63. Miserendino LJ et al: Cutting efficiency of endodontic hand instruments. IV. Comparison of hybrid and traditional instrument design, *J Endod* 14:451, 1989.

64. Morgan LF, Montgomery S: An evaluation of the crown-down pressureless technique, *J Endod* 10:491, 1984.

65. Nygaard-Ostby L: Chelation in root canal therapy, *Odont Tidskr* 65:3, 1957.

66. Pedicord D, ElDeeb ME, Messer HH: Hand versus ultrasonic instrumentation: its effect on canal shape and instrumentation time, *J Endod* 12:375, 1986.

67. Powell SE, Wong PD, Simon JHS: A comparison of the effect of modified and nonmodified instrument tips on apical canal configuration. II, *J Endod* 14:224, 1988.

68. Ram Z: Effectiveness of root canal irrigation, *Oral Surg* 44:306, 1977.

69. Roane JB: Principles of preparation using the balanced force technique. In Hardin J, editor: *Clark's clinical dentistry,* Philadelphia, 1991, JB Lippincott.

70. Roane JB, Sabala CL, Duncanson MG Jr: The "balanced force" concept for instrumentation of curved canals, *J Endod* 11:203, 1985.

71. Sabala CL, Roane JB, Southard LZ: Instrumentation of curved canals using a modified tipped instrument: a comparison study, *J Endod* 14:59, 1988.

72. Sabala CL, Biggs JT: A standard predetermined endodontic preparation concept, *Compend Contin Educ Dent* 12:656-663, 1991.

73. Saunders WP, Saunders EM: Effect of noncutting tipped instruments on the quality of root canal preparation using a modified double flared technique, *J Endod* 18:32, 1992.

74. Schilder H: Periodontically-endodontically involved teeth. In Grossman LI, editor: *Transactions of the Third International Conference on Endodontics,* Philadelphia, 1963 University of Pennsylvania Press.

75. Schilder H: Filling the root canal in three dimensions, *Dent Clin North Am* 11:723, 1967.

76. Schilder H: Cleaning and shaping the root canal, *Dent Clin North Am* 18:269, 1974.

77. Schilder H: Canal debridement and disinfection. In Cohen S, Burns RC, editors: *Pathways of the pulp,* St Louis, 1976, Mosby, p 111.

78. Schilder H: Vertical compaction of warm gutta-percha. In Gerstein H, editor: *Techniques in clinical endodontics,* Philadelphia, 1983, WB Saunders.

79. Schilder H, Goodman A, Aldrich W: The thermomechanical properties of gutta-percha. I. The compressibility of gutta-percha, *Oral Surg* 37:946, 1974.

80. Schilder H, Goodman A, Aldrich W: The thermomechanical properties of gutta-percha. III. Determination of phase transition temperatures for gutta-percha, *Oral Surg* 38:109, 1974.

81. Senia ES, Marshall FJ, Rosen S: The solvent action of sodium hypochlorite on pulp tissue of extracted teeth, *Oral Surg* 31:96, 1971.

82. Sepic AO, Pantera EA, Neaverth EJ, Anderson RW: A comparison of Flex-R files and K-type files for enlargement of severely curved molar root canals, *J Endod* 15:240, 1989.

83. Serene T, Adams JD, Ashok S: *Nickel-titanium instruments applications in endodontics,* St Louis, 1995, Ishiyakau EuroAmerica.

84. Sotokawa T: An analysis of clinical breakage of root canal instruments, *J Endod* 14:75, 1988.

85. Southard DW, Oswald RJ, Natkin E: Instrumentation of curved molar root canals with the Roane technique, *J Endod* 13:479, 1987.

86. Stamos DG et al: An in vitro comparison study to quantitate the debridement ability of hand, sonic, and ultrasonic instrumentation, *J Endod* 13:434, 1987.

87. von der Lehr WN, Marsh RA: A radiographic study of the point of endodontic egress, *Oral Surg* 35:105, 1953.

88. Wade AK, Walker WA, Gough RW: Smear layer removal effects on apical leakage, *J Endod* 12:21, 1986.

89. Walker A: Definite and dependable therapy for pulpless teeth, *J Am Dent Assoc* 23:1418, 1936.

90. Walmsley AD, Williams AR: Effects of constraint on the oscillatory pattern of endosonic files, *J Endod* 15:189, 1989.

91. Walton RE: Current concepts of canal preparation, *Dent Clin North Am* 36:309, 1992.

92. Weine FS: Endodontic therapy, ed 5, St Louis, 1996, Mosby.

93. Weine FS, Kelly RF, Lio PJ: The effect of preparation procedures on original canal shape and on apical foramen shape, *J Endod* 1:255, 1975.

94. Wildey WL, Senia ES: A new root canal instrument and instrumentation technique: a preliminary report, *Oral Surg* 67:198, 1989.

95. Wildey WL, Senia ES, Montgomery S: Another look at root canal instrumentation, *Oral Surg* 74:499, 1992.

96. Williams S, Goldman M: Penetrability of the smeared layer by a strain of *Proteus vulgaris, J Endod* 11:385, 1985.

97. Yahya AS, ElDeeb ME: Effect of sonic versus ultrasonic instrumentation on canal preparation, *J Endod* 15:235, 1989.

Chapter 9

Obturation of the Cleaned and Shaped Root Canal System

James L. Gutmann
David E. Witherspoon

HISTORICAL PERSPECTIVES

In 1924 Hatton indicated that "perhaps there is no technical operation in dentistry or surgery where so much depends on the conscientious adherence to high ideals as that of pulp canal filling."[86] The essence of this statement had been significantly influenced by years of trial and error in both the techniques and materials used to obturate the prepared root canal system. Much of the frustration and challenge that emanated from this concern, however, was due to the lack of development in root canal preparation techniques, coupled with indictments of the "focal infection" craze of that era.[96]

Before 1800 root canal filling, when done, was limited to gold. Subsequent obturations with various metals, oxychloride of zinc, paraffin, and amalgam resulted in varying degrees of success and satisfaction.[108] In 1847 there is evidence that Hill developed the first gutta-percha root canal filling material known as "Hill's stopping."[108] The preparation, which consisted principally of bleached gutta-percha and carbonate of lime and quartz, was patented in 1848 and introduced to the dental profession. In 1867 Bowman made claim before the St. Louis Dental Society of the first use of gutta-percha for canal filling in an extracted first molar.[90]

References to the use of gutta-percha for root canal obturation before the turn of the twentieth century were few and vague. In 1883 Perry claimed that he had been using a pointed gold wire wrapped with some soft gutta-percha (the roots of the present-day core carrier technique?).[148] He also began using gutta-percha rolled into points and packed into the canal. The points were prepared by cutting baseplate gutta-percha into slender strips, warming them with a lamp, laying them on his operating case, and rolling them with another flat surface (a contemporary technique used to custom roll a large cone?). He then used shellac warmed over a lamp and rolled the cones into a point of desired size based on canal shape and length. Before placing the final gutta-percha point, he saturated the tooth cavity with alcohol; capillary attraction let the alcohol run into the canal, softening the shellac so the gutta-percha could be packed (forerunner of a chemical-softening technique?).

In 1887 the S.S. White Company began to manufacture gutta-percha points.[104] In 1893 Rollins introduced a new type of gutta-percha to which he added vermilion.[203] There were many critics of this because vermilion is pure oxide of mercury and dangerous in the quantities suggested by Rollins.

With the introduction of radiographs into the assessment of root canal obturations it became painfully obvious that the canal was not cylindric, as earlier imagined, and that additional filling material was necessary to fill the observed voids. At first, hard-setting dental cements were used but these proved unsatisfactory. It was also thought that the cement used should possess strong antiseptic action, hence the development of many phenolic or formalin type of paste cements. The softening and dissolution of the gutta-percha itself to serve as the cementing agent, through the use of rosins, was introduced by Callahan in 1914.[30] Subsequently a multitude of various pastes, sealers, and cements were created in an attempt to discover the best possible sealing agent for use with gutta-percha.

Over the past 70 to 80 years the dental community has seen attempts to improve on the nature of root canal obturation with these cements and with variations in the delivery of gutta-percha to the prepared canal system. During this era the impetus for these developments was based heavily on the continued belief in the concept of focal infection, elective localization, the hollow tube theory, and the concept that the primary cause for failure of root canal treatment was the apical percolation of fluids, and potentially microorganisms, into a poorly obturated root canal system.[39,153,159] It is from this chronologic perspective of technical and scientific thought that this chapter clarifies and codifies contemporary concepts in the obturation of the cleaned and shaped root canal system.

PURPOSE, RATIONALE, AND IMPORTANCE OF OBTURATION: STANDARD OF CARE

The purposes of obturating the prepared root canal space are well founded in the contemporary art and science of endodontology and can be simply stated as (1) to eliminate all avenues of leakage from the oral cavity or the periradicular tissues into the root canal system and (2) to seal within the system any irritants that cannot be fully removed during canal cleaning and shaping procedures. The rationale for these objectives recognizes that microbial irritants (microorganisms, toxins, and metabolites) along with products of pulp tissue degeneration are the prime causes for pulpal demise and its subsequent extension into the periradicular tissue.[133] Failure to eliminate these etiologic factors and to prevent further irritation via continued contamination of the root canal system are the prime causes for failure with nonsurgical and surgical root canal treatment.[28,67,161,179]

The importance of three-dimensional obturation of the root

canal system cannot be overstated. However, the ability to achieve this goal is primarily dependent on the quality of the canal cleaning and shaping and the skill of the clinician. Even with the most skilled clinician, however, many other factors enter into the ultimate success or failure of each case, such as materials used, how they are used, and radiographic interpretation of process and product. What may loom as the most important attainment is the ultimate coronal restoration of the tooth following canal obturation. There is reasonable evidence to suggest that coronal leakage through improperly placed restorations after root canal treatment[156,167] and failure of the restorative treatment or lack of health of the supporting periodontium are the final determinants of success or failure in treatment[133,201] (Fig. 9-1, A through D).

Contemporary perspectives on the assessment of the quality of root canal obturation have placed an undue reliance on apical leakage studies[211] in addition to two-dimensional radiographic evaluation[107] (Fig. 9-2). This tends to create a false sense of security within the clinician because there is no contemporary root canal obturation technique or material that is impervious to leakage[67] (Fig. 9-3, A and B) and there is a poor correlation between the quality of the root canal obturation (especially an impervious seal) and what is viewed on a buccal radiograph.[41,107] Likewise, it has been shown that when the radiographic appearance of the root canal filling is unacceptable, the likelihood of leakage is high; additionally, when the root filling is radiographically acceptable, the likelihood of leakage is still rather high and failure may occur more than 14% of the time.[28,107] Faced with these dilemmas, the clinician must then choose a path of treatment that will result in the best possible cleaning and shaping of the root canal system coupled with an obturation technique that will provide a high level of three-dimensional seal, apically, laterally, and coronally within the confines of the root canal system. If these technical parameters are achieved, there is a high likelihood that the biologic parameters of ultimate periradicular tissue regeneration will be achieved. These parameters are highlighted by the formation of cementum that forms over and seals the apical foramen and evidences the presence of the insertion of Sharpey's fibers (Fig. 9-4, A and B).

CHARACTERISTICS OF AN IDEAL ROOT CANAL FILLING: STANDARD OF CARE

The American Association of Endodontists has published *Appropriateness of Care and Quality Assurance Guidelines*[5] regarding all aspects of contemporary endodontic treatment.

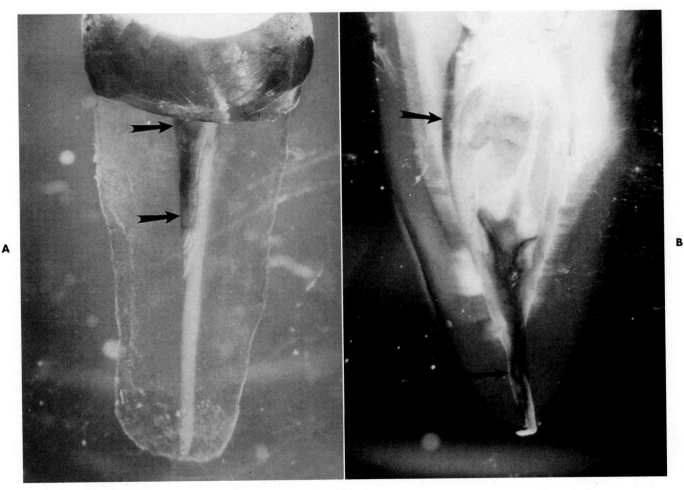

A   B

FIG. 9-1 A, Coronal leakage from beneath a full crown moving apically *(arrows)* along the root canal filling. **B,** Coronal leakage *(arrows)* to the apical foramen in the mesial root of a mandibular molar.

Continued

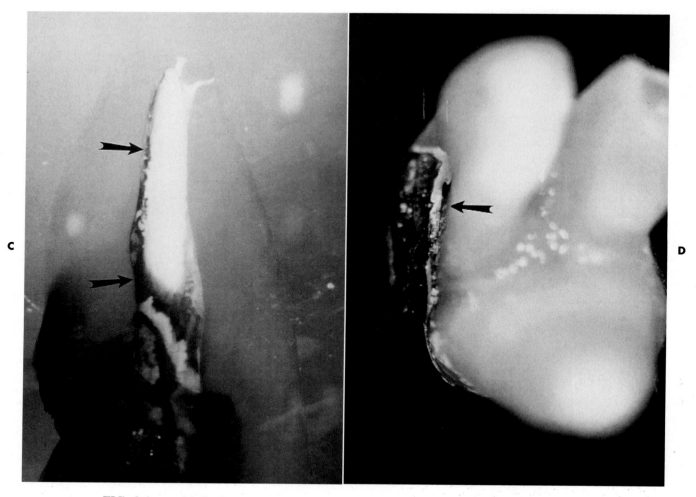

FIG. 9-1, cont'd C, Coronal leakage under a crown on a maxillary molar. Viewed is the palatal root, which shows evidence of leakage down its entire surface *(arrows).* Teeth in **A** through **C** were demineralized, dehydrated, and cleared for viewing. **D,** Artificial crown margins that are conducive to leakage *(arrow).* These avenues must either be prevented or removed if root canal treatment is to be successful.

Root canal obturation is defined and characterized as "the three-dimensional filling of the entire root canal system as close to the cemento-dentinal junction as possible. Minimal amounts of root canal sealers, which have been demonstrated to be biologically compatible, are used in conjunction with the core filling material to establish an adequate seal." Additionally, "use of paraformaldehyde-containing materials for root canal obturation are below the standard for endodontic therapy." Finally with regard to the radiographic assessment of root canal obturation, there should be a "radiographic appearance of a dense, three-dimensional filling which extends as close as possible to the cemento-dentinal junction, *i.e.* without gross overextension or underfilling in the presence of a patent canal." These standards, as stated, should serve as the benchmark for all clinicians who perform root canal treatment, and achievements below these standards must be considered as unacceptable. However, it is only through a cognizant "problem-solving" approach to root canal treatment, that quality assurance can be continually demonstrated in the obturation of the root canal system.[73] This approach demands inspection of the process and elimination of all variables that cause a departure from the standard of care.

Although it is recognized that there is a tremendous variance in the anatomy of the root canal system, the obturated root canal should reflect a shape that is approximately the same shape as the root morphology. Therefore proper cleaning and shaping within the confines of the root canal and in conjunction with the external anatomy of the root is essential. Additionally, the shape of the obturated canal should reflect a continuously tapering funnel preparation without excessive removal of tooth structure at any level of the canal system (Fig. 9-5). Techniques of preparation that encourage excessive removal of coronal root dentin with rotary instruments should be discouraged for three reasons[68] (Fig. 9-6, *A* and *B*). First, the root walls will be weakened. Second, there is a greater likelihood for a lateral or strip perforation in posterior teeth. Third, the gutta-percha/sealer root canal filling, although dense and well compacted in the coronal third, will not strengthen the root or compensate for lost dentin. Additionally, placement of a post in these teeth will not strengthen the root and may predispose to root fracture.[68]

Because of the high degree of variability in radiographic interpretation among clinicians, subtle characteristics of the obturated root canal may go unnoticed. In addition, because of

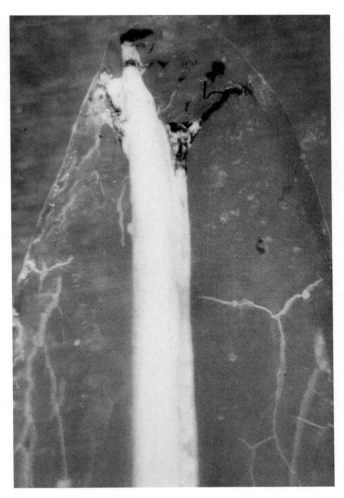

FIG. 9-2 Although the gutta-percha and sealer are well adapted in the apical portion of the canal, there is evidence of leakage into accessory canals. Apical portion of the gutta-percha was softened with chloroform before obturation.

differences in radiopacity in root canal sealer/cements, constituents in specific brands of gutta-percha, interpretation of voids in vivo versus in vitro,[218] the overlying bony anatomy, radiographic angulation, and the limited two-dimensional view of the obturated canal(s), the quality of the obturation may not undergo sufficient assessment as to levels of achievement and quality assurance. For example, one of the most often overlooked aspects in the assessment of root canal obturations is the density of the apical portion of the fill.[71] In essence, the apical third of the canal is filled with a sea of root canal cement and a single uncompacted master cone or poorly condensed mass of previously softened gutta-percha. Radiographically, the apical third of the canal appears less radiodense. An ill-defined outline to the canal wall is evident, along with obvious gaps or voids in the filling material or its adaptation to the confines of the canal (Fig. 9-7, *A* through *D*). In the case of highly radiopaque root canal sealer/cements, the apical portion may only be filled with sealer, giving the clinician the false impression of a dense, three-dimensional obturation with gutta-percha. Therefore it is necessary that the clinician master multiple techniques and become competent in the use of various sealers and cements to ensure the proper management of the wide diversity of anatomic scenarios encountered.

Table 9-1. Requirements for an ideal root canal filling material

Brownlee 1900[26]	Grossman 1940[65]
Easily inserted	Easily introduced
Pliable or moldable	Liquid or semisolid and become solid
Completely fill and seal apex	Seal laterally and apically
Neither expand or contract	Not shrink
Impermeable to fluids	Impervious to moisture
Antiseptic	Bacteriostatic
Not discolor tooth	Not stain tooth
Chemically neutral	Not irritate periapical tissues
Easily removed	Easily removed
Tasteless and odorless	Sterile or sterilizable
Durable	Radiopaque

CHARACTERISTICS OF IDEAL ROOT CANAL FILLING MATERIALS

A plethora of materials have been advocated over the past 150 years for root canal obturation. Historically, gutta-percha has proven to be the material of choice for the successful filling of the canal from its coronal to apical extent. Although not the ideal filling material, it has satisfied the majority of tenets for an ideal root filling material highlighted by Brownlee in 1900 and reiterated by Grossman in 1940 (Table 9-1); its cited disadvantages (i.e., lack of rigidity and adhesiveness, ease of displacement under pressure)[134] do not overshadow its advantages. In light of the shortcomings indicated however, a sealer/cement is always used with the gutta-percha. Therefore contemporary materials of choice are gutta-percha in conjunction with a sealer/cement. Neither substance alone enables canal obturation up to the standard of care regardless of the delivery system or compaction technique. This chapter focuses solely on the use of these materials, highlighting their contemporary use and achievement of success. What must be kept in mind by the clinician is that neither the materials used nor the techniques detailed will be successful without proper cleaning and shaping of the canal as described in Chapter 8. Likewise, the materials and techniques described do not routinely provide for an impervious seal of the canal system; all canals leak to a greater or lesser extent.[67] Therefore it is necessary that the clinician master multiple obturation techniques and become competent with various root canal sealer/cements to manage the diversity of anatomical scenarios encountered.

Gutta-Percha

Gutta-percha is the material of choice as a solid core filling material for canal obturation. It demonstrates minimal toxicity and minimal tissue irritability and is the least allergenic material available when retained within the canal system.[134] In cases of inadvertent gutta-percha cone overextension into the periradicular tissues, it is considered as being well tolerated as long the canal is clean and sealed. Gutta-percha, however, has been shown to produce an intense localized tissue response in subcutaneous tissues when placed in fine particle form or when it has been altered with softening agents (rosin-chloroform).[180] This potential may impact on some advocated obturation techniques.

Chemically pure gutta-percha exists in two distinct, different crystalline forms, alpha and beta.[61] These forms are interchangeable depending on the temperature of the material.

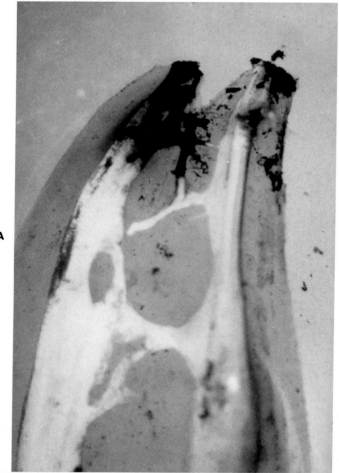

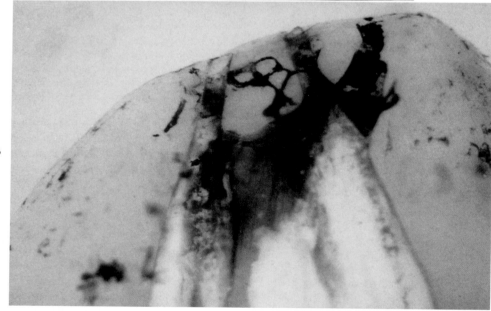

FIG. 9-3 A, Extensive apical leakage into canal anastomosis located between the mesiobuccal and mesiolingual canals of a mandibular molar. **B,** Delta formation at the apex of a mesial root of a mandibular molar. Note the extensive leakage into the apical irregularities regardless of the canal obturation.

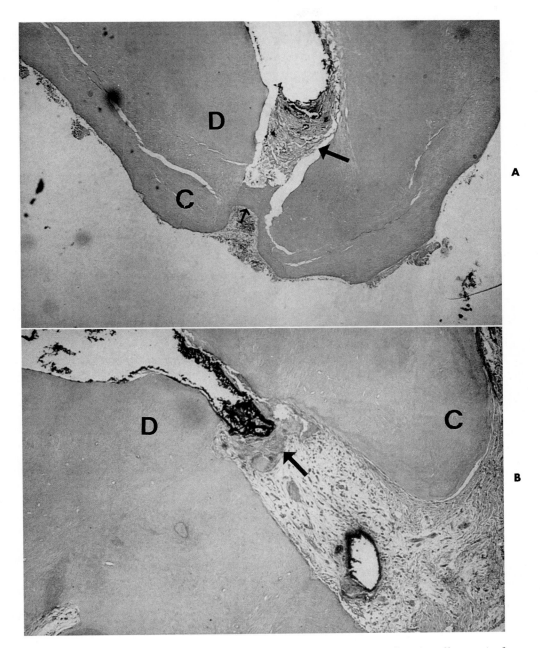

FIG. 9-4 A, Histologic evidence of complete cemental repair and sealing *(small arrow)* of the root canal system regardless of the presence of apical debris *(large arrow)*. Note that the position of the filling material was short of the apical foramen. *C,* Cementum; *D,* dentin. Original magnification ×40. Stain H & E. **B,** Further evidence for apical repair with hard tissue *(arrow)* when the root filling is short of the apical foramen and the apical tissues (periodontal tissues) are protected from damage during instrumentation and obturation. *C,* Cementum; *D,* dentin. Original magnification ×40.

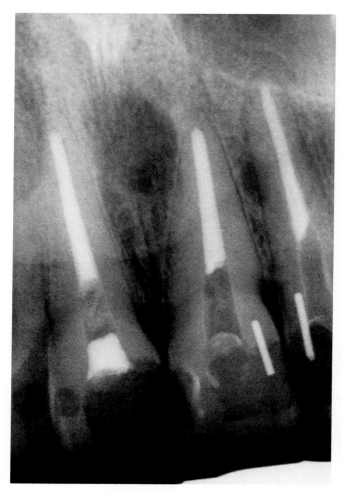

FIG. 9-5 Well-shaped and obturated root canals using gutta-percha, sealer, and lateral compaction.

Whereas most commercially available forms are the beta structure, newer products have adopted the alpha crystalline structure for compatibility with the thermosoftening of the material during obturation. This change has been made because heating of the beta phase (98.6° F; 37° C) causes the crystalline structure to change to the alpha phase (107.6° to 111.2° F; 42° to 44° C) and ultimately into an amorphous melt (132.8° to 147.2° F; 56 to 64° C).[61] Subsequently, the gutta-percha undergoes significant shrinkage during its phase retransformation to the beta state, thereby necessitating thorough compaction during cooling. Produced in the alpha phase, however, the gutta-percha undergoes less shrinkage, and compaction pressures and techniques can better compensate for any shrinkage that may occur.

Gutta-percha can also be softened with chemical solvents to enhance adaptation to the irregularities of the prepared root canal system. Here to, however, shrinkage may occur because of solvent evaporation, or the periradicular tissues may be irritated if either the solvent is expressed beyond the canal or significant amounts of softened gutta-percha are inadvertently placed into the periradicular tissues.[180]

For root canal obturation, gutta-percha is manufactured in the form of cones in both standardized and nonstandardized sizes. The standardized sizes coordinate with the ISO sizes of the root canal files sizes 15 through 140 and are used primarily as the main core material for obturation (Fig. 9-8). The nonstandardized sizes are more tapered from the tip or point to the top and are usually designated as *extra-fine, fine-fine, medium fine, fine, fine medium, medium, medium large, large,* and *extra-large.* With some obturation techniques these cones have been primarily used as accessory or auxiliary cones during compaction, being matched with the shape of the prepared canal space or the compaction instrument. Although the standardized cones have been popular for years since the standardization of the file system,[97] nonstandardized cones have assumed a greater role as the primary core material in the more contemporary obturation techniques. With the development of these techniques, in particular those of vertical compaction with heat softening of gutta-percha, there has be a resurgent interest in the nonstandardized cones. For injectable thermoplastic obturation techniques, gutta-percha may come in either pellet form or in cannules. For some thermomechanical techniques it is available in heatable syringes (Fig. 9-9).

The composition of the available gutta-percha cones is approximately 19% to 22% gutta-percha, 59% to 75% zinc oxide, with the remaining small percentages a combination of various waxes, coloring agents, antioxidants, and metallic salts. The particular percentages of the components vary by manufacturer, with resultant variations in the brittleness, stiffness, tensile strength, and radiopacity of the individual cones primarily because of the gutta-percha and zinc oxide percentages.[45,46] Primarily because of their content of zinc oxide, gutta-percha cones demonstrate definite antimicrobial activity.[129,130] At the very least, however, they should not support microbial growth. The reader is referred to Chapter 14 for more information on gutta-percha.

Sealer/Cements

The use of a sealer during root canal obturation is essential for success. Not only does it enhance the possible attainment of an impervious seal but also serves as a filler for canal irregularities and minor discrepancies between the root canal wall and core filling material. Sealers are often expressed through lateral or accessory canals and can assist in microbial control should there be microorganisms left on the root canal walls or in the tubules.[3,88,149] Sealers can also serve as lubricants to assist in the thorough seating of the core filling material during compaction. In canals in which the smear layer has been removed, many sealers demonstrate increased adhesive properties to dentin, in addition to flowing into the patent tubules.[69,112,138,176,206]

A good sealer should be biocompatible and well tolerated by the periradicular tissues.[186,187] All sealers exhibit toxicity when freshly mixed; however, their toxicity is greatly reduced on setting.[110] All sealers are resorbable when exposed to tissues and tissue fluids.[110] Subsequent tissue healing or repair generally appears unaffected by most sealers, provided their are no adverse breakdown products of the sealer over time.[18,22,23-25] In particular, the breakdown products may have an adverse action on the proliferative capability of periradicular cell populations.[64] Therefore sealers should not be routinely placed in the periradicular tissues as part of an obturation technique.[110]

Sealer/cements can be grouped based on their prime constituent or structure, such as zinc oxide-eugenol, calcium hydroxide, resins, glass ionomers, or silicones. A listing of com-

Text continued on p. 268

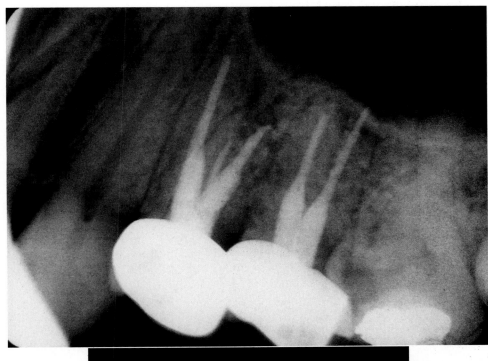

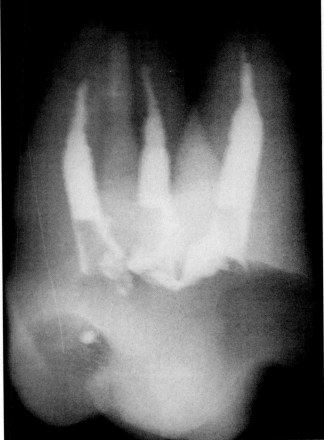

FIG. 9-6 Improper canal shaping that reflects an excessive use of rotary instruments in the coronal two thirds of the canal. The root walls of both teeth have been weakened, and the apical fillings may only be single cones with sealer in the premolar, *top.* Additionally, there has been the failure to achieve proper depth of penetration of the gutta-percha filling in the molar because of the irregular canal preparation, *bottom.*

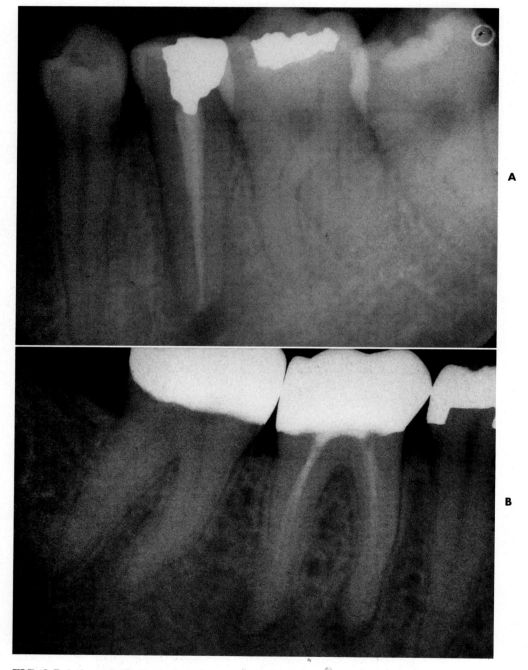

FIG. 9-7 A through **C,** Examples of root canal obturations that lack proper canal shape, in addition to a poorly compacted root canal filling. Voids are seen apically and laterally the length of the fillings. The treatment rendered in each case is below the standard of care, yet was allowed by each clinician that performed the treatment as acceptable. Each case exhibits periradicular pathosis. **D,** Type of void *(arrow)* not always discernible on a dental radiograph. Over time this may contribute to treatment failure.

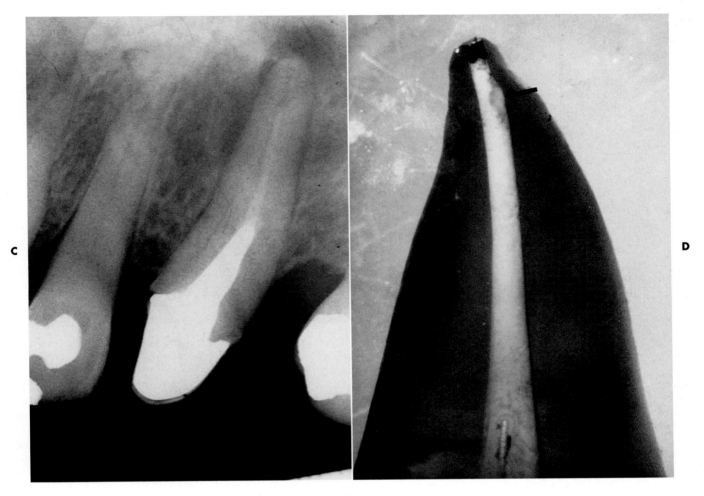

C

D

FIG. 9-7, cont'd For legend see opposite page.

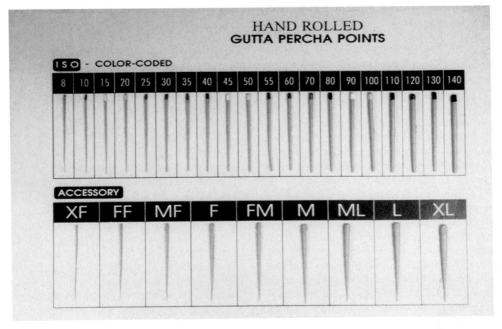

FIG. 9-8 Comparison of standardized gutta-percha cones *(top)* and nonstandardized cones *(bottom)*.

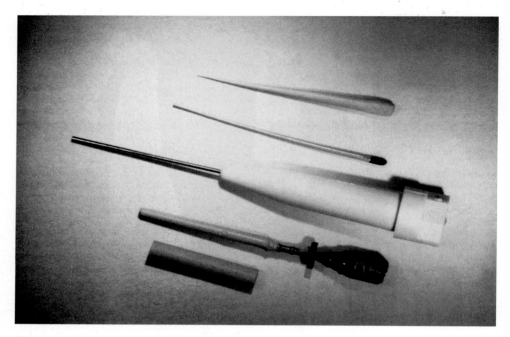

FIG. 9-9 Comprehensive view of the types of gutta-percha available. From top to bottom, nonstandardized cone, standardized point, cannule for thermoplasticized gutta-percha, gutta-percha core carrier, and gutta-percha pellets for thermoplasticized delivery systems.

monly used sealer/cements is found in Table 9-2. However, within this type of grouping, many of the sealer/cements are combinations of components, such as zinc oxide-eugenol and calcium hydroxide (e.g., CRCS and Sealapex). The addition of the calcium hydroxide to the sealers, thereby increasing the pH of the material, is claimed to create a therapeutic material that can be inductive of hard tissue formation. Although an osteogenic response has been observed,[94,183] the solubility of the calcium hydroxide sealers[192,196,197] and the ability of these sealers to sustain a high pH over time[109] have been questioned.

It is recognized that globally, the listings in Table 9-2 are incomplete. However, all effective and safe root canal sealer/cements are of the types listed with minor variations in their constituents. It is necessary that each clinician read the product insert and material safety data sheet (MSDS) for each product purchased before use.

New Directions

With the increased amount of root canal treatment being performed by both the generalist and specialist, there have been renewed efforts to develop better sealer and core obturation materials and techniques. In particular this has focused on the use of glass ionomers,[155] dentin-bonded composite resins[48,112] (Fig. 9-10, *A* and *B*), dentin-bonded apical dentinal plugs,[84] Super EBA and gutta-percha,[47] ultrasonic compaction of gutta-percha,[9] and canal filling under a vacuum with gutta-percha and sealer.[152] To date none have safely reached the highest biologic and technical level. Ideally, future directions should focus on materials that (1) penetrate the patent dentinal tubules, (2) bind intimately to both the organic and inorganic phases of dentin, (3) neutralize or destroy microorganisms and their products, (4) predictably induce a cemental regenerative response over the apical foramen, and (5) strengthen the root system. Needless to say, the delivery system of such materials requires

ease of placement with a rapid and thorough set once in the canal system. Within this futuristic framework, all previous requirements of a root canal sealer/filling material may be inadequate, along with presently used materials.

CONTROVERSIAL CONTEMPORARY ISSUES IN OBTURATION

A multitude of empiric opinions or ideas exist regarding various aspects of root canal obturation. Some are well founded in years of clinical success. Others reflect the entrepreneurial spirit of both generalists and specialists. Some are based on an integration of fact and fiction, whereas other are based on merely a philosophy of "it works well for me"! Before discussing the specific root canal obturation techniques in detail, it is necessary that these ideas be addressed based on a blend of scientific evidence and clinical achievement. This discussion is designed to serve as the basis for the techniques cited and espoused.

Hermetic Seal: Myth or Misconception

Often cited as a major goal of root canal treatment is the achievement of a "hermetic seal." According to accepted dictionary definitions, the word *hermetic* means sealed against the escape or entry of air—or made airtight by fusion or sealing. Yet root canal seals are commonly evaluated for fluid leakage—a parameter used to praise or condemn obturation materials and techniques. This occurs both apically and coronal. Somehow the term *hermetic* has crept into endodontic nomenclature in a manner probably quite similarly as did the invention of an airtight seal. An ancient god of wisdom, learning, and magic in ancient Egypt, Thoth, better known as Hermes Trismegistus (Hermes thrice greatest) is credited with this invention.[154] His significant contribution to civilization allowed the preservation of oils, spices, aromatics, grains, and other ne-

Table 9-2. Commonly used root canal sealer/cements

Name	Manufacturer	Form	ZOE	Ca(OH)$_2$	Resin	GI	Silicone	Work	Set	Specific Indications: Usage Concerns
AH-26 (Thermaseal)	Dentsply, USA/Maillefer, Switzerland	P/L			X			L	L	Allergenic/mutagenic potential; adhesive; formaldehyde release (?); silver containing
AH-Plus* (Topseal)	Dentsply, USA/Maillefer, Switzerland	P/P			X			L	L	Nonmutagenic; no release of formaldehyde; radiopaque; all techniques; low solubility
Sealapex	Kerr Sybron, USA	P/P		X				L	L	Osteogenic (?); possible dissolution; expands on setting
Apexit	Ivoclar-Vivadent, Liechtenstein			X						Softens gutta-percha; good for lateral compaction; viscous; adhesive
CRCS (Calciobiotic)	Hygenic, USA	P/L	X	X				L	L	Silver containing, radiopaque; all techniques
Pulp Canal Sealer	Kerr Sybron, USA	P/L	X					S/M	M/S	Adhesive; good for lateral compaction especially in small canals; softens gutta-percha; good if overextension possible
Wach's Sealex-Extra	Balas Dental Supply	P/L	X					S/M	M	
Grossman-type Stainless										
Roth 801	Roth International, USA	P/L	X					L	L	All techniques; expansion
Roth 811	Roth International, USA	P/L	X					M	M	All techniques
Roth 601	Roth International, USA	P/L	X					S	S	No vertical compaction
Procosol	Procosol Chemical, USA	P/L	X					L/M	L/M	All techniques
Endoseal	Centric Inc, USA	P/L	X					L/M	L/M	All techniques
Tubliseal	Kerr Sybron, USA	P/P	X					S	S	No vertical compaction
Tubliseal-EWT	Kerr Sybron, USA	P/P	X					M	M	All techniques
Grossman-type Silver										
Roth 511	Roth International, USA	P/L	X					L	L	Avoid anterior teeth
Roth 515	Roth International, USA	P/L	X					M	M	Avoid anterior teeth
Ketac-Endo	ESPE-Premier, Germany/USA	Cap				X		S/M	M/S	No compaction; releases fluoride; tubule penetration; bond to dentin?; Strengthen root (?); polymerization shrinkage
Lee Endo Fill	Lee Pharmaceuticals, USA	P/L					X			Shrinkage (?); very dry canal necessary; penetrates tubules

Cap, Capsule; *GI,* glass ionomer; *L,* long; *M,* moderate; *P/L,* powder/liquid; *P/P,* paste/paste; *S,* short; *ZOE,* zinc oxide–eugenol. Data obtainable, however, from studies done at the Universities of Berlin and Munich, Germany.

*No published reports on biocompability or clinical performance.

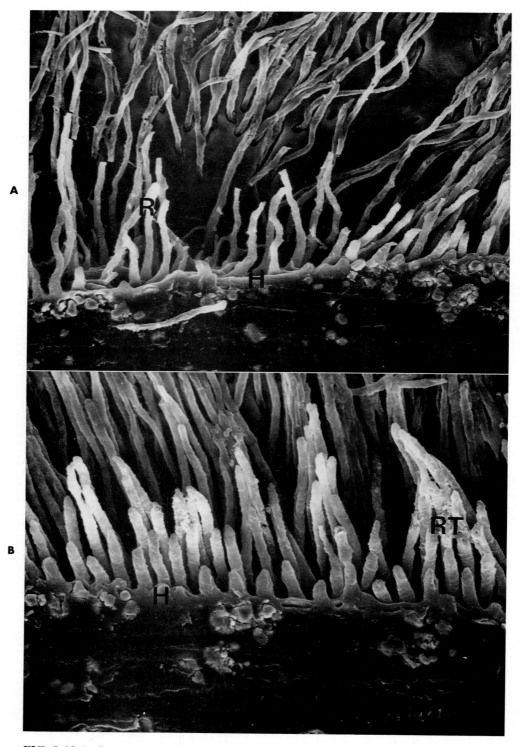

FIG. 9-10 A, Cross-sectional scanning electron microscopic view of the dentine adhesive interface. The hybrid layer *(H)*, resin filling material *(R)*, and demineralized dentin *(D)* are visible with resin tags extending deep into the demineralized tubules. Original magnification ×940. **B,** Cross-sectional scanning electron microscopic view displaying resin tags *(RT)* entering dentine tubules and contiguous with the hybrid layer *(H)*. Original magnification ×660. *(Reproduced by permission from Leonard JE, Gutmann JL, Guo IY: Apical and coronal seal of roots obturated with a dentine bonding agent and resin,* Int Endod J 29:76, 1996.)

cessities in previously porous, earthenware vessels. A simple wax seal of the vessel walls helped to create the "hermetic seal." Endodontically speaking, the term *hermetic* is inappropriate; however, a fluid-tight, fluid-impervious, or bacteria-tight seal would seem more contemporary.

Compaction Versus Condensation

Traditionally, obturation methods were routinely referred to as the condensation (vertical or lateral) of gutta-percha within the root canal space. A closer look at the word condensation provides a very different connotation than that process that occurs during root canal obturation. Although its overwhelming meaning is to make more dense, its prime focus is that of a liquid or a gas with reference to compression, concentration, or reduction. In both the strictest sense and in the clinical sense, gutta-percha cannot be compressed, concentrated, or reduced. The word *compact,* which means to put firmly together, more readily reflects what occurs during root canal obturation. This concept, with regard to gutta-percha, was extensively researched and clearly detailed more than 20 years ago.[171] The fifth edition of *The Glossary—Contemporary Terminology for Endodontics* by the American Association of Endodontists has recognized the importance of that concept and has emphasized the use of the word *compaction* with reference to obturation techniques.[55] This is the word of choice throughout this chapter.

Lateral Versus Vertical Techniques

The literature is replete with studies comparing lateral compaction with vertical compaction, and personal preferences abound. Likewise, endodontic programs have aligned themselves solely with one technique or another, with both authorities claiming superiority. When viewed objectively, many interesting facts emerge regarding this controversy. First, girded with the knowledge of force vectors, it is obvious that pure lateral or vertical compaction rarely occurs. The vectors of force applied during obturation techniques are an integrated blend of forces and result in a composite of forces that are neither true vertical or lateral. Even with the use of differing instruments, such as a spreader with a pointed tip or a plugger with a flattened tip, the vectors of force applied are still a composite. The use of engineering models,[53,169] photoelastic stress models,[83,121] and three-dimensional finite elemental analysis[157,194,214] to determine the nature and location of forces placed during obturation techniques indicates the complexity of this pattern. Second, if there is so much of a difference between the two obturation techniques and specific forces do make a difference, why is lateral compaction chosen as the comparative standard in almost all obturation studies? Third, apparently increases in the compaction pressures do not result in significant differences in apical leakage patterns.[87] Fourth, whether lateral or vertical compaction is performed, obturation can still fall below the standard of care for the same reasons, those being improper canal shaping and lack of competence in the obturation technique chosen. What appears important is the shape of the prepared canal,[53,83,157,194] the recognition that neither obturation technique is a pure technique, and the recognition that excellence with either technique is operator dependent. With proper execution, either manner of canal obturation can be highly successful; the clinician must be able to recognize when the application of either technique, in a pure or modified form, or both techniques will enable the attainment of success on a predictable basis.

Softened Versus Solid Materials

Both Brownlee[26] and Grossman[65] indicated that a softened, pliable, or semisolid filling material would be ideal. Contemporary practices of obturation favor some type of material softening to enable the movement of the material into the canal intricacies,[29] including the dentinal tubules[49,69] (Fig. 9-11, *A* through *E*). However, even these achievements do not guarantee that an impervious seal of the root canal system will be established.[31,47,43,182] Likewise, the dental advertising media are filled with the promotion of techniques via clinical "how-to-do-it" articles that enhance the movement of softened obturation materials into accessory communications. Here too, there is no substantiation as to the levels of success or failure when these accessory channels are filled or unfilled.[204] More importantly, however, is the fact that with softened gutta-percha obturation techniques there has been a greater incidence of material extrusion beyond the confines of the canal[43,118] (see Fig. 9-11, *B*). Although clinically, many cases have been shown to be successful when this occurs, long-term success with root canal treatment is highly predicated on retaining the root filling material within the root.[63,174,180,190] While softening of gutta-percha may be viewed as routinely highly desirable, the selective use of this technique solely or in combination with a solid core of gutta-percha must be at the discretion of the competent clinician when anatomic dictates require this approach.

Use of Solvents for Material Adaptation

Chemical solvents to soften gutta-percha have been used for almost 100 years,[30] and a multitude of variations exist. Uses have ranged from merely dipping the gutta-percha cones into the solvent (1 second) for better canal adaptation to creating a completely softened paste of gutta-percha with the solvent (see Fig. 9-2). What appears to be crucial in the achievement of success with these techniques is the need to allow for dissipation of the chemical solvent, if volatile, or the removal of the excess solvent with alcohol. Failure to do this can result in significant dimensional change in the filling and possible loss of the apical seal.[105] This is possible in the "dip" techniques;[71] however, failure to compact the gutta-percha within a short time period after dipping (15 to 30 seconds) may result in loss of the desired plasticity of the material.[126] What influences the success of these techniques may actually be the shape of the canal as opposed to the presence of residual solvent.[125] Even with softened gutta-percha, the quality of compaction is dependent on the movement of material into canal irregularities.

Small amounts of gutta-percha have also been dissolved in various solvents such as chloroform (chloropercha), chloroform mixed with Canada balsam and zinc oxide (Kloropercha), or eucalyptol (eucapercha) to enhance gutta-percha's adaptation within the canal; however, the efficacy and achievement of these approaches have been both praised[58] and questioned.[78,210] With the advent of thermoplasticized gutta-percha and the availability of gutta-percha in the alpha phase, the need to consider the use of solvents at any time must be questioned. This is not to negate the achievement of success with this approach, but rather to bring about an enhanced focus on the contemporary techniques and the quality of achievement attainable without the use of potentially irritating chemical solvents.[7] The use of solvents, however, may still be considered for a number of challenges the clinician may face in daily practice,[124] such as the custom fitting of master cones in irregular apical preparations or following apexification.[70] Solvents commonly used are chloroform, methychloroformate, halothane, rectified white turpentine, and eucalyptol.[71,102]

Smear Layer Removal Versus Smear Layer Retention

The smear layer is a combination of organic and inorganic debris present on the root canal walls following instrumentation[123] (Fig. 9-12, *A* and *B*). When viewed under scanning electron microscope, the smear layer has an amorphous, irregular, and granular appearance[20,147,213] that represents dentinal shavings, tissue debris, odontoblastic processes, and in previously infected root canals, microbial elements.[123] The appearance of the smear layer is formed by translocating and burnishing the superficial components of the dentinal wall during canal preparation.[10] During the early stages of canal preparation or in irregular anatomic variations of the canal, the smear layer would be predominantly organic in nature before any extensive dentin removal.[32]

The smear layer has been described as being (1) superficial on the dentinal surface and (2) packed into the dentinal tubules. The phenomenon of tubular packing with smear layer debris

has been concluded to be the result of using endodontic instruments during canal preparation, although fluid dynamics and capillary action have also been identified as causative agents.[2,117]

Since the smear layer remaining on the root canal walls has been characterized, the controversy of whether or not to remove this layer before obturation exists.[37] Biologically, the presence of the smear layer has been postulated to be an avenue for leakage and source of substrate for bacterial growth and ingress.[146] The frequency of bacterial penetration in the presence of a smear layer, when canals were obturated with thermoplasticized gutta-percha and sealer, has been shown to be significantly higher than with smear layer removal and obturation.[13] On the other hand, although sophisticated models have demonstrated fluid movement through obturated root canals, bacterial penetration was slight to nonexistent.[212] A further concern is the presence of viable bacteria that may remain in the dentinal tubules and use the smear layer for sustained growth and activity.[20,139] The presence of the smear layer may also prevent or delay the action of disinfectants on bacteria harbored in the dentinal tubules.[141] When the smear layer is not removed, it may slowly disintegrate and dissolve around leak-

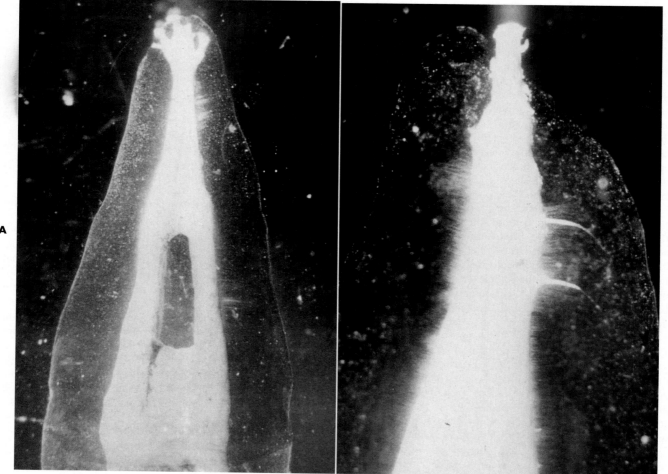

A **B**

FIG. 9-11 A through **D,** Adaptation of gutta-percha and sealer into the canal irregularities, including possibly the dentinal tubules. Smear layer has been removed. (**A** and **B,** Trifecta technique.) (**C** and **D,** ThermaFil technique.) **E,** Scanning electron microscopic view of gutta-percha penetration into the dental tubules during compaction using thermoplasticized gutta-percha. Original magnification ×640. See also Fig. 9-63. Smear layer removed with all techniques.

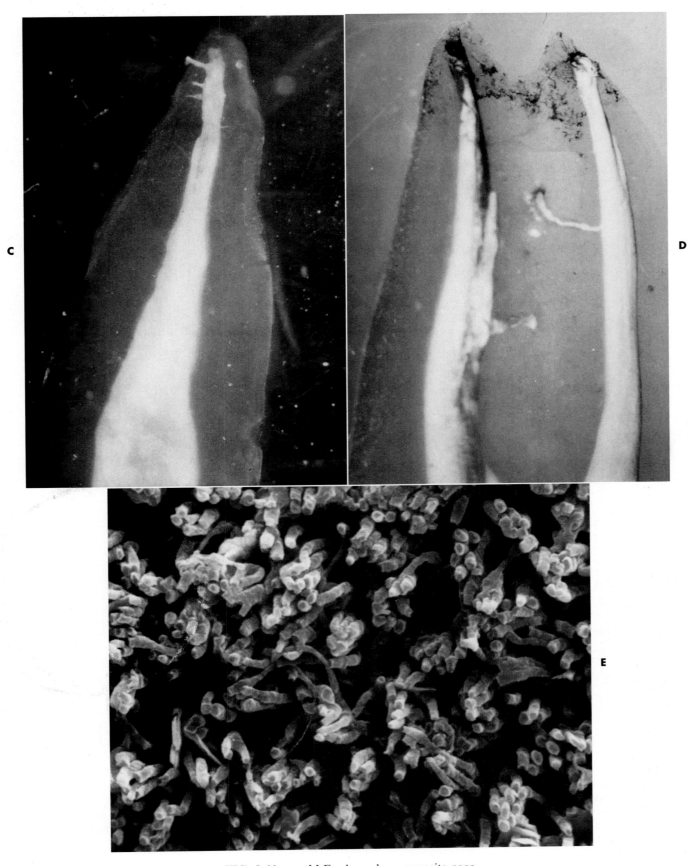

FIG. 9-11, cont'd For legend see opposite page.

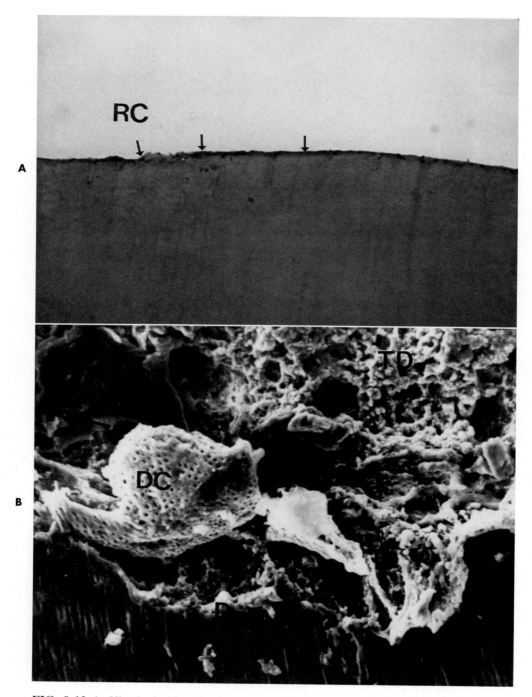

FIG. 9-12 A, Histologic identification of the smear layer on the surface of the cut dentin *(arrows)* in the root canal *(RC)*. Original magnification ×40. Stain H & E. **B,** Scanning electron micrograph of the smear layer. *DC,* Dentin chips; *TD,* tissue debris; *D,* dentin. Original magnification ×480.

ing canal filling materials, or it may be removed by bacterial by-products such as acids and enzymes.[177] Likewise, if the smear layer is removed, there is always the risk of reinfecting the dentinal tubules if the seal does fail.[115]

Technically, the smear layer may interfere with the penetration of gutta-percha into the tubules and the adhesion and penetration of root canal sealers into the dentinal tubules. Significant tubular penetration of gutta-percha and sealers has been shown with thermoplasticized obturations[69,114] (see Fig. 9-11,

E) and experimentally with dentin-bonded composite resins with smear layer removal[112] (see Fig. 9-10, *A* and *B*). Studies have also shown a decreased incidence of microleakage with gutta-percha and sealer obturations when the smear layer was removed and the gutta-percha was chemically or thermally softened before obturation.[50,103] Similar findings were shown with dentin-bonded composite resins.[112] Thus the retention or removal of the smear layer before obturation may influence the quality of the obturation.

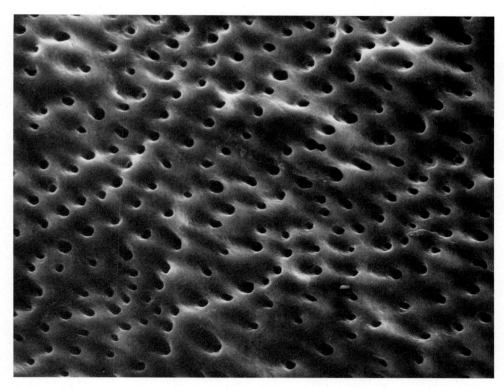

FIG. 9-13 Dentinal tubules following the removal of the smear layer. Note absence of debris seen in Fig. 9-12, *B*. Original magnification ×720.

Table 9-3. Suggested methods for removing the smear layer

Author	Solution		Amount
Goldman et al. (1981)[57]	REDTA*	17%	20 ml
Goldman et al. (1982)[59]	REDTA*	17%	10 ml
	NaOCl	5.25%	10 ml
Yamada et al. (1983)[213]	REDTA*	17%	10 ml
	NaOCl	5.25%	10 ml
White et al. (1984)[207]	REDTA*	17%	10 ml
	NaOCl	5.25%	10 ml
Ciucchi et al. (1989)[35]	NaOCl	3%	1 ml
	EDTA†	15%	2 ml
Gettleman et al. (1991)[52]	EDTA‡	17%	—
	NaOCl	5.25%	—

Reprinted from Gutmann JL: Adaptation of injected thermoplasticized gutta-percha in the absence of the dentinal smear layer, *Int Endod J* 26:87, 1993, by permission.
EDTA, Disodium ethylenediaminetetraacetic acid; *NaOCl,* sodium hypochlorite; *REDTA,* disodium ethylenediaminetetraacetic acid, sodium hydroxide, cetyltrimethylammonium bromide, and water mixture.
*Roth International, Chicago, Ill.
†Largal-Ultra, Septodont, Paris, France.
‡Unknown Source.

Methods for the removal of the smear layer before obturation have primarily focused on the alternating use of a chelating agent (disodium ethylenediaminetetraacetic acid [EDTA]) or weak acid (10% citric acid) followed by thorough canal rinsing with sodium hypochlorite (3% to 5.25%) (Table 9-3; Fig. 9-13). The routine use of these techniques, however, has not been universally advocated, and the long-term value of smear layer removal has not been elucidated. The value of this pro-

cedure before obturation, however, is dependent on the canal cleaning and shaping and the chemical delivery system used (see Chapter 8).

Depth of Instrument Placement During Obturation

The need to compact the gutta-percha and sealer at the apical dentin matrix or constriction of the canal is essential for success. When applying vertical compaction forces or techniques with softened gutta-percha, placement of the compacting instrument short of the apical terminus of canal preparation is advocated. The softened filling material is compacted into the apical preparation in a three-dimensional manner. However, when using the lateral compaction technique, the master gutta-percha cone is already fit into the apical preparation, and compaction of this cone, or adaptation of this cone within the walls of the apical preparation, is essential for a proper seal. This implies the placement of the lateral compaction instrument (spreader) into the apical aspect of the canal. Many authors, however, do not define the parameters of this placement, and many master gutta-percha cones are not compacted in the apical aspect of the canal, which predisposes to leakage.[4] The importance of placing the spreader to within 1 to 2 mm of the prepared apical matrix or constriction has been vividly demonstrated, especially as it relates to canal shape.[4] Even these parameters may fall short of ideal in that failure to place the spreader to the full canal working length may still result in the lack of adaptation and compaction of master gutta-percha cone in the apical portion of the canal[71] (Fig. 9-14, *A* through *G*). This results in a master cone surrounded by a sea of root canal cement that looks acceptable on the radiograph but does not seal the canal.

An argument could be raised that placement of the spreader

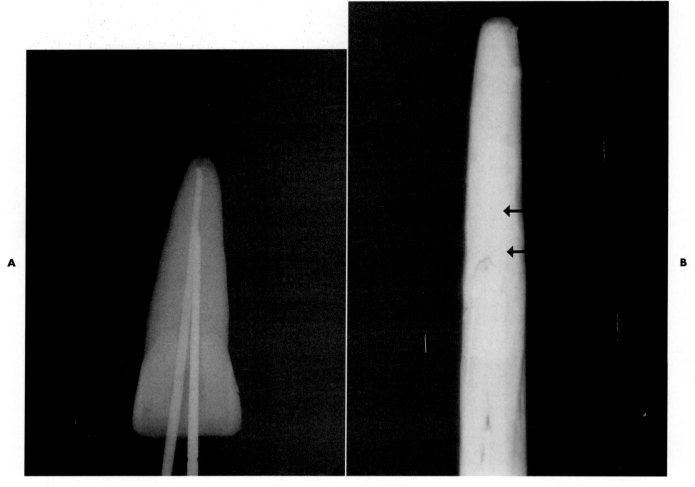

FIG. 9-14 A, Failure to achieve full penetration of a No. 50 spreader. **B,** Note position of spreader in gutta-percha cone *(arrows)* without evidence of apical compaction.

to the working length may result in unnecessarily placed apical forces with the possibility for root fracture.[92,151] Likewise, it may result in the movement of the master cone beyond the confines of the root. In both cases, however, these undesirable outcomes are due to improper canal shaping or the lack of a good apical matrix or stop in sound dentin. Contemporary canal shapes that favor funnel-type preparations from the apical matrix to the coronal orifice as described in Chapter 8 allow for proper placement of the compacting instrument and proper adaptation of the master gutta-percha cone.

Stainless Steel Versus Nickel-Titanium Compactors

Historically, carbon steel or stainless steel compacting instruments were used routinely in the compaction of root canal filling materials. However, potential problems existed in the depth of penetration (especially in curved canals), the potential for wedging and root fractures, and the amount of stress focused on sections of the root walls during compaction. With the advent of nickel-titanium metallic instruments, there are suggestions that many of these problems may be solved, in addition to obtaining root canal fills that have greater density of filling material.[187] Specifically, nickel-titanium compactors (finger spreaders) create significantly less stress in curved ca-

nals than similar stainless steel compactors[40] and are able to penetrate further in curved canals than stainless steel compactors[15] (Fig. 9-15, *A* and *B*). Potential disadvantages include the buckling of the instrument under compaction pressure and the inability to precurve the instrument for ease of canal access. A combination of usage in canals has also been suggested[187] with apical penetration with the nickel-titanium instrument and coronal compaction in the more flared portion of the canal with a stainless steel instrument. Present studies have been limited, however, and long-term usage patterns are nonexistent. Clinician usage also varies and contemporary academic programs are only beginning to incorporate these new instruments into their teaching programs.

Homogeneity of the Canal Filling: Voids in the Root Canal Filling

Ideally, the root canal filling should be a complete homogenous mass that fills the prepared root canal in three dimensions. Often the achievement of this goal cannot be properly ascertained on a postobturation radiograph. Failure to achieve this ideal has been the focus of criticism of the lateral compaction technique unless sealers are used that soften the material and allow for a chemical welding of the gutta-percha cones

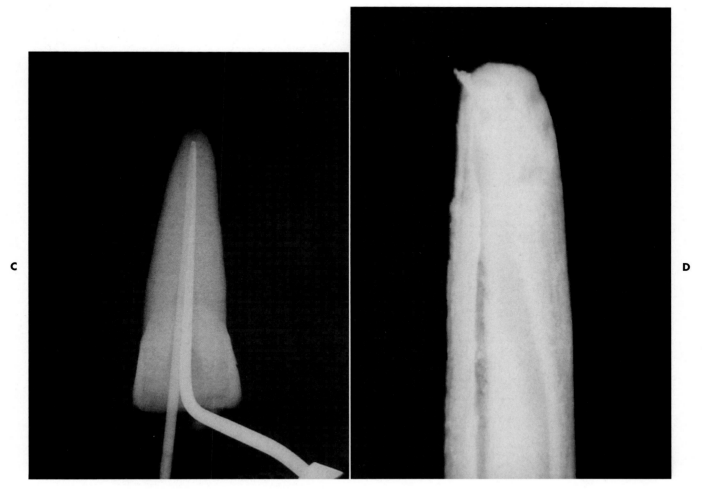

FIG. 9-14, cont'd C, Full penetration of a D11T spreader adjacent to a master cone. **D,** Facial view of compacted gutta-percha cone.   *Continued*

in the canal. Advocates of vertical compaction techniques with heat-softened gutta-percha use this parameter as a claim for technique superiority. However, even in the vertical compaction of thermoplasticized gutta-percha, voids are common and can occur for a number of reasons[71] (Fig. 9-16, *A*).

The prime source of voids in the final root canal obturation is the lack of skill and execution in the obturation technique chosen for a particular canal anatomy, coupled with improper canal shaping. In some cases highly radiopaque root canal sealers mask radiographically the presence of a void in the homogeneity of the root canal filling; in reality this detracts from the quality of the canal obturation. Voids may also be due to the pooling of large amounts of root canal sealers or the improper application of the compaction instrument into the cold or softened gutta-percha (Fig. 9-16, *B*). Voids may exist along the perimeters of the root canal filling or internally within the mass of the gutta-percha. Failure to place additional gutta-percha filling material into spaces created by the compacting instrument is also a prime reason for voids (Fig. 9-16, *C* through *E*). However, the question remains, of what importance is the presence of a void or voids in the final root canal obturation?

The presence of voids in both the apical and coronal portion of the root canal filling may provide avenues for leakage or for fluids to stagnate if leakage should occur. Voids, as evidenced as partly or improperly filled root canals, can give way to bacterial regrowth or reinfection, leading to failures.[149] Voids also detract from the clinician's assessment of the aesthetics of the treatment provided. The importance of this factor, however, is dubious. Voids consistently observed in the root canal fillings may actually stimulate clinicians to seek further experience or alternative techniques in hopes of eliminating the routine presence of voids. Ironically, if the canal system is properly cleaned and shaped and any of the gutta-percha obturation techniques are properly carried out, a well-filled, three-dimensional obturation results. The two-dimensional radiographic determination of this ideal, however, must always be suspect.[107]

Pastes as Root Canal Fillings

The use of paste-type root canal obturation techniques is not advocated in contemporary endodontics for the following reasons.[71,110,134] The components of some pastes may leach into the periradicular tissues, resulting in chronic tissue inflammation or cellular toxicity. Because of porosities in paste fills, most pastes absorb in time, resulting in apical leakage, percolation, and the strong possibility of ultimate treatment failure. Systemically, components of some paste filling materials have

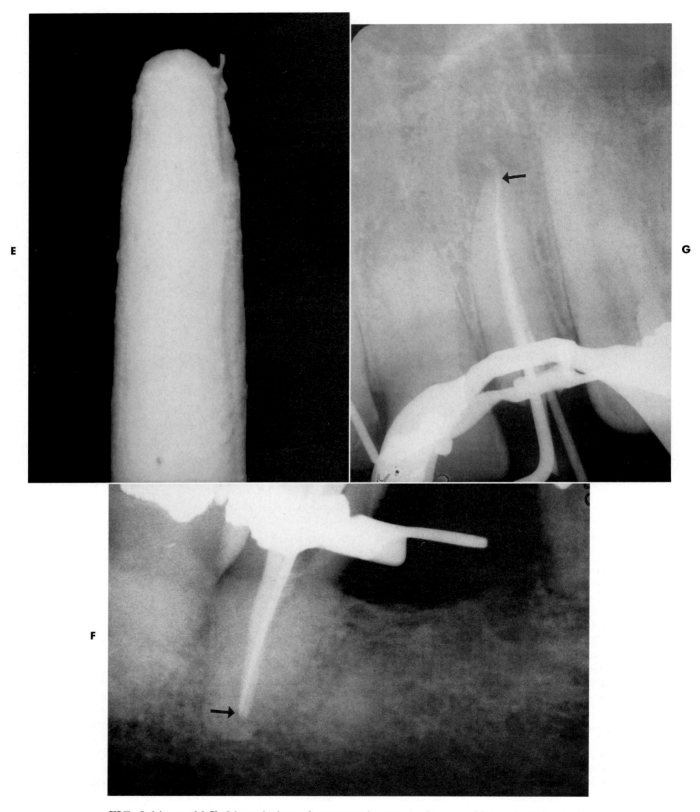

FIG. 9-14, cont'd E, Lingual view of compacted gutta-percha cone. Note adaptation to irregularities of the prepared canal at the apical matrix. **F,** Apical penetration *(arrow)* of a D11T spreader to the apical matrix adjacent to the master cone in a mandibular molar. Depth of penetration is essential for thorough apical compaction. **G,** Similar penetration *(arrow)* of a D11T spreader in a maxillary lateral incisor adjacent to both a master cone and one accessory cone.

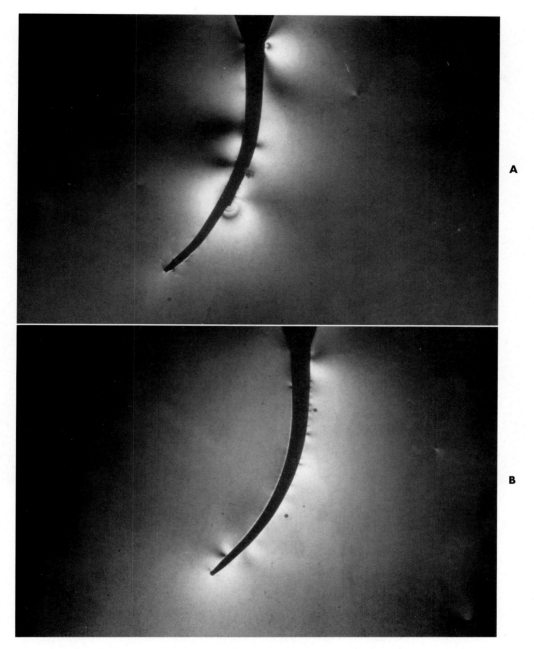

FIG. 9-15 A, Photoelastic stress patterns for a stainless steel finger spreader. Model with a master gutta-percha cone, two accessory cones, and finger spreader under load. Areas of point stress and uneven stress distribution are evident. **B,** Photoelastic stress patterns for a nickel-titanium finger spreader. Model with a master gutta-percha cone, two accessory cones, and finger spreader under load. Areas of point stress are minimal with an even distribution of stress evident. *(Courtesy Dr. Gerald N. Glickman.)*

been shown to be recovered in both blood samples and various vital organs.[17] Chemical components of the paste have been shown to be antigenic, causing immunologic responses.[16] Finally, the apical control of paste fills is all but impossible, especially when no apical matrix is present or a root perforation exists.

Highly Radiopaque Sealers

Some root canal sealers contain significant amounts of radiopacifiers, such as barium sulfate or silver particles. These additives enhance the radiographic appearance of the root canal obturation, especially when the sealer is expressed through accessory or lateral communications. The routine use of these sealers may, however, detract from the quality of the compaction of the solid core material and give a false sense of obturation radiodensity. Likewise, erroneous empiric claims have been made that obturations with highly radiopaque sealers are better than those made with less radiopaque materials, merely based on the radiographic appearance. This type of comparison and claim to superiority is both unfounded and unwar-

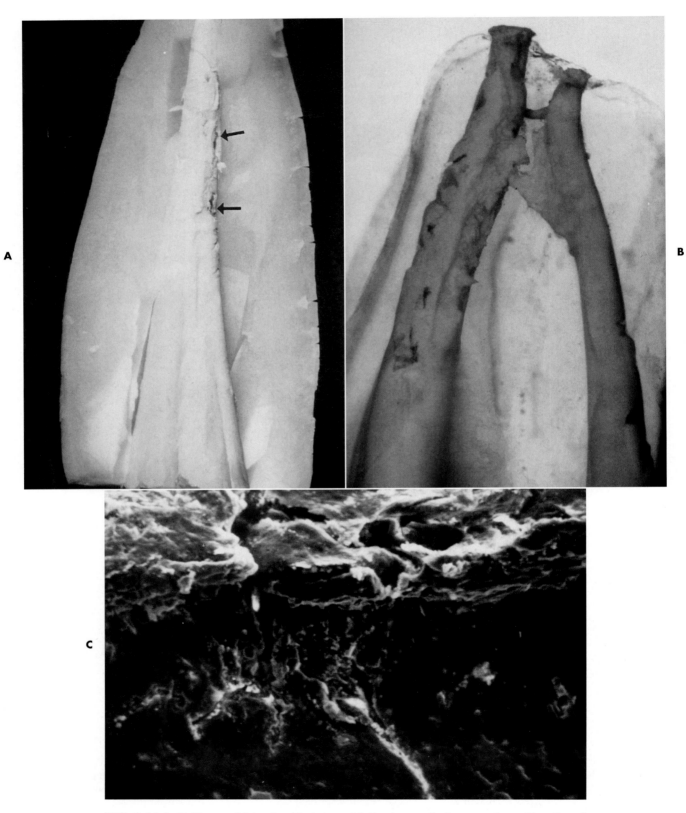

FIG. 9-16 A, Evidence of lateral voids *(arrows)* following vertical compaction with softened gutta-percha. **B,** Further evidence of voids attributed to lack of material softness, flow, and proper compactor penetration. **C,** Scanning electron microscopic evidence of voids and gaps during the vertical compaction of heat-softened gutta-percha. Compactor voids *(CV)* and gutta-percha welds *(GPW)* are visible. These are not discernible radiographically. Magnifications range from ×200 to ×380.

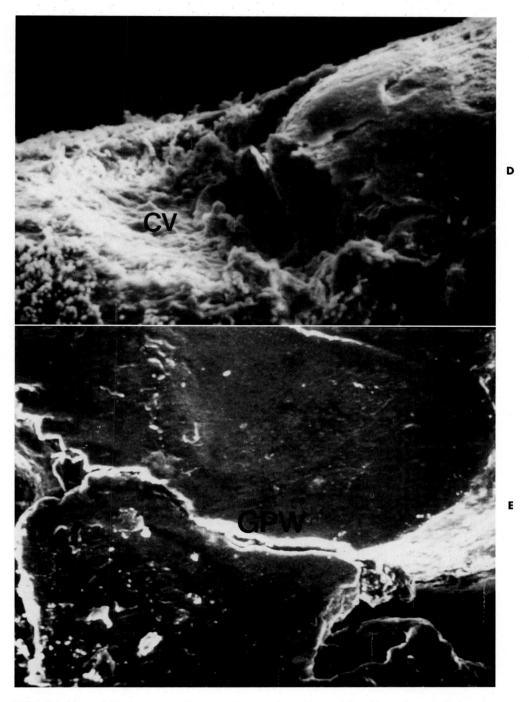

FIG. 9-16 D and **E,** Scanning electron microscopic evidence of voids and gaps during the vertical compaction of heat-softened gutta-percha. Compactor voids *(CV)* and gutta-percha welds *(GPW)* are visible. These are not discernible radiographically. Magnifications range from ×200 to ×380.

ranted and has created divisions among many clinicians. It also demonstrates that undue importance is being placed merely on the radiographic appearance and "aesthetics" of the obturated canal system, as opposed to the necessary attention to detail required during canal cleaning, shaping, and obturation. While it is true that the assessment of the root canal obturation is primarily based on radiographic findings, root canal sealers do not have to be highly radiopaque to be effective.

Apical Position of the Obturation Material

While filling the entire root canal system is the major goal of canal obturation, a major controversy exists as to what constitutes the apical termination of the root canal filling material. Working length determination guidelines often cite the cementodentinal junction or apical constriction as the ideal position for terminating canal cleaning and shaping procedures and the position to which the filling material should be placed[72] (Fig.

9-17). First, the cementodentinal junction is a histologic and not a clinical position in the root canal system. Second, the cementodentinal junction is not always the most constricted portion of the canal in the apical portion of the root. Third, the distance from the apical foramen to the constricture depends on a multitude of factors such as increased cemental deposition or radicular resorption. Both processes are strongly influenced by age, trauma, orthodontic movement, periradicular pathology, or periodontal disease. Especially in periodontal disease states, the cementodentinal junction location has no predictable anatomic appearance or location due to resorptive processes or cemental depositions that may extend well in the root canal[173] (Fig. 9-18). Therefore the foramen and cementodentinal junction position on the root can be highly variable

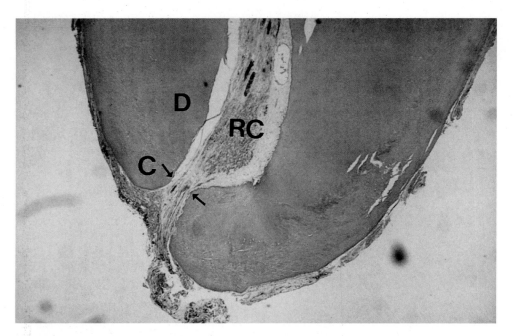

FIG. 9-17 Histologic appearance of the root apex. *C,* Cementum; *D,* dentin; *RC,* root canal. Arrows indicate the narrowest constriction that is not specifically at the cementodentinal junction. Original magnification ×25. Stain H & E.

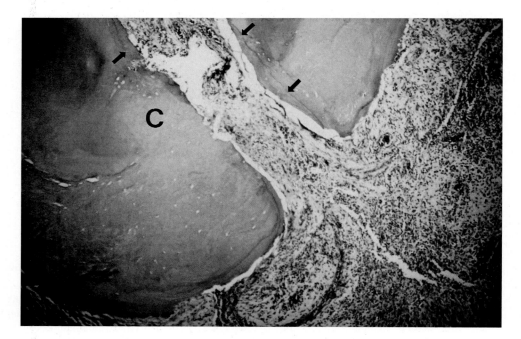

FIG. 9-18 Histologic appearance of a typical root apex. Note the thick layering of the cementum *(C)* in relation to the dentin *(D).* Also note the lack of a discrete cementodentinal junction due to deposition of cementum *(arrows)* along the dentinal wall in the root canal. Original magnification ×40. Stain H & E.

and can exist anywhere from the direct radiographic apex up to 3 mm coronal to the radiographic apex depending on a particular root morphology. These potential anatomic variances have had a major impact on the precise region or location for determining the working length and termination of root canal instrumentation and obturation. These clinical concerns, along with the integrity of the periradicular tissues,[133] have formed the basis for success in prognostic studies that have identified that the optimal result is to end instrumentation and obturation inside the radiographic apex (approximating the cementodentinal junction) (Fig. 9-19, *A* and *B*). When instrumentation and obturation are shorter than this, the success rates drops. When longer than this, especially with filling materials beyond the radiographic apex, an even poorer result is noted[85] (Fig. 9-20). From a realistic viewpoint, however, it is often impossible to know exactly where the apical foramen and apical constriction are located until after the canal has been obturated. Many of the more contemporary obturation techniques advocate canal obturation to within 0.5 mm of the radiographic apex, to the radiographic apex, or beyond, which is confirmed by the presence of a "puff" of filling material. Empiric observations support a high degree of success with these techniques (Fig. 9-21). *However, no long-term prognostic studies have supported this position for the termination of root canal obturations.* Likewise, canals with filling material beyond the confines of the root canal system tend to cause more postoperative discomfort.[82,175]

If a major goal of root canal treatment is to create an environment conducive to the regeneration of cementum over the apical foramen, the periodontium that enters the apical foramen in teeth with vital, yet compromised, pulps should not be challenged with the extrusion of root canal filling materials beyond the end of the canal (Fig. 9-22, *A* and *B*). This concept has been scientifically valid for over 65 years[66,140,181] and is supported by numerous retrospective studies.[63,174,179,190] Even in those cases with periradicular radiolucencies, filling beyond the confines of the canal is less desirable,[174] although filling the root canal as close as possible to its terminus is desirable (Figs. 9-23 and 9-24). Contemporary endodontic practices and long-term evaluative studies favor and support obturation within the confines of the root canal system in all cases in an attempt to prevent further challenge to the already compromised and challenged periradicular tissues.

Apical Seal Versus Coronal Seal: Which is More Important?

Although historically the lack of an apical seal of the root canal system received the most attention as being the prime reason for failure of root canal treatment,[39] contemporary thought and literature documentation emphasize the need to address the thorough seal of the root canal system, both apically and coronally[133] (Fig. 9-25). All techniques used during root canal treatment and the subsequent restoration of the tooth must favor both goals. This implies that compaction of gutta-percha into the root canal system must be complete in all dimensions from the orifice to the apical termination of the filling.

Use of Apical Barriers

A method often used to create an apical stop or matrix for the purpose of obtaining a biologic apical seal supports the placement of dentin chips or other artificial barriers (calcium hydroxide, demineralized dentin, lyophilized bone, tricalcium phosphate, hydroxyapatite, collagen) before canal obturation.[36,160]

This technique is not new, and favorable results were obtained with dentin chips more than 60 years ago.[60] More contemporary studies have supported these findings, provided the dentin chips were uncontaminated by bacteria or their by-products.[95,195,197] Ironically, the packing of chips may occur inadvertently during cleaning and shaping,[217] especially if a patency file is not routinely used.[145] When intentionally placed, the chips are obtained from the coronal dentin using rotary instruments such as Gates-Glidden burs or Peeso reamers after the canal has been cleaned and shaped. Subsequently, the chips are packed in the apical 1 to 3 mm followed by standard canal obturation with guttapercha and sealer.

In addition to possibly creating a biologic seal, the packed chips may assist in confining irrigating solutions to the canal and preventing overfilling, especially when a canal has been overinstrumented;[42] however, they may or may not enhance the seal of the canal apically.[1,217] Regardless, favorable periradicular tissue responses have been noted with enhanced healing, minimal inflammation, and apical cementum deposition.[142]

The use of calcium compounds, in particular calcium hydroxide, as an apical barrier, has also been extensively investigated. Calcium hydroxide in either a moist or dry state is carried to or compacted into the apical 1 to 3 mm of the prepared canal before canal obturation. This process is facilitated with an amalgam carrier, lentula, or syringe with premixed calcium hydroxide. Significant calcifications have been noted at the apical foramen,[150] and the periradicular tissue response in comparison to dentin chips is indistinguishable.[93] Additionally, teeth with apical calcium hydroxide plugs have demonstrated significantly less leakage than teeth without plugs.[205]

Even with promising data that support the potential use of an artificial barrier in the apical portion of the prepared canal, the routine clinical use of this technique does not appear to be the standard of care. If this approach to treatment is to be adopted, a material with predictable inductive capabilities is necessary; one that seals the canal, negates any bacterial influences, and predictably stimulates cementum regeneration across the apical foramen.

Timing of Root Canal Obturation

Historically, root canal treatment was performed in multiple visits to accommodate the need for negative microbial cultures and to ensure the cessation of signs or symptoms. Although the need for cultures is rare, the presence of acute signs or symptoms still exists as a contemporary rationale for not obturating the root canal at the time of cleaning and shaping. Even this dictate has its empiric challenges, although some data exist that support the single-visit management of an acute periradicular abscess.[184] On the other hand, filling of canals that are infected may result in an increase in postoperative discomfort.[98] In fact, the argument for potential postoperative pain following root canal treatment in one visit has been used as a rationale for not obturating at the time of canal cleaning and shaping. On the other hand, studies have shown that postoperative pain is not increased following complete root canal treatment in one visit.[51,132,136,158]

In the absence of significant signs or symptoms, root canal treatment can be completed in one visit. Patients with necrotic pulps and periradicular radiolucencies and patients with draining sinus tracts can receive complete treatment in one visit. Often cases planned for one-visit treatment may have to be completed in more than one visit depending on both patient and clinician factors. Therefore the clinician should consider

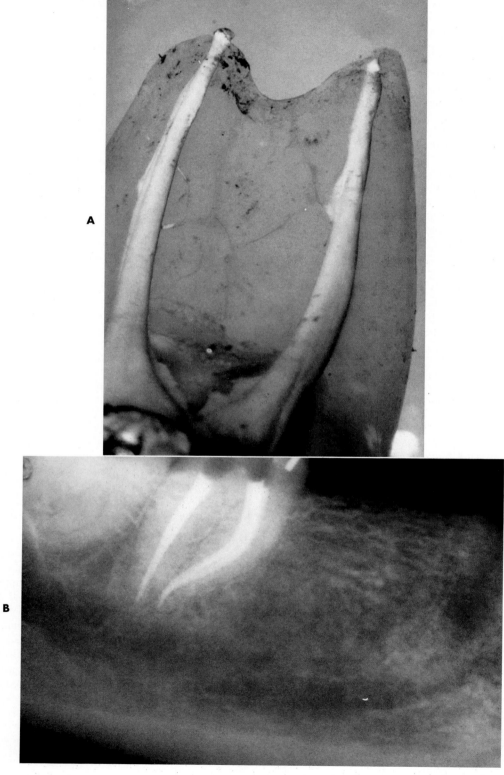

FIG. 9-19 A, Cleared tooth specimen with two canals; the left canal is filled beyond the root end, whereas the right one is filled within the confines of the root. Ideal location is within the root. **B,** Clinical case demonstrating this attainment using vertical compaction of heat-softened gutta-percha. *(**B** courtesy Dr. Constantinos Laghios.)*

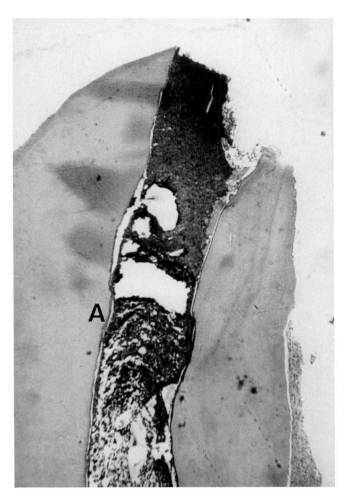

FIG. 9-20 Histologic picture of the damage that is done to the apical constriction when instrumentation is beyond the end of the canal and root. Canal is filled with gutta-percha to level *A* and the remainder of the canal is filled with a blood clot. This environment is not biologically conducive to healing and tissue regeneration. Original magnification ×25. Stain H & E.

the following when planning on canal obturation at the time of canal cleaning and shaping.

- Did the patient have acute signs or symptoms? Do these signs and symptoms indicate that there is significant inflammation or infection beyond the tooth into the bone or soft tissue, or is the acute process located with the confines of the tooth?
- What is the anatomic and technical complexity of the case?
- Is the canal prepared to the optimal size and shape for obturation with the technique chosen? Can spreaders, pluggers, or core carriers be placed to the appropriate depth in the root canal without binding? Can gutta-percha delivery tips or needles be placed in the canal without binding too far away from the prepared apical constriction?
- Is the canal clean and dry? Is there persistent exudate coming from the canal?
- Can the patient tolerate additional treatment time?
- Is the patient amenable to completing the treatment in one visit?

Probably the most crucial and contemporary issue in the tim-

ing of root canal obturation is the prevention of further canal contamination after cleaning and shaping. Often poorly placed temporary restorations fail within hours, and the canal systems are contaminated with oral bacteria. Interappointment endodontic emergencies are often due to the demise of the temporary restoration. Even the use of intracanal medicaments, such as calcium hydroxide, is no guarantee that bacteria will not gain or regain a foothold in the cleaned canal. Therefore in concert with the considerations stated above, the cleaned root canal should be obturated as expediently as possible to avoid further contamination.

Criteria for Determining the Adequacy of Canal Preparation Before Obturation

Although the timing of canal obturation has been discussed in the previous section, a few final issues regarding the technical adequacy of the canal preparation require attention, clarification, and emphasis:

1. The tooth must be properly isolated to eliminate all risks of canal contamination during obturation. This is an extremely important aspect of successful treatment that cannot be overlooked or regarded lightly.
2. Clean, white dentin chips are not a criterion for obturation. The appearance of the dentin chips does not guarantee they are free of bacteria or bacterial products. Likewise, it is all but impossible to sample the entire root canal system on this basis.
3. Preparing the apical portion of the canal three to four times larger than the first file to bind at the apical extent of the canal is not a criterion for obturation. It is highly unlikely that the canal is properly cleaned and shaped using this criterion. It is difficult to get irrigants into the apical portion of small canals, such as No. 20 or 25 without proper canal shaping.
4. All compacting instruments must be prefitted into the canal to determine their depth of penetration, their fit without binding, the location of binding (if any), and their appropriateness for a particular portion of the canal, especially in curved canals.
5. No type of fluid should be present in the canal before obturation. If fluids are present and they are hemorrhagic or purulent in nature, the canal may have been overinstrumented or is unclean; another canal may exist; a residual infection may be present; or the canals may have become contaminated between appointments. In any of the above situations, the source of the problem must be identified and addressed before canal obturation.
6. In multirooted teeth, all efforts must be expended to ensure that the entire canal system has been cleaned and shaped.

METHODS AND TECHNIQUES OF ROOT CANAL OBTURATION

Over the years numerous methods have been advocated to obturate the prepared root canal system, each with their own claims of ease, efficiency, or superiority. Contemporary obturation techniques are no different; although they do reflect a certain degree of sophistication and technologic advancement, contemporary techniques still rely on gutta-percha and sealer to achieve their goal—a three-dimensional filling of the cleaned and shaped root canal space. Therefore this discussion focuses on the basics of root canal obturation, with an empha-

Text continued on p. 294

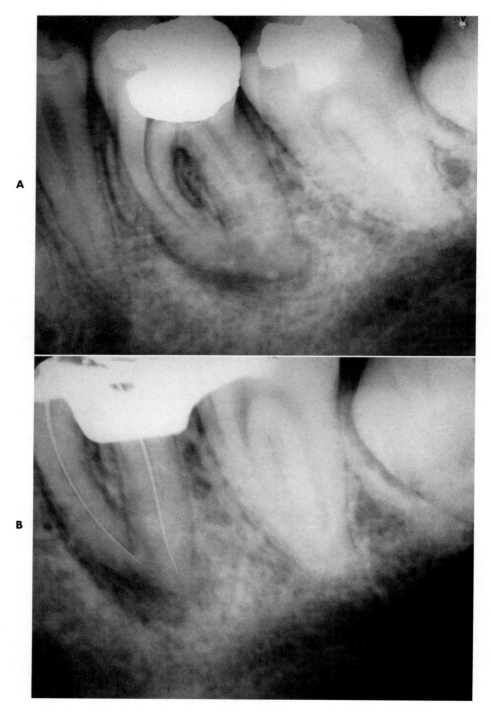

FIG. 9-21 A, Mandibular molar requiring root canal treatment. **B,** Working length determination is short of the root apex. Canals were prepared within the confines of the root.

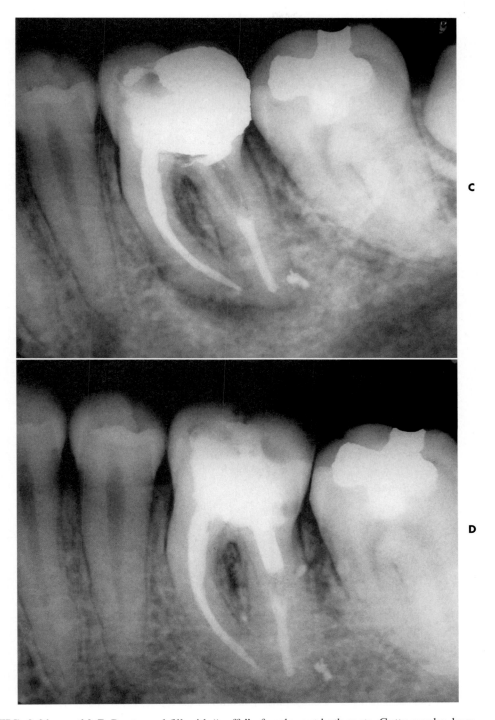

FIG. 9-21, cont'd C, Root canal fill with "puffs" of sealer out both roots. Gutta-percha, however, was retained within the root canal during obturation. **D,** Fifteen-month recall examination shows repair is almost complete, yet the sealer is still present in the periradicular tissues. *(Courtesy Dr. David Rossiter.)*

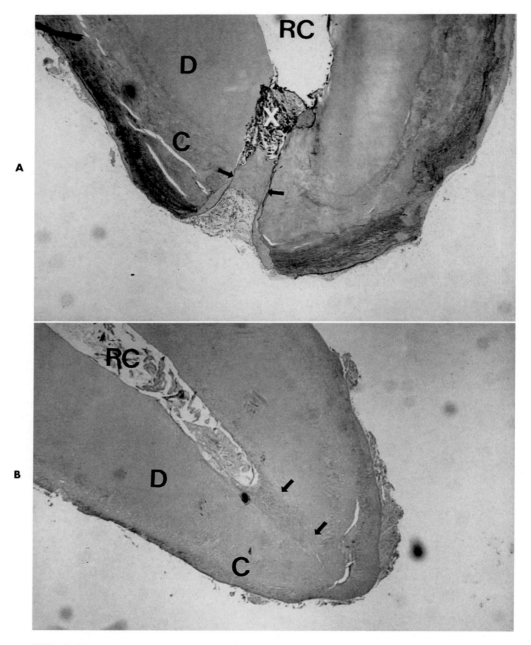

FIG. 9-22 A, Evidence of cemental regeneration *(arrows)* over the obturated root canal when the filling is retained within the root. This is even possible in the presence of debris that was packed apically. *C,* Cementum; *D,* dentin; *X,* debris; *RC,* root canal. Original magnification ×25. Stain H & E. **B,** Repair of the end of the root canal with cementum occupying 3 to 4 mm of the apical portion of the canal adjacent to a short root filling *(arrows).* *C,* Cementum; *D,* dentin; *RC,* root canal. Original magnification ×25. Stain H & E.

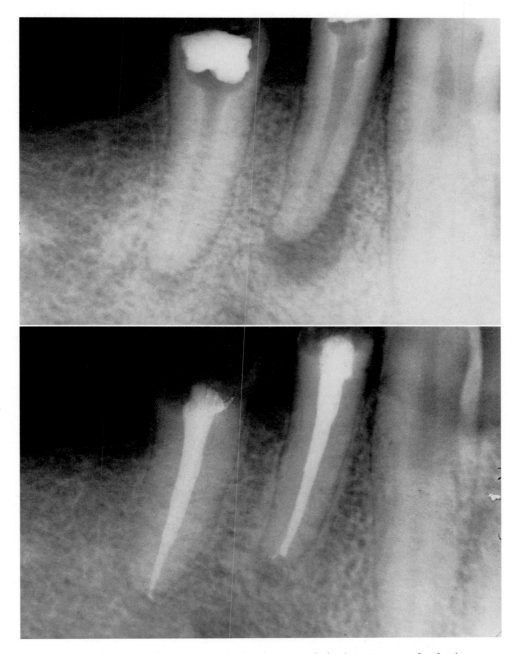

FIG. 9-23 Clinical evidence for periradicular tissue repair in the presence of pulp tissue necrosis and gutta-percha obturations that were short (within the confines of the root).

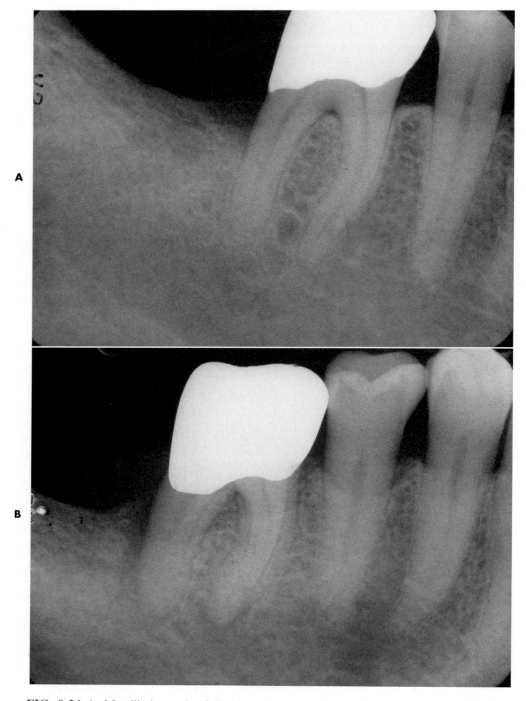

FIG. 9-24 A, Mandibular molar following placement of a gold onlay restoration. Vertical periodontal defect is present on the distal. **B,** Two years later there are radiolucencies around both roots.

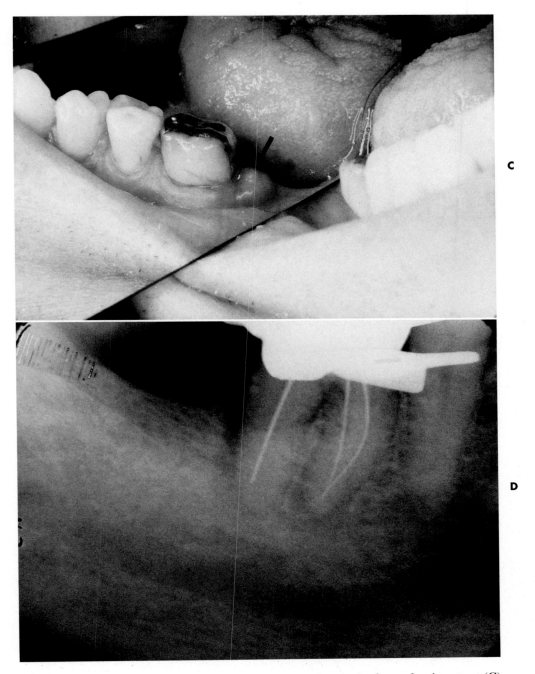

FIG. 9-24, cont'd Distal radiolucency extends to the surface in the form of a sinus tract (**C**) distal to the tooth *(arrow)*. Diagnosis: pulp necrosis with chronic suppurative periradicular periodontitis. **D,** Root canal treatment initiated with working length determination on three canals short of the radiographic apices.

Continued

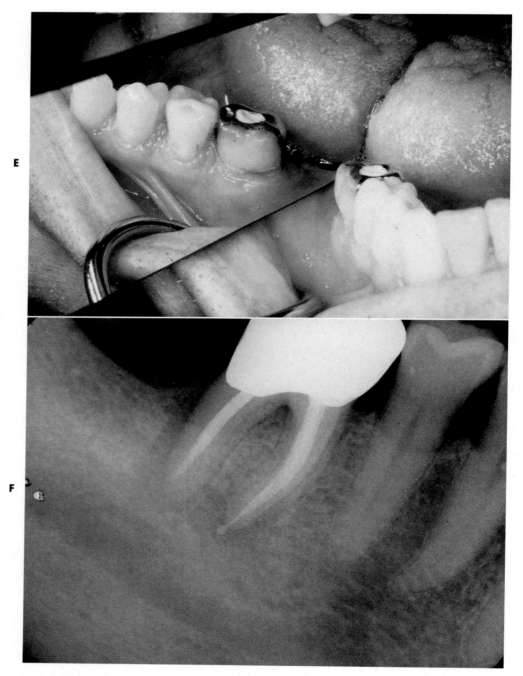

FIG. 9-24, cont'd E, One week following canal debridement shows resolution of the sinus tract. **F,** Root canal obturation with gutta-percha within the confines of the root. Small puff of sealer is extruded on the mesial root.

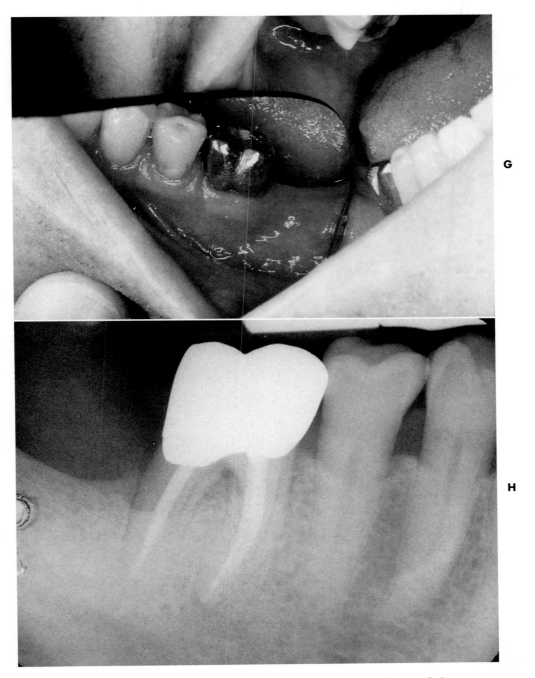

FIG. 9-24, cont'd G, Clinical evidence of repair. **H,** Radiographic evidence of almost complete healing. Patient is symptom free.

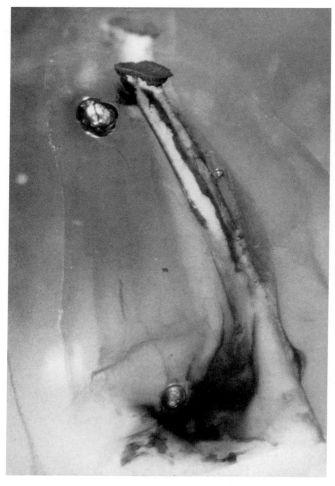

FIG. 9-25 Demineralized, dehydrated, and cleared tooth specimen from a maxillary first molar. There is significant coronal leakage through both the root canal fill and the root-end filling; the latter was placed in an attempt to resolve the patient's continued discomfort after the nonsurgical root canal treatment. Even the root-end filling could not stop the leakage and continued symptoms.

sis on techniques and variations thereof that have proven successful and easy to master.

Four basic techniques exist for the obturation of the root canal system with gutta-percha and sealer: (1) the cold compaction of gutta-percha; (2) the compaction of gutta-percha that has been heat softened in the canal and cold compacted; (3) the compaction of gutta-percha that has been thermoplasticized, injected into the system, and cold compacted; and (4) the compaction of gutta-percha that has been placed in the canal and softened through mechanical means. A multitude of variations on these four basic themes exists, and some of the creative contemporary approaches are highlighted.

Cold Compaction

Most readers identify cold compaction as being synonymous with the lateral compaction of gutta-percha. This technique is applicable to most root canals and requires a continuously tapered funnel canal preparation with an apical matrix in sound dentin.

Brief overview

The basic need for this technique is a master gutta-percha cone that corresponds to the final root canal enlarging instrument that went to the apical extent of the canal (working length). The common compacting instrument is the spreader, which comes in various sizes and should be chosen based on the canal size, length, and curvature (see Table 9-4). The spreader can be a hand or finger instrument (Figs. 9-26 and 9-27). A root canal sealer that can be mixed to a creamy consistency and has ample working time (15 to 30 minutes) is selected. The master cone is placed along with sealer in the canal, and both are compacted with the tapered metallic spreader in a lateral and vertical direction. The space created by the metallic spreader is filled with additional smaller or accessory cones that are also compacted until the canal is completely filled.

Detailed technique

Master cone selection. A master gutta-percha cone is selected based on the final prepared apical size of the root canal system. If standardized K-type and Hedström files are used for canal preparation and the canal is free of debris to the prepared apical matrix, the master cone should fit to the working length or slightly short of it (0.5 mm) (Fig. 9-28). The cone is grasped with cotton pliers at a coronal position that approximates the working length. When placed in the canal, the cone should begin to contact the canals walls in the apical 1 to 3 mm, fit snugly at the designated length, resist movement beyond the apical matrix with coronal pressure, and demonstrate a slight resistance to removal from this position when a withdrawal pressure is applied coronally. If this does not occur, the cone may be carefully trimmed with a sharp scissors, however, a scalpel is preferable,[71,99] removing 0.5 to 1 mm increments until the proper length and snugness is obtained. Sizing gauges for this purpose (Maillefer Instruments SA, Ballaigues, Switzerland) are available to assist in the proper preparation of the master cone if necessary[119] (Fig. 9-29). The final position of the cone within the tooth can be recorded by scoring the cone at the incisal or occlusal reference point with a pointed instrument or by pinching the cone with cotton pliers. Subsequently, the position of the cone is verified radiographically and evaluated as follows:

I. If the cone fits to or within 0.5 mm of the working length, if the cone demonstrates a snugness of fit in the apical 1 to 3 mm, and if there is visible on the radiograph space lateral to the master cone from the junction of the apical and middle third of the canal to the coronal orifice, compaction may proceed.

II. If the cone fits short of the desired length, the following conditions may exist:
   A. Dentin chips may be packed in the apical portion of the canal; this represents inadequate cleaning. These chips must be removed with small files[145] and copious irrigation before refitting the master cone as described in Chapter 8.
   B. The canal may be ledged at a position short of the working length. If this be the case, efforts should be made to renegotiate the canal to the full distance.[54]
   C. There may be a curve in the canal that is not visible on the two-dimensional radiograph. The anatomy of the canal must be verified, and the placement of a curved gutta-percha cone may assist in full canal penetration.   *Text continued on p. 298*

Table 9-4. Root canal spreaders

Root Canal Spreader (RCS) Code	Diameter 1 mm from the Tip (mm)	Diameter 16 mm from the Tip (mm)	Distance from the Tip to the Bend (mm)
RCS3*	0.35	0.88	24.43
RCSD11*	0.50	1.01	22.46
RCSD11S*	0.28	0.80	23.18
RCSD11T*	0.34	1.01	21.50
RCSD11TS*	0.25	1.01	20.40
RCSGP1*	0.24	0.75	20.86
RCSGP2*	0.24	0.82	23.69
RCSGP3*	0.30	0.68	28.35
RCSMA57*	0.22	0.79	26.25
RCSW1S*	0.36	0.91	19.85
RCSW2S*	0.39	0.97	18.92
RCS30*	0.30	0.70	28.10
RCS40*	0.45	0.77	28.10
RCS50*	0.50	0.85	28.10
RCS60*	0.55	0.92	28.10
S20†	0.23	0.52	28.82
S25†	0.30	0.60	28.60
S30†	0.33	0.63	28.76
S40†	0.44	0.73	28.88
S50†	0.42	0.82	28.79
S60†	0.55	0.90	28.72

*Hu-Friedy Co.
†Caulk M-series.

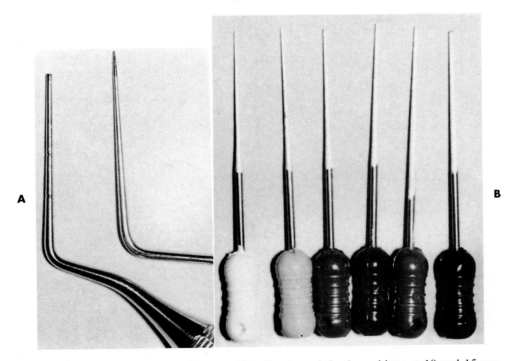

FIG. 9-26 A, *Left,* Root canal plugger with a flat tip and depth markings at 10 and 15 mm from the tip. *Right,* Root canal spreader with a pointed tip (see Tables 9-4 and 9-5). Rubber stops may be placed on the spreader at the proper length for compaction. **B,** Finger spreaders *(left)* and pluggers *(right)* on plastic handles are available from many manufacturers in both stainless steel and nickel-titanium.

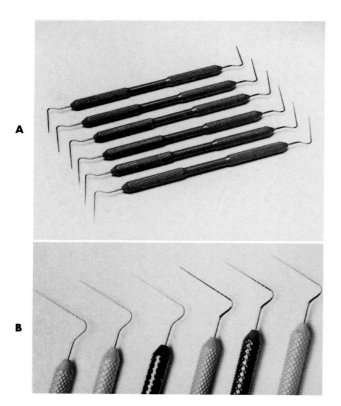

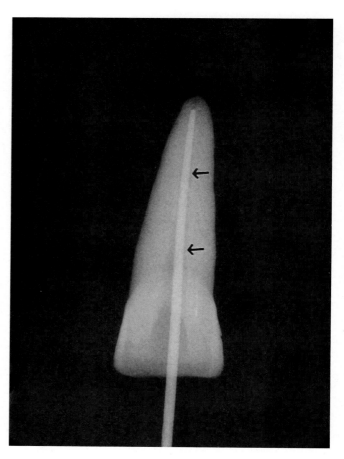

FIG. 9-27 Calibrated color-coded plugger spreaders with sizes and tapers matching the ISO standardization of root canal files. These are referred to as the "M" series as per Dr. Howard Martin. **A,** Sizes Nos. 20, 25, 30, 40, 50, and 60. One end is a spreader for lateral compaction; the other end is a plugger for vertical compaction. **B,** Close-up of the spreader end of the instrument (see Tables 9-4 and 9-5). *(Courtesy Caulk/Dentsply, Milford, Del.)*

FIG. 9-28 Placement of the master gutta-percha cone to the proper depth for lateral compaction. Note also the space visible along the lateral aspects of the cone *(arrows).* This is essential for proper depth of the compacting instrument.

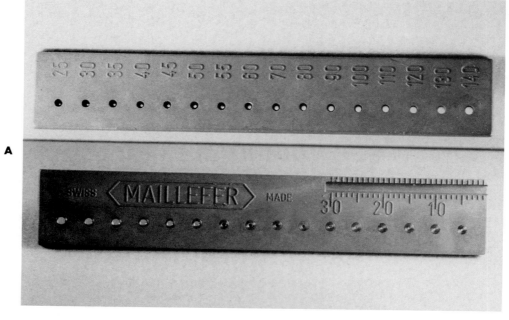

FIG. 9-29 A, Sizing instrument for gutta-percha cones.

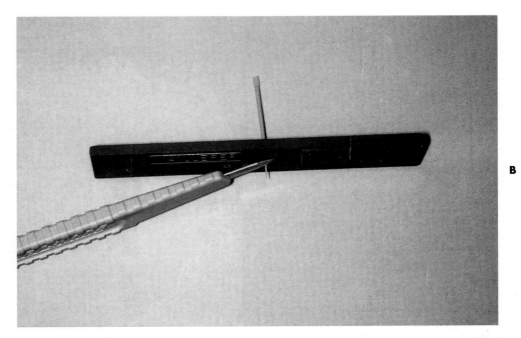

FIG. 9-29, cont'd B, Placement of a cone through the hole that represents the properly sized gutta-percha point for the canal. Excess and improperly tapered tips can be removed carefully with a scalpel blade.

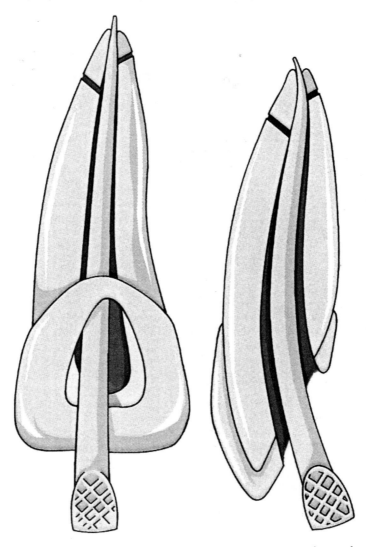

FIG. 9-30 Diagram of a master gutta-percha cone that is too long and must be trimmed or exchanged for a proper fitting cone. This can be accomplished with a scalpel and the sizing instrument.

D. The master cone selected may be too large, and a smaller cone must be selected. Sometimes cones taken from the same container may have different tapers or altered shapes. The use of the sizing instrument is helpful in this situation.

E. The most probable reason for failure to seat the cone to the prepared canal length is improper three-dimensional canal shaping in the apical to middle third of the tooth.[71] Under these circumstances the canal must be reshaped to receive the master cone to the desired length and with the desired snugness of fit.

III. If the cone fits to the proper working length, exhibits snugness of fit, but does not have space lateral to it in the coronal two thirds of the canal, the canal must be reshaped before obturation. Failure to see this space on the radiograph usually indicates that the canal is not properly shaped for adequate spreader penetration during obturation.[71] This usually results in failure to properly seat and compact the cone in the prepared apical seat.

IV. If the master cone goes beyond the working length, the cone can either be cut as previously described or a new, larger cone can be selected (Fig. 9-30). However, with a larger cone also comes a larger taper, that may minimize the amount of lateral space available for spreader penetration in a given canal. Also with the selection of a larger cone in a curved canal, the cone tends to bind too far coronally because of the constricted canal shape at the bend.

V. If the cone goes to length and exhibits snugness of fit clinically yet there is space visible alongside the cone in the apical third but not in the coronal two thirds, either the cone is improperly shaped and sized for the preparation or the canal is not properly shaped in the coronal two thirds of the canal.

VI. If the cone goes to length and radiographically exhibits a wiggly or S-shaped appearance, the cone is too small for the canal and a larger cone must be selected (Fig. 9-31).

Canal preparation. Once the master cone has been properly fit, it is removed from the canal and placed in a sterilizing solution of 70% isopropyl alcohol or 2.5% to 5% sodium hypochlorite (NaOCL). The canal system is then dried with paper points. If the smear layer is to be removed, appropriate solutions are used at this time (refer to Smear Layer Removal Versus Smear Layer Retention). Some authors recommend the removal of all residual moisture by rinsing the canal with 95% ethyl alcohol or 99% isopropyl alcohol.[134] The alcohol is left in the canal for 2 to 3 minutes and then removed with additional sterile paper points.

Compactor selection. Before sealer placement, the compacting instruments are chosen. Sterile (or thoroughly disinfected) compacting instruments should be used during the cleaning and shaping phase to determine if the proper shape has been prepared for depth of instrument placement.

Lateral compaction is achieved with a hand spreader or finger spreader (see Table 9-4). The instrument chosen should be able to reach the canal working length without binding in an empty canal (Fig. 9-32). This implies the need for both proper length and taper of the compacting instrument relative to ca-

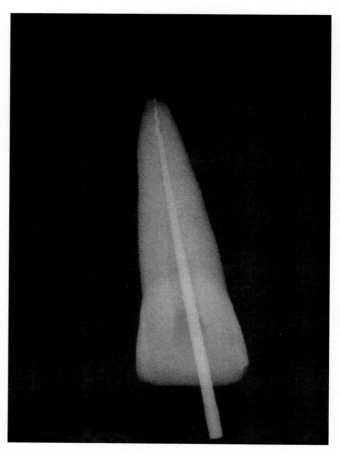

FIG. 9-31 Improperly fit cone that is too small apically. When the irregular appearance is obvious radiographically or clinically a differently sized and shaped cone must be chosen.

nal shape, size, and curvature (Table 9-5). In curved canals a stainless steel instrument can be curved before placement in the canal (Fig. 9-33), or a nickel-titanium instrument can be used (see Fig. 9-15). Whenever possible a rubber stop should be placed on the instrument at the working length. This is not necessary when the metallic instrument is already scored with specific length markers.

Sealer placement. Following the selection of the compacting instrument and the drying of the canal, the root canal sealer is placed in the canal. The effective distribution of root canal sealers throughout the root canal system has been suggested as essential to obtain the best possible root canal seal.[43] Various methods of sealer placement have been identified or evaluated for this purpose, including lentula spirals,[5,91,208] files or reamers,[5,91,208] master gutta-percha cones,[5,208] and ultrasonic instruments.[91,189,208] Evaluation of the efficacy of these techniques has occurred on extracted teeth, using serial sectioning, radiographs, specimen clearing and direct observation, and in the clinical setting. Parameters of sealer distribution used for evaluation have included percentages of dentin walls covered, sealer extrusion beyond the apical foramen, demonstration of accessory canals, and voids in the sealer coverage. Clinician expertise in using a particular placement technique must also be considered.

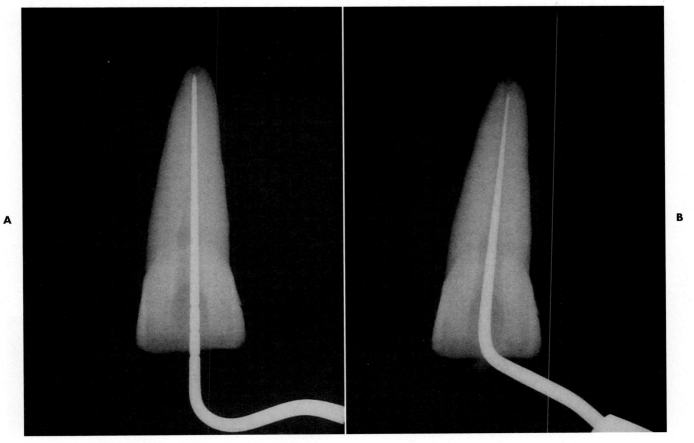

FIG. 9-32 **A,** Improperly fit spreader. Note the instrument occupies the entire canal space and may more than likely wedge between the canal walls. **B,** Properly fit spreader, demonstrating looseness of fit and proper depth of placement.

With cold lateral compaction the use of the master cone, a file, or a lentula to place the sealer is very acceptable (Fig. 9-34). For the best distribution of sealer, however, placement with an ultrasonic instrument may be considered.[188] Whatever vehicle is chosen, it is lightly coated with the sealer and placed in the canal, distributing the sealer evenly over the prepared walls. In larger canals this may have to be done more than once. For lateral compaction the sealer is to be placed to the working length of the canal. The complete filling of the canal with sealer should be avoided, as additional sealer is generally carried to the canal during compaction on the accessory gutta-percha cones. If an ultrasonic file is used, the instrument is lightly coated with the sealer, placed in the canal, and energized for 5 seconds while moving the file in a circumferential motion.[188] Subsequently, a master cone, lightly coated with sealer, is placed directly to the apical matrix (Fig. 9-35).

Master cone placement. Slow insertion of the master gutta-percha cone is necessary for thorough sealer distribution, the dissipation of trapped air, the lateral and coronal movement of the sealer, and the minimization of sealer extrusion beyond the apical foramen. Once in place, as evidenced by the relationship of the scored master cone to the occlusal or incisal reference point, the cone is held in place for 20 to 30 seconds to secure its position apically. If the patient has not been anes-thetized, the movement of trapped air or sealer apically may cause momentary discomfort. Advising the patient ahead of time of the possibility is essential. If there is any doubt as to the position of the master cone and sealer and a slow-setting sealer has been used, radiographic verification can be done at this time. If necessary, the cone can be removed and reposi-tioned according to its desired position.

Master cone compaction. Subsequent to master cone placement, the spreader is slowly inserted alongside the mas-ter cone, either to the working length marked on the spreader or to within 0.5 to 1 mm of this length (Fig. 9-36). As previ-ously discussed, failure to achieve this depth may result in lack of adaptation of the master gutta-percha cone to the prepared apical seat. Although it is recognized that master gutta-percha cones can be elongated and moved apically,[215] there is no tech-nique that can consistently provide for this occurrence because of variations in the shaping of the canal system and the nature of the gutta-percha cones used. The potential of root fracture with this approach has been previously discussed,[92,134,151] and with proper canal shaping and choice of tapered spreader be-fore canal obturation, the wedging forces that have been iden-tified by many authors are insignificant.

As the spreader reaches the desired depth, the master gutta-percha cone is laterally and vertically compacted, moving the

Table 9-5. Suggested spreaders and pluggers corresponding to master gutta-percha cones

Final Apical Size	Recommended Spreader (Hand or Corresponding Finger Spreader)	Recommended Plugger (Hand or Corresponding Finger Plugger)
25	D11S, D11TS, GP1, GP2, W1S, S20, S25 (depending on canal taper and length)	P30, 8, 8A, ⅓ (depending on canal taper, length and desired depth of penetration)
30	Same as for No. 25 except use S30; MA57 or GP3 can be used in long canals >25 mm	P30, 8, 8A, ⅓
35	Same as for No. 25 except use D11T or S35	P30, 8, 8A, ⅓
40	D11T, GP2, W2S, S40	P40, 8, 8A, ⅓
45	D11T, GP2 or GP3, S40	P40, 8½, 8½A, ⅓
50	D11, D11T, GP2 or GP3. S50	P50, 9, 9A or 9½, 9½A, PL1
55	D11, S3, S50	P50, 9, 9A or 9½, 9½A, PL2
60	D11, S3, S60	P60, 9, 9A or 9½, 9½A
70	D11, S3, S70	P70, 9½, 9½A, 10, 10A, 10½, 10½A, 5/7
80	D11, S3, S80	P80, 10, 10A, 10½, 10½A, PL3, 5/7
90	D11, S3, S80	P80, 10, 10A, 10½, 10½A, PL3, 5/7
100	D11, S3, S80	P80, 10, 10A, 10½, 10½A, PL3, 9/11
110	D11, MA 57, S3, S80	PL3 or PL4, 9/11, 11, 11½, 11A, 11½A, or higher

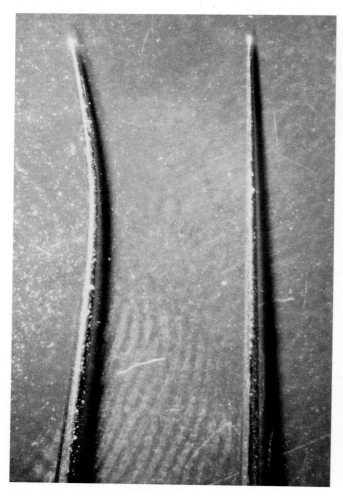

FIG. 9-33 Spreader shapes can be easily changed before entry into curved canals. This facilitates depth of penetration and gutta-percha compaction.

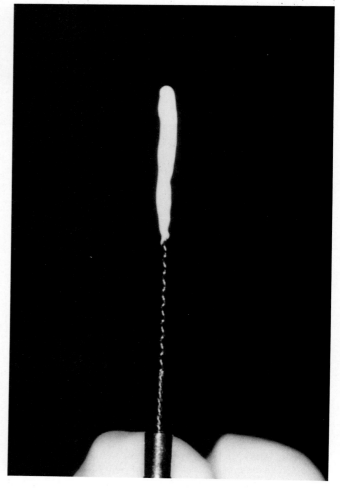

FIG. 9-34 The use of a lentula for the placement of the root canal sealer. Do not use excessive amounts in the canal system with any technique.

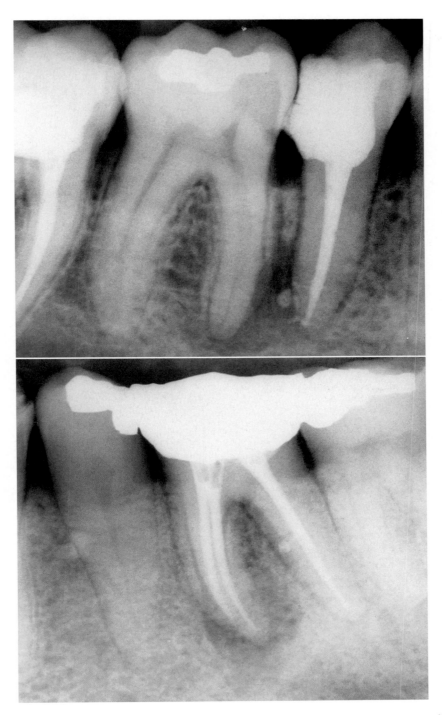

FIG. 9-35 Two examples of root canal obturation in which the smear layer was removed, the sealer was placed with an ultrasonic device, and the canals were obturated using the lateral compaction of gutta-percha. Both cases are filled within the confines of the canal with significant dispersal of sealer into accessory channels. This result can occur with any technique that encourages smear layer removal and the proper dispersion of sealer. *(Courtesy Dr. David Stamos.)*

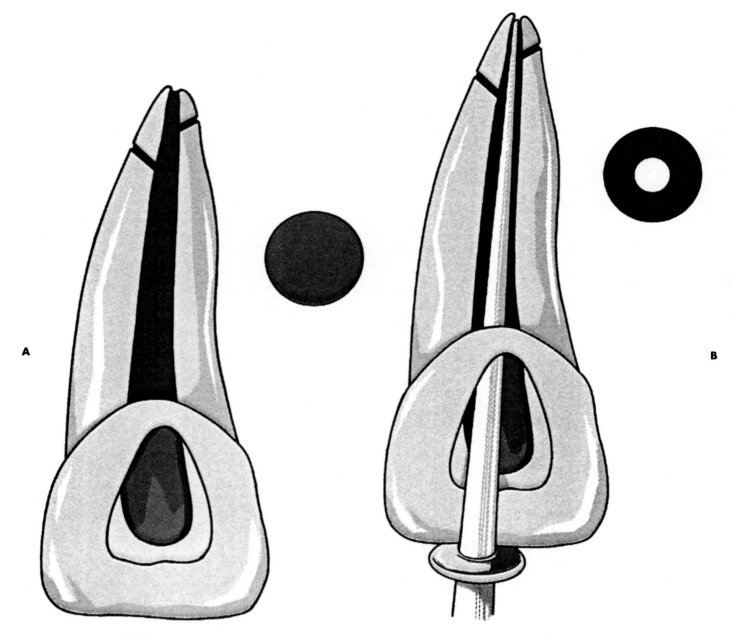

FIG. 9-36 A, Diagram of prepared canal system in the shape of a funnel. **B,** Spreader fit to the proper depth. Note the space available adjacent to the spreader. This instrument must reach the proper apical depth without binding.

instrument in a 180-degree arc. In curved canals this arc is reduced relative to the degree of canal curvature.[71] During this movement the cone is compacted against a particular canal wall while at the same time space is created lateral to the master cone for additional accessory gutta-percha cones (Fig. 9-37).

Placement of accessory cones. Accessory cones are chosen based on the size of the spreader used along with the size of the canal and the position of the space created in the canal (Table 9-6). For example, to the depth of the first spreader penetration, an accessory cone in the range of *extra-fine* to *fine-fine* is used. Both of these cone sizes match well with a D11T or D11TS hand spreader or a No. 25 or 30 finger spreader. Other combinations of spreaders and specific cone sizes also exist and are seen in Table 9-6. The accessory cone is lightly coated with sealer and placed to the same length that the compacting instrument was placed (Fig. 9-38). If this is not possible, the following conditions may be present:

- The accessory cone is too large or is improperly tapered for the space provided.
- The spreader is too small and does not match well with the accessory cone.
- The compaction of the master cone was insufficient to create usable space for an accessory.
- The canal lacks the necessary taper for proper penetration of both the spreader and accessory cone.

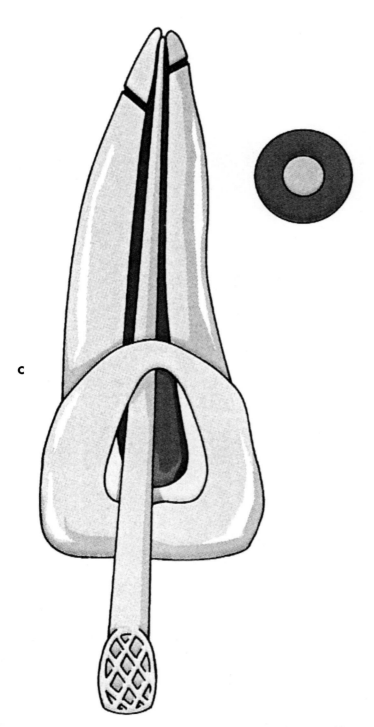

FIG. 9-36, cont'd C, Fit of master gutta-percha cone. Note how this cone binds only in the apical portion of the prepared root.

- The master cone may have been dislodged during the initial compaction.
- The small end of the accessory cone may have curled up or become bent in the canal preventing full penetration of the cone.
- The sealer may have begun to harden, which prevents placement of the accessory cone.

Each of these potential problems with the placement of acces-

Table 9-6. Recommended accessory cone sizes corresponding to the chosen spreader

Spreader	Recommended Accessory Cones
D11TS, GP1 and GP2, S20, MA57	Extra fine or size No. 20
D11TS, D11T, GP3, S25	Fine fine or sizes No. 20 or 25
D11T, S3, W1S, W2S, S30	Fine or size No. 25
D11, S40, S50	Medium fine
Not recommended as accessory cones for lateral compaction	Fine medium, medium, large medium, and large

sory cones must be assessed and corrective action taken when appropriate. Failure to place the accessory cones to the proper depth results in significant voids throughout the canal. These may be discrete radiolucencies or longitudinal voids referred to as spreader tracks. In either case the obturation is below the standard of care outlined earlier in this chapter. If necessary, corrections can be made in most situations by removing the already compacted gutta-percha, recleaning the canal, determining the causative agent for the problem, eliminating it, and refilling the canal.

As the canal becomes obturated with accessory gutta-percha cones apically, the space that is created in the canal moves more coronally (Fig. 9-39). Generally, this space is more tapered and larger accessory cones, such as a *medium fine* or *fine,* may be used depending on the prepared anatomy of the canal. Accessory cones often have very fine tips that may be easily bent, either in their original container or during manipulation. Some clinicians prefer to remove the very fine tip before obturation. Likewise, some clinicians prefer to remove the coronal aspect of the accessory cone before compaction, creating custom accessory cones with lengths appropriate for the canal to be obturated. This is especially helpful in posterior teeth or when access to canals and their orifices are limited.

When removing the spreader from a canal during compaction, the instrument again should be moved in a 180-degree arc,[71] only without compacting pressure. During the movement a light but steady coronal pressure should be applied to loosen the spreader without dislodging the compacted cones. Here also, if the canal is curved, the arc of movement should be limited to approximately 90 degrees or less. Some authors claim that the use of finger spreaders may prevent the dislodging of the gutta-percha because a greater rotation can be used during removal without detriment to the already compacted mass.[178]

Completion of obturation and management of the pulp chamber. The canal is filled with accessory cones until the spreader can penetrate only 2 to 3 mm into the canal orifice (Fig. 9-40). At this point a heated instrument (Glick No. 1 or heater-plugger) or special heating device (Touch n' Heat, EIE/Analytic Technology, San Diego, Calif.) is used to sear off the extended ends of the accessory cones and soften the gutta-percha in the coronal portion of the canal. This is followed by vertical compaction with root canal pluggers (Table 9-7) to adapt the coronal gutta-percha to the canal walls and to enhance the coronal seal of the canal.[11] Pluggers used in this manner must not be wedged between the canal walls. This requires the careful fitting of a plugger into the coronal portion of the canal before obturation. Spreaders are not to be heated and

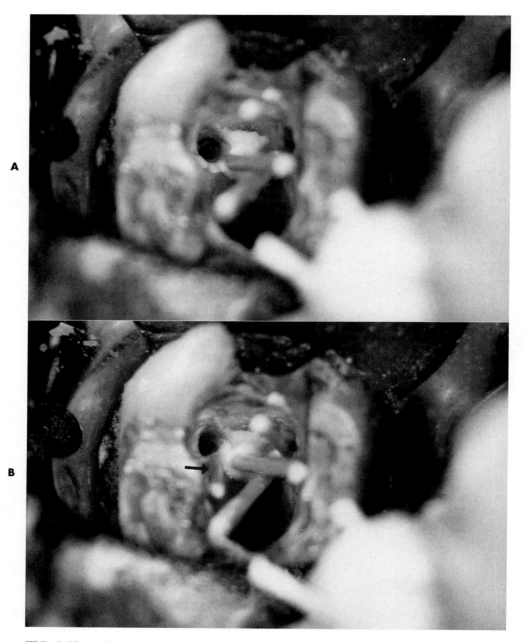

FIG. 9-37 A, Mesiobuccal canal of a mandibular first molar. Master gutta-percha cone has been laterally compacted with sealer. Note how the cone has been moved against the wall of the canal, making room for additional accessory cones. **B,** Following compaction with one accessory cone *(arrow);* note again the space available for additional cones due to the true lateral movement of the gutta-percha during compaction. Failure to do this results in a poorly filled canal.

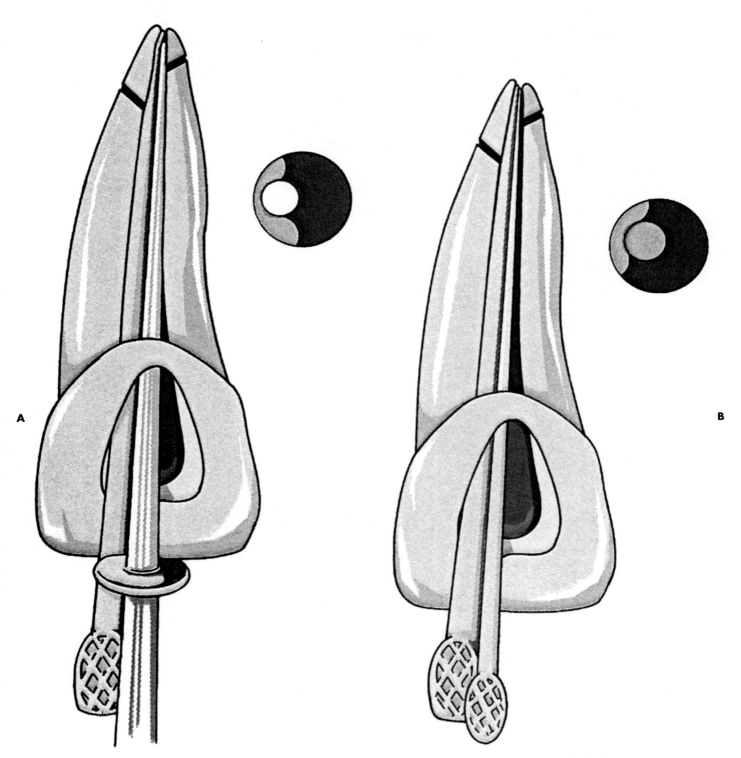

FIG. 9-38 A, Spreader is placed alongside the master cone to the proper apical depth.
B, Following careful removal of the spreader, an accessory cone lightly coated with sealer is
placed to the apical depth created by the spreader.

A

B

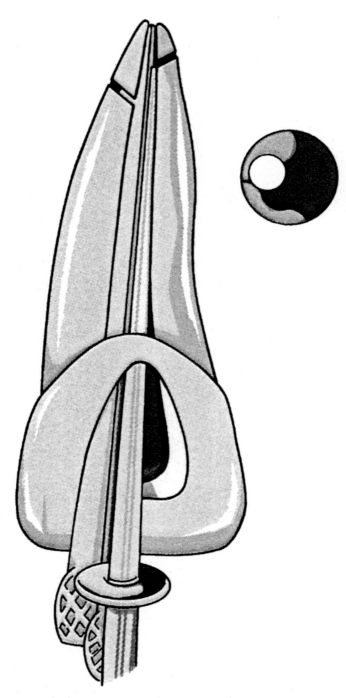

FIG. 9-39 As the obturation process is continued, the depth of apical penetration of the spreader is lessened and the accessory cones gradually obturate the canal.

used to remove the gutta-percha because no effective contemporary spreader made of metal is designed to be heated while at the same time to be used further as a spreader. Likewise, the use of endodontic spoon excavators has also been advocated for this purpose, but these also are not designed to be heated, with their prime purposes being to excavate caries and remove pulp tissue efficiently.

Once the gutta-percha has been compacted coronally, the pulp chamber is cleaned thoroughly with cotton pellets soaked

in alcohol to remove remnants of unset sealer and particles of gutta-percha. A substantial temporary restoration is placed; or in some situations an immediate post space is created (Fig. 9-41) (see Chapter 21), and a permanent restoration is initiated. A final radiograph, without the rubber dam in position, is taken from an angle that adequately demonstrates the obturation of each canal (Figs. 9-42 and 9-43).

Variations in the cold lateral compaction technique. Variations within the above description are common and are usually based on anatomic irregularities, clinician-induced errors, or personal choices. Because of the variations used many of these techniques have become known as "hybrid techniques." Some of the more common variations include the following:

- Apical adaptation techniques for the master cone with solvents. This concept has been discussed previously, and the technique is often referred to as the "direct impression technique."[34] This technique has many variations, some of which are dictated by the size of the apical preparation or canal curvature.[21]
- Canal obturation with lateral compaction in the apical one third only, followed by the searing off of the extended cones and obturation of the coronal portion of the canal with either segments of warmed gutta-percha vertically compacted or the injection of thermally softened gutta-percha and vertical compaction (see subsequent sections).
- Canal obturation with lateral compaction to the canal orifice, followed by a segmental removal of gutta-percha with concomitant vertical compaction to the apical third of the canal. The coronal two thirds is then refilled with either lateral or vertical compaction.
- Placement of artificial barriers as previously discussed that may also include collagen-based sponges, such as Colla-Cote or CollaPlug (CollaTec Inc., Plainsboro, N.J.). This is more common in cases of apexification or when the apical matrix has been destroyed through overinstrumentation.
- Canal obturation with lateral compaction in the apical one third only, followed by the thermomechanical compaction of the accessory cones that extend from the canal.[193]
- Seating of the master cone, removal of the coronal portion of the cone with heat, followed by a vertical compaction of the apical segment. The remainder of the canal is obturated with the standard lateral compaction.[62]
- Placement of the compacting spreader to length adjacent to the master cone and waiting for approximately 1 minute for the master cone to adapt to the apical portion of the canal.[162] This technique is especially advocated when a sealer that contains a gutta-percha softening agent such as eucalyptol is used (see Table 9-2). During the softening of the gutta-percha the pressure applied by the compacting instrument adapts the cone to the canal walls.
- Compaction of gutta-percha with a warm lateral technique using a device known as the Endotec (Caulk/Dentsply, Milford, Del.).[122] As with the chemical softening of specific sealers, this technique favors a more homogeneous mass of compacted gutta-percha.[113] The technique is time consuming relative to other methods of lateral compaction, and the equipment comes with a limited number of sized tips for heat distribution.[89] Even though the tips appear to be similar to a root canal spreader, it is difficult to apply compaction forces with these tips and their use is primarily for heating the gutta-percha cones in the tooth.
- Ultrasonic compaction of gutta-percha cones has also

Text continued on p. 312

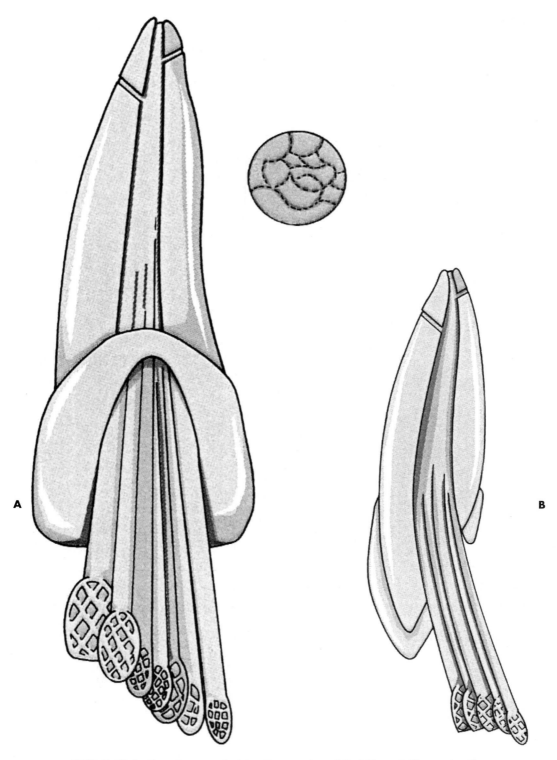

FIG. 9-40 A, Complete canal obturation as viewed facially and, **B,** proximally.

Table 9-7. Root canal pluggers

Root Canal Plugger (RCP) Code	Diameter at the Tip (mm)	Diameter 16 mm from the Tip (mm)	Distance from the Tip to the Bend (mm)
RCP30*	0.33	0.66	27.96
RCP40*	0.41	0.70	27.82
RCP50*	0.53	0.82	27.78
RCP60*	0.63	0.94	27.72
RCP8A*	0.44	1.10	22.50
RCP8½A*	0.48	1.12	21.40
RCP9A*	0.55	1.11	22.00
RCP9½A*	0.66	1.11	22.10
RCP10A*	0.78	1.11	22.50
RCP10½A*	0.91	1.18	22.60
RCP11A*	1.04	1.27	22.60
RCP11½A*	1.18	1.35	22.90
RCP12A*	1.32	1.40	22.40
RCP8*	0.40	1.09	21.38
RCP8½*	0.50	1.20	21.49
RCP9*	0.55	1.18	21.45
RCP9½*	0.65	1.25	22.40
RCP10*	0.82	1.22	22.60
RCP10½*	0.90	1.20	22.30
RCP11*	1.05	1.33	21.75
RCP11½*	1.25	1.30	21.80
RCP12*	1.40	1.40	22.90
RCP*1*/3*	0.42	0.98	21.20
RCP1/*3**	0.52	1.02	21.13
RCP*5*/7*	0.56	1.05	21.21
RCP5/*7**	0.79	1.13	21.13
RCP*9*/11*	1.05	1.33	21.24
RCP9/*11**	1.17	1.32	21.09
RCPL1*	0.51	1.19	18.76
RCPL2*	0.53	1.05	18.80
RCPL3*	0.80	1.29	18.33
RCPL4*	1.07	1.37	16.94
P30†	0.33	0.66	27.39
P40†	0.39	0.72	28.69
P50†	0.52	0.84	28.74
P60†	0.62	0.92	27.59
P70†	0.73	1.02	28.42
P80†	0.80	1.12	28.60

Heat Transfer Instrument Code	Diameter 1 mm from the Tip (mm)	Diameter 16 mm from the Tip (mm)	Distance from the Tip to the Bend (mm)
RCS00P*	0.42	1.03	24.66
RCS0P*	0.38	0.87	22.65

*Hu-Friedy Co.
†Caulk M-series.
Italics and bold indicate end being measured.
RCP8A to RCP12A and RCP8 to RCP12 represent the Schilder-type pluggers. The "A" designation refers to pluggers for anterior teeth; the others are designated for posterior teeth. RCS00P and RCS0P represent the Schilder-type heat transfer instrument.

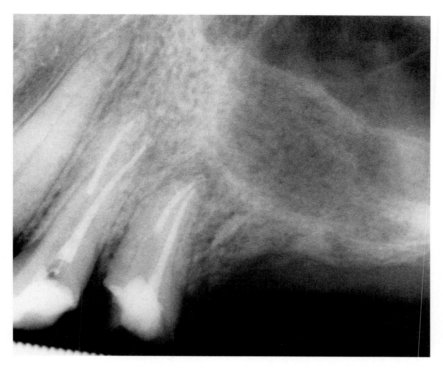

FIG. 9-41 Following lateral compaction, post space is readily made. Immediate restoration of root canal–treated teeth is recommended to prevent coronal leakage and to protect the weakened tooth structure.

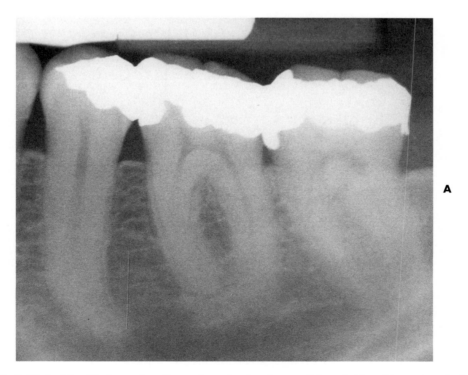

FIG. 9-42 A, Mandibular molar diagnosis as having irreversible pulpitis with acute apical periodontitis.   *Continued*

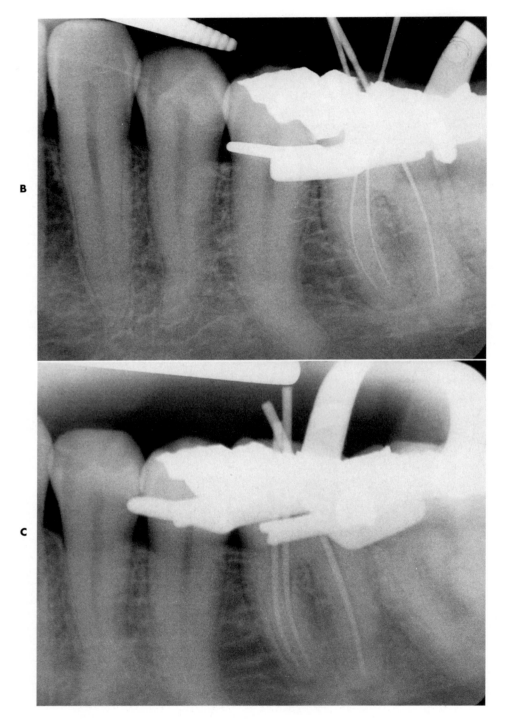

FIG. 9-42, cont'd B, Working length determination within the confines of the root. **C,** Fitting of master cones in all three roots. Note the space adjacent to the length of the cones for the compaction instrument.

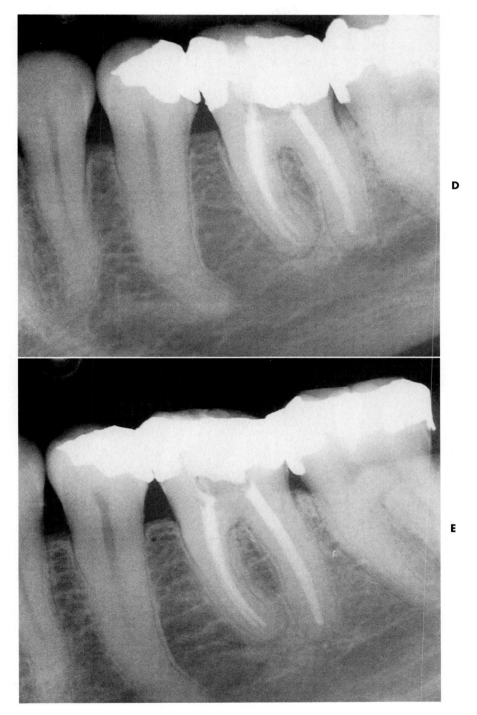

FIG. 9-42, cont'd D, Root canal obturation with lateral compaction and a zinc oxide–eugenol–based sealer; filling material retained within the canal. **E,** Twelve-month recall examination indicating good periradicular healing. Patient is clinically symptom free.

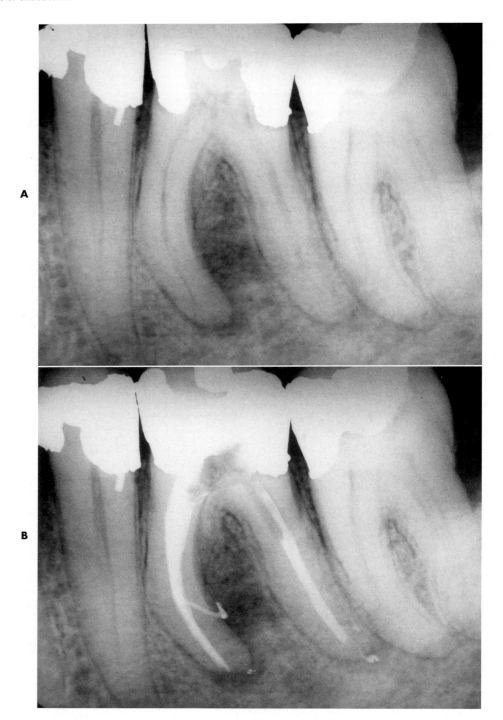

FIG. 9-43 A, Mandibular molar exhibiting significant bone destruction in the periradicular tissues. **B,** Canals were cleaned, shaped, and obturated using lateral compaction, gutta-percha, and a zinc oxide-eugenol–based sealer. Major lateral canal is obturated using this technique. *(Courtesy Dr. David P. Rossiter.)*

been suggested; however, little attention has been paid to developing a standardized and reliable technique with this variation.[9,131]

Anatomic considerations. The anatomic complexities that may demand variations in the delivery of cold laterally compacted gutta-percha deserve a brief mention. These include C-shaped canals that have a wide variation of canal anastomo-

ses, webbings, and irregular communications. Commonly found in second molars, these canal systems are much better obturated using techniques that heat soften the gutta-percha and enhance its movement into the canal irregularities (Fig. 9-44). Hybrid techniques may also be better suited for S-shaped canals (see Fig. 9-19, *B*) because of the double curvature and limited safe penetration with stainless steel compactors. Pri-

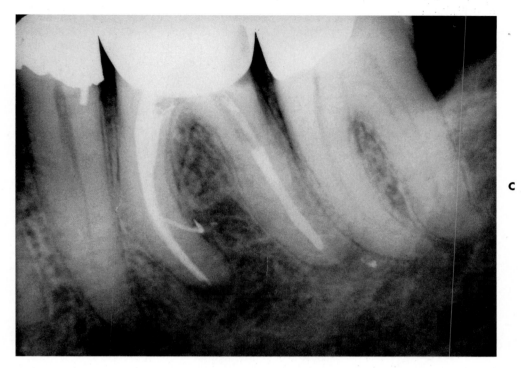

FIG. 9-43, cont'd C, Twelve-month recall indicates that repair is almost complete.

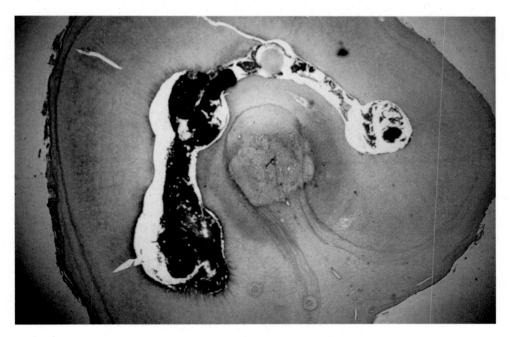

FIG. 9-44 Histologic view of a C-shaped canal. Note the irregularities and visualize how difficult it would be to obturate this type of system with lateral compaction.

marily found in maxillary second premolars, one solution may be to use nickel-titanium spreaders with these anatomic variations or consider a hybrid technique. The nickel-titanium spreaders are also highly recommended with severely curved root canal systems. Internal resorption also poses a challenge for strictly cold lateral compaction. Here again, variations are necessary based on the extent of the defect and often require a segmental warm or injectable warm gutta-percha technique (see subsequent sections) (Fig. 9-45). Root ends with resorptive defects, delta formations, or numerous apical openings may benefit through the use of apical impression techniques in conjunction with cold lateral compaction of gutta-percha.

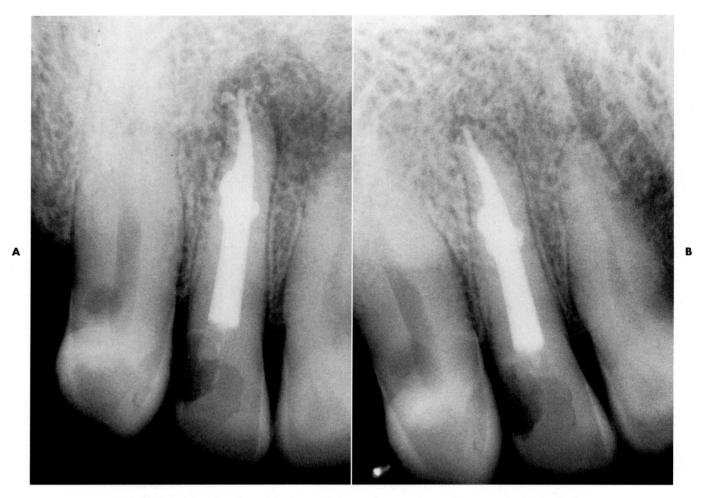

FIG. 9-45 A, Maxillary lateral incisor with internal resorption and large periradicular lesion. Canal was obturated gutta-percha and sealer using primarily lateral compaction. Heat softening of the filling material in the middle third helps to achieve a three-dimensional fill of the resorptive defect. **B,** Eighteen-month recall shows almost complete osseous repair. Patient is symptom free. *(Courtesy Dr. Paul Lovdahl.)*

Finally, obturation of canals following apexification requires a modification of the master gutta-percha cone to better adapt to the irregularly formed apical matrix or barrier. This may be accomplished by heat or chemical softening of commercially available large cones or the creation of a large custom cone. The details of each technique are as follows:

Chemical softening and adaptation. The apical 2 to 3 mm of a slightly oversized master cone is placed in a solvent such as chloroform, methylchloroform, rectified white turpentine, or eucalyptol for about 3 to 5 seconds, removed, and placed into the canal until the working length is achieved with a good apical fit (Fig. 9-46, *A* and *B*). The position of the cone in the canal is marked with regard to depth of placement and orientation to curves. This can be done by scoring the cone with either a cotton forceps or an explorer. It is always best to fit the cone in a canal when an irrigant is present to prevent the adherence of the softened gutta-percha to the canal walls and to moderate the action of the solvent. Once properly fit, the cone is checked radiographically (see Fig. 9-46, *B*), removed, and thoroughly irrigated with sterile water to eliminate any residual solvent. Alcohol can also be used to remove the sol-

vents. Let the master cone dry for 1 or 2 minutes before cementation and compaction.

Heat softening and adaptation. In place of a chemical solvent, heated water can be used to soften the apical portion of the master cone before it is placed in the canal.[71] The cone is dipped into the water (100° F to 120° F; 37.8° to 48.8° C) for 2 to 4 seconds to soften only the outer layers of the apical portion of the cone. The coronal portion of the cone remains firm and serves as a mechanical plunger to seat the softened cone into the prepared apical matrix (Fig. 9-47, *A* through *C*). Radiographic verification of the position of the cone and scoring of the cone for orientation are necessary before the cone is removed from the canal (see Fig. 9-47, *B*). Normal compaction procedures are then instituted, which may be pure cold lateral compaction (see Fig. 9-47, *C*) or a hybrid variation thereof.

Development of custom cone. Two or more cones, either standardized, nonstandardized, or a combination of the two, are chosen depending on the shape of the canal (Fig. 9-48, *A*). The cones are softened with a light amount of heat until they become tacky and adhere to each other (Fig. 9-48, *B*). The cones are rolled and fused together between two glass slabs to the

Text continued on p. 318

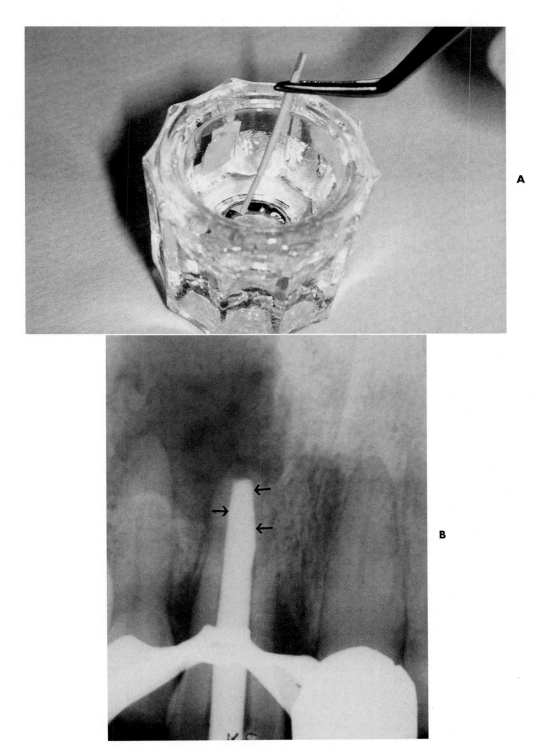

FIG. 9-46 A, Master gutta-percha cone is placed in a solvent for 2 to 3 seconds to soften the external surface of the cone. **B,** Radiographic appearance of the softened cone as it has adapted to the large, irregular canal space *(arrows).*

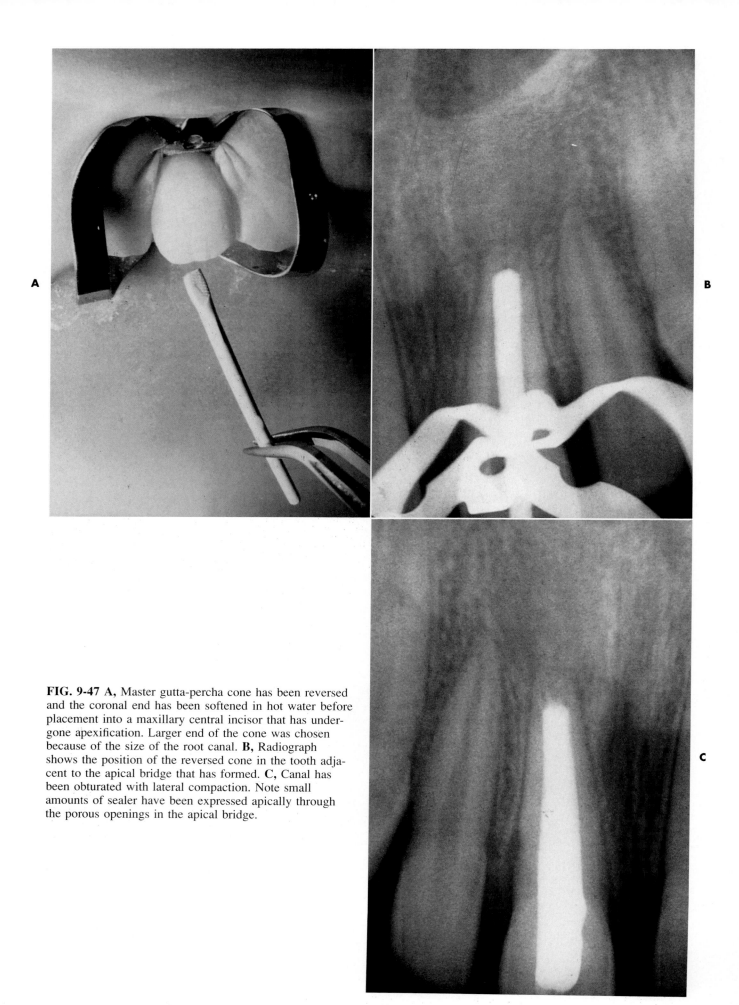

FIG. 9-47 A, Master gutta-percha cone has been reversed and the coronal end has been softened in hot water before placement into a maxillary central incisor that has undergone apexification. Larger end of the cone was chosen because of the size of the root canal. **B,** Radiograph shows the position of the reversed cone in the tooth adjacent to the apical bridge that has formed. **C,** Canal has been obturated with lateral compaction. Note small amounts of sealer have been expressed apically through the porous openings in the apical bridge.

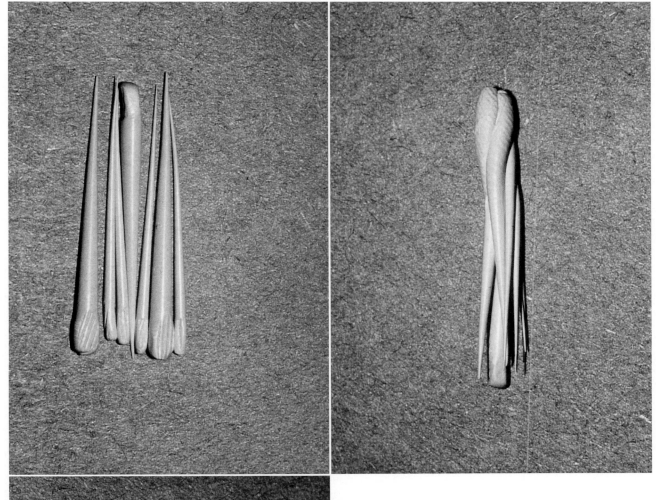

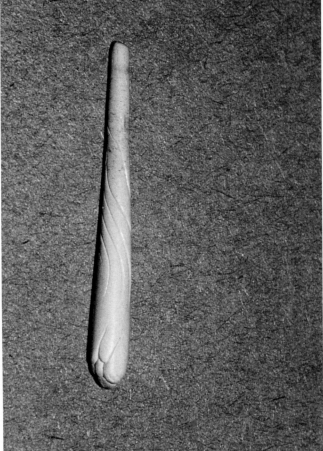

FIG. 9-48 A, Custom cones can be fabricated by fusing multiple cones together, softening the mass, and shaping the newly formed cone to fit the root canal to be obturated. Size and shape of the canal determine the type of cones to be fused. In this case, nonstandardized cones have been selected. **B,** Cones are softened with heat and the fusion begins. With continued warming the mass is rolled between two sterile glass slabs. Angle of the top slab to the bottom slab determines the shape or taper of the canal, whereas the amount of pressure on the slab determines the thickness of the cone at any point along its length. **C,** Example of variably shaped cones.

Continued

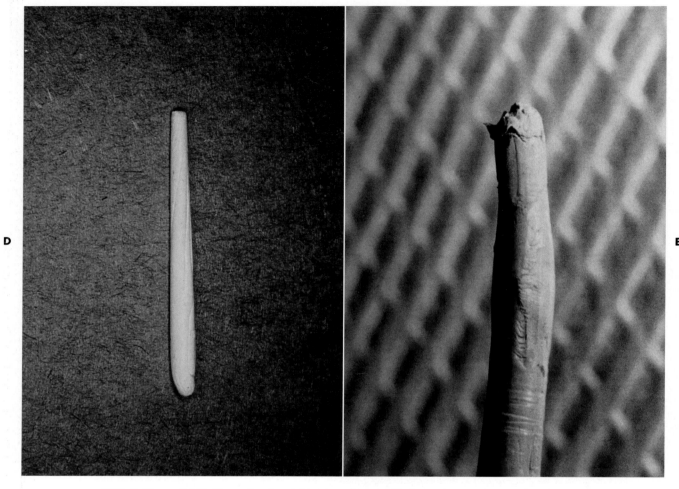

D

E

FIG. 9-48, cont'd D, Example of variably shaped cones. **E,** Once shaped, the apical portion of the cone is softened with heat or chemicals and placed to the apical position within the root canal. Note this cone has been adapted to the canal irregularities both apically and laterally.

desired shape and taper[70,71] (Fig. 9-48, *C* and *D*). Finally, the apical portion of the cone is softened, either with chemicals or heat, and adapted to the irregular shape of the apical portion of the canal (Fig. 9-48, *E*). Subsequent canal obturation can be with either lateral or vertical compaction (Fig. 9-49).

Compaction of Heat-Softened Gutta-Percha

The concept of thermoplasticized compaction is not new and covers any technique that is based entirely on the heat softening of gutta-percha combined primarily with vertical compaction. In its purest form it is similar to lateral compaction, only the material is heated and adapted to the prepared root canal with vertical compaction. In some circles it has been referred to as a warm sectional technique, vertical compaction with warmed gutta-percha, or the Schilder technique.[170] The essential elements of the technique have been with us for almost a century,[202] with entrepreneurial efforts shaping its contemporary evolution and form.[14,170]

Brief overview

A master gutta-percha cone is chosen that approximates the length and shape of the prepared canal. The cone is fit snugly to within 1 to 2 mm of the apical extent of the preparation depending on the nature of the canal anatomy and shape. The common compacting instrument is the plugger, which is chosen based on canal size, length, and curvature (see Figs. 9-26, 9-27, and 9-50) (see Table 9-7). The plugger can be a hand or finger instrument, and the selected instruments are prefitted into the canal to determine the proper depth of penetration without binding against the canal walls. A root canal sealer that can be mixed to a creamy consistency and has ample working time (15 to 30 minutes) is selected. The sealer is placed into the canal to the depth of the master cone position; the master cone is lightly coated on its apical half and placed in the canal. A heated instrument is used to sear off and remove coronal segments of gutta-percha and to transfer heat to the remaining portion of the master cone. A cold plugger is used to compact the softened portion of the cone apically and laterally. This process of heating, removing, and compacting are continued until softened gutta-percha is delivered into the apical 1 to 2 mm of the prepared canal. Subsequently, softened segments are added and compacted to obturate the canal from the apical segment to the canal orifice.

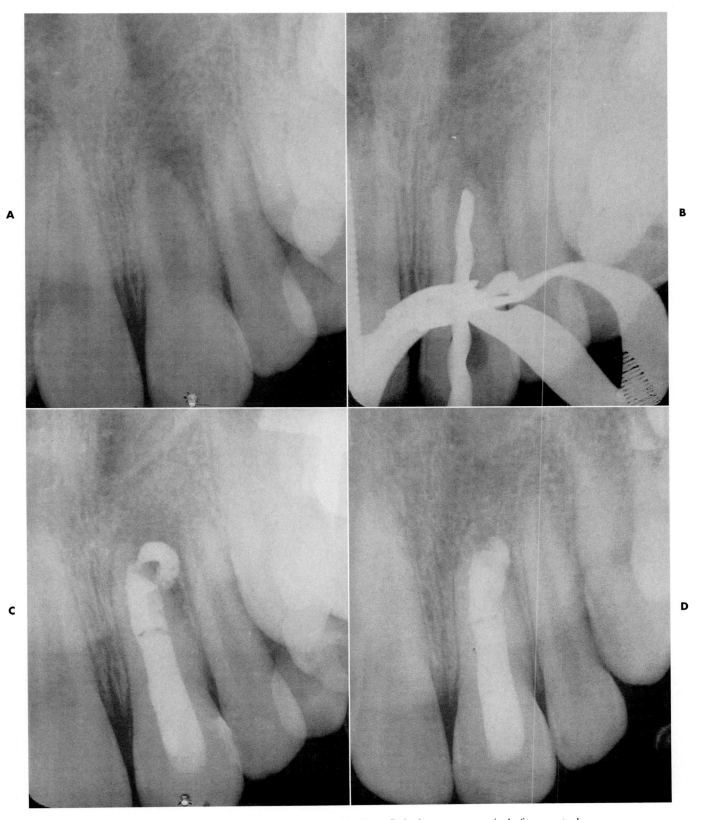

FIG. 9-49 A, Traumatized maxillary central incisor. Pulp became necrotic before root closure. **B,** Root canal system is accessed and cleaned. Working length is maintained within the canal space. **C,** Calcium hydroxide mixed 4 parts to 1 with barium sulfate is placed in and beyond the canal system. Placement beyond gives the clinician important information regarding the nature of the apical bridge that has formed. **D,** Six-month recall examination shows the beginning of osseous repair.
Continued

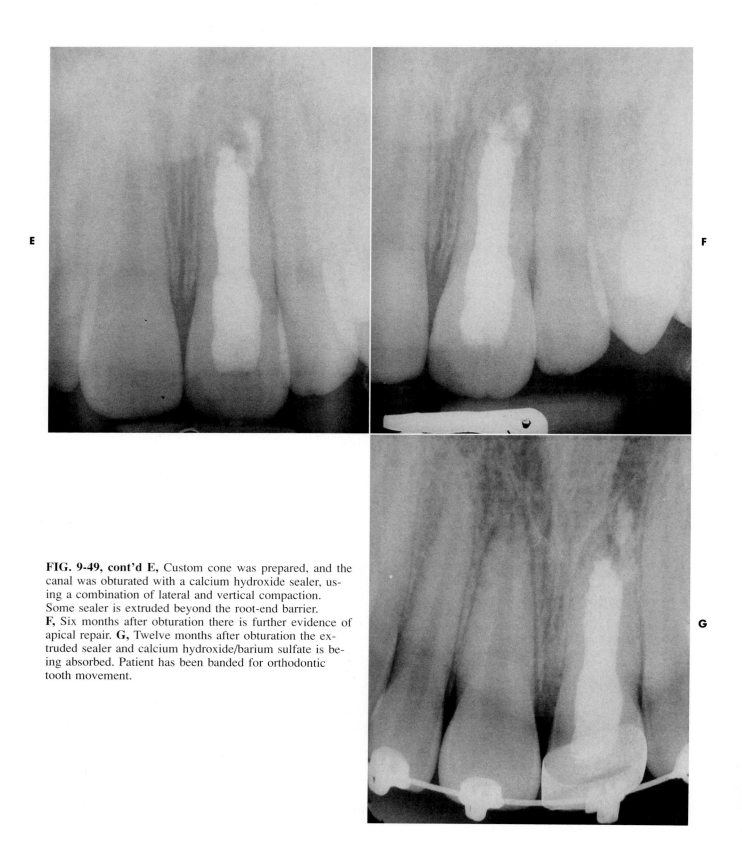

FIG. 9-49, cont'd E, Custom cone was prepared, and the canal was obturated with a calcium hydroxide sealer, using a combination of lateral and vertical compaction. Some sealer is extruded beyond the root-end barrier.
F, Six months after obturation there is further evidence of apical repair. **G,** Twelve months after obturation the extruded sealer and calcium hydroxide/barium sulfate is being absorbed. Patient has been banded for orthodontic tooth movement.

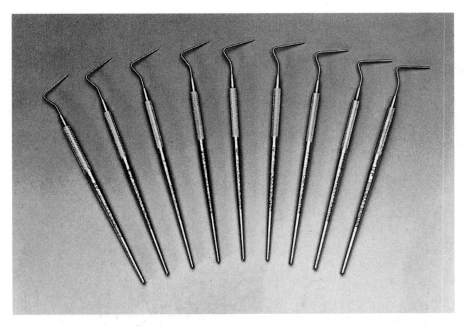

FIG. 9-50 Root canal pluggers used for the vertical compaction of heat softened gutta-percha. These pluggers are often referred to as Schilder pluggers and come in lengths for anterior and posterior teeth (see Table 9-7).

Detailed technique

Master cone selection. A master gutta-percha cone is selected based on the approximate length and shape of the canal. With this technique, the shape of the cone chosen is most important. The choice of cone is a nonstandardized cone, such as *fine, fine medium, medium large,* and so forth. The shape of these cones provides the necessary bulk of gutta-percha for the vertical compaction technique.

The master cone is fit to within 1 to 2 mm of the prepared apical matrix or constriction (Fig. 9-51). The premise for this choice is based on the fact that the softened material moves apically into the prepared canal in a softened state, thereby adapting more intimately to the canal walls. Care must be exercised to ensure that the cone binds only at its apical-most extent and not higher in the canal. This is a function of both proper canal shaping and cone selection. Once the cone is fit to clinical expectations, its position in the canal is verified radiographically and evaluated as follows:

I. If the cone fits to or within 1 to 2 mm of the working length, if the cone demonstrates a snugness of fit at that point, and if the shape of the cone approximates the shape of the canal throughout the canal length, compaction may proceed.

II. If the cone fits short of the desired length, the following conditions may exist (Fig. 9-52):
   A. The cone is binding higher in the canal.
   B. An improperly tapered cone has been chosen.
   C. Dentin chips may be packed in the apical portion of the canal.
   D. Clinician errors, such as a ledge, block, or zip, may be present.
   E. There may be a curve in the canal that is not visible on the two-dimensional radiograph, and the canal preparation narrows rapidly at the curve.

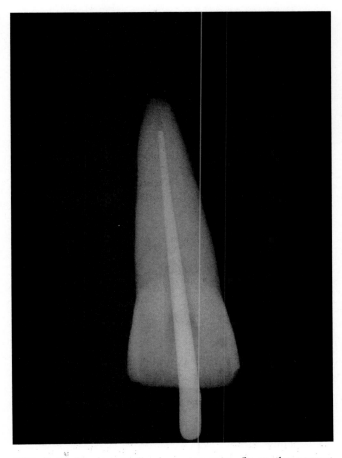

FIG. 9-51 Nonstandardized master cone fit to the correct length for vertical compaction. Note shape of the cone approximates the shape of the prepared canal space.

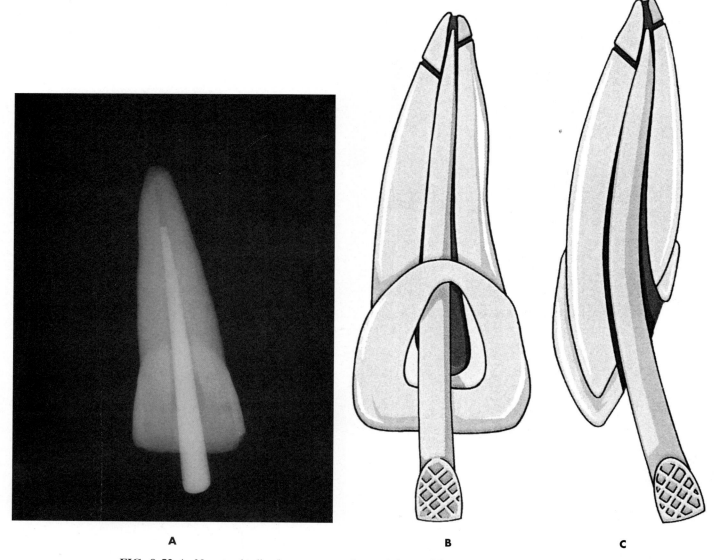

A   B   C

FIG. 9-52 A, Nonstandardized master cone is too large and improperly shaped for the prepared canal. Depth of penetration is insufficient. **B** and **C,** Diagrammatic illustration of this clinical problem.

III. If the cone fits beyond the desired length, the following conditions may exist (Fig. 9-53):
   A. The taper of the cone is insufficient or incorrect.
   B. The apical matrix or constriction has been destroyed through overinstrumentation.
In either case, if the cone is too short or too long, the problem must be assessed and the causative factors removed. This can be done by selecting a new cone, cutting segments from the apical portion of a cone with a scalpel, custom fitting of a cone with chemical or heat softening, or reshaping the canal for a more desirable fit of the cone selected.

Canal preparation. Once the master cone has been properly fitted, it is removed from the canal and placed in a sterilizing solution such as sodium hypochlorite. The canal system is then dried with paper points. If the smear layer is to be removed, appropriate solutions are used at this time (see Smear Layer Removal Versus Smear Layer Retention). If desired, all

residual moisture in the canal may be removed by rinsing the canal with 95% ethyl alcohol or 99% isopropyl alcohol. The alcohol is left in the canal for 2 to 3 minutes and then removed with additional sterile paper points.

Compactor selection. The careful fitting and selection of the compactors used for vertical compaction is crucial to the success of this technique (see Tables 9-5 and 9-7). For many canals, two to three different sizes are necessary to match the tapered, flared canal. One plugger should fit to within a few millimeters of the end of the canal, whereas other pluggers fit at variable distances into the canal (Fig. 9-54). Under no circumstances should any plugger contact the walls of the canal in a wedging manner. This may readily dispose to a vertical root fracture.[171] Therefore the pluggers must be fit to a point where maximal depth is achieved without binding. Pluggers that have markings or are scored at 5 mm increments are desirable. Likewise, rubber stops can be placed on the plugger if

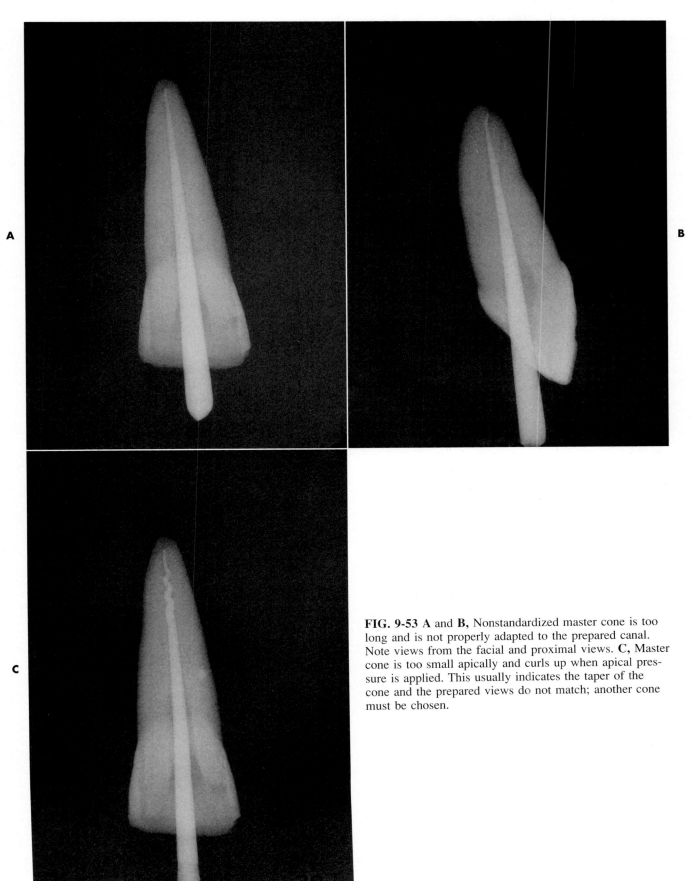

FIG. 9-53 A and **B,** Nonstandardized master cone is too long and is not properly adapted to the prepared canal. Note views from the facial and proximal views. **C,** Master cone is too small apically and curls up when apical pressure is applied. This usually indicates the taper of the cone and the prepared views do not match; another cone must be chosen.

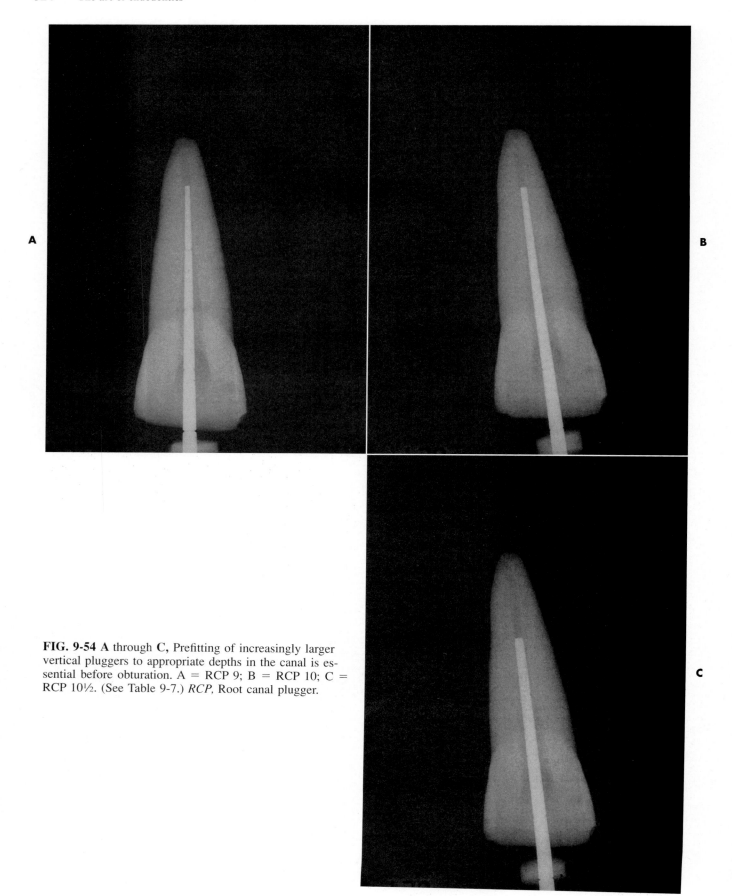

FIG. 9-54 A through **C,** Prefitting of increasingly larger vertical pluggers to appropriate depths in the canal is essential before obturation. A = RCP 9; B = RCP 10; C = RCP 10½. (See Table 9-7.) *RCP,* Root canal plugger.

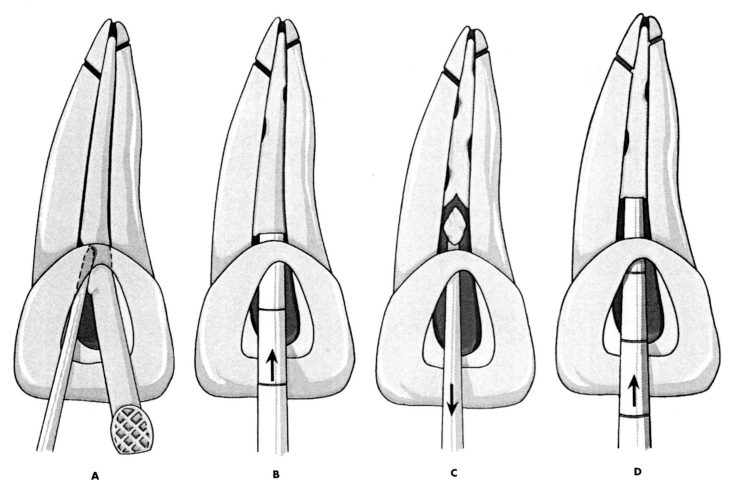

A   **B**   **C**   **D**

FIG. 9-55 A, Removal of the coronal portion of the master cone with a heated instrument. Note the apical position of the cone is short of the working length. **B,** Initial compaction of the coronal portion of the softened gutta-percha. Note the plugger must be of sufficient size to move the material without merely penetrating the softened mass. **C,** Segment of gutta-percha is removed with a heat transfer instrument. **D,** Continued vertical compaction of the softened gutta-percha. **D,** Continued compaction in the middle third of the canal with a properly sized plugger.

Continued

necessary to help control the depth of penetration into the canal.

In addition to selecting pluggers for vertical compaction, a heat transfer instrument (0 or 00, Caulk/Dentsply, Milford, Del.; Hu-Friedy Co., Chicago, Ill.) or a heating instrument (Touch n' Heat, EIE/Analytic Technology, San Diego, Calif.) is chosen to remove segments of the gutta-percha during the compaction apically or to heat and add segments of gutta-percha during the compaction of the coronal portion of the canal.

Sealer placement. As opposed to lateral compaction, the placement of sealer for vertical compaction is minimized in the apical segment of the canal. This prevents excessive movement of the sealer beyond the canal if the foramen is patent and prevents the filling of the apical portion of the canal with sealer only if the foramen is not patent. Therefore using instruments similar to those suggested for cold lateral compaction, a light coating of sealer is placed circumferentially on the canal walls to the approximate depth of the master cone placement. Vertical compaction of the heat-softened gutta-percha

provides for a thin coating of the filling material as it is moved apically and laterally. Likewise, some of the sealer moves coronally in a hydraulic fashion during compaction.

Master cone placement. The properly disinfected master cone is lightly coated with sealer over its apical one third and slowly placed into the canal so as not to force large amounts of the sealer apically. At this point some clinicians choose to expose a radiograph and evaluate the position of the cone before compaction.

Master cone compaction: coronal to apical obturation. The coronal end of the master gutta-percha cone is removed above the canal orifice with a heated instrument (heat transfer instrument or heating device), and the warmed end of the master cone that remains in the canal is compacted, folding it into the coronal portion of the canal (Fig. 9-55, *A*). This is accomplished with the largest plugger that was previously prefit in the canal. The blunted end of the plugger creates a deep depression in the center of the master cone. The outer walls of the softened gutta-percha are then folded inward to fill the central void while at the same time the mass of softened gutta-

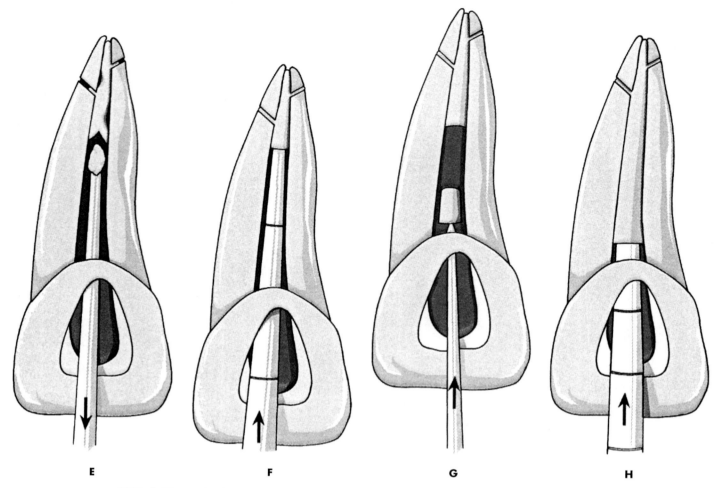

E   F   G   H

FIG. 9-55, cont'd E, Removal of additional gutta-percha segment, followed by apical compaction **(F). G,** Small segment of gutta-percha is heated on the heated transfer instrument and carried to the canal and compacted until the canal is filled to the desired level **(H).**

percha is moved laterally and apically (Fig. 9-55, *B*). Subsequently, the heated instrument is used to remove additional 2 to 3 mm segments of gutta-percha, followed by the compaction of the softened gutta-percha remaining in the canal (Fig. 9-55, *C*). This sequence is repeated until the apical 3- to 4-mm segment of gutta-percha is softened and compacted into the apical preparation. Often it is advisable to expose radiographs during this procedure to monitor the movement of the filling material (Fig. 9-55, *D* through *F*).

Success with the heat softening and apical compaction is predicated on a number of factors within the control of the clinician. Adherence to the following guidelines is therefore very important:

- Use the plugger that has been prefit in each portion or segment of the canal. Larger pluggers are generally applied in the coronal portion, with decreasing sizes used as the compaction proceeds apically. The last plugger used should fit freely in the apical 2 to 3 mm of the canal without contacting the walls.
- The pluggers should be wiped with alcohol or possibly a dry dental cement powder as a separating medium to prevent their sticking to the warmed gutta-percha.

- Do not try to be aggressive and compact the entire remaining segment of the gutta-percha at one time. First of all, the heat applied during the removal of the segments only travels 3 to 4 mm into the remaining gutta-percha. Therefore only the coronal most material is softened sufficiently to obtain quality compaction. Additionally, small incremental heating and compacting provide a fluid movement and adaptation of the gutta-percha to the canal walls and irregularities.
- Controlled application of apical pressure usually results in the best obturation as opposed to rapid and irregular poking at the gutta-percha.
- Once the plugger has reached the depth of 1 to 3 mm into the softened gutta-percha, the plugger is carefully removed and the material on either side of the depression made with the plugger is compacted into the central portion of the canal. Failure to evenly compact this material results in voids in the softened material. This is not a major concern during the coronal to apical compaction but is during the apical to coronal compaction to follow.
- In curved canals it is necessary to curve the pluggers before entry to the approximate shape of the canal. Fortunately,

most of the curves are in the apical one half to one third, and the small pluggers can be easily curved. The best instrument for this is orthodontic pliers or possibly the bending tool that comes with one of the contemporary thermoplasticized gutta-percha delivery units (Obtura II, Obtura Corp., Fenton, Mo.; see following sections).

- Do not try to move the apical segment of gutta-percha into the prepared apical portion of the canal until the apicalmost gutta-percha can be thoroughly softened and carefully adapted to the canal walls and apical constriction or matrix.

Placement of softened segments: apical to coronal obturation. Once the final segment of gutta-percha has been thoroughly compacted, a radiograph is exposed to assess the apical fill. If satisfactory, the root canal appears essentially empty, except at its apical-most extent where a dense apical plug of gutta-percha is located (see Fig. 9-55, *F*). The remaining portion of the canal is obturated with small segments (2 to 4 mm in length) that have been previously prepared to conform to the shape of the pluggers and the canal from the apical segment to the coronal orifice. The segments are speared with the heating instrument and carefully and lightly warmed over a flame to reach a firm yet tacky consistency (Fig. 9-55, *G* through *H*). Subsequently, they are carried to the depth of the gutta-percha in the canal where the tacky segment is lightly touched to the filling material in place. This results in an adherence of the segment to the apical gutta-percha. This is followed by compaction with the prefit pluggers as previously described. Here again, care must be taken to compact the material in all dimensions, folding the gutta-percha in on itself to create a dense mass that fully adheres and is homogeneous with the previously compacted material, otherwise voids are common. This entire process is continued until the canal is fully obturated to the canal orifice or to a specific depth if a post core restoration is planned.

The clinician is cautioned to consider the following:

- Do not overheat the segments of gutta-percha, as they will become too soft to apply or compact or they will easily burn. This aspect of the technique requires practice to achieve a consistent result. Suggestions to enhance heating consistency in the delivery of the segments have been made through the use of controlled heating devices such as the Touch n' Heat and the Endotec.[100]
- Do not apply sealer to the softened segments, as this prevents their adherence to the body of gutta-percha in the canal.
- Compact the material with a light but firm, controlled force.
- Do not use segments larger than 2 to 4 mm in length.
- Use appropriately sized and prefitted pluggers.

On a final note with this technique, the filling of the canal with softened gutta-percha from the apical plug to the coronal orifice has been enhanced significantly with newer injection guttapercha systems (see Technique Variations later in this chapter). However, the technique as presented still provides a high quality of obturation and is the technique of choice of many clinicians (Figs. 9-56 and 9-57).

Completion of obturation and management of the pulp chamber. Once the gutta-percha has been compacted coronally, the pulp chamber is cleaned thoroughly with cotton pellets soaked in alcohol to remove remnants of unset sealer and particles of gutta-percha. A substantial temporary restoration

is placed; in some situations, immediate post space is created (see Chapter 21), and a permanent restoration is initiated. A final radiograph, without the rubber dam in position, is taken from an angle that adequately demonstrates the obturation of each canal.

Technique Variations

Since the inception of the vertical compaction with warm gutta-percha technique in its contemporary format,[14,170] multiple attempts have been made to simplify the approach to heat softening and compaction of gutta-percha. These innovations have focused primarily on enhanced heating systems for intracanal softening of gutta-percha (System B, EIE/Analytic Technology, San Diego, Calif.) before compaction,[27] injectable thermoplasticized gutta-percha systems (Obtura II, Obtura Corp., Fenton, Mo.; UltraFil, Hygenic Corp., Akron, Ohio),[74,127,216] systems designed to heat the material before placement in the canal (SuccessFil, Hygenic Corp., Akron, Ohio),[200] core carrier techniques in which the gutta-percha is coated on a carrier before heating and delivery to the canal (ThermaFil, Tulsa Dental Products, Tulsa, Okla.; Densfil, Caulk/Dentsply, Milford, Del.; SuccessFil, Hygenic Corp., Akron, Ohio),[101] and thermocompaction techniques with rotary instruments (JS Quick-fill, JS Dental, Ridgefield, Conn.).[144,166] Also variations and combinations of the above are available[114,199] (Trifecta, Hygenic Corp., Akron, Ohio; Inject-R-Fill, UBECO, York, Pa.). The most popular of these techniques are discussed in subsequent sections.

Enhanced heated systems

A major improvement in the vertical compaction with warm, softened gutta-percha was the development of the System B heat source. This device can monitor the temperature at the tip of its heat carrier devices and can deliver a precise amount of heat for an indefinite period of time. When the heat carrier is also designed as a plugger, simultaneous heating and compacting can occur; this approach has been referred to as a continuous wave technique.[27] With this system the pluggers have also been designed to match the taper of nonstandardized guttapercha cones. Therefore when a master cone has been properly fitted, the same size plugger can be chosen for heating and compaction. This combination allows compaction of the filling material at exactly the same instant it has been heat softened and creates a single wave of heating and compacting as opposed to the multiple phase approach previously described. An additional advantage includes the compacting of the filling materials at all levels simultaneously throughout the movement of the heating-compacting instrument apically.

In this technique pluggers are fitted to within 5 to 7 mm from the canal terminus. The heat source is set to 392° F ± 50° F (200° C ± 10° C), the canal is thoroughly dried, and the fitted master cone is placed with sealer into the canal. The tip of the plugger is placed into the canal orifice, and the switch on the System B is activated. The plugger is driven through the master cone with in a single motion to a point about 3 mm short of its apical binding position. While pressure on the plugger is maintained, the button on the heating system is released and the plugger is slowed in its apical movement as the its tip cools. When the pluggers stops short of its binding position, pressure is maintained on the plugger until the apical mass of the gutta-percha has set (5 to 10 seconds). This compensates for any material shrinkage during cooling. Then the switch is

Text continued on p. 332

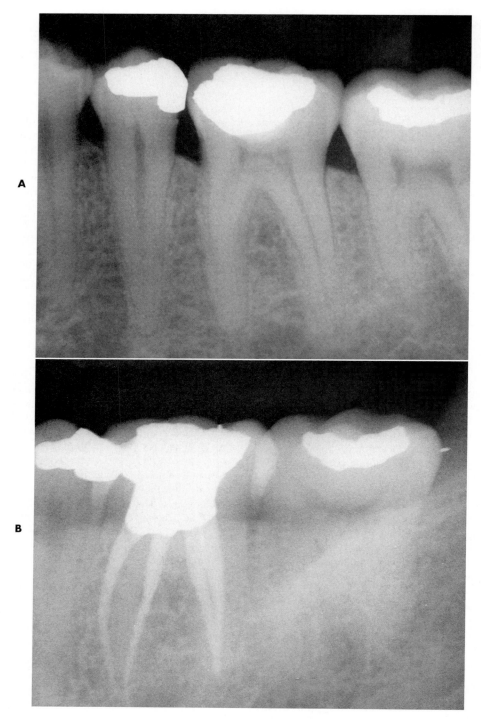

FIG. 9-56 A through **D,** Preoperative and postoperative views of two mandibular molars with four canals, each obturated using vertical compaction with heat-softened gutta-percha. *(Courtesy Dr. James C. Douthitt.)*

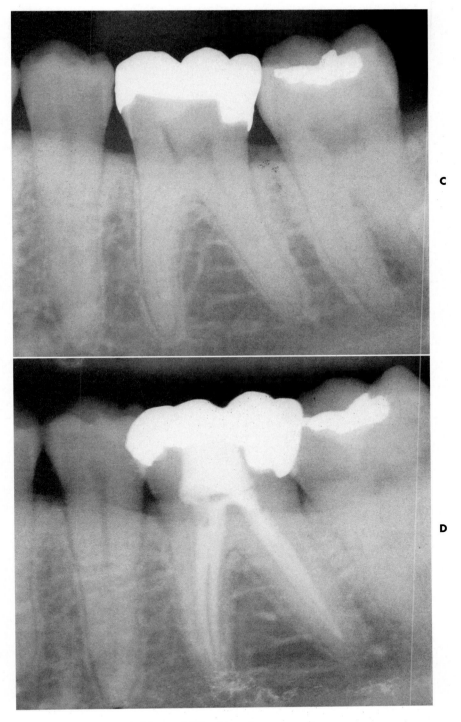

C

D

FIG. 9-56, cont'd For legend see opposite page.

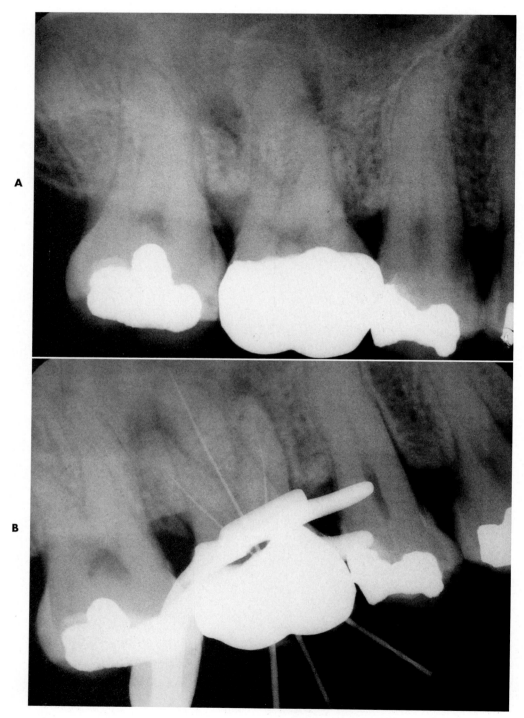

FIG. 9-57 A, Maxillary molar with a necrotic pulp and chronic periradicular periodontitis. **B,** Working lengths determined. *(Courtesy Dr. Constantinos Laghios.)*

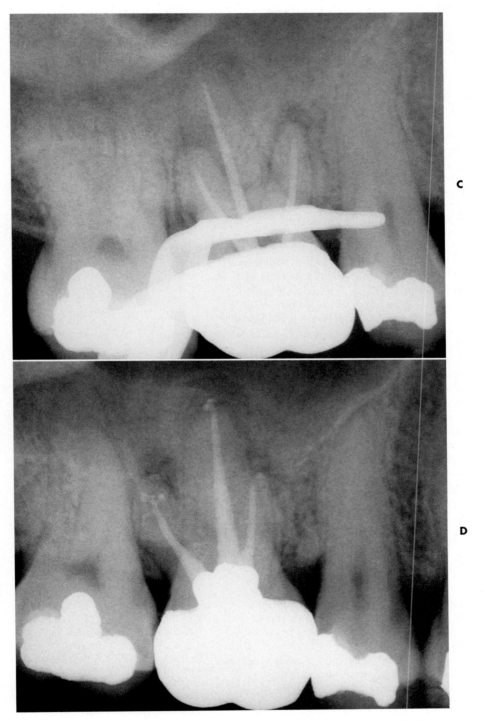

FIG. 9-57, cont'd C, Nonstandardized master cones fit to the appropriate lengths for vertical compaction. **D,** Canals obturated with extrusion of small amounts of sealer through accessory foramina.

reactivated for a short burst of heat (1 second) to release the plugger and surplus gutta-percha. During this short burst the System B is programmed to send a half-second heat surge (572° F; 300° C) to the plugger with a subsequent return to 392° F (200° C). These short bursts should be limited to allow only for removal of the plugger as opposed to heating up the remaining gutta-percha.

The System B is also designed to maintain a stable 392° F (200° C) at the tip of the plugger to ensure constant temperature throughout the apical compaction procedure. If it is too hot, the plugger rapidly drives through the oversoftened gutta-percha and the back pressure necessary for three-dimensional obturation is lost.

Once the apical segment has been obturated, the coronal portion of the canal is backfilled. This can be done with the same system with modified temperatures (212° F; 100° C) or can be done with an injectable gutta-percha technique (see next section). When the System B is used, the plugger is the same as that used for the initial apical compaction with another gutta-percha cone that has the same taper as the master cone and a tip diameter that matches the tip diameter of the plugger. The backfilling cone is prepared at the same time as the original master cone. Sealer is used with the backfilling cone, which is seated in the canal. The cone is warmed without pressure to soften it, followed by a sustained pressure to allow the cone to adapt to the walls and "set" in the canal. Excessive temperatures applied too long must be avoided to prevent the plugger from deeply penetrating the cone and pulling it from the canal. The plugger should be rotated slightly during its removal from the compacted mass. This mass of gutta-percha that was added to the coronal portion can be reheated and compacted as necessary (Fig. 9-58).

Although minimal equipment is required to perform this technique, cost factors in equipment purchase must be considered. Likewise, adaptation of this technique to unusual circumstances and mastery of it with straightforward cases require practice. Presently there are no prospective or retrospective studies to support the safety, efficacy, and long-term success of this technique, nor are there studies that have evaluated the potential effects of the heat generated on the supporting periodontium.

Injectable gutta-percha techniques

The two major injectable gutta-percha techniques available to the clinician are the Obtura II (Obtura Corp., Fenton, Mo.) (Fig. 9-59) and the UltraFil (Hygenic Corp., Akron, Ohio). These techniques have also been routinely referred to as a "high-heat" technique and a "low-heat" technique, respectively. This is mainly due to the temperature required to soften the gutta-percha for delivery into the canal.

Obtura II technique. Canals to be obturated must have a continuously tapering funnel from the apical matrix to the canal orifice.[74] Of significance is a properly shaped canal in the apical to middle transitional area, particularly in curved canals. The proper shaping is essential for the flow of the softened material. Also a definite apical matrix is essential to confine and retain the gutta-percha in the canal system, as filling beyond the end of the root can easily occur.[29,43,118]

Gutta-percha is available in pellets that are inserted into the heated delivery system, which looks like a caulking device (Fig. 9-60). The gutta-percha is heated to approximately 365° to 392° F (185° to 200° C). A needle or applicator tip (gauges

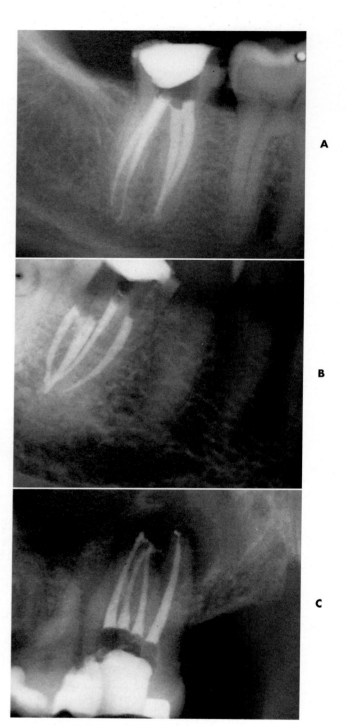

FIG. 9-58 A through **C,** Examples of root canal obturation in molars with vertical compaction using the System B. All teeth have four canals. Note the canal shaping that is necessary and the movement of both sealer and possibly gutta-percha beyond the apical confines or through accessory foramina. *(Courtesy Dr. Constantinos Laghios.)*

20 and 23) designed to deliver the softened gutta-percha is introduced into the canal to the junction of the middle and apical third (Fig. 9-61). The applicator tip is prefitted to ensure that it does not bind against the canal walls. Likewise, the pluggers are also prefitted to determine the proper depth of place-

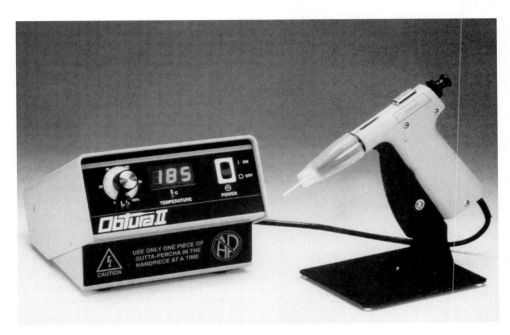

FIG. 9-59 Obtura II thermoplasticized gutta-percha system.

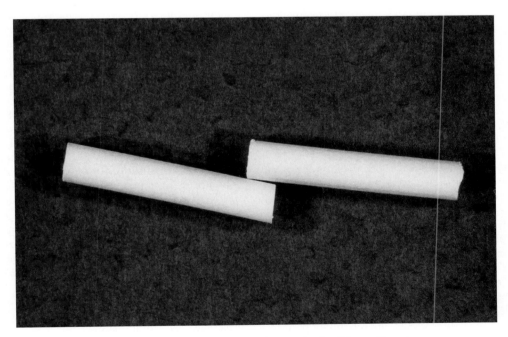

FIG. 9-60 Pellets of gutta-percha for use in the Obtura II system.

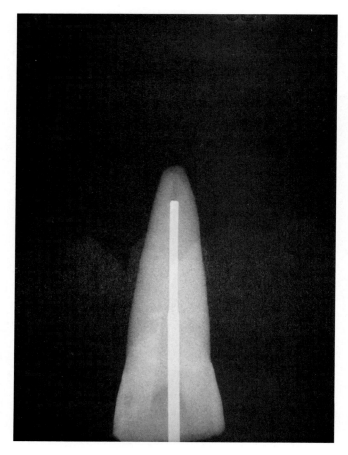

FIG. 9-61 Prefitting of the injection-applicator tip of the Obtura II system into the apical third of the prepared canal without binding is essential for proper delivery and flow of the softened material.

ment for compaction (see Fig. 9-54). If necessary, pluggers can be curved, or newer nickel-titanium pluggers can be used.

Even though the gutta-percha is softened and can be adapted to the intricacies of the prepared canal, root canal sealer is still essential with this technique.[19,43,182] However, sealer must be carefully placed in the canal to prevent its movement beyond the confines of the canal apically and to ensure the placement of gutta-percha at the terminus of the canal system. One to two drops of sealer are placed with an instrument of choice to the approximate depth of the prefitted applicator tip or needle. Do not fill the apical portion of the canal with sealer. A fast-setting sealer is not recommended.

With the needle in its proper position in the canal, the gutta-percha is passively injected into the root canal system, avoiding apical pressure on the needle. In 2 to 5 seconds the softened material fills the apical segment and begins to lift the needle out of the tooth (Fig. 9-62). During this lifting by the softened, flowing mass the middle and coronal portions of the canal are continuously filled until the needle reaches the canal orifice. Controlled compaction of the material follows with prefitted pluggers to adapt the gutta-percha to the prepared canal walls (Fig. 9-62, *B* through *D*). If necessary, additional amounts of gutta-percha can be easily injected to achieve complete obturation. Do not use excessive compaction pressures but fold

the material in on itself as previously described for vertical compaction.

Multiple variations exist with this technique. The softened material can be placed in the apical 2 to 3 mm and compacted at that point (Fig. 9-62, *E* through *G*). Subsequently, the remainder of the canal can be filled as above, or segmental additions can be added and compacted.[198] Control of the apical movement of gutta-percha and sealer appears to be better with this approach.[37] Often this technique is used with the lateral or vertical compaction techniques. Following the compaction of a master cone in the apical 2 to 3 mm, the cone is seared off with a heated instrument and the coronal portion compacted. The Obtura II is then used to backfill the remainder of the canal in either segments or in toto.

With an increased demand for the use of this technique, variations in the consistency of the gutta-percha have become available (Schwed Co. Inc., Kew Gardens, N.Y.). These alterations are designed to improve flow and regulate viscosity. The *regular flow gutta-percha* is a homogenized formulation with superior flow characteristics, whereas the *easy flow gutta-percha* maintains its smooth flow consistency at lower temperatures and has a longer working time. The latter would favor the management of complex cases in which extensive compaction is necessary and cases with small curved canals, in addition to favoring the inexperienced clinician.

The use of the injected thermoplasticized gutta-percha is especially beneficial when managing canal irregularities, such as fins, webs, culs-de-sac, internal resorption, C-shaped canals, accessory or lateral canals, and arborized foramina.[74,120,189,209] The adaptation of the softened gutta-percha to the canal walls has been shown to be significantly better than lateral compaction[29] (Fig. 9-63, *A*), and the removal of the smear layer and obturation of canals with the injectable system result in the movement of gutta-percha and sealer into the dentinal tubules[69] (Figs. 9-11, *E* and 9-63, *B* and *C*). Initial evaluation of clinical success with this technique has also proven favorable[183] (Fig. 9-64). The effective use of this technique, however, is predicated on mastery of its demands and nuances, and application on extracted teeth or models is essential before patient use.[19,74]

In addition to the potential for extrusion of the gutta-percha and sealer beyond the apical foramen (Fig. 9-65), the possibility of heat damage to the periodontium has been identified as a possible drawback to this technique. Temperature rises on the external lateral surface of the roots appear to be negligible with minimal to no tissue damage,[8,74] whereas the apical tissues may experience an inflammatory reaction even to gutta-percha retained within the root canal system.[128] Of importance in these findings is the fact that this data came from an evaluation of the original Obtura system and does not necessarily represent information applicable to the newer Obtura II system, especially with the availability of gutta-percha that can flow at lower temperatures.

UltraFil technique. Canal preparation for this technique has the same requirements as that described for the Obtura II technique. The UltraFil system comes with gutta-percha prepackaged in cannules with attached 22-gauge needles (Fig. 9-66, *A*). The material is prepared in an alpha phase format that softens at a temperature of approximately 158° to 194° F (70° to 90° C) in a special heater (Fig. 9-66, *B*). The warmed cannules are placed in a special sterilizable syringe (Fig. 9-66, *C*) for delivery to the prepared canal.[38,127]

The gutta-percha comes in three different consistencies

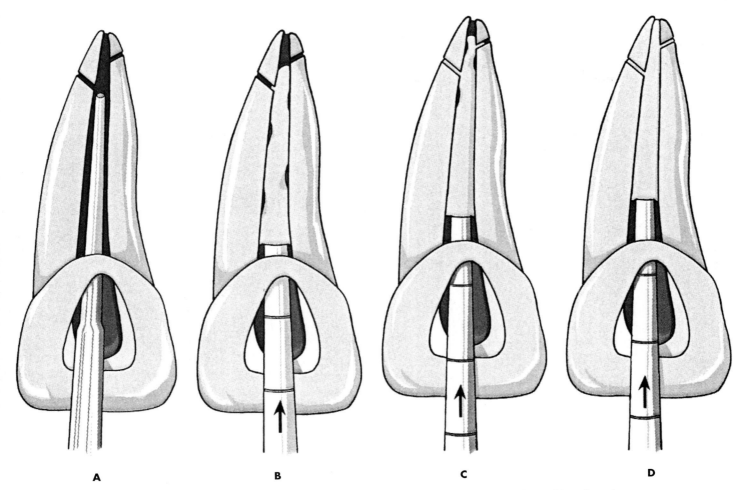

A   **B**   **C**   **D**

FIG. 9-62 A, Prefit of applicator tip. **B,** Canal filled in the coronal two thirds with softened gutta-percha. Properly sized plugger begins the apical movement of the material. **C,** As the plugger penetrates deeper into the canal, the material is folded on itself and compacted apically. **D,** Smaller pluggers are used in the apical portion. *Continued*

based on viscosity; *regular* (low viscosity), *firm set* (moderate viscosity), and *endoset* (high viscosity). Some concern has been identified over the inclusion of crystal-like structures in the regular set material as opposed to the firm set,[56] as implantation testing and tissue reactions to this material have indicated a more accentuated inflammatory response.[219] This was also seen in the periradicular tissues when the regular set material was placed beyond the end of the root.[111] This could be a function of the particle size of the material when in contact with tissues.[180]

Placement of the needle and sealer are somewhat similar to the Obtura II technique. Needle placement is usually farther from the apical matrix, such as 8 to 10 mm. Working time is approximately 60 to 70 seconds. The delivery of the regular set gutta-percha is different from that of the Obtura II. The syringe trigger is squeezed and released and, after a wait of 3 seconds, is squeezed and released again. This sends a bolus of gutta-percha toward the apical preparation. The needle is not withdrawn but left in place until the mass of softened gutta-percha is felt to lift the needle (backflow) from the canal. Further injection continues, allowing the moving gutta-percha to again lift the needle from the canal. The regular set material

cannot be efficiently and effectively compacted because of its soft consistency. Some clinicians have chosen to place a master cone before injection of the regular set material. The cone is compacted to make room for the injectable material, which is then introduced as described. Because of the low viscosity of this material extension beyond the root apex is of major concern, and its use should be restricted to cases with a substantial apical dentin matrix and minimal apical foraminal opening. Likewise, because the regular set material cannot be compacted, the possibility for shrinkage must be considered, and lack of compaction cannot be compensated for by increased amounts of sealer.

With the moderate- to high-viscosity gutta-percha, controlled compaction can follow the injection delivery of the material. Here, as with the Obtura II system, the material can be segmentally or bulk delivered before compaction. The times available for compaction vary based on the material chosen. Variations in this technique are similar to the Obtura II technique, as are the anatomic indications for its applications and the ultimate adaptation to the dentinal walls (Fig. 9-67). Of particular note is the use of the UltraFil system in the Trifecta technique, which is addressed in a subsequent section.

Text continued on p. 341

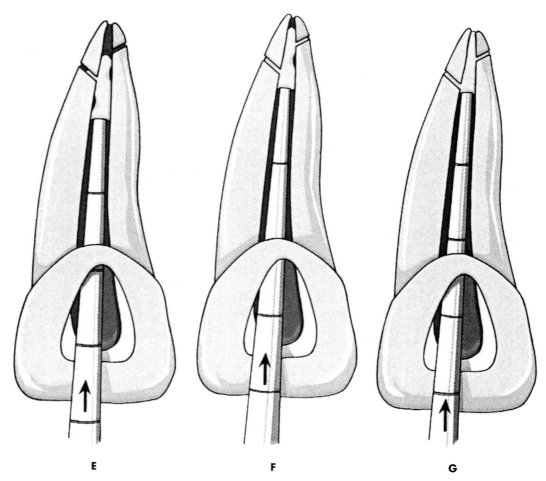

| E | F | G |

FIG. 9-62, cont'd E, Variation of technique. Softened gutta-percha can be placed only in the apical third, followed by compaction with appropriately sized pluggers, which do not bind in the canal (**F** and **G**).

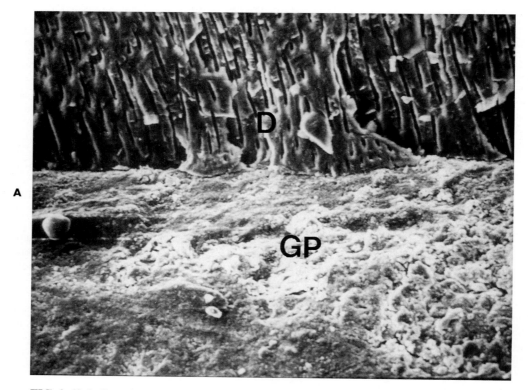

FIG. 9-63 A, Scanning electron microscopic view of the adaptation of thermoplasticized gutta-percha to the dentinal walls. *D,* Dentin; *GP,* gutta-percha.

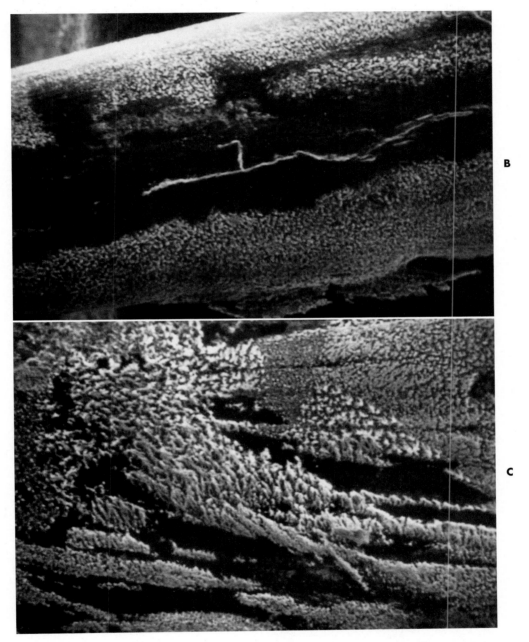

FIG. 9-63, cont'd B and **C,** Penetration of the dentinal tubules (scanning electron micrograph) with thermoplasticized gutta-percha following the removal of the smear layer. Original magnification range from ×76 to ×220.

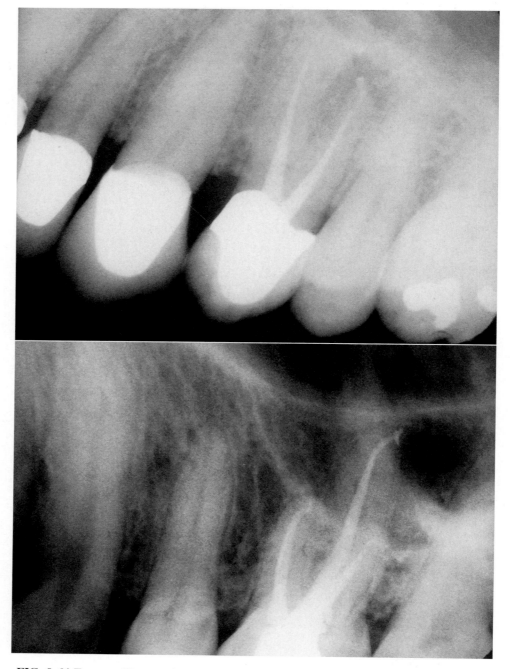

FIG. 9-64 Two maxillary teeth obturated using the original Obtura system of canal filling.

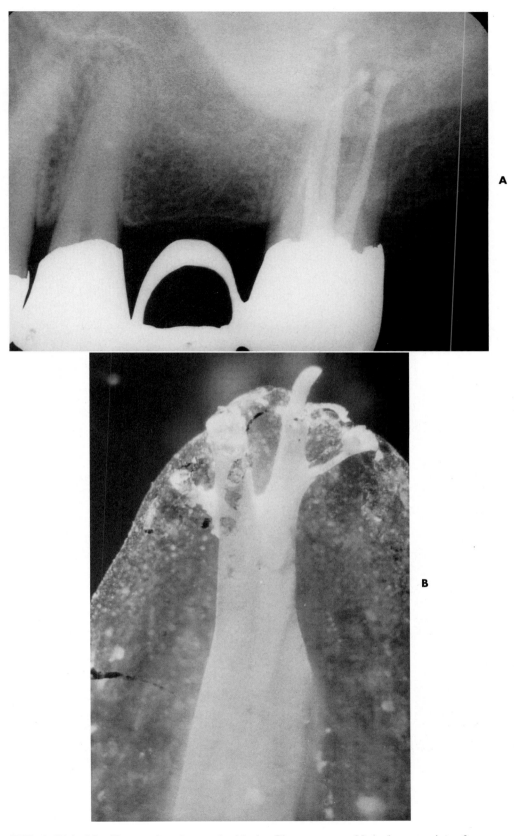

FIG. 9-65 A, Maxillary molar obturated with the Obtura system. Note the extrusion of material beyond the apical foramen in addition to the adaptation of the softened material to canal irregularities and accessory canals. **B,** Magnified view of apical obturation with the original Obtura system. Note the filling of the apical delta and the overfilling of the canal system.

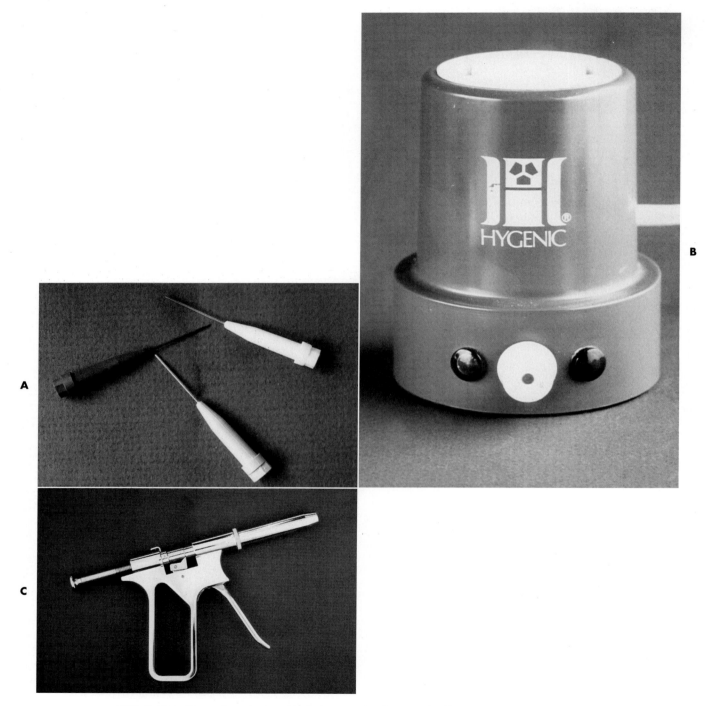

FIG. 9-66 A, Prepackaged gutta-percha in cannules for use with the UltraFil system. **B,** Heater unit for the gutta-percha cannules. **C,** Sterilizable syringe that holds the heated cannules.

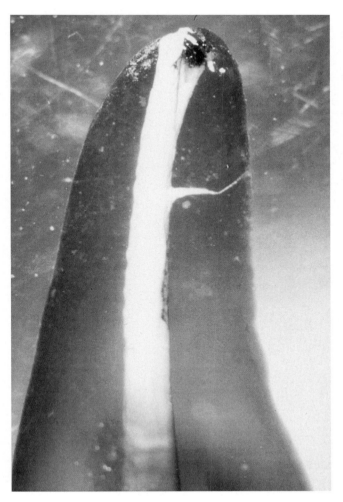

FIG. 9-67 Root canal obturated with the UltraFil system. Note the adaptation of the gutta-percha and the flow of the material into canal irregularities.

Presoftened noninjectable techniques

The development of gutta-percha in different isomeric forms such as alpha and beta phase led to creation of SuccessFil (Hygenic Corp., Akron, Ohio), whereby alpha phase gutta-percha could be heated, placed onto a carrier, and delivered into the canal in the thermoplasticized state without an injection system.

SuccessFil technique. The gutta-percha used in this technique comes in syringes, is of high viscosity, and hardens in 2 minutes. Carriers of titanium or radiopaque plastic are inserted into the syringe to the measured depth of the canal. The gutta-percha is expressed on the carrier, the shape of which is determined by how rapidly the carrier is removed from the syringe. Sealer is lightly coated on the canal walls, avoiding any large apical pooling of material. The carrier with gutta-percha is placed in the canal to the premeasured depth (working length). The gutta-percha can be compacted around the carrier with various instruments depending on the space available. This is followed by the severing of the carrier slightly above the canal orifice with a bur. Few studies have evaluated the efficacy and success of this technique in this form.[200]

Trifecta technique. A variation on the SuccessFil and UltraFil techniques uses the best of both approaches to canal obturation. A small amount (1 to 2 mm) of alpha phase SuccessFil gutta-percha is placed on the tip of a carrier one to two sizes smaller than the final apical canal size. After sealer is placed in the canal, the carrier is placed to the depth of the canal and is slowly rotated counterclockwise and withdrawn from the canal. This is followed by compaction of the small mass of gutta-percha in the canal. The coronal portion of the canal is backfilled with one of the three types of UltraFil gutta-percha, which is compacted if appropriate. Evaluative studies have shown this technique to be quite easily mastered with good adaptability of the gutta-percha and a canal seal comparable to that of other commonly used techniques[114,199] (Fig. 9-68).

Core carrier techniques

The prime core carrier techniques are the ThermaFil Plus (Tulsa Dental Products, Tulsa, Okla.) and Densfil (Caulk/Dentsply, Milford, Del.). For business purposes, Densfil was created under a licensing agreement with the creators of ThermaFil and subsequently can be considered as the same product. Also because SuccessFil required the placement of the softened gutta-percha on the carrier, it was not classified in this section. It should be considered as a variant of the core carrier technique that was developed in 1978 by Johnson.[101] Initially the product was solely designed to use metallic cores on which the gutta-percha was coated. Contemporary technology has resulted in the development of a firm plastic carrier (Fig. 9-69). The discussion to follow focuses primarily on this type of carrier.

ThermaFil technique. As with all other techniques, and this one is no exception, canal shaping is of utmost importance in achieving success. Unique to this technique is the availability of size verification naked plastic cores that are the exact size of the cores covered with gutta-percha (Fig. 9-70). Therefore the size and shape of the canal can be accurately determined before choosing the desired ThermaFil core carrier (Fig. 9-71).

The core carrier is placed in a specific oven (ThermaPrep Plus, Tulsa Dental Products, Tulsa, Okla.) and heated for the specific timeframe designated (Fig. 9-72). During this time the canal is rinsed and dried with paper points. It is suggested that the smear layer be removed with a chelating agent or low-percentage acid (10% citric acid). Removal of the smear layer followed by the placement of a plastic ThermaFil has been shown to significantly decrease coronal bacterial penetration.[13] This is presumably due to the ability of the filling materials to penetrate the patent dentinal tubules. The sealer is applied, lightly coating the walls and avoiding apical pooling. When the ThermaFil carrier is adequately heated, it is removed from the oven and placed into the canal to the predetermined depth marked with a rubber stop on the carrier. The carrier is not twisted during placement, and attempts to reposition the carrier may lead to a disruption of the gutta-percha position in the canal, as the carrier serves to provide both lateral and vertical movement of the softened gutta-percha (Fig. 9-73). The position of the carrier and gutta-percha can be determined radiographically; if the position is satisfactory, the top of the carrier is cut off 1 to 2 mm above the orifice. This is done with a No. 35 or 37 inverted cone while holding the handle with firm apical pressure. If the canal is wide buccolingually, a spreader or plugger

Text continued on p. 345

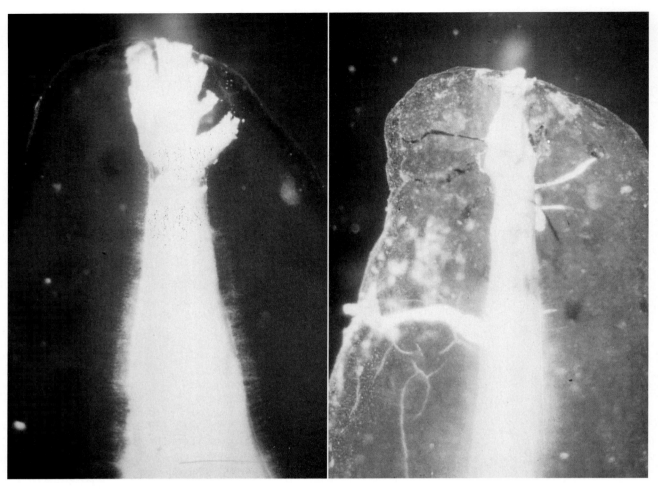

FIG. 9-68 Demineralized, dehydrated, and cleared teeth obturated with the Trifecta technique. The smear layer was removed before obturation. *Left,* Note the filling of the apical delta and possibly the flow of the gutta-percha and sealer into the dentinal tubules. *Right,* Flow of the softened material into the canal irregularities and accessory canals is accentuated.

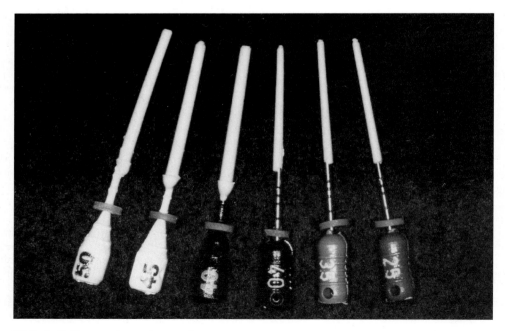

FIG. 9-69 ThermaFil carriers. *Left,* Plastic core. *Right,* Metal cores. Plastic core carriers are recommended.

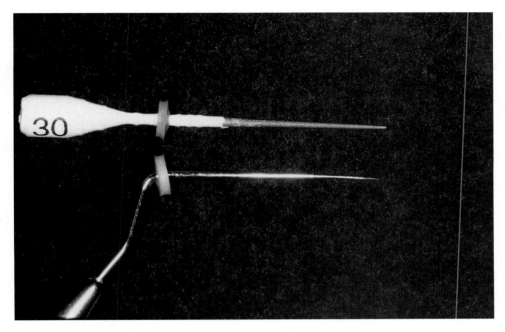

FIG. 9-70 *Top,* Naked ThermaFil plastic carrier can be used to verify the size of the prepared canal. *Bottom,* Comparison with a root canal spreader.

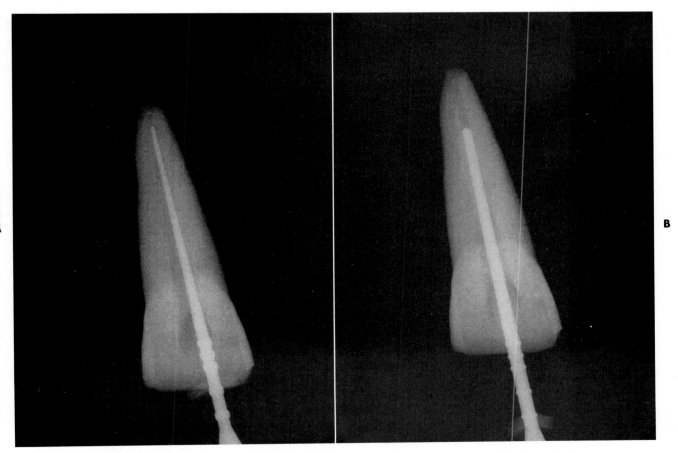

FIG. 9-71 A, Proper fit of the naked ThermaFil plastic carrier. **B,** Improper fit of a naked carrier. Carrier must fit loosely to the appropriate length similarly to the fitting of a root canal spreader.

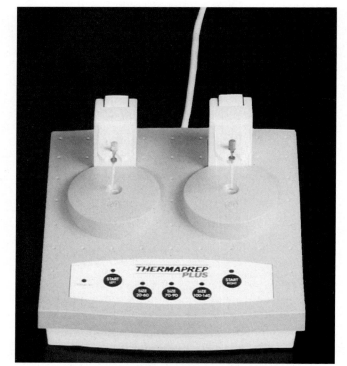

FIG. 9-72 ThermaPrep Plus heating system. *(Courtesy Tulsa Dental Products, Tulsa, Okla.)*

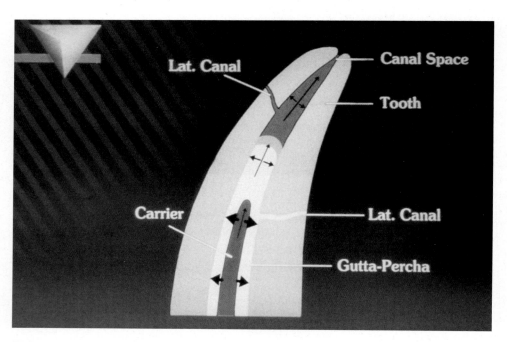

FIG. 9-73 Diagrammatic representation of gutta-percha movement in the root canal system during placement of a plastic ThermaFil core carrier. Note how the carrier can provide both lateral and vertical movement of the heat-softened material. *(Courtesy Tulsa Dental Products, Tulsa, Okla.)*

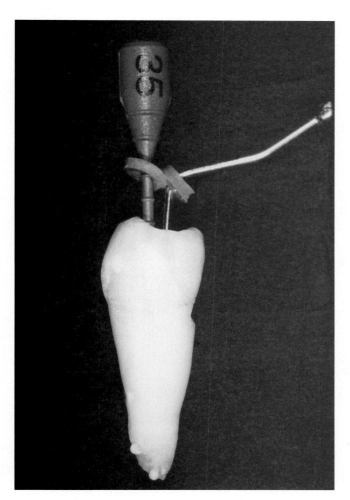

FIG. 9-74 Placement of a root canal spreader adjacent to a heated and positioned ThermaFil core gutta-percha carrier resulted in further compaction and movement of gutta-percha and sealer through root canal foramina. This approach is necessary in wide buccolingual canals and allows for a more three-dimensional obturation.

is inserted alongside the core and the entire mass is compacted, creating space for additional gutta-percha (Fig. 9-74). Accessory cones are added laterally, coupled with concomitant lateral or vertical compaction (Fig. 9-75). If sufficient space is present, an injectable technique can also be used along with appropriate compaction. The cold cones easily become embedded in the softened mass. The gutta-percha reaches its set in about 2 to 4 minutes.

Radiographic assessment of this delivery technique has been shown to be quite favorable[76] (Fig. 9-76), and leakage studies have shown the sealability of the technique to be equal to if not better than lateral compaction.[49,77,172] Adaptation of gutta-percha to the prepared canal walls and irregularities with this method of obturation has been determined to be excellent[77,135] (Fig. 9-77). Clinical parameters of application have also been favorable in its rapidity and efficiency of usage[79,135] (Fig. 9-78).

Post space preparation with this technique has been evaluated and facilitated through the use of various instruments. The space necessary for an intraradicular post can be created immediately or on a delayed basis without altering the apical seal[168] (Fig.

9-79). Effective use of Peeso reamers or Prepi burs (Tulsa Dental Products, Tulsa, Okla.) has resulted in rapid softening and removal of the coronal portion of the plastic carrier and gutta-percha. The reader is referred to Chapter 21 for further details.

Thermomechanical compaction

The thermocompaction of gutta-percha, introduced in 1979, was an innovative approach to heat softening and canal obturation. Using a newly developed instrument called a *McSpadden Compactor,* gutta-percha was softened with the rotary action of the instrument in the canal and moved apically and laterally within the prepared system. Entrepreneurial efforts resulted in the further development of rotary compactors such as the *Condenser* (Maillefer Instruments SA, Ballaigues, Switzerland) and the *Engine Plugger* (Zipperer, VDW, Munich, Germany). Recent developments have resulted in compactors precoated with gutta-percha—*JS Quick-fill* (JS Dental, Ridgefield, Conn.)—and the injectable system of coating compactors similar to the SuccessFil—*Multi-Phase II Pac Mac Compactors* (NT Company, Chattanooga, Tenn.).

Initially there were numerous studies that evaluated the efficacy of this technique of canal obturation. Findings were highly variable but appeared positive. These techniques were rapid, the seal of the canal system appeared adequate, and adaptation of the material was acceptable.[33,81,106,116,163,191] Initial problems included vertical root fractures, cutting of dentin, and breakage of compactors.[137,143] Likewise, the potential for the generation of excessive and deleterious frictional heat levels on the external root surface has been identified.[12,44,80,164,165] Therefore for the technique to be efficacious, slower speeds and low-temperature gutta-percha were identified as necessary to minimize both temperatures and stress on the root canal system during rotary compaction. Likewise, careful canal shaping and careful depth of penetration of the rotary compactor helps to prevent potential problems with this technique.

Because of the multiple variations with this technique, only the essence of the process is presented. The clinician is advised to learn the nuances involved with each technique on extracted teeth or tooth models before patient application.

Thermocompaction technique. A master cone is fit in the canal as has been discussed with previous techniques and placed in the canal with sealer. Good adaptation to the canal length and shape is essential. The rotating compactor is placed in the canal and moved apically with gentle pressure to a point 3 to 4 mm short of the working length or until resistance is met. The compactor is then removed while still rotating and compacting the gutta-percha apically and laterally. If the canal is too wide, the master cone and additional cones may be added before compaction. Following the initial rotary compaction, additional gutta-percha may be added in many different ways.

Variation 1. The master cone in the apical portion of the canal may be laterally or vertically compacted. This is followed by the thermocompaction of the cones in the canal (lateral technique) or the fitting of an additional large cone followed by thermocompaction.

Variation 2. An appropriately sized compactor (0.02 or 0.04 taper) is coated with a beta phase gutta-percha (multiPhase I), which is then overcoated with an alpha phase gutta-percha (multiPhase II) (NT Company, Chatanooga, Tenn.). Sealer is placed on the outer surface of the gutta-percha. The triple-coated compactor is inserted apically slightly short (0.5 mm)

Text continued on p. 349

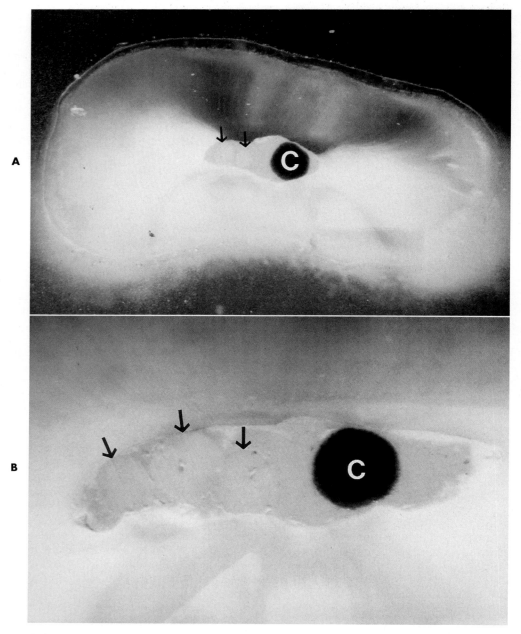

FIG. 9-75 Sectioned distal root of a mandibular first molar. **A,** Section at the junction of the apical and middle thirds following the placement of a plastic ThermaFil carrier and the use of lateral compaction with accessory cones. Arrows indicate position of the accessory cones. Gutta-percha surrounding the plastic core *(C)* is from the carrier. **B,** Section at the junction of the middle and coronal thirds. Three accessory canals *(arrows)* are visible and are embedded in the thermoplasticized gutta-percha of the core carrier *(C).*

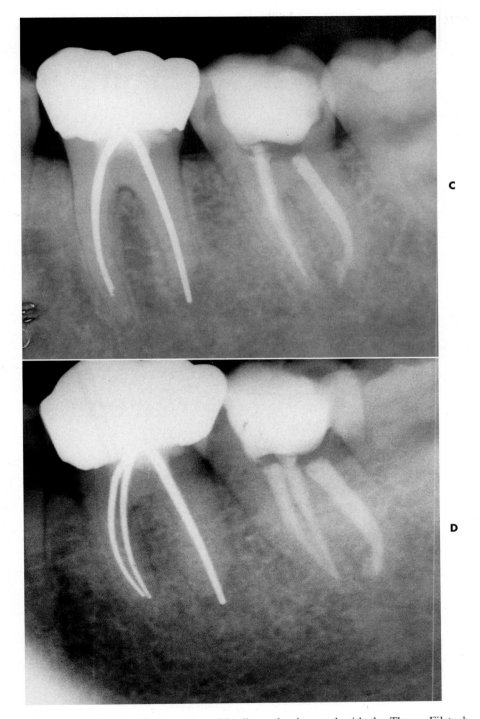

FIG. 9-75, cont'd C, Mandibular molar with all canals obturated with the ThermaFil technique. Distal canal has had additional lateral compaction and the placement of accessory cones. **D,** Mesial view shows the obturation of the wide distal canal and why it is necessary to use additional cones to achieve a three-dimensional fill.

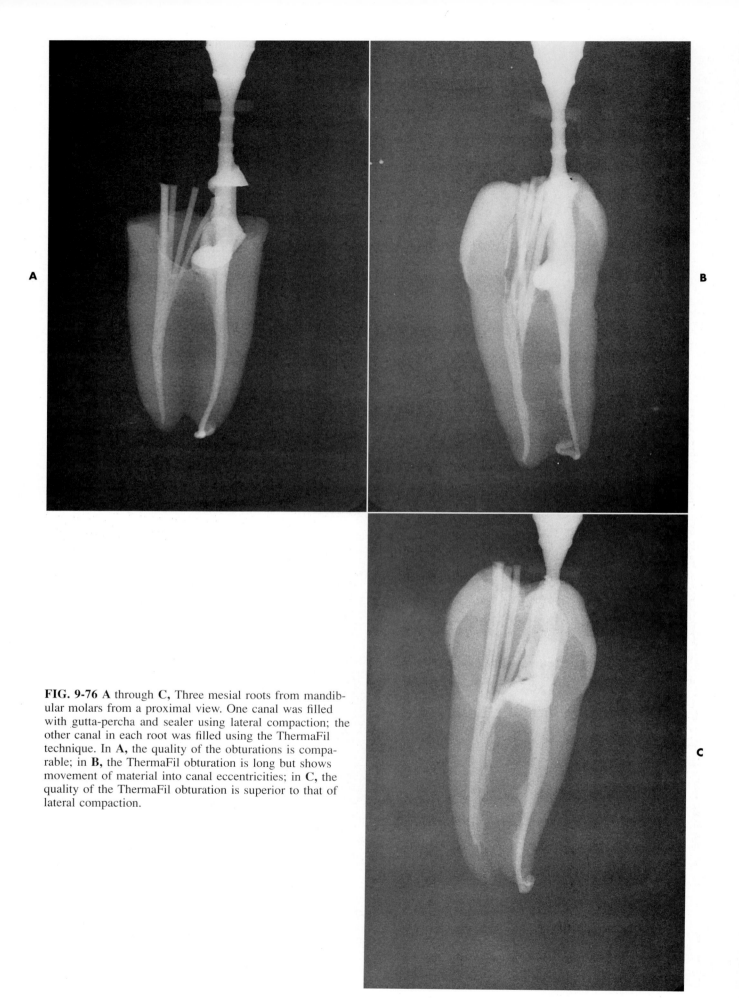

FIG. 9-76 A through **C,** Three mesial roots from mandibular molars from a proximal view. One canal was filled with gutta-percha and sealer using lateral compaction; the other canal in each root was filled using the ThermaFil technique. In **A,** the quality of the obturations is comparable; in **B,** the ThermaFil obturation is long but shows movement of material into canal eccentricities; in **C,** the quality of the ThermaFil obturation is superior to that of lateral compaction.

of the working length as possible without excessive force and without rotation. The force of placement is along the long axis of the compactor. The compactor is rotated at 4000 to 5000 rpm in a special reduction handpiece without exerting apical pressure and resisting back pressure. The compactor is then moved in a circular pattern for 2 seconds and withdrawn slowly while gentle pressure is applied on one side of the canal. Rotation continues until the compactor is fully withdrawn. The chamber may be cleaned of any sealer and gutta-percha as previously discussed.

Variation 3. If the apical foramen is open because of resorption, overinstrumentation, or lack of growth, a bolus of beta phase gutta-percha may be deposited near the foramen and carefully compacted; or an artificial apical barrier may also be placed (refer to Use of Apical Barriers), followed by the delivery of a thermocompacted cone or the presoftened injected-coated compactor obturation.

Variation 4. The use of compactors precoated with cold gutta-percha has also received attention (JS Quick-fill). In this technique sealer is placed to the working length, and the com-

pactor is placed in the canal and rotated at 4000 to 4500 rpm. The compactor is moved apically and withdrawn in a smooth motion while the compactor continues to rotate. The coronal excess of gutta-percha is vertically compacted into the canal. With the smear layer removed, good adaptation of gutta-percha and sealer has been shown with this technique.[144] A 1-year study on coronal leakage with this technique found greater leakage with the JS Quick-fill than with lateral compaction.[162]

Variation 5. The use of ultrasonically softened and compacted gutta-percha has already been addressed in this chapter.

ASSESSMENT OF CANAL OBTURATION AND THE STANDARD OF CARE

As can be seen in the discussion of root canal obturation in this chapter, there are many good contemporary techniques for this purpose. Many techniques are operator sensitive and require a greater learning curve. Others are more straightforward and have stood the test of time for delivering quality, successful obturations. The purpose of this section is to highlight many of the key concepts applicable to all techniques and apply these

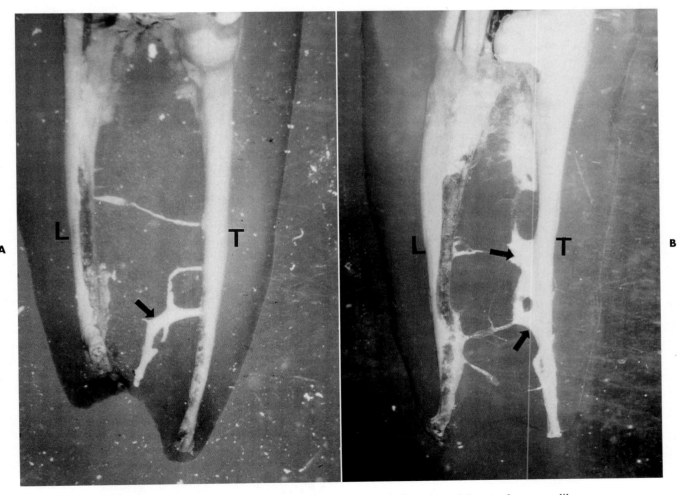

FIG. 9-77 A through **D,** Demineralized, dehydrated, and cleared mesial roots from mandibular molars with canals obturated with either lateral compaction *(L)* or ThermaFil *(T).* All roots are viewed from the proximal view. Generally speaking there is greater movement of both gutta-percha and sealer into the canal irregularities when filled using the ThermaFil technique. Note specifically the areas marked with arrows. *Continued*

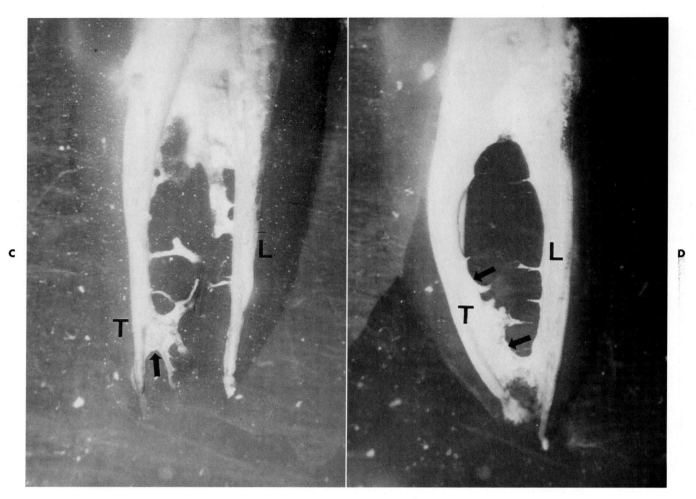

FIG. 9-77, cont'd For legend see previous page.

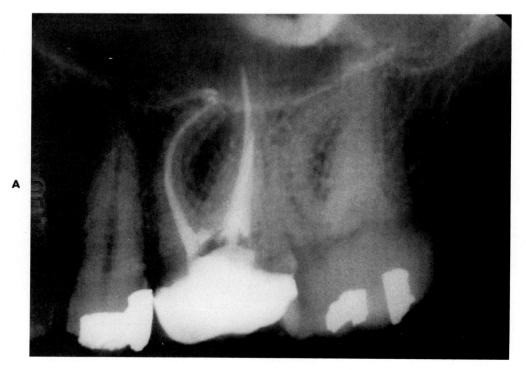

FIG. 9-78 A through **C,** Three clinical cases filled using the ThermaFil technique. Note the ability of the core carrier technique to negotiate curved and irregular canals. Also note the filling of lateral and accessory communications. Minimal amounts of overfilling are present.

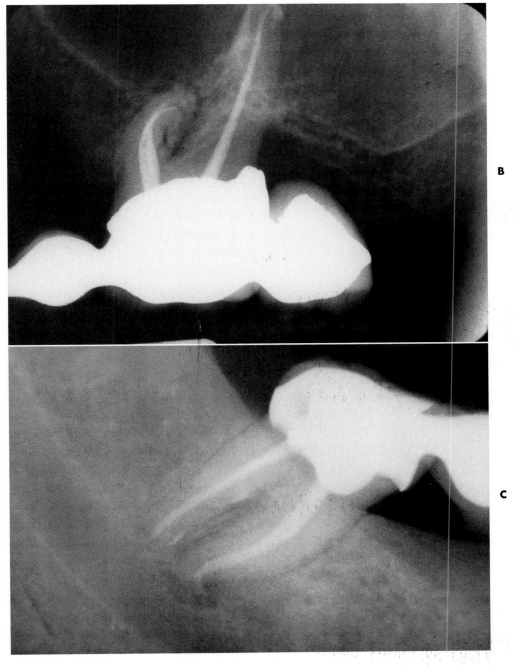

B

C

FIG. 9-78, cont'd For legend see opposite page.

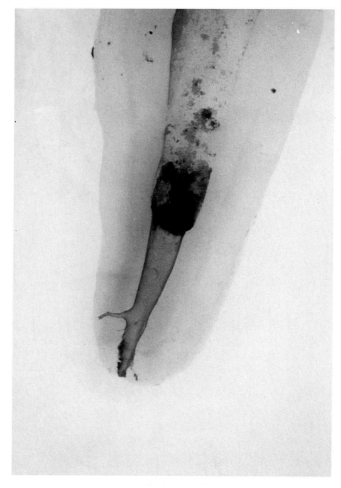

FIG. 9-79 Post space that has been prepared in a canal obturated with a plastic ThermaFil carrier. This can be prepared immediately after canal obturation. *(Courtesy Dr. William P. Saunders.)*

concepts in an integrated fashion in the assessment of treatment rendered, using the principles of the standard of care and quality assurance.

Case 1

A partial pulpectomy was performed on a mandibular second molar because of long-term pain and the presence of a large carious exposure. Little cleaning and shaping was performed on the distal canal, with no attempt being made to instrument and obturate the mesial canals. A gutta-percha cone with sealer was placed halfway down the distal canal, and the access opening was restored with an amalgam (Fig. 9-80). Presently the patient is symptom free. However, there is a significant amount of uncleaned and unfilled canal space. Technically, the treatment rendered falls below the standard of care as stated previously in this chapter. The prognosis is poor based on the etiology for pulpal demise. Quality assurance demands that treatment at the standard of care be provided for the best prognosis. While the patient may be symptom free at present, the possibility for pulpal necrosis or coronal leakage over time will, in all probability, result in a treatment failure and potential patient discomfort. The patient must be informed of this

situation and counseled as to the proper course of action, regardless of the lack of symptoms or signs.

Case 2

A patient has pain in the maxillary first molar. The crown has recently come off during chewing. A radiograph reveals three canals with single gutta-percha cones in place (Fig. 9-81). Technically, the canal obturation is below the standard of care. All clinicians must recognize that single-cone fills are unacceptable and predispose to failure. Coupled with the appearance of the shapes of the cones is the high probability that thorough cleaning and shaping of the canals with the gutta-percha did not occur. There is a high probability also, that significant coronal leakage occurred, as all three roots display periradicular radiolucencies. Likewise, the high incidence of four or more canals in this tooth would indicate that there is additional uncleaned canal space. Retreatment of the root canals must occur before recementing or remaking the crown, whether or not symptoms are present. Failure to do this would constitute negligence on the part of the clinician and would place the patient in an extremely precarious position.

Case 3

The patient is symptom free; however, radiolucencies are present on the mesiobuccal and distobuccal roots of a maxillary first molar (Fig. 9-82). All canals exhibit poor shaping and poor radiographic density of the fillings. The filling in the mesiobuccal canal is off center, indicating in all probability a mesiopalatal canal is present. Technically, the obturation does not meet the standard of care, and the biologic outcomes would support this. The lack of symptoms does not justify acceptance of this level of care, and retreatment is indicated.

Case 4

Two mandibular molars had root canal treatment performed at different times (Fig. 9-83). Each tooth was done by a different clinician. This case can be used to identify subtle shortcomings based on the goals presented in this chapter. First, notice the voids in the fillings in the canals of the second molar compared to the first molar. Notice also the length of the obturated space and the variations in the density of the fills from the orifice to the apex. The key determining factor in this case is not so much the shortcomings in the obturation technique but the lack of proper shaping of the canals in the second molar that in all likelihood prevented a more thorough obturation of the canals. Before any clinician begins to troubleshoot obturation techniques and outcomes, it is necessary to ensure that canal preparation techniques are at the standard of care necessary to achieve the goals cited for canal obturation.

Case 5

A patient had a maxillary premolar that had had root canal treatment and a crown. He wanted a new crown for aesthetic reasons because the recently placed crown had come off. Radiographic examination of the case showed a poorly shaped and obturated root canal, with definite voids and unfilled canal space, both laterally and apically (Fig. 9-84, *A*). When he was advised that a new crown would not be made until the shortcomings in the root canal treatment were rectified, he stated that he had just had the root canal treatment performed 2 months ago and that he had no symptoms. He could not understand why the root canal treatment needed revising. He

Text continued on p. 357

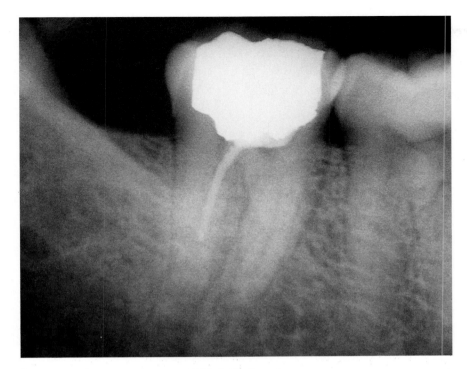

FIG. 9-80 Case 1.

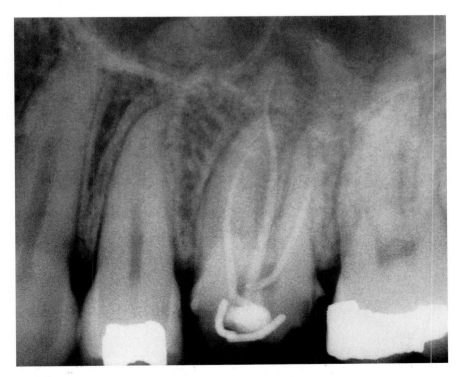

FIG. 9-81 Case 2.

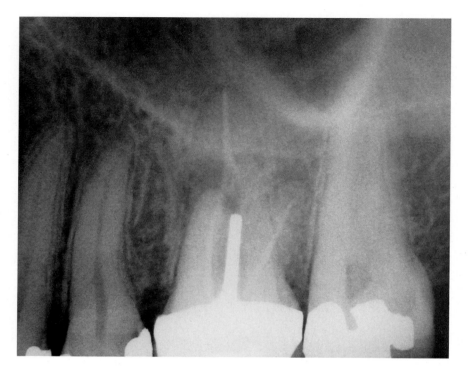

FIG. 9-82 Case 3.

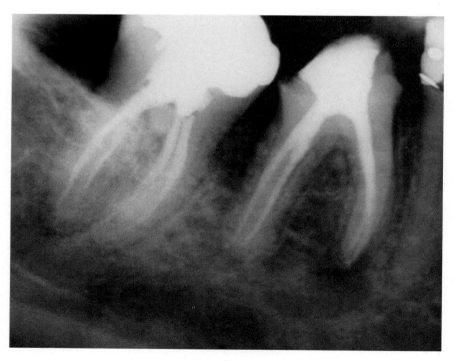

FIG. 9-83 Case 4.

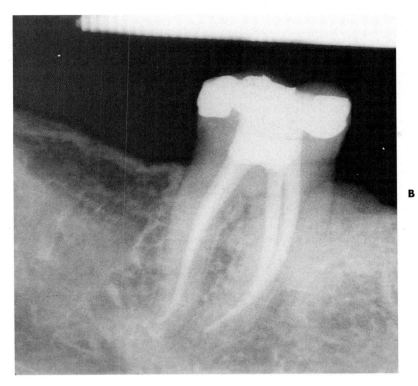

B

FIG. 9-85, cont'd Case 6.

complained to his previous dentist who felt that the root canal treatment was not only acceptable but was at the standard of care. Six weeks later the patient returned with severe pain to percussion and palpation on the maxillary premolar and agreed to have the root canal retreatment. A new working length was established (Fig. 9-84, *B*), and the canal was properly cleaned, shaped, and obturated (Fig. 9-84, *C*). Comparison of the treatment rendered in this case demonstrates the levels of achievement that are necessary to ensure predictable outcomes with endodontic treatment, or as stated in the beginning of this chapter, quality assurance. Achievement of these levels of treatment on a regular basis ensures that the care provided for our patients is at the standard of care.

The final case of this chapter is presented as a standard and a realistic goal that can be routinely achieved by all who choose to do root canal treatment for their patients. This achievement is predicated, however, on a triad of knowledge, application, and assessment, all integrated into a successful outcome.

Case 6

A female patient presented with episodes of spontaneous pain over the past year. The mandibular first molar was tender to bite and often displayed sensitivity to hot and cold. The tooth was determined to have an irreversible pulpitis with acute periradicular periodontitis (Fig. 9-85, *A*). The root canal treatment was begun and completed in one visit. All canals were prepared using .04/.06 rotary nickel-titanium rotary files to an approximate size 30 at the apical extent of the canal, which was determined to be slightly within the confines of the root. Four canals were obturated with warm vertical compaction of a nonstandardized gutta-percha cone and pulp canal sealer, using the System B and Obtura II injectable techniques (Fig. 9-85, *B*). Technically, this case embodies the concepts of con-

temporary endodontics and sets a standard of achievement that should be emulated by all clinicians. (Case courtesy Dr. Myron S. Hilton.)

REFERENCES

1. Adams WR, Patterson SS, Swartz ML: The effect of the apical dentinal plug on broken endodontic instruments, *J Endod* 5:121, 1979.
2. Aktener BO, Cengiz T, Piskin B: The penetration of smear material into dentinal tubules during instrumentation with surface active reagents: a scanning electron microscopic study, *J Endod* 15:588, 1989.
3. Al-Khatib ZZ et al: The antimicrobial affect of various endodontic sealers, *Oral Surg Oral Med Oral Pathol Oral Radiol Endod* 70:784, 1990.
4. Allison DA, Weber CR, Walton RE: The influence of the method of canal preparation on the quality of apical and coronal obturation, *J Endod* 5:298, 1979.
5. Amato R, Goldman M, Tenca J, Burk G: A comparison of the efficiency of various delivery methods on sealer distribution, *J Endod* 10:119, 1984.
6. American Association of Endodontists: *Appropriateness of care and quality assurance guidelines,* 1994, Chicago, The Association.
7. Barbosa SV, Burkard DH, Spångberg LSW: Cytotoxic effects of gutta-percha solvents, *J Endod* 20:6, 1994.
8. Barkhordar RA, Goodis HE, Wantanabe L, Koumdjian J: Evaluation of temperature rise on the outer surface of teeth during root canal obturation techniques, *Quintessence Int* 21:585, 1990.
9. Baumgardner KR, Krell KV: Ultrasonic condensation of gutta-percha: an in vitro dye penetration and scanning electron microscopic study, *J Endod* 16:253, 1990.
10. Baumgartner JC, Mader CL: A scanning electron microscopic evaluation of four root canal irrigations regimens, *J Endod* 13:147, 1987.
11. Baumgardner KR, Taylor J, Walton R: Canal adaptation and coronal leakage: lateral condensation compared to Thermafil, *J Am Dent Assoc* 126:351, 1995.

12. Beatty RG, Vertucci FJ, Hojjatie B: Thermomechanical compaction of gutta-percha: effect of speed and duration, *J Endod* 21:367, 1988.

13. Behrend GD, Cutler CW, Gutmann JL: An in vitro study of smear layer removal and microbial leakage along root canal fillings, *Int Endod J* 29:99, 1996.

14. Berg B: The endodontic management of multirooted teeth, *Oral Surg Oral Med Oral Pathol Oral Radiol Endod* 6:399, 1953.

15. Berry KA, Primack PD, Loushine RJ: Nickel-titanium versus stainless steel finger spreaders in curved canals, *J Endod* 21:221, 1995.

16. Block RM et al: Antibody formation to dog pulp tissue altered by "N2" paste within the root canal, *J Endod* 3:309, 1977.

17. Block RM et al: Systemic distribution of N2 paste containing ^{14}C paraformaldehyde following root canal therapy in dogs, *Oral Surg Oral Med Oral Pathol Oral Radiol Endod* 50:350, 1980.

18. Boiesen J, Brodin P: Neurotoxic effect of two root canal sealers with calcium hydroxide on rat phrenic nerve in vitro, *Endod Dent Traumatol* 7:242, 1991.

19. Bradshaw GB, Hall A, Edmunds DH: The sealing ability of injection-moulded thermoplasticized gutta-percha, *Int Endod J* 22:17, 1989.

20. Brannström M: Smear layer: pathological and treatment considerations, *Oper Dent Suppl* 3:35, 1984.

21. Brilliant JD, Christie WH: A taste of endodontics, *J Acad Gen Dent* 23:29, 1975.

22. Briseño BM, Willerhausen B: Root canal sealer cytotoxicity on human gingival fibroblasts. I. Zinc oxide-eugenol based sealers, *J Endod* 16:383, 1990.

23. Briseño BM, Willerhausen B: Root canal sealer cytotoxicity on human gingival fibroblasts. II. Silicone- and resin-based sealers, *J Endod* 17:537, 1991.

24. Briseño BM, Willerhausen B: Root canal sealer cytotoxicity on human gingival fibroblasts. III. Calcium hydroxide–based sealers, *J Endod* 18:110, 1992.

25. Brodin P, Røed A, Aars H, Ørstavik D: Neurotoxic effects of root filling materials on rat phrenic nerve in vitro, *J Dent Res* 61:1020, 1982.

26. Brownlee WA: Filling of root canals in recently devitalized teeth, *Dominion Dent J* 12(8):254, 1900.

27. Buchanan LS: The continuous wave of obturation technique: "centered" condensation of warm gutta percha in 12 seconds, *Dent Today* 15:60, 1996.

28. Buckley M, Spångberg L: The prevalence and technical quality of endodontic treatment in an American subpopulation, *Oral Surg Oral Med Oral Pathol Oral Radiol Endod* 79:92, 1995.

29. Budd CS, Wleer RN, Kulild JC: A comparison of thermoplasticized injectable gutta-percha obturation techniques, *J Endod* 17:260, 1991.

30. Callahan JR: Rosin, solution for the sealing of the dental tubuli and as an adjuvant in the filling of root canals, *Allied Dent J* 9:53, 110, 1914.

31. Callis PD, Paterson AJ: Microleakage of root fillings: thermoplastic injection compared with lateral condensation, *J Dent* 16:194, 1988.

32. Cameron JA: The use of ultrasound for the removal of the smear layer: the effect of sodium hypochlorite concentrations: SEM study, *Aust Dent J* 33:193, 1988.

33. Chaisrisookumporn S, Rabinowitz JL: Evaluation of ionic leakage of lateral condensation and McSpadden methods by autoradiography, *J Endod* 8:493, 1982.

34. Christie WH, Peikoff MD: Direct impression technique: sealing prepared apical foramen, *J Can Dent Assoc* 46:174, 1980.

35. Ciucchi B, Khettabi M, Holz J: The effectiveness of different endodontic irrigation procedures on the removal of the smear layer: a scanning electron microscopic study, *Int Endod J* 22:21, 1989.

36. Coviello J, Brilliant JD: A preliminary clinical study on the use of tricalcium phosphate as an apical barrier, *J Endod* 5:6, 1979.

37. Czonstkowsky M, Michanowicz A, Vazquez JA: Evaluation of an injection of thermoplasticized low-temperature gutta-percha using radioactive isotopes, *J Endod* 11:71, 1985.

38. Czonstkowsky M, Wilson EG, Holstein FA: The smear layer in endodontics, *Dent Clin North Am* 34:13, 1990.

39. Dow PR, Ingle JI: Isotope determination of root canal failures, *Oral Surg Oral Med Oral Pathol Oral Radiol Endod* 8:1100, 1955.

40. Dwan JJ, Glickman GN: 2-D photoelastic stress analysis of NiTi and stainless steel finger spreaders during lateral condensation, *J Endod* 21:221, 1995.

41. Ebert J, Pawlick H, Petschelt A: Relation between dye penetration and radiographic assessment of root canal fillings in vitro, *Int Endod J* 29:198, 1996.

42. ElDeeb ME, Nguyen TT-Q, Jensen JR: The dentinal plug: its effect on confining substances to the canal and on the apical seal, *J Endod* 9:355, 1983.

43. Evans JT, Simon JHS: Evaluation of the apical seal produced by injected thermoplasticized gutta-percha in the absence of smear layer and root canal sealer, *J Endod* 12:101, 1986.

44. Fors U, Jonasson E, Bergquist A, Berg J-O: Measurements of the root surface temperature during thermomechanical root canal filling in vitro, *Int Endod J* 18:199, 1985.

45. Friedman CE, Sandrik JL, Heuer MA, Rapp GW: Composition and physical properties of gutta-percha endodontic filling materials, *J Endod* 3:304, 1977.

46. Friedman CE, Sandrik JL, Heuer MA, Rapp GW: Composition and mechanical properties of gutta-percha endodontic points, *J Dent Res* 54:921, 1975.

47. Fulkerson MS, Czerw RJ, Donnelly JC: An in vitro evaluation of the sealing ability of Super-EBA cement used as a root canal sealer, *J Endod* 22:13, 1996.

48. Gee JY: A comparison of five methods of root canal obturation by means of dye penetration, *Aust Dent J* 32:279, 1987.

49. Gençoglu N, Samani S, Günday M: Dentinal wall adaptation of thermoplasticized gutta-percha in the absence or presence of smear layer: a scanning electron microscopic study, *J Endod* 19:558, 1993.

50. Gençoglu N, Samani S, Günday M: Evaluation of sealing properties of Thermafil and Ultrafil techniques in the absence or presence of smear layer, *J Endod* 19:599, 1993.

51. Genet JM, Hart AAM, Wesselink PR, Thoden van Velzen SK: Preoperative and operative factors associated with pain after the first endodontic visit, *Int Endod J* 20:53, 1987.

52. Gettleman BH, Messer HH, ElDeeb ME: Adhesion of sealer cements to dentin with and without the smear layer, *J Endod* 17:15, 1991.

53. Gimlin DR, Parr CH, Aguirre-Ramirez G: A comparison of stress produced during lateral and vertical condensation using engineering models, *J Endod* 12:235, 1986.

54. Glickman GN, Dumsha TC: Problems in canal cleaning and shaping. In Gutmann JL, Dumsha TC, Lovdahl PE, Hovland EJ, editors: *Problem solving in endodontics,* ed 3, St Louis, 1997, Mosby.

55. *Glossary: contemporary terminology for endodontics,* ed 5, Chicago, 1994, American Association of Endodontists.

56. Goldberg F et al: Surface architecture of a low-temperature thermoplasticized gutta-percha, *Endod Dent Traumatol* 7:108, 1991.

57. Goldman LB et al: The efficacy of several irrigating solutions for endodontics: a scanning electron microscopic study, *Oral Surg Oral Med Oral Pathol Oral Radiol Endod* 52:197, 1981.

58. Goldman M: Evaluation of two filling methods for root canals, *J Endod* 1:69, 1975.

59. Goldman M et al: The efficacy of several endodontic irrigating solutions: a scanning electron microscopic study: part 2, *J Endod* 8:487, 1982.

60. Göllmer L: Grund der reparativen Fähigkeit der Wurzelhaut (The use of dentin débris as a root canal filling), *Z Stomatol* 34:761, 1936.

61. Goodman A, Schilder H, Aldrich W: The thermomechanical properties of gutta-percha. II. The history and molecular structure of gutta-percha, *Oral Surg Oral Med Oral Pathol Oral Radiol Endod* 37:954, 1974.

62. Goon WWY: The apical push: hermetic seal enhancement using lateral condensation into warm gutta-percha, *Compend Contin Educ Dent* 6:499, 1985.

63. Grahnén H, Hansson L: The prognosis of pulp and root canal therapy: a clinical and radiographic follow-up examination, *Odontol Revy* 12:146, 1961.

64. Granche D et al: Endodontic cements induce alterations in the cell cycle of in vitro cultured osteoblasts, *Oral Surg Oral Med Oral Pathol Oral Radiol Endod* 79:359, 1995.

65. Grossman LI: *Root canal therapy,* Philadelphia, Lea & Febiger, 1940, p 189.

66. Grove CJ: Why root canals should be filled to the dentinocemental junction, *J Am Dent Assoc* 17:293, 1930.

67. Gutmann JL: Clinical, radiographic, and histologic perspectives on success and failure in endodontics, *Dent Clin North Am* 36:379, 1992.

68. Gutmann JL: The dentin-root complex: anatomic and biologic considerations in restoring endodontically treated teeth, *J Prosthet Dent* 67:458, 1992.

69. Gutmann JL: Adaptation of injected thermoplasticized gutta-percha in the absence of the dentinal smear layer, *Int Endod J* 26:87, 1993.

70. Gutmann JL, Heaton JF: Management of the open (immature) apex. II. Non-vital teeth, *Int Endod J* 14:173, 1981.

71. Gutmann JL, Hovland EJ: Problems in root canal obturation. In Gutmann JL, Dumsha TC, Lovdahl PE, Hovland EJ, editors: *Problem solving in endodontics,* ed 3, St Louis, 1997, Mosby.

72. Gutmann JL, Leonard JE: Problem solving in endodontic working length determination, *Comp Contin Educ Dent* 16:288, 1995.

73. Gutmann JL, Lovdahl PE: Problems in the assessment of success and failure, quality assurance and their integration into endodontic treatment planning. In Gutmann JL, Dumsha TC, Lovdahl PE, Hovland EJ, editors: *Problem solving in endodontics,* ed 3, St Louis, 1997, Mosby.

74. Gutmann JL, Rakusin H: Perspectives on root canal obturation with thermoplasticized injectable gutta-percha, *Int Endod J* 20:261, 1987.

75. Gutmann JL, Rakusin H, Powe R, Bowles WH: Evaluation of heat transfer during root canal obturation with thermoplasticized gutta-percha. II. In-vivo response to heat levels generated, *J Endod* 13:441, 1987.

76. Gutmann JL, Saunders WP, Saunders EM, Nguyen L: An assessment of the plastic Thermafil obturation technique. I. Radiographic evaluation of adaptation and placement, *Int Endod J* 26:173, 1993.

77. Gutmann JL, Saunders WP, Saunders EM, Nguyen L: An assessment of the plastic Thermafil obturation technique. II. Material adaptation and sealability, *Int Endod J* 26:179, 1993.

78. Haas SB et al: A comparison of four root canal filling techniques, *J Endod* 15:596, 1989.

79. Haddix JE, Jarrell M, Mattison GD, Pink FE: An in vitro investigation of the apical seal produced by a new thermoplasticized gutta-percha obturation technique, *Quintessence Int* 22:159, 1991.

80. Hardie EM: Heat transmission to the outer surface of the tooth during the thermomechanical compaction technique of root canal obturation, *Int Endod J* 19:73, 1986.

81. Harris GZ, Dickey DJ, Lemon RR, Luebke RG: Apical seal: McSpadden vs lateral condensation, *J Endod* 8:273, 1982.

82. Harrison JW, Baumgartner JC, Svec TA: Incidence of pain associated with clinical factors during and after root canal therapy. II. Postobturation pain, *J Endod* 9:434, 1983.

83. Harvey TE, White JT, Leeb IJ: Lateral condensation stress in root canals, *J Endod* 7:151, 1981.

84. Hasegawa M et al: An experimental study of the sealing ability of a dentinal apical plug treated with bonding agent, *J Endod* 19:570, 1993.

85. Hasselgren G: Where shall the root filling end? *NY State Dent J* 60(6):34, 1994.

86. Hatton EH: Changes produced in the pulp and periapical regions, and their relationship to pulp-canal treatment and to systemic disease, *Dent Cosmos* 66:1183, 1924.

87. Hatton JF, Ferrillo PJ, Wagner G, Stewart GP: The effect of condensation pressure on the apical seal, *J Endod* 14:305, 1988.

88. Heling I, Chandler NP: The antimicrobial effect within dentinal tubules of four root canal sealers, *J Endod* 22:257, 1996.

89. Himel VT, Cain CW: An evaluation of the number of condensor insertions needed with warm lateral condensation of gutta-percha, *J Endod* 19:79, 1993.

90. *History of dentistry in Missouri,* Fulton, Mo, 1938, The Ovid Press, Inc.

91. Hoen MM, LaBounty GL, Keller DL: Ultrasonic endodontic sealer placement, *J Endod* 14:169, 1988.

92. Holcomb J, Pitts D, Nicholls J: Further investigation of spreader loads required to cause vertical root fracture during lateral condensation, *J Endod* 13:277, 1987.

93. Holland GR: Periapical response to apical plugs of dentin and calcium hydroxide in ferret canines, *J Endod* 10:71, 1984.

94. Holland R, de Souza V: Ability of a new calcium hydroxide root canal filling material to induce hard tissue formation, *J Endod* 11:535, 1985.

95. Holland R et al: Tissue reactions following apical plugging of the root canal with infected dentin chips, *Oral Surg Oral Med Oral Pathol Oral Radiol Endod* 49:366, 1980.

96. Hunter W: The role of sepsis and of antisepsis in medicine, *Lancet* 1:79, 1911.

97. Ingle JI: A standardized endodontic technique using newly designed instruments and filling materials, *Oral Surg Oral Med Oral Pathol Oral Radiol Endod* 14:83, 1961.

98. Ingle JI, Zeldow BJ: An evaluation of mechanical instrumentation and the negative culture in endodontic therapy, *J Am Dent Assoc* 57:471, 1958.

99. Jacobsen EL: Clinical aid: adapting the master gutta-percha cone for apical snugness, *J Endod* 10:274, 1984.

100. Jerome CE: Warm vertical gutta-percha obturation: a technique update, *J Endod* 20:97, 1994.

101. Johnson WB: A new gutta-percha technique, *J Endod* 4:184, 1978.

102. Kaplowitz GJ: Evaluation of gutta-percha solvents, *J Endod* 16:539, 1990.

103. Karagöz-Küçükay I, Bayirli G: An apical leakage study in the presence and absence of the smear layer, *Int Endod J* 27:87, 1994.

104. Keane HC: A century of service to dentistry, Philadelphia, 1944, SS White Dental Manufacturing Co.

105. Keane K, Harrington GW: The use of a chloroform-softened gutta-percha master cone and its effect on the apical seal, *J Endod* 10:57, 1984.

106. Kersten HW, Fransman R, Thoden van Velzen SK: Thermomechanical compaction of gutta-percha. I. A comparison of several compaction procedures, *Int Endod J* 19:125, 1986.

107. Kersten HW, Wesselink PR, Thoden van Velzen SK: The diagnostic reliability of the buccal radiograph after root canal filling, *Int Endod J* 20:20, 1987.

108. Koch CRE, Thorpe BL: *A history of dental surgery,* vols 2 and 3, Fort Wayne, Ind, 1909, National Art Publishing Co.

109. Kontakiotis E, Panopoulos P: pH of root canal sealers containing calcium hydroxide, *Int Endod J* 29:202, 1996.

110. Langeland K: Root canal sealants and pastes, *Dent Clin North Am* 18:309, 1974.

111. Langeland K, Liao K, Costa N, Pascon EA: Efficacy of Obtura and Ultrafil root filling devices, *J Endod* 13:135, 1987.

112. Leonard JE, Gutmann JL, Guo IY: Apical and coronal seal of roots obturated with a dentine bonding agent and resin, *Int Endod J* 29:76, 1996.

113. Liewehr FR, Kulild JC, Primack PD: Improved density of gutta-percha after warm lateral condensation, *J Endod* 19:489, 1993.

114. Lloyd A et al: Sealability of the Trifecta technique in the presence or absence of smear layer, *Int Endod J* 28:35, 1995.

115. Love RM, Chandler NP, Jenkinson HF: Penetration of smeared or nonsmeared dentine by *Streptococcus gordonii, Int Endod J* 29:2, 1996.

116. Lugassy AA, Yee F: Root canal obturation with gutta-percha: a scanning electron microscope comparison of vertical compaction and automated thermatic condensation, *J Endod* 8:120, 1982.

117. Mader CL, Baumgartner JC, Peters DD: Scanning electron microscopic investigation of the smeared layer on root canal walls, *J Endod* 10:477, 1984.

118. Mann SR, McWalter GM: Evaluation of apical seal and placement control in straight and curved canals obturated by laterally condensed and thermoplasticized gutta-percha, *J Endod* 13:10, 1987.

119. Marais JT, van der Vyver PJ: Sizing gutta-percha points with a gauge to ensure optimal lateral condensation, *J Dent Assoc South Afr* 51:403, 1996.

120. Marlin J: Injectable standard gutta-percha as a method of filling the root canal, *J Endod* 12:354, 1986.

121. Martin H, Fischer E: Photoelastic stress comparison of warm (Endotec) versus cold lateral condensation techniques, *Oral Surg Oral Med Oral Pathol Oral Radiol Endod* 70:325, 1990.

122. Martin H, LaBounty G: Endotec (warm lateral) vs lateral condensation leakage, *Oral Surg Oral Med Oral Pathol Oral Radiol Endod* 70:325, 1990.

123. McComb D, Smith DC: A preliminary scanning electron microscopic study of root canals after endodontic procedures, *J Endod* 7:238, 1975.

124. McDonald NM, Vire DE: Chloroform in the endodontic operatory, *J Endod* 18:301, 1992.

125. Metzger Z et al: Apical seal by customized versus standardized master cones: a comparative study in flat and round canals, *J Endod* 14:381, 1988.

126. Metzger Z et al: Residual chloroform and plasticity in customized gutta-percha master cones, *J Endod* 14:546, 1988.

127. Michanowicz A, Czonstkowsky M: Sealing properties of an injection-thermoplasticized low-temperature (70°) gutta-percha: a preliminary study, *J Endod* 10:563, 1984.

128. Molyvdas I, Zervas P, Lanbrianidis T, Veis A: Periodontal tissue reactions following root canal obturation with an injection-thermoplasticized gutta-percha technique, *Endod Dent Traumatol* 5:32, 1989.

129. Moorer WR, Genet JM: Antibacterial activity of gutta-percha cones attributed to the zinc oxide component, *Oral Surg Oral Med Oral Pathol Oral Radiol Endod* 53:508, 1982.

130. Moorer WR, Genet JM: Evidence for antibacterial activity of endodontic gutta-percha cones, *Oral Surg Oral Med Oral Pathol Oral Radiol Endod* 53:503, 1982.

131. Moreno A: Thermomechanically softened gutta-percha root canal filling, *J Endod* 3:186, 1977.

132. Mulhern JM, Patterson SS, Newton CW, Ringel AM: Incidence of postoperative pain after one-appointment endodontic treatment of a symptomatic pulpal necrosis in single-rooted teeth, *J Endod* 2:370, 1982.

133. Naidorf IJ: Clinical microbiology in endodontics, *Dent Clin North Am* 18:329, 1974.

134. Nguyen NT: Obturation of the root canal system. In Cohen S, Burns RC, editors: *Pathways of the pulp,* ed 6, St Louis, 1994, Mosby, pp 219-271.

135. Nykaza R, Wong M: Heat softened gutta-percha: an update, *Gen Dent* 39:196, 1991.

136. O'Keefe EM: Pain in endodontic therapy: a preliminary clinical study, *J Endod* 2:315, 1976.

137. O'Neill KJ, Pitts DL, Harrington GW: Evaluation of the apical seal produced by the McSpadden compactor and by lateral condensation with a chloroform-softened primary cone, *J Endod* 9:190, 1983.

138. Oksan T, Aktener BO, Sen BH, Tezel H: The penetration of root canal sealers into dentinal tubules: a scanning electron microscopic study, *Int Endod J* 26:301, 1993.

139. Olgart L, Brannström M, Johnson G: Invasion of bacteria into dentinal tubules: experiments in-vivo and in-vitro, *Acta Odontol Scand* 32:61, 1974.

140. Orban B: Why root canals should be filled to the dentinocemental junction, *J Am Dent Assoc* 17:1086, 1930.

141. Orstavik D, Haapasalo M: Disinfection by endodontic irrigants and dressings or experimentally infected dentinal tubules, *Endod Dent Traumatol* 6:142, 1990.

142. Oswald RJ, Friedman CE: Periapical response to dentin filings, *Oral Surg Oral Med Oral Pathol Oral Radiol Endod* 49:344, 1980.

143. Page ML, Hargreaves KM, ElDeeb M: Comparison of concentric condensation technique with laterally condensed gutta-percha, *J Endod* 21:308, 1995.

144. Pallarés A, Faus V, Glickman GN: The adaptation of mechanically softened gutta-percha to the canal walls in the presence or absence of smear layer: a scanning electron microscopic study, *Int Endod J* 28:266, 1995.

145. Parris J, Wilcox L, Walton R: Effectiveness of apical clearing: histological and radiographic evaluation, *J Endod* 20:219, 1994.

146. Pashley DH: Smear layer: physiological considerations, *Oper Dent Suppl* 3:13, 1984.

147. Pashley DH et al: Scanning electron microscopy of the substructure of smear layers in human dentine, *Arch Oral Biol* 33:265, 1988.

148. Perry SG: Preparing and filling the roots of teeth, *Dent Cosmos* 25:185, 1883.

149. Peters LB, Wesselink PR, Moorer WR: The fate and role of bacteria left in root dentinal tubules, *Int Endod J* 28:95, 1995.

150. Pitts DL, Jones JE, Oswald RJ: A histological comparison of calcium hydroxide plugs and dentin plugs used for the control of gutta-percha root canal filling material, *J Endod* 10:283, 1984.

151. Pitts DL, Matheny HE, Nicholls JI: An in vitro study of spreader loads required to cause vertical root fracture during lateral condensation, *J Endod* 9:544, 1983.

152. Portmann P, Lussi A: A comparison between a new vacuum obturation technique and lateral condensation: an in vitro study, *J Endod* 20:292, 1994.

153. Prinz H: Paper delivered before the St Louis, Missouri Dental Society, Sept 2, 1912.

154. Ramsey WO: Hermetic sealing of root canals: the Greeks had a name for it, *J Endod* 8:100, 1982.

155. Ray H, Seltzer S: A new glass ionomer root canal sealer, *J Endod* 17:598, 1991.

156. Ray HA, Trope M: Periapical status of endodontically treated teeth in relation to the technical quality of the root filling and the coronal restoration, *Int Endod J* 28:12-18, 1995.

157. Ricks-Williamson LJ et al: A three-dimensional finite-element stress analysis of an endodontically prepared maxillary central incisor, *J Endod* 21:362, 1995.

158. Roane JB, Dryden JA, Grimes EW: Incidence of postoperative pain after single- and multiple-visit endodontic procedures, *Oral Surg Oral Med Oral Pathol Oral Radiol Endod* 55:68, 1983.

159. Rosenow EC: Studies on elective localization: focal infection with special reference to oral sepsis, *J Dent Res* 1:205, 1919.

160. Rossmeisl R, Reader A, Melfi R, Marquard J: A study of freeze-dried (lyophilized) cortical bone used as an apical barrier in adult monkey teeth, *Oral Surg Oral Med Oral Pathol Oral Radiol Endod* 53:303, 1982.

161. Rud J, Andreasen JO: A study of failures after endodontic surgery by radiographic, histologic and stereomicroscopic methods, *Int J Oral Surg* 1:311, 1972.

162. Sakkal S, Weine FS, Lemian L: Lateral condensation: inside view, *Compend Contin Educ Dent* 12:796, 1991.

163. Saunders EM: The effect of variation in thermomechanical compaction techniques upon the quality of the apical seal, *Int Endod J* 22:163, 1989.

164. Saunders EM: In vivo findings associated with heat generation during thermomechanical compaction of gutta-percha. I. Temperature levels at the external surface of the root, *Int Endod J* 23:263, 1990.

165. Saunders EM: In vivo findings associated with heat generation during thermomechanical compaction of gutta-percha. II. Histological response to temperature elevation on the external surface of the root, *Int Endod J* 23:268, 1990.

166. Saunders EM, Saunders WP: Long-term coronal leakage of JS Quick-fill root fillings with Sealapex and Apexit sealers, *Endod Dent Traumatol* 11:181, 1995.

167. Saunders WP, Saunders EM: Coronal leakage as a cause of failure in root canal therapy: a review, *Endod Dent Traumatol* 10:105, 1994.

168. Saunders WP, Saunders EM, Gutmann JL, Gutmann ML: An assessment of the plastic Thermafil obturation technique. III. The effect of post space preparation on the apical seal, *Int Endod J* 26:184, 1993.

169. Saw L-P, Messer HH: Root strains associated with different obturation techniques, *J Endod* 21:314, 1995.

170. Schilder H: Filling root canals in three dimensions, *Dent Clin North Am* 11:723, 1967.

171. Schilder H, Goodman A, Aldrich W: The thermomechanical properties of gutta-percha. I. The compressibility of gutta-percha, *Oral Surg Oral Med Oral Pathol Oral Radiol Endod* 37:946, 1974.

172. Scott AC, Vire DE: An evaluation of the ability of a dentin plug to control extrusion of thermoplasticized gutta-percha, *J Endod* 18:52-57, 1992.

173. Seltzer S: *Endodontology: biologic considerations in endodontic procedures*, ed 2, Philadelphia, 1988, Lea & Febiger, pp 25.

174. Seltzer S, Bender IB, Turkenkopf S: Factors affecting successful repair after root canal therapy, *J Am Dent Assoc* 67:651, 1963.

175. Seltzer S, Naidorf I: Flare-ups in endodontics. II. Therapeutic measures, *J Endod* 11:559, 1985.

176. Sen BH, Piskin B, Baran N: The effect of tubular penetration of root canal sealers on dye microleakage, *Int Endod J* 29:23, 1996.

177. Sen BH, Wesselink PR, Türkün M: The smear layer: a phenomenon in root canal therapy, *Int Endod J* 28:141, 1995.

178. Simons J, Ibanez B, Friedman S, Trope M: Leakage after lateral condensation with finger spreaders and D-11-T spreaders, *J Endod* 17:101, 1991.

179. Sjögren U, Hägglund B, Sundqvist G, Wing K: Factors affecting the long-term results of endodontic treatment, *J Endod* 16:498, 1990.

180. Sjögren U, Sundqvist G, Nair PNR: Tissue reaction to gutta-percha particles of various sizes when implanted subcutaneously in guinea pigs, *Eur J Oral Sci* 103:313, 1995.

181. Skillen WG: Why root canals should be filled to the dentinocemental junction, *J Am Dent Assoc* 17:2082, 1930.

182. Skinner RL, Himel VT: The sealing ability of injection-molded thermoplasticized gutta-percha with and without the use of sealers, *J Endod* 13:315, 1987.

183. Sonat B, Dalat D, Günhan O: Periapical tissue reaction to root fillings with Sealapex, *Int Endod J* 23:46, 1990.

184. Southard D, Rooney T: Effective one-visit therapy for the acute apical abscess, *J Endod* 10:580, 1984.

185. Spångberg L: Biologic effect of root canal filling materials, *Odont Tidskr* 77:502, 1969.

186. Spångberg L: Biologic effects of root canal filling materials, *Odontol Revy* 20:133, 1969.

187. Speier MB, Glickman GN: Volumetric and densitometric comparison between nickel titanium and stainless steel condensation, *J Endod* 22:195, 1996.

188. Stamos DE, Gutmann JL, Gettleman BH: In-vivo evaluation of root canal sealer placement and distribution, *J Endod* 21:177, 1995.

189. Stamos DE, Stamos DG: A new treatment modality for internal resorption, *J Endod* 12:315, 1986.

190. Swartz DB, Skidmore AE, Griffin JA: Twenty years of endodontic success and failure, *J Endod* 9:198, 1983.

191. Tagger M, Katz A, Tamse A: Apical seal using the GPII method in straight canals compared with lateral condensation, with or without sealer, *Oral Surg Oral Med Oral Pathol Oral Radiol Endod* 78:225, 1994.

192. Tagger M, Taffer E, Kfir A: Release of calcium and hydroxyl ions from set endodontic sealers containing calcium hydroxide, *J Endod* 14:588, 1988.

193. Tagger M, Tanse A, Katz A, Korzen BH: Evaluation of the apical seal produced by a hybrid root canal filling method, combining lateral condensation and thermatic compaction, *J Endod* 10:299, 1984.

194. Telli C, Gülkan P, Günel H: A critical reevaluation of stresses generated during vertical and lateral condensation of gutta-percha in the root canal, *Endod Dent Traumatol* 10:1, 1994.

195. Torneck CD, Smith JS, Grindall P: Biologic effects of procedures on developing incisor teeth. II. Effect of pulp injury and oral contamination, *Oral Surg Oral Med Oral Pathol Oral Radiol Endod* 35:378, 1973.

196. Tronstad L: Tissue reactions following apical plugging of the root canal with dentin chips in monkey teeth subjected to pulpectomy, *Oral Surg Oral Med Oral Pathol Oral Radiol Endod* 45:297, 1978.

197. Tronstad L, Barnett R, Flax M: Solubility and biocompatibility of calcium hydroxide–containing root canal sealers, *Endod Dent Traumatol* 4:152, 1988.

198. Veis A, Lambrianidis T, Molyvdas I, Zervas P: Sealing ability of sectional injection thermoplasticized gutta-percha technique with varying distance between needle tip and apical foramen, *Endod Dent Traumatol* 8:63, 1992.

199. Vertucci FJ, Hwang CL, Nixon CE: Apical dye penetration associated with three root canal obturation techniques, *J Dent Res* 72:115, 1993.

200. Vertucci FJ, Mattison GD, DeGrood ME, Minden NJ: Apical dye penetration associated with Thermafil and SuccessFil obturations, *J Dent Res* 72:115, 1993.

201. Vire DE: Failure of endodontically treated teeth, *J Endod* 17:338, 1991.

202. Webster AE: Some experimental root canal fillings, *Dominion Dent J* 12:109, 1900.

203. Weinberger BW: *An introduction to the history of dentistry*, St Louis, 1948, Mosby.

204. Weine FS: The enigma of the lateral canal, *Dent Clin North Am* 28:833, 1984.

205. Weisenseel JA Jr, Hicks ML, Pelleu GB Jr: Calcium hydroxide as an apical barrier, *J Endod* 13:1, 1987.

206. Wennberg A, Ørstavik D: Adhesion of root canal sealers to bovine dentine and gutta-percha, *Int Endod J* 23:13, 1990.

207. White RR, Goldman M, Sun Lin P: The influence of the smeared layer upon dentinal tubule penetration by plastic filling materials, *J Endod* 10:558, 1984.

208. Wiemann AH, Wilcox LR: In vitro evaluation of four methods of sealer placement, *J Endod* 17:444, 1991.

209. Wilson PR, Barnes IE: Treatment of internal resorption with thermoplasticized gutta-percha, *Int Endod J* 20:94, 1987.

210. Wong M, Peters DB, Lorton L: Comparison of gutta-percha filling techniques: three chloroform gutta-percha filling techniques: part 2, *J Endod* 8:4, 1982.

211. Wu M-K, Wesselink PR: Endodontic leakage studies reconsidered. I. Methodology, application and relevance, *Int Endod J* 26:37, 1993.

212. Wu M-K et al: Fluid transport and bacterial penetration along root canal fillings, *Int Endod J* 26:203, 1993.

213. Yamada RS et al: A scanning electron microscopic comparison of a high volume final flush with several irrigating solutions: part III, *J Endod* 9:137, 1983.

214. Yaman SD, Alaçam T, Yaman Y: Analysis of stress distribution in a vertically condensed maxillary central incisor root canal, *J Endod* 21:321, 1995.

215. Yared GM, Bou Dagher FE: Elongation and movement of the gutta-percha master cone during initial lateral condensation, *J Endod* 19:395, 1993.

216. Yee FA, Marlin J, Krakow AA, Grøn P: Three-dimensional obturation of the root canal using injection-molded, thermoplasticized dental gutta-percha, *J Endod* 3:168, 1977.

217. Yee RDJ, Newton CW, Patterson SS, Swartz M: The effect of canal preparation on the formation and leakage characteristics of the apical dentin plug, *J Endod* 10:308, 1984.

218. Youngson CC, Nattress BR, Manogue M, Speirs AF: In vitro radiographic representation of the extent of voids within obturated root canals, *Int Endod J* 28:77, 1995.

219. Zmener O et al: Biocompatibility of a thermoplasticized gutta-percha in the subcutaneous connective tissue of the rat, *J Dent Res* 67:616, 1988.

Chapter 10

Records and Legal Responsibilities

Edwin J. Zinman

EXCELLENT ENDODONTIC THERAPY VIA EXCELLENT RECORDS

Importance

Endodontic therapy records serve as an important map, guiding the clinician along the correct road toward diagnosis and treatment. Documentation is essential to attaining endodontic excellence.

Content

Endodontic treatment records should include the following information:

1. Name of patient
2. Date of visit
3. Medical and dental history (periodically updated)
4. Chief complaints
5. Radiographs of diagnostic quality
6. Clinical examination findings
7. Differential and final diagnosis
8. Treatment plan
9. Prognosis
10. Referral, including patient refusals (if any)
11. Progress notes, including complications
12. Completion notes
13. Canceled or missed appointments and stated reasons
14. Emergency treatment
15. Patient concerns and dissatisfactions
16. Planned follow-ups
17. Drug and laboratory prescriptions
18. Patient noncompliance
19. Consent forms
20. Accounting
21. Recalls
22. Name or initial of entrant

Function

Dental records should document the following information:
1. Course of the patient's dental disease and treatment by recorded diagnosis, treatment, and prognosis
2. Communication among the treating dentist and other health care providers, consultants, subsequent treating practitioners, and third-party carriers
3. Official professional business record in dental-legal matters, documenting a sound plan of dental management
4. Necessity and reasonableness of care and treatment for evaluation by peer review and insurance carriers
5. Standard of care followed

Patient Information Form

A patient information form provides data essential for identification and office communication. Name, address, business address, and telephone numbers are needed to contact the patient for scheduling purposes or to inquire about treatment sequelae. Similar information about the patient's spouse, relative, or a close friend who can be notified in an emergency is also required. In the event the patient is a minor, the responsible parent or guardian should provide the information. Often questions about dental insurance and financial responsibility are included to avoid any misunderstandings later and to fulfill federal requirements regarding truth in lending for installment payments of four or more, regardless of interest charges, or any late payment charges.[1,2] Patient information and history forms should be updated periodically or as the need arises (Fig. 10-1).

Health History

Past and present health status should be thoroughly reviewed by the dentist before proceeding so that dental treatment can be safely initiated. Health questionnaires open avenues for discussion about problems of major organ systems, important biochemical mechanisms, such as blood coagulation, and any immunocompromise. As a result of this review, the dentist may suggest or insist that the patient be examined by a physician or tested by a laboratory under medical supervision to determine whether a suspected medical problem may require attention before endodontic therapy proceeds or whether treatment modifications should be made (e.g., because of drug sensitivity or allergy).[3,4]

Every health history form should request information about any current medical therapy and the name of the treating physician to be contacted in the event of emergency. Consultation with the patient's physician may be indispensable to the patient's welfare.

Medical histories must be updated periodically, at least annually. The patient should be asked to review the original history. If there are no changes, the patient should date and sign the original history form. Otherwise, the patient should identify each medical change and date and sign the form as a medical update. If the patient provides an entirely new, updated form (rather than changing data on the old form), earlier medical histories should be retained for future reference. If physi-

---

[1]Morris WO: *Dental litigation,* ed 2, 1977, The Michie Co.
[2]Federal Truth in Lending Act, 15 USC §1601 et seq.
[3]Keeling D: Malpractice claim prevention, *J Calif Dent Assoc* 3(8):55, 1975.
[4]Weichman J: Malpractice prevention and defense, *J Calif Dent Assoc* 3:58, 1975.

PATIENT INFORMATION

Name: _____ Social Security No.: _____ Date: _____

Date of Birth: _____ If Minor, Parents' or Guardians' Names: _____

Marital Status: ☐ Single   ☐ Married   ☐ Separated   ☐ Widowed   ☐ Divorced

Address: _____ Phone: _____ Fax: _____

City: _____ State: _____ Zip Code: _____

REFERRED BY: _____ Patient Driver's License No.: _____

Occupation: _____ Employer: _____ How long: _____

Business Address: _____ Phone: _____

City: _____ State: _____ Zip Code: _____

Name of Spouse: _____

Occupation: _____ Employer: _____ How Long: _____

Business Address: _____ Phone: _____ Fax: _____

City: _____ State: _____ Zip Code: _____

PERSON RESPONSIBLE FOR ACCOUNT: _____

Address (if different from patient): _____

City: _____ State: _____ Zip Code: _____ Phone: _____

Relationship to patient: _____

DENTAL INSURANCE CARRIERS:

_____ Group No.: _____ Local No.: _____

Name of Insured Person: _____ Social Security No.: _____

Relationship to Patient: _____

SECOND DENTAL INSURANCE CARRIER (if dual coverage):

_____ Group No.: _____ Local No.: _____

Name of Insured Person: _____ Social Security No.: _____

Relationship to Patient: _____

Purpose of Visit or Chief Complaint: _____

Date: _____ Signature: _____

FIG. 10-1 Patient information form.

---

cian approval for treatment occurred, record such approval. Also consider verifying approval by fax and letter with copies retained in the chart.

Dental History

The dental history should include past dental difficulties. A positive response may suggest further consultation with the patient and consideration for obtaining the prior treating dentist's written records and radiographs for elucidation.[5,6]

Diagnostic and Progress Records

Diagnostic and progress records often combine the "fill-in" and "check-off" types of forms. *Fill-in* or essay type of forms allow greater latitude of response to a question, resulting in a more detailed description. One drawback, however, is that it also is open to oversights unless a dentist is very conscientious in noting all clinical information by follow up.

An essay type of health history response, alone, is inefficient, since a patient may not distinguish between important versus insignificant signs or symptoms. A *check-off* format is efficient and more practical. Forms with questions that reveal pertinent data alert the clinician to medical or dental conditions that may warrant further consideration or consultation before proceeding. Moreover, such records document missing medical information the patient failed to provide. Therefore at the end of the check-off portion of the medical history, there should be an essay question so that the patient can provide any other pertinent medical information.

[5]Morris WO: *Dental litigation*, ed 2, 1977, The Michie Co.
[6]Terezhalmy G, Bottomley W: General legal aspects of diagnostic dental radiography, *Oral Surg* 48:486, 1979.

Radiographs

Radiographs are essential for diagnosis and also as additional documentation of the pretreatment condition of the patient. A panographic radiograph is not diagnostically accurate for endodontics and therefore is used only as a screening device.[7] Diagnostic quality periapical radiographs are essential aids in diagnosis and midtreatment and completion endodontic therapy, including measuring films, to verify the final result, and for follow-up comparisons at recall examinations. Retain all radiographs.

Evaluation and Diagnosis

Diagnosis includes evaluating the history of the current problem, clinical examination, pulpal testing, and recorded radiographic results. If therapy is indicated, the reasons can be discussed with the patient in an organized way. When other factors affect the prognosis (e.g., strategic importance or restorability of the tooth), the clinician should consider further consultation before initiating any treatment.

Differential Diagnosis

Sound endodontics begins with a proper diagnosis. Otherwise, unnecessary or risky treatment follows. Generally, the following tests should be performed to arrive at a correct and accurate diagnosis:
1. Thermal testing
2. Electrical testing, if possible
3. Percussion
4. Palpation
5. Mobility
6. Periodontal assessment

Negative, as well as positive, pulpal testing results should be recorded. In the mind of a jury, peer review committees, and insurance consultants, if test results were not recorded, the tests may be regarded as not ever having been done, since reasonable dentists should record that testing was done along with test results.

Treatment Plan

Treatment records should contain a written plan that includes all aspects of the patient's oral health. Treatment plans should be coordinated, preferably in writing, with other jointly treating dentists. If another aspect of the patient's dental care not under your direct supervision is not proceeding properly, initiate contact with the other dentist and advise the patient of the problem. For instance, endodontic treatment will probably fail if underlying periodontal pathology is ignored and untreated. Therefore assess and treat the patient's whole mouth, not just the pulp remnants.

If the scope of the examination or treatment is intentionally limited, such as a screening examination or emergency endodontic therapy, the limited scope of the visit should be recorded. Otherwise, the chart appears as if the examination were superficial or the treatment were incomplete and substandard. If a suspicious apical lesion is to be reevaluated, record the future evaluation date and purpose. Otherwise, the chart appears as if the dentist ignored a potential pathologic condition, such as suspected fracture. General soft tissue examination with cancer check is a standard part of any complete dental examination.

---

[7]See Chapter 5.

Consent Form

Following endodontic diagnosis, the benefits, risks, treatment plan, and alternatives to endodontic treatment, including the patient's refusal of recommended treatment, should be presented to the patient or guardian to document acceptance or rejection of the consultation recommendations. The patient (or guardian) should sign and date the consent form, including any video informed consent. Later changes in the proposed treatment plan should also be discussed and initialed by the patient to indicate continued acceptance and to acknowledge understanding of any new risks, alternatives, or referrals.

Treatment Record: Endodontic Chart

A suggested chart is presented herein to facilitate recording of information pertinent to the diagnosis, recommendations, and treatment of the endodontic patient (Fig. 10-2). Systematic acquisition and arrangement of data from the patient questionnaire, and also clinical and radiographic examinations, expedite accurate diagnosis and recording of endodontic treatment in detail with minimal clinician time. Suggested chart format and use are described as follows:

General patient data

Patient name, address, phone number(s), referring doctor, and chief complaint are printed or typed in the corresponding space at the patient's initial office visit.

Appointment schedule and business record

This section is divided into two parts:
1. The first portion is completed by the treating dentist or staff after the diagnosis and treatment plan have been formulated and presented to the patient. Tooth number and quoted fee are posted. Treatment plan is recorded by simply circling the appropriate description. Under *special instructions,* specific treatment requests by the referring dentist are circled. Details of planned adjunctive procedures (e.g., hemisection, root resection) may be written in the adjacent space. Along with information from the patient data section, the dentist can use this for general reference during future treatment. The dental secretary also utilizes this information when scheduling appointments and establishing financial arrangements.
2. The remaining second portion is completed by business personnel. Financial agreements, third-party coverage, account status, and appointment data, including the day, date, and scheduled procedure, are recorded.

Portions of the following diagnosis and treatment sections may be completed by either the dentist or the chairside assistant. The dentist should review and approve entries.

Dental history

Chief complaint should note if the patient is symptomatic at the time of examination. Narrative facts regarding the presenting problem are then recorded. Additional details of the chief complaint obtained during successive questioning are recorded by circling the applicable descriptive adjective within each symptom parameter. The pain intensity index (0 to 10) or pain classification (mild +, moderate + +, severe + + +) should be registered alongside the appropriate description. For accurate assessment of the effects of prior dental treatment pertaining to the examination site, a summary account of such procedures should be documented. All pretreatment signs and symptoms should be described.

FIRST NAME	LAST NAME	AGE

DENTAL HISTORY: CHIEF COMPLAINT   SYMPTOMATIC   ASYMPTOMATIC

SYMPTOMS	Location	Chronology	Quality	Affected By	Prior Tx	Initials: Dr._____ Asst._____
		Inception	sharp intensity	hot palpation	Tx: restorative Yes No	**TOOTH**
			dull + ++ +++	cold manipulation	emergency Yes No	
		Clinical Course:	spontaneous		RCT Yes No	R————————L
			pulsating provoked	biting head position		
localized referred		constant momentary	steady reproducible	chewing activity	Sx Pre-Tx: Yes No	
diffuse radiating		intermittent lingering	enlarging occasional	percussion time of day	Sx Post-Tx: Yes No	

MEDICAL HISTORY

Heart Condition	Anemia / Bleeding	Epilepsy / Fainting	Allergies:	Major Medical Prob:	CONSULTATION:
angina	Diabetes / Kidney	Sinusitis / ENT	penicillin / antibiotics	Females:	Date: Dr.:
coronary	Hepatitis / Liver	Glaucoma / Visual	aspirin / Tylenol	Pregnant _____ mo	Recommendation:
surgery	Herpes	Mental / Neural	codeine / narcotics	Recent Hosp. Operation:	
pacemaker	Thyroid / Hormonal	Tumor / Neoplasms	local anesthetic	Current Medical TX:	
Rheumatic Fever / Murmur	Asthma / Respiratory	Alcoholism / Addictions	N_2O/O_2	Medications:	
Hypertension / Circulatory	Ulcers / Digestive	Infectious Diseases	Latex		
Immunosuppression	Migraine / Headaches	Venereal Disease	other:		Initials: Dr._____ Asst._____

CLINICAL FINDINGS

EXAMINATION	RADIOGRAPHIC	CLINICAL		DIAGNOSTIC TESTS	
Tooth	Attachment Apparatus	Tooth	Soft Tissues	Tooth #	
WNL	PDL normal	WNL	WNL	perio	
caries	PDL thickened	discoloration	extra-oral swelling	mobility	
restoration	alveolar bone, WNL	caries	intra-oral swelling	percussion	
calcification	diffuse lucency	pulp exposure	sinus tract	palpation	
resorption	circumscribed lucency	prior access	lymphadenopathy	cold	
fracture	resorption	attrition / abrasion	TMJ TMD	hot	
perforation / deviation	apical	fracture	perio B	EPT	
prior RCTx/RCF	lateral	restoration		bite / chewing	
separated instrument	hypercementosis	amalgam		date:	
canal obstruction	osteosclerosis	composite	M————D	bruxism: yes_____ no_____	
post / build-up	perio	glass ionomer			
open apex		inlay / onlay		nightguard: yes_____ no_____ Initials: Dr._____ Asst._____
		temporary	L		
		crown			
		abutment			

DIAGNOSIS   PULPAL

PULPAL	PERIAPICAL	ETIOLOGY		PROGNOSIS		
				ENDODONTIC	PERIODONTAL	RESTORATIVE
WNL	WNL	idiopathic trauma		favorable	favorable	favorable
reversible pulpitis	acute apical periodontitis	caries periodontal		questionable	questionable	questionable
irreversible pulpitis	acute apical abscess	restoration orthodontic		poor	poor	poor
necrosis	chronic periapical inflammation	attrition / abrasion prior RCTx				
prior RCTx/RCF	phoenix abscess	developmental intentional				
	osteosclerosis	sinusitis systemic				

PT. CONSULT	___ Examination Findings ___ Periodontal Status ___ Fracture ___ Surgery ___ Prognosis
	___ Treatment Plan ___ Restoration ___ Discoloration ___ Recall ___ Consent Form Initials: Dr._____ Asst._____

TREATMENT	CONS	PRE-TREATMENT	CLEANING / SHAPING	OBTURATION	SURG	Rx									
DATE		pt.	Dr.	local	R.D.	rel oc.	O.D.	access	pulpec.	canal	test	final	G.G.B.	s. file	cotton	temp	G.P.	sealer	tech.	post	post space	B-U	temp	I&D	hemisection	bicuspidization	root resect	S. R.	microsurg. retro.	analgesic	Antibiotic	Ca(OH)2	X-Ray	crown lengthening	bleach	retreatment	doctor initial	chairside init.
mo	day	yr																																				

CANAL	REF	Elec.	X-Ray	Adj.	Final	Size	Rx Date	MEDICATION	DOSE DISP		INSTR.		
B F									x		q	h	
L P									x		q	h	
MB									x		q	h	
ML									x		q	h	
DB									x		q	h	
DL									x		q	h	

FIG. 10-2 Endodontic treatment record.

Medical history

Reference information (e.g., personal physician's name, address, and phone, patient's age, date of last physical examination) are recorded. Obtain a detailed medical history by completing a survey of the common diseases and disorders significant to dentistry along with a comprehensive review of corresponding organ systems and physiologic conditions. Specific entities that have affected the patient are circled. Essential remarks regarding these entries (e.g., details of consultations with the patient's physician) should be documented on an attached blank sheet with dated treatment notes, or the back of this chart (Fig. 10-3). A review of the patient's medical status (including recent or current conditions, treatment, and medications) completes the medical history. Medical histories should be updated at least annually and at reevaluation visits, particularly if evidence of failing endodontic procedures necessitates retreatment.

Examination

Following the dental and medical history, findings obtained from the various phases of the clinical and radiographic examinations are recorded. Lists in each category afford the clinician a systematic format for recording details pertinent to a proper diagnosis. Appropriate descriptions are circled, followed by the necessary notations in the accompanying spaces. Tabular arrangement allows easier recording and comparison of diagnostic test data acquired from one tooth on different dates or from different teeth on one day. As for entries in the dental history, a pain intensity index (0 to 10) or pain classification (mild +, moderate ++, severe +++) should be used whenever possible to document diagnostic test results.

Diagnosis

Careful analysis of accumulated examination data should result in the determination of an accurate pulpal and periapical diagnosis. Clinical conditions are circled, as are the probable etiologic factors for the presenting problem. Alternative modalities of therapy are considered and analyzed. The recommended treatment plan is circled, followed by a prognostic assessment of the intended therapeutic course.

Patient consultation

Patients should be advised of each diagnosis and should consent to the treatment plan before therapy is instituted. Consultation should include an explanation of reasonable alternative treatment approaches and rationales, as well as any preexisting conditions and consequences, including risks from nontreatment or delayed treatment that may affect the outcome of intended therapy. Such discussion is documented by simply completing and endorsing the checklist.

Treatment

All treatment rendered on a given date is documented by placing a check mark (✔) within the designated procedural category. Only the most frequent retreatment procedures are included for tabulation. Descriptions of occasional procedures or explanatory treatment remarks should be entered in writing. A separate dated entry should be made for each patient visit, phone and fax communication (e.g., consultations with the patient or other doctors), and correspondence (e.g., biopsy report, treatment letters). Individual root canal lengths are recorded by (1) circling the corresponding anatomic designation and the method of length

determination (e.g., radiograph and/or electronic measuring device), (2) writing the measurement (in millimeters), and (3) indicating the reference point.

For any medication prescribed, refilled, or dispensed the treatment record should show the date and type of drug, including dosage, quantity, and instructions for use, in the treatment table under *Rx*. Periodic recall intervals, dates, and findings are entered in the spaces provided.

Abbreviations

Abbreviated records can be frustrating if the practitioner is unable to decipher his or her own handwritten entries. Use standard or easily understood abbreviations. Pencil entries are legally valid, but ink entries are less vulnerable to a plaintiff's claim of erasure or record alteration. However, even a short pencil is better than a long memory. Records remember, but patients and dentists alike may forget.

A sample completed endodontic chart (Fig. 10-2 and 10-3) illustrates its proper utilization. An explanatory key listing the standard abbreviations used in the chart is provided in Fig. 10-4.

Computerized Treatment Records

Increasingly, dentists are using computerized record storage. To avoid a claim of record falsification, whatever computer system is used, it should be able to demonstrate that records indicating earlier treatment were not recently falsified. Technology, such as the WORM system, which will identify tampering of computer data, is not foolproof, since it cannot detect tampering where an entire disk of recent origin has been substituted for an earlier version. Periodically a hard copy of data maintained in the computer should be printed out and hand-initialed and dated as written verification of the computer records.

Record Size

Brief records risk incomplete documentation. There is no harm in writing too much but great danger in recording too little. Standard 8½ by 11 inch or larger clinical records possess the advantage of providing the treating dentist adequate space for clinical notes.

Identity of Entry Author

It is inconsequential whether a dentist or an auxiliary records the clinical entries unless otherwise required by state law.[8] What is important is that the correct clinical information is recorded. Each person who makes an entry should record the date and initial the entry. Otherwise, the author's identity may be forgotten should the individual who recorded the entry be needed in a legal proceeding. For instance, initializing the entry makes it easier to identify the particular dentist or auxiliary who, since recording, is now employed elsewhere.

Patient Record Request

Patient requests for records must be honored. It is unethical to refuse to transfer patient records, on patient request, to another treating dentist.[9] Moreover, it is illegal in some states, subjecting the dentist to discipline and fines should the records

---

[8]Calif Bus Prof Code, §1683.
[9]American Dental Association: Principles of ethics and code of professional conduct, §1B.

LAST NAME		FIRST NAME		DR. MR. MISS MRS.	ADDRESS		HOME PHONE	Fax
							BUSINESS PHONE	Fax
REF. DR.					REF. DR. ADDRESS		REF. DR. PHONE	Fax

TOOTH 30   R——L   FEE

CONSULT / EET

TREATMENT PLAN   RCT   AE PE ME

SURGERY   Ca(OH)$_2$

SPECIAL INSTRUCTIONS
POST SPACE
PREFORMED POST/B.U.
COMP. AMAL. TEMP. CR.

Distal Canal Resin

	MIDDLE INITIAL	INSURANCE S D	AMT DUE	REC'D	DATE	DAY	TIME	PRO-CEDURE	X-RAY	REMARKS:
		PRE-AUTH Y N								
		% COVERED								
		VERIFIED								
		FORM SIGNED								
		PT. INFORMED								
		PT. PORTION								
		INS SENT								

DATE MO	DAY	YR	REMARKS	SIGNATURE
2	14	98	*Pt. urged to have a cast metal crown made as soon as possible. Confirming letter to referring doctor.*	Asst. AE Dr. EZ

FIRST NAME / *LAST NAME*

FIG. 10-3 Treatment record section used to detail progress and events.   *Continued*

FIRST NAME	LAST NAME	AGE

DENTAL HISTORY: **CHIEF COMPLAINT** (SYMPTOMATIC) **ASYMPTOMATIC**

Crown placed one week ago. Diffuse pain began The next day - Pt. cannot localize
The pain. Heat, cold and chewing increase the pain.

SYMPTOMS	Location	Chronology	Quality	Affected By	Prior Tx	Initials: Dr. SC Asst.

Left side
V1 — V3

Inception 6 days

Clinical Course:

intensity
+ (++) +++
spontaneous
provoked
steady
enlarging

(sharp) dull
(pulsating)
(reproducible)
occasional

(hot) +
(cold) ++
palpation
manipulation

biting
(chewing)
percussion

head position
activity
time of day

localized   referred   (constant)   momentary
(diffuse)   (radiating)   intermittent   (lingering)

Tx: restorative   (Yes)   No   Crown
emergency   Yes   (No)
RCT   Yes   (No)

Sx Pre-Tx: Yes   (No)
Sx Post-Tx: (Yes)   No

TOOTH
R ———————— L
(19)

MEDICAL HISTORY

				Major Medical Prob:
Heart Condition	Anemia / Bleeding	Epilepsy / Fainting	Allergies:	Females:
angina	(Diabetes) / Kidney	(Sinusitis) / ENT	penicillin / antibiotics	Pregnant _____ mo
coronary	Hepatitis / Liver	Glaucoma / Visual	aspirin / Tylenol	Recent Hosp. Operation:
surgery	Herpes	Mental / Neural	codeine / narcotics	Current Medical TX:
pacemaker	Thyroid / Hormonal	Tumor / Neoplasms	local anesthetic	Medications:
Rheumatic Fever / Murmur	Asthma / Respiratory	Alcoholism / Addictions	N.O/O.	
Hypertension / Circulatory	Ulcers / Digestive	Infectious Diseases	(Latex)	
Immunosuppression	(Migraine) / Headaches	Venereal Disease	other:	Initials: Dr. SC Asst.

CLINICAL FINDINGS

EXAMINATION		RADIOGRAPHIC	CLINICAL		DIAGNOSTIC TESTS

Tooth	Attachment Apparatus	Tooth	Soft Tissues

Tooth #	18	19	20			
perio	WNL	WNL	WNL			
mobility	WNL	WNL	WNL			
percussion	WNL	+	WNL			
palpation	WNL	WNL	WNL			
cold	WNL	+++	WNL			
hot	WNL	++	WNL			
EPT						
bite / chewing	WNL	++	WNL			
date:	2/14/98					
bruxism: yes ✓	no					

Examination Tooth:
WNL
caries
(restoration)   mesial
(calcification)
resorption
fracture
perforation / deviation
prior RCTx/RCF
separated instrument
canal obstruction
post / build-up
open apex

Attachment Apparatus:
PDL normal
(PDL thickened)
alveolar bone, WNL
diffuse lucency
circumscribed lucency
resorption
  apical
  lateral
hypercementosis
osteosclerosis
perio

Clinical Tooth:
WNL
discoloration
caries
pulp exposure
prior access
attrition / abrasion
fracture
(restoration)
amalgam
composite
glass ionomer
inlay / onlay
temporary
(crown)
abutment

Soft Tissues:
(WNL)
extra-oral swelling
intra-oral swelling
sinus tract
lymphadenopathy
TMJ
perio

B 2
M 3 — D 3
L 2

nightguard: yes ✓   no _____   Initials: Dr. SC Asst.

DIAGNOSIS

PULPAL	PERIAPICAL	ETIOLOGY		PROGNOSIS		
				ENDODONTIC	PERIODONTAL	RESTORATIVE

PULPAL:
WNL
reversible pulpitis
(irreversible pulpitis)
necrosis
prior RCTx/RCF

PERIAPICAL:
WNL
(acute apical periodontitis)
acute apical abscess
chronic periapical inflammation
phoenix abscess
osteosclerosis

ETIOLOGY:
idiopathic   trauma
caries   periodontal
(restoration)   orthodontic
attrition / abrasion   prior RCTx
developmental   intentional
sinusitis   systemic

ENDODONTIC: (favorable) questionable poor
PERIODONTAL: (favorable) questionable poor
RESTORATIVE: (favorable) questionable poor

PT. CONSULT	✓ Examination Findings ✓ Periodontal Status ✓ Fracture ✓ Surgery ✓ Prognosis ✓ Treatment Plan ✓ Restoration ___ Discoloration ✓ Recall ✓ Consent Form	Initials: Dr. SC Asst.

TREATMENT	CONS	PRE-TREATMENT	CLEANING / SHAPING	OBTURATION	SURG	Rx				

DATE																															

mo	day	yr	pt.	Dr.	local	R.D.	rel oc.	O.D.	access	pulpec.	canal	test	final	G.G.B.	s. file	cotton	temp	G.P.	sealer	tech.	post	post space	B-U	temp	I&D	REF	hemisection	bicuspidization	root resect	S. R.	analgesic	Antibiotic	Ca(OH)2	X-Ray	crown lengthening	bleach	retreatment	doctor initial	chairside init.
2	14	98	✓	✓	✓	✓			✓	✓	✓	✓	✓	✓			✓	✓	w(I) + glass ionomer core																			SC	

CANAL	REF	Elec.	X-Ray	Adj.	Final	Size	Rx Date	MEDICATION	DOSE DISP	INSTR.
B F							2/14/98	Ibuprofen	600 × 12	1 q 6 h
L P									x	q h
MB		21.0			25				x	q h
ML		20.5			25				x	q h
DB		21.0			30				x	q h
DL		21.0			30				x	q h

FIG. 10-3, cont'd Treatment record section used to detail progress and events.

Ab	=	Antibiotic
ABS	=	Abscess
access	=	Access cavity
analg.	=	Analgesic
apico	=	Apicoectomy
B-U	=	Buildup of tooth
canal	=	Identify canal that has been cleaned and shaped
cotton	=	Placed in pulp chamber between treatments
ENDO	=	Endodontics
EPT	=	Electric pulp test
epin	=	Epinepherine
final	=	Final file
G.G.B.	=	Gates-Glidden bur
G.P.	=	Gutta-percha
I & D	=	Incision and drainage
L.A. or local	=	Local anesthetic
O.D.	=	Open and drain
perio	=	Periodontal
post	=	Preformed, custom, or transilluminated post
pt	=	Patient
pulpec	=	Pulpectomy
R.D.	=	Rubber dam
Rel occ	=	Relieved occlusion
resorp.	=	Resorption
retro	=	Retrograde procedure
S/R	=	Suture removal
s.file	=	Serial filing
S/D	=	Single insurance or dual coverage
sealer	=	Type of sealer used
tech.	=	Technique for canal obturation
temp	=	Temporary restoration
test	=	Test file
WNL	=	Within normal limits
Y/N	=	Insurance preauthorized? Yes or No

FIG. 10-4 Standard abbreviation key.

not be provided to the patient on written request, even if an outstanding balance is owed.[10]

Patient Education Pamphlets

Patient education pamphlets may be used in litigation as evidence that a patient was properly informed and given endodontic alternatives but instead chose extraction. Such pamphlets include the American Dental Association's (ADA's) "Your Teeth Can be Saved by Endodontic Root Canal Treatment" or the American Association of Endodontists (AAE's) "Your Guide to Endodontic Treatment" and "Your Guide to Endodontic Surgery." Indicate in the patient's chart that the patient was shown or given the pamphlet(s), or both.

Recording Referrals

Every dentist, including an endodontic specialist, has a duty to refer under appropriate circumstances. No one is perfect; accordingly, consultations with additional experts or specialists may become necessary. Otherwise, a dentist appears to be the jack-of-all-trades but master of none.

All referrals should be recorded, lest they be forgotten, even if refused. Consider a carbonless, two-part referral card. Provide the original referral slip to the patient to take to the referred dentist and place the copy in the chart. Write on the chart copy that the original was given to the patient along with the date and name of the person who provided the referral card to the patient. If it is mailed, similarly document that a referral card was mailed and/or faxed to the patient. Also send a copy to the referred doctor, so that it may assist the referred doctor, and also as an additional proof that a referral was made in the event the patient fails to keep the referral. Request both the patient and the referred doctor to advise you if referral appointment is not done or cancelled.

Record Falsification

Records must be complete, accurate, legible, and dated. All diagnosis, treatments, and referrals should be recorded. Although undisclosed alterations are always proscribed, subsequent additions may be added to expand, correct, define, modify, or clarify so long as they are dated to indicate a belated entry, rather than entered contemporaneously with associated entry.

To correct an entry, line out but do not erase or obscure the erroneous entry. Place and date the correction on the next available line in the chart. Handwriting and ink experts use infrared technology to prove falsified additions, deletions, or substituted records. If records are proven to be falsified, the dentist may be subject to punitive damages in civil litigation. In addition, the dentist may be subject to license revocation for intentional misconduct.[11] Professional liability insurance policies will likely not indemnify a dentist for the punitive damages portion of a verdict based on fraud or deceit.

---

[10]See, e.g., Calif Health and Safety code, #123110.

[11]Calif Bus Prof Code, §1680(s).

Altered records prove the dentist has not been honest and are done in consciousness of guilt.[13] When patient records have been requested or subpoenaed, it is wise to refrain from examining them, to avoid anxiety and the temptation to clarify an entry. Alteration of records is a cause of large settlements. Dental records are business documents. Do not be cavalier about making belated changes. Insurance carriers may deny renewal of professional liability coverage if the dentist has fraudulently altered dental records.

Records are (1) subject to audits by insurance carriers for documentation that treatment was performed, (2) reviewed by peer review committees, and (3) subject to subpoena by state licensing boards or agencies for disciplinary proceedings. Accordingly, incomplete or missing records expose the dentist not only to civil liability for professional negligence but to criminal penalties for offenses such as insurance fraud.[12]

Spoliation

Spoliation is a tort in which the tortfeasor or wrongdoer alters, changes, or substitutes dental records in an attempt to defeat a civil lawsuit.[13]

It is better to defend a dental negligence lawsuit with poor records rather than altered falsified records. Otherwise, the jury may conclude the defendant dentist acted with consciousness of guilt rather than a mere oversight in maintaining adequate records.

Record alteration may subject the dentist to licensing[14] or ethical discipline, as well as punitive damages for deceitful misconduct. Texaco paid a record settlement of $176 million dollars when tape recordings of company executives revealed a plan to destroy documents evidencing defendant's discriminatory practices as plaintiffs alleged.[15] Additionally, the Texaco executives were criminally prosecuted for obstruction of justice.[16]

Digital radiography may have dental advantages, but because the digital images may be computer manipulated it is legally suspect as unreliable.[17] Therefore hard copies of the digital images should be printed and dated with ink entries to show the informational baseline on which the practitioner based diagnostic or therapeutic decisions. This also protects against computer glitches such as disk drive crashes, electrical power surges, computer virus, or operator delete errors.

Record alteration may be detected by questioned document experts who age-date ink, examine stationery watermarks, or use infrared techniques to show additions or deletions in records.

If an erroneous entry occurs, one can add a late entry, dated as such, to demonstrate later corrected information.

Dental Phobia

Dental phobia may result in patients delaying or avoiding dental care. Frequent cancellations and missed appointments are characteristically associated with fearful dental patients.

Although contributory negligence for patients who do not follow a dentist's treatment recommendations is ordinarily a defense, it may also be used by the patient's advocate to suggest the dentist failed to diagnose dental phobia and therefore appreciate the fearful patient's dilemma in seeking treatment, which the patient may perceive as exacerbating a prior traumatic experience. Referral to practitioners or dental centers who specialize in treating fearful patients should be considered to facilitate dental treatments including endodontics.

LEGAL RESPONSIBILITIES

Malpractice Prophylaxis

Good dentists keep good records. Therefore remember the three *R*s of malpractice prophylaxis: *records, records,* and *records.* Records represent the single most critical evidence a dentist can present in court as confirmation of accurate diagnosis and proper treatment.

Prophylaxis is the cornerstone of good dental care because it provides a healthy dental foundation based on prevention. Likewise, endodontic treatment performed with the requisite standard of care not only saves endodontically treated teeth but also helps insulate the treating dentist from a lawsuit for professional negligence. Sound endodontic principles carefully applied protect both dentist and patient. Careful attention to the principles of due care reduces avoidable or unreasonable risks associated with endodontic therapy.

Standard of Care

Good endodontic practice, as defined by the courts, is the standard of reasonable care legally required to be performed by the treating dentist. The standard of care does not require dental perfection, ideal care, or, by analogy, an A+ grade, in endodontics. Instead, the legal standard is that *reasonable* degree of skill, knowledge, or care ordinarily possessed and exercised by dentists under similar circumstances in diagnosis and treatment.[18]

Although the standard of care is a flexible standard that accommodates individual variations in treatment, it is objectively tested based on what a reasonable dentist would do. Reasonable conduct, at a minimum, constitutes legal due care. Additional precautionary steps that rise above the minimal floor of reasonableness and approach the ceiling of ideal care are laudable but not legally mandated.

HMO Care Versus Standard of Care

Prudent practitioners and not insurance carriers set the standard of care. Third-party payors may limit reimbursement but should not limit access to the quality of care. Practioners have an affirmative duty on behalf of the patient to appeal insurance carrier care denial decisions.[19]

If a carrier denies endodontic therapy or limits endodontics to only certain clinical conditions, a prudent practitioner must provide informed consent to the patient both legally[20] and ethi-

---

[12]Tulsa dentist found guilty of mail fraud, conspiracy, *Tulsa World* Jan 12, 1993.
[13]*Gomez v Acquistapace, et al,* 50 Cal App 4th 740, 57 Cal, Rptr 821 (1996); *Thor v Boska,* 38 Cal App 3d 558, 113 Cal Rptr 296.
[14]California Business and Professions Code, §1680(s).
[15]Holmes S: Texaco settlement could lead to more lawsuits, *San Francisco Examiner,* p A-8, Nov 17, 1996.
[16]*Wall Street Journal,* p A3, Nov 20, 1996.
[17]Jones G, Behrents R, Bailey G: Legal considerations for digitized images, *Gen Dent* 44(3):242, (1996).

[18]*Folk v Kick,* 53 CA3d 176, 185: 126 CR 172, 1975; see also *California Book of Approved Jury Instructions, Civil,* 6.00 et seq.
[19]*Wickline v State of California* 192 Cal App 3d 1630, 239 Cal Rptr 810, 1986; See also Pear R: HMOs see loophole to prevent litigation, *San Francisco Examiner,* p A-6, Nov 17, 1996.
[20]Carroll R: *Risk management handbook for healthcare organizations,* Chicago, 1997, American Hospital Publishing, pp. 307-319.

cally[21] if a tooth may be endodontically treated and retained rather than extracted.

The California Dental Association's recently revised Dental Patient Bill of Rights advises, "You [patient] have the right to ask your dentist to explain all treatment options regardless or coverage or cost."

Dentists may agree to a discounted fee with an HMO carrier but must not discount the quality of care. Peer review and the courts recognize only one standard of care and do not lower the standard or create a double standard for capitation or other reduced-fee HMO plans. Otherwise, HMO would stand for a health maiming organization rather than a health maintenance organization that is designed to improve efficiency but not at the expense of quality care.

Plans that delay treatment approval resulting in endodontic complications or nontreatability may be subject to liability. However, HMO carriers usually argue that the 1974 Employee Retirement Income Security Act (ERISA) preempts state law dental negligence claims against entities who administrate health care benefits to an ERISA plan and shift any blame entirely to the dentist-provider. Case law has produced mixed results regarding carrier liability, but Congress may intervene if the courts continue to exempt ERISA carriers.[22]

Dental Negligence Defined

Dental negligence is defined as a violation of the standard of care (i.e., an act or omission that a reasonably prudent dentist under similar circumstances would not have done).[23] Negligence is equated with carelessness or inattentiveness.[24] Malpractice is a lay term for such professional negligence. Simply stated, dental negligence occurs if a dentist either (1) fails to possess a reasonable degree of education and training to act prudently or (2) despite reasonable schooling, training, and continuing education, acts unreasonably or imprudently or fails to act.

One simple test to determine if a particular treatment outcome results from negligence is to ask the following question: Was the treatment result reasonably avoidable? If the answer is yes, it is probably malpractice. If the answer is no, it is probably an unfortunate misadventure that occurs despite the best of care by other reasonable dentists, but it is not malpractice.

CAVEAT

All examples of negligent endodontic treatment are not included in this chapter, since the myriad of malpractice incidents far exceed the scope of this chapter. Rather, cited examples are elucidated for educational purposes.

Locality Rule

The locality rule, which provides for a different standard of care in different communities, is becoming outdated. Originating in the 19th century, the rule was designed to acknowledge differences in facilities, training, and equipment between rural and urban communities.[25]

The trend across the country is to move from a locally-based standard to a statewide standard, at least for generalists. For endodontists usually a national standard of care is applied, considering that the AAE Board is national in scope. Thus no disparity generally exists between small town and urban endodontics standards, considering advances in communication, transportation, and education.

Peoria dentists should not be any more or less careful than Pittsburgh dentists. A dentist should provide proper endodontic care to a patient regardless of where the treatment is performed. Rather than focusing on different standards for different communities, other more important considerations include endodontic advances, availability of facilities, and whether the dentist is a specialist or general practitioner.

The locality rule has two major drawbacks. In some small population areas dentists may be reluctant to testify as expert witnesses against other local dentists. Also the locality rule allows a small group of dentists in an area to establish a local standard of care inferior to what the law requires of larger urban areas.

Standards of Care: Generalist Versus Endodontist

A general practitioner performing treatment ordinarily performed exclusively by specialists, such as complicated endodontic surgery, advanced periodontal surgery, or full bony impaction surgery, will be held to the specialist's standard of care. A generalist should refer to a specialist rather than perform procedures that are beyond the general practitioner's training or competency, to avoid the likely result that a subsequent treating specialist will regard the generalist's therapy as below the specialist's standard.

Approximately 80% of U.S. general practitioners provide some type of endodontic therapy, and by the year 2000, U.S. endodontic cases are expected to exceed 30 million annually. The expansion of this specialty into the realm of the generalist can be linked to (1) refinements in root canal preparation and filling techniques now taught in dental schools, (2) continuing education courses, and (3) significant improvements in the armamentarium of instruments, equipment, and materials available to dentists.

Higher Standard of Care for Endodontist: Extended Diagnostic and Treatment Responsibilities

Endodontists, as specialists, may be held to a higher standard of skill, knowledge, and care than general practitioners.[26] Endodontists set the standard for routine endodontics. The generalist must therefore meet the specialist's standard.

However, endodontists should not forget their general dentist training. Even though a patient may be referred for a specific procedure or undertaking, the endodontist should not overlook sound biologic principles inherent in the overall treatment. A specialist may also be held liable for failing to conduct an independent examination and instead relying solely on the information referral card or observations of the referring dentist, should the diagnosis or therapeutic recommendations

[21]Improved patient bill of rights unveiled, *California Dental Association Update 15,* Oct 21, 1996.

[22]Labor Secretary Robert Reich interview, *San Francisco Examiner,* p A-6, Nov 17, 1996.

[23]*Mathis v Morrissey,* 11 Cal App 4th 332, 1992; *Folk v Kilk,* 53 Cal App 3d 176, 185, 1975; 126 Cal Rptr 172; Am Jur 2d, Physicians and surgeons and other healers, 138, 1972.

[24]*Webster's Dictionary,* 1987, p 250.

[25]See 18 ALR 4th 603.

[26]*Carmichael v Reitz,* 17 Cal App 3d 958, 1971; Cal BAJI (Book of Approved Jury Instructions), No 6.01.

prove incorrect or the referral card charted the wrong tooth for treatment.

Without performing an independent examination, the endodontist risks misdiagnosis and resulting incorrect treatment. Prevention of misdiagnosis or incorrect treatment requires accurate medical-dental history and clinical examination not only of the specific tooth (or teeth) involved but also the general oral condition. Obvious problems, such as oral lesions, periodontitis, or gross decay, should be noted in the chart and the patient advised regarding a referral for further examination, testing or consultation with the referring dentist.

Radiographs from the referring dentist should be reviewed for completeness, clarity, and diagnostic accuracy. Usually the endodontist takes a new radiograph to verify current status before treatment.

Poor oral hygiene may be indicative of periodontal disease. In such cases endodontic treatment may be compromised unless the associated periodontal condition is brought under control. Referral to a periodontist may be necessary before or after completion of endodontic treatment.

In summary, it is necessary for the endodontist to (1) be alert to any contributory medical or dental condition within the area of endodontic treatment, (2) undertake an independent examination of the treatment area without relying solely on the referring dentist, (3) perform at least a screening general dental examination of the patient's mouth, and (4) advise the patient and referring dentist of findings.

Ordinary Care Equals Prudent Care

Ordinary is commonly understood (outside its legal context) to mean "lacking in excellence" or "being of poor or mediocre quality." As expressed in the context of actions for negligence, however, ordinary care has assumed a technical-legal definition somewhat different from its common meaning. *Black's Law Dictionary,* 4th edition, describes ordinary care as "that degree which persons of ordinary care and prudence are accustomed to use or employ . . . that is, reasonable care."

In adopting this distinction, the courts have defined ordinary care as "that degree of care which people ordinarily prudent could be reasonably expected to exercise under circumstances of a given case."[28] It has been equated with the reasonable care and prudence exercised by ordinarily prudent persons under similar circumstances.[29] It is not extraordinary or ideal care.

Although the standard required of a professional cannot be only that of the most highly skilled practitioner, neither can it be limited to the average member of the profession, since those who have less than median skill may still be competent and qualify.[30] By such an illogical definition, half of all dentists in a community would automatically fall short of the mark and be negligent as a matter of law. "We are not permitted to aggregate into a common class the quacks, the young men who have not practiced, the old ones who have dropped out of practice, the good, and the very best, and then strike an average between

them."[31] Rather, the reasonably prudent dentist is the standard of care and not an arithmetic average or mediocre practitioner. Even if 90% of dentists diagnose or perform a certain treatment unreasonably, no matter how great the number who do it wrong would never make it right.

Customary Practice Versus Negligence

Customary practice may constitute evidence of the standard of care, but it is not the only or exclusive determinant. Moreover, if the customary practice constitutes negligence, it is not reasonable dentistry merely because it is customary practice among a majority of dentists.[32]

Typical negligent custom examples include dentists and hygienists who customarily fail to probe[33] or take diagnostic quality radiographs,[34] do not refer for complicated procedures beyond the ken of their training,[35] disregard aseptic practices such as rubber gloves and face masks,[36] do not employ rubber dams for endodontics,[37] fail to install or periodically check valves in dental units to prevent water retraction suck-back cross-contamination,[38] and routinely diagnose pulpal disease without pulpal testing.[39]

Merely because a majority of practitioners in a community practice a particular method does not establish the standard of care, if such customary practice is unreasonable or imprudent.[40] Ultimately, the courts determine what is or is not reasonable dental practice, considering the available dental knowledge and weighing the risks and benefits of a particular procedure.

The law does not require dental perfection.[41] Instead, the legal yardstick by which such conduct is measured is what a reasonably prudent practitioner would do under the same or similar circumstances regardless of how many or how few practitioners conform to such a standard.

In one case, the evidence was undisputed that virtually no ophthalmologist in the entire state routinely tested for glaucoma patients under the age of 40, since the incidence was only 1 in 25,000 patients. Nevertheless, the Supreme Court of Washington State held that the defendant ophthalmologist was negligent as a matter of law irrespective of customary practice.[42]

There is little excuse for failing to routinely chart periodontal pockets before rendering endodontic therapy, no matter how many other dentists in the community fail to do so. The ben-

---

[27]Howard WW, Parks AL: *The dentist and the law,* p 156; St Louis, 1973, Mosby; *O'Brien v Stover,* (8th Cir) 443 F2d 1013, 1971; *Sinz v Owens,* 33 Cal 2d 749, 205 P.2d 3, 8 ALR 2d 757, 1949.

[28]*Fraijo v Hartland Hospital* 99 Cal App 3d 331, 1979; California BAJI 3.16: *Switzer v Atchison, Topeka, & Santa Fe Railroad Co,* 7 Cal App 2d 661. 666, 47 P 2d 353, 1935; 47 p 2d 353; see 57A Am Jur 2d (Rev ed), Negligence §144 et seq.

[29]Restatement 2d Torts, §283, 289.

[30]Restatement 2d Torts, §299A, Comment (e).

[31]61 Am Jur 2d, Physicians and surgeons and other healers, §110.

[32]*Barton v Owen,* 71 Cal App 3d 484, 492-493, 139 Cal Rptr 494, 1979.

[33]American Academy of Periodontology: *Periodontal screening and recording,* 1992.

[34]Rohlin M et al: Observer performance in the assessment of periapical pathology: a comparison of panoramic with periapical radiography, *Dentomaxillofac Radiogr* 20:127, 1991; Zeider S, Ruttimann U, Webber R: Efficacy in the assessment of intraosseous lesions of the face and jaws in asymptomatic patients, *Radiology* 162:691, 1987.

[35]*Seneris J Hass* 45 Cal 2d 811, 826, 291 P2d 915, 53 ALR 2d 124, 1955.

[36]Recommendations for preventing transmission of human immunodeficiency virus and hepatitis B virus to patients during exposure-prone invasive procedures, *MMWR* 40:1, 1991; Recommended infection practices in dentistry, *MMWR* 35:237, 1986.

[37]*Simpson v Davis,* 219 Kan 584, 549 P2d 950, 1976.

[38]Miller C: Cleaning, sterilization and infection, *J Am Dent Assoc* 48:54, 1993; Williams JF et al: Microbial contamination of dental unit waterlines, *J Am Dent Assoc* 124:59, 1993.

[39]Chapter 1.

[40]*Barton v Owen,* 71 Cal App 3d 484, 492-493, 1977; 139 Cal Rptr 494.

[41]*Gurdin v Dongieux,* 468 So2d 1241, 1985.

[42]*Helling v Carrey,* 83 Wash2d 514, 1974; 519P.2d 981; but see, *Meeks v Marx,* 15 Wash App 571, 556 P2d 1158, 1974.

efit of recognition of periodontal disease by probing and of pulpal disease by testing substantially outweighs the virtually nonexistent risks of conducting these diagnostic procedures. A lame legal defense likely to invoke a jury's wrath is to claim that a necessary diagnostic or prophylactic procedure is "too time consuming," when the dental and medical health of the patient are placed at risk for failure to adopt prudent practices.

Compliance with a safety statute does not conclusively establish due care, since regulations require only minimal care and not necessarily prudent care or what the law regards as due care.[43]

Negligence per se

A civil liability duty of care may be imposed by statutes and safety ordinances. For example, violation of a health safety statute may create a presumption of negligence on the part of the dentist.[44]

Although at trial plaintiff ordinarily has the burden of proving negligence, a rebuttable presumption of negligence is created if the following conditions are met:

1. Violation of a statute, ordinance, or regulation of a public entity occurs;
2. The violation caused injury;
3. Injury resulted from an occurrence that the statute, ordinance, or regulation was designed to prevent; *and*
4. Person suffering injury was one of the persons for whose protection the statute, ordinance, or regulation was adopted.[45]

If plaintiff establishes the presumption of negligence per se, the burden then shifts to the defendant to rebut the plaintiff's case.

Foreseeability of Unreasonable Risk

Each endodontic procedure has some degree of inherent risk. The standard of care requires that the dentist avoid unreasonable risks that may harm the patient. Treatment is deemed negligent when some unreasonable risk of harm to the patient would have been foreseen by a reasonable dentist. Failure to follow the dictates of sound endodontic practice increases the risk of negligence-induced deleterious results. Accordingly, prophylactic endodontic negligence law is designed to prevent foreseeable risks of injury that are reasonably avoidable.

It is not necessary that the exact injuries that occur be foreseeable. Nor is it necessary to foresee the precise manner or circumstances under which the injuries are inflicted. It is enough that a reasonably prudent dentist would foresee that injuries of the same general type would be likely to occur in the absence of adequate safeguards.[46]

Informed Consent Principles

In general

The legal doctrine of informed consent requires that the patient be advised of reasonably foreseeable material risks of endodontic therapy, the nature of the treatment, reasonable alternatives, and the consequences of nontreatment.[47] This doctrine is based on the legal principle that individuals have the right to do with their own bodies as they see fit, including the right to lose teeth, regardless of recommended dental treatment. Thus once the dentist has informed the patient of the diagnosis, recommended corrective treatment or alternative therapy, and the likely risks and prognosis of treatment compared with not proceeding with recommended therapy, an adult of sound mind is entitled to elect to do nothing about existing endodontic disease rather than elect corrective treatment.

To be effective, a patient's consent to treatment must be an informed consent. Accordingly, a dentist has a fiduciary duty to disclose all information *material to the patient's decision.*[48] The scope of a dentist's duty to disclose is measured by the amount of knowledge a patient needs to make an informed choice. Material information is that which the dentist knows or should know would be regarded as significant by a reasonable person in the patient's position when deciding to accept or reject a recommended endodontic procedure.

If a dentist fails to reasonably disclose and a reasonable person in the patient's position would have declined the procedure had adequate disclosure been given, the dentist may be liable if an undisclosed risk manifests. Beyond the foregoing minimal disclosure, a dentist must also reveal such additional information as a skilled practitioner of good standing would provide under similar circumstances. However, a minicourse in endodontics is not required.

Application of standard

Informed consent is a flexible standard that considers the reasonably foreseeable consequences depending on the clinical situation present both before and during treatment. For instance, a fractured endodontic instrument left in the canal presents a varied foreseeable likelihood of root canal failure or impaired success, depending on whether the fracture occurred in the coronal, middle, or apical third of the root canal. Therefore the dentist must advise the patient of relative risks of future failure because of the retained instrument and treatment alternatives available to correct the problem so that the patient can make an intelligent choice among apicoectomy, referral to an endodontist for attempted retrieval, or watchful waiting with close observation at recall visits.

Adequate disclosure includes clinical judgment and experience, which assesses current research and applies it to the clinical needs of each patient. According to the laws of aeronautical engineering, the bumblebee should not fly. Beekeepers, entomologists, flowers, and stung persons know otherwise. So it is with competent clinicians who practice applied dental science in daily practice. Advances in theoretical methods of therapy are great if they "fly" but should be reconsidered if the clinician cannot get off the ground with recommended theoretical treatment, unproven by long-term clinical trials. Today's advances may be tomorrow's retreat if materials, devices, or instruments lacking adequate long-term study of proven safety and efficacy are used. Therefore the dentist should disclose personal clinical failures, if these results are at odds with pub-

[43]*Texas & Pacific Railway Co v Behymer,* 189 US 468, 470, 47 L Ed 905, 23 S Ct622, 1903.
[44]*McGee v Cessna Aircraft Co,* 139 Cal App 3d 179, 188 Cal Rptr 542, 1983.
[45]Calif Evid Code, §669.
[46]Restatement 2d, Torts, §282 et seq.; Witkin BE: *Summary of California law,* §751, 1988.

[47]*Scaria v St Paul Fire & Marine Insurance Co,* 68 Wis 201, 227 NW2d 647, 1975; Zinman E: Informed consent to periodontal surgery: advise before you incise, *J West Soc Periodontol* 24:101, 1976.
[48]*Cobbs v Grant,* 8 Cal 2d 229, 104 Cal Rptr 505, 502 P2d 1, 1972; BAJI 6.11.

lished results of other clinicians, so the patient may make an intelligent choice of therapists.[49]

Material disclosure concerns whether the patient was provided sufficient information for a reasonable patient to achieve a general understanding of the proposed treatment or procedure, including any dentally acceptable reasonable alternatives, predictable nonremote inherent risks of serious injury, and likely consequences should the patient refuse proposed therapy.[50] Informed consent applies only to inherent risks of nonnegligent treatment, since a patient's "consent" to negligent treatment is voidable as contrary to public policy.[51] For instance, a patient who refuses necessary diagnostic radiographs should be refused treatment. Even a superb dentist is not Superman with x-ray vision.

Advice regarding different schools of thought

After advising proper treatment, if other reasonable dentists would disagree or if there are other respectable schools of thought on the correct treatment may be material information that should be disclosed to the patient in the course of obtaining consent.[52] For example, assume for purposes of illustration that there are two schools of thought concerning the optimal treatment for retrofilling and apicoectomy. One school posits that a retrograde with IRM is the appropriate procedure, whereas the minority review asserts that retrograde with super EBA is the preferred treatment. Assume further that an explanation of these two different methods of treatment constitutes material information for the purposes of informed consent. The mere fact that there is a disagreement within the relevant endodontic community does not establish that the selection of one procedure as opposed to the other constitutes negligent endodontic therapy. Since competent endodontists regularly use both procedures, a patient would face an insuperable task in proving dental negligence (i.e., that the endodontist failed "to have the knowledge and skill ordinarily possessed, and to use the care and skill ordinarily used, by reputable specialists practicing in the same field and in the same or a similar locality and under similar circumstances").

On the other hand, the specialist would have a duty under such hypothetical circumstances to disclose the two recognized schools of treatment so that the patient could be sufficiently informed to make the final, personal decision. An endodontist, being the expert, appreciates the risks inherent in the procedure prescribed, the risks of a decision not to undergo the treatment, and the probability of a successful outcome of the treatment. Once this information has been disclosed, this aspect of the endodontist's expert function has been performed. The weighing of these risks against the individual subjective fears and hopes of the patient is not an expert skill. Such evaluation and decision is a nondental judgment reserved for the patient alone.[53] In this hypothetical situation, failure to disclose such material information would deprive the patient of the opportunity to weigh the risks. Consequently, the dentist would have failed in the duty of disclosure.

Avoiding patient claims

If a dentist fails to obtain adequate informed consent, a plaintiff can recover damages even in the absence of any negligent treatment. Therefore discussions of treatment risks with the patient must be documented. Informed consent forms are very helpful, although not legally mandated, since a jury may believe that the patient was informed orally. Equally, if not more, important than consent forms, is a notation in the chart that informed consent risks and alternatives were discussed by the dentist and understood and accepted by the patient. Patients may mentally block out frightening information. Trauma and a potent anesthetic can create retrograde amnesia. Therefore document in your chart risks, benefits, and alternatives provided to the patient.

Follow only the patient-authorized and consented-to treatment plan. If an emergency precludes advising treatment risks to the patient, lack of informed consent is defensible as implied consent, since no reasonable person would refuse necessary nonelective emergency treatment.

Record any recommended but refused treatment and the patient's refusal reason. Such an example follows:

Patient refused endodontic referral for consultation with Dr. Jones since husband was laid off work last month and cannot afford, but understands detrimental risks of delay.

Patients may initial the refusal on the chart, but it is not mandatory.

Reasonable familiarity with a new product or technique is required before it is used. In addition, a patient is entitled to know the dentist's personal experience with a particular modality because the patient has a right to chose between reasonable alternatives, one of which is to seek care from a dentist who has more experience with a particular modality or product. A dentist who fails to obtain informed consent is liable for injury caused by a product or instrument, just as if the dentist's treatment was negligently performed. In other words, the fact that the dentist followed precisely the manufacturer's instructions is no defense if the dentist did not provide adequate information concerning a product or instrument risk to permit the patient to intelligently weigh the information and give informed consent.

Endodontic Informed Consent (Figs. 10-5 and 10-6)

Using statistics presented in national literature regarding success rates for endodontic procedures is insufficient disclosure to fulfill the legal requirements of informed consent if the practitioner's own statistical experience varies significantly from national statistics.[54]

Among specialists, the reported incidence of treatment complications in endodontics is, fortunately, relatively low. Based on a Southwest Endodontic Society retrospective study, a reasonable endodontist or a practitioner with similar abilities should disclose the following facts to patients:[55]

1. Endodontic therapy cannot be guaranteed.
2. Although endodontic therapy is usually successful, a small percentage of teeth are lost despite competent

[49]*Hales v Pittman*, 118 Ariz 305, 576 P 2nd 493, (1978).

[50]Carroll R: *Risk management handbook for healthcare organizations*, Chicago, 1997, American Hospital Publishing, pp 307-319.

[51]*Tunkl v Regents of University of California*, 60 Cal2d 92, 32 Cal Rptr 33, 383 P2d 441, (1963).

[52]*Vandi v Permanente Med. Group*, 7 Cal App 4th 1064, (1992); 9 Cal Rptr 2nd 463.

[53]*Cobbs v Grant*, 8 Cal3d 229, 243, 104 Cal Rptr 505, 502 P2d 1, (1973).

[54]*Hales v Pittman*, 118 Ariz305, 1978; 576 P2d 493, 499-500; *Shelter v Rochelle*, 2 Ariz App at 370, 409 P2d at 86, 1965.

[55]Selbst: Understanding informed consent and its relationship to the incidence of adverse treatment events in conventional endodontic therapy, *J Endod* 16:387, 1990.

ENDODONTIC INFORMED CONSENT

I understand the goal of endodontic root canal treatment is to retain a tooth that may otherwise require extraction. Although endodontic root canal treatment usually has a high degree of clinical success, it is a dental-biological procedure, whose results cannot be guaranteed. Occasionally, endodontic root canal treatment may fail, with resulting tooth loss. A permanent (outside) restoration, such as crown or onlay, will be placed afterwards by my restorative dentist. I agree to notify my restorative dentist immediately following completion of the root canal treatment so that a restoration may be placed over my root canal-filled tooth. Following completion of endodontic root canal treatment, fracture and loss of my root canal-filled tooth due to brittleness may be more likely to occur unless my root canal-filled tooth is restored within a month following completion of endodontics.

Payment

I also acknowledge full responsibility for the payment of such services for my root canal treatment and agree to pay for them, in full, AT or BEFORE COMPLETION, unless other specific arrangements are made with the secretary. One (1) percent interest per month or 12 percent per annum is billed on account balances over 31 days past due.

Insurance Assignment

I authorize my insurance carrier to pay any dental benefits of my plan directly to this dental office. I also authorize release of any information necessary to process my dental insurance claim.

Signed: Patient or Parent _____

Date: _____

Witness: _____

FIG. 10-5 Informed consent form documents the patient's understanding of the proposed endodontic root canal treatment.

PHOTOGRAPHY CONSENT

I, _____, consent to color photography of my teeth or face to be taken by Dr. _____ or his staff for reproduction and viewing by other dentists for scientific or educational purposes in scientific publications or at dental meetings.

Date: _____

_____
Signature of Patient or Legal Guardian

Witness: _____

FIG. 10-6 Photography consent form.

endodontic care, owing to complications or treatment failure.

3. Overfilling or underfilling of root canals occurs in 2% to 4% of cases, which may contribute to treatment failure.
4. Slight to moderate transient postoperative pain may occur; severe postoperative pain occurs in very few cases.
5. Irreparable damage to the existing crown or restoration secondary to endodontic treatment is uncommon.

Video Informed Consent

Animated video informed consent shown to the patient is a dynamic method of providing informed consent. Since the video informed consent is considered part of the dentist's records, in the event the patient disputes having ever been advised of (1) the nature of endodontic disease, (2) the availability of endodontic specialists, or (3) the relative indications for nonsurgical versus surgical endodontic care, the videotape can be played back to the jury as proof that the patient was informed. It is doubtful a jury would believe a forgetful patient who admits having previously viewed the videotape, since the videotape refreshes the stream of memories that may have otherwise faded away into the unconscious.

A patient who can view the videotape is more likely to understand the informed consent disclosure. If a picture is worth a thousand words, a moving picture is worth a thousand pictures. After viewing the videotape and discussing its contents with the dentist, the patient should sign a video consent form, verifying that the video was viewed and all of the patient's questions were answered.

Ethics

Endodontics is one of the seven dental specialties recognized by the ADA. Although any licensed dentist may legally practice endodontics, it is unethical to announce that one specializes in endodontics absent specialty training or being "grandfathered" into endodontic practice. It is ethically unpermissible for a general practitioner to characterize his or her practice as "limited to endodontics."[56] A general practitioner who desires to emphasize or limit his or her practice to endodontics is ethically permitted only to advertise as follows: *General Practitioner—Endodontics.*

Referrals to Other Dentists

Every dental practitioner, including specialists, will at some time need to refer a patient to a specialist for treatment to comply with the standard of care required of a reasonable and prudent dentist.[57]

Generally, if the referral takes place within the same dental practice, the legal doctrine of *respondeat superior* ("let the master answer") may be applicable. Under this rule, a dentist is liable for the dental negligence of a person acting as his agent, employee, or partner.[58] This is determined by whether the principal dentist controls the agent dentist's methodology, regardless of whether such control is actually excercised.

If the referral is made, even within the same physical environment, to an "independent contractor" endodontist who does not diagnose or treat under the direction or supervision of the referring dentist and that referring dentist has no right of control as to the mode of performing the treatment, the principle of agency and responsibility for the acts of another does not apply.[60]

To ensure that the referred dentist is not considered the agent of the referring dentist within the same facility, fees for the referral dentist should not be set by the referring dentist. Nor should the fees be divided equally or shared based on some other arrangement. Also the referral dentist should bill separately and exercise independent diagnostic and therapeutic judgment. Advise the patient that the referred dentist is independent of the referring dentist. Otherwise the referred dentist or specialist may be deemed the ostensible agent, although unintended, and not the actual agent. Thus the legal test for agency is how the facts or circumstances appeared to a reasonable patient, regardless of the dentist's understanding or intent that the other treating dentist be an independent contractor.

Surgical Versus Nonsurgical Endodontics

Litigation to determine whether nonsurgical or surgical endodontics was the proper treatment choice will not be decided by any one clinician, the ADA, AAE, or the ablest of judges. Rather, after considering all of the evidence, including experts, a jury—not of a dentist's peers but of a patient's peers—will decide. Depending on the individual case, the jury may decide that either a combination of nonsurgical and surgical endodontic therapy, rather than one method exclusively, should have been attempted. The jury may also decide that the patient should have been advised of the availability of such alternative therapy. Similarly, the jury may determine that apical surgery should have been done microscopically rather than macroscopically, depending upon expert testimony regarding the relative advantages of each and depending on presenting circumstances such as suspected calcification or separated instrument.

Product Liability

Today's dentist, exploring ways to improve the quality and success of endodontic therapy, is constantly presented with new dental products and techniques.

For prescribing and using drugs or other agents, the ADA's *Principles of Ethics,* Section 10, provides this guideline:

The dentist has an obligation not to prescribe, dispense, or promote the use of drugs or other agents whose complete formulas are not available to the dental profession. He also has the obligation not to prescribe or dispense, except for limited investigative purposes, any therapeutic agent, the value of which is not supported by scientific evidence. The dentist has the further obligation of not holding out as exclusive any agent, method, or technique.

Broken Instruments

Save broken or defective instruments such as a needle whose broken portion becomes lodged in a patient. The instrument manufacturer may be liable because the product was defective rather than the dentist being liable for dental negligence.[61]

---

[56]American Dental Association: *Principles of ethics and code of professional conduct,* §§5-C and 5-D: California Dental Association: *Principle of ethics,* §§8 and 9.
[57]*Simone v Sabo,* 37 Cal2d 253, 231 P2d 19, 1951.
[58]Restatement 2d, Agency, §§228-237.
[59]Restatement 2d, Agency, §§228-237.

[60]*Mission Insurance Co v Worker's Comp Appeals Board,* 123 Cal App 3d 211, 1981.
[61]Restatement 2d, Torts, §402A.

Equipment and Supplies

Keep equipment in good repair and check the condition frequently. Carefully note the manufacturer's instructions and all warnings on both medications and appliances and inform your staff. Infection control in operating dental equipment is mandatory, such as updating and maintaining dental units with check valves to prevent water retraction or suck-back. Inspect check valves monthly and change clogged valves.[62] Water retraction testers, at no charge to the dentist, are available from some manufacturers.[63] Alternatively, disassemble the handpiece, run water through the line for a few seconds, then stop. If a bubble of water is visible at the end of the water hose holes, the check valve is operating properly. If the bubble of water is not visible, water may be sucked back owing to an absent or clogged check valve. An absent or clogged check valve is a source of cross-contamination. Consider filters and disinfectants for flushing dental unit water lines to reduce water tubing biofilm.

Drugs

Exercise extreme caution when administering or prescribing dangerous drugs. For sedative or narcotic drugs write cautionary directions on prescriptions, which the pharmacist should place on the prescription container as a patient reminder. For example, for the appropriate drugs, prepare a prescription rubber stamp or obtain preprinted prescriptions, which state:

Do not drive or operate dangerous machinery after taking medication since drowsiness is likely to occur. Alcohol, sedative, or tranquilizing drugs will cause drowsiness if taken in combination with this prescribed drug.

The ADA and American Medical Association (AMA) provide prescription drug warning pads. Document in the chart each drug information forms provided with the prescription.

Dentist's Liability for Staff's Acts or Omissions

A dentist is liable for the acts or omissions of the dentist's staff under the doctrine of *respondeat superior* ("let the master answer"). This is termed *vicarious liability,* which means that the dentist is responsible not because he or she did anything wrong personally but because the dentist assumes legal responsibility for his or her employees and agents' conduct while they are acting in the course and scope of their employment.

The dentist should instruct the staff in advising patients regarding posttreatment complaints. For example, if the staff ignores signs of infection, such as difficulty in swallowing or breathing and/or elevated temperature, and dismisses the patient's complaints as normal postoperative swelling, the dentist may be held liable for injury to the patient, such as cellulitis, Ludwig's angina, brain abscess, or other complications.

Be cautious when delegating responsibilities. Give clear instructions to ensure that your staff properly represents you and your practice methods. Do not let auxiliaries practice beyond their competency level or license. For example, the dentist should check an assistant-placed restoration before patient dismissal. Staff members should not make final diagnoses or handle patient complaints without the dentist's involvement. Instruct staff to ask appropriate questions and to relay the patient's answers to the dentist so that the dentist can determine what should be done.

Abandonment

Once endodontic treatment is initiated, the dentist is legally obligated to complete the treatment regardless of the patient's payment of any outstanding balance. This requirement is posited on the legal premise that any person who attempts to rescue another from harm must reasonably complete the rescue with beneficial intervention unless another rescuer (dentist) is willing to assume the undertaking.[64] Another view is that should a patient be placed in a position of danger unless further treatment is performed, the dentist must institute reasonable therapeutic measures to ensure that adverse consequences do not result.[65]

A dentist performing endodontic therapy should have reasonable means of communicating with patients after regular office hours to avoid a claim for abandonment. A recorded message is inadequate if the dentist fails to check for recorded messages frequently. Therefore answering services or computer-directed beepers are required by the standard of care.

If the dentist providing endodontic therapy is away from the office for an extended period, a substitute on-call dentist should be available for any endodontic emergency and to answer patients' emergency calls. The endodontic treating dentist should arrange in advance for emergency service with a covering dentist rather than simply leaving a name on the answering machine or with the answering service, without first determining the availability of the covering dentist. Otherwise, the covering dentist may be away and unavailable for emergency care.

To avoid an abandonment claim, several prophylactic measures apply:

1. No legal duty requires a dentist to accept all patients for treatment. A dentist may legally refuse to treat a new patient, despite severe pain or infection, except for racial or handicapped reasons.[66] If treatment is limited to emergency measures only, be certain that the patient is advised that only temporary emergency endodontic therapy is being provided and not complete treatment. Record on the patient's chart, for example:

Emergency palliative treatment only. Patient advised endodontic treatment of tooth number needs to be completed with another dentist or complications likely.

---

[62]Miller C: Cleaning, sterilization and disinfection: basics of microbial killing for infection control, *J Am Dent Assoc* 124:48, 1993.
[63]A-Dec, for instance.

[64]*Lee v Deubre,* Tex Civ App 362 SW 2d 900, 1962; *Clark v Hoek,* 219 Cal Rptr 845, 1985.
[65]*McNamara v Emmons,* 36 Cal App 2d 199, 1939; 97 P2d 503; *Small v Wegner,* Mo 267 SW 2d 26, 50 ALR 2d 170, 1954.
[66]*McNamara v Emmons,* 36 Cal App 2d 199, 1939; 97 P2d 503; *Small v Wegner,* Mo 267 SW 2d 26, 50 ALR 2d 1970, 1954; The Americans with Disabilities Act, Publ No 101-336; Americans with Disabilities Act Title III Regulations, 28 CFR Part 36, Nondiscrimination on the basis of disability by public accommodations and in commercial facilities, US Department of Justice, Office of the Attorney General; and Americans with Disabilities Act Title I Regulations, 29 CFR Part 1630, Equal employment opportunity for individuals with disabilities, US Equal Employment Opportunity Commission.

Also, the patient should acknowledge that treatment is limited to the existing emergency by endorsing an informed consent to emergency endodontics:

I agree to emergency endodontic treatment of my tooth and have been advised that (1) emergency treatment is for temporary relief of pain and (2) further root canal treatment is necessary to avoid further complications, including, but not limited to, pain, infection, fracture, abscess, or tooth loss.

2. No legal duty requires a dentist to continue former patients on recalls or subsequent emergency care once treatment is complete. Thus completion of endodontic treatment for tooth No. 19 at a prior visit does not legally obligate the dentist to initiate endodontic therapy for tooth No. 3, whose endodontic disease began after completing treatment of tooth No. 19.
3. Any patient may be discharged from a practice for any arbitrary reason, except racial or handicap discrimination, so long as all initiated treatment is completed. Accordingly, a former patient who evokes memories of a "frictional" relationship, who is financially irresponsible, or who arrives at the office after an absence of several years with an acute apical abscess in a site where previous care was not rendered may legally be refused treatment.
4. It is not considered abandonment if a patient is given reasonable notice to seek endodontic treatment with another dentist and is willing to seek endodontic services elsewhere.[67] Thus if rapport with the patient dissolves, do not hesitate to suggest that each of you would be better served if any remaining endodontic treatment were performed elsewhere by a different dentist.

Should you wish to discontinue treatment, you may do so, provided it is not done at a time when the patient's dental health will be jeopardized, such as the middle of treatment. Do the following:

1. Notify the patient of the plan to discontinue treatment after a certain date.
2. Allow enough time for the patient to obtain substitute service, usually 30 days.
3. Offer to make emergency service available until a new dentist is obtained.
4. Make records, radiographs, and other information about the patient available to the new dentist.
5. Allow the patient to select a new practitioner or suggest referral by the local dental society if a referral service exists.
6. Document in your records, and send a certified letter to the patient, verifying all of the above.

Expert Testimony

The standard of care that a dentist must possess and exercise is peculiarly within the knowledge of dental experts. However, there are occasional exceptions where the conduct involved is within the common knowledge of laypersons, in which case expert testimony is not required. In determining whether expert testimony is required to establish negligence, one California court commented: "The correct rule on the necessity of expert testimony has been summarized by Bob Dylan: 'You don't need a weatherman to know which way the wind blows.' "[68] Operating on the contralateral side owing to mismounted radiographs or marking the wrong tooth on an endodontic referral card are examples of negligent conduct within the common knowledge of laypersons.

MALPRACTICE INCIDENTS

Screw Posts

Screw posts represent a restorative anachronism. The risk of root fracture is too great compared to the benefit, particularly when reasonable and superior passive alternatives exist (see Chapter 21). Even if the screw post is contemplated to be placed passively, the temptation to turn the screw is too great, considering human nature. Screw posts are not a reasonable and prudent treatment choice.

Paresthesia

Endodontic surgery in the vicinity of the mental foramen or mandibular canal carries with it the risk of irreversible injury to the inferior alveolar and/or mental nerve. Consequently, advise the patient in lay terms, before any surgery near the mental foramen is performed, that there is a risk of temporary or permanent anesthesia or paresthesia. Have the patient execute a written informed consent form confirming that the patient was advised and adequate informed consent was provided.

Failure of Treatment

A dentist should not guarantee success of treatment. It is foolish to assure the patient that you will save a tooth or achieve a perfect result.[69] Endodontic failures may occur despite the best endodontic care.[70] Contributing factors to failure include missed canal, uninstrumented portion of a root canal, infiltrate via a leaky coronal restoration contaminating the root canal filling,[70a] and inadequate isolation of the tooth during instrumentation, such as lack of rubber dam.

To avoid claims based on failed endodontics, the patient should be advised in advance of treatment of the inherent but relatively small risk of failure. It may be adequate to advise the patient of the high statistical probability of success in endodontics so long as the clinical condition of the tooth and the clinician's past success rate warrant such representation.[71] Factors to be considered in avoiding representing the national success rate of endodontics vis-à-vis a particular dentist in a given clinical situation are (1) a tooth whose periodontal status is questionable and (2) a clinician who is known to have an unusually high rate of endodontic failures.

An endodontic treating dentist is also liable for failure to disclose evident pathology in the quadrant being treated. The patient should be advised of any periodontal disease that adversely affects the prognosis of abutment teeth for partial dentures or bridges. A dentist should also advise of cysts, fractures, or lesions of suspected neoplasms. Also be careful not

---

[67]*Murray v US*, Va Civ App, 329 F2d 270, 1964.

[68]*Jorgensen v Beach 'N' Bay Realty, Inc*, 125 Cal App 3d 155, 177 Cal Rptr 882, 1981 quoting "Subterranean Homesick Blues" from *Bringing It All Back Home*. Accord; *Easton v Strassburger*, 152 Cal App 3d 90, 199 Cal Rptr 383, 46 ALR4th 521, 1984.
[69]*Christ v Lipsitz*, 160 Cal Rptr 498; 99 Cal App 3d 894, 1980.
[70]Ingle J, Beveridge E: *Endodontics*, ed 2, Philadelphia, 1976, Lea & Febiger, pp 34, 597; Maloccurrence does not always equal malpractice; see *Gurdin v Dongieux*, 468 So2d 1241, 1985.
[70a]Cheung G: Endodontic failures, Intl Dent J 46:131-138, 1996.
[71]Hales v Pittman, 118 Ariz305, 576 P 22 493, 1978.

to ignore any evident pathology which, if untreated, may adversely affect the dental or medical health of the patient. A dentist who fails to plan treatment properly plans for treatment to fail.

The doctrine of informed consent protects both the dentist and the patient so there will be no surprises or patient disappointment if an adverse result occurs. Should a nonnegligent failure or poor result occur, the availability of a signed informed consent form may serve as a reminder to the patient that the risk of complications was discussed in advance of treatment and that, unfortunately, the patient's endodontic treatment came out on the wrong end of the statistical curve.

Slips of the Drill

A slip of the drill, like a slip of the tongue, may be unintentional, but nevertheless cause harm. When a cut tongue or lip occurs, it is usually the result of operator error. To paraphrase Alexander Pope, to err is human, but to forbear divine. To increase the likelihood that a patient will forbear from filing suit because of a cut lip or tongue, the clinician should follow these steps:

1. Inform the patient that you indeed regret the injury to the patient. This is not a legal admission of guilt but rather an admission that you are a compassionate human being.
2. Repair the injured tissue yourself or refer the patient to an oral or plastic surgeon, depending on the extent of the injury and whether a plastic revision due to scarring is likely.
3. Advise the patient that you will pay the bill for the referred treatment of the oral or plastic surgeon. Indeed, have the oral or plastic surgeon send the bill directly to you for payment. Send the oral or plastic surgeon's bill to your professional liability carrier. Most carriers will pay the claim under the medical payments provisions of the general liability policy for an "accident" rather than as a malpractice incident compensable under the professional liability policy. Call the patient periodically to check on healing and recovery.

Electrosurgery

Electrosurgery can cause problems if mishandled. Damage to the oral cavity caused by poor use of electrosurgical devices consists primarily of gingival and osseous necrosis and sloughing distal to the surgical field and pulpal necrosis of affected teeth.

All equipment should be properly maintained and certified to meet American National Standard/American Dental Association Specification No. 44 on Electrical Safety Standards. Check current equipment to see that units meet ANSI standards and that electrical cords and other components are in good repair. Electrical receptacles should meet the requirements of the National Electrical Code for circuit grounding and ground fault protection. During use, the dispersive electrode plate should be well away from metal parts of the dental chair and the patient's clothing. Skin contact can cause burns. Use of plastic mirrors, saliva ejectors, and evacuator tips is strongly recommended.

Reasonable Versus Unreasonable Errors of Judgment

Although a dentist is legally responsible for unreasonable errors in judgment, mistakes occasionally do happen despite adherence to the standards of reasonable care. Maloccurrence

does not alone prove malpractice unless the maloccurrence is caused by a malpractice error.[72]

For example, accessory or fourth canals on molar teeth are frequently difficult to locate and tax the best of operators. Failure to locate an accessory or fourth canal does not conclusively constitute an unreasonable error of judgment. Rather, this may represent a reasonable error of judgment in the performance of endodontics. Nevertheless, if the additional canal was readily apparent radiographically, the existence of a fourth canal should have been considered and treatment should have extended to it.

Treatment of the Incorrect Tooth

A reasonable, nonnegligent mistake of judgment may occur owing to difficulty in localizing the source of endodontic pain. Vital pulps may on occasion be sacrificed in an attempt to diagnose the source of pain. Nevertheless, it is unreasonable, and therefore inexcusable, to treat the wrong tooth because it is recorded incorrectly on the referral slip or because the radiographs are mounted incorrectly or reversed.

If the wrong tooth is treated because of an unreasonable mistake of judgment, the dentist should be sympathetic, waive payment for all endodontic treatment, and offer to pay the fee for crowning the unnecessarily treated tooth.

Swallowing of an Endodontic Instrument

Use of a rubber dam in endodontics is mandatory.[73] Even if the endodontically treated tooth is broken down and cannot be clamped, a rubber dam, regardless of required modification, should be used in all instances (see Chapter 5). Not only is microbial contamination thereby reduced, but also the risk of a patient's aspirating or swallowing an endodontic instrument (Fig. 10-7).

If a patient swallows a file, it is likely because of the dentist's failure to observe the standard of care. If such an incident does occur, (1) advise the patient that you regret what occurred, (2) refer the patient for immediate medical care, including radiography, to determine if it is lodged in the bronchus or stomach so that appropriate measures are taken to remove it, and (3) offer to pay for the patient's out-of-pocket medical expenses.

Overfill of a Canal

A very slight overfill of a root canal with conventional sealants can occur without violating the standard of care (Chapter 9). Gross overfills usually indicate faulty technique. Nevertheless, so long as the overfill is not in contact with vital structures, such as the mandibular nerve or sinuses, permanent harm is unlikely, unless the root canal is filled with a paraformaldehyde-containing sealant causing chemical burn–type injury.

If, however, severe postoperative pain is foreseeable as a result of the overfilling, the patient should be advised of the likelihood of postoperative discomfort because of contact of the sealant material with the surrounding tissue. Similarly, if the overfill is slight or increased postoperative pain is unlikely, the patient need not be advised, lest it cause unnecessary alarm. However, a note should be made on the patient's chart of the overextension—and of the reason for not informing the patient. Fortu-

---

[72]*Gurdin v Dongieux,* 468 So 2d 1241, 1985; *Tropani v Holzer,* 158 Cal App 2d 1, 321 P2d 803.
[73]*Simpson v Davis,* 219 Kan584; 549 P2d 950, 1976.

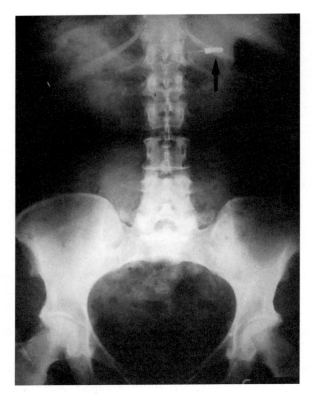

FIG. 10-7 Swallowed endodontic instrument demonstrates the wisdom of using a rubber dam.

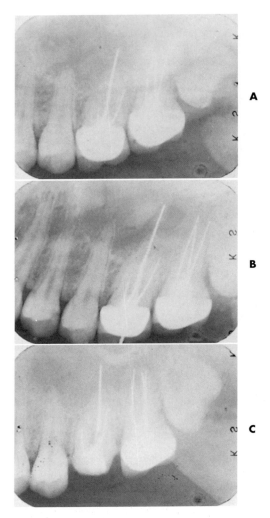

FIG. 10-8 Gross overfill into sinus with a silver point, which ultimately caused sinusitis and loss of tooth No. 14 as a result of endodontic failure.

nately, slight to moderate overfillings with inert conventional endodontic sealers like gutta-percha with Grossman's paste usually repair themselves and produce no irreversible changes.

Current Usage of Silver Points

Use of silver points in lieu of gutta-percha or other conventional endodontic filling materials represents a departure from the current standard of care. Fig. 10-8 represents gross overfilling with a silver point that ultimately caused the loss of tooth No. 14 as a result of endodontic failure.

Use of N-2 (Sargenti Paste)

Dental literature reports that permanent paresthesias are associated with gross overfilling with paraformaldehyde sealant (N-2) but are not reported with conventional sealants[73a] (Fig. 10-9). Current use of paraformaldehyde-containing endodontic sealants is not merely the result of a philosophic difference between two respectable schools of thought. Rather, the distinction is between the reasonable and prudent school of thought that advocates conservative conventional endodontics, and the imprudent, radical school of paraformaldehyde providers who risk permanent, deleterious injury with N-2 overfills. Stated otherwise, no matter how many N-2 practitioners use this technique and unsafe material, their sheer number does not make it right.

A dentist may be liable for fraudulent concealment or intentional misrepresentation, or as a co-conspirator, if obvious dental disease due to the negligence of another dentist is detected and the patient is falsely advised that none exists. For instance, if a gross overfill of a paraformaldehyde sealant is evident radiographically and the patient reports that another dentist caused the overfill, which resulted in paresthesia, a subsequent treating dentist may be liable for fraudulent or negligent concealment if he or she defends such gross negligence by advising the patient that the paresthesia will probably disappear shortly and that using N-2 merely reflects a philosophic difference rather than substandard practice.

The federal Food, Drug, and Cosmetic Act, enacted in 1938 and amended in 1962, prohibits interstate shipment of an unapproved drug or individual components used to compound the drug.[74] On February 12, 1993, the FDA dental advisory panel confirmed that N-2's safety and effectiveness remain unproven. N-2 may not be shipped interstate nor may it be distributed

---

[73a]Kleirer D, Averbach R; painful dysesthesia of the inferior alveolar nerve following use of a para formaldehyde-containing root canal sealer, *Endod Dent Traumatol* 4:46-48, (1988); Neaverth E: Disabling complications following inadvertent overextension of a root canal filling material, *J. Endod* 15:135-138, (1989).

[74]USCA, §§301 et seq.

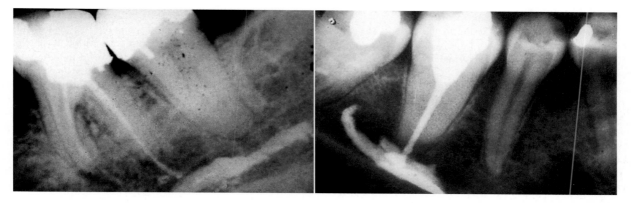

FIG. 10-9 Overextensions of Sargenti paste filling the inferior alveolar canal. Both cases could have been avoided if the practitioners had selected a conventional sealing material and used a technique that emphasizes length control.

intrastate if any of the N-2 ingredients were acquired interstate. Mail order shipments of N-2 from out-of-state pharmacies in quantities greater than for single-patient use are considered a bulk sales order rather than a prescription, thus violating FDA regulations.[75] A San Francisco jury awarded punitive damages against the N-2–distributing New York pharmacy for knowingly shipping N-2 in violation of FDA regulations and with deliberate disregard for patient safety.[76]

PROPHYLACTIC ENDODONTIC PRACTICE

Periodontal Examination

Competent endodontic treatment begins with adequate diagnostic procedures, as discussed in Chapters 1 and 2. An adequate periodontal evaluation must accompany each endodontic diagnosis, which requires a diagnostic radiograph, clinical visualization, evaluation of the periodontal tissues, and probing for periodontal pockets with a calibrated periodontal probe, particularly in furcation areas.[77]

Although endodontic treatment may be successful, tooth loss may nevertheless result from progress of any residual untreated periodontitis. Consequently, periodontal evaluation and prognosis are mandatory so that the patient and dentist can make an informed and intelligent choice about whether to proceed with endodontics, a combination of periodontal and endodontic treatment, or extraction.

Each tooth undergoing endodontic therapy, as well as adjacent teeth, should be probed with a calibrated periodontal instrument to obtain six measurements per tooth. Pockets of 4 mm or greater should be recorded on the patient's chart. If no pockets exist, *WNL* (within normal limits), or a similar abbreviation, should be noted. Mobility should also be charted and designated class I, II, or III. Gingival recession, furcations, and mucogingival deficiencies should be recorded.

A dentist who treats with endodontic success but ignores loss of periodontal attachment may misdiagnose or fail to appreci-

ate the risk of failure because of poor periodontal prognosis. The endodontic treating dentist should not assume that a periodontal evaluation has been performed by another dentist, even the referring dentist. Instead, an independent periodontal evaluation should be done.

If clinically significant periodontal disease is present, the endodontic treating dentist should consult with the restorative dentist to determine whether the periodontal disease will be properly treated or referred in conjunction with endodontic treatment. A patient should be advised of any compromise of the endodontically treated tooth's periodontal status to comply with required informed consent disclosure.

Preoperative and Postoperative Radiographs

1. A current preoperational diagnostic periapical radiograph is mandatory.
2. Working films are necessary to verify canal length (if an electronic canal-measuring device is not used) and the apical extent of the gutta-percha fill.
3. Posttreatment radiographs are essential for determining the adequacy of the endodontic seal, as discussed in Chapter 9.

Patient Rapport

Good patient relations are 15% dependent on your competency to cure and 85% on demonstrating to the patient that you care enough to always give your professional best.

Rapport between dentist and patient reduces the likelihood the patient will sue. Develop rapport by demonstrating genuine interest in the patient and making the patient feel like the most valued one in the practice.

Patients feel important if they are seated in the operatory within a reasonable time after arriving. The longer a patient is kept waiting, the more frustration and animosity build up. If the patient cannot be seen within a reasonable time, a staff member should communicate the reason and, if appropriate, offer to reschedule the appointment. Staff or doctor should telephone the patient at the end of the day following any difficult procedure or surgery as a patient reminder to follow postoperative instructions and to check on the patient's status. Any patient complaints and symptoms should be recorded, as well as noncompliance with instructions, the latter as evidence of the patient's contributory negligence.

[75]*Cedars N Towers Pharm, Inc v USA*, Fla Fed Dist Ct No 77-4965, Aug 18, 1978.

[76]*Irsheid v Elbee Chemists and Available Products, Inc*, San Francisco Super Ct, Docket No 908373, 1992.

[77]McFall W et al: Presence of periodontal data in patient records of general practices: patient records, *J Periodontol* 59:445, 1988.

Rapport Building Blocks

Sir William Osler advised, "Listen to the patient. He's trying to tell you what's wrong with him." The best communicators listen more than they speak. When they do speak, it is mostly to clarify what the patient has said. Difficult doctor-patient relationships create poor communications. Improved understanding of the patient's complaints fosters better rapport, aids treatment, and reduces the likelihood of litigation.

In handling the patient's complaints ask, "What do *you* think is causing the problem?" Otherwise, you may solve the patient's dental problem but not the patient's perceived problem. Failing to clarify the patient's expectations about diagnoses and recommended treatment leaves the patient with unresolved worries and concern. For instance, a patient may fear that a retained endodontic file is carcinogenic unless this fear is allayed with a careful explanation.

Do not rush the visit. Full attention to the patient's complaints, good eye contact, and respectful addressing of the patient gains rapport, improves communication, and prevents lawsuit. Care more, not less, lest you be judged careless.

Avoid questions that require a yes or no answer. Instead, ask what are the patient's problems. Rephrase the patient's complaints to prevent miscommunication. Then ask if you have summarized the patient's complaints accurately. Summarizing clarifies understanding by repeating important points. Inquire if there are any remaining questions. Nonverbal communication can be a powerful tool. For instance, shake hands initially or comfort with an outstretched hand if pain is provoked.

Emotions are the dominant force behind most malpractice claims. Patients who feel misled, betrayed, or abandoned become angry and may seek vindication of their rights more than financial compensation. Thus maintain a tactful and courteous approach and be attentive to the patient's needs and complaints. Always make sure that your communications with the patient are clear, even to the point of being repetitious, by asking if the patient has any questions. Never abandon a patient in the middle of a course of treatment and always be available to provide follow-up care. Avoid telephone diagnosis. If you do so, follow-up with a chart note.

Good telephone communication is a matter of asking the right questions, such as asking a postoperative patient if there is difficulty breathing or swallowing, as well as the degree and location of swelling. In cases of suspected infection, remain at a telephone where you can be reached until the patient or family member calls you back with a temperature reading to verify the patient is afebrile.

Do not make off-the-cuff diagnoses. One dentist dismissed a patient's party guest's endodontic problem as sensitivity due to gum recession and recommended a desensitizing toothpaste. A lawsuit resulted from inadequate diagnosis and recommended follow-up despite mere cocktail chatter.

Keep conversations professional. Making light of a minor occurrence, like the dropping of an instrument, with a quip about your "one-drink-too-many" at lunch, may seem funny at the time you said it but may not sound so funny if the patient soberly reiterates your quip to the jury.

Do not let a patient's flattery of your abilities undermine your best professional judgment. Heroic measures usually result in treatment failures, a dissatisfied patient, and ultimately a law suit for uninformed consent despite the patient's virtually hopeless prognosis.

A patient dissatisfied with prior treatment, such as a patient with a bag full of dentures or bridges made by other competent dentists, should signal a waving red flag to stop rather than proceeding with treatment. Young practitioners are more apt to walk into traps of a patient's request for unreasonable treatment where more experienced practitioners fear to tread.

A compassionate and concerned dentist who is able to demonstrate that the patient is cared about, as well as cared for, avoids many malpractice actions. Thus when an iatrogenic mishap occurs, it behooves the clinician to be frank and forthright with the patient. Moreover, concealment of negligence may extend the statute of limitations, since most states with discovery statutes construe discovery as the date on which the patient discovered the negligent cause of the injury and not the date of the injury itself.[78] Furthermore, belated discovery of injury from another dentist evokes a feeling of betrayal in the patient and destroys any rapport that would otherwise dissuade the patient from instituting litigation.

Fees

Clarify fees and payment procedures before initiating treatment. If the dental treatment becomes more extensive than originally planned, discuss the increased charges and reasons with the patient before continuing treatment. Resist charging for untoward complications such as extended postoperative visits or retrieving broken instruments.

An overzealous receptionist who places payment pressure on a dissatisfied patient, or the dentist who sues to collect a fee from an already displeased patient, may invite a countersuit for malpractice. Refunding fees or paying for the treatment fee of the subsequent treating dentist under the general liability rather than professional liability portion of your insurance policy is usually much less expensive than a week in court and a jury award for a patient's pain and suffering. If you do sue for your fee, do so only if your treatment is beyond reproach and your records substantiate proper diagnosis, treatment, and informed consent options.

Post Perforation

Post selection is important for avoiding perforations. Generally, posts should not exceed one third of the mesiodistal width of a tooth and should follow the canal anatomy. Excessively large posts violate these guidelines and unreasonably increase the risk of perforation or tooth fracture.

Ordinarily, a prudent practitioner performing endodontic therapy should reasonably be able to avoid post perforations. If post perforation occurs, early diagnosis and treatment is important, since belated diagnosis and treatment substantially increase the risk of endodontic failure. If perforation is relatively small in size (such as 1 mm or less) and promptly diagnosed at the time of the post perforation, immediate treatment with intracanal sealants in the area of the perforation will probably succeed. Delayed diagnosis and treatment result in bacterial contamination in the area surrounding the perforation. Periodontal-endodontic lesions or lateral periodontal abscesses secondary to delayed diagnosis prognosticate a substantially high risk of failure associated with delayed perforation repair therapy.

---

[78]*Dolan v Borelli*, 13 Cal App 4th 816, 1993; *Franklin v Albert*, 411 NE2d 458 Mass, 1980. Note, 38 Mont L Rev 399, 1977; Annot, 80 ALR 2d 368, §7b, 1961.

Cores

Incorrect choice of cores can contribute to failure including fractures. For instance, some manufacturers, such as ESPE Premeir for Ketac silver, recommend against use of their core material unless at least two thirds of the tooth remains before buildup. Failure to follow the manufacturer's directions can be considered by an expert concerning whether the standard of care was met.

Resin-reinforced post and core systems show promise for structurally weakened incisors, but long-term longevity has not been reported. A ferrule or other counterrotational core design is an important consideration for fracture resistance and retention,[79] although not proven as statistically significant for the resin-reinforced dowel systems.[80]

Posttrauma Therapy

Following a traumatic incident, splinting may be necessary if the teeth are mobile. Splinting is usually unnecessary in the absence of mobility. If reversible type of splints such as bonding or other noninvasive splinting procedures are done, despite nonmobility, no harm will likely result, although splinting was probably unnecessary.

Following traumatic complete tooth avulsion, the earlier the tooth is replanted, the greater is the prognosis for salvageability. Additionally, the choice of storage media before replantation is an important factor for increased salvageability. Most patients do not have a readily available sterile solution, or if the avulsed tooth is placed underneath the tongue, the risk of swallowing the tooth may occur. Therefore placement of the tooth in a sealed plastic zipper-locked type of container or sandwich bag is a convenient and readily available storage source for many patients.[81]

Continuing Education

A dentist is legally obligated to maintain current knowledge in the field of endodontics. Otherwise, the dentist may have only 1 year of knowledge repeated 30 times during the span of a 30-year career.

Examples of recent endodontic advancements include improved shaping or filling and packing techniques. A variable tapered file system and heat pluggers are but some examples of technologic advancements.

By not maintaining continuing education knowledge a practitioner may condemn otherwise salvageable teeth. For instance, a thin-walled incisor historically had a guarded prognosis, particularly when the post placement was close to the labial surface creating an unesthetic result.[82] Newer translucent posts transilluminate light unlike opaque metal posts. Moreover, dentin-bonded resin composite for intraradicular rehabilitation more nearly approach elastic limits of dentin for improved tensile and shearing stress resistance compared with

prefabricated or cast posts dowel and core systems. The latter system does not add strength to a structurally weakened root, whereas improved resin reinforcement materials do improve strength.[83-84]

Advances in Endodontics

Technologic advances are touted as ideal endodontics. However, the standard of care is a minimal standard of reasonably acceptable practice rather than the ideal. Thus the reasonable and prudent practitioner is not required to know and use all of the latest technologic advances in endodontics. On the other hand, the reasonable and prudent practitioner must keep current with available advances.

Microsurgical endodontics is an example of so-called cutting-edge endodontics. Nonetheless, the great expense of this technique and the fact that most endodontics can be accomplished successfully without superpower optics do not mean that standard of care always requires microsurgical endodontics. Use of magnifying loupes or similar devices may prove to be adequate. This standard is changing and may represent at the least an informed consent patient choice.

If studies demonstrate significantly superior results for some alternative to surgical endodontics, the informed consent standard of care may require that the patient be advised of the alternative technique, even if it is more expensive. There may be more than one path to success. So long as the dentist uses reasonably acceptable techniques and informs the patient of reasonable alternatives, the standard of care is met. Moreover, today's surgical advance may be tomorrow's retreat. Breast and temporomandibular joint implants are two examples of inadequately tested technology that proved disastrous.[85] Microscopic apical surgery is gaining increasing acceptance and utilization.

Other Dentist's Substandard Treatment

Do not be overly protective of blatant examples of another dentist's substandard dental treatment. On discovery of a gross violation of the minimal standard of dental care, a dentist has an ethical responsibility to report the matter to one's local dental society peer review or the dental licensing board or agency.[86] If you do not and the patient later discovers poor treatment, you could be sued as a co-conspirator to fraudulent concealment of another practitioner's neglect.

Corroborate your suspicion of prior care deficiencies by obtaining the patient's written authorization for transfer of a copy of the prior dentist's records including radiographs. If still in doubt after obtaining and reviewing the records, consider speaking with the prior dentist to learn what occurred previously, after first obtaining the patient's consent.

Peer Review

If despite good rapport, candid disclosure, and an offer to pay corrective medical or surgical bills the patient is still un-

[79]Hunt P, Gogarnoiu D.: Evaluation of post and core systems, *J Esthetic Dent* 8(2):74-83, 1996.

[80]Saupe W, Gluskin A, Radke R: A comparative study of fracture resistance between morphologic dowel and cores and resin-reinforced dowel system in the intraradicular restoration of structurally compromised roots, *Quintessence Int* 27:483, 1996.

[81]Andreasen JO, Andreasen FM: Essentials of traumatic injuries to the teeth, Cambridge, 1991, Munksgaard, p 119; see also AAE *Recommended guidelines for treatment of the avulsed tooth.*

[82]Freedman G, Glassman G, Serotta K: Endoaesthetics. I. Intraradicular rehabilitation, *Ontario Dent* 69:28, 1992.

[83]Lui JL: Composite resin reinforcement of flared canals using light-transmitting plastic posts, *Quintessence Int* 25:313, 1994.

[84]Saupe et al, *supra.*

[85]Federal Register 58:43442-43445, Aug 16, 1993; Randall T: Antibodies to silicone detected in patients with severe inflammatory reactions, *JAMA* 268:14, 1992.

[86]ADA principles of ethics and code of professional conduct. I-G. Justifiable criticism, *J Am Dent Assoc* 123:102, 1992.

DENTAL AUXILIARY CONFIDENTIALITY AGREEMENT

I, _____, have been informed by
(Dental Assistant)

_____, DDS, that all dental, medical, and
(Dentist Name)

financial information concerning patients is confidential.

As a condition of employment, I agree to maintain the confidentiality of all oral and written information, including treatment charts, and to not disclose such information to any unauthorized outside persons, including any family members, except upon request and authorization by the patient, the patient's agent, or supervising dentist.

I understand and agree that breach of this employment agreement shall constitute good cause for my discharge from employment. I acknowledge that I may by personally liable for any violation of a patient's privacy or civil rights committed by me without consent of the patient, or the patient's agent, or approval by above-named dentist.

Date: _____

Witness: _____

Signature of Dental Assistant

FIG. 10-10 Dental auxiliary confidentiality agreement.

satisfied, the clinician should consider referring the patient to peer review. Peer review committees award damages only for out-of-pocket losses, not for pain and suffering or lost wages. Consequently, even if the committee's decision is adverse to the dentist, the damage award will probably be less than a jury's verdict. If peer review finds for the dentist, the patient may be discouraged from proceeding further with litigation. Peer review proceedings, including the committee's decision, are not admissible at trial for either side.[87]

Insurance carriers usually honor and pay a peer review committee award, since a fair adjudication of the merits has been determined. The award is usually less than a jury would award. Also, defense costs, including attorney's fees, are saved.

Human Immunodeficiency Virus (HIV) and Endodontics

A dentist may not ethically refuse to treat an HIV-seropositive patient solely because of such diagnosis.[88] Although in the 1980s no federal law had clearly extended the protection of the handicapped laws to patients with acquired immunodeficiency syndrome (AIDS), federal congressional action in 1990 extended this protection to the dental office setting with the passage of the Americans with Disabilities Act.[89] Many states already offer additional protection under state law.[90]

Confidentiality for patients disclosing their HIV status is important, since an inadvertent disclosure to an insurance carrier or to other third parties, without any need to know, may result in cancellation of the patient's health, disability, or life insurance, resulting in a claim against the dentist whose office disclosed such information without authorization. Therefore employees should sign the confidentiality agreement contained in Fig. 10-10. In signing, the staff may be alerted to appreciate the seriousness and importance of maintaining the confidentiality of patient health histories, since the medical history may document AIDS, venereal disease, or other socially stigmatizing diseases.

Should a patient request the dentist not to inform the staff of the patient's HIV status, the dentist should refuse to treat, since this information is essential to staff members. For example, an accidental needlestick with HIV-infected blood, which carries a risk of approximately one chance in 250 of seroconversion, may occur. Current medical protocol includes prophylactic administration of zidovudine (AZT) either to prevent or to slow the manifestation of AIDS for deep-penetrating, accidental needlestick exposure.

Although a treating dentist risks devastating a dental practice by informing patients that the dentist has contracted AIDS, the legal risk of not informing the patient is also great indeed. The health care provider may be required to advise patients of positive HIV test results under the doctrine of informed consent (advising of a known risk of harm, i.e., accidental exposure).[91] Even if the patient never contracts AIDS, the patient may nonetheless bring an action for intentional concealment as a variant of informed consent and seek to recover emotional distress and punitive damages. Conversely, patients may be legally liable for lying on their health history regarding their HIV status.[92]

Infective Endocarditis

If warranted by the patient's medical history, consult with the patient's physician to determine the necessity of antibiotic prophylaxis against infective endocarditis in accordance with

[87]Calif Evid Code, §1157.

[88]Davis M: Dentistry and AIDS: an ethical opinion, *J Am Dent Assoc* (suppl 9-5), 1989.

[89]Americans with Disabilities Act, Pub L 101-336.

[90]Decision and order of the New York City Commission on Human Rights, *Whitmore v The Northern Dispensary,* Aug 17, 1988; California court upholds ban on AIDS discrimination, *ADA News* 5 Feb 1990.

[91]*Doe v US Attorney General*, ND Calif Dec 28, 1992, No c-88-3820.

[92]*Boulais v Lustig,* Los Angeles Super Ct BC038105 [\$102,500 jury verdict to an ungloved surgical technician].

current American Heart Association (AHA) Guidelines.[93] If the physician does not appear knowledgeable about those guidelines, provide a copy of the guidelines to the physician. If the physician advises that deviation from AHA guidelines is appropriate, ask the physician why. Record your discussions with the physician in the patient's chart. Confirm in writing by letter to the physician your discussion and the physician's recommendation.

Communications with the physician should be specific, since the physician may not appreciate dental treatment. The following format might be used by fax and letter:

Dear Doctor:

Your patient requires dental treatment that will result in transient bacteremia. Does the patient have a heart valve defect that increases the risk of infective endocarditis? If so, please advise of the diagnosed defect and recommended prophylactic antibiotic and dosage.

---

[93]Dajani AS, Taubert KA, Wilson W, Bolger AF, Bayer A, Ferrieri P, Gluitz MH, Shulman ST, Nouri S, Newburger JW, Hutto C, Pallasch TJ, Gage TU, Levison ME, Peter G, Zuccaro G Jr.; Prevention of bacterial endocarditis: recommendations by the Amer Heart Assoc, *JAMA* 277:1794, 1997.

Please also advise if your recommendation is in accordance with the enclosed American Heart Association current guidelines concerning bacterial endocarditis relating to dental treatment.

Thank you for your anticipated cooperation.

Enclosure: 1997 American Heart Association Guidelines

Patient with joint prostheses require premedication only at the orthopedist's discretion. There are no ADA, AHA, or American Academy of Orthopedic Surgeons mandatory requirements. Generally none is required.

CONCLUSION

If the dentist performs endodontics within the standard of care, as described in this chapter, there should be little concern that a lawsuit for professional negligence will be successful. "Prophylactic" measures are suggested in this chapter to help reduce the chances of litigation by reducing avoidable risks associated with endodontic care.

Both the patient and dentist benefit from risk reduction. It is far better for the dentist to take the extra minute to *do it right* rather than to subject a patient to a lifetime of misery for an expedient but risky wrong.

PART TWO

THE SCIENCE OF ENDODONTICS

Chapter **11**

Pulp Development, Structure, and Function

Henry O. Trowbridge
Syngcuk Kim

The pulp is a soft tissue of mesenchymal origin with specialized cells, the odontoblasts, arranged peripherally in direct contact with dentin matrix. The close relationship between odontoblasts and dentin is one of several reasons why dentin and pulp should be considered as a functional entity, sometimes referred to as the *pulp-dentin complex.* Certain peculiarities are imposed on the pulp by the rigid mineralized dentin in which it is enclosed. Thus it is situated within a low-compliance environment that limits its ability to increase in volume during episodes of vasodilation and increased tissue pressure. Since the pulp is relatively incompressible, the total volume of blood within the pulp chamber cannot be greatly increased, although reciprocal volume changes can occur between arterioles, venules, lymphatics, and extravascular tissue. In the pulp therefore careful regulation of blood flow is of critical importance.

The dental pulp is in many ways similar to other connective tissues of the body, but its special characteristics deserve serious consideration. Even the mature pulp bears a resemblance to embryonic connective tissue. The pulp houses a number of tissue elements, including nerves, vascular tissue, connective tissue fibers, ground substance, interstitial fluid, odontoblasts, fibroblasts, antigen-presenting cells, and other minor cellular components.

The pulp is actually a microcirculatory system whose largest vascular components are arterioles and venules. No true arteries or veins enter or leave the pulp. Unlike most tissues the pulp lacks a true collateral system and is dependent on the rela-

tively few arterioles entering through the root foramina. Since with age there is a gradual reduction in the luminal diameters of these foramina, the vascular system of the pulp decreases progressively.

The primary role of the pulp is to produce dentin, but it is also a rather unique sensory organ. Being encased in a protective layer of dentin, which in turn is covered with enamel, it might be expected to be quite unresponsive to stimulation; yet despite the low thermal conductivity of dentin, the pulp is undeniably sensitive to thermal stimuli such as ice cream and hot drinks. Later in this chapter we consider the unusual mechanism that allows the pulp-dentin complex to function as such an exquisitely responsive sensory system.

Following tooth development the pulp retains its ability to form dentin throughout life. This enables the vital pulp to partially compensate for the loss of enamel or dentin caused by mechanical trauma or disease. How well it serves this function depends on many factors, but the potential for regeneration and repair is as much a reality in the pulp as in other connective tissues of the body.

It is the purpose of this chapter to bring together what is known about the development, structure, and function of the dentin-pulp complex in the hope that this knowledge will provide a firm biologic basis for clinical decision making.

DEVELOPMENT

Embryologic studies have shown that the pulp is derived from the cephalic neural crest. Neural crest cells arise from

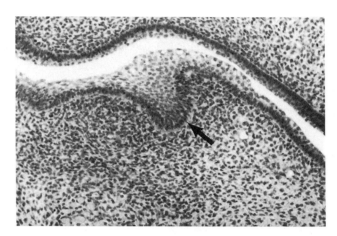

FIG. 11-1 Dental lamina *(arrow)* arising from the oral ectoderm.

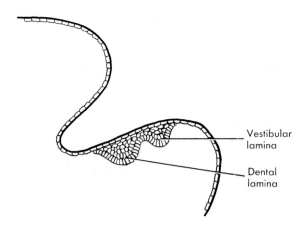

Vestibular lamina

Dental lamina

FIG. 11-2 Diagram showing formation of the vestibular and dental lamina from oral ectoderm.

the ectoderm along the lateral margins of the neural plate and migrate extensively. Those that travel down the sides of the head into the maxilla and mandible contribute to the formation of the tooth germs. The dental papilla, from which the mature pulp arises, develops as ectomesenchymal cells proliferate and condense adjacent to the dental lamina at the sites where teeth will develop (Fig. 11-1). It is important to remember the migratory potential of ectomesenchymal cells, for later in this chapter we consider the ability of pulp cells to move into areas of injury and replace destroyed odontoblasts.

During the sixth week of embryonic life, tooth formation begins as a localized proliferation of ectoderm associated with the maxillary and mandibular processes. This proliferative activity results in the formation of two horseshoe-shaped structures, one on each process, that are termed the primary dental laminae. Each primary dental lamina splits into a vestibular and a dental lamina (Fig. 11-2).

Numerous studies have indicated that the embryonic development of any tissue is promoted by interaction with an adjacent tissue. The complex epithelial-mesenchymal interactions during tooth development have been studied extensively. Cell-to-cell and cell–to–extracellular matrix (ECM) interactions direct the differentiation of ameloblasts and odontoblasts by causing these cells to change gene expression.

The timing and position of epithelium and mesenchyme are thought to reside in the sequential expression of cell transmembrane linkage molecules such as integrin, cell adhesion molecules (CAMs), and substrate adhesion molecules (SAMs). CAMs mediate morphogenesis through controlled cell proliferation, specific cell-to-cell adhesion, and migration. Cells contain membrane proteins called integrins, which are specific receptors for CAMs. Laminin is the CAM of basement membranes. It contains binding domains for heparan sulfate, type IV collagen, and cells. SAMs carry out cell-to-ECM interactions. The best-studied SAMs of the ECM are the fibronectins, a family of glycoproteins that bind to fibrin, collagen, heparan sulfate, and cell surfaces.

Growth factors are polypeptides produced by cells that initiate proliferation, migration, and differentiation of a variety of cells. It can be assumed that growth factors are involved in signaling during epithelial-mesenchymal interactions that regulates tooth morphogenesis and cell differentiation. For ex-

ample, epidermal growth factor (EGF) has been shown to play a role in tooth development by stimulating proliferation of cells in the enamel organ and preodontoblasts.[111] It has been hypothesized that transforming growth factor-β_1 (TGF-β_1) may regulate changes in the composition and structure of ECM.[105] A fibroblast growth factor may also be involved in the determination and differentiation of odontoblasts.

From the onset of tooth formation, a dental basement membrane (DBM) exists between the inner dental epithelium and the dental mesenchyme. The DBM consists of a thin basal lamina, which is formed by the epithelial cells, and a layer of ECM derived from the dental mesenchyme. The basal lamina is composed of an elastic network composed of type IV collagen, which has binding sites for other basement membrane constituents such as laminin, fibronectin, and heparan sulfate proteoglycans. Laminin binds to type IV collagen and also to receptors on the surface of preameloblasts and ameloblasts. The DBM also contains mesenchyme-derived type I and type III collagen, hyaluronate, heparan sulfate, and chondroitin 4- and 6-sulfates. Odontoblast cell surface proteoglycans function as receptors for matrix molecules. Signals from components of the matrix influence the migration and differentiation of odontoblasts. The composition of the DBM changes during tooth development, and these alterations appear to modulate the successive steps in odontogenesis. With the differentiation of odontoblasts, type III collagen disappears from the predentin matrix, and fibronectin, which surrounds preodontoblasts, is restricted to the apical pole of mature odontoblasts.[67]

The initial stage of development of the dental papilla is characterized by proliferative activity beneath the dental lamina at sites corresponding to the positions of the prospective primary teeth. Even before the dental lamina begins to form the enamel organ, a capillary vascular network develops within the ectomesenchyme, presumably to support the increased metabolic activity to the presumptive tooth buds. This primordial vascularization is thought to play a key role in induction of odontogenesis.

Stages of Development

Although formation of the tooth is a continuous process, as a matter of convenience the process has been divided into three stages: bud, cap, and bell (Fig. 11-3). The *bud stage* is the ini-

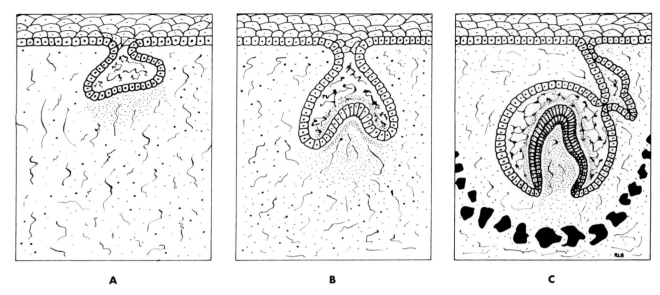

A   **B**   **C**

FIG. 11-3 Diagrammatic representation of, **A,** the bud, **B,** the cap, and, **C,** the bell stages of tooth development.

tial stage of tooth development, wherein the epithelial cells of the dental lamina proliferate and produce a budlike projection into the adjacent ectomesenchyme. The *cap stage* is reached when the cells of the dental lamina have proliferated to form a concavity that produces a caplike appearance. The outer cells of the "cap" are cuboidal and constitute the outer enamel epithelium. The cells on the inner or concave aspect of the "cap" are somewhat elongated and represent the inner enamel epithelium. Between the outer and inner epithelia is a network of cells termed the stellate reticulum because of the branched reticular arrangement of the cellular elements. The rim of the enamel organ (i.e., where the outer and inner enamel epithelia are joined) is termed the cervical loop. As the cells forming the loop continue to proliferate, there is further invagination of the enamel organ into the mesenchyme. The organ assumes a bell shape, and tooth development enters the *bell stage* (Fig. 11-4). During the bell stage the ectomesenchyme of the dental papilla becomes partially enclosed by the invaginating epithelium. Also during this stage the blood vessels become established in the dental papilla.

The condensed ectomesenchyme surrounding the enamel organ and dental papilla complex forms the dental sac and ultimately develops into the periodontal ligament (see Fig. 11-4). As the tooth bud continues to grow, it carries a portion of the dental lamina with it. This extension is referred to as the lateral lamina. During the bell stage the lateral lamina degenerates and is invaded and replaced by mesenchymal tissue. In this way the epithelial connection between the enamel organ and the oral epithelium is severed. The free end of the dental lamina associated with each of the primary teeth continues to grow and form the successional lamina. It is from this structure that the tooth germ of the succedaneous tooth arises. As the maxillary and mandibular processes increase in length, the permanent first molar arises from posterior extensions of the dental lamina. After birth the second and third molar primordia appear as the dental laminae proliferate into the underlying mesenchyme.

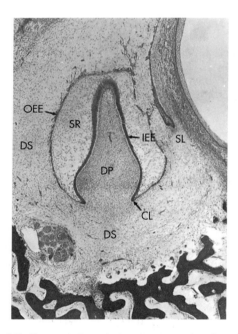

FIG. 11-4 Bell stage of tooth development showing the outer enamel epithelium *(OEE)*, stellate reticulum *(SR)*, inner enamel epithelium *(IEE)*, dental papilla *(DP)*, cervical loop *(CL)*, successional lamina *(SL)*, and dental sac *(DS)*.

Differentiation of Odontoblasts

Differentiation of epithelial and mesenchymal cells into ameloblasts and odontoblasts, respectively, occurs during the bell stage of tooth development. This differentiation is always more advanced in the apex of the "bell" (the region where the cusp tip will develop) than in the area of the cervical loop. From the loop upward toward the apex the cells appear progressively more differentiated. The preameloblasts differentiate at a faster rate than the corresponding odontoblasts so that at any given level mature ameloblasts appear before the odontoblasts have fully matured. In spite of this difference in rate of maturation, dentin matrix is formed before enamel matrix.

During the bell stage of development there is still mitotic activity among the relatively immature cells of the inner enamel epithelium in the region of the cervical loop. As they commence to mature into ameloblasts, mitotic activity ceases and the cells elongate and display the characteristics of active protein synthesis (i.e., an abundance of rough endoplasmic reticulum [RER], a well-developed Golgi complex, and numerous mitochondria).

As the ameloblasts undergo differentiation, changes are taking place across the basement membrane in the adjacent dental papilla. Before differentiation of odontoblasts, the dental papilla consists of sparsely distributed polymorphic mesenchymal cells with wide intercellular spaces (Fig. 11-5). With the onset of differentiation a single layer of cells, the presumptive odontoblasts (preodontoblasts), align themselves along the basement membrane separating the inner enamel epithelium from the dental papilla. These cells stop dividing and elongate into short columnar cells with basally situated nuclei (Fig. 11-6). Several cytoplasmic projections from each of these cells extend toward the basal lamina. At this stage the preodontoblasts are still relatively undifferentiated.

As the odontoblasts continue to differentiate, they become progressively more elongated and take on the ultrastructural characteristics of protein-secreting cells. Cytoplasmic processes from these cells extend through the DBM toward the basal lamina, and more and more collagen fibrils appear within the ECM. The first formed collagen fibers pass between the preodontoblasts and extend toward the basal lamina to form large, fan-shaped bundles 1000 to 2000 Å in diameter, often referred to as *von Korff fibers*. These fibers stain with silver stains and are associated with a high content of proteoglycans. Some smaller collagen fibers approximately 500 in diameter also pass between the odontoblasts and are thought to arise deeper in the dental papilla.[9]

A study on collagen gene expression during rat molar tooth development found both types I and III collagen mRNA in developing odontoblasts.[22] Levels of type I collagen mRNA increased with the progression of odontoblast differentiation while type III collagen gene expression decreased as dentinogenesis proceeded. Both type I and type III collagen mRNA were detected in dental pulp mesenchyme.

Dentinogenesis first occurs in the developing tooth at sites where the cusp tips or incisal edge will be formed. It is in this region that odontoblasts reach full maturity and become tall columnar cells, at times attaining a height of 50 μm or more (see Fig. 11-6). The width of these cells remains fairly constant at approximately 7 μm. Production of the first dentin matrix involves the formation, organization, and maturation of collagen fibrils and proteoglycans. As more collagen fibrils accumulate subjacent to the basal lamina, the lamina becomes discontinuous and eventually disappears. This occurs as the collagen fibers become organized and extend into the spaces between the ameloblast processes. Concurrently the odontoblasts extend several small processes toward the ameloblasts. Some of these become interposed between the processes of ameloblasts, resulting in the formation of enamel spindles (dentinal tubules that extend into the enamel). Membrane-bound vesicles bud off from the odontoblast processes and be-

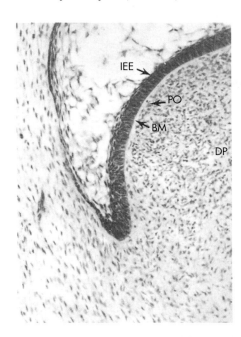

FIG. 11-5 Bell stage shows preodontoblasts *(PO)* aligned along the basement membrane *(BM)* separating the inner enamel epithelium *(IEE)* from the dental papilla *(DP)*.

come interspersed among the collagen fibers of the dentin matrix. These vesicles subsequently play an important role in the initiation of mineralization (this subject is discussed later). With the onset of dentinogenesis the dental papilla becomes the dental pulp.

As predentin matrix is formed, the odontoblasts commence to move away toward the central pulp, depositing matrix at a rate of approximately 4 to 8 μm per day in their wake. Within this matrix a process from each odontoblast becomes accentuated and remains to form the primary odontoblast process. It is around these processes that the dentinal tubules are formed.

Root

Root development commences after the completion of enamel formation. The cells of the inner and outer enamel epithelia, which comprise the cervical loop, begin to proliferate and form a structure known as the Hertwig epithelial root sheath (Fig. 11-7). This sheath determines the size and shape of the root or roots of the tooth. As in the formation of the crown, the cells of the inner enamel epithelium appear to influence the adjacent mesenchymal cells to differentiate into preodontoblasts and odontoblasts. As soon as the first layer of dentin matrix mineralizes, gaps appear in the root sheath, allowing mesenchymal cells from the dental sac to move into contact with the newly formed dentin. These cells then differentiate into cementoblasts and deposit cementum matrix on the root dentin.

Epithelial Rests of Malassez

The epithelial root sheath does not entirely disappear with the onset of dentinogenesis. Some cells persist within the periodontal ligament and are known as epithelial rests of Malassez. Although the number of these rests gradually decreases with age, it has been shown that at least some of them retain the

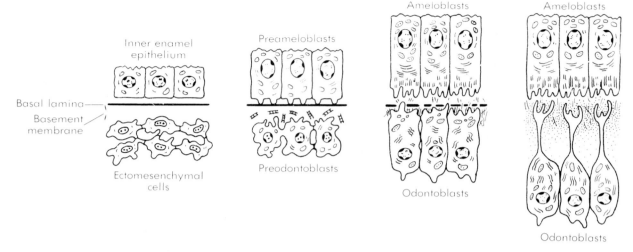

FIG. 11-6 Diagrammatic representation of the stages of odontoblast differentiation.

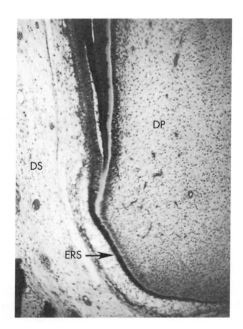

FIG. 11-7 Root development showing dental pulp *(DP)*, dental sac *(DS)*, and epithelial root sheath *(ERS)*.

ability to undergo cell division[117] (Fig. 11-8). *If in later life a chronic inflammatory lesion develops within the periapical tissues as a result of pulp disease, proliferation of the epithelial rests may produce a periapical (radicular) cyst.*

Accessory Canals

Occasionally during formation of the root sheath a break develops in the continuity of the sheath, producing a small gap. When this occurs, dentinogenesis does not take place opposite the defect. The result is a small "accessory" canal between the dental sac and the pulp. An accessory canal can become established anywhere along the root, thus creating a periodontal-endodontic pathway of communication and a possible portal of entry into the pulp if the periodontal tissues lose their integrity. *In periodontal disease the development of a periodontal pocket may expose an accessory canal and thus allow microorganisms or their metabolic products to gain access to the pulp.*

DENTIN

Fully mature dentin is composed of approximately 70% inorganic material and 10% water. The principal inorganic component consists of $Ca_{10}(PO_4)_6(OH)_2$ (hydroxyapatite). Organic matrix accounts for 20% of dentin, of which about 91% is collagen. Most of the collagen is type I, but there is a minor component of type V. Noncollagenous matrix components include phosphoproteins, proteoglycans, γ-carboxyglutamate–containing proteins (gla-proteins), acidic glycoproteins, growth factors, and lipids. The elasticity of dentin provides flexibility for the overlying brittle enamel.

Dentin and enamel are closely bound together at the dentin-enamel junction (DEJ), and dentin joins cementum at the cemento-dentinal junction (CDJ). Electron microscopy has revealed that the hydroxyapatite crystals of dentin and enamel are intermixed in the area formerly occupied by the basal lamina of the inner enamel epithelium. Since the basal lamina is dissolved before the onset of dentinogenesis, no organic membrane separates the crystals of enamel from those of dentin. It is well known clinically that the DEJ is an area of considerable sensitivity. The reason for this is not clear, but it is thought that the branching of the dentinal tubules in the region of the DEJ may play a role.

Types

Developmental dentin is that which forms during tooth development. That formed physiologically after the root is fully developed is referred to as *secondary dentin*. Developmental dentin is classified as *orthodentin*, the tubular form of dentin found in the teeth of all dentate mammals. Mantle dentin is the first formed dentin and is situated immediately subjacent to the enamel or cementum. It is typified by its content of the thick fan-shaped collagen fibers deposited immediately subjacent to the basal lamina during the initial stages of dentino-

mer collagens. Noncollagenous elements consist of several proteoglycans (dermatan sulfate, heparan sulfate, hyaluronate, keratan sulfate, chondroitin 4-sulfate, chondroitin 6-sulfate), glycoproteins, glycosaminoglycans (GAGs), gla-proteins, and *phosphophoryn* (dentin phosphoprotein). Phosphophoryn is a highly phosphorylated, tissue-specific molecule that is unique to the odontoblast cell lineage.[14] It is produced by the odontoblast and transported to the mineralization front. It is thought to bind to calcium and play a role in mineralization. In addition, growth factors such as TGF-β, insulin-like growth factors, and platelet-derived growth factor have been identified in dentin.

Mineralization

Mineralization of dentin matrix commences within the initial increment of mantle dentin. Calcium phosphate crystals begin to accumulate in matrix vesicles within the predentin. Presumably these vesicles bud off from the cytoplasmic processes of odontoblasts. Although matrix vesicles are distributed throughout the predentin, they are most numerous near the basal lamina. The hydroxyapatite crystals grow rapidly within the vesicles, and in time the vesicles rupture. The crystals thus released mix with crystals from adjoining vesicles to form advancing crystal fronts that merge to form small globules. As the globules expand, they fuse with adjacent globules until the matrix is completely mineralized.

Apparently matrix vesicles are involved only in mineralization of the initial layer of dentin. As the process of mineralization progresses, the advancing front projects along the collagen fibrils of the predentin matrix. Hydroxyapatite crystals appear on the surface and within the fibrils and continue to grow as mineralization progresses, resulting in an increased mineral content of the dentin.

Dentinal Tubules

A characteristic of human dentin is the presence of tubules that occupy from 20% to 30% of the volume of intact dentin. These tubules house the major cell processes of odontoblasts. Tubules form around the odontoblast processes and thus traverse the entire width of the dentin from the DEJ or CDJ to the pulp. They are slightly tapered, with the wider portion situated toward the pulp. This tapering is the result of the progressive formation of peritubular dentin, which leads to a continuous decrease in the diameter of the tubules toward the enamel.

In coronal dentin the tubules have a gentle **S** shape as they extend from the DEJ to the pulp. The **S**-shaped curvature is presumably a result of the crowding of odontoblasts as they migrate toward the center of the pulp. As they approach the pulp, the tubules converge because the surface of the pulp chamber has a much smaller area than the surface of dentin along the DEJ.

The number and diameter of the tubules at various distances from the pulp have been determined (Table 11-1).[36] Investigators[2] found the number and diameter of dentinal tubules to be similar in rats, cats, dogs, monkeys, and humans, indicating that mammalian orthodentin has evolved amazingly constantly.

Lateral tubules containing branches of the main odontoblastic processes have been demonstrated by other researchers,[57] who suggested that they form pathways for the movement of materials between the main processes and the more distant matrix. It is also possible that the direction of the branches influ-

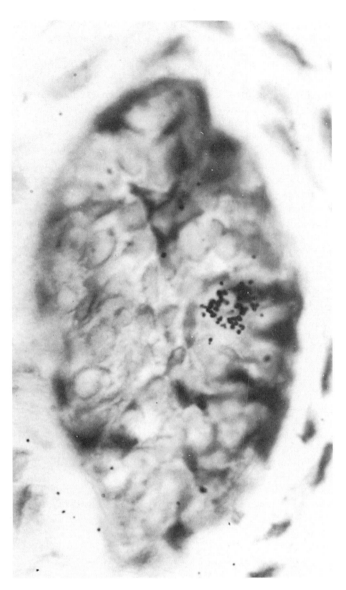

FIG. 11-8 Radioautograph of an epithelial rest cell showing ^{3}H-thymidine labeling of the nucleus, indicating that the cell is preparing to divide. *(From Trowbridge HO, Shibata F: Periodontics 5:109, 1967.)*

genesis. These fibers run roughly perpendicular to the DEJ. Spaces between the fibers are occupied by smaller collagen fibrils lying more or less parallel with the DEJ or CDJ.

Circumpulpal dentin is formed after the layer of mantle dentin has been deposited, and it constitutes the major part of developmental dentin. The organic matrix is composed mainly of collagen fibrils, approximately 500 Å in diameter, that are oriented at right angles to the long axis of the dentinal tubules. These fibrils are closely packed together and form an interwoven network.

Predentin

Predentin is the unmineralized organic matrix of dentin situated between the odontoblast layer and the mineralized dentin. Its macromolecular constituents include type I and type II tri-

ences the orientation of the collagen fibrils in the intertubular dentin.

Near the DEJ the dentinal tubules ramify into one or more terminal branches (Fig. 11-9). This is due to the fact that during the initial stage of dentinogenesis the differentiating odontoblasts extended several cytoplasmic processes toward the DEJ, but as the odontoblasts withdrew, their processes converged into one major process (see Fig. 11-6).

Peritubular Dentin

Dentin lining the tubules is termed *peritubular dentin,* whereas that between the tubules is known as *intertubular dentin* (Fig. 11-10). Presumably precursors of the dentin matrix that is deposited around each odontoblast process are synthesized by the odontoblast, transported in secretory vesicles out into the process, and released by reverse pinocytosis. With the formation of peritubular dentin there is a corresponding reduction in the diameter of the process.

Peritubular dentin represents a specialized form of orthodentin not common to all mammals. The matrix of peritubular dentin differs from that of intertubular dentin in having relatively fewer collagen fibrils and a higher proportion of sulfated proteoglycans. Because of its lower content of collagen, peritubular dentin is more quickly dissolved in acid than is intertubular dentin. By preferentially removing peritubular dentin, acid etching agents used during dental restorative procedures enlarge the openings of the dentinal tubules, thus making the dentin more permeable.

Peritubular dentin is more highly mineralized and therefore harder than intertubular dentin. The hardness of peritubular dentin may provide added structural support for the intertubular dentin, thus strengthening the tooth.

Intertubular Dentin

Intertubular dentin is located between the rings of peritubular dentin and constitutes the bulk of circumpulpal dentin (see Fig. 11-10). Its organic matrix consists mainly of collagen fibrils having diameters of 500 to 1000. These fibrils are oriented approximately at right angles to the dentinal tubules.

Dentinal Sclerosis

Partial or complete obturation of dentinal tubules may occur as a result of aging or develop in response to stimuli such as attrition of the tooth surface or dental caries. When tubules become filled with mineral deposits, the dentin becomes sclerotic. Dentinal sclerosis is easily recognized in histologic ground sections because of its translucency, which is due to the homogeneity of the dentin, since both matrix and tubules are mineralized. Studies using dyes, solvents, and radioactive ions have shown that sclerosis results in decreased permeabil-

Table 11-1. Mean number and diameter per square millimeter of dentinal tubules at various distances from the pulp in human teeth

Distance from Pulp (mm)	Number of Tubules (1000/mm²)		Tubule Diameter (μm)	
	Mean	Range	Mean	Range
Pulpal wall	45	30-52	2.5	2.0-3.2
0.1-0.5	43	22-59	1.9	1.0-2.3
0.6-1.0	38	16-47	1.6	1.0-1.6
1.1-1.5	35	21-47	1.2	0.9-1.5
1.6-2.0	30	12-47	1.1	0.8-1.6
2.1-2.5	23	11-36	0.9	0.6-1.3
2.6-3.0	20	7-40	0.8	0.5-1.4
3.1-3.5	19	10-25	0.8	0.5-1.2

From Garberoglio R, Brännström M: *Arch Oral Biol* 21:355, 1976.

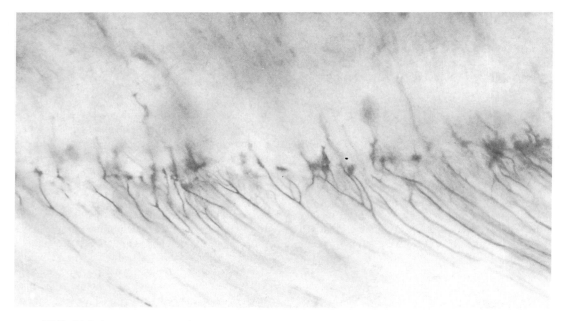

FIG. 11-9 Ground section of a tooth demonstrating branching of the dentinal tubules near the DEJ. This branching may account for the increased clinical sensitivity at the DEJ.

ity of dentin. Thus dentinal sclerosis, by limiting the diffusion of noxious substances through the dentin, helps to shield the pulp from irritation.

One form of dentinal sclerosis is thought to represent an acceleration of peritubular dentin formation. This form appears to be a physiologic process, and in the apical third of the root it develops as a function of age.[102] Dentinal tubules can also become blocked by the precipitation of hydroxyapatite and

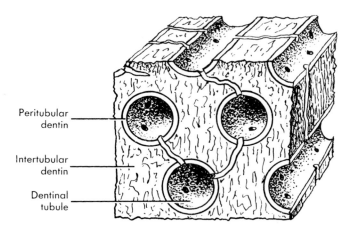

Peritubular dentin

Intertubular dentin

Dentinal tubule

FIG. 11-10 Diagram illustrating peritubular and intertubular dentin. *(From Trowbridge HO: Dentistry 82 2(4):22-29, 1982.)*

whitlockite crystals within the tubules. This type occurs in the translucent zone of carious dentin and in attrited dentin and has been termed pathologic sclerosis.[125]

Interglobular Dentin

The term *interglobular dentin* refers to organic matrix that remains unmineralized because the mineralizing globules fail to coalesce. This occurs most often in the circumpulpal dentin just below the mantle dentin where the pattern of mineralization is more likely to be globular than appositional. In certain dental anomalies (e.g., vitamin D–resistant rickets and hypophosphatasia) large areas of interglobular dentin are a characteristic feature (Fig. 11-11).

Dentinal Fluid

Free fluid occupies about 22% of the total volume of dentin. This fluid is an ultrafiltrate of blood in the pulp capillaries, and its composition resembles plasma in many respects. The fluid flows outward between the odontoblasts into the dentinal tubules and eventually escapes through small pores in the enamel. It has been shown that the tissue pressure of the pulp is approximately 14 cm H_2O (10.3 mm Hg).[20] Consequently, there is a pressure gradient between the pulp and the oral cavity that accounts for the outward flow of fluid. Exposure of the tubules by tooth fracture or during cavity preparation often results in the outward movement of fluid to the exposed dentin surface in the form of tiny droplets. This outward movement of fluid can be accelerated by dehydrating the surface of

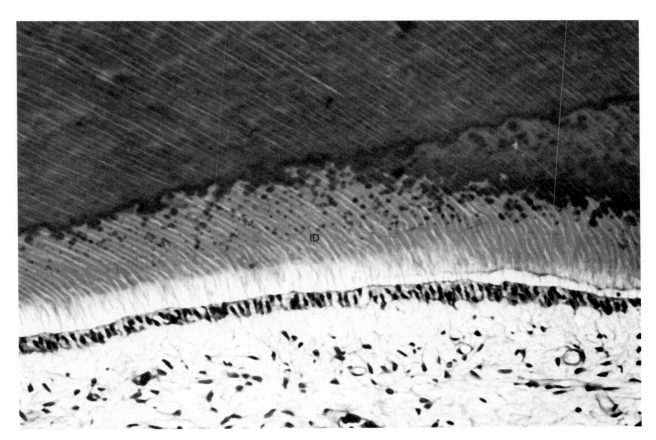

FIG. 11-11 Section showing interglobular dentin *(ID)* in a deciduous incisor from a 3-year-old boy with childhood hypophosphatasia.

the dentin with compressed air, dry heat, or the application of absorbent paper. Rapid flow of fluid through the tubules is thought to be a cause of dentin sensitivity (see pp. 407-408).

Bacterial products or other contaminants may be introduced into the dentinal fluid as a result of dental caries, restorative procedures, or growth of bacteria beneath restorations.[11,12] Dentinal fluid may thus serve as a sump from which injurious agents can percolate into the pulp, producing an inflammatory response.

Dentin Permeability

The permeability of dentin has been well characterized.[88-90] Dentinal tubules are the major channels for fluid diffusion across dentin. Since fluid permeation is proportional to tubule diameter and number, dentin permeability increases as the tubules converge on the pulp (Fig. 11-12). The total tubular surface near the DEJ is approximately 1% of the total surface area of dentin,[90] whereas close to the pulp chamber the total tubular surface may be nearly 45%. Thus from a clinical standpoint it should be recognized that dentin beneath a deep cavity preparation is much more permeable than dentin underlying a shallow cavity.

One study[33] found that the permeability of radicular dentin is much lower than that of coronal dentin. This was attributed to a decrease in the density of the dentinal tubules from approximately 42,000/mm^2 in cervical dentin to about 8000/mm^2 in radicular dentin. These investigators found that fluid movement through outer radicular dentin was only approximately 2% that of coronal dentin. The low permeability of outer radicular dentin should make it relatively impermeable to toxic substances such as bacterial products emanating from plaque.

Factors modifying dentin permeability include the presence of odontoblast processes in the tubules and the sheathlike lamina limitans that lines the tubules. Collagen fibers have also been observed in some tubules. Thus the functional or physiologic diameter of the tubules is only about 5% to 10% of the anatomic diameter (i.e., the diameter seen in microscopic sections).[77]

In dental caries an inflammatory reaction develops in the pulp long before the pulp actually becomes infected.[114] This indicates that bacterial products reach the pulp in advance of the bacteria themselves. Dentinal sclerosis beneath a carious lesion reduces the permeation by obstructing the tubules, thus decreasing the concentration of irritants that are introduced into the pulp.

The cutting of dentin during cavity preparation produces microcrystalline grinding debris that coats the dentin and clogs the orifices of the dentinal tubules. This layer of debris is termed the smear layer. Because of the small size of the particles, the smear layer is capable of preventing bacteria from penetrating dentin.[79] Removal of the grinding debris by acid etching greatly increases the permeability of the dentin by decreasing the surface resistance and widening the orifices of the tubules. Consequently, the incidence of pulpal inflammation may be increased significantly if cavities are treated with an acid cleanser, unless a cavity liner, base, or dentin-bonding agent is used.

When researchers exposed the dentin surface of vital and nonvital teeth to the oral environment for 150 days, bacterial invasion of dentinal tubules occurred more rapidly in the nonvital teeth.[79] Presumably this was due to the resistance offered by the presence of dentinal fluid and odontoblast processes in the tubules of vital teeth. It is also possible that antibodies or

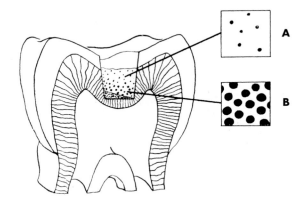

FIG. 11-12 Diagram illustrating the difference in size and density of tubules in the dentinal floor between a shallow (**A**) and a deep (**B**) cavity preparation. *(From Trowbridge HO:* Dentistry 82 *22(4):22-29, 1982.)*

other antimicrobial agents may be present within the dentinal fluid of teeth with vital pulps.

MORPHOLOGIC ZONES OF THE PULP

Odontoblast Layer

The outermost stratum of cells of the healthy pulp is the odontoblast layer (Figs. 11-13 and 11-14). This layer is located immediately subjacent to the predentin; the odontoblast processes, however, pass on through the predentin into the dentin. Consequently, the odontoblast layer is actually composed of the cell bodies of odontoblasts. Additionally, capillaries, nerve fibers, and dendritic cells may be found among the odontoblasts.

In the coronal portion of a young pulp the odontoblasts assume a tall columnar form. The tight packing together of these tall slender cells produces the appearance of a palisade. The odontoblasts vary in height; consequently, their nuclei are not all at the same level and are aligned in a staggered array. This often produces the appearance of a layer three to five cells in thickness. Between odontoblasts there are small intercellular spaces approximately 300 to 400 Å in width.

The odontoblast layer in the coronal pulp contains more cells per unit area than in the radicular pulp. Whereas the odontoblasts of the mature coronal pulp are usually columnar, those in the midportion of the radicular pulp are more cuboidal (Fig. 11-15). Near the apical foramen the odontoblasts appear as a flattened cell layer. Since there are fewer dentinal tubules per unit area in the root than in the crown of the tooth, the odontoblast cell bodies are less crowded and are able to spread out laterally.

Between adjacent odontoblasts there are a series of specialized cell-to-cell junctions (junctional complexes) including desmosomes (zonula adherens), gap junctions (nexuses), and tight junctions (zonula occludens). Spot desmosomes located in the apical part of odontoblast cell bodies mechanically join odontoblasts together. Numerous gap junctions provide low-resistance pathways through which electrical excitation can pass between cells (Fig. 11-16). These junctions are most numerous during the formation of primary dentin. Gap junctions and desmosomes have also been observed joining odontoblasts to the processes of fibroblasts in the subodontoblastic area. Tight junctions are found mainly in the apical part of odontoblasts in young teeth. These structures consist of linear ridges

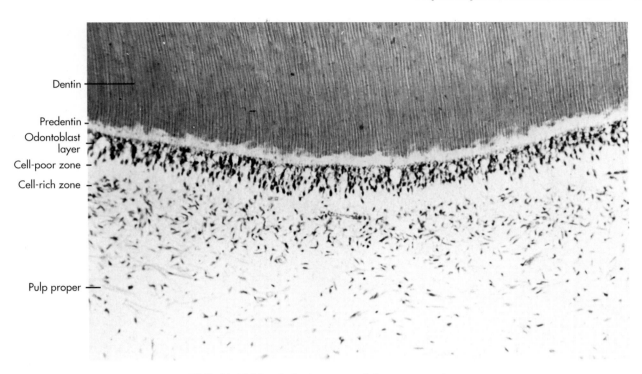

FIG. 11-13 Morphologic zones of the mature pulp.

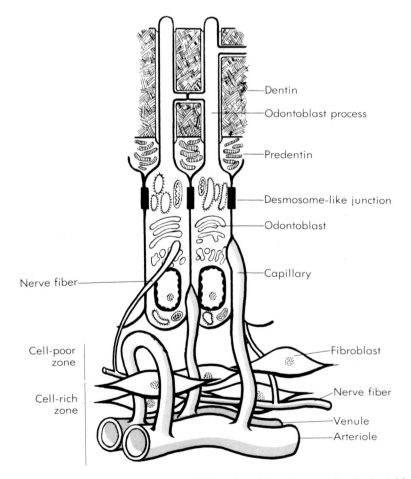

FIG. 11-14 Diagrammatic representation of the odontoblast layer and subodontoblastic region of the pulp.

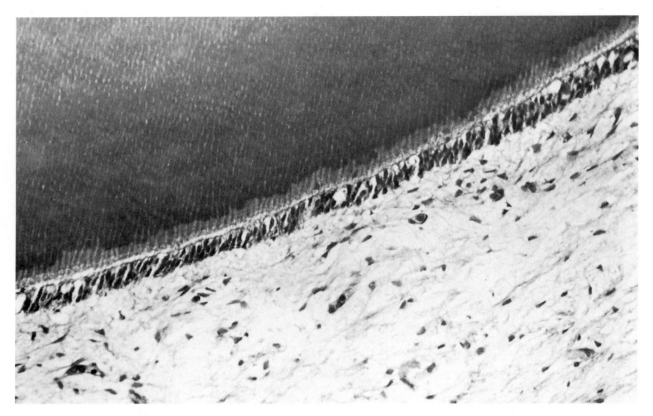

FIG. 11-15 Low columnar odontoblasts of the radicular pulp. The cell-rich zone is inconspicuous.

and grooves that close off the intercellular space. It appears that tight junctions determine the permeability of the odontoblast layer by restricting the passage of molecules, ions, and fluid between the extracellular compartments of the pulp and predentin.[120]

Cell-Poor Zone

Immediately subjacent to the odontoblast layer in the coronal pulp, there is often a narrow zone approximately 40 μm in width that is relatively free of cells (see Fig. 11-13). It is traversed by blood capillaries, unmyelinated nerve fibers, and the slender cytoplasmic processes of fibroblasts. The presence or absence of the cell-poor zone depends on the functional status of the pulp. It may not be apparent in young pulps, where dentin forms rapidly, or in older pulps, where reparative dentin is being produced.

Cell-Rich Zone

Usually conspicuous in the subodontoblastic area is a stratum containing a relatively high proportion of fibroblasts compared with the more central region of the pulp (see Fig. 11-13). It is much more prominent in the coronal pulp than in the radicular pulp. Beside fibroblasts, the cell-rich zone may include a variable number of macrophages and lymphocytes.

On the basis of evidence obtained in rat molar teeth, it has been suggested[37] that the cell-rich zone forms as a result of peripheral migration of cells populating the central regions of the pulp, commencing at about the time of tooth eruption. Although cell division within the cell-rich zone is a rare occurrence in normal pulps, death of odontoblasts causes a great in-

crease in the rate of mitosis. Since irreversibly injured odontoblasts are replaced by cells that migrate from the cell-rich zone onto the inner surface of the dentin,[32] this mitotic activity is probably the first step in the formation of a new odontoblast layer.

Pulp Proper

The pulp proper is the central mass of the pulp (see Fig. 11-13). It contains the larger blood vessels and nerves. The connective tissue cells in this zone are fibroblasts, or pulpal cells.

CELLS OF THE PULP

Odontoblast

Because it is responsible for dentinogenesis both during tooth development and in the mature tooth, the odontoblast is the most characteristic cell of the pulp-dentin complex. During dentinogenesis the odontoblasts form the dentinal tubules, and their presence within the tubules makes dentin a living tissue.

Dentinogenesis, osteogenesis, and cementogenesis are in many respects quite similar. Therefore it is not surprising that odontoblasts, osteoblasts, and cementoblasts have many similar characteristics. Each of these cells produces a matrix composed of collagen fibers and proteoglycans that is capable of undergoing mineralization. The ultrastructural characteristics of odontoblasts, osteoblasts, and cementoblasts are likewise similar in that each exhibits a highly ordered RER, a prominent Golgi complex, secretory granules, and numerous mitochondria. In addition, these cells are rich in RNA, and their

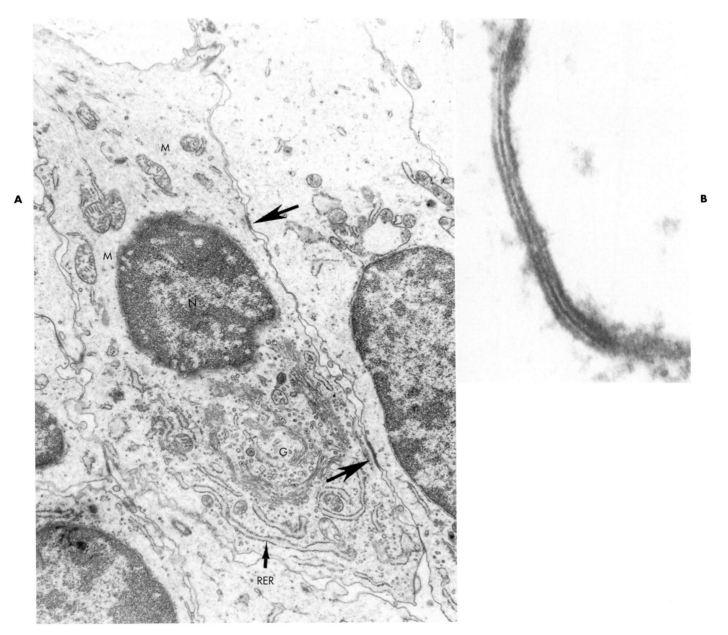

FIG. 11-16 A, Electron micrograph of a mouse molar odontoblast demonstrating gap junctions *(arrows)*, nucleus *(N)*, mitochondria *(M)*, Golgi complex *(G)*, and rough endoplasmic reticulum *(RER)*. **B,** High magnification of a section fixed and stained with lanthanum nitrate to demonstrate a typical gap junction. *(Courtesy Dr. Charles F. Cox, School of Dentistry, University of Michigan.)*

nuclei contain one or more prominent nucleoli. These are the general characteristics of protein-secreting cells.

Perhaps the most significant differences between odontoblasts, osteoblasts, and cementoblasts are their morphologic characteristics and the anatomic relationship between the cells and the structures they produce. Whereas osteoblasts and cementoblasts are polygonal to cuboidal in form, the fully developed odontoblast of the coronal pulp is a tall columnar cell. In bone and cementum some of the osteoblasts and cementoblasts become entrapped in the matrix as osteocytes or cementocytes, respectively. The odontoblasts, on the other hand, leave behind cellular processes to form the dentinal tubules.

Lateral branches between the major odontoblast processes interconnect the processes through canals just as osteocytes and cementocytes are linked together through the canaliculi in bone and cementum. This provides for intercellular communication as well as circulation of fluid and metabolites through the mineralized matrix.

The ultrastructural features of the odontoblast have been the subject of numerous investigations. The cell body of the active odontoblast has a large nucleus that may contain up to four nucleoli (Fig. 11-17). The nucleus is situated at the basal end of the cell and is contained within a nuclear envelope. A well-developed Golgi complex, centrally located in the supranuclear

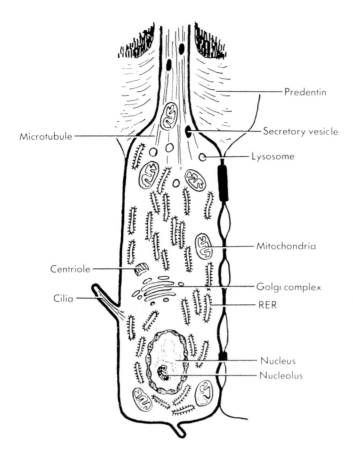

Predentin

Secretory vesicle

Microtubule

Lysosome

Mitochondria

Centriole

Cilia

Golgi complex

RER

Nucleus

Nucleolus

FIG. 11-17 Diagram of a fully differentiated odontoblast.

cytoplasm, consists of an assembly of smooth-walled vesicles and cisternae. Numerous mitochondria are evenly distributed throughout the cell body. RER is particularly prominent, consisting of closely stacked cisternae forming parallel arrays that are dispersed diffusely within the cytoplasm. Numerous ribosomes closely associated with the membranes of the cisternae mark the sites of protein synthesis. Within the lumen of the cisternae filamentous material probably representing newly synthesized protein can be observed.

Apparently the odontoblast synthesizes mainly type I collagen, although small amounts of type V collagen have been found in the ECM. In addition to proteoglycans and collagen, the odontoblast secretes dentin sialoprotein and phosphophoryn, a highly phosphorylated phosphoprotein involved in extracellular mineralization. Phosphophoryn is unique to dentin and is not found in any other mesenchymal cell lines. The odontoblast also secretes alkaline phosphatase, an enzyme that is closely linked to mineralization but whose precise role is yet to be illuminated.

In contrast to the active odontoblast, the resting or inactive odontoblast has a decreased number of organelles and may become progressively shorter. These changes can begin with the completion of root development.

Odontoblast Process

A dentinal tubule forms around each of the major processes of odontoblasts. The odontoblast process occupies most of the

space within the tubule and somehow mediates the formation of peritubular dentin. Fine cytofilaments are the other structures found in the process.

Microtubules and microfilaments are the principal ultrastructural components of the odontoblast process and its lateral branches.[49] Microtubules extend from the cell body out into the process. These straight structures follow a course that is parallel with the long axis of the cell and impart the impression of rigidity. Although their precise role is unknown, theories as to their functional significance suggest that they may be involved in cytoplasmic extension, transport of materials, or simply the provision of a structural framework. Occasionally mitochondria can be found in the process where it passes through the predentin.

The plasma membrane of the odontoblast process closely approximates the wall of the dentinal tubule. Localized constrictions in the process occasionally produce relatively large spaces between the tubule wall and the process. Such spaces may contain collagen fibrils and fine granular material, which presumably represents ground substance. The peritubular dentin matrix lining the tubule is circumscribed by an electron-dense limiting membrane.[107] A space separates the limiting membrane from the plasma membrane of the odontoblast process. This space is usually narrow except in areas where, as mentioned previously, the process is constricted.

In restoring a tooth, preparation of a cavity or crown often disrupts odontoblasts. Consequently, it would be of considerable clinical importance to establish conclusively the extent of the odontoblast processes in human teeth. With this knowledge the clinician would be in a better position to estimate the impact of the restorative procedure on the underlying odontoblasts. The extent to which the process extends outward in the dentin has been a matter of considerable controversy. It has long been thought that the process is present throughout the full thickness of dentin. However, ultrastructural studies using transmission electron microscopy have described the process as being limited to the inner third of the dentin.[48,107] This could possibly be the result of shrinkage occurring during fixation and dehydration during histologic processing. Other studies employing scanning electron microscopy have described the process extending further into the tubule, often as far as the DEJ.[38,58,129] However, it has been suggested that what has been observed in scanning electron micrographs is actually an electron-dense structure, the lamina limitans, that lines the surface of the tubule.[106,107]

In an attempt to resolve this issue, monoclonal antibodies directed against microtubules were used to demonstrate tubulin in the microtubules of the process. Immunoreactivity was observed throughout the dentinal tubule, suggesting that the process extends throughout the entire thickness of dentin.[99,100] However, a more recent study employing fluorescent carbocyanine dye and confocal microscopy found that odontoblast processes in rat molars do not extend to the outer dentin or DEJ except during the early stages of tooth development.[17] Obviously this problem warrants further study.

The odontoblast is considered to be a fixed postmitotic cell in that once it has fully differentiated, it apparently cannot undergo further cell division. If this is indeed the case, the life span of the odontoblast coincides with the life span of the viable pulp.

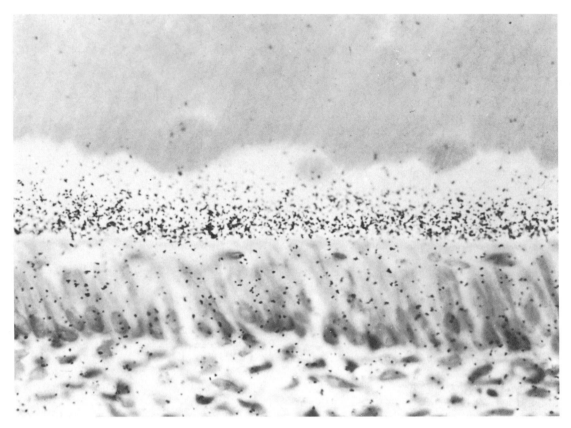

FIG. 11-18 Radioautograph demonstrating odontoblasts and predentin in a developing rat molar 1 hour after intraperitoneal injection of ³H-proline.

Relationship of Odontoblast Structure to Function

Isotope studies have shed a great deal of light on the functional significance of the cytoplasmic organelles of the active odontoblast.[127] In experimental animals the intraperitoneal injection of collagen precursors such as ³H-proline is followed by autoradiographic labeling of the odontoblasts and predentin matrix (Fig. 11-18). Rapid incorporation of the isotope in the RER soon leads to labeling of the Golgi complex in the area where the procollagen is packed and concentrated into secretory vesicles. Labeled vesicles can then be followed along their migration pathway until they reach the base of the odontoblast process. Here they fuse with the cell membrane and release their tropocollagen molecules into the predentin matrix by the process of reverse pinocytosis. It is now known that collagen fibrils precipitate from a solution of tropocollagen and that the aggregation of fibrils occurs on the outer surface of the odontoblast plasma membrane. Fibrils are released into the predentin and increase in thickness as they approach the mineralized matrix. Whereas fibrils at the base of the odontoblast process are approximately 150 in diameter, fibrils in the region of the calcification front have attained a diameter of about 500 Å.

Similar tracer studies[126] have elucidated the pathway of synthesis, transport, and secretion of the predentin proteoglycans. The protein moiety of these molecules is synthesized by the RER of the odontoblast, whereas sulfation and addition of the GAG moieties to the protein molecules take place in the Golgi complex. Secretory vesicles then transport the proteoglycans to the base of the odontoblast process, where they are secreted into the predentin matrix. Proteoglycans, principally chondroitin sulfate, accumulate near the calcification front. The role of the proteoglycans is speculative, but mounting evidence suggests that they act as inhibitors of calcification by binding calcium. It appears that just before calcification the proteoglycans are removed, probably by lysosomal enzymes secreted by the odontoblasts.[25]

Pulp Fibroblast

The most numerous cells of the pulp, fibroblasts appear to be tissue-specific cells capable of giving rise to cells that are committed to differentiation as odontoblast-like cells, given the proper signal. These cells synthesize types I and III collagen, as well as proteoglycans and GAGs. Thus they produce and maintain the matrix proteins of the ECM. Since they are also able to phagocytose and digest collagen, fibroblasts are responsible for collagen turnover in the pulp.

Although distributed throughout the pulp, fibroblasts are particularly abundant in the cell-rich zone. The early-differentiating fibroblasts are polygonal and appear to be widely separated and evenly distributed within the ground substance. Cell-to-cell contacts are established between the multiple processes that extend out from each of the cells. Many of these contacts take the form of gap junctions, which provide for electronic coupling of one cell to another. Ultrastructurally the organelles of the immature fibroblasts are generally in a rudimentary stage of development, with an inconspicuous Golgi complex, numerous free ribosomes, and sparse RER. As they mature, the cells become stellate in form and the Golgi complex enlarges, the RER proliferates, secretory vesicles appear, and the fibroblasts take on the characteristic appearance of protein-secreting cells. Along the outer surface of the cell body, collagen fibrils commence to appear. With an increase in the number of blood vessels, nerves, and fibers there is a relative decrease in the number of fibroblasts in the pulp.

A colleague once remarked that the fibroblasts of the pulp are very much like Peter Pan in that they never grow up. There may be an element of truth in this statement, for these cells do seem to remain in a relatively undifferentiated modality as compared to fibroblasts of most other connective tissues.[42] This perception has been fortified by the observation of large numbers of reticulin-like fibers in the pulp. Reticulin fibers have an affinity for silver stains and are similar to the argyrophilic fibers of the pulp. However, in a careful review of the subject, Baume[4] concluded that because of distinct histochemical differences, reticulin fibers, such as those of gingiva and lymphoid organs, are not present in the pulp. He suggested that these pulpal fibers be termed *argyrophilic collagen fibers*. The fibers apparently acquire a GAG sheath, and it is this sheath that is impregnated by silver stains. In the young pulp the nonargyrophilic collagen fibers are sparse, but they progressively increase in number as the pulp ages.

Many experimental models have been developed to study wound healing in the pulp, particularly dentinal bridge formation following pulp exposure or pulpotomy. One study[32] demonstrated that mitotic activity preceding the differentiation of replacement odontoblasts appears to occur primarily among fibroblasts.

Macrophage

Tissue macrophages, or histiocytes, are monocytes that have left the bloodstream, entered the tissues, and differentiated into macrophages. They are usually found in close proximity to blood vessels. These cells are quite active in endocytosis and phagocytosis. Because of their mobility and phagocytic activity they are able to act as scavengers, removing extravasated red blood cells, dead cells, and foreign bodies from the tissue. Ingested material is destroyed by the action of lysosomal enzymes.

In addition, a proportion of macrophages, when primed by cytokines, participate in immune reactions by processing antigen and presenting it to lymphocytes. The processed antigen is bound to class II (Ia) histocompatibility antigens on the macrophage, where it can interact with specific receptors present on immunocompetent T cells. Such interaction is obligatory for induction of cell-mediated immunity. When activated by the appropriate inflammatory stimuli, macrophages are capable of producing a large variety of soluble factors including interleukin-1, tumor necrosis factor, growth factors, and other cytokines.

Dendritic Cell

Dendritic cells, like macrophages, are accessory cells of the immune system. Similar cells are found in the epidermis and mucous membranes, where they are called *Langerhans' cells*. Dendritic cells are primarily found in lymphoid tissues, but they are also widely distributed in connective tissues, including the pulp[56,86] (Fig. 11-19). These cells are termed *antigen-*

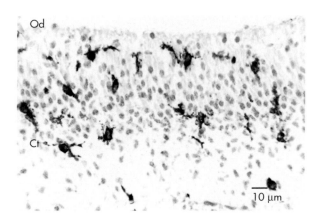

FIG. 11-19 Class II antigen-expressing dendritic cells in the odontoblast layer *(Od)* and subodontoblastic connective tissue *(Ct)* in normal rat incisor pulp, as demonstrated by immunocytochemistry. *(From Jontell M et al: J Dent Res 67:1263, 1988.)*

presenting cells and are characterized by dendritic cytoplasmic processes and the presence of cell surface class II antigens. Like macrophages, they phagocytose and process antigens but are otherwise only weakly phagocytic. Together with macrophages and lymphocytes, dendritic cells are believed to participate in immunosurveillance in the pulp.

Lymphocyte

Hahn et al.[40] reported finding T lymphocytes in normal pulps from human teeth. T8 (suppressor) lymphocytes were the predominant T-lymphocyte subset present in these pulps. Lymphocytes have also been observed in the pulps of impacted teeth.[65] The presence of macrophages, dendritic cells, and T lymphocytes indicates that the pulp is well equipped with cells required for the initiation of immune responses.

Mesenchymal Cell

Some authors are of the opinion that primordial mesenchymal cells persist in adult tissues as "undifferentiated" mesenchymal cells. However, during wound healing well-differentiated fibroblasts undergo rapid serial division to give rise to new fibroblasts. Similarly, replacement odontoblasts are derived from mature fibroblasts. Consequently, there is no need to postulate that in the pulp new mesenchymal cells arise from cells other than pulpal fibroblasts.

Mast Cell

Mast cells are widely distributed in connective tissues, where they occur in small groups in relation to blood vessels. Their presence in the normal pulp tissue has been a matter of controversy, although they are routinely found in chronically inflamed pulps. This cell has been the subject of considerable attention because of its dramatic role in inflammatory reactions. The granules of mast cells contain heparin, an anticoagulant, as well as histamine, an important inflammatory mediator.

METABOLISM

The metabolic activity of the pulp has been studied by measuring the rate of oxygen consumption and the production of carbon dioxide or lactic acid by pulp tissue in vitro.[28,31,93] A later investigation[41] employed the radiospirometry method.

Because of the relatively sparse cellular composition of the pulp the rate of oxygen consumption is low in comparison to that of most other tissues. During active dentinogenesis, metabolic activity is much higher than following the completion of crown development. As would be anticipated, the greatest metabolic activity is found in the region of the odontoblast layer.

In addition to the usual glycolytic pathway, the pulp has the ability to produce energy through a phosphogluconate (pentose phosphate) shunt type of carbohydrate metabolism,[29] suggesting that the pulp may be able to function under varying degrees of ischemia. This could explain how the pulp manages to withstand periods of vasoconstriction resulting from the use of infiltration anesthesia employing epinephrine-containing local anesthetic agents.[61]

Several commonly used dental materials (e.g., eugenol, zinc oxide–eugenol, calcium hydroxide, silver amalgam) have been shown to inhibit oxygen consumption by pulp tissue, indicating that these agents may be capable of depressing the metabolic activity of pulpal cells.[30,55] One study[41] found that application of orthodontic force to human premolars for 3 days resulted in a 27% reduction in respiratory activity in the pulp.

GROUND SUBSTANCE

Connective tissue is a system consisting of cells and fibers, both embedded in the pervading ground substance. Cells that produce connective tissue fibers also synthesize the major constituents of ground substance. Whereas the fibers and cells have recognizable shapes, ground substance is described as being amorphous. It is generally regarded as a gel rather than a sol and so is considered to differ from tissue fluids. The term *extracellular matrix* (ECM) is used to describe ground substance, regarding it as the material into which fibers are deposited. Because of its content of polyelectric polysaccharides, the ECM is responsible for the water-holding properties of connective tissues.

Nearly all proteins of the ECM are glycoproteins. Proteoglycans are an important subclass of glycoproteins. These molecules support cells, provide tissue turgor, and mediate a variety of cell interactions. They have in common the presence of GAG chains and a protein core to which the chains are linked. Except for heparan sulfate and heparin, the chains are composed of disaccharides. The primary function of GAG chains is to act as adhesive molecules that can bond to cell surfaces and other matrix molecules.

Fibronectin is a major surface glycoprotein that, together with collagen, forms an integrated fibrillary network that influences adhesion, motility, growth, and differentiation of cells. Laminin, an important component of basement membranes, binds to type IV collagen and cell surface receptors. Tenascin is another substrate adhesion glycoprotein.

In the pulp the principal proteoglycans include hyaluronic acid,* dermatan sulfate, heparan sulfate, and chondroitin sulfate.[73] The proteoglycan content of pulp tissue decreases approximately 50% with tooth eruption.[70] During active dentinogenesis, chondroitin sulfate is the principal proteoglycan, particularly in the odontoblast-predentin layer, where it is somehow involved with mineralization; with tooth eruption

hyaluronic acid and dermatan sulfate increase, and chondroitin sulfate decreases greatly.

The consistency of a connective tissue such as the pulp is largely determined by the proteoglycan components of the ground substance. The long GAG chains of the proteoglycan molecules form relatively rigid coils constituting a network that holds water, thus forming a characteristic gel. Hyaluronic acid in particular has a strong affinity for water and is a major component of ground substance in tissues with a large fluid content, such as Wharton's jelly. The water content of the pulp is very high (approximately 90%); thus the ground substance forms a cushion capable of protecting cells and vascular components of the tooth.

Ground substance also acts as a molecular sieve in that it excludes large proteins and urea. Cell metabolites, nutrients, and wastes pass through the ground substance between cells and blood vessels. In some ways ground substance can be likened to an ion-exchange resin, since the polyanionic changes of the GAGs bind cations. Additionally, osmotic pressures can be altered by excluding osmotically active molecules. Thus proteoglycans can regulate the dispersion of interstitial matrix solutes, colloids, and water and in large measure determine the physical characteristics of a tissue such as the pulp.

Degradation of ground substance can occur in certain inflammatory lesions in which there is a high concentration of lysosomal enzymes. Proteolytic enzymes, hyaluronidases, and chrondroitin sulfatases of lysosomal and bacterial origin are examples of the hydrolytic enzymes that can attack components of the ground substance. The pathways of inflammation and infection are strongly influenced by the state of polymerization of the ground substance components.

CONNECTIVE TISSUE FIBERS OF THE PULP

Two types of structural proteins are found in the pulp: collagen and elastin. Elastin fibers are confined to the walls of arterioles and, unlike collagen, are not a part of the ECM.

A single collagen molecule, referred to as tropocollagen, consists of three polypeptide chains, designated as either α-1 or α-2 depending on their amino acid composition and sequence. The different combinations and linkages of chains making up the tropocollagen molecule has allowed collagen fibers and fibrils to be classified into a number of types. Type I is found in skin, tendon, bone, dentin, and pulp. Type II occurs in cartilage. Type III is found in most unmineralized connective tissues. It is a fetal form found in the dental papilla and the mature pulp. In the bovine pulp it comprises 45% of the total pulp collagen during all stages of development. Types IV and VII collagen are components of basement membranes. Type V collagen is a constituent of interstitial tissues. Type I collagen is synthesized by odontoblasts and osteoblasts; fibroblasts synthesize types I, III, V, and VII.

In collagen synthesis the protein portion of the molecule is formed by the polyribosomes of the RER of connective tissue cells. The proline and lysine residues of the polypeptide chains are hydroxylated in the cisternae of the RER, and the chains are assembled into a triple-helix configuration in the smooth endoplasmic reticulum. The product of this assembly is termed procollagen, and it has a terminal unit of amino acids known as the telopeptide of the procollagen molecule. When these molecules reach the Golgi complex, they are glycosylated and packaged in secretory vesicles. The vesicles are transported to the plasma membrane and secreted via exocytosis into the ex-

---

*Since there is still some doubt as to whether hyaluronic acid is linked to protein, it should probably be referred to as a GAG rather than a proteoglycan.

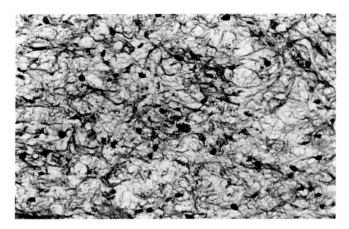

FIG. 11-20 Delicate network of pulpal collagen fibers as demonstrated by the Pearson silver impregnation method.

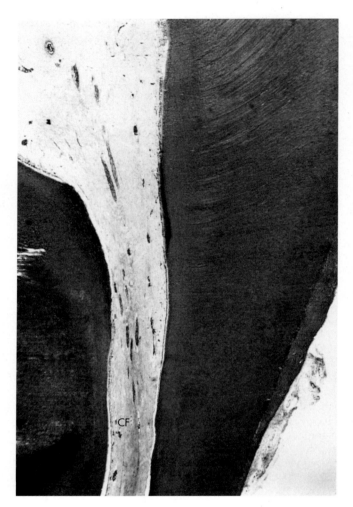

FIG. 11-21 Histologic section of pulp stained with Masson trichrome stain showing abundance of collagen fibers *(CF)* in the radicular pulp as compared with the coronal pulp.

tracellular milieu, thus releasing the procollagen. Here the terminal telopeptide is cleaved by a hydrolytic enzyme, and the tropocollagen molecules begin aggregating to form collagen fibrils. It is believed that aggregation of tropocollagen is somehow mediated by the GAGs. The conversion of soluble collagen into insoluble fibers occurs as a result of cross-linking of tropocollagen molecules.

In the young pulp, small collagen fibers stain black with silver impregnation stains and are thus referred to as *argyrophilic fibers* (Fig. 11-20). They are very similar, if not identical to, reticular fibers in other loose connective tissues in that they are not arranged in bundles and tend to form delicate networks. The presence of collagen fibers passing from the dentin matrix between odontoblasts into the dental pulp has been reported in fully erupted teeth.[9] Larger collagen fiber bundles are not argyrophilic but can be demonstrated with special histochemical methods such as the Masson trichrome stain or Mallory's triple connective tissue stain (Fig. 11-21). These fibers are much more numerous in the radicular pulp than in the coronal pulp. The highest concentration of these larger fiber bundles is usually found near the apex (Fig. 11-22). Thus Torneck[113] advised that during pulpectomy if the pulp is engaged with a barbed broach in the region of the apex, this generally affords the best opportunity to remove it intact.

INNERVATION

Pain is a complex phenomenon that involves not only sensory response but also emotional, conceptual, and motivational aspects of behavior. Nevertheless, it is the evoked potentials in the tooth that initiate signals to the brain, and therefore control of dental pain should be based on an understanding of the origin of these pain signals.

The sensory system of the pulp appears to be well suited for signaling potential damage to the tooth. The tooth is innervated by a large number of myelinated and unmyelinated nerve fibers. (The number of axons entering a human premolar may reach 2000 or more.)

Regardless of the nature of the sensory stimulus (i.e., thermal change, mechanical deformation, injury to the tissues), all afferent impulses from the pulp result in the sensation of pain. The innervation of the pulp includes both *afferent neurons,* which conduct sensory impulses, and *autonomic fibers,* which

Table 11-2. Classification of nerve fibers

Type of Fiber	Function	Diameter (μm)	Conduction Velocity (m/sec)
Aα	Motor, proprioception	12-20	70-120
Aβ	Pressure, touch	5-12	30-70
Aγ	Motor, to muscle spindles	3-6	15-30
Aδ	Pain, temperature, touch	1-5	6-30
B	Preganglionic autonomic	<3	3-15
C dorsal root	Pain	0.4-1.0	0.5-2.0
sympathetic	Postganglionic sympathetic	0.3-1.3	0.7-2.3

provide neurogenic modulation of the microcirculation and perhaps regulate dentinogenesis.

In addition to sensory nerves, sympathetic fibers from the superior cervical ganglion appear with blood vessels at the time the vascular system is established in the dental papilla. In the adult tooth sympathetic fibers form plexuses, usually around pulpal arterioles. Stimulation of these fibers results in constriction of the arterioles and a decrease in blood flow. Both adren-

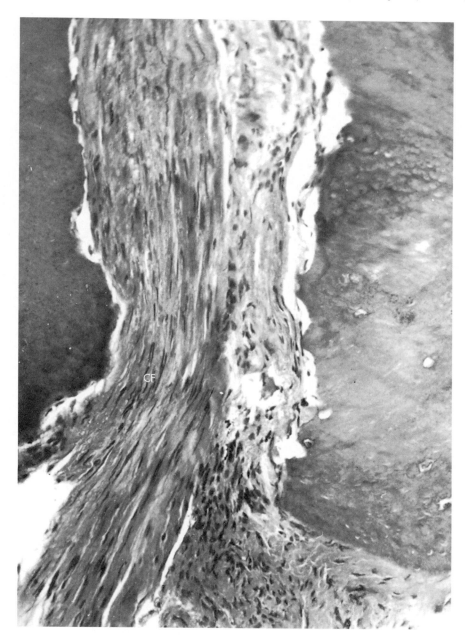

FIG. 11-22 Dense bundles of collagen fibers (CF) in the apical pulp.

Table 11-3. Characteristics of sensory fibers

Fiber	Myelination	Location of Terminals	Pain Characteristics	Stimulation Threshold
Aδ	Yes	Principally in region of pulp-dentin junction	Sharp, pricking	Relatively low
C	No	Probably distributed throughout pulp	Burning, aching, less bearable than Aδ fiber sensations	Relatively high, usually associated with tissue injury

ergic and cholinergic fibers have been found in close relation to odontoblasts.[51]

Nerve fibers are usually classified according to their diameter, conduction velocity, and function as shown in Table 11-2. In the pulp there are two types of sensory nerve fibers, *myelinated* (A fibers) and *unmyelinated* (C fibers).

The A fibers include both A beta (Aβ) and A delta (Aδ) fibers. The Aβ fibers may be slightly more sensitive to stimulation than the Aδ fibers, but functionally these fibers are grouped together. Approximately 90% of the A fibers are Aδ fibers. The principal characteristics of these fibers are summarized in Table 11-3.

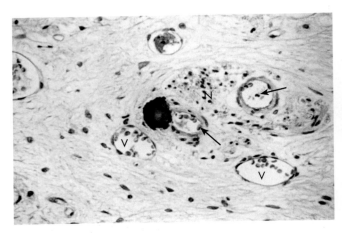

FIG. 11-23 Cross section of the apical pulp of a human premolar, demonstrating nerve fiber bundle *(N)*, arterioles *(arrows)*, and venules *(V)*. Note presence of a small pulp stone projecting outward from the wall of an arteriole.

During the bell stage of tooth development, "pioneer" nerve fibers enter the dental papilla following the path of blood vessels. Although only unmyelinated fibers are observed in the dental papilla, a proportion of these fibers are probably A fibers that have not yet become myelinated. Myelinated fibers are the last major structures to appear in the developing human dental pulp. The number of nerve fibers gradually increases, and some branching occurs as the fibers near the dentin; during the bell stage very few fibers enter the predentin.

The sensory nerves of the pulp arise from the trigeminal nerve and pass into the radicular pulp in bundles via the foramen in close association with arterioles and venules (Fig. 11-23). Each of the nerves entering the pulp is invested within a Schwann cell, and the A fibers acquire their myelin sheath from these cells. With the completion of root development the myelinated fibers appear grouped in bundles in the central region of the pulp (Fig. 11-24). Most of the unmyelinated C fibers entering the pulp are located within these fiber bundles; the remainder are situated toward the periphery of the pulp.[92]

Investigators[52] found that in the human premolar the number of unmyelinated axons entering the tooth at the apex reached a maximal number shortly after tooth eruption. At this stage they observed an average of 1800 unmyelinated axons and more than 400 myelinated axons, although in some teeth fewer than 100 myelinated axons were present. The number of A fibers gradually increased to more than 700 five years after eruption. *The relatively late appearance of A fibers in the pulp may help to explain why the electric pulp test tends to be unreliable in young teeth.*[35]

A quantitative study of nerve axons 1 to 2 mm above the root apex of fully developed human canine and incisor teeth has been conducted.[53] It reported a mean of 361 and 359 myelinated axons in canines and incisors, respectively. The number of unmyelinated axons was much greater, with means of 2240 for canines and 1591 for incisors. Thus approximately 80% of the nerves were unmyelinated fibers. However, some myelinated fibers may lose their sheaths before entering the

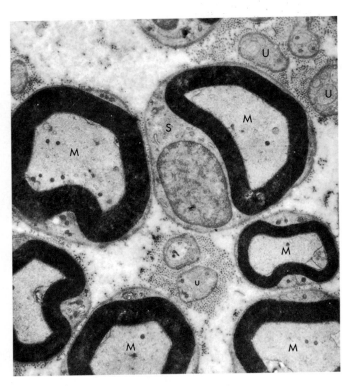

FIG. 11-24 Electron micrograph of the apical pulp of a young canine tooth, showing in cross section myelinated nerve axons *(M)* within Schwann cells *(S)*. Smaller, unmyelinated axons *(U)* are enclosed singly and in groups by Schwann cells. *(Courtesy Dr. David C. Johnsen, School of Dentistry, Case Western Reserve University.)*

apex or, in young teeth, they may not yet have acquired a sheath. Consequently, it has been difficult to accurately assess the true proportion of myelinated and unmyelinated fibers entering the pulp.

The nerve bundles pass upward through the radicular pulp together with blood vessels. Once they reach the coronal pulp, they fan out beneath the cell-rich zone, branch into smaller bundles, and finally ramify into a plexus of single-nerve axons known as the plexus of Raschkow (Fig. 11-25). Full development of this plexus does not occur until the final stages of root formation.[26] It as been estimated that each fiber entering the pulp sends at least eight branches to the plexus of Raschkow. There is prolific branching of the fibers in the plexus, producing a tremendous overlap of receptor fields.[43] It is in the plexus that the A fibers emerge from their myelin sheaths and, while still within Schwann cells, branch repeatedly to form the subodontoblastic plexus. Finally, terminal axons exit from their Schwann cell investiture and pass between the odontoblasts as free nerve endings (Figs. 11-26 and 11-27).

The extent to which dentin is innervated has been the subject of numerous investigations. With the exception of the intratubular fibers discussed above, dentin is devoid of sensory nerve fibers. This offers an explanation as to why pain-producing agents such as acetylcholine and potassium chloride do not elicit pain when applied to exposed dentin. Similarly,

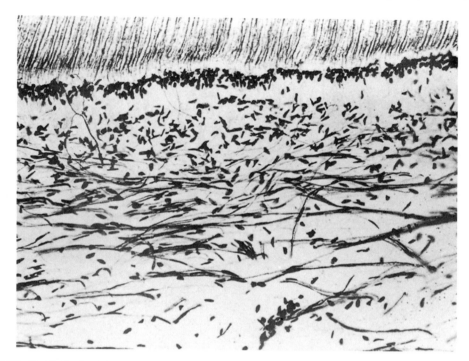

FIG. 11-25 Parietal layer of nerves (plexus of Raschkow) below the cell-rich zone. *(From Avery JK:* J Endod *7:205, 1981.)*

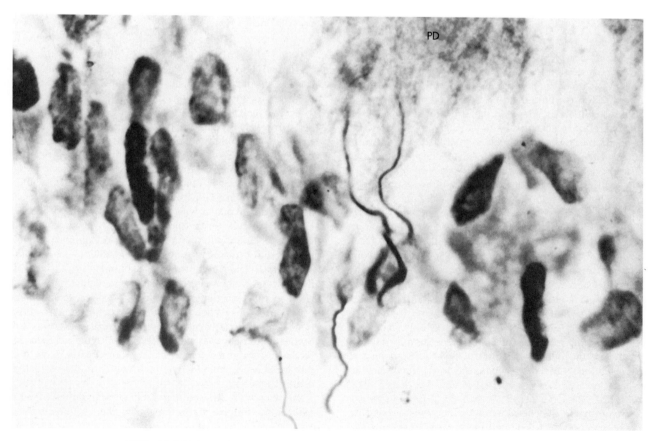

FIG. 11-26 Nerve fibers passing between odontoblasts to the predentin *(PD)*.

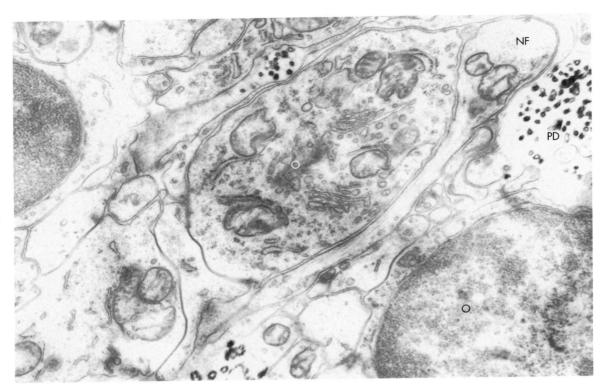

FIG. 11-27 Unmyelinated nerve fiber *(NF)* without a Schwann cell covering located between adjacent odontoblasts *(O)* overlying pulp horn of a mouse molar tooth. Predentin *(PD)* can be seen at upper right. Within the nerve there are longitudinally oriented fine neurofilaments, microvesicles, and mitochondria. *(From Corpron RE, Avery JK: Anat Rec 175:585, 1973.)*

application of topical anesthetic solutions to dentin does not decrease its sensitivity.

One investigator[39] studied the distribution and organization of nerve fibers in the pulp-dentin border zone of human teeth. On the basis of their location and pattern of branching, he described several types of nerve endings (Fig. 11-28). He found simple fibers that run from the subodontoblastic nerve plexus toward the odontoblast layer but do not reach the predentin. These fibers terminate in extracellular spaces in the cell-rich zone, the cell-poor zone, or the odontoblast layer. Other fibers extend into the predentin and run straight or spiral through a dentinal tubule in close association with an odontoblast process. Most of these intratubular fibers extend into the dentinal tubules for only a few μm, but a few may penetrate as far as 100 or so μm. The area covered by a single such terminal complex often reach thousands of square microns.

Intratubular nerve endings are most numerous in the area of the pulp horns where as many up to 40% of the tubules contain fibers.[68] The number of intratubular fibers decreases in other parts of the dentin, and in root dentin only about one tubule in a hundred contains a fiber. The anatomic relationships between the odontoblast processes and sensory nerve endings have led to much speculation as to the functional relationships between these structures, if any. The nerve fibers lie in a groove or gutter along the surface of the odontoblast process, and toward their terminal ends they twist around the process like a corkscrew. The cell membranes of the odontoblast process and the nerve fiber are closely approximated and run closely parallel for the length of their proximity but are not synaptically linked.[50]

Although it may be tempting to speculate that the odontoblasts and their associated nerve axons are functionally interrelated and that together they play a role in dentin sensitivity, evidence for this is lacking. If the odontoblast were acting as a receptor cell,* it would synapse with the adjacent nerve fiber. However, researchers have been unable to find synaptic junctions that could functionally couple odontoblasts and nerve fibers together. With regard to the membrane properties of odontoblasts, it has been reported that the membrane potential of the odontoblast is low (around −30 mV) and that the cell does not respond to electrical stimulation.[64,128] Thus it would appear that the odontoblast does not possess the properties of an excitable cell. Furthermore, the sensitivity of dentin is not diminished following disruption of the odontoblast layer.[13,69]

In addition to sensory nerves, sympathetic fibers from the superior cervical ganglion appear with blood vessels at the time the vascular system is established in the dental papilla. In the adult tooth sympathetic fibers form plexuses, usually around pulpal arterioles. When stimulated, these fibers cause constriction of the arterioles, resulting in a decrease in blood flow. Sympathetic fibers have also been found lying independent of blood vessels in the region of the odontoblasts. It is thought that these nerve endings may be involved in the regulation of dentin formation.

Another study showed that a reduction in pulpal blood flow induced by stimulation of sympathetic fibers leading to the pulp

---

*A receptor cell is a nonnerve cell capable of exciting adjacent afferent nerve fibers. Synaptic junctions connect receptor cells to afferent nerves.

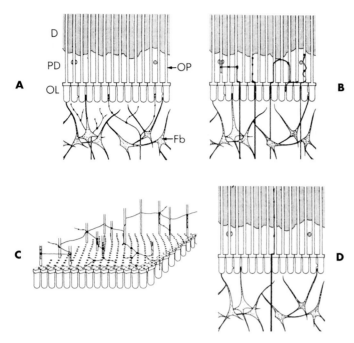

FIG. 11-28 Schematic drawing showing distribution of nerve fibers in the pulp-dentin border zone. **A,** Fibers running from the subodontoblastic plexus to the odontoblast layer. *D,* Dentin; *Fb,* fibroblast; *OL,* odontoblast layer; *OP,* odontoblast process; *PD,* predentin. **B,** Fibers extending into the dentinal tubules in the predentin. **C,** Complex fibers that branch extensively in the predentin. **D,** Intratubular fibers extending into the dentin. *(Courtesy T. Gunji, Niigata University, Japan.)*

results in depressed excitability of pulpal A fibers.[23] The excitability of C fibers is less affected than that of A fibers by a reduction in blood flow.[112]

Of considerable clinical interest is the evidence that nerve fibers of the pulp are relatively resistant to necrosis.[24,78] This is apparently due to the fact that nerve bundles in general are more resistant to autolysis than other tissue elements. Even in degenerating pulps, C fibers might still be able to respond to stimulation. Furthermore, it may be that C fibers remain excitable even after blood flow has been compromised in the diseased pulp, for C fibers are often able to function in the presence of hypoxia.[112] This may offer an explanation as to why instrumentation of the root canals of apparently nonvital teeth sometimes elicits pain.

Pulp Testing

The electric pulp tester delivers a current sufficient to overcome the resistance of enamel and dentin and stimulate the sensory A fibers at the pulp-dentin border zone. C fibers of the pulp do not respond to the conventional pulp tester because significantly more current is needed to stimulate them.[81] Bender et al.[5] found that in anterior teeth the optimal placement site of the electrode is the incisal edge of anterior teeth, as the response threshold is lowest at that location and increases as the electrode is moved toward the cervical region of the tooth.

Cold tests using carbon dioxide (CO_2) snow or liquid refrigerants and heat tests employing heated gutta-percha or hot water activate hydrodynamic forces within the dentinal tubules,

which in turn excite the intradental A fibers. C fibers are not activated by these tests unless they produce injury to the pulp. It has been shown that cold tests do not injure the pulp.[35] Heat tests have a greater potential to produce injury; but if the tests are used properly, injury is not likely.

Sensitivity of Dentin

The mechanisms underlying dentin sensitivity have been the subject of keen interest in recent years. How are stimuli relayed from the peripheral dentin to the sensory receptors located in the region of the pulp-dentin border zone? Converging evidence indicates that *movement of fluid in the dentinal tubules is the basic event in the arousal of pain.*[115] It now appears that pain-producing stimuli such as heat, cold, air blasts, and probing with the tip of an explorer have in common the ability to displace fluid in the tubules.[10] This is referred to as the hydrodynamic mechanism of dentin sensitivity. Thus fluid movement in the dentinal tubules is translated into electrical signals by sensory receptors located within the tubules or subjacent odontoblast layer. Researchers[75,123] were able to demonstrate a positive correlation between rate of fluid flow in the tubules and discharge evoked in intradental nerves. It was found that outward flow of fluid produced a much stronger nerve response than inward movement.

In experiments on humans, brief application of heat or cold to the outer surface of premolar teeth evoked a painful response before the heat or cold could have produced temperature changes capable of activating sensory receptors in the underlying pulp.[119] The evoked pain was of short duration, 1 or 2 seconds. The thermal diffusivity of dentin is relatively low; yet the response of the tooth to thermal stimulation is rapid, often less than a second. How best can this be explained? Evidence suggests that thermal stimulation of the tooth results in a rapid movement of fluid into the dentinal tubules. This results in activation of the sensory nerve terminal in the underlying pulp. Presumably heat expands the fluid within the tubules, causing it to flow toward the pulp, whereas cold causes the fluid to contract, producing an outward flow. The rapid movement of fluid across the cell membrane of the sensory receptor deforms the membrane and activates the receptor. All nerve cells have membrane channels through which charged ions pass, and this current flow, if great enough, can stimulate the cell and cause it to transmit impulses to the brain. Some channels are activated by voltage, some by chemicals, and some by mechanical pressure. In the case of pulpal nerve fibers that are activated by hydrodynamic forces, pressure would increase the flow of sodium and potassium ions through pressure-activated channels, thus initiating generator potentials.

The dentinal tubule is a capillary tube having an exceedingly small diameter.* Therefore the effects of capillarity are significant, as the narrower the bore of a capillary tube, the greater the effect of capillarity. Thus if fluid is removed from the outer end of exposed dentinal tubules by dehydrating the dentinal surface with an air blast or absorbent paper, capillary forces produce a rapid outward movement of fluid in the tubule (Fig. 11-29). According to Brännström[11] desiccation of dentin can theoretically cause dentinal fluid to flow outward at a rate of 2 to 3 mm/sec. In addition to air blasts, dehydrating solutions containing hy-

---

*To appreciate fully the dimensions of dentin tubules, understand that the diameter of the tubules is much smaller than that of red blood cells.

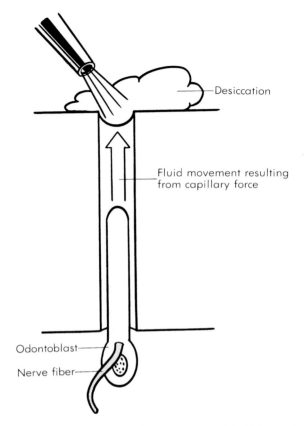

Desiccation

Fluid movement resulting
from capillary force

Odontoblast

Nerve fiber

FIG. 11-29 Diagram illustrating movement of fluid in the dentinal tubules resulting from the dehydrating effect of a blast of air from an air syringe.

perosmotic concentrations of sucrose or calcium chloride can produce pain if applied to exposed dentin.

Investigators have shown that it is the A fibers rather than the C fibers that are activated by stimuli such as heat, cold, and air blasts applied to exposed dentin.[83] However, if heat is applied long enough to increase the temperature of the pulp-dentin border several degrees Celsius, the C fibers may respond, particularly if the heat produces injury. It seems that the A fibers are only activated by a very rapid displacement of the tubular contents.[82] Slow heating of the tooth produced no response until the temperature reached 43.8°C, at which time C fibers were activated, presumably because of heat-induced injury to the pulp.

It has also been shown that pain-producing stimuli are more readily transmitted from the dentin surface when the exposed tubule apertures are wide and the fluid within the tubules is free to flow outward.[54] For example, other researchers found that acid treatment of exposed dentin to remove grinding debris opens the tubule orifices and makes the dentin more responsive to stimuli such as air blasts and probing.[47]

Perhaps the most difficult phenomenon to explain is pain associated with light probing of dentin. Even light pressure of an explorer tip can produce strong forces.* Presumably these forces mechanically compress the openings of the tubules and

cause sufficient displacement of fluid to excite the sensory receptors in the underlying pulp. Considering the density of the tubules in which hydrodynamic forces would be generated by probing, thousands of nerve endings would be simultaneously stimulated, thus producing a cumulative effect.

Another example of the effect of strong hydraulic forces that are created within the dentinal tubules is the phenomenon of odontoblast displacement. In this reaction the cells bodies of odontoblasts are displaced upward in the dentinal tubules, presumably by a rapid movement of fluid in the tubules produced when exposed dentin is desiccated, as with the use of an air syringe or cavity-drying agents (Fig. 11-30). Such displacement results in the loss of odontoblasts, since cells thus affected soon undergo autolysis and disappear from the tubules. (Displaced odontoblasts may eventually be replaced by cells that migrate from the cell-rich zone of the pulp, as discussed later.)

The hydrodynamic theory can also be applied to an understanding of the mechanism responsible for hypersensitive dentin. Hypersensitive dentin is associated with the exposure of dentin normally covered by cementum. The thin layer of cementum is frequently lost as gingival recession exposes cementum to the oral environment. Cementum is subsequently worn away by brushing, flossing, or the use of toothpicks. Once exposed, the dentin may respond to the same stimuli that any exposed dentin surface responds to (mechanical pressure, dehydrating agents, etc.). Although the dentin may at first be very sensitive, within a few weeks the sensitivity usually subsides. This desensitization is thought to occur as a result of gradual occlusion of the tubules by mineral deposits, thus reducing the hydrodynamic forces. Additionally, deposition of reparative dentin over the pulpal ends of the exposed tubules probably also reduces sensitivity.

Currently the treatment of hypersensitive teeth is directed toward reducing the functional diameter of the dentinal tubules so as to limit fluid movement. To accomplish this objective, there are several possible treatment modalities[116]: (1) formation of a smear layer on the sensitive dentin by burnishing the exposed root surface; (2) application of agents such as oxalate compounds that form insoluble precipitates within the tubules; (3) impregnation of the tubules with plastic resins; and (4) application of dentin bonding agents to seal off the tubules.

Neuropeptides

Of immense current interest is the presence of neuropeptides in sensory nerves. Pulpal nerve fibers contain neuropeptides such as calcitonin gene-related peptide (CGRP), substance P (SP), neuropeptide Y, neurokinin A, and vasoactive intestinal polypeptide (VIP).[71,87,124] In rat molars the largest group of intradental sensory fibers contains CGRP. Some of these fibers also contain other peptides such as SP and neurokinin A.[15] Release of these peptides can be triggered by such things as tissue injury, complement activation, antigen-antibody reactions, or antidromic stimulation of the inferior alveolar nerve. Once released, vasoactive peptides produce vascular changes that are similar to those evoked by histamine and bradykinin (i.e., vasodilation). In addition to their neurovascular properties, SP and CGRP contribute to hyperalgesia and promote wound healing.

It has been reported[75] that mechanical stimulation of dentin produces vasodilation within the pulp, presumably by causing the release of neuropeptides from intradental sensory fibers. Electrical stimulation of the tooth has a similar effect.[45]

---

*A force of 10 g (0.022 pound) applied to an explorer having a tip 0.002 inch in diameter would produce a pressure of 7000 psi on the dentin.

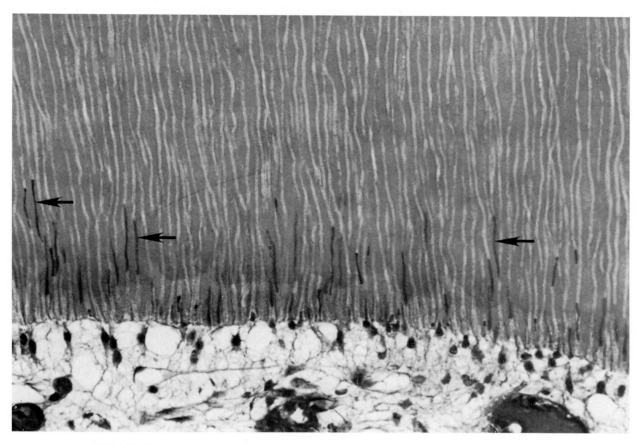

FIG. 11-30 Nuclei of odontoblasts *(arrows)* displaced upward into the dentinal tubules.

Plasticity of Intradental Nerve Fibers

Within the past few years it has become apparent that the innervation of normal rat molars is a dynamic complex in which the number, size, and cytochemistry of nerve fibers can change during aging and after tooth injury.[16,34] For example, nerve fibers sprout into inflamed tissue surrounding sites of pulpal injury, and the content of CGRP and SP increases in these sprouting fibers.[18] When inflammation subsides there is a decrease in the number of sprouts. Fig. 11-31 compares the normal distribution of CGRP-immunoreactive sensory fibers in an adult rat molar with those beneath a shallow cavity preparation. Regulation of such change appears to be a function of nerve growth factor (NGF). NGF receptors are found on intradental sensory fibers and Schwann cells. Evidence indicates that NGF is synthesized by fibroblasts in the coronal subodontoblastic zone (cell-rich zone), particularly in the tip of the pulp horn.[19] Maximal sprouting of CGRP- and SP-containing nerves fibers corresponds to areas of the pulp where there is increased production of NGF.

Hyperalgesia

Three characteristics of hyperalgesia are spontaneous pain, a decreased pain threshold, or an increased response to a painful stimulus. It is recognized that hyperalgesia can be produced by sustained inflammation, as in the case of sunburned skin. Clinically, it has been observed that the sensitivity of dentin is often increased when the underlying pulp becomes acutely inflamed, and the tooth may be more difficult to anesthetize. Although a precise explanation for this hyperalgesia is lacking,

apparently localized elevations in tissue pressure that accompany acute inflammation play an important role.[103] Clinically, we know that when a pulp chamber of a painful tooth with an abscessed pulp is opened, drainage of pus soon produces a reduction in the level of pain. This suggests that pressure may contribute to hyperalgesia.

In addition, certain mediators of inflammation such as bradykinin, 5-hydroxytryptamine (5-HT) and prostaglandin E_2 are capable of producing hyperalgesia. For example, 5-HT and CGRP are able to sensitize intradental fibers to hydrodynamic stimuli such as cold, air blasts, and osmotic stimulation.[84] Unmyelinated fibers are activated by a number of inflammatory mediators. Bradykinin, for example, produces a dull, aching pain when placed in a deep cavity in a human tooth.

Leukotriene B_4 (LTB_4) was shown to have a long-lasting sensitizing effect on intradental nerves, suggesting that it may potentiate nociceptor activity during pulpal inflammation.[72] Both LTB_4 and complement component C5a stimulate neutrophils to secrete a pain-producing leukotriene, 8(R),15(S)-diHETE.

Painful Pulpitis

From the foregoing it is apparent that pain associated with the simulation of the A fibers does not necessarily signify that the pulp is inflamed or that tissue injury has occurred. A fibers have a relatively low threshold of excitability, and painful pulpitis is more likely to be associated with nociceptive C fiber activity. The clinician should carefully examine symptomatic teeth to rule out the possibility of hypersensitive dentin, cracked fillings,

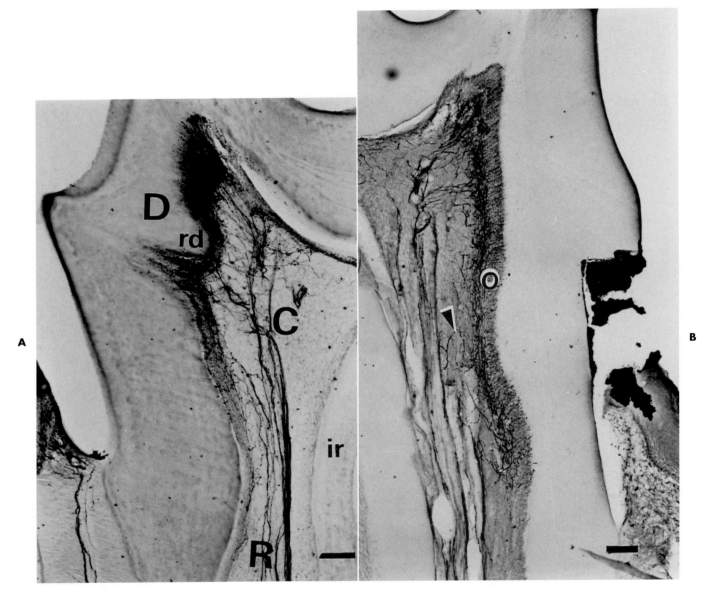

FIG. 11-31 A, Normal distribution of CGRP-immunoreactive sensory fibers in adult rat molar. Nerve fibers typically are unbranched in the root *(R)*, they avoid interradicular dentin *(ir)*, and form many branches in coronal pulp *(C)* and dentin *(D)*. Nerve distribution is often asymmetric, with endings concentrated near the most columnar odontoblasts, in this case on the left side of the crown. When reparative dentin *(rd)* forms, it alters conditions so that dentinal innervation is reduced. **B,** Shallow class I cavity preparation on the cervical root of a rat molar was made 4 days earlier. Primary odontoblast layer *(O)* survived, and many new calcitonin gene-related peptide (CGRP)–immunoreactive terminal branches spread beneath and into the injured pulp and dentin. Terminal arbor can be seen branching *(arrowhead)* from a larger axon and growing into the injury site. Scale bar: 0.1 mm. **A,** ×75; **B,** ×45. *(From Byers MR:* Arch Oral Biol *39(suppl):13S, 1994.)*

or tooth fracture, each of which may initiate hydrodynamic forces, before establishing a diagnosis of pulpitis.

Pain associated with an inflamed or degenerating pulp may be either provoked or spontaneous. The hyperalgesic pulp may respond to stimuli that usually do not evoke pain, or the pain may be exaggerated and persist longer. On the other hand, the tooth may commence to ache spontaneously in the absence of any external stimulus. There is not a satisfactory explanation

as to why a pulp that has been inflamed but asymptomatic for weeks or months suddenly begins to ache at 3 AM. Such unprovoked pain manifests itself as a dull, aching, poorly localized sensation qualitatively different from the brief, sharp, well-localized sensation associated with the hydrodynamic mechanism of dentin sensitivity.

Närhi[80] has done much to elucidate the role of hydrostatic pressure changes in the activation of pulpal nerve fibers. In his

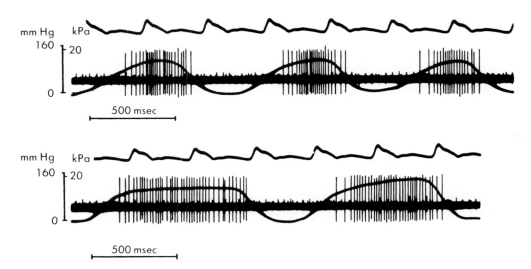

FIG. 11-32 Response of a single dog pulp nerve fiber to repeated hydrostatic pressure stimulation pulses. Lower solid wavy line of each recording indicates the stimulation pressure applied to the pulp. Upper line *(kPa)* is the femoral artery blood pressure curve recorded to indicate the relative changes in the pulse pressure and the heart cycle. *(From Närhi M:* Proc Finn Dent Soc *74[suppl 5]:1, 1978.)*

experiments involving cats and dogs both positive and negative pressure changes were introduced into the pulp by means of a cannula inserted into the dentin. Using single-fiber recording techniques, he found a positive correlation between the degree of pressure change and the number of nerve impulses leaving the pulp. He theorized that the pressure changes produced local deformities in the pulp tissue, resulting in a stretching of the sensory nerve fibers (Figs. 11-32 and 11-33).

VASCULAR SUPPLY

Blood from the dental artery enters the tooth via arterioles having diameters of 100 μm or less. These vessels pass through the apical foramen or foramina in company with nerve bundles (see Fig. 11-23). Smaller vessels may enter the pulp via lateral or accessory canals. The arterioles course up through the central portion of the radicular pulp and give off branches that spread laterally toward the odontoblast layer, beneath which they ramify to form a capillary plexus (Fig. 11-34). As the arterioles pass into the coronal pulp, they fan out toward the dentin, diminish in size, and give rise to a capillary network in the subodontoblastic region (Fig. 11-35). This network provides the odontoblasts with a rich source of metabolites.

Capillary blood flow in the coronal portion of the pulp is nearly twice that in the root portion.[60] Moreover, blood flow in the region of the pulp horns is greater than in other areas of the pulp.[76] In young teeth, capillaries commonly extend into the odontoblast layer, thus assuring an adequate supply of nutrients for the metabolically active odontoblasts (Fig. 11-36).

The subodontoblastic capillaries are surrounded by a basement membrane, and occasionally fenestrations (pores) are observed in capillary walls.[91] These fenestrations are thought to provide rapid transport of fluid and metabolites from the capillaries to the adjacent odontoblasts.

Blood passes from the capillary plexus first into postcapillary venules (Fig. 11-37) and then into larger venules. Venules in the pulp have unusually thin walls, which may facilitate the movement of fluid in or out of the vessel. The muscular coat

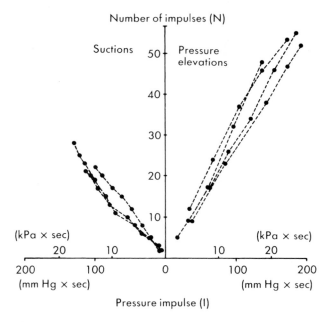

FIG. 11-33 Relationship between the number of nerve impulses *(N)* and the pressure impulse *(I)* of a small group of pulpal cat nerve fibers with three suction stimuli and four pressure elevations. Pressure impulse is labeled as both *mm Hg × sec* and *kPa × sec*. *(From Närhi M:* Proc Finn Dent Soc *74[suppl 5]:1, 1978.)*

of these venules is thin and discontinuous. The collecting venules become progressively larger as they course to the central region of the pulp. The largest venules have a diameter that may reach a maximum of 200 μm; thus they are considerably larger than the arterioles of the pulp. According to one study[63] the principal venous drainage in multirooted teeth sometimes flows down only one root canal or courses out

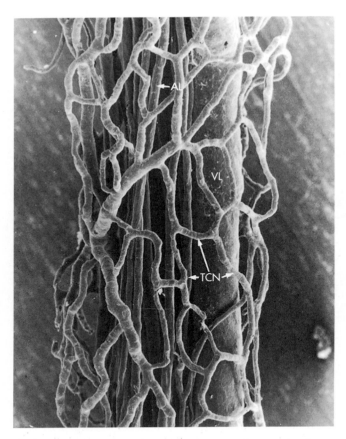

FIG. 11-34 High-power scanning electron micrograph of vascular network in the radicular pulp of a dog molar showing the configuration of the subodontoblastic terminal capillary network *(TCN)*. Venules *(VL)* and arterioles *(AL)* are indicated. *(Courtesy Dr. Y. Kishi, Kanagawa Dental College, Kanagawa, Japan.)*

through an accessory canal in the bifurcation or trifurcation area of the tooth.

Arteriovenous anastomoses (AVAs) may be present in both the coronal and radicular portions of the pulp, particularly in the latter.[104] Such vessels provide a direct communication between arterioles and venules, thus bypassing the capillary bed. The AVAs are relatively small venules, having a diameter of approximately 10 μm.[63] It is hypothesized that the AVAs play an important role in the regulation of the pulp circulation. Theoretically they could provide a mechanism for shunting blood away from areas of injury where damage to the microcirculation may result in thrombosis and hemorrhage.

It has been reported that the fraction of blood in the coronal pulp of cat canines is 14.4%.[122] The average capillary density was found to be 1404/mm², which is higher than in most other tissues of the body.

Among the oral tissues, the pulp has the highest volume of blood flow, but it is substantially lower than blood flow in the major visceral organs (Fig. 11-38). This reflects the fact that the respiratory rate of pulp cells is relatively low. As would be anticipated, pulpal blood flow is greater in the peripheral layer of the pulp (i.e., the subodontoblastic capillary plexus) than in the central area.[63]

Regulation of Pulpal Blood Flow

Several systems are involved in the regulation of pulpal blood flow, including sympathetic adrenergic vasoconstriction,[62] β-adrenergic vasodilation,[109] a sympathetic cholinergic vasoactive system,[1] and an antidromic vasodilation system involving sensory nerves, including axon reflex vasodilation.[95] It has been shown that a parasympathetic vasodilator mechanism is not present in cat dental pulp.[96] However, the presence of cholinergic nerve endings among odontoblasts in mouse and monkey pulps has been reported, along with the suggestion that these fibers may influence dentinogenesis.[3]

The walls of arterioles and venules are associated with smooth muscle that is innervated by unmyelinated sympathetic fibers. When stimulated, these fibers transmit impulses that cause the muscle fibers to contract, thus decreasing the diameter of the vessel (vasoconstriction). It has been shown experimentally that electrical stimulation of sympathetic fibers leading to the pulp results in a decrease in pulp blood flow.[23] Activation of α-adrenergic receptors by the administration of epinephrine-containing local anesthetic solutions may result in a marked decrease in pulpal blood flow.[59]

One investigation measured tissue and intravascular pressures in the pulps of cats.[111] The tissue pressure was estimated to be approximately 6 mm Hg. Pressure in the arterioles, capillaries, and venules was 43, 35, and 19 mm Hg, respectively (Fig. 11-39).

Blood circulation in an inflamed pulp involves very complex pathophysiologic reactions that have not been fully elucidated, in spite of numerous studies.[46,60] A unique feature of the pulp is that it is rigidly encased within dentin. This places it in a low-compliance environment, much like the brain, bone marrow, and nail bed. Thus pulp tissue has limited ability to expand, so vasodilation and increased vascular permeability evoked during an inflammatory reaction result in an increase in pulpal hydrostatic pressure.[121] Presumably any sudden rise in intrapulpal pressure would be distributed equally within the area of pressure increase, including the blood vessels. Theoretically if tissue pressure increases to the point that it equals the intravascular pressure, the thin-walled venules would be compressed, thereby increasing vascular resistance and reducing pulpal blood flow.[59] This could explain why injection of vasodilators such as bradykinin into an artery leading to the pulp results in a reduction rather than an increase in pulpal blood flow.[109,110] However, Heyeraas et al.[45] observed that an increase in intrapulpal tissue pressure promoted absorption of tissue fluid back into the blood and lymphatic vessels, thereby reducing the pressure. Thus it would appear that blood flow can increase, in spite of an elevation in tissue pressure. Obviously a combined multidisciplinary approach is needed to better understand the intricate circulatory changes occurring during the development of pulpal inflammation.

Using the laser Doppler technique to study pulpal blood flow in dogs, Sasano et al.[94] suggested that an increase or decrease in pulpal blood flow is more dependent on systemic blood pressure than on local vasoconstriction or vasodilation.

Lymphatics

The existence of lymphatics in the pulp has been a matter of debate, since it is not easy to distinguish between venules and lymphatics by ordinary light microscopic techniques. However, studies using light and electron microscopy

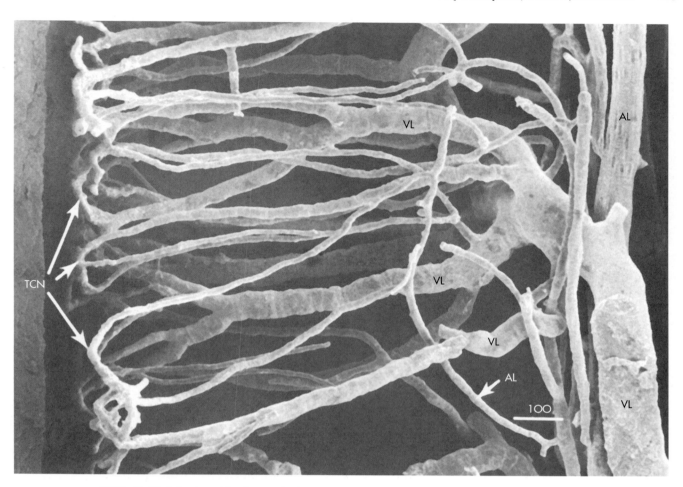

FIG. 11-35 Subodontoblastic terminal capillary network *(TCN)*, arterioles *(AL)*, and venules *(VL)* of young canine pulp. Dentin would be to the far left and the central pulp to the right. Scale bar: 100 μm. *(From Takahashi K et al:* J Endod *8:131, 1982.)*

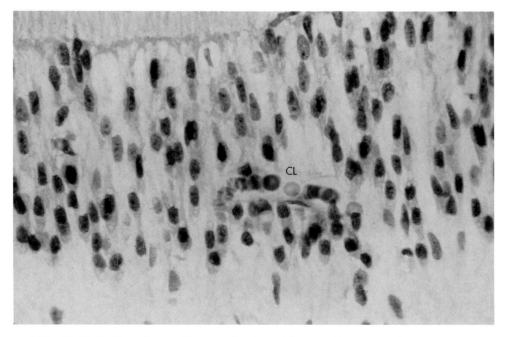

FIG. 11-36 Capillary loop *(CL)* extending into the odontoblast layer of a young pulp.

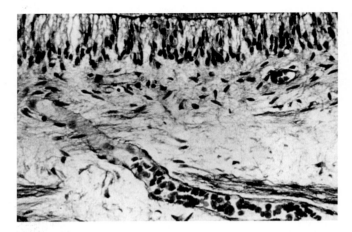

FIG. 11-37 Postcapillary venule draining blood from subodontoblastic capillary plexus.

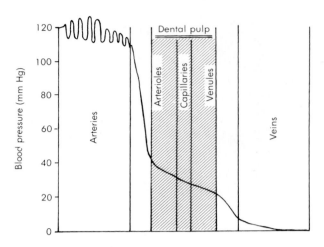

FIG. 11-39 Blood pressure fall along extrapulpal and intrapulpal blood vessels. *(Modified from Heyeraas KJ: J Dent Res 64(special issue):585, 1985.)*

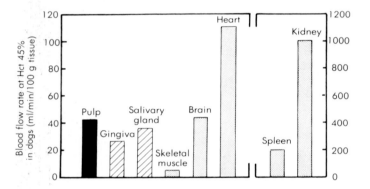

FIG. 11-38 Blood flow per 100 g tissue weight for various organs and tissues at 45% hematocrit *(Hct)* in dogs. *(From Kim S: J Endod 11:465, 1985.)*

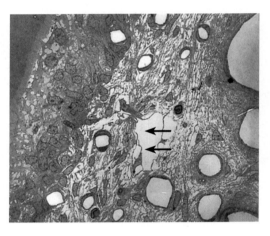

FIG. 11-40 Electron micrograph showing lymphatic vessel *(arrows)* in a cat dental pulp. *(From Bishop MA, Malhotra M: Am J Anat 187:247, 1990.)*

have described lymphatic capillaries in human and in cat dental pulps[8,74] (Fig. 11-40).

REPAIR

The inherent healing potential of the dental pulp is well recognized. As in all other connective tissues, repair of tissue injury commences with debridement by macrophages followed by proliferation of fibroblasts, capillary buds, and the formation of collagen. Local circulation is of critical importance in wound healing and repair. An adequate supply of blood is essential to transport inflammatory elements into the area of pulpal injury and to provide the young fibroblasts with nutrients from which to synthesize collagen. Unlike most tissues the pulp has essentially no collateral circulation; and for this reason it is theoretically more vulnerable than most other tissues. Thus in the case of severe injury, healing would be impaired in teeth with a limited blood supply. It seems reasonable to assume that the highly cellular pulp of a young tooth, with a wide-open apical foramen and rich blood supply, has a much better healing potential than does an older tooth with a narrow

foramen and a restricted blood supply. However, proof of this is lacking.

Dentin that is produced in response to the death of primary odontoblasts has been known by several different names:

Irregular secondary dentin

Irritation dentin

Tertiary dentin

Reparative dentin

The term most commonly applied to irregularly formed dentin is *reparative dentin,* presumably because it so frequently forms in response to injury and appears to be a component of the reparative process. It must be recognized, however, that this type of dentin has also been observed in the pulps of normal unerupted teeth without any obvious injury.[85]

It will be recalled that secondary dentin is deposited circumpulpally at a very slow rate throughout the life of the vital tooth. In contrast, the formation of reparative dentin occurs at the pulpal surface of primary or secondary dentin at sites corresponding to areas of irritation. For example, when a carious lesion has invaded dentin, the pulp usually responds by deposit-

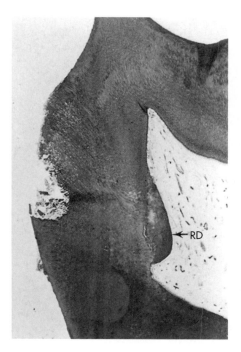

FIG. 11-41 Reparative dentin *(RD)* deposited in response to a carious lesion in the dentin. *(From Trowbridge HO: J Endod 7:52, 1981.)*

ing a layer of reparative dentin over the dentinal tubules of the primary or secondary dentin that communicate with the carious lesion (Fig. 11-41). Similarly when occlusal wear removes the overlying enamel and exposes the dentin to the oral environment, reparative dentin is deposited on the pulpal surface of the exposed dentin. In general, the amount of reparative dentin formed in response to caries or attrition of the tooth surface is proportional to the amount of primary dentin that is destroyed. Thus the formation of reparative dentin allows the pulp to retreat behind a barrier of mineralized tissue.

Compared to primary dentin, reparative dentin is less tubular and the tubules tend to be more irregular with larger lumina. In some cases no tubules are formed. The cells that form reparative dentin are not as columnar as the primary odontoblasts of the coronal pulp and are often cuboidal (Fig. 11-42). The quality of reparative dentin (i.e., the extent to which it resembles primary dentin) is quite variable. If irritation to the pulp is relatively mild, as in the case of a superficial carious lesion, the reparative dentin formed may resemble primary dentin in terms of tubularity and degree of mineralization. On the other hand, reparative dentin deposited in response to a deep carious lesion may be relatively atubular and poorly mineralized with many areas of interglobular dentin. The degree of irregularity of reparative dentin is probably determined by factors such as the amount of inflammation present, the extent of cellular injury, and the state of differentiation of the replacement odontoblasts.

The poorest quality of reparative dentin is usually observed in association with marked pulpal inflammation. In fact, the dentin may be so poorly organized that areas of soft tissue are entrapped within the dentinal matrix. In histologic sections these areas of soft tissue entrapment impart a Swiss cheese appearance to the dentin (Fig. 11-43). As the entrapped soft tis-

sue degenerates, products of tissue degeneration further contribute to the inflammatory stimuli assailing the pulp.

It has been reported[21] that trauma caused by cavity preparation that is too mild to result in the loss of primary odontoblasts does not lead to reparative dentin formation, even if the cavity preparation is relatively deep. This evidence would suggest that reparative dentin is formed by new odontoblast-like cells. For many years it has been recognized that destruction of primary odontoblasts is soon followed by increased mitotic activity within fibroblasts of the subjacent cell-rich zone. It has been shown that the progeny of these dividing cells differentiate into functioning odontoblasts.[32] Other investigators[130] have studied dentin bridge formation in the teeth of dogs and found that pulpal fibroblasts appeared to undergo dedifferentiation and revert to undifferentiated mesenchymal cells (Fig. 11-44). These cells divided, and the new cells then redifferentiated in a new direction to become odontoblasts. Recalling the migratory potential of ectomesenchymal cells from which the pulpal fibroblasts are derived, it is not difficult to envision the differentiating odontoblasts moving from the subodontoblastic zone to the area of injury to constitute a new odontoblast layer.

The similarity of primary odontoblasts to replacement odontoblasts was established by D'Souza et al.[22] These researchers were able to show that cells forming reparative dentin synthesize type I but not type III collagen and are immunopositive for dentin sialoprotein.

Baume[4] has suggested that the formation of atubular "fibrodentin" results in the secondary induction of odontoblast differentiation, provided a capillary plexus develops beneath the fibrodentin. This is consistent with the observation made by other researchers[132] that the newly formed dentin bridge is composed first of a thin layer of atubular dentin on which a relatively thick layer of tubular dentin is deposited. The fibrodentin* was lined by cells resembling mesenchymal cells, whereas the tubular dentin was associated with cells closely resembling odontoblasts.

Still other researchers[101] studied reparative dentin formed in response to relatively traumatic experimental class V cavity preparations in human teeth. They found that seldom was reparative dentin formed until about the 30th postoperative day, although in one case dentin formation was observed on day 19. The rate of formation was 3.5 μm/day for the first 3 weeks after the onset of dentin formation. Then it decreased markedly. By postoperative day 132, dentin formation had nearly ceased. Assuming that most of the odontoblasts were destroyed during cavity preparation, as was likely in this experiment, it is probably that the lag phase between cavity preparation and the onset of reparative dentin formation represented the time required for the proliferation and differentiation of new replacement odontoblasts.

Does reparative dentin protect the pulp, or is it simply a form of scar tissue? To serve a protective function, it would have to provide a relatively impermeable barrier that would exclude irritants from the pulp and compensate for the loss of developmental dentin. The junction between developmental and reparative dentin has been studied. Using a dye diffusion technique, Fish[27] noted the presence of an atubular zone situated between primary dentin and reparative dentin (Fig. 11-45).

---

*Actually, the term *osteodentin* was used rather than *fibrodentin*.

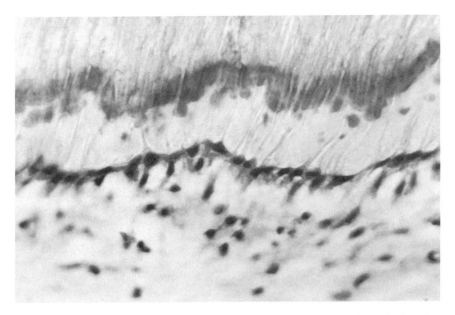

FIG. 11-42 Layer of cells forming reparative dentin. Note the decreased tubularity of reparative dentin as compared to the developmental dentin above.

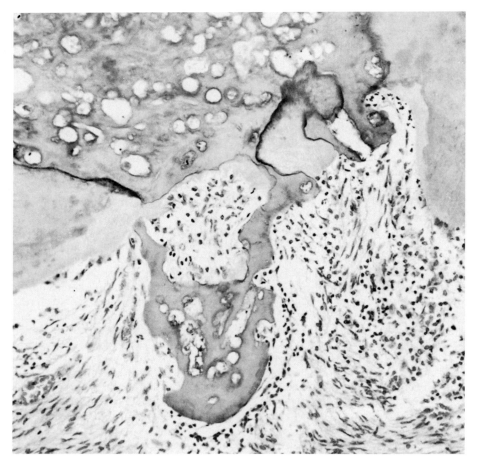

FIG. 11-43 Swiss cheese type of reparative dentin. Note the numerous areas of soft tissue inclusion and infiltration of inflammatory cells in the pulp.

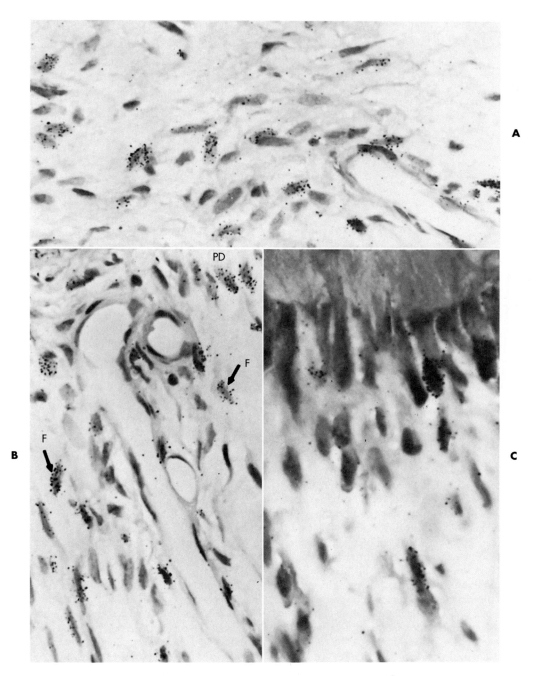

FIG. 11-44 Autoradiographs from dog molars illustrating uptake of ^{3}H-thymidine by pulp cells preparing to undergo cell division following pulpotomy and pulp capping with calcium hydroxide. **A,** Two days after pulp capping. Fibroblasts, endothelial cells, and pericytes beneath the exposure site are labeled. **B,** By the fourth day fibroblasts *(F)* and preodontoblasts adjacent to the predentin *(PD)* are labeled, which suggests that differentiation of preodontoblasts occurred within 2 days. **C,** Six days after pulp capping, new odontoblasts are labeled and tubular dentin is being formed. (Tritiated thymidine was injected 2 days after the pulp capping procedures in **B** and **C.**) *(From Yamamura T et al:* Bull Tokyo Dent Coll *21:181, 1980.)*

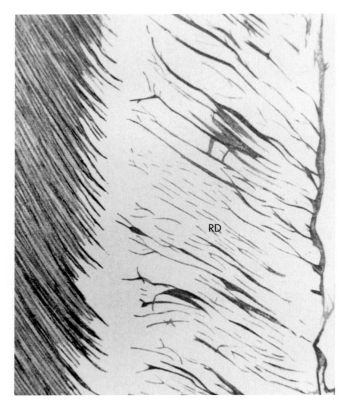

FIG. 11-45 Diffusion of dye from the pulp into reparative dentin. Note atubular zone between reparative dentin *(RD)* and primary dentin on the left. *(From Fish EW:* Experimental investigation of the enamel, dentin, and dental pulp, *London, 1932, John Bale Sons & Danielson, Ltd.)*

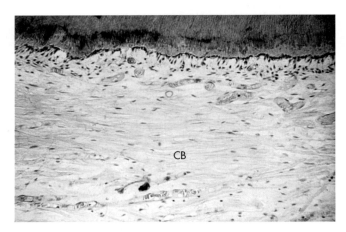

FIG. 11-46 Fibrosis of dental pulp showing replacement of pulp tissue by large bundles of collagen *(CB)*.

root planning frequently result in reparative dentin formation along the pulpal wall subjacent to the instrumented root surface.

Fibrosis

Not uncommonly the cellular elements of the pulp are largely replaced by fibrous connective tissue. It appears that in some cases the pulp responds to noxious stimuli by accumulating large fiber bundles of collagen rather than by elaborating reparative dentin (Fig. 11-46). However, fibrosis and reparative dentin formation often go hand in hand, indicating that both are expressions of a reparative potential.

PULPAL CALCIFICATIONS

Calcification of pulp tissue is a very common occurrence. Although estimates of the incidence of this phenomenon vary widely, it is safe to say that one or more pulp calcifications are present in at least 50% of all teeth. In the coronal pulp calcification usually takes the form of discreet, concentric pulp stones (Fig. 11-47), whereas in the radicular pulp calcification tends to be diffuse (Fig. 11-48). Some authors believe that pulp calcification is a pathologic process related to various forms of injury, whereas others regard it as a natural phenomenon. (Perhaps the greatest endodontic significance of pulp calcification is that it may hinder root canal shaping.)

Pulp stones range in size from small, microscopic particles to accretions that occupy almost the entire pulp chamber (Fig. 11-49). The mineral phase of pulp calcifications has been shown to consist of carbonated hydroxyapatite.[118] Histologically, two types of stones are recognized: (1) those that are round or ovoid with smooth surfaces and concentric laminations (see Fig. 11-47) and (2) those that assume no particular shape, lack laminations, and have rough surfaces (Fig. 11-50). Laminated stones appear to grow by the addition of collagen fibrils to their surface, whereas unlaminated stones develop via the mineralization of preformed collagen fiber bundles. In the latter type the mineralization front seems to extend out along the coarse fibers, making the surface of the stones appear fuzzy (Fig. 11-51). Often these course fiber bundles appear to have undergone hyalinization, thus resembling old scar tissue.

Pulp stones that form around epithelial cells (remnants of Hertwig's epithelial root sheath) are termed denticles. Presumably the epithelial remnants induce adjacent mesenchymal cells

Scott and Weber[97] found, in addition to a dramatic reduction in the number of tubules, that the walls of the tubules along the junction were thickened and often occluded with material similar to peritubular matrix. These observations would indicate that the junctional zone between developmental and reparative dentin is an atubular zone of low permeability.

One group[108] studied the effect of gold foil placement on human pulp and found that this was better tolerated in teeth in which reparative dentin had previously been deposited beneath the cavity than in teeth that were lacking such a deposit. It would thus appear that reparative dentin can protect the pulp, but it must be emphasized that this is not always the case. It is well known that reparative dentin can be deposited in a pulp that is irreversibly injured and that its presence does not necessarily signify a favorable prognosis (see Fig. 11-43). The quality of the dentin formed, and hence its ability to protect the pulp, to a large extent reflects the environment of the cells producing the matrix.

Periodontally diseased teeth have smaller root canal diameters than do teeth that are periodontally healthy.[66] The root canals of such teeth are narrowed by the deposition of large quantities of reparative dentin along the dentinal walls.[98] The decrease in root canal diameter with increasing age, in the absence of periodontal disease, is more likely to be the result of secondary dentin formation.

In one study,[44] it was shown in a rat model that scaling and

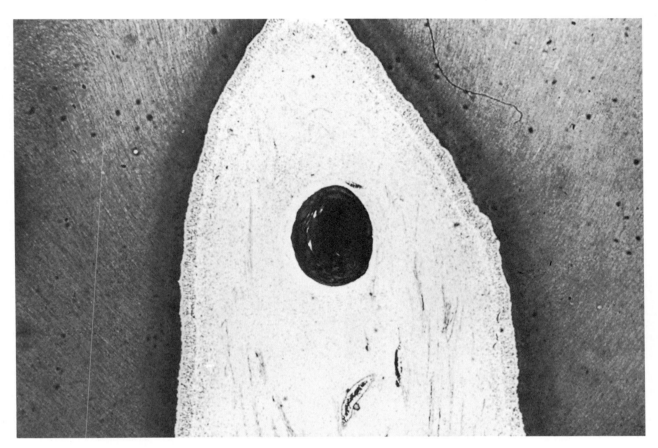

FIG. 11-47 Pulp stone with a smooth surface and concentric laminations in the pulp of a newly erupted premolar extracted in the course of orthodontic treatment.

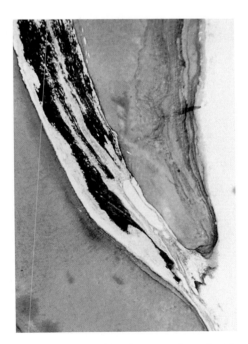

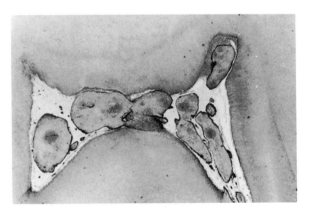

FIG. 11-49 Pulp stones occupying much of the pulp chamber.

FIG. 11-48 Diffuse calcification near the apical foramen.

to differentiate into odontoblasts. Characteristically these pulp stones are found near the root apex and contain dentinal tubules.

Quite frequently, small mineralizations are observed in association with the walls of arterioles, even in normal pulps of young teeth (see Fig. 11-23). Such deposits usually project outward from the vessel wall and do not encroach on the lumen. *The cause of pulpal calcification is largely unknown.*

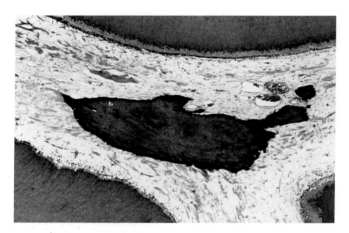

FIG. 11-50 Rough surface form of pulp stone. Note hyalinization of collagen fibers.

Calcification may occur around a nidus of degenerating cells, blood thrombi, or collagen fibers. Many authors believe this represents a form of dystrophic calcification. In this type calcium is deposited in tissues where degenerate, calcium phosphate crystals may be deposited within the cell, initially within the mitochondria, because of the increased membrane permeability to calcium that results from a failure to maintain active transport systems within the cell membranes. Thus degenerating cells serving as a nidus may initiate calcification of a tissue. In the absence of obvious tissue degeneration the cause of pulpal calcification is enigmatic. It is often difficult to assign the term *dystrophic calcification* to pulp stones, since they so often occur in apparently healthy pulps, suggesting that functional stress need not be present for calcification to occur. Calcification in the mature pulp is often assumed to be related to the aging process. However, in a study involving 52 impacted canines from patients between 11 and 76 years of age Nitzan et al.[85] found that concentric denticles demonstrated a constant incidence for all age groups, indicating no relation to aging. Diffuse calcifications, on the other hand, increased in incidence to age 25 years and thereafter remained constant in successive age groups.

At times, numerous concentric pulp stones are seen in all the teeth of a young individual with no apparent cause. In such cases the appearance of pulp stones may be ascribed to individual biologic characteristics (as with torus, cutaneous nevi, etc.).[85]

Although soft tissue collagen does not usually calcify, it is

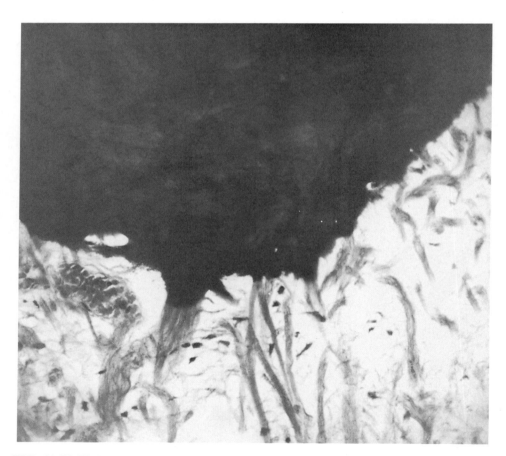

FIG. 11-51 High-power view of a pulp stone from Fig. 11-50 showing the relationship of mineralization fronts to collagen fibers.

not at all uncommon to find calcification occurring in old hyalinized scar tissue in the skin. This may be due to the increase in the extent of cross-linking between collagen molecules, since increased cross-linkage is thought to enhance the tendency for collagen fibers to calcify. There may thus be a relationship between pathologic alterations in collagen molecules within the pulp and pulpal calcification.

Calcification replaces the cellular components of the pulp and may possibly embarrass the blood supply, although concrete evidence for this is lacking. Pain has frequently been attributed to the presence of pulp stones; but because calcification so often occurs in pathologically involved pulps, it is difficult to establish a cause-and-effect relationship, particularly since pulp stones are so frequently observed in teeth lacking a history of pain.

Calcific Metamorphosis

Luxation of teeth as a result of trauma may result in calcific metamorphosis, a condition that can in a matter of months or years lead to partial or complete radiographic obliteration of the pulp chamber. The cause of radiographic obliteration is excessive deposition of mineralized tissue resembling cementum or occasionally bone on the dentin walls (Fig. 11-52). Histologic examination invariably reveals the presence of some soft tissue, and cells resembling cementoblasts can be observed lining the mineralized tissue.

Clinically, the crowns of teeth affected by calcific metamorphosis may show a yellowish hue as compared with adjacent normal teeth. This condition usually occurs in teeth with incomplete root formation. Trauma results in disruption of blood vessels entering the tooth, thus producing pulpal infarction. The wide periapical foramen allows connective tissue from the periodontal ligament to proliferate and replace the infarcted tissue, bringing with it cementoprogenitor and osteoprogenitor cells capable of differentiating into either cementoblasts or osteoblasts, or both.

AGE CHANGES

Continued formation of secondary dentin throughout life gradually reduces the size of the pulp chamber and root canals. In addition, certain regressive changes in the pulp appear to be related to the aging process. There is a gradual decrease in the cellularity as well as a concomitant increase in the number and thickness of collagen fibers, particularly in the radicular pulp. The thick collagen fibers may serve as foci for pulpal calcification (see Fig. 11-51). The odontoblasts decrease in size and number and may disappear altogether in certain areas of the pulp, particularly on the pulpal floor over the bifurcation or trifurcation areas of multirooted teeth.

With age there is a progressive reduction in the number of nerves and blood vessels.[6] There is also evidence that aging results in an increase in the resistance of pulp tissue to the action of proteolytic enzymes,[131] as well as hyaluronidase and sialidase,[7] suggesting an alteration of both collagen and proteoglycans in the pulps of older teeth.

The main changes in dentin associated with aging are an

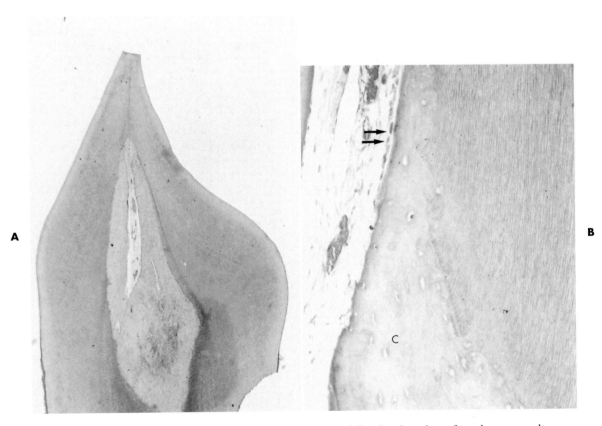

FIG. 11-52 A, Calcific metamorphosis of pulp tissue following luxation of tooth as a result of trauma. Note presence of soft tissue inclusion. **B,** High-power view showing cementoblasts *(arrows)* lining cementum *(C),* which has been deposited on the dentin walls.

increase in peritubular dentin, dentinal sclerosis, and the number of dead tracts.* Dentinal sclerosis produces a gradual decrease in dentinal permeability as the dentinal tubules become progressively reduced in diameter.

REFERENCES

1. Aars H, Brodin P, Anderson E: A study of cholinergic and β-adrenergic components in the regulation of blood flow in the tooth pulp and gingiva of man, *Acta Physiol Scand* 148:441, 1993.
2. Ahlberg K, Brännström M, Edwall L: The diameter and number of dentinal tubules in rat, cat, dog and monkey: a comparative scanning electronic microscopic study, *Acta Odontol Scand* 33:243, 1975.
3. Avery JK, Cox CF, Chiego DJ Jr: Presence and location of adrenergic nerve endings in the dental pulps of mouse molars, *Anat Rec* 198:59, 1980.
4. Baume LJ: The biology of pulp and dentine. In Myers HM, editor: *Monographs in oral science*, vol 8, Basel, 1980, S Karger AG.
5. Bender IB et al: The optimum placement-site of the electrode in electric pulp testing of the 12 anterior teeth, *J Am Dent Assoc* 118:305, 1989.
6. Bernick S, Nedelman C: Effect of aging on the human pulp, *J Endod* 1:88, 1975.
7. Bhussary BR: Modification of the dental pulp organ during development and aging. In Finn SB, editor: *Biology of the dental pulp organ: a symposium*, Birmingham, 1968, University of Alabama Press.
8. Bishop MA, Malhotra MP: A investigation of lymphatic vessels in the feline dental pulp, *Am J Anat* 187:247, 1990.
9. Bishop MA, Malhotra M, Yoshida S: Interodontoblastic collagen (von Korff fibers) and circumpulpal dentin formation: an ultrathin serial section study in the cat, *Am J Anat* 191:67, 1991.
10. Brännström M: The transmission and control of dentinal pain. In Grossman LJ, editor: *Mechanisms and control of pain*, New York, 1979, Masson Publishing USA.
11. Brännström M: *Dentin and pulp in restorative dentistry*, Nacka, Sweden, 1981, Dental Therapeutics AB.
12. Brännström M: Communication between the oral cavity and the dental pulp associated with restorative treatment, *Oper Dent* 9:57, 1984.
13. Brännström M, Åström A: A study of the mechanism of pain elicited from the dentin, *J Dent Res* 43:619, 1964.
14. Butler WT et al: Recent investigations on dentin specific proteins, *Proc Finn Dent Soc* 88(suppl 1):369, 1992.
15. Byers MR: Dynamic plasticity of dental sensory nerve structure and cytochemistry, *Arch Oral Biol* 39(suppl):13S, 1994.
16. Byers MR, Schatteman GC, Bothwell MA: Multiple functions for NGF-receptor in developing, aging and injured rat teeth are suggested by epithelial, mesenchymal and neural immunoreactivity, *Development* 109:461, 1990.
17. Byers MR, Sugaya A: Odontoblast process in dentin revealed by fluorescent Di-I, *J Histochem Cytochem* 43:159, 1995.
18. Byers MR, Taylor PE: Effect of sensory denervation on the response of rat molar pulp to exposure injury, *J Dent Res* 72:613, 1993.
19. Byers MR, Wheeler EF, Bothwell M: Altered expression of NGF and p75 NGF-receptor mRNA by fibroblasts of injured teeth precedes sensory nerve sprouting, *Growth Factors* 6:41, 1992.
20. Cuicchi B et al: Dentinal fluid dynamics in human teeth, in vivo, *J Endod* 21:191, 1995.
21. Diamond RD, Stanley HR, Swerdlow H: Reparative dentin formation resulting from cavity preparation, *J Prosthet Dent* 16:1127, 1966.
22. D'Souza RN et al: Characterization of cellular responses involved in reparative dentinogenesis in rat molars, *J Dent Res* 74:702, 1995.
23. Edwall L, Kindlová M: The effect of sympathetic nerve stimulation on the rate of disappearance of tracers from various oral tissues, *Acta Odontol Scand* 29:387, 1971.
24. England MC, Pellis EG, Michanowicz AE: Histopathologic study of the effect of pulpal disease upon nerve fibers of the human dental pulp, *Oral Surg* 38:783, 1974.
25. Engström C, Linde A, Persliden B: Acid hydrolases in the odontoblast-predentin region of dentinogenically active teeth, *Scand J Dent Res* 84:76, 1976.
26. Fearnhead RW: Innervation of dental tissues. In Miles AEW, editor: Structure and chemical organization of teeth, vol 1, New York, 1967, Academic Press.
27. Fish EW: *Experimental investigation of the enamel, dentin, and dental pulp*, London, 1932, John Bale Sons & Danielson, Ltd.
28. Fisher AK: Respiratory variations within the normal dental pulp, *J Dent Res* 46:24, 1967.
29. Fisher AK, Walters VE: Anaerobic glycolysis in bovine dental pulp, *J Dent Res* 47:717, 1968.
30. Fisher AK et al: Effects of dental drugs and materials on the rate of oxygen consumption in bovine dental pulp, *J Dent Res* 36:447, 1957.
31. Fisher AK et al: The influence of the stage of tooth development on the oxygen quotient of normal bovine dental pulp, *J Dent Res* 38:208, 1959.
32. Fitzgerald M, Chiego DJ, Heys DR: Autoradiographic analysis of odontoblast replacement following pulp exposure in primate teeth, *Arch Oral Biol* 35:707, 1990.
33. Fogel HM, Marshall FJ, Pashley DH: Effects of distance of the pulp and thickness on the hydraulic conductance of human radicular dentin, *J Dent Res* 67:1381, 1988.
34. Fried K: Changes in pulp nerves with aging, *Proc Finn Dental Soc* 88(suppl 1):517, 1992.
35. Fuss Z et al: Assessment of reliability of electrical and thermal pulp testing agents, *J Endod* 12:301, 1986.
36. Garberoglio R, Brännström M: Scanning electron microscopical investigation of human dentinal tubules, *Arch Oral Biol* 21:355, 1976.
37. Gotjamanos T: Cellular organization in the subodontoblastic zone of the dental pulp. II. Period and mode of development of the cell-rich layer in rat molar pulps, *Arch Oral Biol* 14:1011, 1969.
38. Grossman ES, Austin JC: Scanning electron microscope observations on the tubule content of freeze-fractured peripheral vervet monkey dentine *(Cercopithecus pygerythrus)*, *Arch Oral Biol* 28:279, 1983.
39. Gunji T: Morphological research on the sensitivity of dentin, *Arch Histol Jpn* 45:45, 1982.
40. Hahn C-L, Falkler WA Jr, Siegel MA: A study of T cells and B cells in pulpal pathosis, *J Endod* 15:20, 1989.
41. Hamersky PA, Weimer AD, Taintor JF: The effect of orthodontic force application on the pulpal tissue respiration rate in the human premolar, *Am J Orthod* 77:368, 1980.
42. Han SS: The fine structure of cells and intercellular substances of the dental pulp. In Finn SB, editor: *Biology of the dental pulp organ*, Birmingham, 1968, University of Alabama Press.
43. Harris R, Griffin CJ: Fine structure of nerve endings in the human dental pulp, *Arch Oral Biol* 13:773, 1968.
44. Hattler AB, Listgarten MA: Pulpal response to root planing in a rat model, *J Endod* 10:471, 1984.
45. Heyeraas KJ, Jacobsen EB, Fristad I: *Vascular and immunoreactive nerve fiber reactions in the pulp after stimulation and denervation: proceedings of the International Conference on Dentin/Pulp Complex*, Tokyo, 1996, Quintessence, pp 162-168.
46. Heyerass KJ, Kvinnsland I: Tissue pressure and blood flow in pulpal inflammation, *Proc Finn Dent Soc* 88(suppl 1):393, 1992.
47. Hirvonen T, Närhi M: The excitability of dog pulp nerves in relation to the condition of dentine surface, *J Endod* 10:294, 1984.
48. Holland GR: The extent of the odontoblast process in the cat, *J Anat* 121:133, 1976.
49. Holland GR: The odontoblast process: form and function, *J Dent Res* 64(special issue):499, 1985.

---

*The term *dead tract* refers to a group of dentinal tubules in which odontoblast processes are absent. Dead tracts are easily recognized in ground sections, since the empty tubules refract transmitted light and the tract appears black in contrast to the light color of normal dentin.

50. Holland GR: Morphological features of dentine and pulp related to dentine sensitivity, *Arch Oral Biol* 39(suppl):3S, 1994.

51. Inoue H, Kurosaka Y, Abe K: Autonomic nerve endings in the odontoblast/predentin border and predentin of the canine teeth of dogs, *J Endod* 18:149, 1992.

52. Johnsen DC, Harshbarger J, Rymer HD: Quantitative assessment of neural development in human premolars, *Anat Rec* 205:421, 1983.

53. Johnsen D, Johns S: Quantitation of nerve fibers in the primary and permanent canine and incisor teeth in man, *Arch Oral Biol* 23:825, 1978.

54. Johnson G, Brännström M: The sensitivity of dentin: changes in relation to conditions at exposed tubule apertures, *Acta Odontol Scand* 32:29, 1974.

55. Jones PA, Taintor JF, Adams AB: Comparative dental material cytotoxicity measured by depression of rat incisor pulp respiration, *J Endod* 5:48, 1979.

56. Jontell M, Bergenholtz G: Accessory cells in the immune defense of the dental pulp, *Proc Finn Dent Soc* 88(suppl 1):345, 1992.

57. Kaye H, Herold RC: Structure of human dentine. I. Phase contrast, polarization, interference, and bright field microscopic observations on the lateral branch system, *Arch Oral Biol* 11:355, 1966.

58. Kelley KW, Bergenholtz G, Cox CF: The extent of the odontoblast process in rhesus monkeys *(Macaca mulatta)* as observed by scanning electron microscopy, *Arch Oral Biol* 26:893, 1981.

59. Kim S: Neurovascular interactions in the dental pulp in health and inflammation, *J Endod* 14:48, 1990.

60. Kim S, Schuessler G, Chien S: Measurement of blood flow in the dental pulp of dogs with the ^{133}xenon washout method, *Arch Oral Biol* 28:501, 1983.

61. Kim S et al: Effects of local anesthetics on pulpal blood flow in dogs, *J Dent Res* 63:650, 1984.

62. Kim S et al: Effects of selected inflammatory mediators in blood flow and vascular permeability in the dental pulp, *Proc Finn Dent Soc* 88(suppl 1):387, 1992.

63. Kramer IRH: The distribution of blood vessels in the human dental pulp. In Finn SB, editor: *Biology of the dental pulp organ*, Birmingham, 1968, University of Alabama Press.

64. Kroeger DC, Gonzales F, Krivoy W: Transmembrane potentials of cultured mouse dental pulp cells, *Proc Soc Exptl Med* 108:134, 1961.

65. Langeland K, Langeland LK: Histologic study of 155 impacted teeth, *Odontol Tidskr* 73:527, 1965.

66. Lantelme RL, Handleman SL, Herbison RJ: Dentin formation in periodontally diseased teeth, *J Dent Res* 55:48, 1976.

67. Lesot H, Osman M, Ruch JV: Immunofluorescent localization of collagens, fibronectin and laminin during terminal differentiation of odontoblasts, *Dev Biol* 82:371, 1981.

68. Lilja J: Innervation of different parts of the predentin and dentin in a young human premolar, *Acta Odontol Scand* 37:339, 1979.

69. Lilja J, Noredenvall K-J, Brännström M: Dentin sensitivity, odontoblasts and nerves under desiccated or infected experimental cavities, *Swed Dent J* 6:93, 1982.

70. Linde A: The extracellular matrix of the dental pulp and dentin, *J Dent Res* 64(special issue):523, 1985.

71. Luthman J, Luthman D, Hökfelt T: Occurrence and distribution of different neurochemical markers in the human dental pulp, *Arch Oral Biol* 37:193-208, 1992.

72. Madison S et al: Effect of leukotriene B$_4$ on intradental nerves, *J Dent Res* 68(special issue)243:494, 1989.

73. Mangkornkarn C, Steiner JC: In vivo and in vitro glycosaminoglycans from human dental pulp, *J Endod* 18:327, 1992.

74. Marchetti C, Piacentini C: Examin au microscope photonique et au microscope electronique des capilaries lymphatiques de al pulpe dentaire humaine, *Bulletin du Groupement International Pour la Récherche Scientifque en Stomatologie et Odontologie* 33:19, 1990.

75. Matthews et al: *The functional properties of intradental nerves: proceedings of the International Conference on Dentin/Pulp Complex*, Tokyo, 1996, Quintessence pp 146-153.

76. Meyer MW, Path MG: Blood flow in the dental pulp of dogs determined by hydrogen polarography and radioactive microsphere methods, *Arch Oral Biol* 24:601, 1979.

77. Michelich V, Pashley DH, Whitford GM: Dentin permeability: a comparison of functional versus anatomical tubular radii, *J Dent Res* 57:1019, 1978.

78. Mullaney TP, Howell RM, Petrich JD: Resistance of nerve fibers to pulpal necrosis, *Oral Surg* 30:690, 1970.

79. Nagaoka S et al: Bacterial invasion into dentinal tubules of human vital and nonvital teeth, *J Endod* 21:70, 1995.

80. Närhi M: Activation of dental pulp nerves of the cat and the dog with hydrostatic pressure, *Proc Finn Dent Soc* 74(suppl 5):1, 1978.

81. Närhi M et al: Electrical stimulation of teeth with a pulp tester in the cat, *Scand J Dent Res* 87:32, 1979.

82. Närhi M et al: Activation of heat-sensitive nerve fibers in the dental pulp of the cat, *Pain* 14:317, 1982.

83. Närhi M et al: Role of intradental A- and C-type nerve fibers in dental pain mechanisms, *Proc Finn Dent Soc* 88(suppl 1):507, 1992.

84. Ngassapa D, Närhi M, Hirvonen T: The effect of serotonin (5-HT) and calcitonin gene-related peptide (CGRP) on the function of intradental nerves in the dog, *Proc Fin Dent Soc* 88(suppl 1):143, 1992.

85. Nitzan DW et al: The effect of aging on tooth morphology: a study on impacted teeth, *Oral Surg* 61:54, 1986.

86. Okiji T et al: An immunohistochemical study of the distribution of immunocompetent cells, especially macrophages and Ia antigen-presenting cells of heterogeneous populations, in normal rat molar pulp, *J Dent Res* 71:1196, 1992.

87. Olgart L et al: Release of substance P–like immunoreactivity from the dental pulp, *Acta Physiol Scand* 101:510, 1977.

88. Pashley DH: Dentin permeability: theory and practice. In Spangberg L, editor: *Experimental endodontics,* Boca Raton, Fla, 1989, CRC Press.

89. Pashley DH: Dentin permeability and dentin sensitivity, *Proc Finn Dent Soc* 88(suppl 1):31-38, 1992.

90. Pashley DH: Dentin conditions and disease. In Lazzari G, editor: *CRC handbook of experimental dentistry,* Boca Raton, Fla, 1993, CRC Press.

91. Rapp R et al: Ultrastructure of fenestrated capillaries in human dental pulps, *Arch Oral Biol* 22:317, 1977.

92. Reader A, Foreman DW: An ultrastructural qualitative investigation of human intradental innervation, *J Endod* 7:161, 1981.

93. Sasaki S: Studies on the respiration of the dog tooth germ, *J Biochem* 46:269, 1959.

94. Sasano T, Kuriwada S, Sanjo D: Arterial blood pressure regulation of pulpal blood flow as determined by laser Doppler, *J Dent Res* 68:791, 1989.

95. Sasano T et al: Axon reflex vasodilatation in cat dental pulp elicited by noxious stimulation of the gingiva, *J Dent Res* 73:1797, 1994.

96. Sasano T et al: Absence of parasympathetic vasodilatation in cat dental pulp, *J Dent Res* 74:1665, 1995.

97. Scott JN, Weber DF: Microscopy of the junctional region between human coronal primary and secondary dentin, *J Morphol* 154:133, 1977.

98. Seltzer S, Bender IB, Ziontz M: The interrelationship of pulp and periodontal disease, *Oral Surg* 16:1474, 1963.

99. Sigal MJ et al: A combined scanning electron microscopy and immunofluorescence study demonstrating that the odontoblast process extends to the dentinoenamel junction in human teeth, *Anat Rec* 210:453, 1984.

100. Sigal MJ et al: The odontoblast process extends to the dentinoenamel junction: an immunocytochemical study of rat dentine, *J Histochem Cytochem* 32:872, 1984.

101. Stanley HR, White CL, McCray L: The rate of tertiary (reparative) dentin formation in the human tooth, *Oral Surg* 21:180, 1966.

102. Stanley HR et al: The detection and prevalence of reactive and physiologic sclerotic dentin, reparative dentin and dead tracts beneath various types of dental lesions according to tooth surface and age, *J Oral Pathol* 12:257, 1983.

103. Stenvik A, Iverson J, Mjör IA: Tissue pressure and histology of normal and inflamed tooth pulps in Macaque monkeys, *Arch Oral Biol* 17:1501, 1972.

104. Takahashi K, Kishi Y, Kim S: A scanning electron microscope study of the blood vessels of dog pulp using corrosion resin casts, *J Endod* 8:131, 1982.

105. Thesleff I, Vaahtokari A: The role of growth factors in determination and differentiation of the odontoblast cell lineage, *Proc Finn Dent Soc* 88(suppl 1):357, 1992.

106. Thomas HF: The extent of the odontoblast process in human dentin, *J Dent Res* 58(D):2207, 1979.

107. Thomas HF, Payne RC: The ultrastructure of dentinal tubules from erupted human premolar teeth, *J Dent Res* 62:532, 1983.

108. Thomas JJ, Stanley HR, Gilmore HW: Effects of gold foil condensation on human dental pulp, *J Am Dent Assoc* 78:788, 1969.

109. Tönder KJH: Effect of vasodilating drugs on external carotid and pulpal blood flow in dogs: "stealing" of dental perfusion pressure, *Acta Physiol Scand* 97:75, 1976.

110. Tönder KJH, Naess G: Nervous control of blood flow in the dental pulp in dogs, *Acta Physiol Scand* 104:13, 1978.

111. Topham RT et al: Effects of epidermal growth factor on tooth differentiation and eruption. In Davidovitch Z, editor: *The biological mechanisms of tooth eruption and root resorption,* Birmingham, Ala, 1988, Ebsco Media.

112. Torebjörk HE, Hanin RG: Perceptual changes accompanying controlled preferential blocking of A and C fiber responses in intact human skin nerves, *Exp Brain Res* 16:321, 1973.

113. Torneck CD: Dentin-pulp complex. In Ten Cate AR, editor: *Oral histology: development, structure, and function,* ed 4, St Louis, 1994, Mosby.

114. Trowbridge HO: Pathogenesis of pulpitis resulting from dental caries, *J Endod* 7:52, 1981.

115. Trowbridge HO: Intradental sensory units: physiological and clinical aspects, *J Endod* 11:489, 1985.

116. Trowbridge HO: Review of current approaches to in-office management of tooth hypersensitivity, *Dent Clin North Am* 34:561, 1990.

117. Trowbridge HO, Shibata F: Mitotic activity in epithelial rests of Malassez, *Periodontics* 5:109, 1967.

118. Trowbridge HO, Stewart JCB, Shapiro IM: *Assessment of indurated, diffusely calcified human dental pulps: proceedings of the International Conference on Dentin/Pulp Complex,* Tokyo, 1996, Quintessence pp 297-300.

119. Trowbridge HO et al: Sensory response to thermal stimulation in human teeth, *J Endod* 6:6405, 1980.

120. Turner DF: Immediate physiological response of odontoblasts, *Proc Finn Dent Soc* 88(suppl 1):55, 1992.

121. van Hassel HJ: Physiology of the human dental pulp, *Oral Surg* 32:126, 1971.

122. Vongsavan N, Matthews B: The vascularity of dental pulp in cats, *J Dent Res* 71:1913, 1992.

123. Vongsavan N, Matthews B: The relation between fluid flow through dentine and the discharge of intradental nerves, *Arch Oral Biol* 39(suppl):140S, 1994.

124. Wakisaka S: Neuropeptides in the dental pulp: their distribution, origins and correlation, *J Endod* 16:67, 1990.

125. Weber DF: Human dentine sclerosis: a microradiographic study, *Arch Oral Biol* 19:163, 1974.

126. Weinstock A, Weinstock M, Leblond CP: Autoradiographic detection of ^{3}H-fucose incorporation into glycoprotein by odontoblasts and its deposition at the site of the calcification front in dentin, *Calcif Tiss Res* 8:181, 1972.

127. Weinstock M, Leblond CP: Synthesis, migration and release of precursor collagen by odontoblasts as visualized by radioautography after ^{3}H-proline administration, *J Cell Biol* 60:92, 1974.

128. Winter HF, Bishop JG, Dorman HL: Transmembrane potentials of odontoblasts, *J Dent Res* 42:594, 1963.

129. Yamada T et al: The extent of the odontoblast process in normal and carious human dentin, *J Dent Res* 62:798, 1983.

130. Yamamura T: Differentiation of pulpal wound healing, *J Dent Res* 64(special issue):530, 1985.

131. Zerlotti E: Histochemical study of the connective tissue of the dental pulp, *Arch Oral Biol* 9:149, 1964.

Chapter 12

Periapical Pathology

James H.S. Simon

The inflammatory response associated with periapical pathology has been traditionally taught similar to an inflammatory response anywhere in the body. For example, when a splinter (irritant or antigen) is lodged in the skin, there is an immediate acute inflammatory response. If the splinter is not removed, chronic inflammatory cells infiltrate the site and fibroblasts isolate and wall off the reaction with a fibrous capsule. However, if the irritant is removed, healing either by repair or regeneration occurs. This has been assumed to occur also with a periapical lesion. Once bacteria and their products reach the apical area, they encounter polymorphonuclear neutrophil leukocytes (PMNs) and macrophages. If this process is allowed to continue, chronic inflammatory cells, lymphocytes, plasma cells, and fibroblasts wall off the irritating agents. If the irritant is removed (i.e., the canal is cleaned, shaped, and filled), healing should occur similar to healing after the splinter is removed. The process, however, is not this simple.

Historically, when x-ray films first began to reveal dark areas at the apexes of teeth, wholesale extraction of these "bags of infection" was recommended. This was the beginning of the focal infection era. In an early attempt to disprove the focal infection theory, Fish[13] implanted viable bacteria in the jaws of guinea pigs. He took a culture of *Staphylococcus aureus* on cotton wool and placed it in a hole drilled into the mandible. The guinea pigs were killed from 4 to 40 days later. Histologic results showed that the infection remained localized regardless of the virulence of the organism or its invasive capacity. The bacteria were confined by PMNs to the *zone of infection*. The next area, the *zone of contamination* contained chronic round cells but no bacteria. Surrounding this zone was the *zone of irritation* with histiocytes as the predominant cell in addition to osteoclasts. Finally, there was the *zone of stimulation* with mostly fibroblasts, capillary buds, and osteoblasts. This confirmed his view that despite the abnormal x-ray appearance of the periapical lesion and the heavy round cell infiltration, bacteria could not be shown histologically beyond the *zone of infection*. This experiment has been used to describe periapical lesions of teeth. The lucency is caused by the body's response to bacteria and their products located within the canal. It was felt that bacteria only leaked past the apical foramen in an acute alveolar abscess, where the body is temporarily overwhelmed by the bacteria. Fish's study was duplicated with a strain of *S. aureus*. Osteomyelitis occurring up to 21 days after inoculation was shown histologically. Viable bacteria were found well beyond what Fish would have considered to be the *zone of infection*.

Until the mid-1970s it was believed that endodontic pathology was caused mostly by aerobic staphylococci and streptococci. However, with the advent of practical methods for anaerobic culturing, it became apparent that endodontic disease begins as polymicrobial infections dominated by anaerobic species.[35] Kantz and Henry[20] introduced a new technique for anaerobic culturing that allowed for the identification of anaerobes in the pulpal and periapical tissues. Also Sundquist[16,41] was the first to correlate symptoms (pain and suppuration) with the specific bacteria black-pigmented *Bacteroides*. Nair[32] believes that periapical lesions are infected only when they are acute and causing symptoms. Periapical bacteria have also been shown to penetrate cementum.[21] This body of research clearly implicates bacteria as the culprit in the disease process.

ARE PERIAPICAL LESIONS INFECTED?

Whether periapical lesions are infected has been a controversial question over the years. Other than the acute alveolar abscess, *histologic* studies in general have not been able to demonstrate viable bacteria in periapical lesions.[7,17,25,34,52] These findings persist up to the present time.[51] However, a body of evidence is now forming that indicates many of these lesions may indeed be infected before and after endodontic treatment. In a recent study Iwu et al.[18] showed 88% or 14 of 16 periapical granulomas were positive for bacteria when they were homogenized and *cultured*. Wayman et al.[53] studied 58 cases of periapical lesions. They cut these lesions in half and examined one half histologically and cultured the other half. In only 8 of 58 could they *histologically* demonstrate bacteria. However, when the other half of the lesion was *cultured,* 51 of 58 results were positive. They found 133 isolates, of which 87 were strict anaerobes, 37 were facultative anaerobes, and only 9 were aerobes. The bacteria[3] were found not only in periapical abscesses but also in granulomas and cysts.

With the demonstration of bacteria in periapical lesions it is not surprising to find reported cases of failure of nonsurgical endodontic therapy because of the persistence of bacteria. Researchers[1,2,15,39,49,50] demonstrated the presence of live bacteria past the apexes of endodontically treated teeth. Happonen[15] found, in 16 cases verified immunocytochemically, 13 had *Actinomyces israelii,* 10 had *Arachnia propionica,* 6 had *Actinomyces naeslundii,* and 9 had multiple bacteria. Therefore it is apparent that the bacteria can leak past the apex of a tooth and may *survive* in the periapical tissues in spite of good nonsurgical endodontic therapy (Figs. 12-1, 12-2, and 12-3).

At one time it was considered better to have these irritants outside the tooth, where the blood supply is richer and the body's own defense mechanism can neutralize the antigenic material. With the persistence of a periapical lesion after conventional endodontic therapy, it becomes apparent that the body's own defense mechanism may not always be capable of healing these lesions. Since the etiologic agent is now outside

Text continued on p. 434

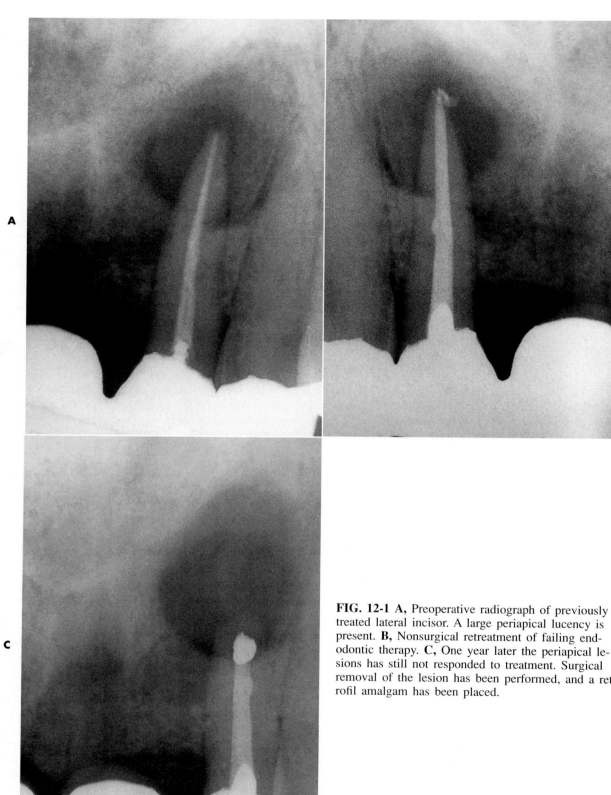

FIG. 12-1 A, Preoperative radiograph of previously treated lateral incisor. A large periapical lucency is present. **B,** Nonsurgical retreatment of failing endodontic therapy. **C,** One year later the periapical lesions has still not responded to treatment. Surgical removal of the lesion has been performed, and a retrofil amalgam has been placed.

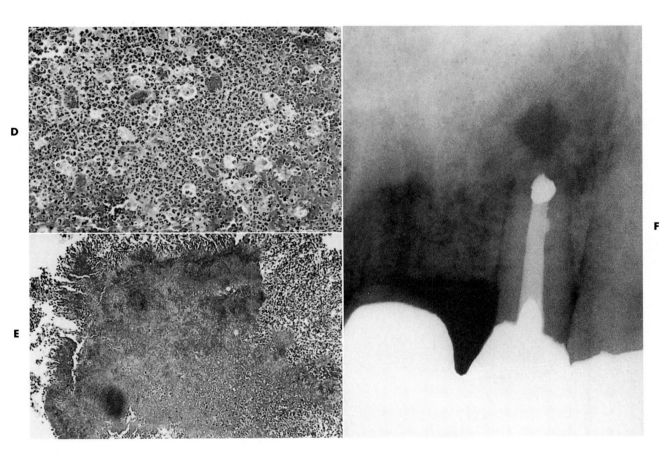

FIG. 12-1, cont'd D, Histologic section of lesion showing polymorphonuclear neutrophil leukocytes (PMNs) and microphages (stain H & E). **E,** Another section of the lesion showing "sulfur granules" or the presence of actinomycosis. **F,** One year recall showing healing by the formation of an apical scar.

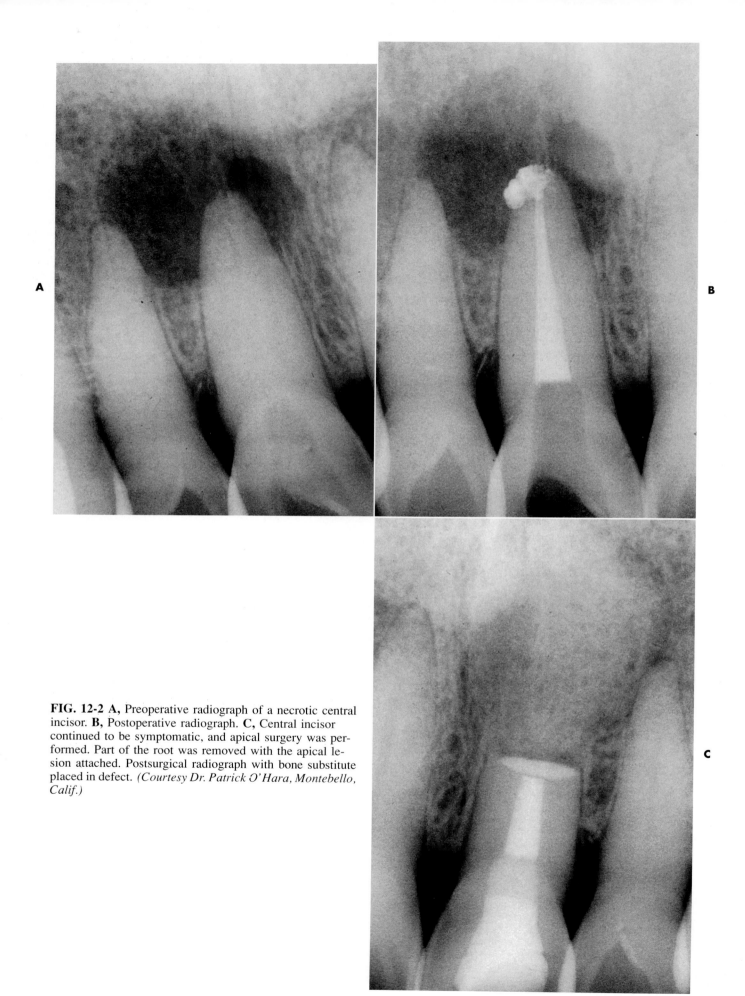

FIG. 12-2 A, Preoperative radiograph of a necrotic central incisor. **B,** Postoperative radiograph. **C,** Central incisor continued to be symptomatic, and apical surgery was performed. Part of the root was removed with the apical lesion attached. Postsurgical radiograph with bone substitute placed in defect. *(Courtesy Dr. Patrick O'Hara, Montebello, Calif.)*

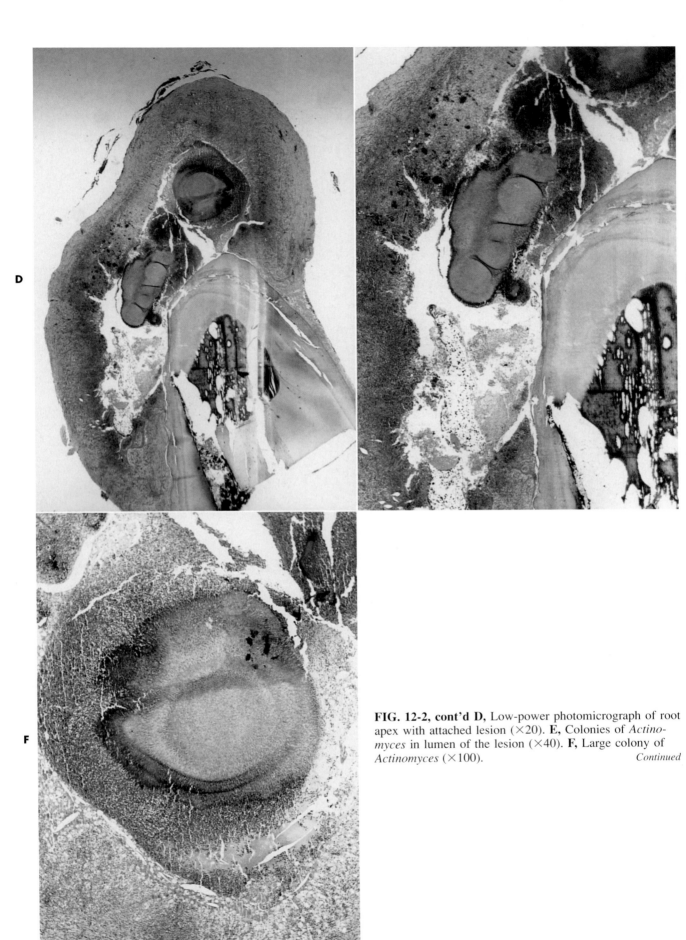

FIG. 12-2, cont'd D, Low-power photomicrograph of root apex with attached lesion (×20). **E,** Colonies of *Actinomyces* in lumen of the lesion (×40). **F,** Large colony of *Actinomyces* (×100).   *Continued*

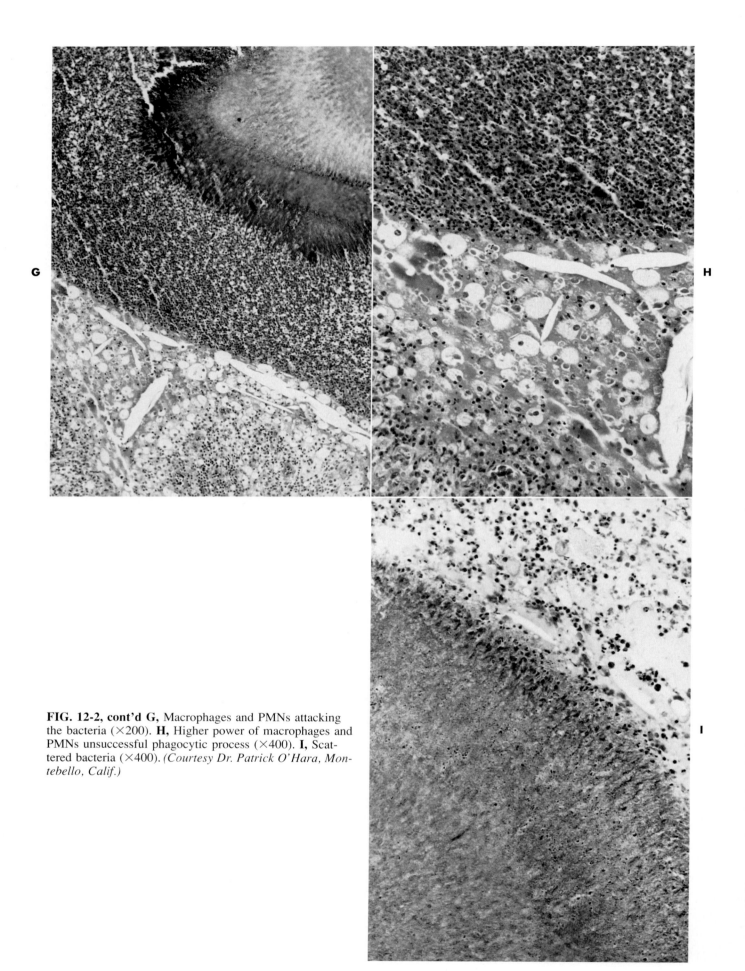

FIG. 12-2, cont'd G, Macrophages and PMNs attacking the bacteria (×200). **H,** Higher power of macrophages and PMNs unsuccessful phagocytic process (×400). **I,** Scattered bacteria (×400). *(Courtesy Dr. Patrick O'Hara, Montebello, Calif.)*

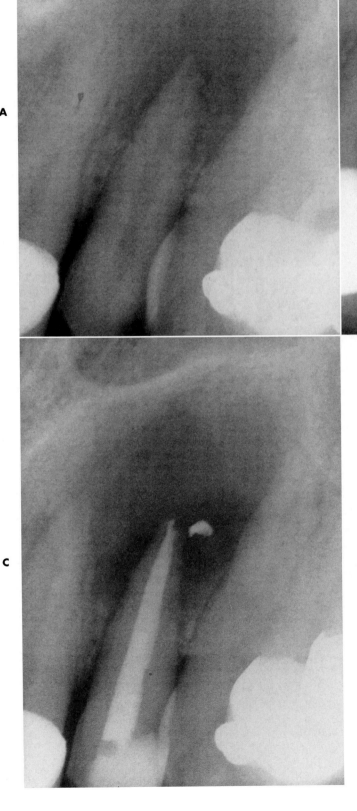

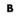

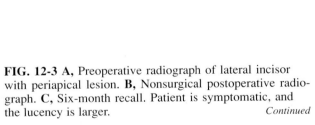

FIG. 12-3 A, Preoperative radiograph of lateral incisor with periapical lesion. **B,** Nonsurgical postoperative radiograph. **C,** Six-month recall. Patient is symptomatic, and the lucency is larger. *Continued*

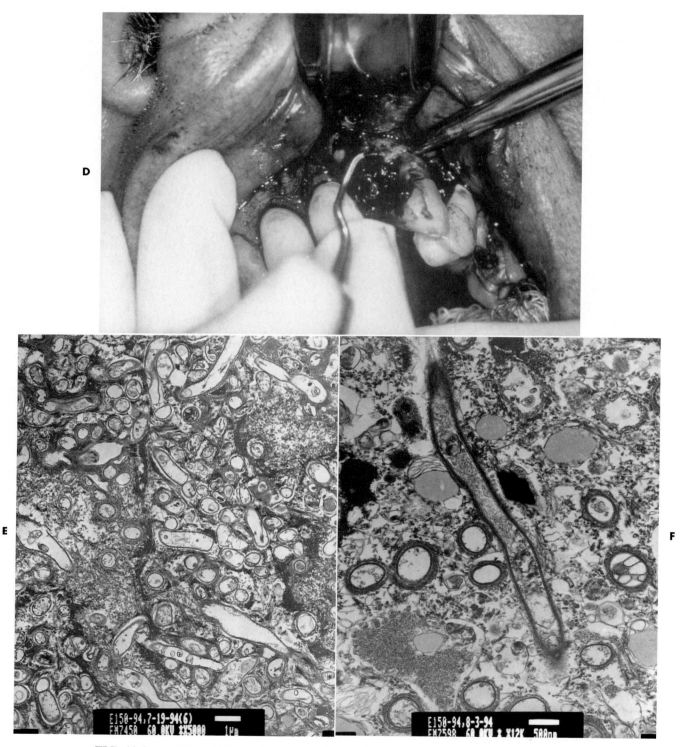

FIG. 12-3, cont'd D, At time of surgery and extraction, a small green ball was removed and placed in glutaraldehyde. **E,** Transmission electron micrograph of growing hyphae of a fungus. **F,** Higher power micrograph of hyphae.

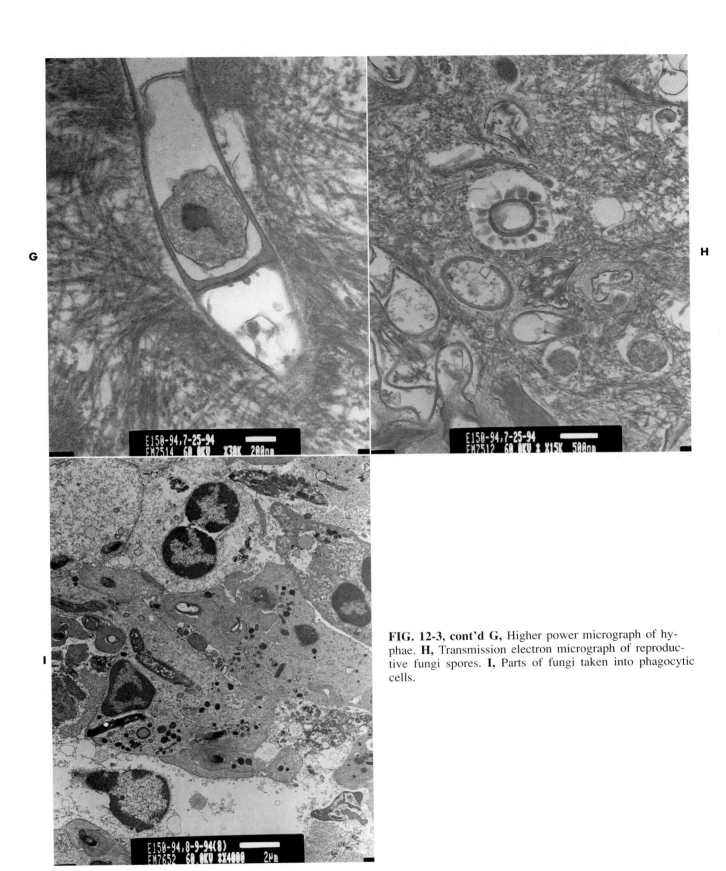

FIG. 12-3, cont'd G, Higher power micrograph of hyphae. **H,** Transmission electron micrograph of reproductive fungi spores. **I,** Parts of fungi taken into phagocytic cells.

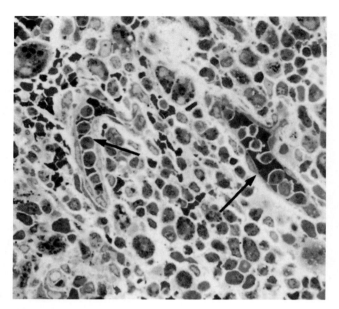

FIG. 12-4 Photomicrograph of an area of inflammation with two capillaries showing white and red blood cells flowing through the vessels *(arrows)* (×400).

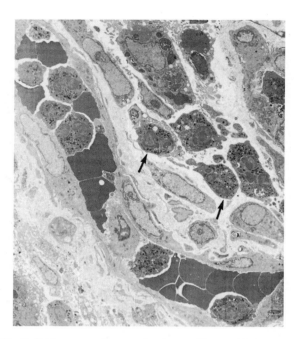

FIG. 12-5 Electron micrograph of a capillary with PMNs and erythrocytes inside. Note PMNs in the extravascular tissue *(arrows)* (×3450).

the canal, nonsurgical endodontic treatment may not be sufficient to effect healing.[9] Once past the foramen, viable bacteria, endotoxin,[12,54] fungi, and foreign bodies[22] may require surgery to remove them. With current testing procedures it is now possible to demonstrate viable bacteria and fungi in the periapex. With improved techniques it is entirely possible that in the next decade we may find virus and virus particles in the periapex as etiologic agents.

The response to periapical pathology is complex. Our tendency has been to oversimplify the process because of our lack of complete understanding of the processes involved.

PERIAPICAL PATHOLOGY

Endodontic pathology is a bacterial disease.[14,35] The periapex of the tooth becomes involved when bacteria invade the pulp, rendering it partially to totally necrotic. This was shown graphically in a classic study by Kakehashi et al.[19] on gnotobiotic (germ-free) rats. They exposed the pulps of normal rats and left them open to the oral environment. Necrosis of the pulp ensued, followed by periapical inflammation and lesion formation. However, when the same procedure was performed on germ-free rats, not only did the pulps remain vital and relatively uninflamed, but the bur holes were repaired with dentin by the 36th day. The study demonstrated that without bacteria and their products, periapical lesions of endodontic origin *do not* occur. Confirmation came from a study by Moeller et al.[27] on nine monkeys. It was shown that noninfected necrotic pulp tissue did not induce periapical lesions or inflammatory reactions. However, if the pulp tissue was then infected, periapical lesions and inflammation in the apical tissues ensued. Additionally, Korzen et al.[23] demonstrated it is a mixed infection and not a monoinfection that results in the more florid disease process. Thus it is well established that periapical pathology is the result of bacteria, their products, and the host's response to them.

HOST RESPONSE

Inflammation

The basic disease process in both pulp and periapical disease is infection. The host responds to the infection with inflammation. Many definitions of inflammation exist but none is precise. Menkin[26] defined inflammation as the complex vascular, lymphatic, and local tissue reaction of a higher organism to an irritant. Because inflammation is the host's response to an infection, the terms *inflammation* and *infection* are not interchangeable. The host can have an inflammatory response without the presence of infection (i.e., sunburn).

Vascular Changes

The initial vascular change in inflammation is a transient contraction of the microcirculation followed by an almost immediate dilation (Figs. 12-4 and 12-5). As the vessels dilate, the blood flow slows. The red blood cells move to the middle of the vessel (rouleaux formation), and the white blood cells move to the periphery and stick to the endothelial wall (margination) (Fig. 12-6). The vasculature in the postcapillary venules becomes leaky because of contraction of endothelial cells under the influence of histamine, which allows plasma to escape into the tissue spaces. Because of this leakage, edema results, causing increased tissue pressure.

The immediate transient vascular response is most likely mediated by histamine, whereas the delayed vascular response is mediated by other vasoactive amines such as bradykinin. In addition, other plasma proteins such as fibrinogen pass into the tissues and contribute to the inflammatory response. Fibrinogen is converted to fibrin when it contacts the tissue collagen and forms a meshwork to isolate the reaction (Fig. 12-7). The white blood cells that now line the endothelial wall of the vessels squeeze through the endothelial gaps and into the tissue by ameboid movement. This movement is called diapedesis.

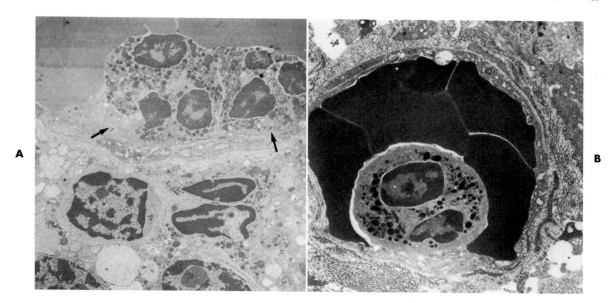

FIG. 12-6 A, Electron micrograph of a portion of a large vessel showing margination of two leukocytes *(arrows)* (×11,000). **B,** Smaller vessel with PMN about to squeeze through the wall.

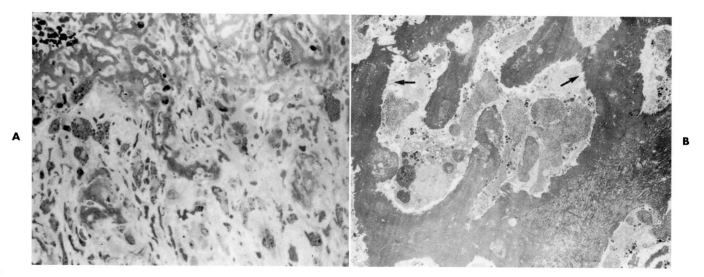

FIG. 12-7 A, One-micrometer section showing fibrin in the tissues walling off the resection. **B,** Ultrastructural picture of fibrin in the tissue *(arrows).*

Acute Inflammation

In acute inflammation the PMNs are the first cells to emigrate to the site of infection (Fig. 12-8). They are drawn there by chemotactic agents that are either expressed by the bacteria itself or by other mediators of inflammation. The monocytes are next attracted to the site. When these cells enter the tissues, they are called tissue macrophages or histiocytes (Fig. 12-9). Neutrophils survive for hours, whereas macrophages last for days to months. The neutrophil is characterized by its lobulated nucleus, whereas the macrophage has a single large nucleus. Both have extensive cytoplasmic granules containing lysosomal enzymes. In the inflammatory process both PMNs and macrophages function as phagocytes (Fig. 12-10). The process of phagocytosis includes attaching, ingesting, and then destroying the bacteria.

Microscopically the picture includes PMNs, macrophages, and the tissue response as a result of chemical mediators. On the clinical level we can now account for the five cardinal signs of inflammation (Figs. 12-11 and 12-12):

1. Redness: Increased dilation of the vessels
2. Swelling: Escape of vascular fluid into the tissues causing edema
3. Pain: Release of pain mediators such as bradykinin and tissue pressure due to hyperemia and edema
4. Heat: Increased blood supply to the injured tissues
5. Loss of function: Due to pain and swelling

The diagnosis of acute inflammation is both a histologic and clinical diagnosis. Histologically, PMNs and macrophages constitute the predominant acute inflammatory cells, but clinically the presence of pain usually denotes an acute condition. The

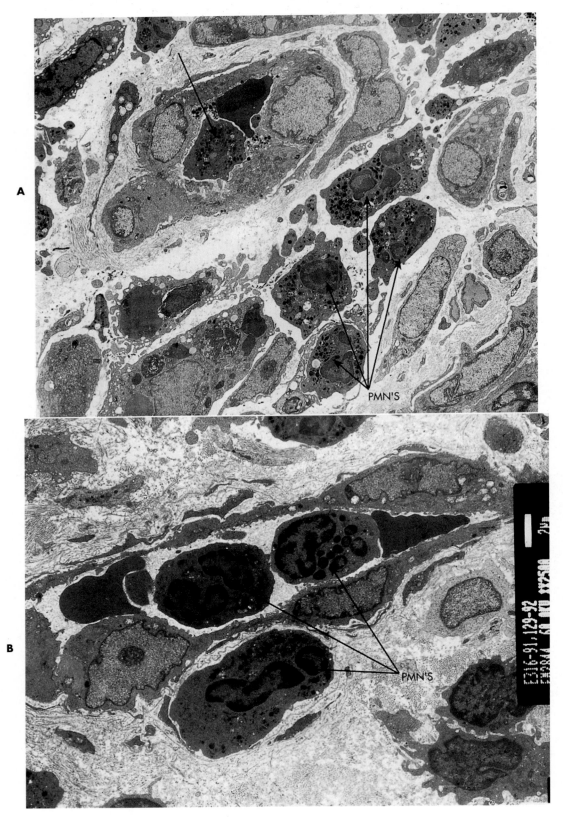

FIG. 12-8 A, Electron micrograph of a capillary containing a red blood cell and a PMN with numerous PMNs in the surrounding tissue. This is the beginning of acute inflammation. **B,** Longitudinal cut of a capillary with PMNs in the lumen and a PMN in the tissue.

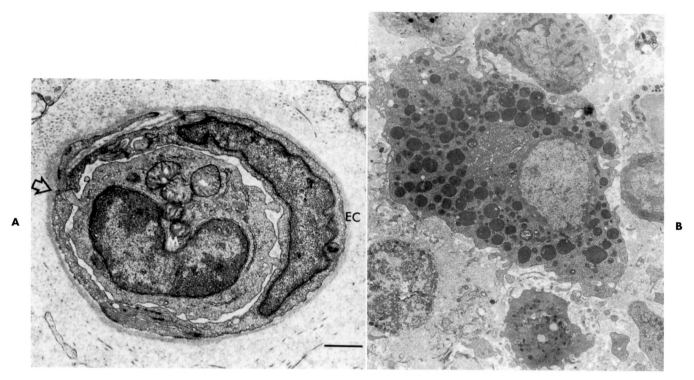

FIG. 12-9 A, Monocyte *(M)* in a capillary with three pseudopods extended (×12,900). One pseudopod *(upper left)* is beginning to squeeze through the intercellular gap *(arrow)*. Note the prominent endothelial cells *(EC)*. **B,** Electron micrograph of a macrophage now out in the tissue.

other cardinal signs of acute inflammation may also be present (i.e., swelling, heat, redness, and loss of function).

ACUTE APICAL PERIODONTITIS

Acute apical inflammation is a very painful response that occurs before alveolar bone is resorbed. Apically the vascular response to the antigens within the pulp produces edema. The edema and PMNs rapidly fill the periodontal ligament between the tooth and bone. Because the fluid is not compressible, any external pressure on the tooth forces the fluid against already sensitized nerve endings, resulting in exquisite pain. The tooth is painful to percussion until the bone begins to resorb and space is created to accommodate the edema fluid. The patient may also complain of the tooth feeling elevated in the socket, but no lesion is demonstrable on the radiograph.

ACUTE APICAL ABSCESS

An acute apical abscess may result when large numbers of bacteria leak past the apex and elicit a severe inflammatory response. This response is acute with the dominating cell being the PMN. With the release of PMN lysosomal enzymes into the tissue space and the concomitant tissue degradation, an abscess is formed (see Figs. 12-11 and 12-12). An abscess is defined as a localized collection of pus, which microscopically is composed of dead cells, debris, PMNs, and macrophages. Clinically, varying degrees of swelling occur with or without pain. The patient complains that the tooth feels elevated out of the socket. Elevated temperature and malaise may follow. The body responds to this insult by trying to isolate the abscess or establish drainage either intraorally or extraorally.

If drainage is not effected, the abscess may spread into fascial planes or spaces of the head and neck, forming a cellulitis.

Phoenix Abscess

If a periapical radiolucency is present and an acute inflammatory response is superimposed on this preexisting chronic lesion, it is termed a phoenix abscess. It is an acute exacerbation of an existing chronic inflammation (Fig. 12-13).

ACUTE OSTEOMYELITIS

Acute osteomyelitis can arise directly from an endodontic infection. Live bacteria pass the apex and multiply in the marrow spaces and soft tissue of the bone. Osteomyelitis may be a serious progression of periapical infection that results in a diffuse spread through the medullary spaces, ultimately leading to necrosis of bone. Acute osteomyelitis may be localized or spread throughout large areas of bone.[36] The patient usually has severe pain, an elevated temperature, and palpable lymph nodes. Although the teeth are loose and sore in the early stages, there may be no swelling, and radiographic changes are difficult to detect (Fig. 12-14). Microscopically the medullary spaces are filled predominantly with neutrophils. There may or may not be pus formation. Other microscopic findings include bone resorption due to vigorous activity of the osteoclasts and the lack of osteoblasts.

If untreated the acute form may progress to chronic. Clinically, chronic suppurative osteomyelitis is the same as the acute form except the symptoms are milder and radiographically diffuse bone resorption is evident. Osteomyelitis is a very serious extension of periapical disease and must be treated

Text continued on p. 441

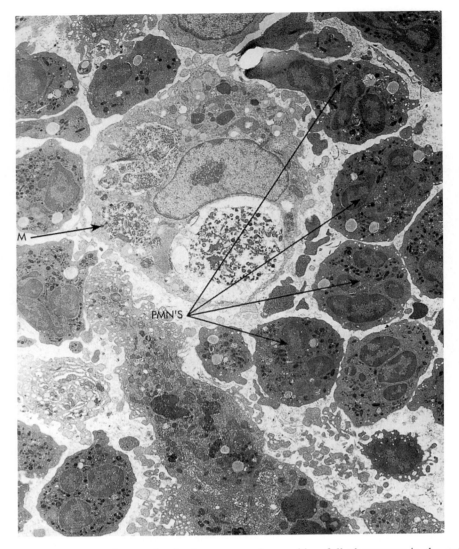

FIG. 12-10 Electron micrograph of a large macrophage with a full phagosome in the cytoplasm. Cell is surrounded by PMNs.

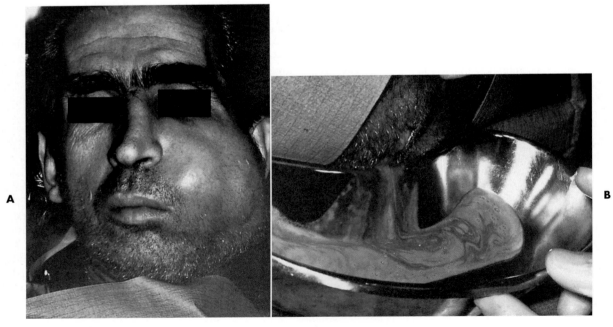

FIG. 12-11 A, Clinical photograph of an acute apical abscess. B, Pus and blood draining externally into a basin from the incised abscess.

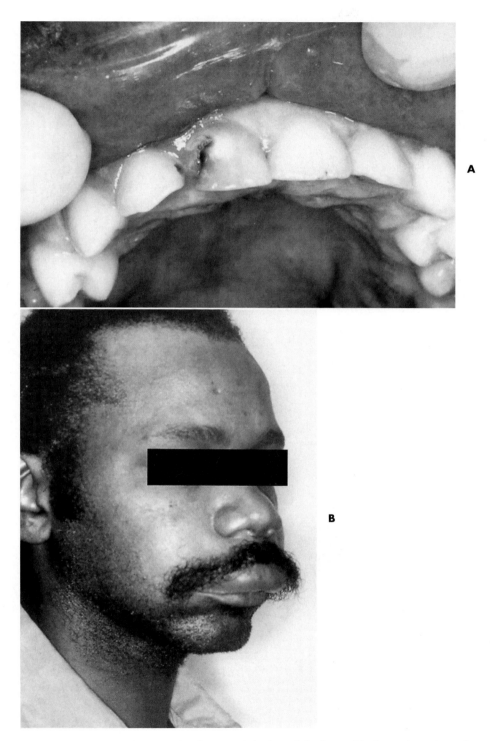

FIG. 12-12 A, Clinical photograph of upper right lateral incisor with decay into the pulp.
B, Acute abscess with cellulitis of upper lip.

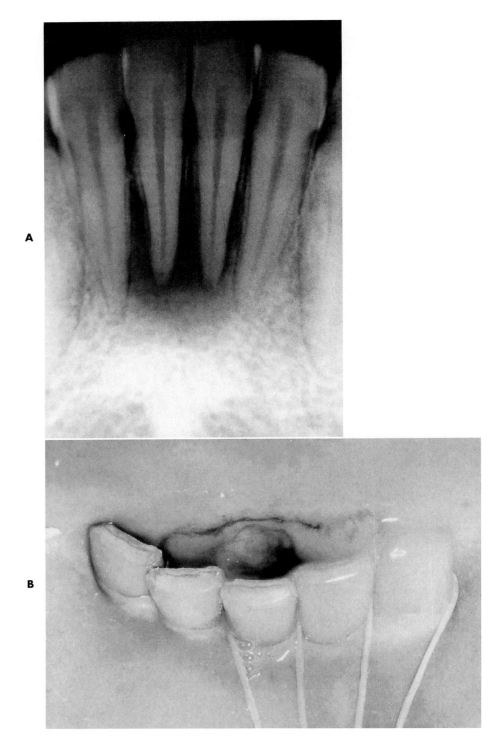

FIG. 12-13 A, Radiograph of lower anterior teeth with periapical lucency. **B,** On opening the central incisors, copious amounts of pus drained through the canals. Diagnosis is phoenix abscess.

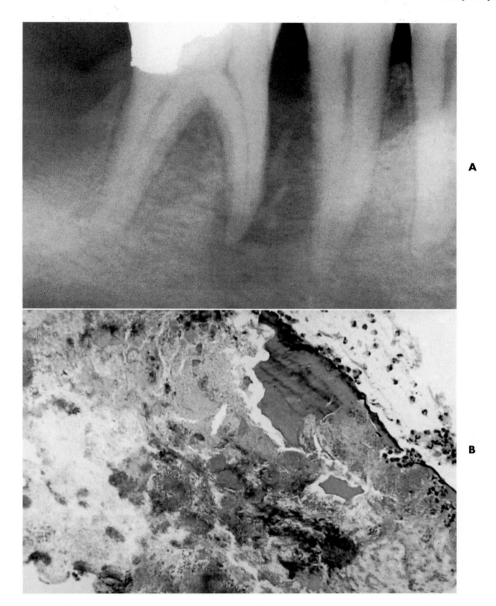

FIG. 12-14 A, Radiograph of lower first molar area with a diffuse radiolucency. Molar was necrotic and did not respond to pulp testing procedures. **B,** Biopsy of the area reveals dead avascular bone, debris, and bacteria. Diagnosis is acute osteomyelitis.

promptly and aggressively (Fig. 12-15). This can be a disease of endodontic origin; however, the etiologic agent (bacteria) is beyond the confines of the pulp and in the surrounding tissues. Endodontic therapy or extraction may not be effective treatment options. More extensive surgical intervention, hyperbaric oxygen, and antibiotic therapy may be required.

Chronic Inflammation

If the acute process is not treated and does not heal but continues, the response becomes chronic. This is a change in both time and cell population. The acute inflammatory process is an *exudative* response, whereas chronic is a *proliferative* response. Microscopically, proliferation of fibroblasts and vascular elements and the infiltration of macrophages and lymphocytes are characteristic. In addition to the chronic inflammatory response, macrophages and lymphocytes elicit an immune response. The purpose of the immune system is to neutralize, inactivate, or destroy a stimulus (antigen or bacteria). This is accomplished by the following:

1. Direct neutralization by antibody binding to the stimulus or destruction of the stimulus by sensitized lymphocytes leading to blast lymphocytes to plasma cells producing antibodies (Figs. 12-16 and 12-17)
2. Activation of biochemical and cellular mediator systems that can destroy the antigen

People are either immunocompetent or immunodeficient. Immunocompetence is the ability to generate an immune response that can overcome many diseases and infections. Immunodeficient people cannot make this response and are thus afflicted with many inflammatory and infectious diseases. The

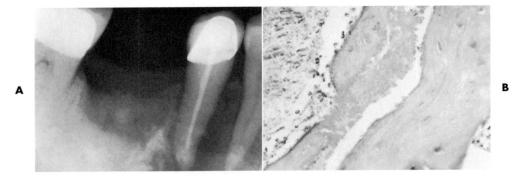

FIG. 12-15 A, Radiograph of chronic osteomyelitis showing extensive bone destruction in the mandible. **B,** Histologic section of necrotic bone with bacterial colonies.

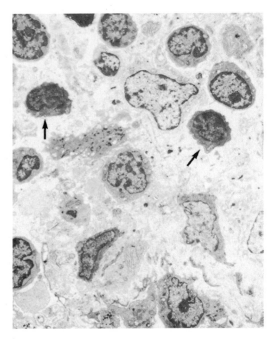

FIG. 12-16 Electron micrograph of numerous lymphocytes *(arrows)* in the lymphoblast stage transforming into plasma cells. Note the presence of a macrophage ($\times$5240).

host's ability to respond to an antigen has a genetic predisposition. This was formerly referred to as host resistance. Diseases, immunosuppressive medications, etc., can also alter the host's ability to mount an immune response.

Immunopathologies

The immunopathologies are hypersensitivity reactions of the immune system that produce injury to the host.[45,46,48] These can be considered in two broad groups: antibody mediated (types I, II, and III) and T-cell mediated (type IV).[40]

   I. Antibody-mediated hypersensitivities: These reactions are mediated by antibodies that have sensitized basophils or mast cells.
     A. Type I: The primary exposure of the host to an antigen sensitizes the mast cells or basophils. The anti-

body, IgE primes the mast cells or basophils for the next exposure to the antigen. When that occurs, massive degranulation of these sensitized cells results in the release of histamine and the production of arachidonic acid metabolites with their resulting biologic effects.
     B. Type II: IgG or IgM react with cell surface antigens to have a cytotoxic effect by either activating complement, which ultimately results in cell lysis, or phagocytosis by macrophages, PMNs, or K cells in a process known as antibody-dependent-cell-mediated cytotoxicity (ADCC).
     C. Type III: Type III hypersensitivities are also mediated by IgG and IgM and involve the fixation of complement. Free antigen (not cell or tissue bound) forms immune complexes with the antibodies.[30,47] This elicits the complement cascade. Complement components C5a and C567 are chemotactic for PMNs and macrophages. These subsequently phagocytize the immune complexes and release their lysosomal enzymes, which ultimately leads to tissue destruction of the host. The Arthus reaction is this type of hypersensitivity.
   II. T-cell–mediated hypersensitivities:
     A. Type IV: These reactions develop slowly and reach their peak between 24 and 72 hours. Typically what happens is a sensitized individual encounters the antigen again. The accessory cell presents the antigen to the sensitized T cell and the T cell undergoes blast transformation. The T cell expresses lymphokines, and the macrophage releases lysosomal enzymes that damage the host tissues.

Evidence indicates that all these inflammatory and immune processes may take place in the pulp and periapical tissues. Therefore in the following descriptions all these reactions may be occurring. This results in a microscopic picture that we label as chronic inflammation.

PERIAPICAL EXTENSION OF PULPAL INFLAMMATION

Periapical inflammation may begin before the pulp is totally necrotic. Bacterial products, mediators of inflammation, and deteriorating pulp tissue leak past the apex and evoke a chronic inflammatory response from the vessels in the periodontal liga-

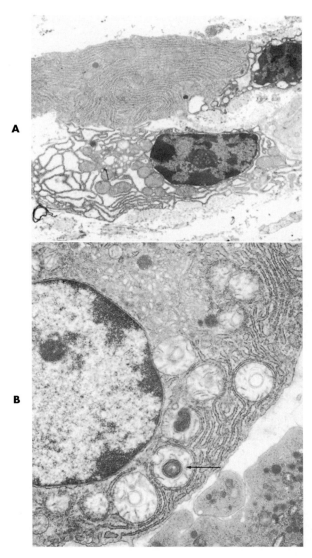

FIG. 12-17 A, Electron micrograph of two plasma cells, one with normal rough endoplasmic reticulum and the other with very dilated rough endoplasmic reticulum. This dilation is thought to indicate immunoglobulin production and synthesis (×3450). **B,** High-power electron micrograph of part of a plasma cell showing the rough endoplasmic reticulum with ribosomes on the surface and myelin figures in the Golgi apparatus *(arrow)* (×23,700).

ment. This explains why it is possible to have a periapical radiolucency and still have some vital tissue remaining in the apical canal (Fig. 12-18). The periapical inflammatory response is an extension of the pulpal inflammation and necrosis.

Condensing Osteitis (Focal Sclerosing Osteomyelitis)

A very low-grade, subclinical inflammatory response may lead to an increase in bone density rather than resorption and lucency. This response is dependent on the quality, duration, and virulence of the irritants. This lesion may be clinically asymptomatic or possess the range of pulpal symptomatology. Radiographically there is increased bone density and opacity

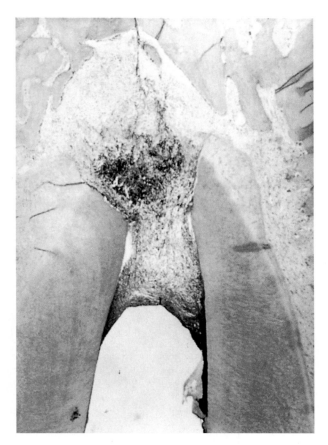

FIG. 12-18 Histologic section showing vital pulp tissue remaining in the canal with inflammation at the foramen and periapical bone resorption. *(Courtesy Dr. Jacob Valderhaug, Univ. of Oslo, Norway.)*

at the apex. Since this is a lesion of endodontic origin, there must be a cause for the pulpal disease.

Microscopically, dense bone with growth lines is prevalent with a mild chronic inflammatory infiltrate in the marrow spaces. If there is an altered or necrotic pulp, endodontic treatment is indicated (Fig. 12-19). The opacity may or may not heal. The differential diagnosis is as follows:

1. Focal osteopetrosis
2. True cementoblastoma
3. Stage III osseous dysplasia

If the involved tooth is a virgin tooth or has a "normal" pulp, the diagnosis is focal osteopetrosis or periapical osteosclerosis. This is *not* a lesion of endodontic etiology, and no treatment is necessary.

CHRONIC APICAL PERIODONTITIS (GRANULOMA)

Chronic apical inflammation is a relatively low-grade, long-standing response to canal bacteria and irritants. Clinically, this lesion is usually asymptomatic and is detected by an apical radiolucency. Microscopically the lesion is characterized by a predominance of lymphocytes, plasma cells, and macrophages surrounded by a relatively uninflamed fibrous capsule made up of collagen, fibroblasts, and capillary buds (Fig. 12-20). In the inflammatory area large amorphous circles with very pale staining may be seen. These are Russell bodies and are thought

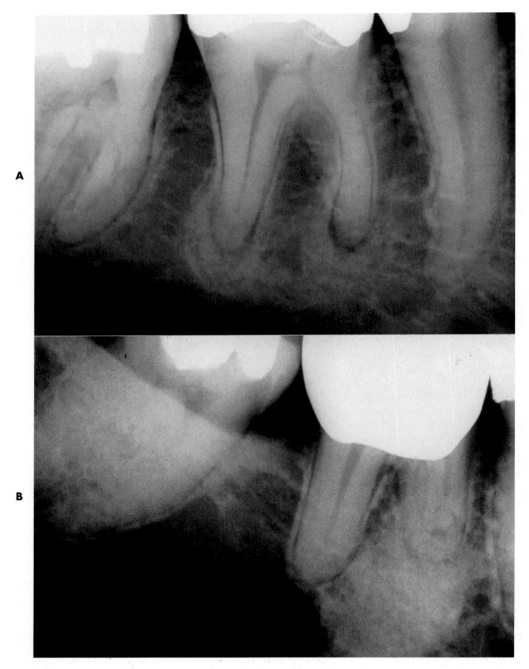

FIG. 12-19 A and **B,** Necrotic mandibular molars with periapical radiopaque lesions.

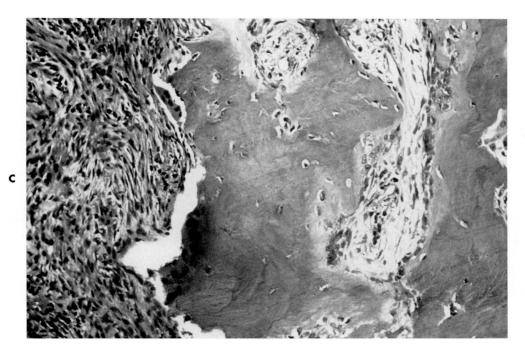

FIG. 12-19, cont'd C, Histologic section of condensing osteitis showing low-grade chronic inflammation, osteoblasts, and osteoid formation.

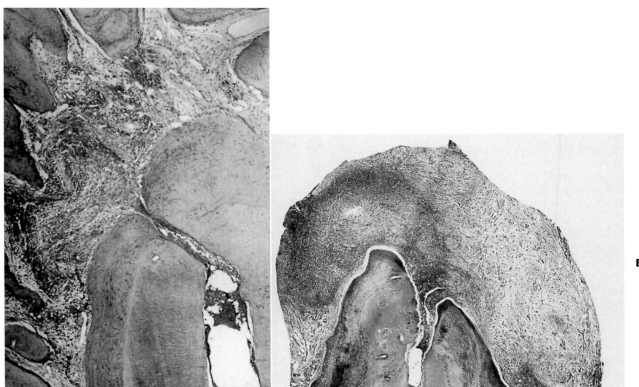

FIG. 12-20 A, Histologic section of necrotic canal with beginning periapical (granuloma) lesion formation. **B,** Histologic section of necrotic canal with chronic (granuloma) inflammatory lesion. (**A,** *Courtesy Dr. Jacob Valderhaug, Univ. of Oslo, Norway.*)

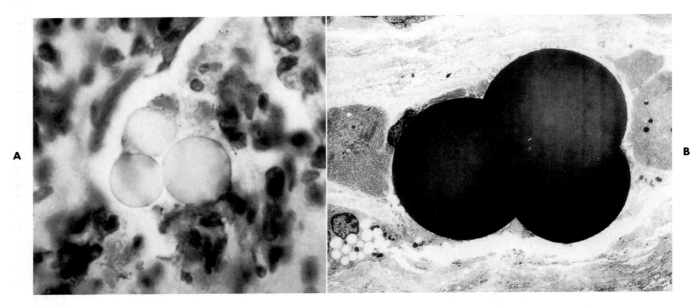

FIG. 12-21 A, Histologic section of granuloma showing three circular amorphous Russell bodies (stain H & E ×400). **B,** Electron micrograph of three Russell bodies that have coalesced. Note rough endoplasmic reticulum of associated plasma cell.

to be associated with plasma cells that no longer have the capability to produce antibodies (Fig. 12-21). Cords or strands of proliferating epithelium may or may not be present. This lesion is usually not purely chronic in nature, as some PMNs may be seen scattered throughout the lesion.

SUPPURATIVE APICAL PERIODONTITIS (GRANULOMA WITH FISTULATION)

An apical lesion that has established drainage through a sinus tract is termed suppurative inflammation (Fig. 12-22). Clinically, the patient may complain of a "gumboil" or a bad taste in the mouth. Pus may be expressed through the opening by gentle pressure. A radiograph should be taken with a gutta-percha probe or silver point inserted into the tract to determine the cause of the lesion. Microscopically the tract may be filled with PMNs or pus. Chronic inflammatory cells may line the periphery, and in later stages epithelium may be present (Fig. 12-23). Studies estimate that epithelium lines the tract 10% to 30% of the time. Valderhaug has stated that the longer the tract exists, the greater is the chance it will have an epithelial lining.[50a]

FOREIGN BODY REACTION

A foreign body response may occur to many types of substances. The reaction can be acute or chronic. What usually distinguishes these lesions microscopically is the presence of multinucleated giant cells surrounding a foreign material (Fig. 12-24). If the material is soluble in the solutions used to prepare the histologic section, the giant cells appear to be surrounding a space.[22] Usually the giant cells are surrounded by a chronic inflammatory infiltrate. The giant cells are thought to be formed by the fusion of several macrophages creating a multinuclear cell (Fig. 12-25). These lesions may or may not be symptomatic. The etiologic agent is now beyond the apical foramen, and therefore surgery may be necessary to remove the offending foreign material and effect healing.

ROLE OF EPITHELIUM

One of the normal components of the lateral and apical periodontal ligament is the epithelial rests of Malassez. The term *rests* is misleading in that it evokes a vision of discrete islands of epithelial cells.

It has been shown that these rests are actually a fishnetlike, three-dimensional, interconnected network of epithelial cells. In many periapical lesions, epithelium is not present and therefore is presumed to have been destroyed.[37] If the rests remain, they may respond to the stimulus by proliferating in an attempt to wall off the irritants coming through the apical foramen. The epithelium is surrounded by chronic inflammation and is termed an epitheliated granuloma (a granuloma containing epithelium) (Fig. 12-26, *A*). If this lesion is not treated, the epithelium continues to proliferate in an attempt to wall off the source of irritation (i.e., bacteria and products from the apical foramen). The term *bay cyst* has been coined for the microscopic representation of this situation[38] (Fig. 12-26, *B*). This is a chronic inflammatory lesion that has epithelium lining the lumen, but the lumen has a direct communication with the root canal system through the foramen. It is not a true cyst because a true cyst is a three-dimensional, epithelium-lined cavity with no communication between the lumen and the canal system (Fig. 12-26, *C*). The true cyst is the completion of the epithelial proliferative lesion.

When periapical lesions are studied in relation to the root canal, completely epithelium-lined cavities are found.[31,38] These are termed "true" cysts. There has been some confusion in the diagnosis when lesions are studied only on curetted biopsy material. Since the tooth is not attached to the lesion, orientation to the apex is lost. Therefore the criterion used for diagnosis of a cyst is "a strip of epithelium that appears to be lining a cavity." It is apparent that curetting both a "bay" cyst and a "true" cyst could give the same microscopic diagnosis. A "bay" cyst could be sectioned in such a way that it could resemble or give the appearance of a "true" cyst.

Text continued on p. 453

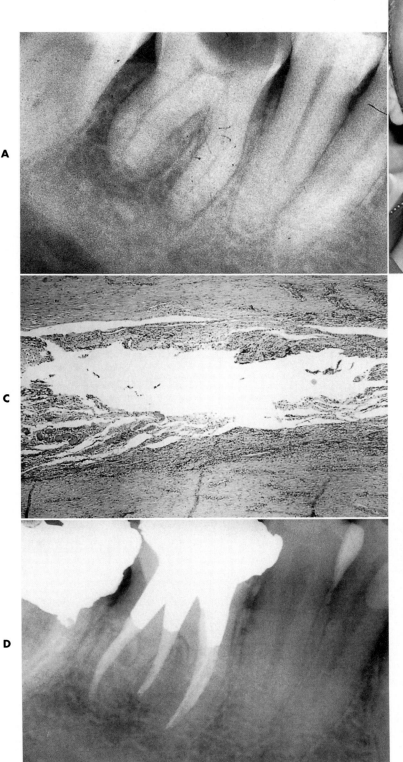

A

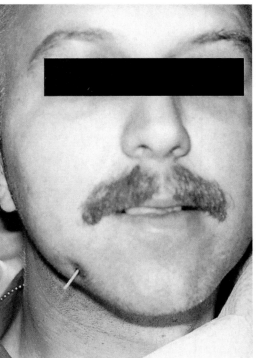

B

C

D

FIG. 12-22 A, Preoperative radiograph showing necrotic lower first molar. **B,** Clinical photograph of extra oral fistula with a gutta-percha cone inserted into the tract that led to the necrotic first molar. **C,** Histologic section of the fistulous tract showing acute and chronic inflammation, but no epithelium. **D,** One year recall after nonsurgical endodontic therapy and surgical removal of the sinus tract.

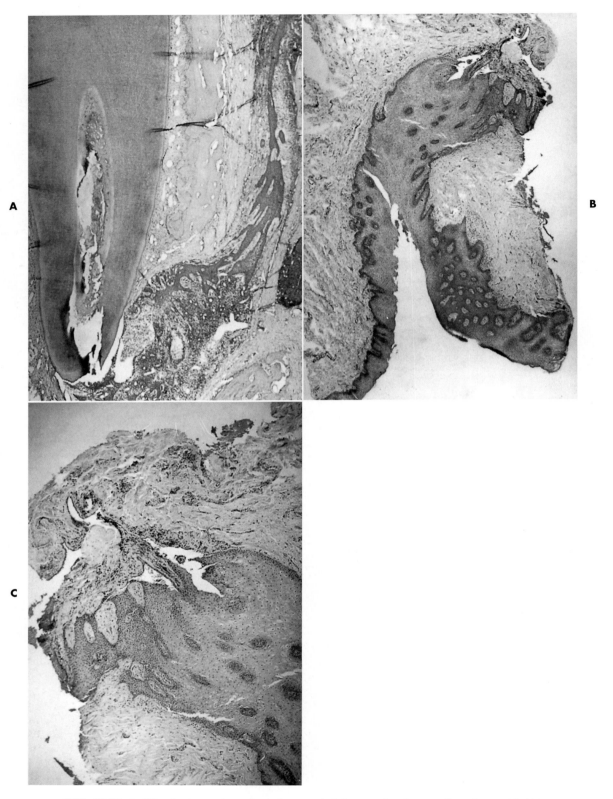

FIG. 12-23 A, Histologic section of monkey tooth left open for 1 year. Complete epithelial lining of fistulous tract. **B,** Human fistulous tract showing oral epithelium growing into the tract. **C,** High-power photomicrograph shows oral epithelium meeting epithelium from the rests of Malassez.

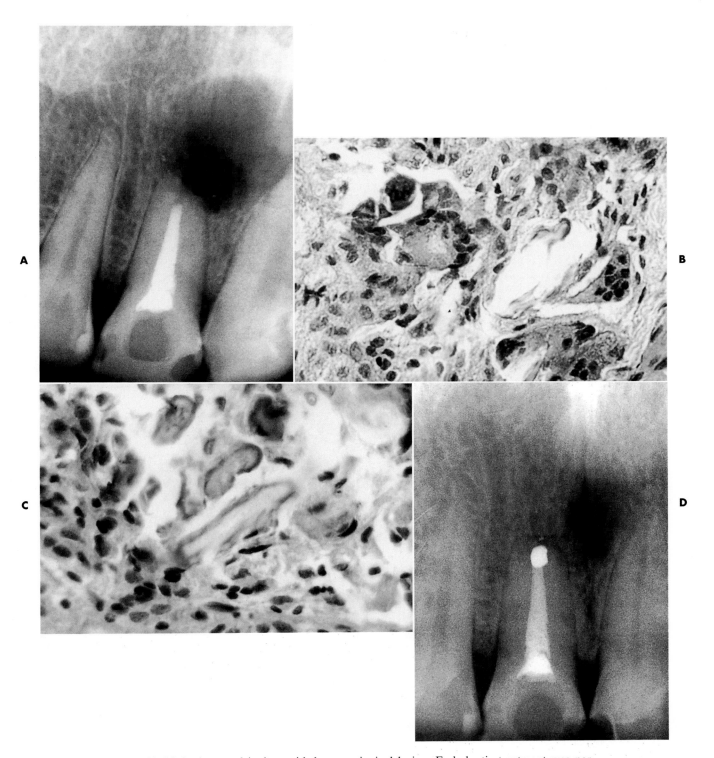

FIG. 12-24 A, A central incisor with large periapical lesion. Endodontic treatment was performed 27 years ago. **B,** Histologic section of lesion showing giant cells and foreign bodies. **C,** High-power photomicrograph of foreign body particles. **D,** After surgical removal, healing occurs 1 year later.

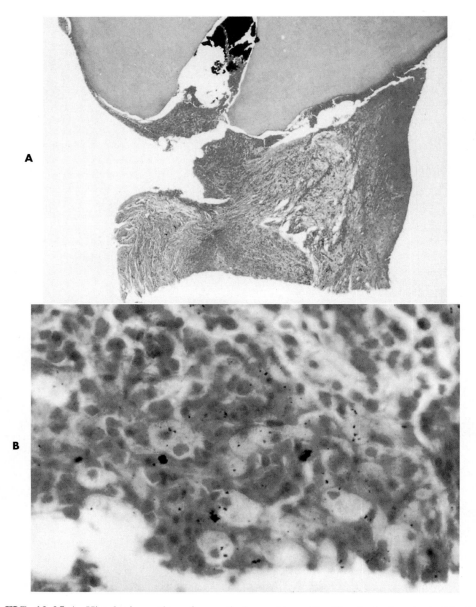

FIG. 12-25 A, Histologic section of necrotic lower bicuspid with attached periapical lesion. Note black foreign material in the canal. **B,** High-power photomicrograph of central part of the lesion showing black foreign body particles and large macrophages.

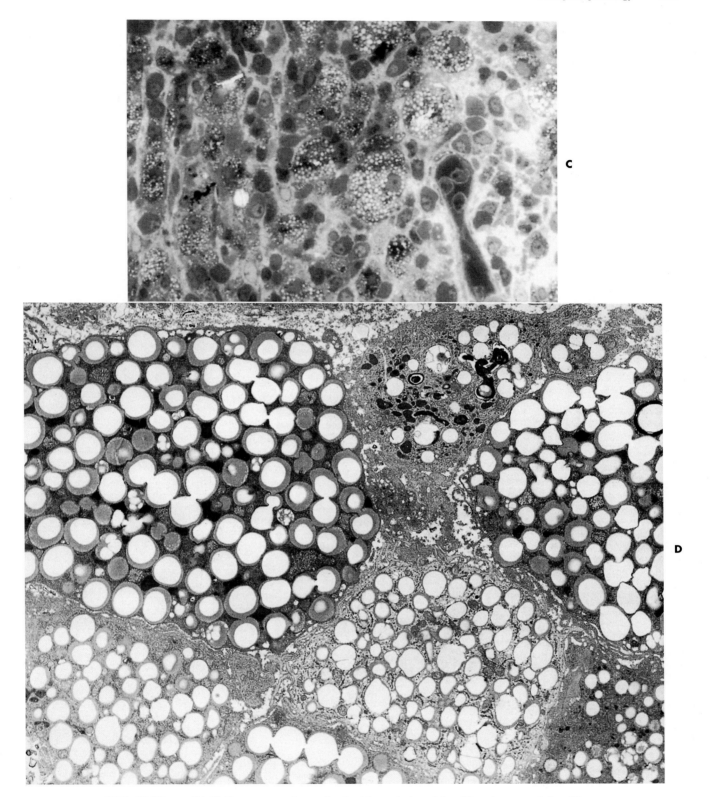

FIG. 12-25, cont'd C, One-μm section stained with methylene blue. Note large particles filling the cytoplasm of the macrophages. **D,** Transmission electron micrograph showing the entire cytoplasm of the macrophages full of foreign material. No cellular organelles are visible.

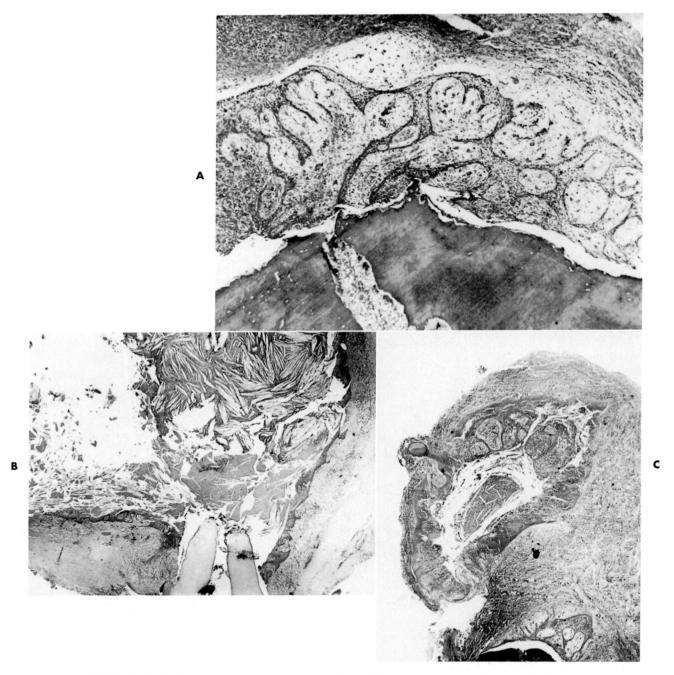

FIG. 12-26 **A,** Chronic apical periodontitis with proliferating cords of epithelium. **B,** Low-power photomicrograph of a bay cyst or apical periodontal pocket. Root canal opens directly into the lumen of this epithelium-lined lesion. **C,** Low-power photomicrograph of a true cyst. This is a cavity completely lined with epithelium and does not communicate with the root canal system.

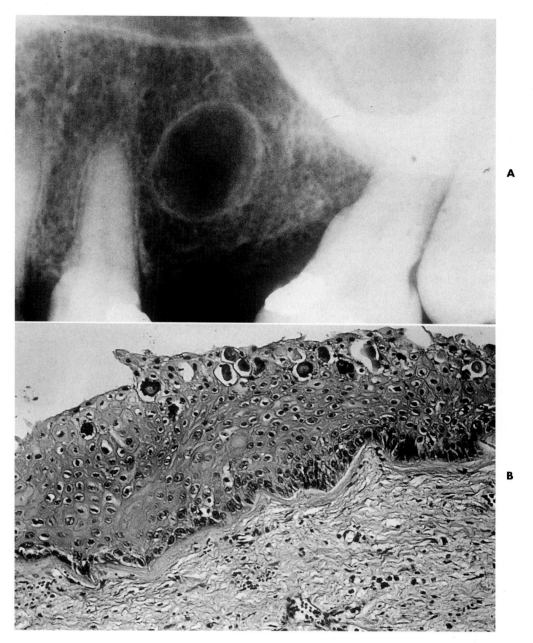

FIG. 12-27 A, Circular radiolucency in bone. **B,** Histologic section of inflamed cyst lining. Diagnosis was residual cyst.

This distinction between a "bay" and a "true" cyst is important from the standpoint of healing.[11] Endodontists state that some cysts heal with nonsurgical root canal treatment, whereas surgeons state that cysts must be surgically excised.* It may be that "true" cysts must be surgically removed, but "bay" cysts that communicate with the root canal may heal with nonsurgical root canal therapy. Since root canal therapy can directly affect the lumen of the "bay" cyst, the environmental change may bring about resolution of the lesion. The "true" cyst is independent of the root canal system; therefore conventional therapy may have no effect on the "true" cyst. This would ex-

plain the discrepancy between the endodontic and surgical opinions on the treatment of cysts. The formation of a cyst and its progression from a bay cyst to a true cyst occurs over time. Valderhaug showed that in monkeys no cysts were formed until at least 6 months after the canal contents became necrotic.[50b] Thus the longer a lesion has been present, the greater is the chance of becoming a "true" cyst. However, the incidence of "true" cysts is probably less than 10%.[35,38]

The final stage of epitheliated inflamed lesions is the residual cyst (Fig. 12-27). These are inflamed cysts found in the jawbones after tooth extraction. If there is a true cyst at the apex of a tooth with a necrotic canal and the tooth is extracted, the true cyst may be left behind and thus forms a residual cyst. This is the only odontogenic inflamed cyst found in the jaws.

References 5, 6, 7, 8, 24, 29, 35, 42, 44.

The implications for healing are profound. Extracting the tooth removes all the etiologic agents in the pulp and canal. (It is the ultimate root canal!) If the cause was restricted to the root canal, extraction would remove the etiologic agent completely; therefore there would be no such entity as a residual cyst. Since it is taught to curette the socket at the time of extraction of a tooth or root with a lucency, the incidence of residual cysts has decreased dramatically. However, a residual cyst thus substantiates the concept of the cause beyond the apical foramen.

It has been suggested that if an apical cyst is suspected or in all cases of periapical lucencies, a size No. 20 file should be placed several millimeters past the apical foramen.[6] The object is to puncture the cyst wall and set up an acute inflammatory reaction to destroy the epithelial lining.

Cohen[10] has shown that acute inflammatory cells are a normal component of cyst epithelium and that they travel from the connective tissue to the lumen through channels in the epithelium; they do not destroy the epithelial lining but pass through into the lumen without causing any damage. Fig. 12-28 shows the pathway of the acute cells into the lumen. If an acute alveolar abscess was created, it would probably destroy the epithelium, but this is a radical way to treat an epithelial lining.

Another microscopic finding in epithelium is the occurrence of Rushton bodies. These have been described as "hyaline" (glasslike) bodies that only occur within the epithelium (Fig. 12-29). Formerly, they were thought to be packed red blood cells. However, studies now show that they are not composed of erythrocytes but are probably an epithelial secretion. Their function is unknown.

HEALING

Healing can occur by either regeneration or repair. This distinction is important when considering what type of tissue forms after the antigenic agents are gone. If the tissue returns to its original state, it is called regeneration. If the original tissue is replaced with dense fibrous connective tissue, it is called repair or scarring.

Several cell types are involved in healing. Macrophages clean up the debris, fibroblasts repair the damage, and differentiated or undifferentiated cells regenerate the damaged tissues. Because of the increased oxygen demands during healing, proliferation of capillary buds also occurs.

APICAL SCAR

Healing of periapical disease may lead to scar formation. This occurs when the tissue that was originally present is replaced with dense fibrous connective tissue after the irritant has been destroyed.[34] Scar formation may also occur after surgical intervention takes place where both the buccal and the lingual cortical plates have been lost (Fig. 12-30). This shows as a radiolucency but does not require treatment. For all intents and purposes this lesion has "healed." Microscopically there is an abundance of dense collagen bundles with some fibroblasts. In the earlier stages of healing, macrophages, fibroblasts, and capillary buds may be present (see Fig. 12-30).

In summary, periapical pathology is caused by combinations of bacteria usually anaerobic, bacterial products and the host's response (inflammation) to them. The different periapical diagnoses are only different stages in the inflammatory response. These lesions are not static but are capable of undergoing constant change. They are only static under the microscope.

ACKNOWLEDGMENTS

A special acknowledgment to Sant Sekhon, Ph.D., and Nora L. Tong, M.A., of the Department of Veterans Affairs Medical Center, Long Beach, California, for the transmission electron microscopic work displayed in this chapter.

Text continued on p. 462

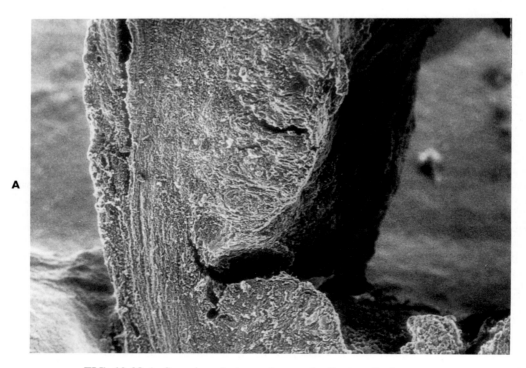

FIG. 12-28 A, Scanning electron micrograph of cut wall of a true cyst.

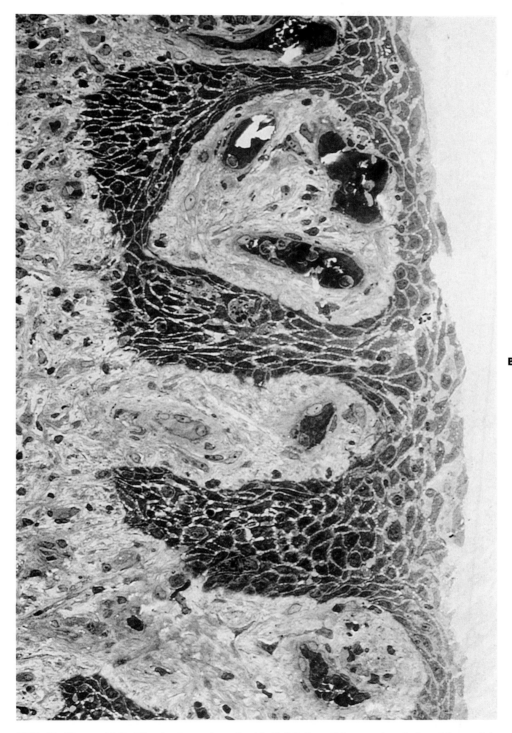

FIG. 12-28, cont'd B, Histologic section of epithelial lining of the cyst (methylene blue stain).

Continued

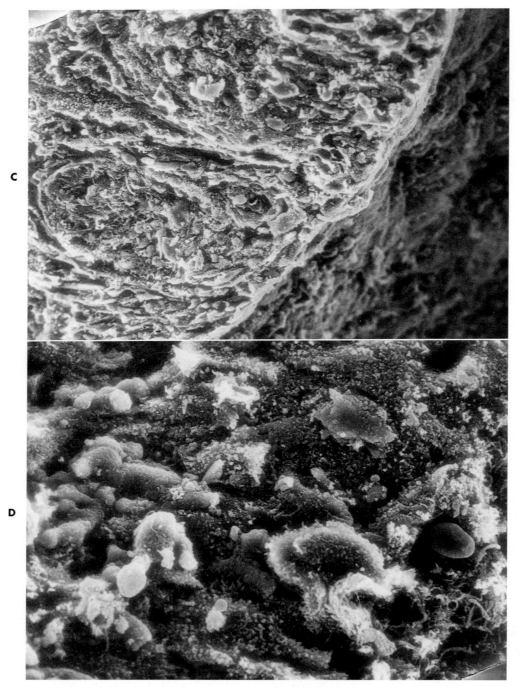

FIG. 12-28, cont'd C, Same area under the scanning electron microscope. Note lumen. **D,** Higher power photomicrograph of epithelium. Small white dots are the desmosomes.

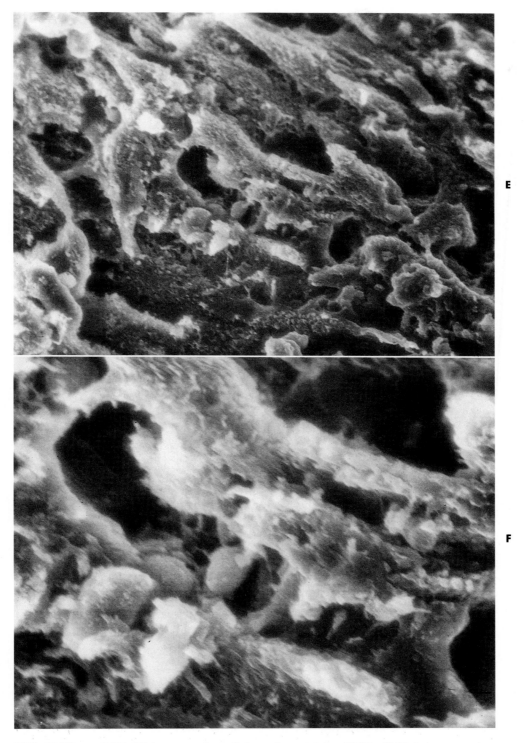

FIG. 12-28, cont'd E, High-power view of channels containing PMNs. **F,** Higher power view
of channels.   *Continued*

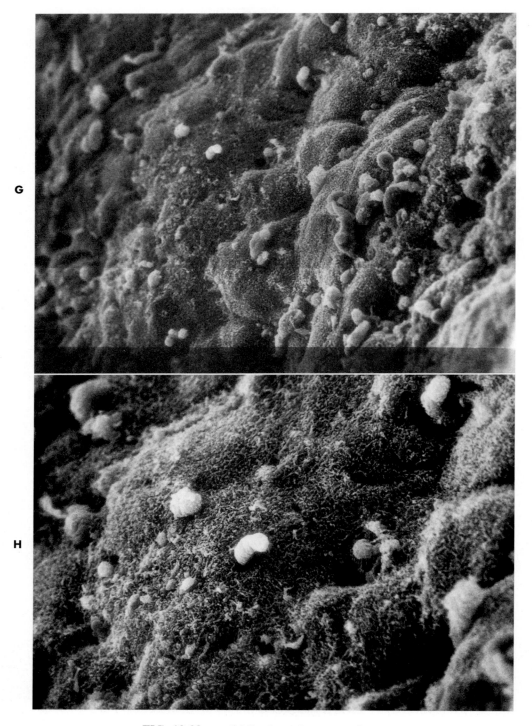

FIG. 12-28, cont'd For legend see opposite page.

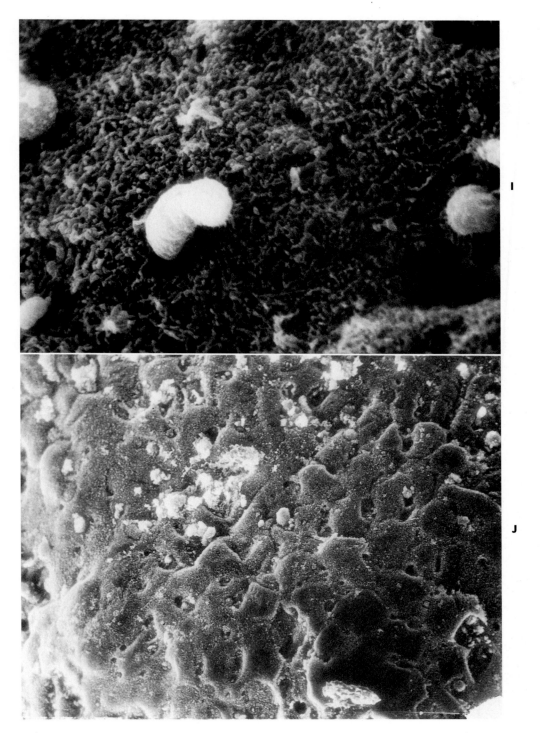

FIG. 12-28, cont'd G to **I,** Flat lumenal surface of cyst epithelium with PMNs coming through pores (channels) into the lumen. Note epithelial surface covered with microvilli. **J,** Different area of lumenal surface showing overlapping of epithelial cells and opening of the channels (pores).

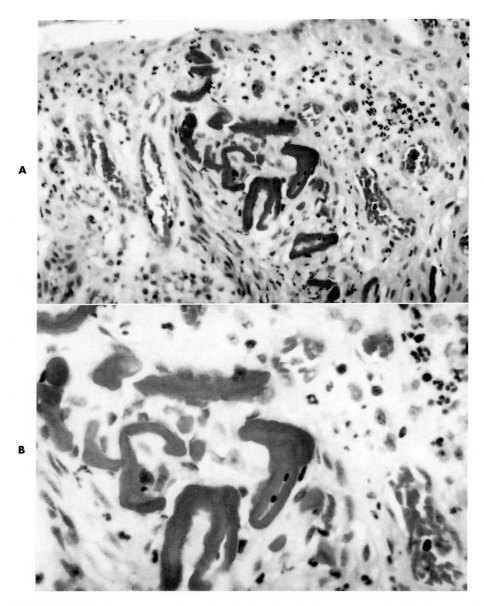

FIG. 12-29 A, Low-power photomicrograph of epithelium containing Rushton bodies. **B,** High-power photomicrograph of hyaline bodies.

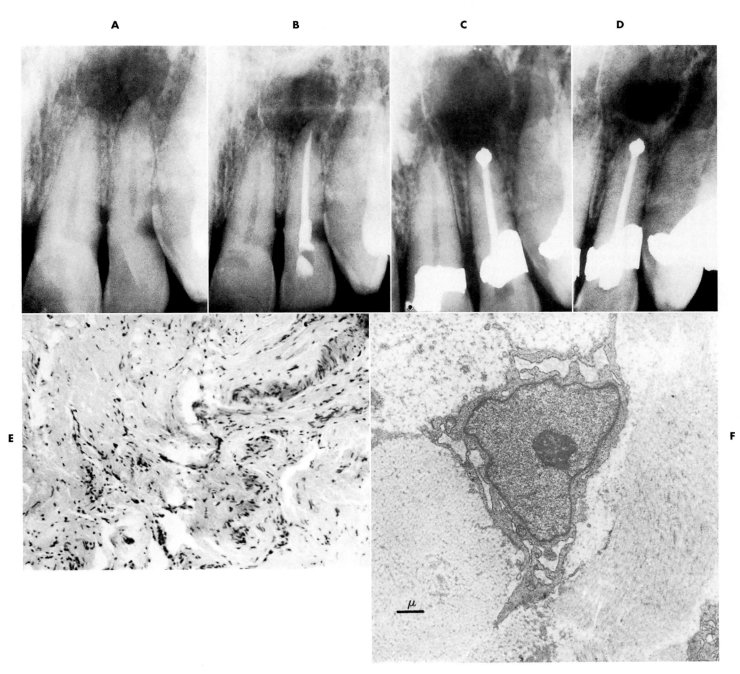

FIG. 12-30 A, Preoperative. **B,** Postoperative. **C,** Six months later. **D,** Six-year recall. Note the apparent periapical healing. **E,** Biopsy of the lesion revealed dense connective tissue with scattered inflammatory cells. Diagnosis was an apical scar (×2200). **F,** Fibroblast surrounded by dense collagen fibers (×12,400).

REFERENCES

1. Barnett F et al: Ciprofloxacin treatment of periapical *Pseudomonas aeruginosa* infection, *Endodont Dent Traumatol* 4:132-137, 1988.
2. Barnett F et al: Demonstration of *Bacteroides intermedius* in periapical tissue using indirect immunofluorescence microscopy, *Endodont Dent Traumatol* 6:153-156, 1990.
3. Baumgartner JC, Falkler WA Jr: Bacteria in the apical 5 mm of infected root canals, *Endodont* 17:380-383, 1991.
4. Baumgartner JC, Falkler WA: Reactivity of IgG from explant cultures of periapical lesions with implicated microorganisms, *Endodont* 17:207-212, 1991.
5. Bhaskar SN: Periapical lesions: types, incidence, and clinical features, *Oral Surg* 21:657, 1966.
6. Bhaskar SN: Nonsurgical resolution of radicular cysts, *Oral Surg* 38:458, 1972.
7. Block RM et al: A histopathologic, histobacteriologic, and radiographic study of periapical endodontic surgical specimens, *Oral Surg* 42(5):656, 1976.
8. Brynolf I: A histologic and roentgenologic study of the periapical region of human upper incisors, *Odont Rev* 18(suppl 2):1, 1976.
9. Bystrom A et al: Healing of periapical lesions of pulpless teeth after endodontic treatment with controlled asepsis, *Endodont Dent Traumatol* 3:58-63, 1987.
10. Cohen M: Pathways of inflammatory cellular exudate through radicular cyst epithelium: SEM study, *J Oral Pathol* 8:369, 1979.
11. Cymerman JJ et al: Human T lymphocyte subpopulations in chronic periapical lesions, *Endodont* 10:9, 1984.
12. Dwyer TG, Torabinejad M: Radiographic and histologic evaluation of the effect of endotoxin on the periapical tissues of the cat, *J Endod* 7:31, 1981.
13. Fish EW: Bone infection, *J Am Dent Assoc* 26:691-712, 1939.
14. Fouad A et al: Induced periapical lesions in ferret canines: histologic and radiographic evaluation, *Endodont Dent Traumatol* 8:56-62, 1992.
15. Happonen RP: Periapical actinomycosis: a follow-up study of 16 surgically treated cases, *Endodont Dent Traumatol* 2:205-209, 1986.
16. Hasioka K et al: The relationship between clinical symptoms and anaerobic bacteria from infected root canals, *J Endod* 18:558-561, 1992.
17. Hedman WJ: An investigation into residual periapical infection after pulp canal therapy, *Oral Surg* 4:1173-1179, 1951.
18. Iwu C et al: The microbiology of periapical granulomas, *Oral Surg* 69:502-505, 1990.
19. Kakehashi S, Stanley HR, Fitzgerald RJ: The effects of surgical exposure of dental pulps in germ-free and conventional laboratory rats, *Oral Surg* 20:340, 1965.
20. Kantz WE, Henry CA: Isolation and classification of anaerobic bacteria from intact pulp chambers of non-vital teeth in man, *Arch Oral Biol* 19:91-96, 1974.
21. Kirya T et al: Bacteria invading periapical cementum, *J Endod* 20:169-172, 1994.
22. Koppang HS et al: Cellulose fibers from endodontic paper points as an etiologic factor in post-endodontic periapical granulomas and cysts, *J Endod* 15:369-372, 1989.
23. Korzen BH, Krakow AA, Green DB: Pulpal and periapical tissue responses in conventional and noninfected gnotobiotic rats, *Oral Surg* 37:782, 1974.
24. Lalonde ER, Luebke RG: The frequency and distribution of periapical cysts and granulomas, *Oral Surg* 25:861, 1968.
25. Langeland K, Block RM, Grossman LI: A histopathologic and histobacteriologic study of 35 periapical endodontic surgical specimens, *J Endod* 3:8, 1977.
26. Menkin V: *Dynamics of inflammation,* New York, 1940, Macmillan.
27. Moeller AJR et al: Influence on periapical tissues of indigenous oral bacteria and necrotic pulp tissue in monkeys, *Scand J Dent Res* 890:475-484, 1981.
28. Molven O, Halse A, Grung B: Incomplete healing (scar tissue) after periapical surgery: radiographic findings 8 to 12 years after treatment, *J Endod* 22:264-268, 1966.
29. Mortensen H, Winther JE, Birn H: Periapical granulomas and cysts: an investigation of 1600 cases, *Scand J Dent Res* 78:141, 1971.
30. Morton TH, Clagett JA, Yavorsky JD: Role of immune complexes in human periapical periodontitis, *J Endod* 3:261, 1977.
31. Nair PNR, Pajarola G, Schroeder HE: Types and incidence of human periapical lesions obtained with extracted teeth, *Oral Surg* 81:93-101, 1996.
32. Nair R: Light and electron microscopic studies of root canal flora and periapical lesions, *J Endod* 13:29-39, 1987.
33. Nobuhara W, Del Rio C: Incidence of periradicular pathoses in endodontic treatment failures, *J Endod* 19:315-318, 1993.
34. Patterson SS, Shafer WG, Healey HJ: Periapical lesions associated with endodontically treated teeth, *J Am Dent Assoc* 68:191, 1964.
35. Ranta K, Haapasalo M, Ranta H: Monoinfection of root canals with *Pseudomonas aeruginosa, Endodont Dent Traumatol* 4:269-272, 1988.
36. Roane JB, Marshall, FJ: Osteomyelitis: a complication of pulpless teeth, *Oral Surg* 34:257, 1972.
37. Seltzer S, Soltanoff W, Bender IB: Epithelial proliferation in periapical lesions, *Oral Surg* 27:111, 1969.
38. Simon JHS: Incidence of periapical cysts in relation to the root canal, *J Endod* 6:845, 1980.
39. Sjogren U et al: Survival of *Arachnia propionica* in periapical tissue, *Int Endod J* 21:277-282, 1988.
40. Stabholz A, McArthur WP: Cellular immune response of patients with periapical pathosis to necrotic dental pulp antigens determined by release of LIF, *J Endod* 4:282, 1978.
41. Sundquist G, Johansson E, Sjogren U: Prevalence of black-pigmented *Bacteroides* species in root canal infections, *J Endod* 15:13-19, 1989.
42. Tani-Ishii N et al: Histological findings of human leprosy periapical granulomas, *J Endod* 22:120-122, 1966.
43. Ten Cate AR: The epithelial cell rests of Malassez and the genesis of the dental cyst, *Oral Surg* 34:957, 1972.
44. Toller P: Origin and growth of cysts of the jaws, *Ann R Coll Surg Engl* 40:306, 1967.
45. Torabinejad M, Bakland LK: Immunopathogenesis of chronic periapical lesions, *Oral Surg* 46:685, 1978.
46. Torabinejad M, Bakland LK: Prostaglandins: their possible role in the pathogenesis of pulpal and periapical disease (parts I and II). *J Endod* 6:733, 769, 1980.
47. Torabinejad M, Kettering JD: Detection of immune complexes in human dental periapical lesions by anticomplement immunofluorescence technique, *Oral Surg* 48:256, 1979.
48. Torabinejad M et al: Concentrations of leukotriene B$_4$ in symptomatic and asymptomatic periapical lesions, *Endodont* 18:205-208, 1992.
49. Tronstad L et al: Extraradicular endodontic infections, *Endodont Dent Traumatol* 3:86-90, 1987.
50. Tronstad L et al: Periapical bacterial plaque in teeth refractory to endodontic treatment, *Endodont Dent Traumatol* 6:73-77, 1990.
50a. Valderhaug J: Histologic study of experimentally induced vadicular cysts, *Int J Oral Surg* 1:137-147, 1972.
50b. Valderhaug J: Histologic study of experimentally produced intraoral odontogenic fistulae in monkeys, *Int J Oral Surg* 2:54-61, 1973.
51. Walton RE, Ardjmand K: Histological evaluation of the presence of bacteria in induced periapical lesions in monkeys, *Endodont* 18:216-221, 1992.
52. Walton RE, Garnick JJ: The histology of periapical inflammatory lesions in permanent molars in monkeys, *Endodont* 12:49-53, 1986.
53. Wayman B et al: A bacteriological and histological evaluation of 58 periapical lesions, *J Endod* 18:152-155, 1992.
54. Wesselink PR, Thoden van Velzen SK, Makkes PC: Release of endotoxin in an experimental model simulation of the dental root canal, *Oral Surg* 45(5):789, 1978.

Chapter 13

Microbiology and Immunology

James D. Kettering
Mahmoud Torabinejad

Pulpal and periradicular pathosis are usually induced as a result of direct or indirect involvement of oral bacteria. This was demonstrated nearly a century ago and has been confirmed with more advanced bacteriologic and immunologic tests. Based on present knowledge, it appears that most changes in pulpal and periradicular tissues are of bacterial origin and must be dealt with as infectious processes. Because bacteria play a major role in the pathogenesis of pulpal and periradicular lesions, a fundamental knowledge of endodontic microbiology is needed to understand (1) the role of bacteria in these diseases, (2) pathways of pulpal and periradicular infections, (3) the responses of pulpal and periradicular tissues to bacterial infection, and (4) the methods used to control and eradicate root canal infections during root canal therapy. Tronstad[92] has summarized recent developments in endodonic research, relating how these principles apply to the management of patients with endodontic problems.

ROLE OF BACTERIA IN PULPAL AND PERIRADICULAR DISEASES

The intact hard tissues of the tooth normally protect the pulp by acting as physical barriers. These tissues can also be viewed as structures, which, while protecting, can physically restrict pulpal inflammation during tissue injuries. Any pulpal injury can result in inflammation and its consequences such as increased vascular permeability, vasodilation, pain, hard tissue resorption, and pulpal necrosis. Although irritants can be physical, thermal, or chemical in nature, microorganisms are considered to be the main cause of pulpal and periradicular pathosis.

In 1890 Miller[53] demonstrated the presence of bacteria in necrotic human pulp tissue. A number of studies have since implicated bacteria as prerequisite for pulpal and periradicular diseases.[11,51] Most studies investigated the flora of infected root canals and have reported the presence of numerous species of bacteria. The predominant species frequently found in infected root canals were streptococci and micrococci and a small percentage of anaerobic bacteria.[105] Depending on the culture media and techniques for bacterial identification, types and number of isolated organisms have varied significantly. Early investigations found a small incidence of anaerobic bacteria, whereas later studies have reported a prevalence as high as 90% of these bacteria in the infected root canals.[38,82]

To demonstrate the importance of bacteria, Kakehashi et al.[37] exposed the dental pulps of conventional and germ-free (gnotobiotic) rats to their own flora, which resulted in the development of pulpal and periradicular lesions in conventional rats but failed to create lesions in germ-free rats.

One investigation[43] studied the effects of normal oral flora and monoinfection (Streptococcus mutans) on the pulp and periradicular tissues of conventional and gnotobiotic rats. Its results showed that the severity of pulpal and periradicular inflammation was directly related to the quantity of microorganisms in the root canals and to how long these tissues were exposed to the microorganisms. Furthermore, it showed that the degree of inflammation was less severe with monoinfection than with mixed infection. Until the early 1970s, most microbiologic studies on root canal flora reported primarily the presence of facultative bacteria in this system. However, technologic advances in the isolation of anaerobes and increased awareness of the medical and dental progressions of the role of anaerobes in various diseases caused significant changes in medical and dental bacteriology. Based on the results of more recent studies, it appears that root canal infections are multibacterial and that anaerobic organisms, namely Bacteroides species, play a significant role in clinical signs and symptoms of pulpal and periradicular disease.[82] Bacteroides species have recently undergone classification changes. New genus names, Porphyromonas and Prevotella, have been assigned to many of the Bacteroides organisms routinely mentioned in endodontic research and clinical reports. Since both genera names are still encountered, we list both for clarity.

Other investigators, in a series of experiments, examined the importance of bacteria in the development of periradicular lesions, composition of root canal flora, and the influence of a combination of oral bacteria on periradicular tissues of monkeys. In one study[56] the researchers severed the pulps of teeth in monkeys. The amputated pulps were either immediately sealed aseptically or left open to be contaminated with indigenous oral flora for 1 week and then sealed. After 6 to 7 months, clinical, radiographic, and histologic examinations of the teeth that were sealed aseptically showed no pathologic changes in their periradicular tissues. In contrast, teeth with infected root canals had inflammatory reactions in their tissues. In another experiment[24] the investigators mechanically devitalized the pulps of monkeys, left them exposed to oral flora for 1 week, and then sealed them for 3, 6, and 35 months. Bacteriologic examinations of infected root canals at the end of these observation periods showed that 85% to 98% of the isolated bacteria were anaerobic. The most frequently found anaerobic species were Bacteroides and gram-positive anaerobic rods. A small percentage of facultative anaerobic bacteria was also isolated from the infected root canals.

Like most bacteria, anaerobes require specific environmental factors for their growth. Several investigators have shown that anaerobic bacteria, such as *Bacteroides*, are usually isolated from mixed infections and acquire some of their nutritional needs from their accompanying infective organisms.[74,81] One study[26] reported that hemin and vitamin K were essential elements for the growth of certain strains of *Prevotella melaninogenica (Bacteroides melaninogenicus)*.

Socransky and Gibbons[74] showed in an animal study that these substances could be provided to *Prevotella melaninogenica (Bacteroides melaninogenicus)* by gram-positive bacteria in mixed infections. Later studies[48] suggest that presence of hemin or succinates significantly increases the virulence of *Porphyromonas (Bacteroides) gingivalis*.

Schifferle et al.[68] showed that protoporphyrin IX and inorganic iron can replace the hemin growth requirement of *Porphyromonas (Bacteroides) gingivalis*. Their studies concluded that in vivo protophophyrin availability may modulate host cellular membrane protein expression and, in turn, affect host immune responses against *Porphyromonas (Bacteroides) gingivalis*.

Fabricius et al.[23] inoculated 75 root canals of monkeys with 11 bacterial species separately, or in combinations, and sealed the access cavities for a period of 6 months. Their bacteriologic and histologic examinations showed that mixed infections have a greater capacity to cause apical lesions than do monoinfections. Furthermore, they reported that the *Bacteroides* strain did not survive in the root canals when inoculated as pure cultures. Enterococci survived as pure cultures, and facultative streptococci induced small periradicular lesions. Sundqvist[82] demonstrated a high correlation between the presence of *Prevotella melaninogenica (Bacteroides melaninogenicus)* and clinical and radiographic signs and symptoms of periradicular pathosis. Griffee et al.[29] also found a similar correlation between the presence of this organism and pain, sinus tract formation, and foul odor. Other researchers[108] found that *Peptococcus magnus* and *Bacteroides* species were commonly associated with symptomatic cases, whereas oral streptococci and enteric bacteria were isolated from asymptomatic cases. Haapasalo[32] reported on the bacteriology of 62 infected human root canals, giving special attention to the *Bacteroides* species. His results confirmed the findings of previous investigations: almost all root canal infections are mixed, and acute symptoms are usually related to the presence of specific anaerobes, such as *Porphyromonas (Bacteroides) gingivalis*, *Porphyromonas (Bacteroides) endodontalis*, and *Prevotella (Bacteroides) buccae*.

Brook et al.[7] confirmed the polymicrobial nature of bacteria isolated from aspirates of periradicular abscesses in 39 patients, with anaerobic isolates being present in more than 70% of the bacteria recovered. Wasfy et al.[100] obtained similar results in the microbiologic evaluation of periradicular infections when they found that anaerobic bacteria were the predominant flora in specimen cultures. Anaerobes comprised 73% (190 of 259) of cultivable bacteria.

Gomes et al.[27] found significant associations between individual clinical features and the following pairs of species: (a) pain (37 cases) and *Peptostreptococcus* species/*Prevotella* species, *Peptostreptococcus* species/*Prevotella melaninogenica*, *Peptostreptococcus micros*/*Prevotella melaninogenica* (all $P < 0.01$); (b) swelling (23 cases) and *Peptostreptococcus micros*/*Prevotella* species ($P < 0.01$); "wet" canal (57 cases) and *Prevotella* species/*Eubacterium* species ($P < 0.01$), *Peptostreptococcus* species/*Eubacterium* species ($P < 0.05$). The authors suggested from this study that statistically significant associa-

tions exist between individual symptoms and signs and particular combinations of specific bacteria.

PATHWAYS OF PULPAL AND PERIRADICULAR INFECTIONS

Under normal circumstances, pulp tissue and its surrounding dentin are protected by the enamel and cementum. Anything that causes the loss of natural enamel or cementum (including caries or iatrogenic etiologic agents) exposes the dentin (and eventually the pulp tissue) to the injurious effects of mechanical, chemical, and microbial irritants. The major pathways of pulpal contamination are exposed dentinal tubules, direct pulp exposure, lateral and apical foramen, and blood-borne bacteria.

Dentinal Tubules

Following loss of enamel or cementum the dentinal tubules become exposed to the bacteria present in the oral cavity. The dentinal tubules extend from the pulp to the dentinoenamel and cementodentinal junctions. The diameters of these tubules are approximately 2.5 μm near the pulp and about 1 μm at the dentinoenamel and cementodentinal junctions. Although an actual quantitation of the dentinal tubules has not been performed, their numbers are large: approximately 15,000 dentinal tubules in a square millimeter of dentin near the cementodentinal junction. Because of the size and numbers of tubules in the dentin, microorganisms can enter, multiply, and invade numerous exposed tubules.

A number of investigators have shown the presence of bacteria within the exposed dentinal tubules of vital and pulpless teeth. Experiments in vivo and in vitro show that dentinal tubules of viable dentin are not easily invaded by oral microorganisms.[58] Slow invasion of viable dentin by bacteria might be due to the presence of natural resistance factors in the dentin and the pulp tissue.

Hoshino et al.[35] used anaerobic procedures to demonstrate the early bacterial invasion of unexposed dental pulps, which were covered by clinically sound dentin beneath the carious lesions. Six of nine teeth had bacterial invasion, with the predominant organisms being obligate anaerobes. The authors concluded that the organisms isolated in this study had passed through some individual dentinal tubules on the way to invasion of the dental pulp.

One investigator[18] who demonstrated bacteria in the dentinal tubules of pulpless teeth attributed their presence to the invasion of these tubules after pulpal necrosis. Presence of bacteria, their by-products, and other irritants in the dentinal tubules usually results in inflammatory responses in pulpal tissue. Pulpal inflammation can also occur when dentinal tubules transport irritants from incipient caries to the pulp or when the tubules contain and permit passage of microorganisms present beneath the restorative dental materials or next to periodontal pockets.[6,50] Leakage studies[6] indicate that bacterial penetration around dental materials may contribute more to pathogenic changes in pulpal tissue than do the chemicals present in these materials. Another study[1] examined the presence of bacteria in the dentin of periodontally involved teeth and compared it with that of teeth with a healthy periodontium. They found more microorganisms in the dentin and pulpal tissue of the periodontally involved teeth than in those of normal teeth. Removal of cementum during periodontal therapy can expose numerous dentinal tubules to oral flora, which can allow the penetration of microorganisms into the pulp tissue. Production of a smear layer during root manipulation and calcium and phosphate ions in saliva can delay invasion of the dentinal tubules by oral microorganisms.

Sen et al.[70] define the smear layer as an amorphous, irregular, and granular appearing layer of material composed of dentin, remnants of pulp tissue and odontoblastic processes, and sometimes bacteria. When root canals are instrumented during endodontic therapy, this layer is always formed on the canal walls. It has been shown that this layer is not a complete barrier to bacteria, and it delays but does not abolish the action of endodontic disinfectants. The removal of the smear layer is apparently controversial at this time, and the presence or absence may affect the durability of the apical and coronal seal. The authors point out that once this layer is removed, there is risk of reinfecting dentinal tubules if the seal fails. Further studies are needed to establish the clinical importance of the absence or presence of the smear layer.

Infection by dentinal tubules is generally thought to occur as an advancing bacterial front, and it is therefore slow. Most authors believe that acid-producing bacteria (with gram-positive organisms predominating) invade the tubules and demineralize the walls. Proteolytic species follow, acting on the organic matrix, which is denuded in the enlarged dentinal tubules. The acids and other metabolites and toxic products diffuse faster than the bacteria, so that the odontoblasts are affected, possibly leading to their breakdown. If the advancing bacteria are eliminated, healing may occur. Dental caries is the most common cause of pulp injury, and many pulp reactions may be long-standing infections from dentinal tubules, originating from the cavity bottom and walls as a result of leaky filling materials. If untreated, bacteria finally reach pulp tissue, and the inflammation ensues. Bacterial numbers increase, polymorphonuclear neutrophil leukocytes (PMNs) infiltrate, and abscesses form, leading to the death of the pulp tissue. This route of infection appears to be selective for only a few bacterial strains, mostly facultative anaerobic bacteria found in the oral flora.

Siqueira et al.[73] evaluated the ability of anaerobic bacteria commonly isolated from endodontic infections to penetrate dentinal tubules and determined that all bacterial strains tested were able to penetrate into tubules, although to different extents. Love[47] found that the pattern of bacterial invasion of the dentinal tubules of the cervical and midroot areas had a heavy infection of bacteria, penetrating as deep as 200 μm. Invasion of the apical dentin was significantly different, with a mild infection and maximal penetration of 60 μm.

Pulp Exposure

In addition to contaminated dentinal tubules, direct pulpal exposure as a result of traumatic injuries or tooth decay can obviously cause contamination of pulpal tissue.

As a consequence of pulpal exposure to oral flora, the pulp and its surrounding dentin can harbor bacteria and their byproducts. Depending on the virulence of the bacteria, host resistance, amount of circulation, and degree of drainage, pulp tissue may stay inflamed for an extended period of time, or it may rather rapidly become necrotic. After pulpal necrosis the entire root canal system becomes infected with various species of bacteria, which can diffuse from this system into the periodontal ligament through the apical foramen or lateral canals. Bacteria within the root canal system usually results in

the development of periradicular and sometimes lateral lesions.

If the pulp is exposed, as with caries for example, the pulp is exposed to the entire oral flora. α-Hemolytic streptococci, enterococci, and lactobacilli are most often found; other facultatively anaerobic organisms are present in smaller numbers. As the depth of the necrotic pulp increases, more species of obligately anaerobic bacteria become established. These include anaerobic gram-positive cocci and gram-negative rods and are favored by the low oxygen tension found in the necrotic parts of the pulp. The mixed complex of mainly anaerobic flora present can influence the symptoms that patients may experience.

Periodontal Ligament

Although a clear cause-and-effect relationship exists between root canal infection and periradicular or lateral lesions, penetration of bacteria in the opposite direction (toward the pulp) during periodontal disease is a subject of controversy and current investigation. Theoretically, patent lateral canals and apical foramina adjacent to periodontal pockets should provide access for oral microorganisms to the root canal system. When the pulp is infected through the apical foramen, it appears that an impaired state of the pulp is always a prerequisite for infection. Only a few species of facultatively anaerobic streptococci appear to be involved. Grossman[31] applied *Serratia marcescens* over the labial gingiva of dogs' and monkeys' teeth and traumatized them with a metal weight. After recovering the same organism from pulpal tissue, he concluded that the periodontal ligament provided pathways for passage of these organisms into the pulpal tissue.

Kiryu et al.[42] investigated whether microorganisms are able to invade periapical cementum from the adjacent periapical lesions. They isolated seven obligate anaerobes and one aerotolerant anaerobe from cementum samples taken from 10 amputated tooth roots at the time of apicoectomy. These included the genera of *Prevotella, Peptostreptococcus, Eubacterium, Fusobacterium,* and the aerotolerant *Campylobacter.* The authors concluded that bacteria could successfully invade cementum via periapical periodontal tissue and that such bacteria could play a significant role in chronic periapical pathosis.

Anachoresis

Another possible source of pulpal contamination and infection is anachoresis. This phenomenon is defined as a positive attraction of blood-borne microorganisms to inflamed or necrotic tissue during a bacteremia. In 1939 Csernyei[19] demonstrated for the first time the anachoretic effect of periradicular inflammation in dogs. After an application of croton oil to the pulp tissues of rats' teeth and injection of microorganism into the bloodstream, Robinson and Boling[64] localized the same organism that was applied to the pulp tissues of rats' teeth and injected into the bloodstream in the damaged tissues. Later other investigators confirmed their results histopathologically.[10] It has been long reported that dental extractions, and even toothbrushing, can produce bacteremia.[69] During bacteremia, circulating microorganisms can be attracted to and can be localized in inflamed or necrotic pulps. Despite its occurrence in experimental animals, the contribution of anachoresis as a major source of pulpal infection in human beings has not been clearly demonstrated.

Regardless of their pathways, after entering the pulp tissue the bacteria colonize, multiply, and contaminate the entire root canal system and possibly the periradicular tissues. Depending on the level of oxygen tension and the presence or absence of essential nutrients in the root canal system, specific groups of bacteria survive and establish the flora of infected root canals.

Flora of Root Canal and Periradicular Lesions

Most root canal infections appear to be multibacterial. At the present time, a number of investigators have been or are attempting to define the role of specific microorganisms or groups of bacteria in pathogenesis of pulpal and periradicular lesions.

Dark-field microscopy[85] represents a limited methodology for identifying these organisms. Yet the technique has demonstrated that cocci, rods, filaments, spirochetes, and motile organisms are present and have all been identified in infected root canals. Trope et al.[93] suggested that a dark-field microscopic spirochete count of lesion exudates may be useful to differentiate between an endodontic lesion or a periodontal lesion. This could be significant, since successful treatment results depend on an accurate diagnosis. More sophisticated studies are required to conclusively identify individual or groups of bacteria as causative agents. At the same time, it has also been suggested that some pulpless teeth appear to be sterile, including those that show radiographic evidence of periradicular pathosis. This has been used to question the exact role of microorganisms in pathologic changes in the pulp and periradicular diseases. In view of the recent reports, however, the basis of such uncertainty lies in the limited technology and interpretation of experiments in these studies.

Early studies[105] generally reported a predominance of facultative organisms over obligately anaerobic species. *Streptococcus* (α and γ) species, gram-negative cocci, and lactobacilli were most often recovered, with a variety of anaerobes (varying in their resistance to atmospheric oxygen) usually found in numbers that constituted less than 50% of the total isolates reported. Through the use of improved techniques, a large variety of bacteria (genera and species) have been isolated from root canals and periradicular lesions. Exemplar studies[38,104] have given information that allows us to recognize a few generalities. Organisms most often found appear to be normal or usual flora of the oral cavity; only rarely is a bacterium recovered that can be shown to originate from other parts of the body. The composition of the microbiota from different infected root canals shows a great variability.[104] The variations that are reported relate to the distribution of anaerobes versus facultative organisms and the different bacterial forms and species. In those cases where quantitation was attempted, the total count of bacteria varied from tooth to tooth.[104]

In general, a mixed flora of bacteria can be isolated in the various studies. This mixture usually comprises five to eight species. Studies[32,82] have suggested that several *Bacteroides* species are more likely to be involved rather than just one species. Such reports must be viewed in comparison with the more than 300 known bacterial species that are known to reside in the oral cavity. Obviously the organisms that do eventually become involved in root canal infections have to survive a harsh selection process. Although finding several different species at once is common, it is usual for one or two of the species to dominate the mixture. Table 13-1 shows a range of bacteria that have been isolated from earlier studies, circa 1980 to 1982.

A number of organisms have been identified to a species level; however, it is not uncommon to find results reporting

Table 13-1. Typical bacteriologic report of organisms identified (circa 1980 to 1982)

Organism	Relative No.
Aerobic	
Streptococcus salivarius	3
α-Hemolytic streptococci	2
γ-Hemolytic streptococci	1
Anaerobic	
Gram-positive cocci	
Peptococcus constellatus	3
Peptococcus intermedius	2
Peptococcus species	3
Peptostreptococcus micros	4
Microaerophilic streptococci	5
Gram-negative cocci	
Veillonella parvula	44
Gram-positive bacilli	
Actinomyces species	3
Eubacterium species	1
Lactobacillus species	3
Gram-negative bacilli	
Bacteroides bivius	1
Bacteroides corrodens	3
Bacteroides melaninogenicus asaccharolyticus	2
Bacteroides melaninogenicus intermedius	1
Bacteroides melaninogenicus melaninogenicus	2
Bacteroides melaninogenicus species	4
Bacteroides ochraceus	1
Bacteroides oralis	3
Bacteroides species	3
Fusobacterium nucleatum	3
Fusobacterium species	2

Modified from Brook I, Grimm S, Kielich RB: *J Endod* 7:380, 1981.

only different members of specific genera. Although the explanations for this limited identification are probably varied, a prime reason may be the limited capabilities of such identification processes that were available in the respective research laboratories or even clinical laboratories. Nevertheless, the combined data clearly demonstrate the variations in types and numbers of microorganisms that were isolated and identified in this period.

As more studies are published, we are better able to appreciate the multibacterial etiology that most likely exists in endodontic problems. Debelian et al.[20] recovered *Propionibacterium acnes* from root canals and blood samples taken during and after patient treatment. *Actinomyces israelii* was isolated from an unusual case of a persistent infection related to a root-filled tooth.[25] *Streptococci mutans* (NCTC 10832) was reported to be noncariogenic in monoinfected gnotobiotic rats by Watts and Paterson,[102] but the same organism was associated with extensive periradicular inflammation 28 days after the creation of untreated pulpal exposures.

Other studies[45,104] have taken advantage of improved procedures and sampling methodologies to accurately sample anaerobic niches and maintain microorganism viability. Improved identification procedures, often with mechanized systems using a computer-based microorganism library, now enable investigators routinely to identify organisms to the species level. Table 13-2 contains a typical list of bacteria that have

Table 13-2. Identity of bacterial strains isolated from 50 acute peripheral abscesses

	No. of Isolates
Facultative Anaerobes	
Actinomyces meyeri	1
Actinomyces naeslundii	1
Actinomyces odontolyticus	1
Arachnia propionica	1
Capnocytophaga ochraceus	1
Eikenella corrodens	1
Haemophilus parainfluenzae	2
Lactobacillus fermentum	2
Lactobacillus salivarius	1
Streptococcus milleri	25
Streptococcus mitior	3
Streptococcus mitis	3
Streptococcus mutans	1
TOTAL	43
Strict Anaerobes	
Bacteroides capillosus	1
Bacteroides distasonis	1
Bacteroides gingivalis	14
Bacteroides intermedius	5
Bacteroides melaninogenicus	12
Bacteroides oralis	20
Bacteroides ruminicola	6
Bacteroides uniformis	1
Bacteroides ureolyticus	1
Eubacterium lentum	1
Fusobacterium mortiferum	1
Fusobacterium nucleatum	6
Peptococcus species	32
Peptostreptococcus species	14
Propionibacterium acnes	1
Streptococcus constellatus	1
Streptococcus intermedius	3
Veillonella parvula	3
TOTAL	123

Modified from Lewis MAO, McFarlane TW, McGowan DA: *J Med Microbiol* 21:101, 1986.

been reported in these later studies; and Table 13-3 presents a current report on bacterial species recovered from periradicular lesions with possible oral cavity communication and with no obvious communication.[103]

The black-pigmented *Bacteroides* species have gained special prominence in the search for etiologic organisms associated with endodontic infections.[80] This genus is a rather heterogeneous group of microorganisms. These were divided into eight separate species, including *B. asaccharolyticus, B. corporis, B. denticola, B. endodontalis,*[96] *B. gingivalis, B. intermedius, B. melaninogenicus,* and *B. loeschei.* These organisms are able to produce abscesses that are severe and spread rapidly. *B. intermedius* and *B. endodontalis* appear to produce localized abscesses.[8] Current classification names for these organisms include *Porphyromonas (gingivalis* and *endodontalis)* and *Prevotella (melaninogenica* and *intermedia).*

Little or no information is available regarding the virulence of the other black-pigmented *Bacteroides* species. Haapsalo[32] has summarized the frequency of isolation of these species in human dental root canal infections.

In contrast to the presence of numerous studies on root canal flora, information on the microbiota of periradicular tissues subsequent to root canal infection is both limited and controversial. Grossman[30] states that although a tooth with a granuloma may have an infected root canal, it usually has sterile periradicular tissue. *"A granuloma is not an area in which bacteria live, but in which they are destroyed."* The relative sterility of periradicular lesions of pulpal origin has been claimed by some investigators.[44,75] However, others have supported the concept that bacteria are present in periradicular lesions and that their presence initiates and perpetuates such lesions.[86]

The location of and certain combinations of organisms are starting to be recognized as significant. Baumgartner and Falkler[4] examined the apical 5 mm of root canals from 10 freshly extracted teeth. Of the 50 bacterial isolates, 34 (68%) were strict anaerobes, demonstrating the predominance of such organisms in this site. Walton and Ardjmand[99] found bacterial masses at the apical foramen of induced periradicular lesions in monkeys and concluded that such masses could contaminate periradicular tissues during surgery or extraction and could give a false-positive result on microbiologic sampling. Watts and Paterson[101] found bacteria in only a minority of sections of root canals and periradicular tissues of albino rats, with and without traumatic pulpal exposures. More research must be conducted to clearly delineate this situation.

Sato et al.[67] investigated the bacterial composition of necrotic pulps of human teeth by sampling the split surfaces of freshly extracted teeth and culturing for microorganisms using reliable anaerobic techniques. Of the 276 bacterial isolates, 251 (91%) were obligate anaerobes. The genera *Peptostreptococcus* (25%), *Propionibacterium* (19%), *Eubacterium* (17%), and *Fusobacterium* (13%) were most commonly recovered. *Bifidobacterium* (2%), *Lactobacillus* (1%), *Actinomyces* (1%), and *Veillonella* (0.7%) were also recovered. The microflora of necrotic pulps of human deciduous teeth was, in the authors' conclusions, similar to that reported for the deep layers of dentinal lesions of adults.

Studies recognizing synergy or a positive correlation between species are also available. Simonson et al.[72] reported a highly significant synergistic relationship between *Treponema denticola* and *Porphyromonas (Bacteroides) gingivalis,* whereas Sundqvist[78] found strong positive correlations between *Fusobacterium nucleatum* and *Peptostreptococcus micros* and *Porphyromonas (Bacteroides) endodontalis, Selenomonas sputigena,* and *Wolinella recta.* Such results are consistent with the concept of a special and selective environment in the root canal that is due in part to the cooperative and antagonistic nature of the relationships between bacteria in the root canal. A greater response of the dental pulp to combinations of *Lactobacillus plantarium* and *Streptococcus mutans* (NTCC 10919) has also been reported.[60]

Microorganisms and their products have been shown to be directly responsible for tissue damage or immunologic responses. Extracts of *Porphyromonas (Bacteroides) gingivalis* were found to be toxic to cultivated human pulpal cells and L929 cells.[61] Extensive bone loss was associated with a periradicular infection with this organism and complement activation by lipopolysaccharides purified from gram-negative bacteria isolated from infected root canals.[34] Sundqvist[79] reviewed the selective pressures in the bacterial interrelations and the nutritional supply from the root canal. He accurately noted that endodontic treatment, apart from directly eliminating bacteria,

Table 13-3. Bacterial species recovered from periradicular lesions with possible oral cavity communication (C) and with no obvious communication (N)

Species	Anaerobes		Facultative Anaerobes		Aerobes	
	C	N	C	N	C	N
Gram-positive cocci						
Gamella morbillorum			1	1		
Peptostreptococcus anaerobius	1					
Peptostreptococcus magnus	1					
Peptostreptococcus micros	10	4				
Staphylococcus aureus			1			
Staphylococcus auricularis				1		
Staphylococcus capitis			1	2		
Staphylococcus epidermidis			5	7		
Staphylococcus hominis					1	
Staphylococcus warneri			1			
Streptococcus anginosus constellatus			1	1		
Streptococcus constellatus			1			
Streptococcus intermedius	3			3		
Streptococcus MG intermedius			1			
Streptococcus milleri			1			
Streptococcus mitis			1			
Streptococcus mutans			1			
Streptococcus salivarius			1			
Streptococcus sanguis II			2	1		
Group F β-streptococcus					1	
Gram-negative cocci						
Moraxella osloensis					1	
Veillonella parvula	1	3				
Gram-positive rods						
Actinomyces israelii	2					
Actinomyces meyeri		1				
Actinomyces odontolyticus	2	1				
Bacillus pumilus				1		
Bacillus species				1		
Bifidobacterium		1				
Corynebacterium pyogenes					1	
Corynebacterium species					4	1
Eubacterium lentum	3					
Lactobacillus acidophilus	1					
Lactobacillus casei		1				
Propionibacterium acnes	4	4				
Gram-negative rods						
Bacteroides buccae	4					
Bacteroides distasonis		1				
Bacteroides fragilis		1				
Bacteroides gracilis	4	3				
Bacteroides intermedius	6					
Bacteroides loeschei		1				
Bacteroides melaninogenicus	2	1				
Bacteroides oris	1					
Bacteroides porphomonas gingivalis		1				
Centers for Disease Control (CDC) group M-S		1				
Fusobacterium necrophorum	2					
Fusobacterium nucleatum	8	5				
Fusobacterium varium	1					
Fusobacterium species		1				
Pseudomonas aeruginosa					1	1
TOTAL	56	30	18	18	9	2

Modified from Wayman BE et al: *J Endod* 18:152, 1992.

can disrupt the delicate ecology and deprive persisting bacteria of their nutritional source.

RESPONSES OF PULPAL AND PERIRADICULAR TISSUES TO BACTERIAL INFECTION

Dental pulp and periradicular tissues react to bacterial infections as do other connective tissues elsewhere in the body. The extent of damage depends on the virulence factors of participating bacteria and the resistance factor of the host tissues. The degree of pulpal and periradicular response to bacterial irritants varies from slight tissue inflammation to complete pulpal necrosis or acute periradicular osteomyelitis with systemic signs and symptoms of severe infection.

Dental caries contain numerous species of bacteria, such as *Streptococcus mutans,* lactobacilli, and actinomyces.[49] The population of microorganisms decreases to few or none in the deepest layers of the carious dentin.[106]

As a result of the presence of microorganisms in the dentin, a variety of immunocompetent cells can be recruited to the dental pulp. The pulp is initially infiltrated by chronic inflammatory cells, such as macrophages, lymphocytes, and plasma cells. The concentration of these cells increases as the decay progresses toward the pulp. PMNs are the predominant cells at the site of pulp exposure.

Pulp studies have shown the presence of immunocompetent cells and cells that recognize foreign antigens.[36] As a result of the interaction of microorganisms and their by-products, various mediators of inflammation, such as neuropeptides, vasoactive amines, kinins, complement components, and arachidonic acid metabolites, are released.[87]

Neuropeptides are proteins generated from somatosensory and autonomic nerve fibers following injury. They include substrate P, calcitonin gene-related peptides, and neurokinins originating from the sensory nerve fibers, as well as dopamine β-monooxygenase and neuropeptide Y originating from sympathetic nerve fibers. These substances, which participate in the process of inflammation and pain transmission, were recently demonstrated in intrapulpal nerve fibers using immunohistochemistry.[12,97]

The importance of vasoactive amines, such as histamine, in the pathophysiology of pulpal inflammation has been demonstrated by the presence of histamine-like substances in the walls of blood vessels in experimentally induced pulpitis.[88] High concentrations of kinins have been found in symptomatic human periapical abscesses.[87] Kinins are considered the main mediators of the pain associated with inflammatory responses. The complement system, when activated, causes enhanced phagocytosis, increased vascular permeability, and lysis of cellular antigens. The presence in inflamed pulp of the C3 complement fragment suggests that this system participates in the pathogenesis of pulpitis.[87]

Arachidonic acid is released from the phospholipids of cell membranes as a result of cell damage. When metabolized through the cyclooxygenase or lipoxygenase pathway, various prostaglandins, thromboxanes, and leukotrienes are produced. These metabolites have been identified in experimentally induced pulpitis, and their concentrations have been significantly reduced by the use of nonsteroidal antiinflammatory medications.[87]

Specific immune reactions can also initiate and perpetuate pulpal diseases. Various classes of immunoglobulins have been found in inflamed human dental pulp and in periradicular lesions.[87] An interaction between these immunoglobulins and antigens, such as bacteria or their by-products present in dental caries, can trigger antibody-mediated responses.[33,84] Bergenholtz et al.[5] have induced Arthus type of reactions in the pulp tissue of sensitized monkeys. Bridging of IgE molecules on mast cells in the dental pulp by antigens can initiate type I (anaphylactic) reactions in this tissue.

Although lymphocyte subtypes present in inflamed pulpal tissues have not yet been extensively identified, it is likely that some of these cells are T lymphocytes that participate in the cell-mediated immunologic response. The degree of pulpal inflammation is dependent on the outcome of the interaction of microorganisms, their by-products, and the resistance factors present in pulpal tissue. Based on present evidence, it appears that *Bacteroides* species play an important role in pathogenesis and in clinical signs and symptoms of pulpal and periradicular diseases. Proteinases released from these microorganisms can degrade several important defensive proteins, such as immunoglobulins and complement components.[17,57,80]

Mild infections usually do not result in significant changes in the pulp. However, moderate-to-severe insults can cause a significant release of inflammatory mediators, which results in increased vascular permeability, vascular stasis, and migration of leukocytes to this tissue. The disturbed blood flow, combined with lysosomal enzymes released from disintegrated leukocytes, can cause small abscesses and necrotic foci in the pulp. Uncontrolled pulpal infection or aberrant inflammatory reactions can result in total pulp necrosis and colonization of bacteria in the root canal system.[87] Egress of these organisms or their by-products from the root canal system into the periapical tissues is the main cause for the development of periradicular lesions.

Numerous studies have shown that the root canal system can act as a pathway for host sensitization. As in human pulpal lesions, pathologic changes associated with human periradicular lesions are also mediated by nonspecific inflammatory reactions or specific immunologic responses[87] (Fig. 13-1).

Mast cells are normally found in connective tissues and have been found in human periradicular lesions.[87] Degranulation of these mast cells is usually stimulated by antigens bridging IgE molecules on the mast cells, with the subsequent release of vasoactive amines such as histamine. Mast cells discharging vasoactive amines into the periradicular tissues can, in turn, initiate an inflammatory response or aggravate an existing inflammatory process.[87]

C3 complement components have been found in human periradicular lesions.[87] The inciting activators of the classic and alternate pathways of the complement system include IgM and IgG, bacteria and their by-products, lysosomal enzymes from PMNs, and clotting factors. Most of these activators have been found in pathologically involved periradicular lesions. Activation of the complement system in periradicular tissues can contribute to bone resorption either by destruction of the bone or by inhibition of new bone formation.[87]

Data from several studies indicate that immune responses contribute to the formation and perpetuation of human periradicular lesions. Altered host tissue, bacteria, and their toxins and by-products present in pathologically involved root canals have the antigenic potential to initiate such responses.[87]

The presence of potential allergens, IgE molecules, and mast cells in human periradicular tissues indicates that all the components of an IgE-mediated reaction are present in apical le-

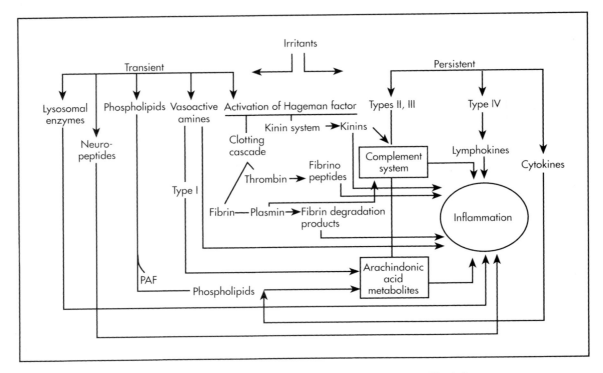

FIG. 13-1 Pathways of inflammation and bone resorption by nonspecific inflammatory mediators and specific immune reactions.

sions and that type I immunologic reactions can occur in these tissues. The presence of various classes of immunoglobulins and immunocompetent cells and the detection of immune complexes and C3 fragments in human apical lesions indicate that type II and type III immune reactions can also occur in periradicular tissues.[87]

In addition to B cells and their by-products (immunoglobulins), cell-mediated reactions also participate in pathogenic changes in periradicular tissues. Natural killer cells as well as other T cells have been found in chronic human apical lesions.[40,89]

By using an indirect immunoperoxidase technique, we examined the presence and relative concentration of B cells and T lymphocytes and their subpopulations in human periradicular lesions.[89] Our findings showed that there were numerous B cells, suppressor T cells, and helper T cells in these lesions and that the T cells outnumbered the B cells significantly (p = 0.0001). These findings have been confirmed by other investigators who have shown that T cells are more numerous than B cells.[83]

Subpopulations of T lymphocytes have been examined in humans and experimental animals. Stashenko and Yu[76] enumerated helper and suppressor T cells in developing rat periradicular lesions. Their findings indicate that helper T cells are predominant during the active phase of lesion development, whereas suppressor T cells are associated with chronic lesions. The presence of different types of lymphocytes in human periradicular lesions suggests that various types of immune reactions participate in the pathogenesis of these lesions.[87] Based on present knowledge, it appears that nonspecific inflammatory and specific immune reactions contribute significantly to the protection—and under certain circumstances—to the destruction of pulpal and periradicular tissues.

In addition to well-defined mediators of inflammation such as neuropeptides, fibrinolytic peptides, kinins, lysosomal enzymes, complement components, and arachidonic acid metabolites,[87] a number of less well-characterized substances are released by a variety of cells. These soluble substances, which are capable of activating other cells, are referred to collectively as *cytokines.* When released from lympcytes they are called *lymphokines;* when released by monocytes, they are referred to as *monokines.* Interleukins are substances that mediate communication between leukocytes. This heterogeneous group of proteins have several common features. Cytokines are glycoproteins secreted as a result of cellular stimulation and have low molecular weights. They are not stored within cells, are produced locally, have very short half-lives, and are extremely potent. They interact with cell surface receptors, which leads to a change in the patterns of cellular RNA and protein synthesis and cell behavior.

The major cytokines include interleukins, interferons, tumor necrosis factor (TNF), and colony-stimulating factors. Most interleukins cause T- or B-cell proliferation, or both, and can stimulate differentiation and proliferation of other inflammatory cells. Among interleukins, IL-1 and IL-6 are proinflammatory and chemotactic for inflammatory cells. Bone resorptive activity of IL-1 is probably due to its effect on osteoclast differentiation from hematopoietic progenitor cells and formation of osteoclast-like giant cells in cultured bone marrow.[87] TNF consists of two proteins (TNF-α and TNF-β) with similar biologic functions. TNF-α is produced mainly by macrophages, whereas TNF-β (lymphotoxin) is the product of activated lymphocytes. Both TNF molecules are potent stimulators of bone resorption and inhibit collagen formation.[87]

TNF has been found in periradicular tissue exudates of teeth with apical periodontitis.[65] IL-1 has also been found in human dental pulps of symptomatic carious teeth and third molars with pericoronitis,[21] human chronic apical lesions,[3] and symptomatic apical lesions.[46] Studies[77] in a rat model system have shown that higher levels of bone resorptive activity are present during the active phase of periradicular lesion expansion than in the chronic phase, and this activity may be due mainly to the presence of molecules in the cytokine molecular weight range of IL-1 and TNF.

METHODS OF CONTROL AND ERADICATION OF ROOT CANAL INFECTIONS

Because bacteria initiate and perpetuate most pulpal and periradicular diseases, disinfection of pathologically involved root canal systems is considered to be paramount in endodontic therapy. The steps involved in the disinfection of root canals are the isolation of the involved teeth, sanitation of the field of operation, and use of sterile instruments, as well as the removal of bacteria, their by-products, and debris. Special precautions taken to prevent recontamination of the cleaned root canal include obturation of the root canal in three dimensions and placement of leak-resistant permanent restorations. Lack of asepsis during root canal therapy, or its poor application, can result in complications for the patient, clinician, and dental auxiliaries.[14]

The presence of bacteria in the root canal system should be dealt with as an infectious process. Like other infectious sites in the body, root canal infections must be debrided mechanically, and under special circumstances supportive measures such as the systemic use of antibiotics should be considered. Unlike causative agents of infections elsewhere in the body, those of root canal infections are within hard tissues and cannot be easily reached by defensive cells of the body. Because of its anatomic location and its complexity, disinfection of the root canal system is performed mainly by mechanical means and is aided by chemical substances.

Isolation and Sanitation of the Field of Operation

Use of physical barriers, such as gloves and the rubber dam, during root canal therapy reduces the incidence of reinfection and lessens the chance of cross-contamination. Human saliva contains numerous species of bacteria. Like other bodily fluids, saliva, gingival fluid, and more importantly blood should be considered infective and sources for the transmission of pathogenic bacteria and viruses. As described previously in Chapter 5, protective barrier techniques such as safety glasses, masks, plastic face shields, and gloves *must* be used to reduce the chance of cross-contamination. Regarding the use of gloves in dental practice, the U.S. Department of Health and Human Services has made the following recommendations[94]:

Gloves must always be worn when touching blood, saliva, or mucous membranes . . . . When all work is completed on one patient, the hands must be washed and regloved before performing procedures on another patient. Repeated use of a single pair of gloves is not recommended, since such use is likely to produce defects in the glove material which will diminish its value as an effective barrier.

Despite these recommendations, some dental professionals still use no gloves at all or use rewashed gloves. An investigation has shown that rewashed gloves remain contaminated even after several washings.[107]

In addition to advocating the use of protective barriers, the U.S. Department of Health and Human Services has made strict recommendations regarding sterilization and disinfection of handpieces and other dental materials and equipment and has specifically recommended the use of rubber dams and high-speed vacuums to minimize generation of droplets and spatter.[94,95] An investigation tested the permeability of three weights of dental rubber dam materials to Phi-X-174 virus particles and *Escherichia coli* bacteria.[9] Results showed that in the absence of manufacturer's defects, rubber dams are capable of providing adequate physical barriers during dental procedures.

Irrigants and Intracanal Medications

Because of the complexity of root canals, cleaning and shaping them by presently available instruments is almost impossible. To aid disinfection, irrigants and sometimes intracanal medications are used during root canal therapy. An ideal intracanal irrigant is a lubricant that can dissolve organic debris, has low toxicity and low surface tension, and is an effective disinfectant or sterilizer. A number of solutions, from distilled water to caustic acids, have been suggested as intracanal irrigants.

Despite its drawbacks, such as tissue toxicity and its limitations in penetrating into the irregularities of the root canal system,[59,71] sodium hypochlorite is the most commonly used intracanal irrigant during root canal therapy. Bystrom and Sundqvist[15] have shown that the use of sodium hypochlorite reduces the bacterial population significantly. This property of sodium hypochlorite is partly due to its antibacterial effect and to its flushing action as an intracanal irrigant.[63,71] In addition, the combination of ultrasound-energized intracanal instruments and constant irrigation has been advocated to enhance cleaning and disinfection of the root canal system.[16]

Some bacteria survive after "complete cleaning and shaping" and therefore can grow in the empty root canal when no intracanal medicament is used between appointments.[13,15] Because of our inability to completely eradicate microorganisms during cleaning and shaping and the inability of present temporary filling materials to provide a bacteria-proof seal between appointments, the use of intracanal medications have been advocated to further reduce the number of microorganisms after cleaning and shaping and before obturation of the root canal system if the case cannot be completed in one visit. Many chemicals (phenolics, aldehydes, antibiotics, steroids, and recently calcium hydroxide) have been used to disinfect the root canal, reduce pain, or render inert the root canal contents.[62] Because of the anatomic configurations of the root canal system and the inherent properties of these medications, such as their toxicity and allergenicity, their routine use and their value as adjuncts to cleaning and shaping have been questioned.[98] Many studies have shown the bactericidal effect of calcium hydroxide against several species of bacteria.[32,66] A recent study has also demonstrated the ability of calcium hydroxide to dissolve organic tissues and debris.[52] *Based on present knowledge of the properties of calcium hydroxide, as an intracanal medication it is preferable to other medications.* Calcium hydroxide paste can be placed into the cleaned root canal by injection or by intracanal instruments and can be flushed out by irrigating the root canal with sodium hypochlorite, alcohol, or sterile water.

Culturing and Identification Techniques

The aim of endodontic treatment is to eliminate the bacteria from the root canals of involved teeth and then to allow for resolution and repair of any damaged periradicular tissues. At one time, various methods were used to check the sterility produced by routine endodontic treatment regimens. Currently this routine culturing is not generally followed because today's standard techniques have been shown to be effective in eliminating the majority of these microorganisms. This has reduced the need to spend a great deal of time and money, which such techniques would require.

There are still several situations wherein bacterial sampling of root canals might be beneficial. Occasionally conventional root canal therapy does not eliminate the symptoms of endodontic infection. If unusual pathogens are present, culturing along with antibiotic-sensitivity testing may be the only way to determine accurately their presence and to select the most appropriate antibiotic.

A number of patients today may require more precise bacteriologic monitoring. These include patients (1) who are undergoing immunosuppressive therapy, (2) who are at high risk for endocarditis, or (3) who have heart valve prostheses may require a sampling at an early appointment to determine whether an antimicrobial susceptibility test may be needed. The wide range of microorganisms that may be encountered in infected root canals may not necessarily be treatable empirically.

Finally, a sterility-check test culture may be taken as a teaching device. Such a sample placed in a medium supporting a wide growth of microorganisms simply requires a *growth-no-growth analysis* to see if the operator has maintained an aseptic technique in the field or operation. The actual process of sampling for microbial culture must be well understood if the results are to be interpreted with confidence.

The role of the endodontic microflora in pulpal disease and in endodontic treatment failures is well established. A recent study[28] evaluated the need for effective microbial control by means of the biomechanical procedures routinely used in such treatments, examining whether the efficacy of this stage of treatment might be dependent on the vulnerability of the involved species, which might not be uniform. In the examination of 42 root canals, microbiologic samples were collected before and after instrumentation, and the bacterial findings were compared for 15 cases of "primary" root canal treatments and 27 cases of "secondary" treatment. When all 42 cases were evaluated, significant decreases were found between first and second samples for anaerobes ($P = 0.0117$) and for gram-positive species ($P = 0.008$), especially *Peptostreptococcus* species ($P = 0.02$). The authors concluded that certain species are more resistant to biomechanical procedures than others.

Taking the Culture

The collecting of root canal samples requires the use of techniques that allow both facultative and anaerobic bacteria to grow. The clinician must keep in mind that contamination with normal oral flora as a result of contact with saliva or careless handling causes false culturing results.

Good aseptic technique in the collection process is an absolute requirement. Next in importance is getting the sample to a microbiologic laboratory where it may be processed with as little delay as possible. A carrier medium should be used that maintains viability of all the organisms in the sample. The actual sampling technique is not difficult to master. It is important to remember that the initial preparation of the site, in large part, determines the success or failure of a good culture sample.

A question might arise as to whether a clinician can collect proper and acceptable microbiologic samples if these are needed only occasionally. Molander et al.[54] evaluated the results of root canal culturing among general dental practitioners within the city of Gothenburg, Sweden, by examining 25 years of laboratory records. Most use of microbiologic root canal sampling (MRS) appeared to be directed toward selection of special cases, and the results of culturing revealed a predominance of facultative bacteria being identified. The authors concluded that although evidence of contamination was found, the practitioners frequently appeared to produce valid microbiologic samples. The same investigators[55] questioned 240 general dentists concerning certain practice characteristics and attitudes to MRS. The data showed that MRS was mainly performed by dentists working with adult patients in private practice and, again, was applied in selected cases. The main reason for not using MRS appeared to be a perceived lack of relative advantage over conventional treatment strategies.

It is essential in the teeth to be sampled that they are first isolated and the crown and rubber dam are disinfected. Any dressing should be removed and discarded. Care should also be taken to remove any excess disinfectant that might contaminate the bacteriologic sample. Antibacterial chemicals should not be placed into the root canal before sampling. Once the root canal is exposed, a sterile absorbent point is inserted into the canal to remove any trace of medication that might be present. This is then discarded. A fresh sterile absorbent point is inserted into the root canal and allowed to remain in place to absorb as much exudate (if any) as possible. If the canal is dry, it can be moistened with transport medium added to the canal, using a soaked sterile paper point. This point is removed, using sterilized cotton pliers, and placed as quickly as possible in a medium or transport solution. Speed of handling and careful choice of medium increase the chances of isolating the more fastidious microorganisms.

In sampling an orofacial lesion or a submucosal abscess the surface area must be disinfected. This sample can be collected by penetrating the lesion with a sterile needle and drawing the fluid into a sterile syringe. Air can be expelled from the syringe after withdrawal, and the needle can be plugged by carefully sticking it into a rubber stopper. This procedure can be used to maintain an anaerobic atmosphere for sample transport, or the material can be transferred to a transport medium, as described above.

Once the sample is collected, it is important to get it to the microbiology laboratory as quickly as possible to ensure successful culturing results. Most dentists are not directly associated with a laboratory capable of isolating and identifying microorganisms from these samples. If such a laboratory is available, proper media and incubation procedures should be used to get both facultative and anaerobic organisms to grow.

Attempts to identify and quantify the different bacteria isolated increase the amount of work that will be required. If a hospital clinical laboratory or commercial laboratory is to be used, it is important to communicate the dentist's specific needs to the personnel involved in sample analysis. Such laboratories often report normal oral flora only in general terms. Once the laboratory realizes that a specific identification is needed, the normal or usual flora can be specifically named and reported.

If antimicrobial testing is needed, it should be done only on pure cultures not on mixtures of microorganisms. Final results are usually available in 4 to 7 days. One advantage of using a clinical or commercial laboratory is that many now use sophisticated, automatic identification systems that rely on computer-based data systems to identify bacterial isolates. Such identities and antibiotic susceptibility tests done with these machines can often produce results in less than 24 hours.

The techniques used to study and identify bacteria are essentially familiar and common. Gram stain examination of an original sample shows the presence or absence of microbes (and identifies gram-positive and gram-negative species) and cells (epithelial, erythrocytes, PMNs). This technique is limited in the information it can express, however. No specific identification of genus or species is possible, and live organisms are not distinguished from dead microbes. It gives only an overview of the bacteria involved and the host's response to the infection.

The media that are routinely used in most diagnostic laboratories easily support the growth of the oral bacteria usually identified as causing endodontic infections. Blood agar enriched to support *Brucella* species growth can serve as an excellent medium for both facultative and fastidious anaerobic microorganisms. Broth media (fluid thioglycolate or chopped meat broth) likewise allow the growth of both. Media that accommodate specific needs for organisms such as yeast, molds, or *Mycobacterium* species can be obtained readily and used as determined by the microbiologist. Specific identification of a wide range of oral microorganisms can be readily achieved. Rare or unusual species may require media or techniques available only in the research laboratory setting.

In determining a final bacterial identification, immunologic techniques combined with standard identification procedures can increase accuracy and decrease the time factor.[88] Fluorescent antibody techniques use a chemical (fluorescein isothiocyanate [FITC]) that can be attached to antibodies (polyclonal or monoclonal). A specific antibody-antigen (bacterial) complex is easily seen when viewed with a fluorescence microscope. Such techniques have been used by several investigators.[2,39]

The enzyme-linked immunosorbent assay (ELISA) uses different labels that can be attached to antibodies instead of FITC. Such labels include horseradish peroxidase or alkaline phosphatase. ELISA tests can be used to identify antigens (bacteria) or to measure antibodies to known antigens. These are well-established procedures and have been used to study the involvement of specific bacteria in the development of pulpal and apical lesions.[41,90]

Because some endodontic treatments are performed in two or more appointments, temporary restorations are used to seal the access cavity preparations between appointments. The most commonly used temporary restorations in root canal therapy are zinc oxide–eugenol (e.g., IRM) and Cavit. One study[22] has shown that IRM was less leakproof than Cavit ($P < 0.05$) and TERM ($P < 0.05$); thermocoupling introduced on the fourth day of the experiment increased percolation of IRM and decreased tightness of Cavit, whereas TERM remained leakproof.

Obturation of the root canal system in three dimensions and consequent elimination of spaces for bacterial growth are the final steps in eradication of infected root canals. Proper condensation of gutta-percha in conjunction with a root canal sealer usually provides an adequate seal after cleaning of the root canals. To avoid recontamination of the root canals and to ensure long-term success, the access cavity to the obturated root canal must be sealed with permanent filling materials within 30 days.

Coronal leakage can occur when root-filled canals are exposed to the oral cavity. After cleaning and shaping and then obturation of 45 root canals, we purposely put the coronal por-

tion of the filling materials in contact with *Staphylococcus epidermidis* or *Proteus vulgaris*.[91] The number of days required for these bacteria to penetrate the entire root canals was measured. Results revealed that more than 50% of the root canals were completely contaminated after 19 days of exposure to *Staphylococcus epidermidis,* and about 50% of the root canals were also totally contaminated when their coronal surfaces were exposed to *Proteus vulgaris* for 42 days. The results of this investigation show the importance of a timely strong coronal seal after completion of root canal therapy.

REFERENCES

1. Adriaens PA, De Boever JA, Loesche WJ: Bacterial invasion in root cementum and radicular dentin of periodontal diseases teeth in humans: a reservoir of periodontopathic bacteria, *J Periodont* 59:222, 1988.
2. Assed S et al: Anaerobic microorganisms in root canals of human teeth with chronic apical periodontitis detected by indirect immunofluoresence, *Endodont Dent Traumatol* 12:66, 1996.
3. Barkhordar RA, Hussain MZ, Hayashi C: Detection of the IL-1β in human periapical lesions, *Oral Surg* 73:334, 1992.
4. Baumgartner JC, Falkler WA: Bacteria in the apical 5 mm of infected root canals, *J Endodont* 17:380, 1991.
5. Bergenholtz Z, Ahlstedt S, Lindhe J: Experimental pulpitis in immunized monkeys, *Scand J Dent Res* 85:396, 1977.
6. Bergenholtz Z et al: Bacterial leakage around dental restorations: its effect on the dental pulp, *Oral Surg* 11:439, 1982.
7. Brook I, Frasier EH, Gher ME: Aerobic and anaerobic microbiology of periapical abscesses, *Oral Microbiol Immunol* 6:123, 1991.
8. Brook I, Grimm S, Kielich RB: Bacteriology of acute periapical abscess in children, *J Endodont* 7:380, 1981.
9. Buoncristiani J, Burch P, Torabinejad M: *Permeability of common dental barriers to small virus particles: student table clinic,* 1988, Loma Linda University.
10. Burke GW, Knighton HT: The localization of microorganisms in inflamed dental pulps of rats following bacteremia, *J Dent Res* 39:205, 1960.
11. Burket LW: Recent studies relating to periapical infection, including data obtained from human necroscopy studies, *J Am Dent Assoc* 25:260, 1938.
12. Byers MR et al: Effects of injury and inflammation on pulpal and periapical nerves, *J Endodont* 16:78, 1990.
13. Bystrom A, Claesson R, Sundqvist G: The antibacterial effect of camphorated paramonochlorophenol, camphorated phenol and calcium hydroxide in the treatment of infected root canals, *Endodont Dent Traumatol* 1:170, 1985.
14. Bystrom A, Sundqvist G: Bacteriologic evaluation of the efficacy of mechanical root canal instrumentation in endodontic therapy, *Scand J Dent Res* 89:321, 1981.
15. Bystrom A, Sundqvist G: The antibacterial action of sodium hypochlorite and EDTA in 60 cases of endodontic therapy, *Int Endodont J* 18:35, 1985.
16. Cameron JA: The use of ultrasonics in the removal of smear layer: a scanning electron microscope study, *J Endod* 9:289, 1983.
17. Carlsson J et al: Degradation of the human proteinase inhibitors alpha$_1$-antitrypsin and alpha$_2$-macroglobulin by *Bacteroides gingivalis,* *Infect Immun* 43:644, 1984.
18. Chrinside I: Bacterial invasion of non-vital dentin, *J Dent Res* 40:134, 1961.
19. Csernyei AJ: Anachoretic effect of chronic periapical inflammation, *J Dent Res* 18:527, 1939.
20. Debelian GJ, Olsen I, Tronstad L: Profiling of *Propionibacterium acnes* recovered from root canal and blood during and after endodontic treatment, *Endodont Dent Traumatol* 8:248, 1992.
21. Desouza R et al: Detection and characterization of IL-1 in human dental pulps, *Arch Oral Biol* 34:307, 1989.
22. Deveaux E et al: Bacterial leakage of Cavit, IRM and TERM, *Oral Surg* 74:634, 1992.

23. Fabricius L et al: Influence of combinations of oral bacteria on periapical tissues of monkeys, *Scand J Dent Res* 90:200, 1982.

24. Fabricius L et al: Predominant indigenous oral bacteria isolated from infected root canals after varied times of closure, *Scand J Dent Res* 90:134, 1982.

25. Figures KH, Douglas CWI: *Actinomyces* associated with a root-treated tooth: report of a case, *Int Endodont J* 24:326, 1991.

26. Gibbons RJ, MacDonald JB: Hemin and vitamin K compounds as required factors for the cultivation of certain strains of *Bacteroides melaninogenicus, J Bacteriol* 80:164, 1980.

27. Gomes BPFA, Lilley JD, Drucker DB: Associations of endodontic symptoms and signs with particular combinations of specific bacteria, *Int Endodont J* 29:69, 1996.

28. Gomes BPFA, Lilley JD, Drucker DB: Variations in the susceptibilities of components of the endodontic microflora to biomechanical procedures, *Int Endodont J* 29:235, 1996.

29. Griffee MB et al: The relationship of *Bacteroides melaninogenicus* to symptoms associated with pulpal necrosis, *Oral Pathol* 50:457, 1980.

30. Grossman LI: Bacteriologic status of periapical tissue in 150 cases of infected pulpless teeth, *J Dent Res* 38:101, 1959.

31. Grossman LI: Origin of microorganisms in traumatized pulpless sound teeth, *J Dent Res* 46:551, 1967.

32. Haapsalo M: *Bacteroides* spp in dental root canal infections, *Endodont Dent Traumatol* 5:1, 1989.

33. Hahn CL, Falkler WA: Antibodies in normal and diseased pulps reactive with microorganisms isolated from deep caries, *J Endod* 18:28, 1991.

34. Horiba N et al: Complement activation by lipopolysaccharides purified from gram-negative bacteria isolated from infected root canals, *Oral Surg* 74:648, 1992.

35. Hoshino E et al: Bacterial invasion of non-exposed dental pulp, *Int Endodont J* 25:2, 1992.

36. Jontell M et al: Dendritic cells and macrophages expressing class II antigens in the normal cat incisor pulp, *J Dent Res* 67:1263, 1988.

37. Kakehashi S, Stanley HR, Fitzgerald RJ: The effects of surgical exposures of dental pulps in germ-free and conventional laboratory rats, *Oral Surg* 20:340, 1965.

38. Kantz WE, Henry CA: Isolation and classification of anaerobic bacteria from intact pulp chamber of non-vital teeth in man, *Arch Oral Biol* 19:91, 1974.

39. Kettering J, Payne W, Prabhu S: Antibody levels against eleven oral microorganisms in an endodontic population, *J Dent Res* 67:202, 1988.

40. Kettering JD, Torabinejad M: Presence of natural killer cells in human chronic periapical lesions, *Int Endodont J* 26:344, 1993.

41. Kettering J, Torabinejad M, Jones S: Identification of bacteria involved in pathogenesis of human periapical lesions by the ELISA technique, *J Endod* 14:198, 1988.

42. Kiryu T, Hoshino E, Iwaku M: Bacteria invading periapical cementum, *J Endod* 20(4):169, 1994.

43. Korzen B, Krakow A, Green D: Pulpal and periapical tissue responses in conventional and monoinfected gnotobiotic rats, *Oral Surg* 37:783, 1974.

44. Langeland K, Block RM, Grossman LI: A histobacteriologic study of 35 periapical endodontic surgical specimens, *J Endod* 3:8, 1977.

45. Lewis MAO, McFarlane TW, McGowan DA: Quantitative bacteriology of acute dento-alveolar abscesses, *J Med Microbiol* 21:101, 1986.

46. Lim GC et al: Interleukin-1-beta in symptomatic and asymptomatic human periradicular lesions, *J Endod* 20(5):225, 1994.

47. Love RM: Regional variation in root dentinal tubule infection by *Streptococcus gordonii, J Endod* 22(6):290, 1996.

48. Maryland D, McBride BC: Ecological relationship of bacteria involved in a simple, mixed anaerobic infection, *Infect Immun* 27:44, 1980.

49. McKay GS: The histology and microbiology of acute occlusal dentin lesions in human permanent premolar teeth, *Arch Oral Biol* 21:51, 1976.

50. Mejare B, Mejare I, Edwardsson S: Acid etching and composite restorations: a culturing and histologic study on bacterial penetration, *Endodont Dent Traumatol* 3:1, 1987.

51. Melville TH, Birch RH: Root canal and periapical floras of the infected teeth, *Oral Surg* 23:93, 1967.

52. Metzler RS, Montgomery S: The effectiveness of ultrasonics and calcium hydroxide for debridement of human mandibular molars, *J Endod* 15:373, 1989.

53. Miller WD: Microorganisms of the human mouth, Philadelphia, 1890, SS White Dental Co, p 96.

54. Molander A, Reit C, Dahlen G: Microbiological root canal sampling: diffusion of a technology, *Int Endodont J* 29:163, 1996.

55. Molander A, Reit C, Dahlen G: Reasons for dentist's acceptance or rejection of microbiological root canal sampling, *Int Endodont J* 29:168, 1996.

56. Moller AJR: Influence on periapical tissues of indigenous oral bacteria and necrotic pulp tissue in monkeys, *Scand J Dent Res* 89:475, 1981.

57. Nilsson T, Carlsson J, Sundqvist G: Inactivation of key factors of the plasma proteinase cascade systems by *Bacteroides gingivalis, Infect Immun* 50:467, 1985.

58. Olgart L, Brannstrom M, Johnson G: Invasion of bacteria into dentinal tubules: experiments in vivo and in vitro, *Acta Odontol Scand* 32:61, 1974.

59. Pashley E et al: Cytotoxic effects of NaOCl on vital tissue, *J Endod* 11:525, 1985.

60. Paterson RC, Watts A: Pulp responses to two strains of bacteria isolated from human carious dentine (*L. plantarium*—NCTC 1406) and *Streptococcus mutans* (NCTC 10919) *Int Endodont J* 25:134, 1992.

61. Pissiotis E, Spangberg LSW: Toxicity of sonicated extracts of *Bacteroides gingivalis* on human pulpal cells and L929 cells in vitro, *J Endod* 17:553, 1991.

62. Pumarola J et al: Antimicrobial activity of seven root canal sealers, *Oral Surg* 74:216, 1992.

63. Ram Z: Effectiveness of root canal irrigation, *Oral Surg* 44:306, 1977.

64. Robinson HBG, Boling LR: The anachoretic effect in pulpitis. I. Bacteriologic studies, *J Am Dent Assoc* 28:268, 1941.

65. Safavi K, Rossomado L: TNF identified in periapical tissue exudates of teeth with apical periodontitis, *J Endod* 17:12, 1991.

66. Safavi K et al: Comparison of antimicrobial effects of calcium hydroxide and iodine-potassium iodide, *J Endod* 11:454, 1985.

67. Sato T, Hoshino E, Uematsu H, Noda T: Predominant obligate anaerobes in necrotic pulps of human deciduous teeth, *Microb Ecol Health Dis* 6:269, 1993.

68. Schifferle RE et al: Effect of protoporphyrin IX limitation on *Porphyromonas gingivalis, J Endod* 22(7):352, 1996.

69. Sconyers JR, Crawford JJ, Moriarty JD: Relationship of bacteremia to toothbrushing in patients with periodontitis, *J Am Dent Assoc* 87:616, 1973.

70. Sen BH, Wesselink PR, Turkun M: The smear layer: a phenomenon in root canal therapy, *Int Endodont J* 28(3):141, 1995.

71. Senia ES, Marshall FJ, Rosen S: The solvent action of sodium hypochlorite on pulp tissue of extracted teeth, *Oral Surg* 31:96, 1971.

72. Simonson LG et al: Bacterial synergy of *Treponema denticola* and *Porphyromonas gingivalis* in a multinational population, *Oral Microbiol Immunol* 7:111, 1992.

73. Siqueira JF, Uzeda MD, Fonseca MEF: A scanning electron microscopic evaluation of in vitro dentinal tubule penetration by selected anaerobic bacteria, *J Endod* 22(6):308, 1996.

74. Socransky SS, Gibbons RJ: Required role of *Bacteroides melaninogenicus* in mixed anaerobic infections, *J Infect Dis* 115:247, 1965.

75. Spångberg L, Engstrom B, Langeland K: Biologic effects of dental materials. 3. Toxicity and antimicrobial effect of endodontic antiseptics in vitro, *Oral Surg* 36:856, 1973.

76. Stashenko P, Yu SM: T helper and T suppressor cell reversal during the development of induced rat periapical lesions, *J Dent Res* 68:830, 1989.

77. Stashenko P, Yu SM, Wang CY: Kinetics of immune cell and bone resorptive responses to endodontic infections, *J Endod* 18:422, 1992.

78. Sundqvist G: Associations between microbial species in dental root canal infections, *Oral Microbiol Immunol* 7:257, 1992.

79. Sundqvist G: Ecology of the root canal flora, *J Endod* 18:427, 1992.

80. Sundqvist G, Johansson E, Sjogren U: Prevalence of black-pigmented *Bacteroides* species in root canal infections, *J Endod* 15:13, 1989.

81. Sundqvist G et al: Capacity of anaerobic bacteria from necrotic dental pulps to induce purulent infections, *Infect Immun* 25:685, 1979.

82. Sundqvist G et al: Degradation of human immunoglobulins G and M and complement factors C3 and C5 by black-pigmented *Bacteroides*, *J Med Microbiol* 19:85, 1985.

83. Tani N et al: Comparative histological identification and relative distribution of immunocompetent cells in sections of frozen or formalin-fixed tissue from human periapical inflammatory lesions, *Endodont Dent Traumatol* 8:163, 1992.

84. Tani N et al: Immunobiological activities of bacteria isolated from the root canals of post endodontic teeth with persistent periapical lesions, *J Endod* 18:58, 1992.

85. Thilo B et al: Dark-field observation of the bacterial distribution in root canals following pulp necrosis, *J Endod* 12:202, 1986.

86. Torabinejad M: Mediators of pulpal and periapical pathosis, *Calif Dent Assoc J* 14:21, 1986.

87. Torabinejad M: Mediators of acute and chronic periradicular lesions, *Oral Surg* 78:511, 1994.

88. Torabinejad M, Bakland LK: Prostaglandins: their possible role in pathogenesis of pulpal and periapical diseases. II, *J Endod* 6:769, 1980.

89. Torabinejad M, Kettering JD: Identification and relative concentration of B and T lymphocytes in human chronic periapical lesions, *J Endod* 11:122, 1985.

90. Torabinejad M, Kettering JD: Immunological techniques in endodontal research. In Spångberg LS, editor: *Experimental endodontics,* Boca Raton, Fla, 1990, CRC Press, pp 155-172.

91. Torabinejad M et al: Factors associated with endodontic interappointment emergencies of teeth with necrotic pulps, *J Endod* 14:261, 1988.

92. Tronstad L: Recent development in endodontic research, *Scand J Dent Res* 100:52, 1992.

93. Trope M, Rosenberg E, Tronstad L: Darkfield microscopic spirochete endodontic and periodontal abscesses, *J Endod* 18:82, 1992.

94. US Department of Health and Human Services: Recommended infection-control practices for dentistry, *MMWR* 35:1, 1986.

95. US Department of Health and Human Services: Recommendations for prevention of HIV transmission in health care settings, *MMWR* 36:75, 1987.

96. van Winkelhoff AJ, van Steenberg JM, de Graaf J: *Porphyromonas (Bacteroides) endodontalis:* its role in endodontal infections, *J Endod* 18:431, 1992.

97. Wakisaka S: Neuropeptides in the dental pulp: distribution, origin, and correlation, *J Endod* 16:67, 1990.

98. Walton RE: Intracanal medicaments, *Dent Clin North Am* 28:783, 1984.

99. Walton RE, Ardjmand K: Histological evaluation of the presence of bacteria in induced periapical lesions in monkeys, *J Endod* 18:216, 1992.

100. Wasfy MO et al: Microbiological evaluation of periapical infections in Egypt, *Oral Microbiol Immunol* 7:100, 1992.

101. Watts A, Paterson RC: Detection of bacteria in histological sections of the dental pulp, *Int Endodont J* 23:1, 1990.

102. Watts A, Paterson RC: Pulp response to, and cariogenicity of, a further strain of *Streptococcus mutans* (NTCC 10832), *Int Endodont J* 25:142, 1992.

103. Wayman BE et al: A bacteriological and histological evaluation of 58 periapical lesions, *J Endod* 18:152, 1992.

104. Williams BL, McCann GF, Schoenknecht FD: Bacteriology of dental abscesses of endodontic origin, *J Clin Microbiol* 18:770, 1983.

105. Winkler KC, van Amerongen J: Bacteriologic results from 4,000 root canal cultures, *Oral Surg* 12:857, 1959.

106. Wirthlin MR: Acid-reacting stains, softening and bacterial invasion in human carious dentin, *J Dent Res* 49:42, 1970.

107. Yetter CG, Torabinejad M, Torabinejad A: An investigation on the safety of rewashed gloves, *J Dent Hyg* 63:358, 1989.

108. Yoshida M et al: Correlation between clinical symptoms and microorganisms isolated from root canals of teeth with periapical pathosis, *J Endod* 13:24, 1987.

Chapter 14

Instruments, Materials, and Devices

Larz S. W. Spångberg

Many instruments, materials, and devices are required for adequate endodontic treatment. This chapter provides a broad orientation to these various groups without providing more than general instruction in their use during endodontic treatment. The reader is referred to the various chapters of this book that discuss treatment. In recent years many new devices and instruments have been brought forward, and it is therefore important that the clinician approaches these with some caution as few have yet been tried by time or scientific assessment. The outline of this chapter follows the natural progression of endodontic treatment.

DIAGNOSTIC MATERIALS AND DEVICES

Radiography is an essential part of endodontic diagnosis. Modern technology is rapidly shifting toward digital filmless imaging. It is important that the endodontist is well informed in this diagnostic field as modern technology has opened up new image enhancing methods.[24,99,125,140,159,165]

Materials for Thermometric Evaluation

Pulp stimulation with heat or cold is the oldest method to evaluate pulpal health and the pulp's ability to respond to external stimulation. This evaluation of pulpal response must not be confused with vitality testing, which requires the evaluation of pulpal circulation.

Heating of the pulp is commonly achieved by applying heated gutta-percha that may reach a temperature of 168.8° F (76° C). Special care should be taken not to damage the pulp with excessive heat. Other methods for conducting the heat test are described in Chapter 1.

Cold test is commonly done by applying ice, a liquid refrigerant, or dry ice. Ice (32° F, 0° C) is limited because it is normally only effective on intact teeth in the anterior part of the mouth. Ethyl chloride (Fig. 14-1) and liquid refrigerant such as dichlorodifluoromethane (Endo Ice, Hygienic Corp., Akron, Ohio) (−21° F, −30° C) provide good sources for lowering the tooth temperature.[45] They are normally not sufficient for the stimulation of a tooth with very extensive restorations or full crown coverage. In these cases dry ice (−108° F, −78° C) is an excellent stimulant (Figs. 14-2 and 14-3). Cold water baths are another effective method described in Chapter 1.

Although both the levels of heat (168.8° F, 76° C) and cold (−108° F, −78° C) are extreme, it has been demonstrated that the effect on the pulp does not jeopardize the health of the pulp if used with care.[178] The understanding of pain responses to thermometric pulp testing has its basis in the hydrodynamic theory for the sensitivity of dentin. Thus the pain sensation the patient experiences requires that the hydrodynamic mechanisms are intact, as the nerves in the pulp do not respond to

heat or cold stimulation. In other words, hot or cold sensation on stimulation is dependent on that a part of a morphologically intact pulp still exists.

Electrometric Pulp Testers

"The basic requirements are an adequate stimulus, an adequate technique of applying this to the teeth and a careful interpretation of the result."[156] This exactly describes the problems and difficulties with electric pulp testing, which is often overused and poorly understood.

Evaluation of responding nerve endings can be done with an electrical pulp tester (Figs. 14-4 and 14-5). Several such instruments are available on the commercial market. An electrical pulp tester, however, is only as good as the person interpreting the patient responses. The sensation the patient may feel when electrical current is passed through the tooth is the result of direct nerve stimulation. There is no reasonable assurance, however, that these nerves are located in an intact pulp. Necrotic and disintegrating pulp tissue often leaves an excellent electrolyte in the pulp space. This electrolyte can easily conduct the electrical current to nerves further down into the pulp space, simulating normal pulp response. This becomes even more complicated in a multirooted tooth, where the health status of the pulp may vary in each root. Positive response to electrometric recordings should not be used for differential diagnosis of pulpal disease.[121] Provided the examination was conducted properly, a lack of response suggests the lack of responding nerve endings. In most cases this means pulp necrosis. If the nerves to the pulp have been transected during surgery, the pulp could still be vital. Pulp tissue is much more sensitive to electrical stimulation than gingival and periapical tissues.[30] Most modern pulp testers cannot put out high enough energies to stimulate periradicular tissues.

Several pulp testers with different characteristics are commercially available. It has been shown that pulsating direct current with a duration of 5 to 15 ms provides the best nerve stimulation.[30,156] The optimal stimulation is achieved when the cathode is used for tooth stimulation. The faster the current is rising, the more effective is the stimulation and the less compensation takes place in the nerves. Somewhat simplified, Ohm's law ($E = R \times I$) is applicable to electrical pulp testing, although the phenomenon most likely is a combination of impedance and resistance. Understanding this explains many phenomena occurring during electrometric pulp testing. Pulp testers operates at a relatively high potential difference (several hundred volts) but at a very low current (μA). Enamel and dentin constitute a very high resistance (Ω) in the electrical circuit through the tooth. Of these, enamel has the highest resistance. In dentin the lowest resistance is parallel with the-

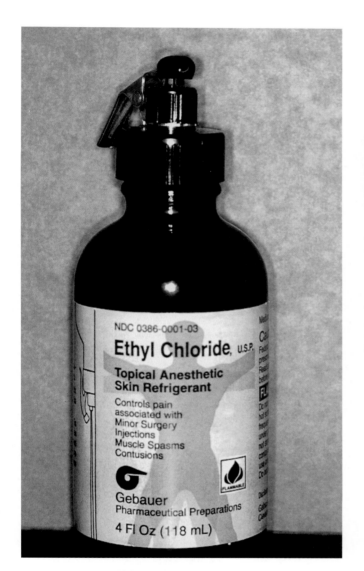

FIG. 14-1 Ethyl chloride.

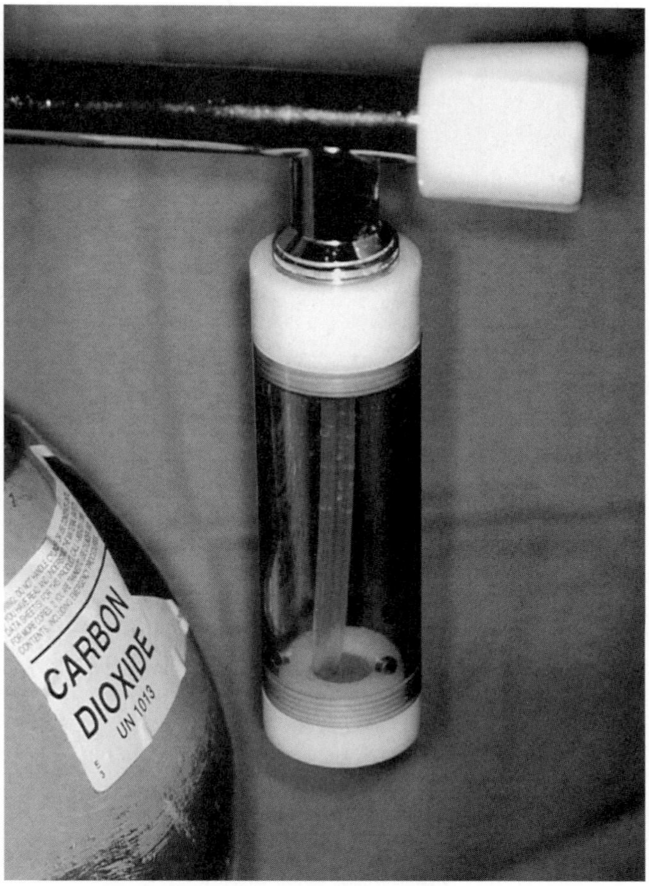

FIG. 14-2 Dry ice maker.

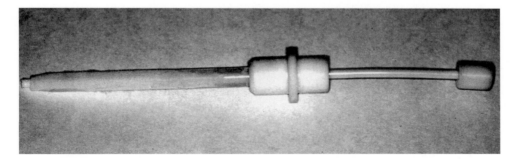

FIG. 14-3 Dry ice stick with holder and plunger.

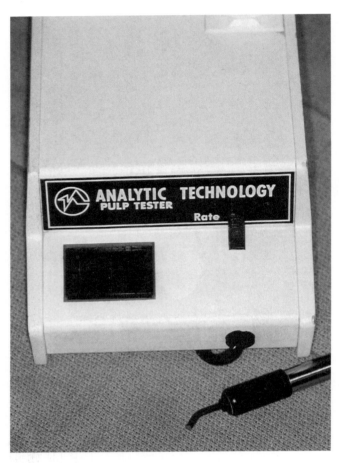

FIG. 14-4 Electrical pulp tester (Analytic Technology, Redmond, Wash.).

tubules. It is the product of E and I (E × I) that results in nerve response. This energy can be "consumed" in the hard tissue part of the tooth, leaving too low a level of stimulation for the pulpal nerves. Therefore to be able to compare recordings on the same tooth at different times it is very important that the tooth electrode is applied at the same location and with the same conduction each time. This is practically impossible under clinical conditions. Electrometric recording is often used when monitoring traumatic injuries to the teeth. Under these conditions it must be understood that the need to increase stimulation from one observation time to another very often suggests increased hard tissue formation in the pulp space ($\Uparrow \Omega$) and not real changes in the pulp's ability to respond.

It is also very important that the tooth is kept very dry when performing electrometric recording. Due to the high electrical potential used, the current tends to creep along any wet external tooth surface to the gingiva, creating a short circuit and leaving too little energy for the pulp through the very high resistance of the tooth. This is also the reason why critical recordings must be done after the teeth are isolated from the saliva with rubber dam and insulated from each other by inserting mylar strips through the contact points.

Based on this relative shortcoming, the electrometric pulp tester should not be the primary instrument of choice when assessing pulpal health. A positive cold test provides a more accurate response that is easier to interpret. Neither of these tests assure vitality of the pulp if the results are positive.

Pulp Vitality Testing

Vitality testing requires the measurement of pulpal blood flow. There are several devices regularly applied in medicine for the evaluation of circulatory changes. Several of these have been used for the experimental evaluation of pulpal health. Gazelius et al.[77] reported the successful application of laser Dop-

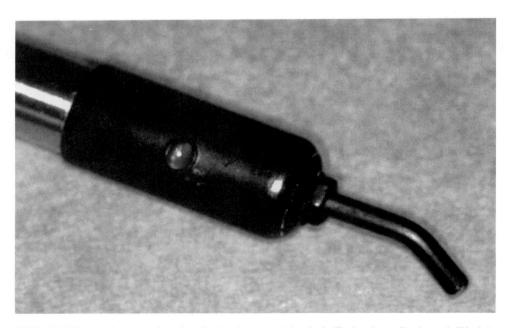

FIG. 14-5 Tooth electrode for electrical pulp tester (Analytic Technology, Redmond, Wash.).

pler flowmetry for the study of human pulpal blood flow. The value of this method has been well documented but the practical difficulty of its clinical use and the high cost have slowed its application.[105,106,175,188]

Pulse oximeter is another nondestructive method for monitoring pulp vitality by recording the oxygenation of pulpal blood flow. It was evaluated as a clinical tool in a preliminary investigation and found to perform satisfactorily.[198] Special sensors were developed to study blood flow and blood oxygenation in vitro.[59,160] Further careful attempts to apply the technology to a clinically useful device have been disappointing.[109]

Photoplethysmography of pulpal blood flow has also been evaluated for the assessment of pulp vitality.[58]

Although all these methods are successfully applied in medicine and in dental research, they have been less successfully applied to routine endodontic care. This is due to the fact that the circulatory system of the pulp is encased in a rigid structure and is therefore difficult to study without tissue removal. Thus the need for an absolute rigid observation point when using the Doppler phenomenon and the interference of extra pulpal circulatory systems when using the pulse oximetry and photoplethysmography have limited the introduction of these interesting methods to endodontic practice.

Tooth Slooth

The tooth slooth (Fig. 14-6) has proven very useful for the differential diagnosis of various stages of incomplete crown fractures (cracks). It is designed in such way that chewing force can be applied selectively on one cusp at a time, thereby evaluating weaknesses in defined areas of a tooth. This device is much more effective than cotton rolls or wooden sticks, which are often suggested for this important examination to establish a differential diagnosis.

MATERIALS FOR ENDODONTIC FIELD ISOLATION

The reader is referred to Chapter 5.

ENDODONTIC INSTRUMENTS

Although most instruments used in general dentistry are applicable to endodontic work, some hand instruments are unique for endodontic procedures. In addition, there are many different instrument types for procedures performed inside the pulp space. They are hand-operated instruments for root canal preparation, engine-driven and energized instruments for root canal preparation, instruments for root canal obturation, and rotary instruments for post space preparation.

During the last 25 years extensive work has been done to standardize instruments to improve quality. Internationally, the International Standards Organization (ISO) has been working with the Federation Dentaire Internationale (FDI) in the Technical Committee 106 Joint Working Group (TC-106 JWG-1). The American Dental Association (ADA) has been involved in this international development, together with the American National Standards Institute (ANSI) but has also independently developed American standards that have later been conforming with the international standard. There are two ISO/FDI standards pertaining to instruments. ISO/FDI No. 3630/1 deals with K-type files (ANSI/ADA No. 28), Hedström files (ANSI/ADA No. 58), and barbed broaches and rasps (ANSI/ADA No. 63). ISO/FDI No. 3630/3 deals with condensers, pluggers, and spreaders (ANSI/ADA No. 71).

Hand Instruments

Except for the mirror, all regular hand instruments used in endodontics are different from their regular dental counterparts. Thus the endodontic explorer has two straight and very sharp

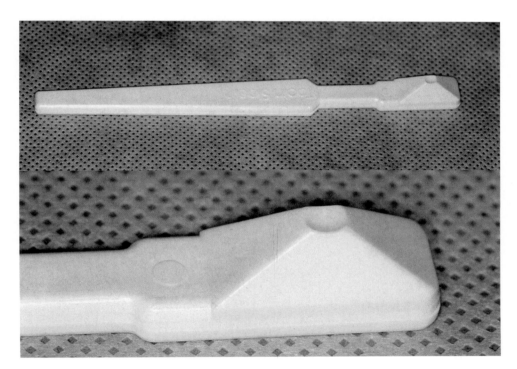

FIG. 14-6 Tooth slooth.

ends angulated in two different directions from the long axis of the instrument (Fig. 14-7).

There are several different types of endodontic spoons. They have a much longer offset than regular spoons—from the long axis of the instrument for better reach. They are intended for pulp tissue excision and should therefore be kept well sharpened (see Fig. 14-7).

The locking pliers with grooves for holding paper and gutta-percha points are an important instrument for rapid and secure transfer during endodontic work with a chairside assistant (Fig. 14-8). This instrument is always superior to the College or Perry pliers for work with points. The latter, however, is also needed for work within small pulp chambers, as the working ends of the "points plier" often are too large.

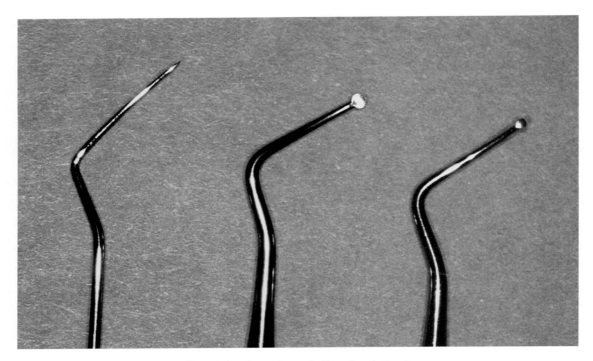

FIG. 14-7 Endodontic explorer *(left)* and endodontic spoons.

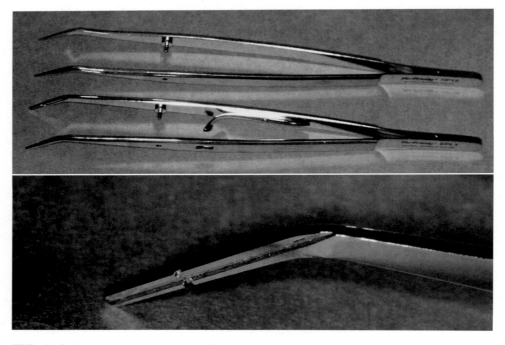

FIG. 14-8 Endodontic pliers. Nonlocking and locking pliers for gutta-percha and absorbent points. Note how the working part has grooves for holding of points.

Instruments for Pulp Space Preparation

The classification of endodontic instruments for root canal preparation is subdivided into three groups. Group I includes hand/finger-operated instruments such as barbed broaches and K-type and H-type instruments. Group II includes engine-driven instruments of a similar type as group I but with the handles replaced with attachments for a latch type of handpiece. In the past few instruments have been in this group, as rotary root canal files were rarely used. In recent years, however, the nickel-titanium rotary instruments have become popular, and instruments like ProFile, LightSpeed, and Quantec, although not standardized, could be included in this grouping. Group III includes the low-speed instruments where the latch type of attachment is in one piece with the working part. Typical instruments in this group are Gates-Glidden burs and Peeso reamers.

Hand/finger-operated instruments

This group of instruments comprises all instruments that generally are included in the group of instruments called files. Barbed broach, rasps and K-type and Hedström files are the old type of instruments in this category. Many new instrument designs have been brought to the market in recent years. These design changes affect the stiffness of the instrument, its efficiency, and the form of the cutting tip.

Traditionally, root canal instruments were manufactured from carbon steel. Its tendency to corrode due to the use of corrosive chemicals such as iodine and chlorine and during steam sterilization (Fig. 14-9) was a significant problem until stainless steel became the standard. Stainless steel has proven to be very valuable and has provided an improved quality of instruments (Fig. 14-10).[158,230]

As part of the attempts to improve the qualities of endodontic files new metal alloys have also been introduced. The alloy with most promise at this time is nitinol, which is an equi-atomic alloy of nickel-titanium.[247] Nickel-titanium alloy has a very low elastic modulus providing very good elastic flexibility to instruments. This alloy is expensive and difficult to manufacture and mill. It belongs to a category of alloys called "shape memory alloys" that have some extraordinary qualities. The most important characteristic of this alloy, applicable to its use in endodontic instruments, is its ability to recover from plastic strain when unloaded (pseudoelasticity). The alloy normally exists in an austenitic crystalline phase. On stressing at a constant temperature, the austenitic phase transforms to a martensitic structure. If the stress is released, the structure recovers to an austenitic phase and its original shape. This phenomenon is not similar to conventional elastic deformation but totally related to a stress-induced thermoelastic transformation from austenitic phase to martensitic phase. In the martensitic phase only a light force is required for bending. There are, however, limits. When yield stress of the martensitic phase is reached, deformation occurs and fracture results. Thus this alloy differs from the traditionally used stainless steel in that it may be strained much further than steel before it is permanently deformed. Resistance to fracture, however, measured as angular deflection before fracture, is higher for stainless steel instruments than for nickel-titanium instruments.[42] The alloy undergoes significant phase changes during stress. These can be slow thermoelastic or burst type of martensite. During these crystal changes the nickel-titanium instrument is very prone to fracture. This is of special concern when used for rotary instruments. Attempts to improve the nitinol alloy are ongoing,

and it was shown that the surface hardness could be greatly improved through the implantation of boron in the alloy.[127]

Barbed broach and rasps. The barbed broach and the rasp are the oldest endodontic intracanal instruments still being manufactured (Fig. 14-11). There are specifications for both the barbed broach and the rasp (ANSI No. 63; ISO No. 3630-1). Although similar in design, there are some significant differences in taper and barb size. Thus the broach has a taper of 0.007 to 0.010 mm/mm, and the rasp, 0.015 to 0.020 mm/mm. The barb height is much larger in the broach than in the rasp. As the barb comes out of the instrument core, the broach is a much weaker instrument than the rasp. The broaches and rasps

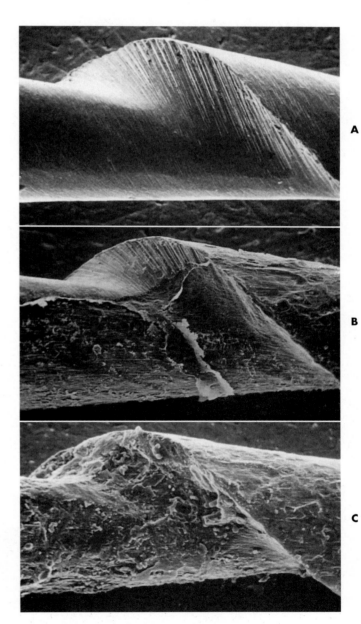

FIG. 14-9 Effect of chlorine and steam sterilization on carbon steel file. **A,** Untreated file. **B,** Five minutes exposure to 5% sodium hypochlorite followed by water rinse, drying, and autoclave sterilization. **C,** Same treatment as in **B** but repeated three times. Severe damage to the file. *(Courtesy Dr. Evert Stenman.)*

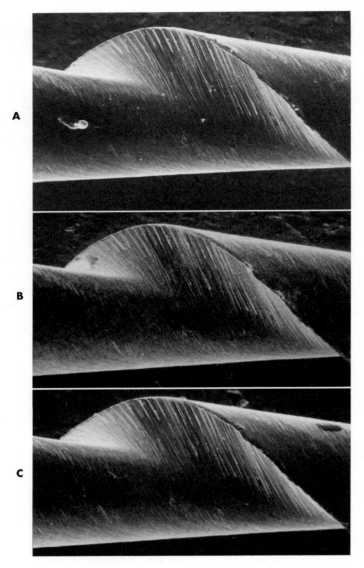

FIG. 14-10 Effect of chlorine and steam sterilization on stainless steel file. **A,** Untreated file. **B,** Five minutes exposure to 5% sodium hypochlorite followed by water rinse, drying, and autoclave sterilization. **C,** Same treatment as in **B** but repeated three times. No damage to the file. *(Courtesy Dr. Evert Stenman.)*

were designed to extract pulp tissue from the root canal simply by attaching to the tissue remnants. This was especially useful when removing arsenic or paraformaldehyde devitalized pulps, which become very fibrous when coagulated. Vital pulps, low in collagen, are not easy to remove with a broach. Furthermore, it is impossible with these instruments to sever the pulp in a calculated way. Therefore they have lost their usefulness in contemporary endodontics. A barbed broach does not cut or machine dentin; however, it is an excellent tool for the removal of cotton or paper points that have accidentally been lodged in the root canal.

K-type instruments. The K-type file and reamer (originally from Kerr Manufacturing Co.; 1915) are the oldest useful instruments for cutting and machining of dentin (ANSI No. 28; ISO No. 3630/1) (Figs. 14-12 and 14-13). The instruments are made from a steel wire that is ground to a tapered square or triangular cross section. This wire is then twisted to generate a file or a reamer. During this process the steel is work hardened. The file has more flutes per length unit than the reamer. If the core is twisted more or the instrument is thicker, the work hardening increases. This changes the physical properties of the file, making the reamer, that is less twisted, more flexible than a comparable file. The K-type instrument is useful for the penetration of root canals and increasing their size. The instrument primarily works by crushing the dentin when turned into a canal slightly smaller than the diameter of the instrument. Thus the apical enlargement with a K-type instrument is not an abrasive action but mainly a compression-and-release destruction of the dentin surrounding the canal.[206] Because of its dull flutes (rakes) and shallow concavities between the flutes, the K-type instrument does not easily thread itself deep into the dentin when used in rotary motion (compared to the H-type file). Although the reamer has fewer cutting rakes per length unit, it is as effective as a file in crushing and removing dentin, as there is more space between the flutes allowing better transport of dentin debris. The K-type instrument is poor in removing bulk dentin. Because of its working motion (rotation and pull) a K-type instrument used in a reaming motion causes little transport of the root canal, as the instrument tends to be self-centered in the canal. This is not true, however, if the K-type instrument is used in a filing motion.[245] The K-type file is strong and can easily be precurved to a desired form for filing. An advantage of the K-type design is that it is often obvious when a file has been stressed to permanent deformation. When this happens, the flutes on the working part of the file are wound tighter or opened up wider (Fig. 14-14). This sign is

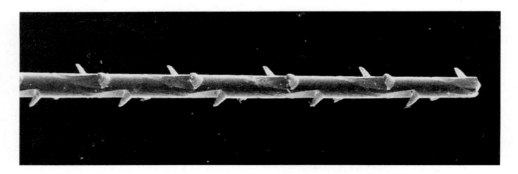

FIG. 14-11 Barbed broach (Union Broach, York, Pa.).

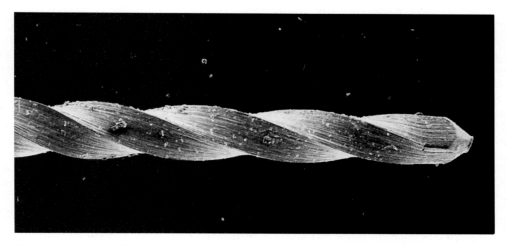

FIG. 14-12 K-type file (Kerr Manufacturing Co., Romulus, Mich.). Instrument fresh from a box displays significant amount of debris. This is not an uncommon observation in many brands of instruments. Therefore new instruments should be cleaned before being sterilized and used. Tip is blunted.

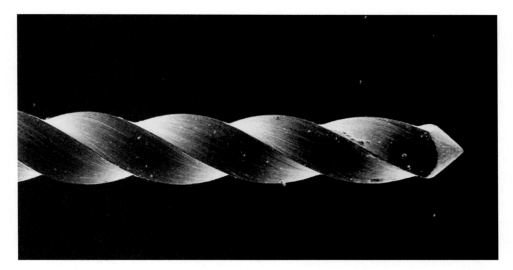

FIG. 14-13 K-type file No. 40 (Maillefer Instruments SA, Ballaiques, Switzerland). Note the clean surface and the well-rounded tip.

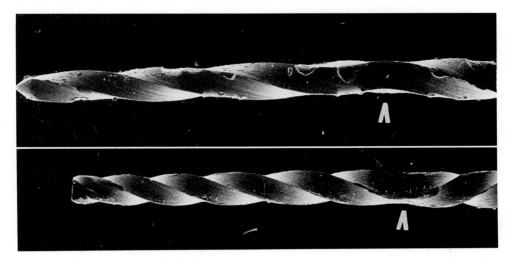

FIG. 14-14 K-type files stressed to deformation during clockwise and counterclockwise twisting. The deformed areas are marked with an arrow. These instruments are close to fracture.

a clear indication that the file has been permanently deformed and must be discarded. The K-type instrument and the hybrid files with the twisted K-type pattern fracture during clockwise motion after plastic deformation.[93] In counterclockwise motion little plastic deformation occurs before a brittle fracture occurs.[44] These files have a similar torsional strength regardless if used in clockwise or counterclockwise motions. In counterclockwise rotation breakage occurs in half or less of the rotations required for breakage in clockwise rotation.[44,120,124] Thus this type of instrument should therefore be operated more carefully when forced in counterclockwise direction.

Hedström file. The H-type instrument (ANSI No. 58; ISO No. 3630/1) is a more aggressive instrument than the K-type instrument. The H-type file is ground from a round steel blank. Modern computer-assisted machining technology has made it possible to develop H-type instruments with very complex forms. This technique makes it possible to adjust the rake angle and the helical angle. The edge that is facing the handle of the instrument can therefore be made rather sharp (Figs. 14-15 and 14-16). The H-type file machines the root

canal wall when the instrument is pulled but has no abrasive effect when pushed. The sharpness of these edges allows the file to self-thread into the root canal walls when turned clockwise. Combined with the compressibility of the dentin it is easy for the inexperienced user to enter into a situation where the file is so far into the dentin that it cannot be pulled or unscrewed but will fracture. This rarely happens with a K-type file or reamer. Due to these characteristics, a H-type file is less useful for reaming of a root canal but ideal for bulk removal of dentin.

In the design of an H-type file the rake angle and the distance between the flutes are important for the working of the file. The rake angle may be seen as the direction of the cutting edge if visualized as a surface (Figs. 14-17 and 14-18). If this surface is turned in the same direction as the force applied, the rake angle is positive. On the other hand, if the blade performs a scraping action faced away from the direction of the force, the rake angle is said to be negative. Most endodontic instruments have a slightly negative rake angle. If the rake angle is positive, the instrument actually works like a shaver

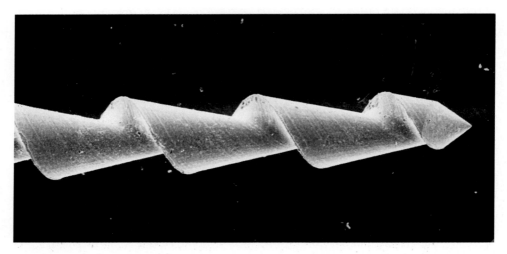

FIG. 14-15 Hedström file No. 45 (Maillefer Instruments SA, Ballaiques, Switzerland).

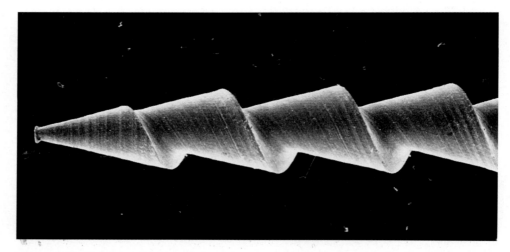

FIG. 14-16 Hedström file No. 50 (Antaeos, Vereinigte Dentalwerke, München, Germany). Steeper helical angle than file in Fig. 14-15. Note the blunted tip that is a common result of force used during attachment of handle.

on the dentin surface. Under such circumstances the instrument may dig itself into the dentin. Therefore the ideal instrument has a neutral or slightly positive rake for maximal effectiveness. The area between the flutes fills with dentin when the file is pulled over the root canal surface. The larger this groove, the longer the file is effective. When the groove is filled with dentin shavings, the instrument lifts off the surface and no longer planes effectively. Thus a file with a positive rake angle and a deep groove between the flutes is the most effective in removing dentin. This reduces the thickness of the core, however, making the instrument less stiff and more prone to fractures. The desire to have an aggressive instrument must therefore be balanced with the expectation of strength and must be

considered seriously when choosing a brand. Contrary to K-type instruments, the Hedström file is difficult to bend to the desired curvature without sharp nicks. The instrument may break through the development of cracks, followed by ductile failure.[93] Clinically, this happens without any physical external signs of stress like the flute changes observed on K-type instruments (see Fig. 14-14).

Hybrid instruments. Many new designs of files are simply modifications of the K-type and H-type files. These files are not made to any national or international standards, but their size designation often follows the specifications for K-type or H-type files. By changing the cross-sectional geometry of a K-type instrument from a square to rhomboid, it has

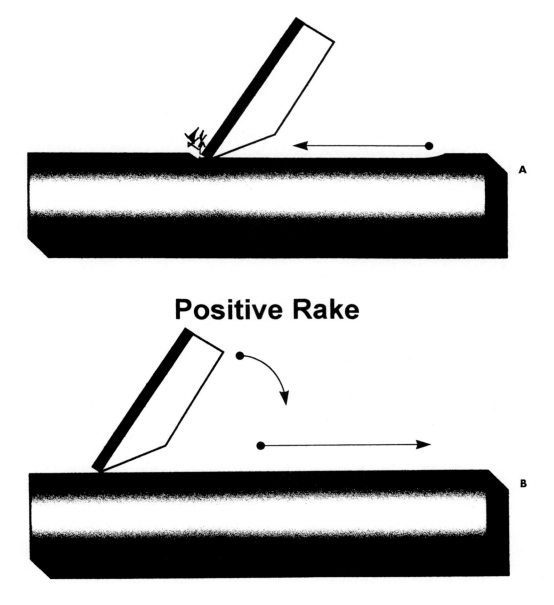

Positive Rake

Negative Rake

FIG. 14-17 Rake angle. **A,** Positive rake angle planes the substrate surface. **B,** Negative angle scrapes the surface.

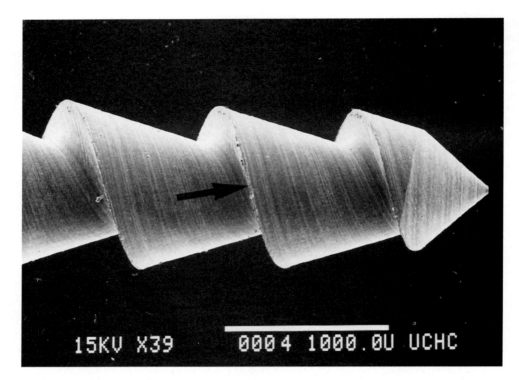

FIG. 14-18 Hedström file No. 100 (CC Cord, Roydent, Rochester Hills, Mich.). Rake angle close to neutral *(arrow)* makes this instrument very efficient during machining strokes.

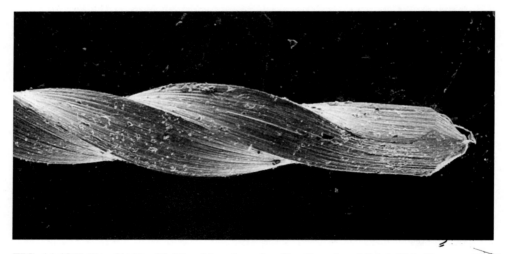

FIG. 14-19 K-Flex file No. 35 (Kerr Manufacturing Co., Romulus, Mich.). This file resembles a classic K-file with its twisted pattern (compare Figure 16). The crossection of the blank is rhomboid giving the instrument a small and a large diameter that can be seen clearly in this figure. Note the untwisted tip.

been possible to create an instrument, using classic K-file manufacturing technique, that is more flexible because one cross section is smaller than the cross section determining the size. It also allows more space for dentin shavings between the root canal wall and the instrument. These types of files are known as "flex files" (Fig. 14-19). Using modern computer-assisted grinding technology, it has also been possible to fabricate from a round blank files similar to the K-type file. These files can be made with much sharper flutes to increase the machining qualities and with much deeper space between the

flutes to allow for transport of more dentin shavings (Figs. 14-20 and 14-21). In regard to strength this type of instrument is more similar to H-type files than K-type files. Because of the sharper rake of ground K-type files, they also tend to more easily become lodged in the root canal walls and break on unscrewing or removal.[205] These milled K-type instruments are also available in nickel-titanium alloy (Figs. 14-22 and 14-23).

There are also many modifications of the H-type file. Thus several brands now supply H-type files with double-helix configuration (Figs. 14-24 and 14-25). Although this doubles the

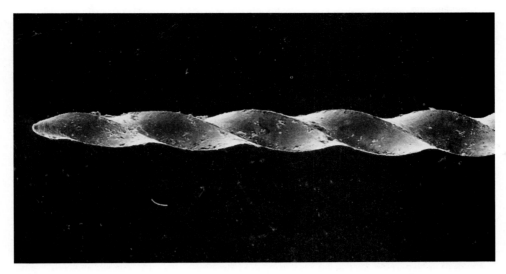

FIG. 14-20 Flex-R file (Union Broach, York, Pa.). This is a milled K-type instrument. The flutes are sharper with a less negative rake than a traditional twisted K-type file. The tip is well rounded.[179]

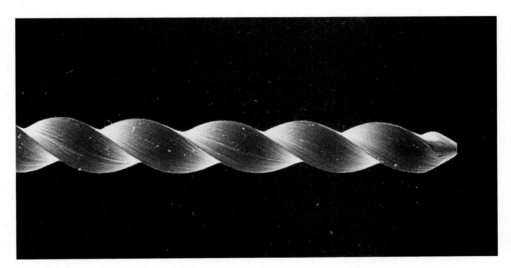

FIG. 14-21 FlexoFile (Maillefer Instruments SA, Ballaiques, Switzerland). Milled K-type instrument. Note the smooth surface and well-formed tip.

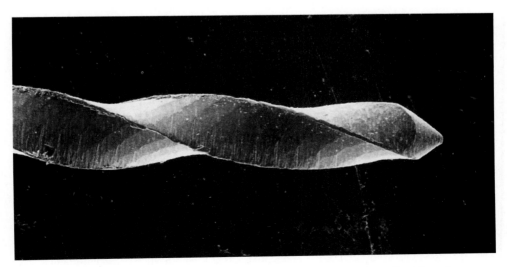

FIG. 14-22 Ultra Flex No. 30 (Texeed). Milled K-type nickel-titanium file. Note the course surface, which is a typical result of milling in nickel-titanium alloy. The flutes are less sharp than a steel counterpart and are often rolled over the edge.

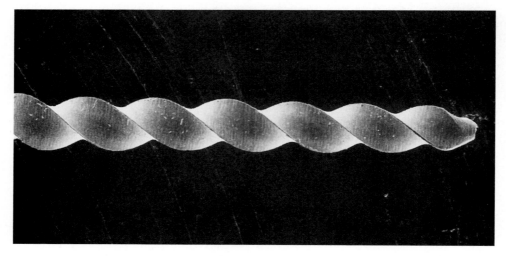

FIG. 14-23 Sureflex No. 30 (Caulk/Dentsply, Milford, Del.). Milled K-type nickel-titanium file with a higher helical angle than Ultra Flex (see Fig. 14-22). Compare design with the FlexoFile (see Fig. 14-21).

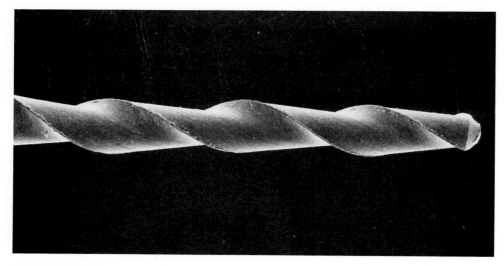

FIG. 14-24 Hyflex X-file (Hygenic Corp., Akron, Ohio). Hedström type nickel-titanium file with double helix.

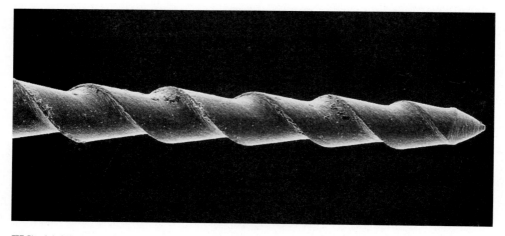

FIG. 14-25 Mity Turbo (JS Dental, Ridgefield, Conn.). Hedström type nickel-titanium file with tighter double helix than the Hyflex X-file. This file is much less efficient in machining a substrate than the Hyflex X-file seen in Fig. 14-24.[114]

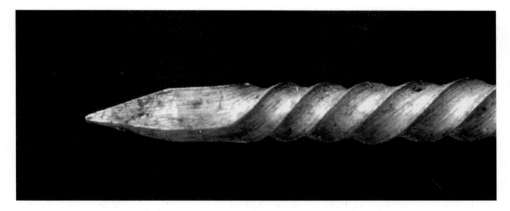

FIG. 14-26 K-type instrument with aggressive pyramid type of tip.

number of machining edges, the space between the edges is radically decreased; therefore overall effectiveness is not enhanced compared to conventional Hedström files.[114] Modified H-type files with continuously variable helical angle are also available.

Tip design. It was observed by Weine et al.[251] that the abrasive effect of the instrument tip had an important effect on the control of the root canal preparation. In a study of cutting efficiency of some endodontic files, where the files were performing a quarter turn reciprocal drilling action in a Giromatic handpiece under 1000 g pressure, it was also found that the tip design had an effect on what was called "cutting efficiency."[149,150] These results are not surprising, as the instruments used in the study were larger than the predrilled hole they had to penetrate. Therefore the only way the instruments could advance is by using abrasive planes on the tip.

Abrasive tips may be helpful when penetrating canals smaller than the file. If steel files are used, however, the inherent stiffness of these files enhances the machining of dentin on the concave side of the curvature, resulting in some ledging. Much has been written about the importance of various sophisticated tip modifications to prevent such ledging, but there is no scientific proof that any one design is better than the other during clinical work.[115,171,172,179,182,183] The original K-type file had a tip that resembled a pyramid (Fig. 14-26). It was therefore very capable of lateral and apical machining. Practically all contemporary file designs have an acceptable nonaggressive tip design, and there should be little concern over tip geometry in the selection of files if they are within the ANSI/ISO guidelines (Fig. 14-27).

Rotary instruments

Many types of rotary instruments are used during endodontic treatment procedures. In addition to regular burs, adapted for endodontics, there are various types of root canal reamers for preparation of the root canal or for the removal of root canal filling materials and preparation for post space.

Burs. In addition to conventional burs, there are burs with extended shanks useful for preparation in the pulp space. Many burs are available in surgical length (26 mm) and some in extra long shank (34 mm) for low-speed contraangle handpieces (Fig. 14-28). This latter model is exceptionally helpful in deep preparation in the pulp chamber and root canals, as it allows good visibility and control.

After access has been achieved, there is little need for high-

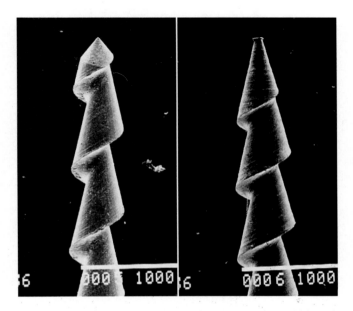

FIG. 14-27 Hedström files with different tip designs. Although sold as standardized files, these files (of the same size) display very different tips.

speed preparation in the pulp chamber. Low-speed preparation with sharp burs is as effective as high-speed preparation and allows a better tactile control during this critical phase of preparation.

Reamers. Gates-Glidden burs and Peeso reamers are examples of common rotary reamers. The Gates-Glidden bur is commonly used during initial root canal preparation for opening of orifices and coronal root canal preparation. This reamer is available both in a 32-mm length and a shorter 28-mm length for posterior teeth (Fig. 14-29).

The risk for perforation with Gates-Glidden reamers is less than with other types of reamers, as the short head is less self-guiding (Fig. 14-30). It is self-centering in the root canal, however. This may result in unexpected thinning of the furcation wall of root canals when larger sizes are used. This is especially pronounced on the furcation sides of mesial roots of molars. Gates-Glidden instruments are also available in nickel-titanium (Fig. 14-31).

The Peeso reamer is an instrument mostly used for post

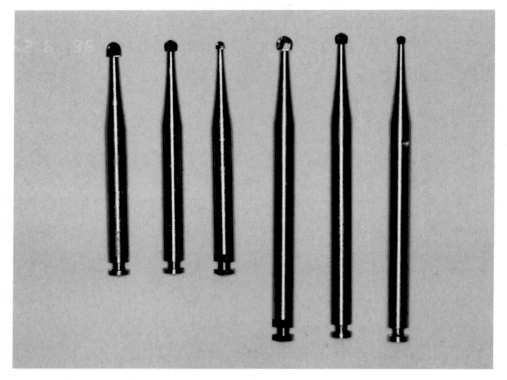

FIG. 14-28 Round burs for endodontic use. Surgical burs *(left)* have a length of 26 mm, whereas the burs to the right are 32 mm long. This extra length allows direct view around the head of the handpiece during pulp chamber preparation.

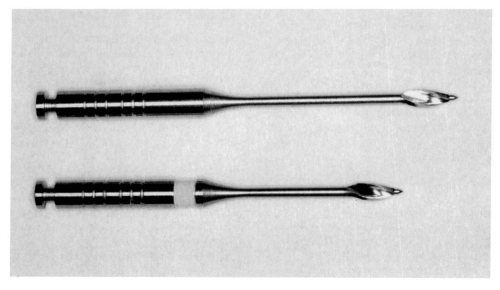

FIG. 14-29 Gates-Glidden burs (stainless steel) (Union Broach, York, Pa.). Normal length (32 mm) and short length (28 mm).

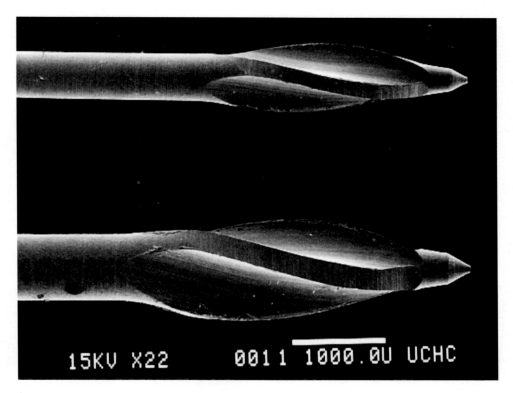

FIG. 14-30 Working part of Gates-Glidden bur (stainless steel). Note the rounded safety tip and the lack of sharp cutting edges. The instrument has a marginal land to center the drill in the canal and more safely machine the canal walls.

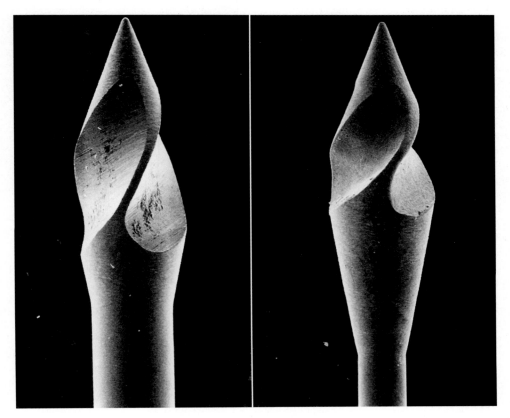

FIG. 14-31 Working part of nickel-titanium Gates-Glidden bur (Tulsa Dental Products, Tulsa, Okla.). Small size to the left and a large instrument to the right. Compare design with the LightSpeed rotary instrument in Fig. 14-38.

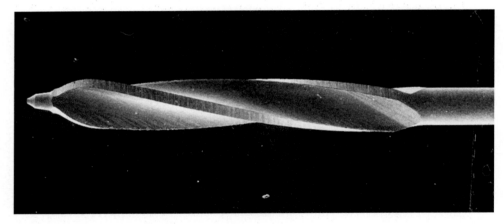

FIG. 14-32 Peeso reamer (Union Broach, York, Pa.). Note safety tip and guiding marginal lands on machining surfaces.

space preparation (Fig. 14-32). It is a stiff instrument and therefore does not follow the root canal if there is a slight curvature. This reamer easily cuts laterally, causing perforations, despite the "safety tip." The inexperienced user should be especially careful when using the Peeso reamers.

Rotary root canal instruments. With the advent of nickel-titanium for endodontic files the idea of a safe rotary file was born. Attempts to use conventional steel files for mechanical instrumentation of root canals have been ongoing for many years with little success. The steel file does not have the flexibility to be used for rotary movements in a curved root canal without significantly altering the canal configuration and perforating the canal wall. In addition, the design of the instruments was such that they easily became overstressed and fractured. The rotary instrument device that best survived through many years was the Giromatic handpiece. This provided a quarter turn reciprocal movement of the instruments used. Most common for Giromatic handpieces were the rasps and barbed broaches, but K-type and H-type instruments were also used. The Giromatic handpiece was an ineffective instrument that never became an important addition to the endodontic armamentarium. With nickel-titanium it became practical to develop a file type of instrument that could be effectively used as a rotary root canal instrument in moderately curved root canals. Presently there are three major instruments available that provide useful alternatives. They are ProFile (Tulsa Dental Products, Tulsa, Okla.), LightSpeed (Light Speed Technology, Inc., San Antonio, Tex.), and Quantec (NT Co., Chattanooga, Tenn.). Although different in design, all three have some basic similarities in the use of a radial land. The radial land prevents the instrument from cutting into the canal walls in an uncontrolled fashion and causing unwanted transportation. The land also contributes significantly to the strength of the instrument by the relatively large peripheral mass. This peripheral strengthening has been further accentuated in the Quantec instrument. Rotary nickel-titanium instruments require constant speed to prevent stress fractures. Although it may sometimes be possible to operate these nickel-titanium instruments with an air-driven handpiece, it is highly recommended that an electrical handpiece (Fig. 14-33) be used, as the speed can be maintained more evenly and at the right rpm.

ProFile: ProFile comes in ten sizes (Nos. 1 through 10) and in two different tapers (Fig. 14-34). The standard taper is 0.04

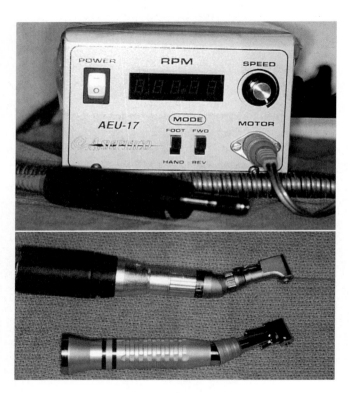

FIG. 14-33 Electrical handpiece with different gear reductions and motor controller (Aseptico, Kirkland, Wash.).

mm/mm. In addition, the instrument is available in 0.06 mm/mm taper. This instrument is not sized in the ISO/ANSI standard but is sized by the standard introduced by the manufacturer. Because of the large taper the instrument becomes rather stiff before the apical preparation has been sufficiently enlarged (Nos. 5 through 6). This places some limitations on its use in narrow, curved root canals. The instrument is well manufactured and true to design at all sizes (Fig. 14-35 and 14-36). The ProFile group also has an orifice opener (Fig. 14-37). The rotational speed used for ProFile is in the range of 150 to 300 rpm.

LightSpeed: LightSpeed resembles the Gates-Glidden reamer with a long shaft and a short flame-formed cutting head

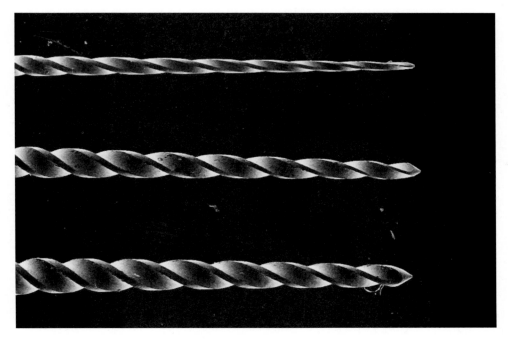

FIG. 14-34 Rotary ProFile Series 29 nickel-titanium instruments (Tulsa Dental Products, Tulsa, Okla.). Sizes Nos. 3, 5, and 6. The instruments have marginal lands that guide the instrument in the center of the canals and around curvatures.

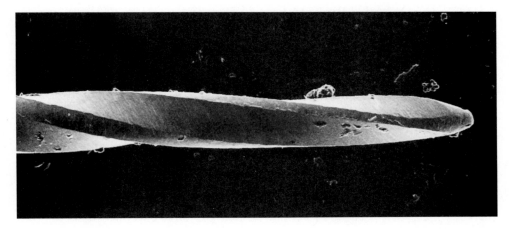

FIG. 14-35 Rotary ProFile Series 29 nickel-titanium instruments (Tulsa Dental Products, Tulsa, Okla.). Size No. 3.

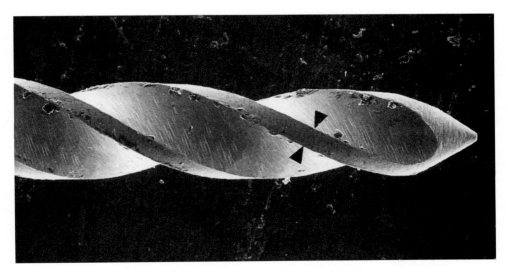

FIG. 14-36 Rotary ProFile Series 29 nickel-titanium instruments (Tulsa Dental Products, Tulsa, Okla.). Size No. 5. Note the wide marginal land of the instrument *(arrows)*.

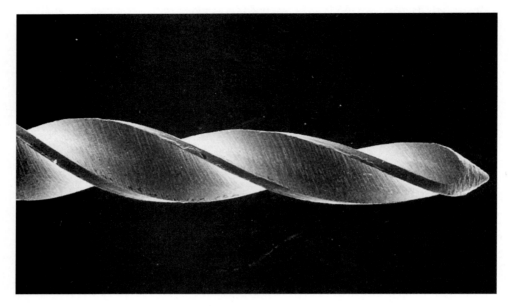

FIG. 14-37 Rotary ProFile Series 29 nickel-titanium orifice opener (Tulsa Dental Products, Tulsa, Okla.). The instrument has a larger taper than regular ProFile 0.04 instruments.

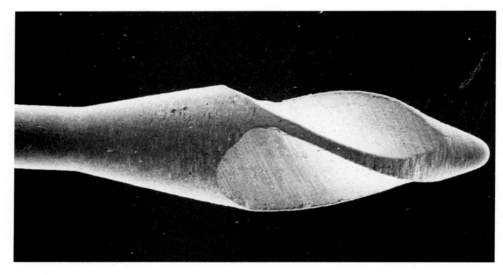

FIG. 14-38 LightSpeed rotary nickel-titanium instruments (LightSpeed Technologies, San Antonio, Tex.). Size No. 90. Well-outlined instrument head with radial lands.

(Fig. 14-38). It comes in sizes from No. 020 up to No. 140 (according to ISO/ANSI). It also includes "half" sizes such as No. 0225, No. 0275, etc., up to No. 060). In the smaller sizes the head is less well defined (Fig. 14-39). The design has been shown to vary with the instrument size.[135] With careful use this instrument is not more prone to fracture than other nickel-titanium rotary instruments. It is of essence, however, that the manufacturers' instructions are followed to the letter and that no sizes are skipped during preparation when increasing the canal size. The instrument works very well and prepares ideal canals with little or no transportations. The excessive number of instruments for a complete instrumentation is a strain, however. The rotational speed used for LightSpeed is in the range of 1500 to 2000 rpm.

Quantec: Quantec is a relatively new development. This is a set of 10 instruments to be used with some variation depend-

ing on the root canal anatomy. The first instrument is an orifice opener with a taper of 0.06 mm/mm (Fig. 14-40). Then come three instruments Nos. 15, 20, and 25 with a taper of 0.02 mm/mm (ISO/ANSI). These three instruments establish the apical preparation to No. 25. The following four instruments have an apical size of No. 25 but increasing taper (0.03, 0.04, 0.05, and 0.06 mm/mm). These four instruments provide the backfilling of bulk dentin removal and flare the root canal. The remaining two instruments have a standard taper of 0.02 mm/mm but an apical size of Nos. 40 and 45. In many aspects the design of the Quantec and ProFile instruments are similar. The choices of sizes and tapers are different, however. The lands of the Quantec instrument are also much wider with a modification that provides enhanced strength to the instrument (Fig. 14-41). The tip design of the Quantec file appears very aggressive (Figs. 14-40 and 14-41). During milling of nitinol

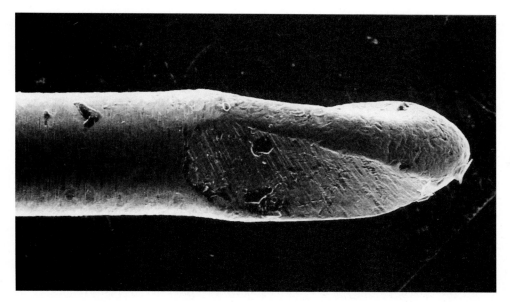

FIG. 14-39 LightSpeed rotary nickel-titanium instruments (LightSpeed Technologies, San Antonio, Tex.). Size No. 20. Working head is slightly larger than the shaft. Radial lands are poorly defined.

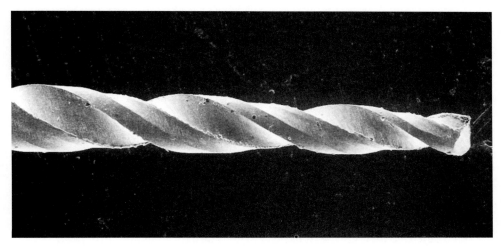

FIG. 14-40 Quantec rotary nickel-titanium instrument (NT Company, Chattanooga, Tenn.). Orifice opener No. 1. Taper 0.06 mm/mm. Note the blunt and sharp tip of the instrument.

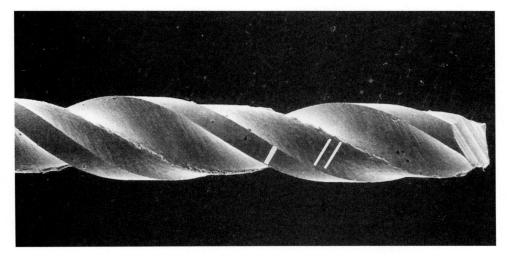

FIG. 14-41 Quantec rotary nickel-titanium instrument (NT Company, Chattanooga, Tenn.). Size No. 10. Taper 0.02 mm/mm. Note the typical double land that characterizes the Quantec instrument. Higher marginal land performs the machining *(wide white bar)* of the root canal, whereas the lower reduced peripheral surface *(double white bars)* contributes to peripheral strength. Note the sharp and blunt tip.

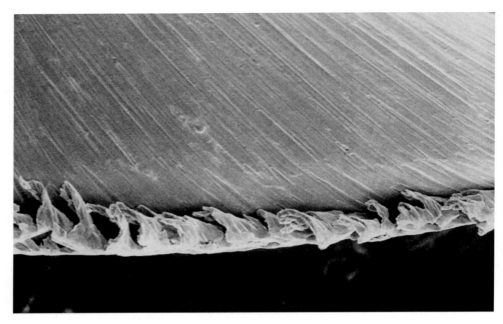

FIG. 14-42 Quantec rotary nickel-titanium instrument (NT Company, Chattanooga, Tenn.). High magnification of edge between the reduced peripheral surface and the U-groove. Because of the difficulties in milling nickel-titanium alloys edges are often "rolled over" like this. Similar rollover can be seen when nickel-titanium instruments wear (see Fig. 14-22).

there is always a certain degree of rollover at sharp edges (Fig. 14-42).

Sonic and ultrasonic instruments

A radically different way of instrumenting root canals was introduced when files were activated with electromagnetic ultrasonic energy.[177] Today, piezoelectrical ultrasonic units are also available for this purpose. These units activate an oscillating sinusoidal wave in the file with a frequency around 30 kHz.

There are principally two different types of devices: the ultrasonic device (25 to 30 kHz; CaviEndo [magnetostrictive; Fig. 14-43] and ENAC [piezoelectrical; Fig. 14-44]) and the sonic at 2 to 3 kHz (Sonic Air MM1500, Megasonic 1400, Endostar). The ultrasonic devices use regular type of instruments (K-type files), whereas the sonic devices use special instruments known as Rispi Sonic, Shaper Sonic, Trio Sonic, and (Heli Sonic) files.

Although similar in function, the piezoelectrical design has advantages over the magnetostrictive systems. Little heat is generated, and therefore no cooling is needed for the electrical handpiece. In addition, the piezoelectrical transducer transfers more energy to the file than the magnetostrictive system, making it more powerful.[10] The magnetostrictive system generates a large amount of heat, and a special cooling system is needed in addition to the irrigation system for the root canal (see Fig. 14-43).

The file in an ultrasonic device vibrates in a sinus wave–like fashion. In a standing wave there are areas with maximal displacement (antinodes) and areas with no displacement (nodes). The tip of the instrument exhibits an antinode. If powered too high, the instrument may break because of the intense vibration. Therefore files must be used only a short time and with careful setting of power. The frequency of breakage in

files used for more than 10 minutes may be as high as 10% and normally occurs at the nodes of vibrations.[3]

The ultrasonic devices have a very efficient system for irrigation into the pulp space during operation. During free ultrasonic vibration in a fluid two significant physical effects are observed: *cavitation* and *acoustic streaming*. During the oscillation in a fluid a positive pressure is followed by a negative pressure in the fluid. If the tensile strength of the fluid is exceeded during this oscillation of pressure gradients, a cavity is formed in the fluid in the negative phase. During the following positive pressure phase the cavity implodes with great force. This is *cavitation*. The power of dental ultrasonic units is too low during normal clinical conditions to create significant mechanical cavitation effects on the dentin walls.[7,8] *Acoustic streaming* creates small intense circular fluid movement (eddy flow) around the instruments. The eddying occurs closer to the tip than in the coronal end of the file, with an apically directed flow at the tip. Acoustic streaming increases the cleaning effect of the irrigant in the pulp space through hydrodynamic shear stress. Increased amplitude occurring at smaller file sizes enhances the acoustic streaming.[6] This has proven to be of great value in the cleaning of root canals, as conventional irrigation solutions do not penetrate small spaces well.[174,187,203] Acoustic streaming has little direct antimicrobial effect.[4,9] Both cavitation and acoustic streaming are dependent on the free vibration of the file. The limits of the space in a root canal significantly inhibit the practical utility of ultrasonic devices for root canal cleaning. Depending on size and power the file tip may have an amplitude of 20 to 140 μm, requiring a canal size of a No. 30 through 40 file for free oscillation. Any contact with the root canal walls dampens oscillation. As the contact with the canal wall increases, the oscillation is dampened and too weak to maintain acoustic

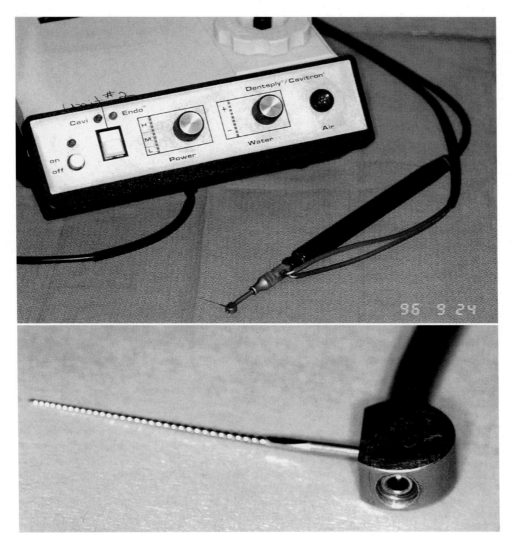

FIG. 14-43 Cavi-Endo ultrasonic device (Caulk/Dentsply, Milford, Del.). The unit allows setting for endodontic work or periodontal scaling. The top lid covers a container for irrigation solution. Power and irrigation rate can be adjusted. The irrigation and cooling drain are attached close to the working head. Files are attached with a hexscrew.

streaming. Small file size with minimal contact to the root canal wall provides optimal cleaning conditions.[11]

The ultrasonic devices are slightly disappointing as instruments to enhance the removal of dentin from the root canal walls.[148,169] Through acoustic streaming, however, these devices enhance the ability to clean the pulp space and difficult-to-debride areas.[16,50,51,253] It is unclear, however, if this can be achieved during regular preparation when the file is actively dampened and little acoustic streaming takes place.[229,248,249] Cleaning is further enhanced by the excellent irrigation systems provided in some of the devices. Applying a freely oscillating file with sodium hypochlorite irrigation for a couple of minutes to aid in the pulp space disinfection is therefore believed to be useful, after good biomechanical instrumentation of the pulp space.[208]

Sonic devices are more useful for true hard tissue removal during root canal preparation.[148,260] Since the files operate like a conventional handpiece, the file vibrations are less likely to be dampened by contact with the root canal walls. Therefore

the special files used in these systems are true bulk dentin removers. The Rispi Sonic file is less aggressive than the Shaper Sonic file. The instruments come in lengths from 17 mm to 29 mm and in various sizes from No. 010 and up. Because of the rasplike design of the instruments, they tend to leave a rougher canal surface than many other mechanical devices. The working length and the apical part of the root canal are normally prepared with conventional files, after which the sonic files are used. Both sonic and ultrasonic instruments are prone to cause canal transport if used carelessly.[5,117,133] Various, often conflicting, techniques for using these instruments have been described, and the individual user should take time to be acquainted with the instrument for optimal use.

National and international standards for instruments

As a result of concerns nearly 40 years ago, efforts were made to standardize endodontic files and root filling materials. This resulted in an international standard for endodontic files known in the United States as the ANSI No. 58 for Hedström

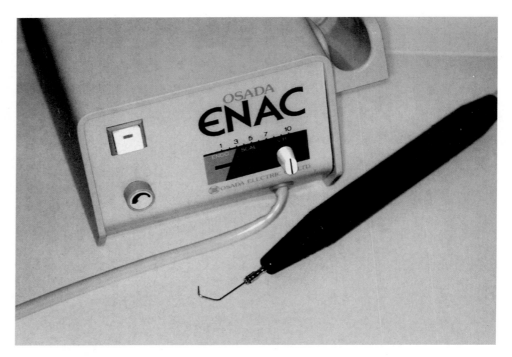

FIG. 14-44 ENAC piezoelectrical ultrasonic device (Osada, Tokyo, Japan). The handpiece has adapters for periodontal scaling or endodontic work. Power and water flow can be adjusted.

Table 14-1. Dimensions of standardized K-type file, H-type file, and gutta-percha cones (ANSI Nos. 28, 58, and 78)*

Size	D_0	D_{16}	Color
006	*0.06*	*0.38*	*No color assigned*
008	*0.08*	*0.40*	*No color assigned*
010	0.10	0.42	Purple
015	0.15	0.47	White
020	0.20	0.52	Yellow
025	0.25	0.57	Red
030	0.30	0.62	Blue
035	0.35	0.67	Green
040	0.40	0.72	Black
045	0.45	0.77	White
050	0.50	0.82	Yellow
055	0.55	0.87	Red
060	0.60	0.92	Blue
070	0.70	1.02	Green
080	0.80	1.12	Black
090	0.90	1.22	White
100	1.00	1.32	Yellow
110	1.10	1.42	Red
120	1.20	1.52	Blue
130	1.30	1.62	Green
140	1.40	1.72	Black

*Sizes denoted in italics are only for files, commercially available but not part of ANSI No. 28 or No. 58. Colors on instrument handles or gutta-percha cones are not mandatory. The size must be printed on the handles. The tolerance for files is ± 0.02 mm and for gutta-percha cones is ± 0.05 mm. Length for the gutta-percha cones is ≥ 30 mm ± 2 mm.

files and ANSI No. 28 for K-type files (Table 14-1). There are several similarities in these standards but there are also some important differences. Fig. 14-45 illustrates the important measurements dictated by the standard. The size designation is derived from the projected diameter at the tip of the instrument. This is an imaginary measurement and is not reflected in the real size of the working part of the instrument. The taper of the instruments are prescribed to be 0.02 mm/mm of length starting at the tip. Thus the working diameter is the product of taper and the length of the tip. Three standard lengths are available at 21 mm, 25 mm, and 31 mm. The working part of the instrument must be at least 16 mm.

This system of numbering files with at least 15 different sizes replaced the old, somewhat imperfect system that numbered the sizes from Nos. 0 through 6. Although the new standard includes many sizes, rational clinicians may compose the proper collection of fewer instrument sizes for their special work habit.

In recent years suggestions to change the numbering system for files with different sizes have been implemented by several manufacturers. One system has introduced "half" sizes in the range of Nos. 15 through 60. Thus there are instruments in sizes Nos. 15, 17.5, 20, 22.5, etc. Considering the fact that most manufacturers already are unable to size their instruments within accepted range (Fig. 14-46),[234] the introduction of "half" sizes makes no rational sense. It is reasonable, however, if standards are strictly adhered to, to use "half" sizes for instrument systems like the LightSpeed, where the strength of the instrument is so low that full-size increments may generate stresses beyond the tolerance of the instrument.

Another manufacturer (Tulsa Dental Products, Tulsa, Okla.) has introduced the concept of dimensional increments in percent (29%) of diameter instead of real increments (in 0.05 mm).

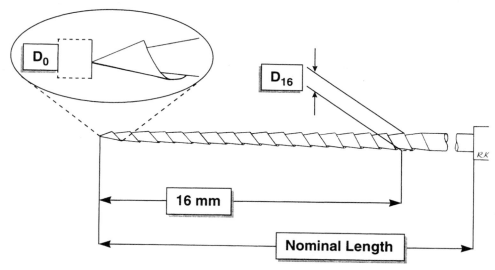

FIG. 14-45 Measuring points for ANSI/ADA No. 28 and No. 58 for K-type and H-type instruments. The measuring point for the diameter of the instrument *(size)* is imaginary (D_0) and projects the taper of the instrument at the tip. Thus an instrument with a short tip is more true to its size than instruments with long tip. D_{16} represents the diameter at the end of the working part that must be at least 16 mm long.

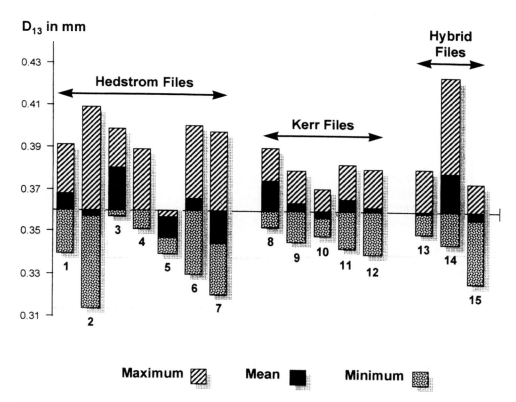

FIG. 14-46 Results from a study of the size of standardized root canal instruments (No. 030). Measurements made 3 mm from the tip where a conforming instrument should measure 0.36 ±0.02 mm. Mean marked in black. Shaded areas indicate maximal and minimal values. Few instruments conform to the standard. For details see Stenman and Spångberg.[234] *1,* Antaeos; *2,* Hygenic; *3,* Miltex; *4,* Maillefer; *5,* J.S. Dental; *6,* Union Broach; *7,* Brasseler; *8,* Antaeos; *9,* Miltex; *10,* Maillefer; *11,* J.S. Dental; *12,* Brasseler; *13,* S-File; *14,* K-Flex; *15,* Flex-R.

These files are numbered in a system of Nos. 1 through 13 (ProFile Series 29). No objective literature available demonstrates the advantage of this system over the nationally and internationally accepted ANSI/ISO system.

Effectiveness and wear of instruments

Although the advertising literature is rich in claims of various forms of superiority of file designs, few claims can be verified in objective endodontic literature.

There are no standards for the cutting or machining effectiveness of endodontic files, neither are there clear requirements regarding resistance to wear. When studying the effectiveness of instruments, there are two measurements to investigate. One is the instrument's effectiveness in cutting or breaking loose dentin, and the other is the effectiveness in machining dentin. These two measurements are radically different. There are methods to quantitate machining, but as of now there is no good method that measures cutting. Some studies have attempted evaluation of cutting, but the methodologies have involved the drilling motion with K-type instruments and at high speed compared to clinical use.[69,246] There are studies of machining, however, that evaluate the effectiveness of an instrument when used in a linear movement.[113,114,157,231-233,250] They show that instruments are very different when comparing brands and types but also within one brand and type. For K-type files the effectiveness varies 2 to 12 times between files

of the same brand. The variation for Hedström files is larger and varies between 2.5 to more than 50 times.[146,232] The greater variation among Hedström files is easy to understand as the H-type file is the result of more individual grinding during manufacturing than the conventional K-type file, which is difficult to alter much during manufacturing. During the grinding of a Hedström file it is possible to modify the rake angle to neutral or even slightly positive. This is impossible to achieve with a K-type file. The Hedström file is therefore approximately 10 times more effective in removing dentin than the K-type file (Fig. 14-47). In the machining process the rake edge shaves off dentin that accumulates in the grooves between the rake edges. The deeper and larger this space is, the longer the stroke can be before the instrument is riding on its own debris and therefore making it ineffective. These design variations and the rake angle of the edges determine the effectiveness of a Hedström file. Of the hybrid files the K-Flex file, which is a modified K-type file, shows variables similar to K-type files. The Flex-R file, which is a ground instrument, is more similar to H-type files in its variation in effectiveness. It is also much more effective in substrate removal than the K-type files but cannot measure up to the H-type files' ability to machine.

Nickel-titanium alloy instruments are as effective or better than comparable stainless steel instruments in machining dentin.

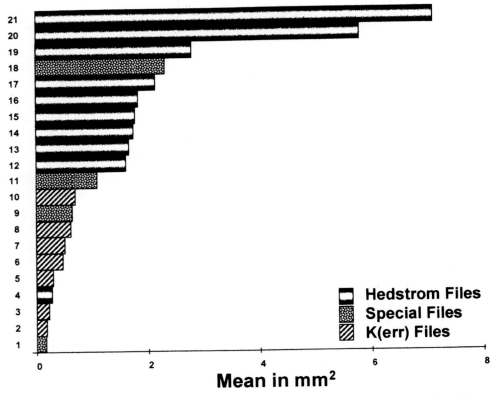

FIG. 14-47 Comparison of effectiveness of various endodontic instruments in machining. Substrate removal measured in mm². Hedström files are in general much more efficient than K-type instruments. For details see Stenman and Spångberg.[233] *1*, Trio-Cut; *2*, Miltex; *3*, Brasseler; *4*, Brasseler; *5*, Healthco Delux; *6*, JS Dental; *7*, Aristocrat; *8*, Antaeos; *9*, K-Flex; *10*, Maillefer; *11*, Flex-R; *12*, Union Broach; *13*, Maillefer; *14*, Miltex; *15*, J.S. Dental; *16*, Healthco Delux; *17*, Hygenic; *18*, S-File; *19*, Aristocrat; *20*, Zipperer; *21*, Antaeos.

Steel files wear significantly when used on dentin.[113] Thus after 300 pull strokes on dentin the instruments may lose up to 55% of their original effectiveness. Nickel-titanium files also wear noticeably, but they are much more resistant to wear than the steel files (Figs. 14-48 and 14-49).[114] The nickel-titanium file is significantly more expensive than the steel file, and it is important from a cost-effective point of view to decide what instruments to use.

Modern endodontic stainless steel instruments are fabricated from excellent metal alloys, and their resistance to fracture is great. With careful application of force and a strict program to discard instruments after use, few instrument fractures should occur. Stainless steel files are so inexpensive that adequate cleaning and sterilization for reuse of files in sizes up to No. 60 may not be cost effective. Therefore files in the range up to No. 60 should be considered disposable instruments. Fig. 14-50 suggests a file setup that provides efficient overview of the instruments. In a file disposable system the sponge, holding the instruments used during the treatment, will be disposed of, including the files.

Devices for Root Canal Length Measurements

Traditionally, measurements during root canal instrumentation have been made by exposing radiographs with a root canal file in place in the canal. Based on this information the working length has normally been determined.

Sundada[235] suggested that the apical foramen could be lo-calized with the use of an electrical current. This early, often imperfect, technique has undergone significant and successful modifications. Today, the apex locator has developed to an accurate tool for the determination of working length.[70-74] Apex locators are still sensitive to individual interpretation, however, and the user must carefully train with the instrument to be proficient. In addition, many instruments are very sensitive to the type of tissue or fluid content of the root canal.

Two of the best modern apex locators are Endex or Apit (Osada Electric Co., Tokyo, Japan) and Root ZX (J. Morita Co., Kyoto, Japan).[74,123] These devices, which are easy to use and less sensitive to the root canal content, measure the electrical impedance between the file and the mucosa. Normally two electrical currents at different frequency are emitted, and the apex is related to the place of maximal difference calculated by subtraction or division. The Endex device uses 1 and 5 kHz and provides apex location based on subtraction. The Root ZX emits currents at frequencies of 8 and 0.4 kHz and provides apex location based on the resulting quotient. When the file tip reaches the apical foramen area, the instrument gives some type of signal. There are typically three parts to an apex locator. They are the lip clip, the file clip, and the instrument itself, which has a display indicating the advancement of the file toward the apex (Fig. 14-51).

On average the best of these instruments provides accurate measurements to within 0.5 mm of the apex.[74,123] Therefore to achieve a "safe" measurement, 1 mm should be subtracted

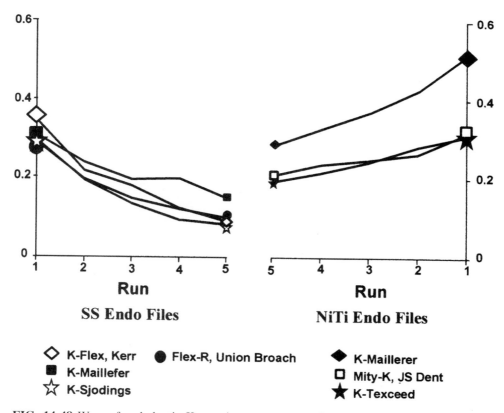

FIG. 14-48 Wear of endodontic K-type instruments manufactured in stainless steel *(SS)* or nitinol *(NiTi)*. The machining efficiency measured in mm². The efficiency measured after one, two, three, four, and five runs in dentin. The files lose their efficiency as they wear after contact with dentin. Nickel-titanium instruments maintain their abrasive efficiency better than stainless steel files.

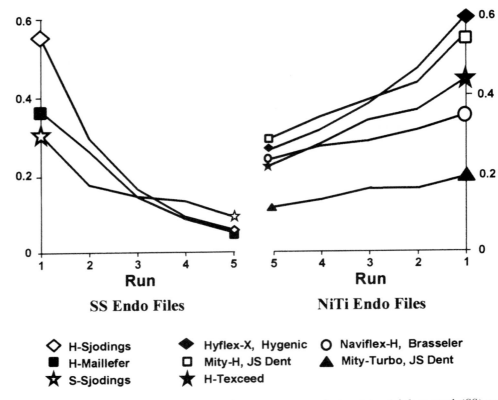

FIG. 14-49 Wear of endodontic H-type instruments manufactured in stainless steel *(SS)* or nitinol *(NiTi)*. The machining efficiency measured in mm^2. The efficiency measured after one, two, three, four, and five runs in dentin. The files lose their efficiency as they wear after contact with dentin. Nickel-titanium instruments maintain their abrasive efficiency better than stainless steel files.

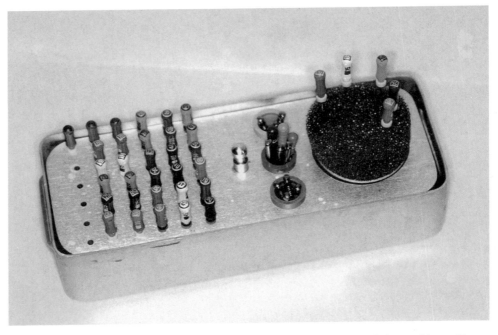

FIG. 14-50 Simple file box for organization of endodontic files, extended round burs, Gates-Glidden burs, and finger spreaders and pluggers (Union Broach).

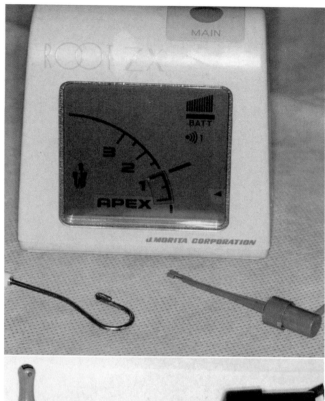

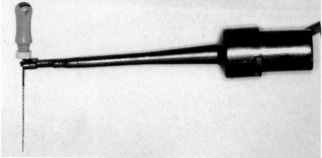

FIG. 14-51 Root ZX apex locator with lip clip and file holder (J Morita, Kyoto, Japan).

Table 14-2. Size designation for auxiliary gutta-percha cones*

Designation	D_3	D_{16}	Taper
XF†	0.20	0.45	0.019
FF	0.24	0.56	0.025
MF‡	0.27	0.68	0.032
F	0.31	0.80	0.038
FM	0.35	0.88	0.041
M	0.40	1.10	0.054
ML§	0.43	1.25	0.063
L	0.49	1.55	0.082
XL	0.52	1.60	0.083

*The cones are pointed. The diameters 3 mm (D_3) and 16 mm (D_{16}) from the tip are prescribed. Tolerance is ± 0.05 mm. Length is ≥ 30 mm ± 2 mm.
†*X*, Extra; *F*, fine.
‡*M*, Medium.
§*L*, Large.

from the instruments' measurement. The final measurement can then be established with a radiograph. Electronic measurements provide more accurate estimates of working length than the normal subtraction of 2 mm from a preoperative radiograph. In a recent study comparing the radiographic method of apex location with the Endex apex locator, it was found that the electronic device was slightly more reliable.[173]

Instruments for Root Canal Obturation

When the root canal has been properly cleaned and enlarged, the space is obturated with a man-made material. A number of obturation methods are practiced, but the lateral and vertical condensations are the two most common.

There are a great number of specialized instruments for each method practiced. The gutta-percha cones are best handled with a grooved endodontic pliers, allowing a firm and controlled grip of the cones (see Fig. 14-8). The pliers are also available with a lock to accommodate various working preferences. Other significant instruments for obturation are spreaders and pluggers. The spreader is a tapered and pointed instrument intended to laterally displace gutta-percha for insertion of addi-

tional accessory gutta-percha cones. The plugger is a similar instrument but with a blunt end. In smaller sizes the spreader and the plugger are often used interchangeably. These instruments are available as a handled instrument or as a finger-held instrument (Fig. 14-52). The handled instruments are potentially dangerous instruments, as the tip of the working end is offset from the long axis of the handle. This arrangement results in strong lateral wedging forces on the working end if the instrument is not firmly operated. The risk of inducing vertical damage to the root is greatly reduced with finger spreaders and pluggers. Each operator must choose the appropriate spreader and plugger according to personal working preferences. There are standardized instruments with the same taper as the files (0.02 mm/mm). Considering the greater taper of standardized accessory gutta-perch cones (Table 14-2) it may sometimes be better to use nonstandardized spreaders with a larger taper to better accommodate the gutta-percha.

In recent years spreaders and pluggers have become available in nickel-titanium. In curved canals these instruments are superior, as they easily follow canal curvatures and are less likely to be deformed during use (Fig. 14-53).

Heat carriers are used for vertical condensation obturation techniques. Traditionally, heat carriers are handled instruments similar to pluggers. They are used to transfer heat to the gutta-percha in the root canal, allowing apical and lateral displacement of the gutta-percha. Electrical heat carriers such as Endotec (Caulk/Dentsply, Milford, Del.) and Touch'N Heat (Analytic Technologies, Redmond, Wash.) are also available. These devices have heat carriers that can be heated to controlled levels. Some also have various tips for different endodontic applications (Fig. 14-54).

For the placement of the sealer/cement and calcium hydroxide dressings a lentulo spiral is a necessity (Fig. 14-55). This spiral drives the paste into the root canal in an effective way. It is necessary, however, for optimal effect that the spiral is as large as possible. The paste is forced forward as the material is squeezed between the canal walls and the spiral. The lentulo spiral is a safe instrument if used correctly. It must be operated clockwise in the handpiece and never started or stopped in the root canal. If not, it will cut into the wall of the root canal and break.

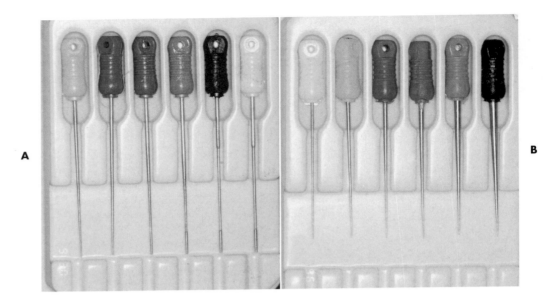

FIG. 14-52 Sets of finger spreaders and pluggers made of nickel-titanium alloy (HyFlex; Hygenic, Akron, Ohio). **A,** Spreaders in sizes extra fine, fine-fine, medium-fine, fine, and medium. **B,** Pluggers in sizes Nos. 20, 25, 30, 35, 40, and 45.

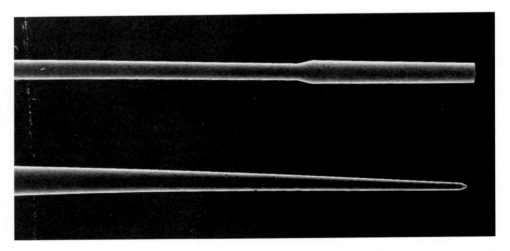

FIG. 14-53 HyFlex nickel-titanium finger spreader and plugger. Note the very smooth surfaces.

Devices for Removal of Root Canal Obstructions

The reader is referred to Chapter 25.

MATERIALS FOR DISINFECTION OF THE PULP SPACE

Irrigation Materials

Instrumentation of the root canal system must always be supported by an irrigation system capable of removing pulp tissue remnants and dentin debris.[87] In modern treatment systems the irrigation fluid is delivered with a fine-caliber needle[2,81] in large volume,[18] and the debris is aspirated with a good suction device. The effervescence occurring when sodium hypochlorite is mixed with hydrogen peroxide has been used for the removal of debris from the root canal but has poor effectiveness.[2,238] Liberal amounts of irrigation are essential for the effective

function of the files. Many anecdotal descriptions of the lubricating effect of irrigation fluids are merely the mistaken effect of debris transportation. Without irrigation, instruments rapidly become ineffective because of accumulation of debris. Irrigation cleans the instrument, making it more effective. Irrigation is very essential for the reduction of the numbers of bacteria in an infected root canal, but it has only a minimal effect on the infected root canal walls and is therefore not capable of rendering the pulp space free of bacteria. Consequently, the antimicrobial effect of an irrigation fluid should not be the only concern when choosing among suitable compounds. The surface tension and cleaning effectiveness are equally important qualities when searching for the ideal irrigant.

Quaternary ammonium compounds that have a low surface tension have been extensively used as irrigation fluid. They are detergents and therefore an effective aid in pulp space cleaning,

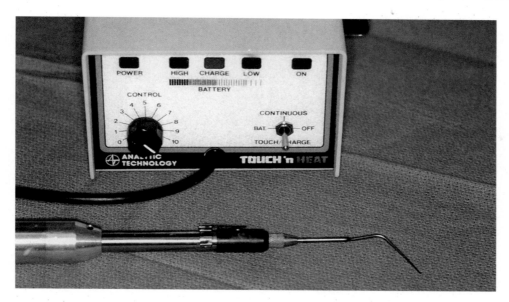

FIG. 14-54 Touch 'N Heat device for heating various endodontic instruments for obturation or gutta-percha removal (Analytic Technology, Redmond, Wash.). Spreader attached to the handpiece.

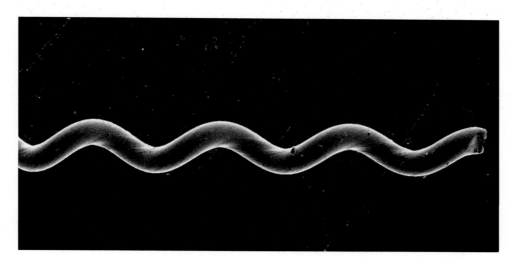

FIG. 14-55 Lentulo spiral.

as they remove lipid pulp breakdown products. Because of their toxicity their use is now less common.[23] Quaternary ammonium compounds are still used as additive to ethylenediaminetetraacetic acid (EDTA) in EDTAC (EDTA and cetrimide) to provide some antimicrobial effect. The irrigation fluid that has dominated endodontic treatment in North America is sodium hypochlorite, which is now the irrigant of choice globally. It has a strong proteolytic effect and therefore serves as an excellent aid during mechanical instrumentation. Chlorhexidine has also been suggested as an irrigant, but there are few advantages to its use during instrumentation beside an antimicrobial effect that is not yet satisfactorily assessed under clinical conditions.[162,166]

Proteolytic materials

The most common proteolytic irrigation material is sodium hypochlorite. Potassium hypochlorite was first suggested as a presurgical hand-washing agent in the middle of the nineteenth century. Sodium hypochlorite (NaOCl) became an important

agent for the treatment of infected wounds in the early twentieth century.[43,52,53] Necrotic tissue and debris are dissolved through a complex biochemical process. The amount of free chlorine is important for this breakdown of the proteins into amino groups.[61] Increased temperature also potentiates the antimicrobial and tissue-dissolving effect of sodium hypochlorite.[47,49,128]

The original concentration suggested by Dakin[52,53] was 0.5%, but the concentration used in dentistry has been as high as 5.25%. A 1% concentration, however, provides sufficient tissue dissolution and antimicrobial effect if used freely. Higher concentrations of sodium hypochlorite affect living tissue and do not improve the reduction of bacteria during endodontic treatment[36,37] (Fig. 14-56). Sodium hypochlorite has an antimicrobial effect as long as free chlorine is available in the solution. Since free chlorine is the important component that is consumed during tissue breakdown, it is essential that the sodium hypochlorite is replenished frequently, especially when low concentrations are used. This becomes more important

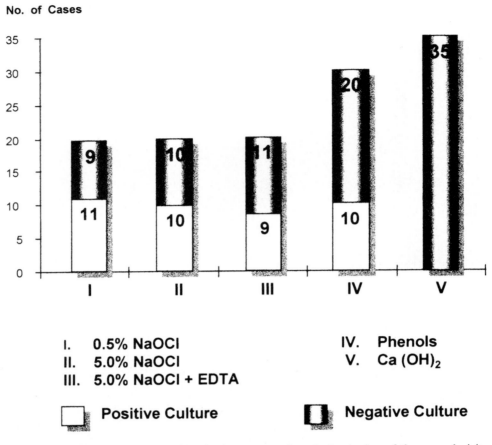

No. of Cases

I. 0.5% NaOCl
II. 5.0% NaOCl
III. 5.0% NaOCl + EDTA
IV. Phenols
V. Ca (OH)₂

☐ Positive Culture   ▣ Negative Culture

FIG. 14-56 Result of root canal disinfection measured at the beginning of the second visit. **I,** Instrumented with 0.5% sodium hypochlorite, no dressing between visits. **II,** Similar treatment as in **I** but using 5% sodium hypochlorite. **III,** Similar treatment as in **I** but using 5% sodium hypochlorite and EDTA. **IV,** Instrumented with sodium hypochlorite followed by dressing with camphorated phenol or paramonochlorphenol. **V,** Similar treatment as in **IV** but using calcium hydroxide as dressing.

when the root canals are narrow and small. Sodium hypochlorite does not wet dentin well, and small canals and canal extensions are poorly irrigated.[174,187,203] Attempts to change the surface tension of sodium hypochlorite have been made without significant success.[1,48] Sodium hypochlorite has been shown to also deplete dentin of organic compounds and to significantly increase the permeability of dentin.[21]

Pure sodium hypochlorite is a USP preparation and may be purchased from a pharmacy. It is common, however, that dentists use commercial 5.25% sodium hypochlorite (bleach, Chlorox, etc.). At this concentration it is highly toxic, meaning that it unnecessarily necrotizes wound surface areas that should remain unharmed. The literature is rich in suggestions that there are no differences in postoperative pain following the use of high concentrations of sodium hypochlorite.[94,97,98] This proves little, as there are poor correlations between tissue damage and clinical symptoms. Commercial sodium hypochlorite is buffered to a pH of approximatively 12 to 13. This adds another toxic component to that of sodium hypochlorite to make the solution even more caustic. Therefore if commercial bleach is used as a base for preparing a 1% irrigation solution, it is better to use sterile 1% sodium bicarbonate as a diluent instead of water. This helps in adjusting the pH to a less caustic level.

Diluted and buffered sodium hypochlorite has a limited shelf-life and should be stored in a dark and cool place no longer than 1 to 2 weeks.

There are few clinical complications to the use of sodium hypochlorite. The most common complication is accidental injection of sodium hypochlorite into periradicular tissue.[22,182] This results in excruciating pain, periapical tissue bleeding, and extensive swelling. The pain normally subsides within a couple of hours. The swelling increases for the first day, after which healing occurs. The prognosis is good.

Detergents

Detergents are often used as irrigation solutions, as they are very effective in removing fatty tissue residues that are by-products of tissue necrosis. The more common materials used are in the family of quaternary ammonium compounds. These compounds were once considered optimal for antimicrobial therapy and effective in very low concentrations. This has proven wrong, and the preparations have a toxicity comparable to other irrigation solutions and a rather narrow bactericidal spectrum.[23,181] Quaternary ammonium antiseptics are normally used in water solution at 0.1% to 1%. Zephiran Chloride is a compound that has been commonly used as an end-

Table 14-3. Tissue irritation of antiseptics used for intracanal dressings*

Dilution	IKI 2%	CP	FC	Cresatin	CPC
1:16	26.9 ± 3.0	—	—	—	—
1:32	2.9 ± 0.3	—	—	—	—
1:64	3.3 ± 0.4	33.8 ± 3.1	21.6 ± 0.8	—	—
1:128	1.6 ± 0.2	16.1 ± 1.4	15.7 ± 1.0	29.7 ± 2.2	33.4 ± 2.7
1:256	1.6 ± 0.1	2.1 ± 0.1	17.0 ± 3.5	19.9 ± 2.2	28.2 ± 2.4
1:512	1.1 ± 0.1	1.1 ± 0.1	11.1 ± 1.7	12.2 ± 0.8	23.0 ± 1.8
1:1024	—	—	4.5 ± 0.9	0.5 ± 0.2	1.9 ± 0.5
1:2048	—	—	1.6 ± 0.4	—	—

IKI, Iodine potassium iodide; *CP*, camphorated phenol; *FC*, formocresol; *CPC*, camphorated parachlorophenol.
*Measurement of enhanced vascular permeability after intradermal injection of 0.1 ml of the diluted antiseptic. Figures indicate leaked albumine measured after 3 hr as μg of Evans blue. Normal values <3 μg. Formocresol causes inflammation when diluted 1000 times; formocresol, cresatin, and camphorated parachlorophenol when diluted 500 times; and camphorated phenol at a dilution of 128 times. Iodine potassium iodide is the least irritating antiseptic. M ± SD. See Spångberg et al.[225] for details.

odontic irrigation solution. Considering its toxicity and low antimicrobial effectiveness, there are no reasons to use this detergent rather than a mild (1% or less) sodium hypochlorite solution.

Another group of antimicrobial agents with detergent effects are the iodophores. Wescodyne and Iodopax are common products in this line of antiseptics. These organic iodine products are not allergenic and are effective at low concentrations. They are antimicrobially effective at an iodine concentration of 0.05% (volume/volume). Detergents have also been mixed with calcium hydroxide for irrigation.[20]

Decalcifying materials

During mechanical preparation of the root canal a smear layer is formed. There is no clear scientifically based understanding if this smear layer must be removed or can be left. There are, however, a multitude of opinions on both sides of this question. In addition to weak acids, solutions for the removal of the smear layer include carbamide peroxide, aminoquinaldinium diacetate (Salvizol), and EDTA. In objective studies carbamide peroxide and Salvizol appear to have little effect on the smear layer buildup.[25,180] A 25% citric acid solution also failed to provide reliable smear layer removal.[261]

EDTA is often suggested as an irrigation solution, as it has the capability to chelate and remove the mineralized portion of smear layers.[79,80,138,139,161] It also can decalcify up to a 50-μm thin layer of the root canal wall if used liberally.[244,252] EDTA is normally used in a concentration of 17%. It removes smear layers in less than 1 minute if the fluid is able to reach the root canal wall surface. Under clinical conditions reports suggest that the fluid should be kept in the root canal for at least 15 minutes to obtain optimal results. The decalcifying process is self-limiting, as the chelator is used up. To achieve continuous effect the EDTA must be replaced through frequent irrigation.[80] For root canal preparation, it has limited value as an irrigation fluid. It may open up a hair-fine canal if given the time to soften the 50 μm it is capable of. This amount, at two opposite canal walls, results in 100 μm. This is equivalent to the tip of a No. 010 file.

The smear layer consists of both an organic and an inorganic component. To effectively remove this smear layer it is normally insufficient to use EDTA only. A proteolytic component such as sodium hypochlorite must also be added for removal of the organic components of the smear layer.[82]

A commercially available product, EndoDilator N-Ø (Union Broach, York, Pa.), is a combination of EDTA and a quaternary ammonium compound. Such irrigation fluid has a slight detergent effect mixed with the chelating effect.

Intracanal Disinfection Materials

Biomechanical instrumentation and irrigation with an antimicrobial solution is essential for the disinfection of the pulp space, but some suggest it may not be sufficient for the complete elimination of microorganisms in a necrotic pulp space.[36,37,87] Therefore further disinfection with an effective antimicrobial agent might be necessary (see Fig. 14-56). The most commonly used intracanal disinfectants belong to the family of phenol or phenol derivatives. Antiseptics on a chlorine or iodine base are also common. In recent years more attention has been given to the use of calcium hydroxide as intracanal dressing for the treatment of infected pulp necrosis. Conventional antiseptics are generally toxic, and care must be taken not to induce undue tissue damage (Table 14-3).

Phenolic preparations

Phenol (C_6H_5OH) or carbolic acid is one of the oldest antimicrobial agents used in medicine. Despite its severe toxicity, derivatives of phenol, such as paramonochlorphenol (C_6H_4OHCl), thymol ($C_6H_3OHCH_3C_3H_7$), and cresol ($C_6H_4OHCH_3$), are still in common use for endodontic treatment. Phenol is a nonspecific protoplasm poison having optimal antibacterial effect at 1% to 2%. Many dental preparations use much too high concentration of phenol in the range of 30%. At such concentration the antimicrobial effect in vivo is lower than optimal and of very short duration.[143] Derivatives of phenol are stronger antiseptics and toxins than phenol alone. The phenolic compounds are often available as camphorated solutions. Camphoration results in a less toxic phenolic compound because of a slower release of toxins to the surrounding tissues.

Studies in vitro have shown that phenol and phenol derivatives are highly toxic to mammalian cells and that the antimicrobial effectiveness of phenol and phenol derivatives does not correspond favorably to their toxicity.[222,223] Experimentation in vivo also demonstrated that phenol and phenol derivatives induce inflammatory changes at much lower concentrations than many other antimicrobial agents.[225]

Phenols are ineffective antiseptics under clinical conditions. Two weeks of intracanal dressing, where the canals were filled with camphorated phenol or camphorated parachlorophenol, failed to eliminate intracanal bacteria in a third of the cases studied[36] (see Fig. 14-56). Phenolic compounds are also unable to release an effective antimicrobial vapor and are therefore ineffective when placed on a cotton pellet in the pulp space.[60,225]

Formaldehyde

Formaldehyde has been extensively used in endodontic therapy and still enjoys great popularity despite its high toxicity and mutagenic potential.[130] The compound of interest when discussing pulp space disinfection is formocresol. The formaldehyde component of formocresol may vary substantially between 19% formaldehyde to 37% formaldehyde. Tricresol formalin is another formaldehyde preparation containing 10% (tri)cresol and 90% formaldehyde. Thus all these preparations contain formaldehyde well above the 10% normally used for fixation of pathologic specimens. Formaldehyde is volatile and therefore releases antimicrobial vapors if applied on a cotton pellet for pulp chamber disinfection. All these formaldehyde preparations are potent toxins with an antimicrobial effectiveness much smaller than their toxicity.[65,223,225] The formaldehyde in contact with tissue in the pulp and periapical tissues is transported to all parts of the body.[15,33] Considering the outright toxic and tissue destructive effect and the mutagenic and carcinogenic potential *there is no clinical reason to use formocresol as an antimicrobial agent for endodontic treatment.* The alternatives are many better antiseptics with significant lower toxicity.

Halogens

Chlorine has been used for many years for irrigation of root canals. It is also sometimes used as intracanal dressing in the form of Chloramine-T.[63,65]

Iodine, in the form of iodine potassium iodide, is a very effective antiseptic solution[166,222] with a low tissue toxicity.[63,65,223,225] It was shown in vitro that iodine potassium iodide (IKI 2%) penetrated more than 1000 μm of dentin in 5 minutes.[166] It is an effective disinfectant for infected dentin, and it is capable of killing bacteria in infected dentin in 5 minutes in vitro.[187] Iodine potassium iodide releases vapors that have a strong antimicrobial effect.[60,225] This solution can be prepared by mixing 2 g of iodine in 4 g of potassium iodide. This mixture is then dissolved in 94 ml of distilled water. Tincture of iodine (5%) has also proven to be one of the few reliable agents for the disinfection of rubber dam and tooth surfaces during the preparation of an aseptic endodontic working field.[152]

Calcium hydroxide

The use of calcium hydroxide (Ca(OH)$_2$) in endodontics was introduced by Hermann in 1920.[100] Although well documented for its time, the clinical applications during the following 25 years were not well known.[101] Calcium hydroxide cannot be categorized as a conventional antiseptic, but it does kill bacteria in the root canal space. It has been routinely used by many endodontists during the last 40 years. The value of calcium hydroxide in endodontic treatment of necrotic infected teeth is now well documented.[36,207] Calcium hydroxide is normally used as a slurry of calcium hydroxide in a water base. At body temperature, less than 0.2% of the calcium hydroxide is dissolved into Ca^{++} and OH$^-$ ions. Calcium hydroxide needs water to dissolve. Therefore it is most advantageous to use water

as the vehicle for the calcium hydroxide paste. In contact with air calcium hydroxide forms calcium carbonate (CaCO$_3$). This is an extremely slow process, however, and of little clinical significance. Calcium hydroxide paste with a significant amount of calcium carbonate feels granular, as the carbonate has a very low solubility. It has been suggested to use Cresatin or camphorated parachlorophenol as the mixing vehicle. Mixing with Cresatin results in the formation of calcium cresylate and acetic acid, whereas mixing with camphorated parachlorophenol results in calcium parachlorphenolate. In both instances the hydrolysis is inhibited, and the advantageous high pH is not reached.[14]

Calcium hydroxide is a slowly working antiseptic. Direct contact experiments in vitro require a 24-hour contact period for complete kill of enterococci.[187] In clinical experimentation 1 week of intracanal dressing has been shown to safely disinfect a root canal system.[207] In addition to killing the bacteria calcium hydroxide has an extraordinary quality in its ability to hydrolyze the lipid moiety of bacterial lipopolysaccharides and thereby inactivates the biologic activity of the lipopolysaccharide.[185,186] This is a very desirable effect, as dead cell wall material remains after killing of the bacteria that causes the root canal infection. Calcium hydroxide not only kills the bacteria but also reduces the effect of the remaining cell wall material lipopolysaccharide (LPS).

Calcium hydroxide may be mixed with sterile water or saline but is also available commercially (Fig. 14-57). It should be mixed to a thick mixture to carry as much calcium hydroxide particles as possible. This slurry is best applied with a lentulo spiral. For maximal effectiveness it is important that the root canal is filled homogeneously to the working length.

Saturated calcium hydroxide solution mixed with a detergent is an effective antimicrobial agent suitable for irrigation.[21]

ROOT CANAL FILLING MATERIALS

After the pulp space has been appropriately prepared, it must be obturated with a material that is capable of completely preventing communication between the oral cavity and the periapical tissue wound. The prepared apical connective tissue wound area cannot heal with epithelium. Therefore the root filling, placed against this wound, serves as an alloplastic implant. These expectations regarding physical and biologic properties make the selection of a good obturation material critical. The materials commonly used for root canal fillings can normally be divided into a solid phase and a cementing medium—a sealer.

Solid Materials

Gutta-Percha

Gutta-percha is the most commonly used material. Gutta-percha is the dried juice of the Taban tree (*Isonandra percha*). It was first introduced to the Royal Asiatic Society of England in 1843 by Sir Jose d'Almeida and was introduced into dentistry in the late 1800s. It occurs naturally as 1,4-polyisoprene and is harder, more brittle, and less elastic than natural rubber. A linear crystalline polymer like gutta-percha melts at a set temperature, and a random but distinct change in structure results. The crystalline phase appears in two forms: alpha phase and beta phase. The forms differ only in the molecular repeat distance and single-bond form. The alpha form is the material that comes from the natural tree product. The processed form, called beta form, is used in gutta-percha for root fillings.[194]

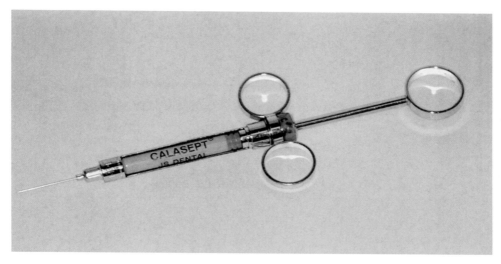

FIG. 14-57 Calasept (J.S. Dental, Ridgefield, Ct.) loaded in carpule syringe for dispensing into pulp chamber.

When heated, gutta-percha undergoes phase transitions. Thus when the temperature increases, there is a transition from beta phase to alpha phase at around 115° F (46° C). This then changes to an amorphous phase around 130 to 140° F (54° to 60° C). When cooled very slowly (1° F per hour), it crystallizes to the alpha phase. Normal cooling returns the gutta-percha to the beta phase. Gutta-percha cones soften at a temperature above 147° F (64° C).[83,194] It can easily be dissolved in chloroform and halothane.

Modern gutta-percha cones for root fillings contain only about 20% gutta-percha (Table 14-4). The major content is zinc oxide, which constitutes 60% to 75% of the material. The zinc oxide content provides a major part of the radiopacity of endodontic gutta-percha. The remaining 5% to 10% consists of various resins, waxes, and metal sulfates. The specific content is normally a manufacturing secret.

Gutta-percha cone material, 1-mm thick, has a radiopacity corresponding to 6.44 mm aluminum.[29]

Because gutta-percha cannot be heat sterilized, other methods for decontamination must be used. The most practical method is to *disinfect the gutta-percha in sodium hypochlorite before use.* This can be done in 1 minute if submerged in a 5% solution of sodium hypochlorite.[204] It is imperative, however, after this disinfection that the gutta-percha is rinsed in ethyl alcohol to remove crystallized sodium hypochlorite before obturation. Crystals of sodium hypochlorite on the gutta-percha cones impair the obturation seal.

Gutta-percha is normally applied using some form of condensation pressure. It has been shown, however, that real compression of gutta-percha is practically impossible.[195] Thus compression during root canal filling procedures cannot be expected to compress gutta-percha but dislodge gutta-percha points to a more complete fill of the root canal. Gutta-percha may also be plasticized with a solvent or through heating to better fit the pulp space for the obturation. Both methods result in a slight shrinkage of approximately 1% to 2% when the gutta-percha has solidified.[141,257,258] It has been suggested that shrinkage in warmed gutta-percha may be prevented if not heated above 113° F (45° C). This is, however, practically impossible when performing vertical warm condensation.[84,90,91,196] It is impor-

Table 14-4. Composition of gutta-percha for endodontic use

Gutta-Percha Cones	
Gutta-percha	19-22%
Zinc oxide	59-75%
Heavy metal salts	1-17%
Wax or resin	1-4%

tant, however, to carefully control the temperature during warm condensation to prevent focal areas of unnecessary high temperatures. The first line of defense would be to use devices that can provide better temperature control than an open flame.[108] Several such electrically controlled heating devices are available (see Fig. 14-54).

Gutta-percha oxidizes in air and exposure to light and becomes brittle.[163] It should therefore be stored in a cool dry place for better shelf-life. Methods to rejuvenate such aged gutta-percha have been suggested.[214]

Gutta-percha cannot be used as the sole filling material because it lacks the adhering quality that is necessary to seal the root canal space. Several techniques have been described to use heat or solvents to adapt the gutta-percha to the canal space better, but a sealer/cement is always needed for the final seal. Gutta-percha cannot seal, as it lacks adhesive properties.

Endodontic gutta-percha is sold as cones in a variety of shapes and tapers (Fig. 14-58). There are two types: "core" points used as master cones and "auxiliary" points used for lateral condensation. There is an accepted international standard for gutta-percha points. Thus the sizing of gutta-percha core points (master cones) is based on similar size and taper standards as the endodontic files (ANSI/ADA No. 78) (see Table 14-1). It is very important to realize, however, that the tolerance is much less stringent for gutta-percha. An endodontic file must be manufactured with a tolerance of ± 0.02 mm, but the gutta-percha must only measure up to ± 0.05 mm. The consequence is that at the same size of instrument and gutta-percha point, there could be a 0.07 mm difference (greater than

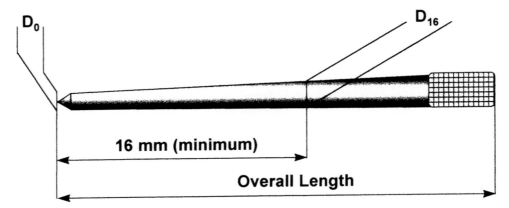

FIG. 14-58 Gutta-percha cone measurement points according to ADA/ANSI No. 78.

one file size) in diameter. This discrepancy could be even larger in the (usual) cases when the standards are not strictly followed by the manufacturer.[234] The auxiliary points have a larger taper and a pointed tip. They are also standardized but in a very different system (see Table 14-2). They are normally supplied in sizes such as fine, fine medium, medium fine, medium, medium large, etc. These gutta-percha cones are usually used as accessory points during lateral condensation. Although core points often are used as master cones for obturation, there are also applications where the auxiliary cone is more suited.

Antibacterial gutta-percha is a 10% iodoform formulation, newly developed by Martin. ABGP is activated, releasing free iodine for bactericidal activity, whenever or wherever there is any leakage within the root canal system and tissue fluid, exudate, or salivary contamination comes into contact with the ABGP. Although unpublished in vitro studies show greater than a tenfold inhibition of various microorganisms (e.g., *Staphylococcus aureus*, *Streptococcus viridans*, *Bacteroides fragilis*) compared to regular gutta percha, it cannot be recommended until long-term studies confirm its safety and efficacy. The ABGP remains inert, similar to regular gutta percha, if no leakage or contamination is present. ABGP theoretically acts as insurance against failure due to subsequent leakage and bacterial contamination.

Silver cones

Pure silver molded in a conical shape has also been used for root canal fillings since the 1930s.[107,242]

The use of silver cones is becoming increasingly rare. It was often used for the obturation of very narrow canals. Because of the stiffness of silver, this technique was easier than using gutta-percha. In recent years stainless steel files have often purposely been used for root canal obturation in clinical situations with heavily calcified, dilacerated narrow canals as a better substitute for silver.

Obtaining good obturation with silver is difficult, as it cannot be made to conform with the pulp space like gutta-percha. Most silver cones contain small amounts of other trace metals (0.1% to 0.2%) such as copper and nickel. This adds to the corrosion of silver cones that is a very common complication in clinical cases[34,96,116,266] (Fig. 14-59). Other reasons for the corrosion of silver in situ are the presence of metal restorations and posts that may have been used in teeth in the area. The silver corrosion products are highly toxic and may in themselves cause severe tissue injury.[78,202] Corrosion has been sug-

gested as a reason for the failure of many silver cone root fillings; but despite numerous reports of silver corrosion in situ, it is not clear if the high failure rate of silver root fillings is associated with the corrosion or simply is the result of poor obturation with such rigid material.

Like all solid materials available today, silver cones or stainless steel files also have the technical drawback that they cannot independently seal the root canal, as these materials do not stick to the dentin walls. Therefore the metal core material must always be used with a cementing material—an endodontic sealer.

Sealers/Cements

Endodontic sealers

In the root canal filling the sealer plays a very important role. Thus the sealer fills all the space the gutta-percha is unable to fill because of gutta-percha's physical limitations. A good sealer must have adhesive strength both to the dentin and to the core material, which usually is gutta-percha. In addition, the sealer must have cohesive strength to hold the obturation together. The sealers are usually a mixture that hardens through a chemical reaction. Such reaction normally includes the release of toxic material, making the sealer less biocompatible. In general, the sealer is the critical part when assessing the toxicity of materials used.

Several sealer/cements such as AH26, Ketac-Endo, and Diaket may be used as the sole filling material, as they have sufficient volume stability to maintain a seal. Under such use preventing excess is often very difficult, as the sealer is applied with a lentulo spiral.

The sealer is expected to have some degree of radiopacity to be clearly visible on adequately exposed radiographs. Additives being used to enhance radiopacity are silver, lead, iodine, barium, and bismuth. Compared to gutta-percha cones most sealers have a slightly lower radiopacity.

There are a variety of sealers among which to choose, and the clinician must be careful to evaluate all characteristics of a sealer before selecting.

Zinc oxide–eugenol cements

Many endodontic sealers are simply zinc oxide–eugenol cements that have been modified for endodontic use. The mixing vehicle for these materials is mostly eugenol. The powder contains zinc oxide that is finely sifted to enhance the flow of

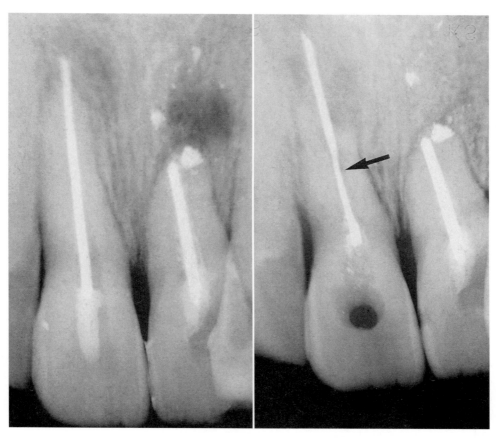

FIG. 14-59 Silver cone root filling. Poorly performed silver cone obturation shows extensive corrosion *(arrow)* 2 years after placement.

the cement. Setting time is adjusted to allow for adequate working time. One millimeter of zinc oxide–eugenol cement has a radiopacity corresponding to 4 to 5 mm of aluminum, which is slightly lower than gutta-percha.[29] These cements easily lend themselves to the addition of chemicals, and paraformaldehyde is often added for antimicrobial and mummifying effects, germicides for antiseptic action, rosin or Canada balsam for greater dentin adhesion, and corticosteroids for suppression of inflammatory reactions. Zinc oxide is a valuable component in the sealer (Table 14-5). It is effective as an antimicrobial agent[237] and has been shown to provide cytoprotection to tissue cells. The incorporation of rosins in sealers may initially have been for the adhesive properties.[89] Rosins (colophony), which are derived from a variety of conifers, are composed of approximatively 90% resin acid. The remaining parts are volatile and nonvolatile compounds such as terpene alcohol, aldehydes, and hydrocarbons. Resin acids are monobasic carboxylic acids with the basic molecular formula $C_{20}H_{30}O_2$. Resin acids are amphiphilic, with the carbon group being lipophilic, affecting the lipids in the cell membranes. This way the resin acids have a strong antimicrobial effect that on mammalian cells is expressed as cytotoxicity. The resin acids work very similar to quaternary ammonium compounds by increasing the cell membrane permeability of the affected cell. Although toxic, the combination of zinc oxide and resin acids may be overall beneficial. The antimicrobial effect of zinc oxide in both gutta-percha cones and in many sealers brings a low level

of long-lasting antimicrobial effect. The resin acids are both antimicrobial and cytotoxic, but the combination with zinc oxide exerts a significant level of cytoprotection.[212,236]

Resin acids may under certain conditions react with zinc, forming resin acid salt (resinate). This matrix-stabilized zincresinate is only slightly soluble in water.[137,213] Therefore zinc oxide–eugenol cements with resin components are less soluble than regular zinc oxide–eugenol cements.

The setting of zinc oxide–eugenol cements is a chemical process combined with physical embedding of zinc oxide in a matrix of zinc eugenolate. Particle size of zinc oxide, pH, and the presence of water regulate the setting and other additives that might be included in special formulas. The formation of eugenolate constitutes the hardening of the cement. Free eugenol always remains in the mass and acts as an irritant. Some more common zinc oxide–eugenol cements are Rickert's sealer (Kerr, Romulus, Mich.), Proco-Sol (Star Dental, Conshohocken, Pa.), U/P-Grossman's sealer (Sultan Chemists, Englewood, N. J.), Wach's sealer (Sultan Chemists), Tubli-Seal (Kerr), Endomethasone (Septodont, Saint-Maur, France), and N2 (Agsa, Locarno, Switzerland). Zinc oxide–eugenol cements lose some volume with time because of dissolution in tissues with the release of eugenol and zinc oxide. This volume loss was measured in pure zinc oxide–eugenol cements over a 180-day period and found to be over 11%.[111] It can be expected that the addition of resin acids to the zinc oxide–eugenol cement significantly reduces this dissolution.[137]

Table 14-5. Composition of some common zinc oxide–eugenol endodontic cements

	Kerr Sealer (Rickert's)	Proco-Sol	Proco-Sol (Nonstaining)	Grossman's Sealer	Wach's Paste	Tubli-Seal
Powder						
Zinc oxide	34.0-41.2	45.0	40.0	42.0	61.3	57.4-59.0
Silver (molecular/precipitated)	25.0-30.0	17.0				
Oleoresins	16.0-30.0					18.5-21.3
Resin (hydrogenated)		36.0				
Staybelite resin			30.0	27.0		
Dithymoliodide	11.0-12.8					
Magnesium oxide U.S.P.		2.0				
Calcium phosphate					12.3	
Bismuth subcarbonate			15.0	15.0		
Bismuth subnitrate					21.5	
Bismuth subiodide					1.8	
Bismuth trioxide						7.5
Barium sulfate			15.0	15.0		
Sodium borate (anhydrous)				1.0		
Heavy magnesium oxide					3.1	
Thymol iodide						3.8-5.0
Oils and waxes						10.0-10.1
Liquid						
Oil of cloves	78.0-80.0				22.2	
Eugenol		90.0	83.3	100.0		*
Canada balsam	20.0-22.0	10.0			74.2	
Sweet oil of almond			16.7			
Eucalyptol					1.8	
Beechwood creosote					1.8	
Polymerized resin						*
Annidalin						*

*Proportions of components not disclosed.

Table 14-6. Composition of two zinc oxide–eugenol endodontic cements with formaldehyde

	Endomethasone*			
	Type A	Type B	Type C	N2 and RC-2B
Powder				
Zinc oxide	+	+	+	62.0-69.0
Bismuth subcarbonate				5.0-9.0
Bismuth subnitrate	+	+	+	2.0-4.0
Barium sulfate				2.0-3.0
Dexamethasone	+	+	+	
Hydrocortisone acetate			+	
Hydrocortisone				1.2
Prednisolone				0.2
Tetraiodothymol	+	+	+	
Paraformaldehyde		+	+	6.5
Titanium dioxide				2.0-3.0
Phenylmercuric borate				0.16
Lead tetroxide				11.0-12.0
Liquid				
Eugenol	+	+	+	92.0-100.0
Geraniol				8.0

*Amounts are not disclosed by the manufacturer; + indicates part of formula.

For a long time it has been common to mix formaldehyde into endodontic sealers. The most common combinations have been zinc oxide–eugenol cements mixed with formaldehyde (Table 14-6). This is an undesirable additive to any sealer, as it only adds to the already toxic effect of eugenol and prevents or delays healing. The use of endodontic materials with formaldehyde content has been popular because formaldehyde necrotizes the nerve endings in the tissue area and thus masks inflammatory processes. Thus despite the necrotic effect of formaldehyde, the patients have few immediate symptoms and the damage is only clinically noticeable years later.

Chloropercha

Chloropercha (Moyco, Union Broach, York Pa.) is another type of sealer that has been in use for many years. It is made by mixing white gutta-percha (alba) with chloroform. This will allow a gutta-percha root filling to fit better in the canal. It is important to recognize, however, that chloropercha has no adhesive properties. Another commercial form of chloropercha, called Kloroperka N-Ø (N-Ø Therapeutics, Oslo, Norway), contains resins and Canada balsam, thereby providing better adhesive properties (Table 14-7). Various forms of chloropercha have a radiodensity (1 mm thick) corresponding to only 1.2 to 2.7 mm of aluminum, which is much less than 1 mm of gutta-percha at 6.4 mm of aluminum.[29] These sealers appear vague on a radiograph. The general problem with most chloropercha products is their shrinkage during the evaporation or disappearance of the chloroform. Some brands, like the Kloroperka N-Ø, contain filler particles such as zinc oxide to

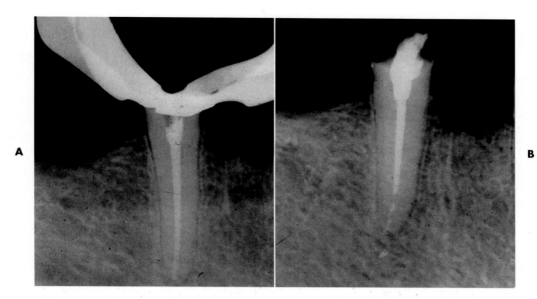

FIG. 14-60 Root filling performed with a resin chloroform dip method. Too much chloroform has been used. Obturation seems good at time of filling (**A**), but at a follow-up 2 weeks later (**B**), when the chloroform had evaporated, the gutta-percha mass has lost significant volume and "dropped" into the periapical tissue.

Table 14-7. Composition of gutta-percha sealers*

	Kloroperka N-Ø	Chloropercha
Powder		
Canada balsam	19.6	
Resin	11.8	
Gutta-percha	19.6	9.0
Zinc oxide	49.0	
Liquid		
Chloroform	100.0	91.0

*Chloropercha is a premixed sealer. Kloroperka N-Ø is a powder/liquid mixture.

reduce the shrinkage. Zinc oxide also increases radiopacity. Another variation on the chloropercha technique is to use a mixture of 5% to 8% of rosins in chloroform.[39] A rosin chloroform wash of the root canal leaves a very adhesive residue. This residue in combination with dipping of the gutta-percha cone in resin chloroform provides the sealer in this technique. This is a difficult technique, as there is no sealer to fill areas where there are voids between the gutta-percha cones. Chloroform technique for obturation requires that the operator has good basic skills with various obturation techniques, as the technique is very sensitive to proper manipulations (Fig. 14-60). When the chloroform technique is correctly used, the shrinkage is not greater than when gutta-percha is plasticized by heat.[258]

The use of chloroform has been sharply curtailed in recent years because of its projected toxicity. In endodontics, however, the amounts used are normally insignificant and cause no health hazard. One must, however, take prudent steps to reduce the vaporization during use, as chloroform is highly volatile. Thus when used for softening of gutta-percha during revision of old root fillings, the chloroform should be dispensed

through a syringe and hypodermic needle. For other uses the *exposure time, amounts used,* and *chloroform surface exposed* should all be kept to a minimum. There are some chloroform substitutes in use such as halothane and turpentine. Halothane is less effective in softening gutta-percha than chloroform, is hepatotoxic like chloroform, and has a higher local toxicity than chloroform (Table 14-8). Therefore halothane is not a good substitute. Turpentine is not carcinogenic but is reported to easily cause allergic reactions. It has a high local toxicity and dissolves gutta-percha poorly. Therefore there are presently no good substitutes to the use of chloroform in endodontic treatment procedures. With careful workplace hygiene there is little risk associated with the occasional use of miniscule amounts of chloroform in endodontics.[19,134]

Calcium hydroxide sealers

Recently several calcium hydroxide ($Ca(OH)_2$)–based sealers have been brought to the market. Examples of such sealers are Sealapex (Kerr), CRCS (Hygenic Corp., Akron, Ohio), and Apexit (Vivadent, Schaan, Liechtenstein). These sealers are promoted as having therapeutic effect because of the calcium hydroxide content (Box 14-1). No such convincing results from scientific trials have been shown. To be therapeutically effective calcium hydroxide must be dissociated into Ca^{++} and OH^-. Therefore to be effective, an endodontic sealer based on calcium hydroxide must dissolve and the solid consequently lose content. Thus one major concern is that the calcium hydroxide content may dissolve, leaving obturation voids. This would ruin the function of the sealer, as it would disintegrate in the tissue. These sealers also have poor cohesive strength.[255] There is no objective proof that a calcium hydroxide sealer provides any advantage for root canal obturations or has any of the desirable biologic effects of calcium hydroxide paste. In a study of diffusion of hydroxyl ions into surrounding dentin after root filling with Sealapex and Apexit, no traces were found in teeth filled with Apexit. Some hydroxyl ions could be detected in the dentin

Table 14-8. Toxic effect of gutta-percha solvents on L929 cells in vitro*

Time	Control	Chloroform	Halothane	Turpentine
Air Evaporation				
Fresh mix	7.2 ± 0.7	94.4 ± 3.0	102.5 ± 7.5	87.3 ± 2.2
1 day	10.1 ± 0.4	11.3 ± 1.8	12.6 ± 0.9	66.6 ± 5.3
7 days	9.5 ± 0.4	11.6 ± 0.9	14.8 ± 1.0	12.5 ± 2.8
Liquid Evaporation				
Fresh mix	7.2 ± 0.7	102.1 ± 6.4	98.4 ± 6.6	87.0 ± 2.1
1 day	10.1 ± 0.4	89.1 ± 6.7	103.9 ± 9.0	71.8 ± 4.7
7 days	9.5 ± 0.4	11.6 ± 5.8	10.1 ± 2.8	64.2 ± 3.9

From Barbosa SV et al: *J Endod* 20:6, 1994.
*Gutta-percha (2.5 g) was dissolved in either chloroform, halothane, or turpentine (5 ml). The cell response was measured as radiochromium release at various times after mixing. The solvents were allowed to evaporate in air or through a liquid layer. The higher the release, the higher is the toxicity. M ± SD.

BOX 14-1.
CONTENT OF CALCIUM HYDROXIDE SEALERS: SEALAPEX, CRCS, AND APEXIT*

Sealapex

Base

Calcium hydroxide	25.0%
Zinc oxide	6.5%

Catalyst

Barium sulfate	18.6%
Titanium dioxide	5.1%
Zinc stearate	1.0%

CRCS

Powder

Calcium hydroxide
Zinc oxide
Bismuth dioxide
Barium sulfate

Liquid

Eugenol
Eucalyptol

Apexit

Base

Calcium hydroxide	31.9%
Zinc oxide	5.5%
Calcium oxide	5.6%
Silicon dioxide	8.1%
Zinc stearate	2.3%
Hydrogenized colophony	31.5%
Tricalcium phosphate	4.1%
Polydimethylsiloxane	2.5%

Activator

Trimethyl hexanedioldisalicylate	25.0%
Bismuth carbonate basic	18.2%
Bismuth oxide	18.2%
Silicon dioxide	15.0%
1.3-Butanedioldisalicylate	11.4%
Hydrogenized colophony	5.4%
Tricalcium phosphate	5.0%
Zinc stearate	1.4%

*Proportions are unavailable for CRCS and incomplete for Sealapex.

---

close to the root filling with Sealapex.[228] In a similar study of calcium and hydroxyl ion release from Sealapex and CRCS negligible release was noted from CRCS. Sealapex released more ions but disintegrated in the process.[240] Studies in vivo of Sealapex and CRCS have demonstrated that Sealapex and CRCS easily disintegrates in the tissue.[211] They both cause chronic inflammation.[212,243] Considering the alternatives, calcium-containing sealers are not a practical choice of material.

Polymers

New sealers are mostly polymers (Table 14-9). The more common brands are Endofill (Lee Pharmaceuticals, South El Monte, Calif.), AH26 (Caulk/Dentsply, Milford, Del.), and Diaket (ESPE, Seefeld, Germany). AH26 is an epoxy resin that initially was developed to serve as a single filler material.[199,201] Because of its good handling characteristics it has been extensively used as a sealer. It has a good flow, seals well to dentin walls, and allows for a sufficient working time.[132,201] One millimeter of AH26 has a radiopacity corresponding to 6.66 mm of aluminum and thus very similar to gutta-percha.[29] Like most sealers, AH26 is very toxic freshly prepared.[167,216-220] This toxicity decreases rapidly during the setting, and after 24 hours the cement has one of the lowest toxicities of endodontic sealers. The reason for the toxicity of the AH26 sealer is the release of a very small amount of formaldehyde as a result of the chemical setting process. This amount of brief release of formaldehyde, however, is thousands of times lower than the long-term release from conventional formaldehyde-containing sealers such as N2.[226] After the initial setting AH26 exerts little toxic effect in vitro or in vivo.[26,27,167,200,254]

Diaket is a polyketone compound containing vinyl polymers that, mixed with zinc oxide and bismuth phosphate, forms an adhesive sealer.[197] Small amounts of camphor and phenol interact negatively with the setting process and must be care-

Table 14-9. Composition of resin-type endodontic sealers

	Resins		
	AH26	**Diaket**	**Riebler's Paste**
Powder			
Silver powder	10%		
Zinc oxide		98.0%	*
Bismuth oxide	60%		
Bismuth phosphate		2.0%	
Hexamethylenetetramine	25%		
Titanium oxide	5%		
Formaldehyde (polymerized)			*
Barium sulfate			*
Phenol			*
Liquid			
Bisphenoldiglycidyl ether	100%		
2.2′-Dihydroxy 5.5′-dichlorodiphenylmethane		*	
Propionylacetophenone		*	
Triethanolamine		*	
Caproic acid		*	
Copolymers of vinyl acetate, vinyl chloride, and vinyl isobutylether		*	
Formaldehyde			*
Sulfuric acid			*
Ammonia			*
Glycerin			*

*Proportions not available.

fully removed before obturation. The material sets quickly in the root canal at body temperature but remains soft longer at room temperature. The volume stability is good and the solubility low.[88,102,103] It is highly toxic in vitro and causes extensive tissue necrosis. The irritation is long lasting.[167,216-220]

Glass-ionomer cement

Recently glass-ionomer cements have been introduced as endodontic sealers (Ketac-Endo, EPPE). Glass-ionomer cements are known to cause little tissue irritation.[264,265] It also has a low toxicity in vitro.[170] There are little biologic data available relative to its use as an endodontic sealer, so safety and efficacy have not been established.

There are questions about the quality of the seal with Ketac-Endo because of observed dentin-sealer adhesive failures.[56,210]

Formaldehyde-containing sealers

A large group of endodontic sealer/cements have substantial additives of paraformaldehyde. Some of the more common are Endomethasone, Kri paste, Riebler's paste, and N2. Although not much different in content as far as toxicity is concerned, N2 has been the material most commonly focused on when discussing this phenomenon. This material is also known as RC 2B or the "Sargenti technique." Throughout the years it has been heavily commercialized. It is difficult to understand that anyone can subscribe to the idea that treating the apical pulp wound with a strong tissue-coagulating toxic material may enhance healing.

N2 is basically a zinc oxide–eugenol sealer. Its composition has been varied extensively throughout the years. The significant content of lead oxide[62,256] and smaller amount of organic

mercury (Fig. 14-61) that formerly were major toxic components of N2 are often missing in recent formulas. It still contains large amounts of formaldehyde. It seals well in combination with a core.[35,86] Since it contains 6% to 8% paraformaldehyde and sometimes hydrocortisone and prednisolone, it loses substantial volume when exposed to fluid.[88] It also absorbs more than 2% of fluid during the first week in situ.[102]

N2 is very toxic in experiments in vitro[224] and in animal experiments.[92,122,216-221] The tissue reaction normally observed is a coagulation necrosis within a very short time, reaching its maximum in less than 3 days. The coagulated tissue is altered to such an extent that it cannot undergo any repair for months, since it is formaldehyde impregnated. With time the formaldehyde is washed out of the necrotic tissue,[15,32] allowing either bacteria to be established in the necrosis or, if the blood supply is adequate, repair to take place.[216-221] In clinical applications this untoward tissue reaction can be seen as localized inflammatory reactions in the periapical tissue.[64]

Standards and Properties

Physical properties

ADA/ANSI document No. 57 outlines various test methods for the evaluation of physical properties of endodontic sealer filling materials. Sealers are classified into two categories (types) depending on intended usage: type I materials are intended to be used with core material, and type II materials are intended for use with or without core material or sealer. Type I materials are divided into three classes. Class 1 includes materials in the form of powder and liquid that set through a nonpolymerizing process. Class 2 includes materials in the form of two pastes that set through a nonpolymerizing process. Finally, class 3 includes polymer and resin systems that set through polymerization. The subclasses for type II materials are the same as for type I materials, except that metal amalgams are also included. Document No. 57 describes testing methods for working time, setting time, flow, film thickness, solubility, and disintegration. There is also a specific requirement for radiodensity.[29]

Despite these often detailed requirements there are still significant disagreements on ideal properties. Therefore most of these expectations are guidelines that have not significantly affected the industry.

Biologic properties

ADA/ANSI document No. 41 recommends various protocols for the biologic evaluation of dental materials. This document outlines recommended test protocols for various dental materials including certain guidelines for endodontic filling materials. These methods include general toxicity assessments (LD_{50}), cytotoxicity assessments in vitro, sensitization assays, mutagenicity assays, implantation tests, and usage tests. For each of these items there are several test methods to choose from depending on type of material.

Root canal filling materials are generally toxic and none fulfills the expectations that document No. 41 requires. In an attempt to select more biologically acceptable materials it is possible, however, to use methods described in document No. 41 to distinguish more toxic from less toxic materials. This results in a less intensive or long-lasting chemical insult to the remaining apical pulp or apical periodontium. If the wound

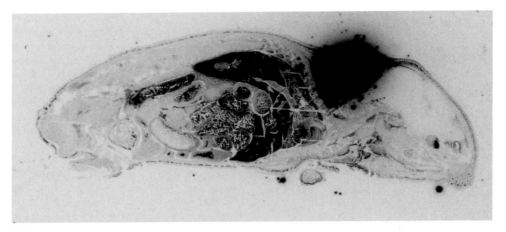

FIG. 14-61 N2. Freshly mixed paste of N2 was injected in the neck skin of newborn mouse. Mercury in the powder had been made radioactive. Twenty-four hours after injection the mouse was instantly frozen and sectioned. This figure shows the autoradiogram resulting from such section. Neck area where the injection was done is highly radioactive but practically all parts of the body are radioactive *(black)* to some degree. This shows that any zinc oxide–eugenol cement introduced into the tissue allows leakage of components that are transported to all parts of the body.

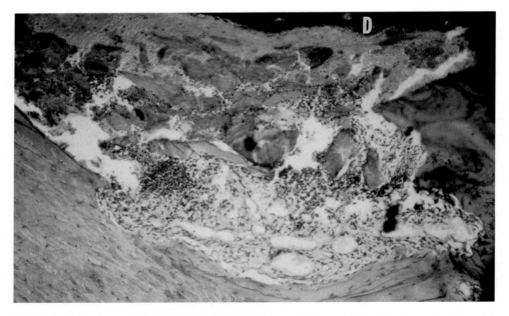

FIG. 14-62 Implant of Diaket (ESPE, Seefeld, Germany) in mandible of guinea pig. Material has necrotized the surrounding bone that contains sequestered bone and severe accumulation of all forms of inflammatory cells. Diaket at *D*.

area is free from bacteria when the initial chemical necrosis occurs, there is no reason to believe that tissue repair would not take place as the initial irritant decreases in intensity. There may be some tissue irritation due to phagocytosis of particles of the material, but the result would not be an expanding lesion.[209] Discounting paraformaldehyde-containing endodontic materials, endodontic sealers should not be implicated as the cause for the development of a periradicular bone lesion. When the tissue in the apical root area is not sterile, however, a chemical pulp or periapical necrosis is a good area for microbial expansion. Thus materials that cause extensive tissue ne-

crosis, either inside the root canal or when extruded as an excess of filling material, are in fact vehicles for the development of a failing endodontic treatment (Fig. 14-62). This supports the idea that treatment should focus on the proper application of asepsis and antisepsis and use materials that cause as few tissue injuries as possible.

Gutta-percha as a root canal filling material has been extensively investigated and found to be biocompatible. In comparison with sealers used for root canal obturations it clearly has the lowest tissue toxicity (Fig. 14-63). In implantation studies ranging up to 6 months in length, gutta-percha has been shown

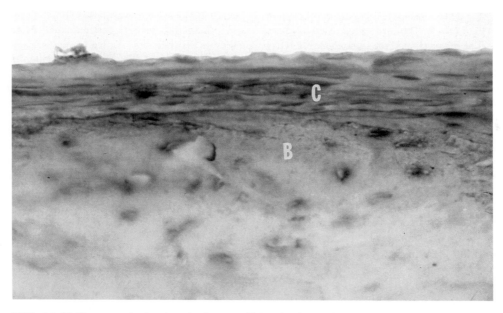

FIG. 14-63 Gutta-percha implant in the mandible of guinea pig. Twelve weeks. Gutta-percha implant *(on top)* has healed in well with a thin connective tissue interface *(C)* between the healed bone *(B)* and the implant that was lost during histologic preparation. Compare tissue reaction with Fig. 14-62.

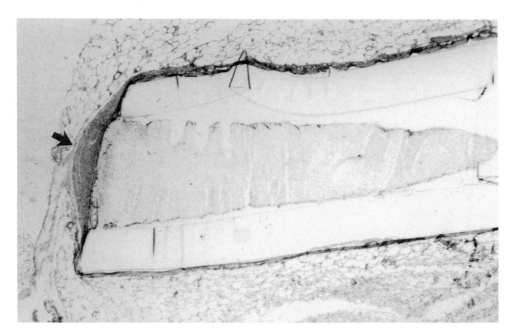

FIG. 14-64 Gutta-percha implant in subcutaneous connective tissue of guinea pig. Twelve weeks. Material was implanted in a Teflon tube. The tissue has responded with a connective tissue capsule *(arrow)* that is thicker than tissue surrounding the tube. No sign of inflammatory cells.

to heal in well with minimal irritation.* Similar findings were reported from implantation in humans. After implantation the gutta-percha is normally surrounded by a defined capsule rich in cells but without significant presence of inflammatory cells but some presence of macrophages (Fig. 14-64). Results from

more sensitive assays in vitro supports the in vivo results, suggesting that gutta-percha for root canal fillings have a low toxicity.[167,216-219,224] Gutta-percha in the form of small particles induces an intensive foreign body reaction with massive accumulation of mononucleated and multinucleated macrophages.[209] This is not surprising, however, as material normally considered inert, such as Teflon, causes similar reactions when presented to the tissues as an irregular surface or particles.[41]

*References 26-28, 67, 68, 104, 151, 209, 215-220

Sealers and cements are the very toxic component of a gutta-percha root filling (Fig. 14-65). Therefore great care must be given to the selection of materials and the understanding what each material may contribute to a disease process. Zinc oxide–eugenol cements have a significant drawback in their release of free eugenol and loss of volume during the hydrolysis that takes place after setting. Several of the polymer materials have a high toxicity during the polymerization phase (AH26, Diaket, Endofill) but may become practically inert when polymerized (AH26, Endofill) (Fig. 14-66). Sealers with inclusions of dissolvable components such as calcium hydroxide lose these components in the tissue with a compromise of the integrity of the fill.

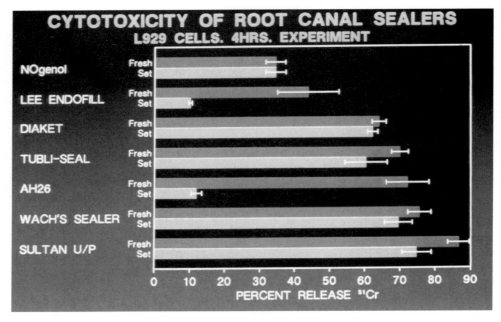

FIG. 14-65 Cytotoxic effect of endodontic sealers on L929 fibroblasts in vitro. Toxicity measured as release of ^{51}Cr. The more release the more cytotoxic is the material. Freshly prepared sealers are always more toxic than set sealers. Many sealers stay toxic even after setting.

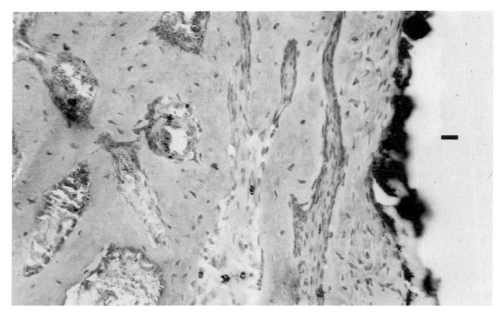

FIG. 14-66 Implant of AH26 in the mandible of the guinea pig. Twelve weeks. Bone has grown up and integrated with the implant (at *I*). Remnants of the AH26 implant, that was lost during histologic preparation, can be seen as a black area at the top. Complete healing observed without signs of inflammation.

DELIVERY SYSTEMS FOR ROOT CANAL FILLING MATERIALS

The search for simplification and increased proficiency has led to the development of many new hybrid materials. All hybrids available today are based on gutta-percha. The differences focus on alternative methods to introduce the gutta-percha into the root canal system with maintained control. The methods presently in use are either injection techniques or gutta-percha cones attached to a more rigid skeleton.

Most hybrid obturation methods require modification in the outline of the root canal preparation. Therefore before attempting hybrid obturation methods, considering technique variations for optimal results is important.[257]

A comparison of the more commonly practiced obturation methods with an objective and sensitive dye penetration method failed to show any major difference in the quality of the obturation (Fig. 14-67).[55]

Rigid Systems

ThermaFil (Tulsa Dental Products, Tulsa, Okla.; Densfil, Caulk/Dentsply, Milford, Del.) is an obturation system where the gutta-percha is preapplied to a core skeleton that resembles an endodontic file (Fig. 14-68). The gutta-percha obturator is heated in a special heater (ThermaPrep Oven, Tulsa Dental Products, Tulsa Okla.; Fig. 14-69) to appropriate softness and the obturation is done with the complete device (gutta-percha + core). A sealer must be used for complete obturation. These devices are available with a plastic, stainless steel, or titanium core. The larger size plastic core material can, if needed, be softened with chloroform for easy removal. These obturators offer an alternative method for obturation with gutta-percha.

Injection Techniques

Several techniques have been described for introducing gutta-percha into the root canal system after the gutta-percha has been plasticized with heat. There are principally two methods.

UltraFil (Hygenic) is a system where the heated (158° F, 70° C) and modified gutta-percha is injected, under pressure, into the carefully prepared root canal (Figs. 14-70 and 14-71).[145] A similar system, Obtura II (Texeed, Costa Mesa, Calif.),[262] dispenses a heavier form of gutta-percha heated to a higher temperature (302° to 338° F, 150° to 170° C) than UltraFil (158° to 194° F, 70° to 90° C). The UltraFil line has been expanded to a complex system with accessory components. Thus an apical plug can be created with SuccessFil using the Trifecta system. The canal system can then be backfilled with the Endoset or Firmset gutta-percha in the UltraFil system. Obtura is more a delivery system for gutta-percha and is most often used in the vertical condensation obturation technique.

Although the temperature of the gutta-percha in the Obtura injection gun is as high as 302° to 338° F (150° to 170° C), the temperature of the extruded material may vary between 140° to 176° F (60° to 80° C)[90,91] and 280.04° F (137.8° C).[59] The UltraFil gutta-percha leaves the injection at a temperature of 145.22° F (62.9° C).[59] The intracanal temperatures after de-

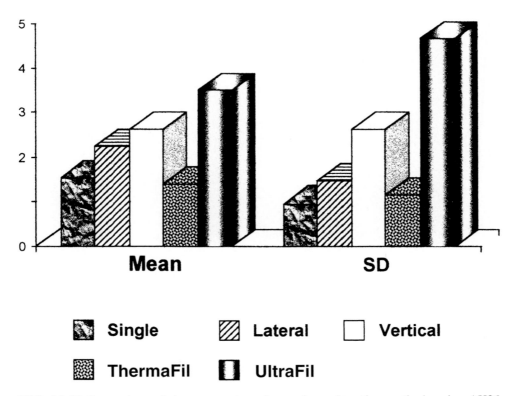

FIG. 14-67 Comparison of dye penetration after various obturation methods using AH26 sealer. Dye was delivered with a vacuum method. Measured as millimeters of leakage. Single cone technique and ThermaFil resulted in the least leakage followed by lateral condensation, vertical condensation, and UltraFil. Standard deviation is high, as is common for leakage studies, reflecting the variability in the obturation method. The less complicated the obturation method, the lower is the standard deviation.

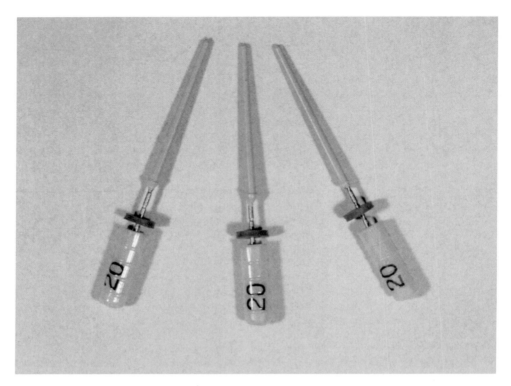

FIG. 14-68 ThermaFil obturators (Tulsa Dental Products, Tulsa, Okla.).

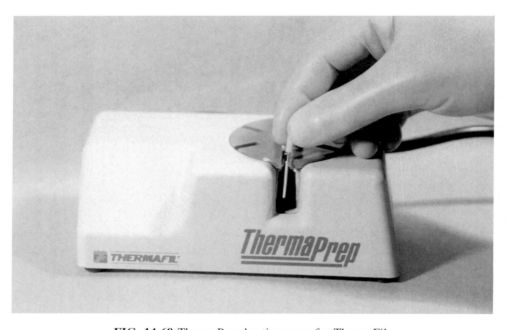

FIG. 14-69 ThermaPrep heating oven for ThermaFil.

livery of these two gutta-percha systems have been measured, with intracanal thermocouples, to be 107.6° to 192.2° F (42° to 89° C) with the Obtura system and 77° to 113° F (25° to 45° C) with the UltraFil system.[59] With the high temperatures resulting from injection of gutta-percha with the Obtura system, periodontal injuries have been reported after endodontic treatment of teeth in the ferret and the dog.[153,190,191]

Shrinkage of gutta-percha in these injectable gutta-percha systems does not appear to be different from the shrinkage of normal gutta-percha. When plasticized by heat, gutta-percha has a volume loss of approximatively 2% when cooling.[85]

Rotary Techniques

Heat softening of gutta-percha can be achieved using frictional heat. This was first suggested with the introduction of the McSpadden compactor instrument. This technique has seen

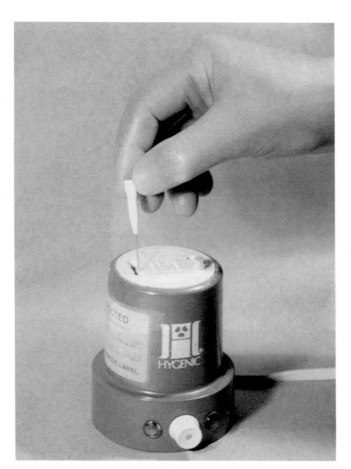

FIG. 14-70 UltraFil heating oven (Hygenic, Akron, Ohio). Single dose of gutta-percha is being loaded in the heater.

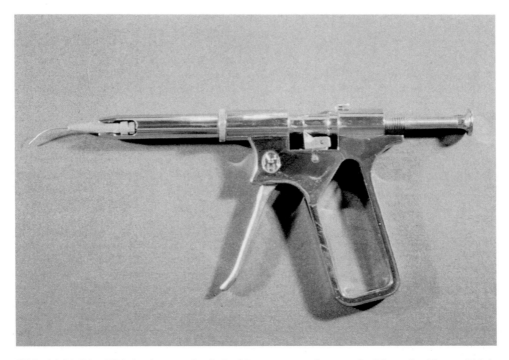

FIG. 14-71 UltraFil injection gun loaded with a gutta-percha carpule (Hygenic, Akron, Ohio).

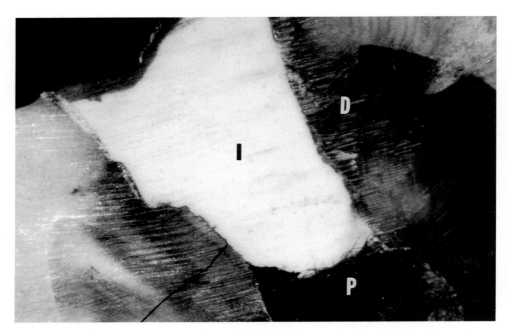

FIG. 14-72 Temporary filling of IRM (white at *I*). Dye has penetrated the margins and dyed the content of the pulp chamber *(P)*. Dentin *(D)* has been stained by the dye penetrating the margins.

many variations[189,239] and the development of several compaction instruments. The generated heat may exceed safe levels as for other heat compaction techniques.[190,191] One device called Quickfil (J.S. Dental, Ridgefield, Conn.) is commercially available. The ability to obturate root canals with this device and friction heating was found to be as good as lateral condensation.[192] Volumetric changes in the gutta-percha after friction heat compaction are similar to other types of gutta-percha condensations using heat.[46]

TEMPORARY CEMENTS

If endodontic therapy cannot be completed in one visit, the pulp space must be closed with a sealing temporary cement. This cement must be capable of providing a satisfactory seal to prevent bacteria and fluid products from the oral cavity from contaminating the pulp space. This cement must have enough structural strength to withstand the masticatory forces and retain the seal. The most common materials are IRM (L.D. Caulk, Milford, Del.), TERM (L.D. Caulk, Milford, Del.), and Cavit (ESPE, Seefeld, Germany). IRM is a reinforced zinc oxide cement available in powder or liquid but also in single-dose mixing capsules. Cavit is a ready-mixed material composed of zinc oxide, calcium sulfate, glycol and polyvinyl acetate, polyvinyl chloride, and triethanolamine. It sets on contact with water. TERM is a filled composite resin that is light activated. Of these, TERM and Cavit provide better seal than IRM at any thickness of the restorations.[12,95,112] IRM has extensive marginal leakage of fluid, whereas Cavit seems to absorb fluid into the entire body of the restoration. These findings are surprising; however, IRM may, due to its eugenol content, provide a bacterial barrier but allows leakage of other liquid substances (Figs. 14-72 and 14-73). Therefore if Cavit or other types of relatively soft temporary cements are used, they must be placed at a thickness of at least 4 to 5 mm. If a more robust temporary restoration is required for a longer time period than 1 week, the soft cement must be covered with a harder cement such as IRM or glass ionomer cement.

RETROGRADE ENDODONTIC TREATMENT

Root End Preparation

Root end preparation has classically been done with rotary instruments. Because of the restriction in available space in the periapical area, special handpieces have been developed (Fig. 14-74). In recent years there has been extensive use of ultrasonic and sonic preparation of the root end. Such preparation can be done more conservatively than preparation with a bur. It also requires less angulated resection of the root apex. Because of their higher strength the piezoelectrical units have a clear advantage as this type of preparation requires power (Figs. 14-75 and 14-76). A serious concern was raised, however, reporting a high frequency of apical cracks of the dentin in the resected area.[126,193] This cracking was especially pronounced at higher power settings. This phenomenon requires further careful assessment, as initial crack lines may years later propagate a more extensive fracture.

Root End Filling Materials

The choice of root end filling materials is a subject of great controversy among endodontic surgeons. The classic material was silver amalgam, but it was suggested that the zinc normally found in the alloy may cause tissue damage.[164] This would be due to the precipitation of toxic zinc carbonate in the tissue associated with such root end amalgam filling. Despite the lack of more solid information regarding zinc in amalgam and its consequences it has become a standard to use zinc-free alloys for root end fillings. More recent studies of the possible formation of zinc carbonate in the tissue has been unsuccessful. Thus there is no solid evidence that zinc-containing amalgams would be less suitable for retrograde obturations[118,119,131,136] (Figs.

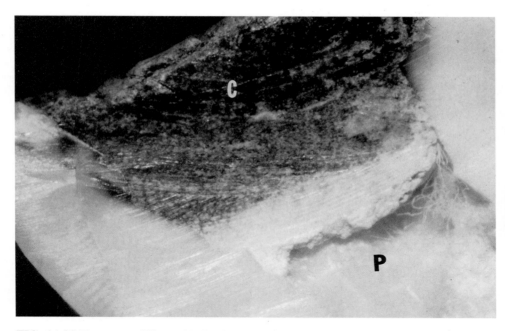

FIG. 14-73 Temporary filling with Cavit. Dye has been absorbed into the body of the restoration *(C)* but not penetrated to the pulp chamber *(P)* that is filled with white cotton. Inner part of the Cavit has no stain.

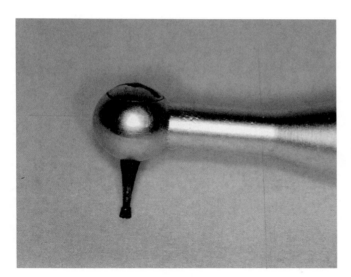

FIG. 14-74 Miniature contraangle handpiece for root end preparation.

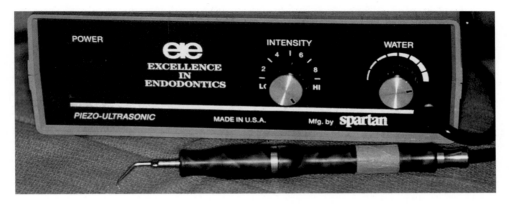

FIG. 14-75 Spartan piezoelectrical ultrasonic device with sterilizable handpiece. Power and irrigation flow can be adjusted.

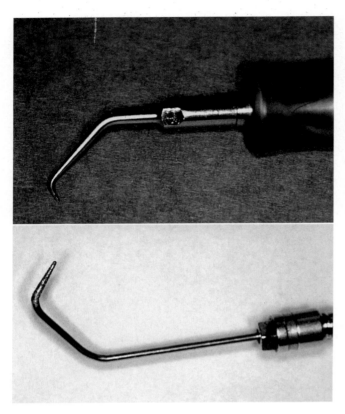

FIG. 14-76 Working tips for root end preparation. Upper figure is a Spartan steel tip. Lower figure is a diamond-coated tip for an Enac unit.

14-77 and 14-78). Zinc is toxic in excess, however, and the tissue tolerance is rather low. Thus in evaluations in vitro amalgams containing zinc are slightly more toxic than zinc-free amalgams (Table 14-10).

Because of various concerns about the use of silver amalgam other materials such as zinc oxide–eugenol cements (IRM, Super EBA), glass-ionomer cements, composite resins, and Cavit have been used. The attempt to use Cavit as a retrograde obturation material was unsuccessful.[70]

Glass-ionomer cements have generally been evaluated and compared to amalgam and gutta-percha with some success.[40,54,110,263,264] Silver glass-ionomer cement (Ketac-Silver) was evaluated and compared to zinc oxide–eugenol and amalgam and found to be superior in in vitro and in vivo applications.[31,170]

All these materials have been used as alternatives to silver amalgam, but no clear and objective preferential material can be found. Results are highly variable after root end obturations, and it is possible to find data in the literature to support most of these materials including silver amalgam. It is therefore reasonable to believe that, within the scope of the reviewed materials, the material may be just one of several factors that determine success or failure after root end surgery.

LASERS

Laser applications in endodontics are still in their infancy. It remains unclear if the use of laser technology will ever mature to have a practical application in this field of dentistry. Numerous papers have been written on the subject but mostly with inadequate documentation. Presently there is little support for the unbounded enthusiasm found in many commercial brochures and professional publications.

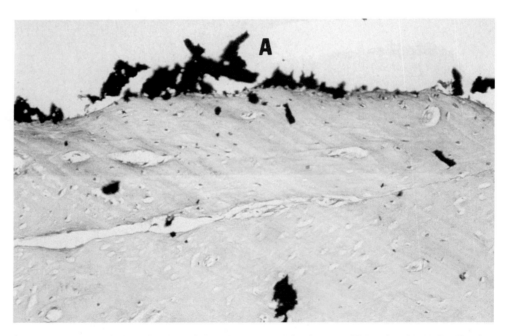

FIG. 14-77 Dispersalloy implanted freshly prepared in the mandible of guinea pig. Twelve weeks. Remnants of the amalgam *(A)*, which were removed during the histologic preparation, are black. Bone has healed and integrated with the amalgam without any layer of soft connective tissue.

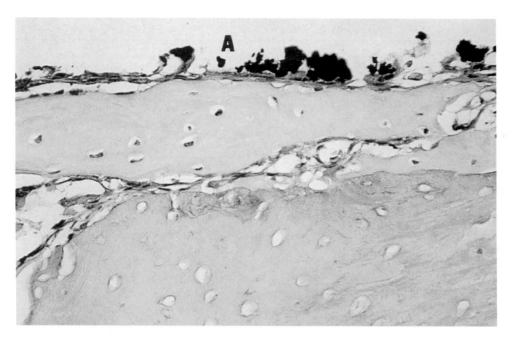

FIG. 14-78 Zinc-free amalgam implanted freshly prepared in the mandible of guinea pig. Twelve weeks. Remnants of the amalgam *(A)*, which were removed during the histologic preparation, are black. Bone has healed and integrated with the amalgam without any layer of soft connective tissue.

The lasers most commonly applied in endodontic research are carbon dioxide laser (10,600 nm wavelength), Nd:YAG laser (1064 nm), argon laser (418 to 515 nm), and xenon chloride Excimer laser (308 nm). There are many factors affecting laser-tissue interaction. One significant factor is the relationship between wavelength and tissue absorption of the energy. Thus the wavelength of a carbon dioxide laser is highly absorbed by water in the tissues. Nd:YAG laser is almost transparent to water but absorbed in pigmented tissue and hemoglobin. Therefore it may cause deeper damage to tissue than a carbon dioxide laser. Refraction and diffuse scattering of radiation is another serious concern when operating in crystalline structures such as teeth.

Some of the attempted applications in endodontics have been related to lowering dentin permeability, instrumenting, cleaning and disinfecting root canals, and root end surgery.

Various attempts have been made to decrease dentin permeability by fusing the dentin surface with carbon dioxide and Nd:YAG lasers. Lowered permeability after treatment with carbon dioxide and Nd:YAG lasers has been reported,[147,241] but increased permeability has also been reported.[168] Xenon chloride Excimer laser has been shown to occlude dentin tubules.[227]

The use of lasers for root canal preparation has not been successful. Levy[129] suggested that it was possible to effectively clean root canals with a water and air cooled Nd:YAG laser. The illustrations in the publication, however, did not support the claims as they did not demonstrate root canal walls but dentin cut parallel to the dentin tubules. Another study using an Nd:YAG laser showed that the heat generation during laser treatment of the root canals in the teeth of dogs resulted in necrosis of periodontal tissue and subsequent ankylosis.[17] Some Nd:YAG lasers have air and water cooling to decrease the heat buildup. It is highly questionable, however, if it is advisable to force water at a pressure of 2 psi and air at 10 psi down the pulp space to control temperature increases.[147]

Argon laser as an adjunct to regular instrumentation and irrigation was shown to improve the cleanliness of the root canal walls.[154] Root canal disinfection with Nd:YAG laser has been attempted with poor results.[155] Superficially infected root canals were lased in attempts to disinfect the canals. The laser was found to reduce the number of bacteria in the root canal. The laser treatment was much less effective, however, than a 2-minute dressing with 1% sodium hypochlorite, which killed all bacteria.

Argon, Nd:YAG, and carbon dioxide lasers have been tried for the softening of gutta-percha during root canal obturation.[13] During these procedures significant temperature increases were found on the external root surfaces. Depending on the type of laser and procedure the increases were recorded between 50.54° to 57.92° F (10.3° and 14.4° C). In an in vivo situation this would correspond to 117.14° to 124.52° F (47.3° to 51.4° C) in the periodontal tissues. This is uncomfortably close to a temperature of 127.4° F (53° C) that has been reported as dangerous for bone tissues.[66] Furthermore, these recordings were in vitro without the tissue absorption that occurs because of pigments and scattered radiation.

Lasers have also been used for root end surgery but with poor results.[75,176,259]

Another potential problem with significant consequences is the observation that smoke generated by laser treatment may carry infectious agents present in the burned area.[142]

Table 14-10. Toxicity of two amalgams for root end filling*

| | Cell Material Contact Time | | | |
| | 4 hr | | 24 hr | |
	Experiment	Control	Experiment	Control
Kerr Zinc-Free Amalgam				
In vitro				
Fresh	12.1 ± 0.9	7.7 ± 0.4	34.9 ± 1.2	25.7 ± 0.8
Set 1 day	7.7 ± 0.4	7.7 ± 0.4	28.7 ± 1.9	24.7 ± 1.8
Set 7 days	—	—	31.9 ± 1.8	25.7 ± 0.8
Implanted				
Retrieved	9.0 ± 0.3	9.4 ± 0.5	25.1 ± 1.0	25.4 ± 1.2
Corroded	—	—	45.6 ± 10.2	26.7 ± 0.8
Repolished	6.9 ± 0.6	7.5 ± 0.5	30.7 ± 1.9	25.7 ± 0.8
Dispersalloy				
In vitro				
Fresh	37.1 ± 1.0	6.0 ± 0.8	—	—
Set 1 day	9.8 ± 0.2	7.4 ± 0.1	67.9 ± 0.8	24.5 ± 0.8
Set 7 days	7.4 ± 0.5	6.0 ± 0.8	61.8 ± 3.0	28.9 ± 0.6
Implanted				
Retrieved	9.7 ± 1.8	9.4 ± 0.5	49.0 ± 7.6	25.4 ± 1.2
Corroded	—	—	44.8 ± 7.0	26.7 ± 0.8
Repolished	7.3 ± 0.4	7.5 ± 0.5	31.5 ± 1.3	25.7 ± 0.8

*Cytotoxicity measured as release of radiochromium from L929 cells in vitro. The amalgams were prepared and tested immediately, after 1 day and after 1 week. Amalgam samples were also prepared and implanted subcutaneously in guinea pigs for 3 months, retrieved, and tested for cytotoxicity. Samples were also corroded in saline for 3 months and tested for cytotoxicity. The samples were then polished and once again tested for cytotoxicity. The zinc-free amalgam showed a slightly lower cytotoxicity than the amalgam containing zinc. M ± SD.

SUMMARY

The reader is urged to use only instruments, materials, and devices that are supported by long-term independent studies to be safe and effective for the intended applications.

REFERENCES

1. Abou-Rass M, Patonai FJ: The effects of decreasing surface tension on the flow of irrigating solutions in narrow root canals, *Oral Surg Oral Med Oral Pathol* 53:524, 1982.
2. Abou-Rass M, Piccinino MV: The effectiveness of four clinical irrigation methods on the removal of root canal debris, *Oral Surg Oral Med Oral Pathol* 54:323, 1982.
3. Ahmad M: An analysis of breakage of ultrasonic files during root canal instrumentation, *Endodont Dent Traumatol* 5:78, 1989.
4. Ahmad M: Effect of ultrasonic instrumentation on *Bacteroides intermedius*, *Endodont Dent Traumatol* 5:83, 1989.
5. Ahmad M, Pitt Ford TR: A comparison using macroradiography of canal shapes in teeth instrumented ultrasonically and by hand, *J Endod* 15:339, 1989.
6. Ahmad M, Pitt Ford TR, Crum LA: Ultrasonic debridement of root canals: acoustic streaming and its possible role, *J Endod* 13:490, 1987.
7. Ahmad M, Pitt Ford TR, Crum LA: Ultrasonic debridement of root canals: an insight into the mechanisms involved, *J Endod* 13:93, 1987.
8. Ahmad M, Pitt Ford TR, Crum LA, Walton AJ: Ultrasonic debridement of root canals: acoustic cavitation and its relevance, *J Endod* 14:486, 1988.
9. Ahmad M, Pitt Ford TR, Crum LA, Wilson RF: Effectiveness of ultrasonic files in the disruption of root canal bacteria, *Oral Surg Oral Med Oral Pathol* 70:328, 1990.
10. Ahmad M, Roy RA, Ghanikamarudin A, Safar M: The vibratory pattern of ultrasonic files driven piezoelectrically, *Int Endodont J* 26:120, 1992.
11. Ahmad M, Roy RA, Kamarudin AG: Observations of acoustic streaming fields around an oscillating ultrasonic file, *Endodont Dent Traumatol* 8:189, 1992.
12. Anderson RW, Powell BJ, Pashley DH: Microleakage of three temporary endodontic restorations, *J Endod* 14:497, 1988.
13. Anić I, Matsumoto K: Dentinal heat transmission induced by a laser-softened gutta-percha obturation technique, *J Endod* 21:470, 1995.
14. Anthony DR, Gordon TM, del Rio CE: The effect of three vehicles on the pH of calcium hydroxide, *Oral Surg Oral Med Oral Pathol* 54:560, 1982.
15. Araki K, Isaka H, Ishii T, Suda H: Excretion of ^{14}C-formaldehyde distributed systemically through root canal following pulpectomy, *Endodont Dent Traumatol* 9:196, 1993.
16. Archer R, Reader A, Nist R, Beck M, Meyers WJ: An in vivo evaluation of the efficacy of ultrasound after step-back preparation in mandibular molars, *J Endod* 18:549, 1992.
17. Bahcall J, Howard P, Miserendino L, Walia H: Preliminary investigation of the histological effects of laser endodontic treatment on the periradicular tissues in dogs, *J Endod* 18:47, 1992.
18. Baker NA, Eleazer PD, Averbach RE, Seltzer S: Scanning electron microscopic study of the efficacy of various irrigating solutions, *J Endod* 1:127, 1975.
19. Barbosa SV, Burkard DH, Spångberg LSW: Cytotoxic effect of gutta-percha solvents, *J Endod* 20:6, 1994.
20. Barbosa SV, Safavi KE, Spångberg LSW: Influence of sodium hypochlorite on the permeability and structure of cervical human dentine, *Int Endodont J* 27:309, 1994.
21. Barbosa SV, Spångberg LSW, Almeida D: Low surface tension calcium hydroxide solution is an effective antiseptic, *Int Endodont J* 27:6, 1994.
22. Becker GL, Cohen S, Borer R: The sequelae of accidentally injecting sodium hypochlorite beyond the root apex, *Oral Surg Oral Med Oral Pathol* 38:633, 1974.

23. Bengmark S, Rydberg B: Cytotoxic action of cationic detergents on tissue growth in vitro, *Acta Chir Scand* 134:1, 1968.

24. Benz C, Mouyen F: Evaluation of the new RadioVisioGraphy system image quality, *Oral Surg Oral Med Oral Pathol* 72:627, 1991.

25. Berg MS, Jacobsen EL, BeGole EA, Remeikis NA: A comparison of five irrigating solutions: a scanning electron microscopic study, *J Endod* 12:192, 1986.

26. Bergdahl M, Wennberg A, Spångberg L: Biologic effect of polyisobutylene on bony tissue in guinea pigs, *Scand J Dent Res* 82:618, 1974.

27. Bergdahl M, Wennberg A, Spångberg L: Biologic effect of polyisobutylene on HeLa cells and on subcutaneous tissue in guinea pigs, *Scand J Dent Res* 82:613, 1974.

28. Bernhardt H, Eulig HG: Die Reaktion des Knochengewebe auf in die Markhöhle bei Meerschweinchen implantierte Gutta-percha, *Dtsch Zahnärztl* 7:295, 1953.

29. Beyer-Olsen EM, Ørstavik D: Radiopacity of root canal sealers, *Oral Surg Oral Med Oral Pathol* 51:320, 1981.

30. Björn H: Electrical excitation of teeth, *Svensk Tandläk T* 39(suppl): 1946.

31. Blackman R, Gross M, Seltzer S: An evaluation of the biocompatibility of a glass ionomer-silver cement in rat connective tissue, *J Endod* 15:76, 1989.

32. Block RM et al: Systematic distribution of N2 paste containing ^{14}C paraformaldehyde following root canal therapy in dogs, *Oral Surg Oral Med Oral Pathol* 50:350, 1980.

33. Block RM et al: Systemic distribution of [^{14}C]-labeled paraformaldehyde incorporated within formocresol following pulpotomies in dogs, *J Endod* 9:175, 1983.

34. Brady JM, del Rio CE: Corrosion of endodontic silver cones in humans: a scanning electron microscope and x-ray microprobe study, *J Endod* 1:205, 1975.

35. Brown BDK, Kafrawy AH, Patterson SS: Studies of Sargenti technique of endodontics: autoradiographic and scanning electron microscope studies, *J Endod* 5:14, 1979.

36. Byström A, Claesson R, Sundqvist G: The antimicrobial effect of camphorated paramonochlorphenol, camphorated phenol, and calcium hydroxide in the treatment of infected root canals, *Endodont Dent Traumatol* 1:170, 1985.

37. Byström A, Sundqvist G: Bacteriological evaluation of the effect of 0.5 percent sodium hypochlorite in endodontic therapy, *Oral Surg Oral Med Oral Pathol* 55:307, 1983.

38. Byström A, Sundqvist G: The antibacterial action of sodium hypochlorite and EDTA in 60 cases of endodontic therapy, *Int Endodont J* 18:35, 1985.

39. Callahan JR: Rosin solution for the sealing of the dentinal tubuli and as an adjuvant in the filling of root canals, *J Allied Dent Society* 9:53, 1914.

40. Callis PD, Santini A: Tissue response to retrograde root fillings in the ferret canine: a comparison of a glass ionomer cement and gutta percha with sealer, *Oral Surg Oral Med Oral Pathol* 64:475, 1987.

41. Calnan J: The use of inert plastic material in reconstructive surgery, *Br J Plast Surg* 16:1, 1963.

42. Canalda-Sahli C, Brau-Aguadé E, Berástegui-Jimeno E: A comparison of bending and torsional properties of K-files manufactured with different metallic alloys, *Int Endodont J* 29:185, 1996.

43. Carrel A: Abortive treatment of wound infection, *Br Med J* 2:609, 1915.

44. Chernick LB, Jacobs JJ, Lautenschlager EP, Heuer MA: Torsional failure of endodontic files, *J Endod* 2:94, 1976.

45. Cohen HP, Cha BY, Spångberg LSW: Endodontic anesthesia in mandibular molars: a clinical study, *J Endod* 19:370, 1993.

46. Cohen BD, Combe EC, Lilley JD: Effect of thermal placement techniques on some physical properties of gutta-percha, *Int Endodont J* 25:292, 1992.

47. Cunningham WT, Balekjian AY: Effect of temperature on collagen-dissolving ability of sodium hypochlorite endodontic irrigant, *Oral Surg Oral Med Oral Pathol* 49:175, 1980.

48. Cunningham WT, Cole JS, Balekjian AY: Effect of alcohol on the spreading ability of sodium hypochlorite endodontic irrigant, *Oral Surg Oral Med Oral Pathol* 53:333, 1982.

49. Cunningham WT, Joseph SW: Effect of temperature on the bactericidal action of sodium hypochlorite endodontic irrigant, *Oral Surg Oral Med Oral Pathol* 50:569, 1980.

50. Cunningham WT, Martin H: A scanning electron microscope evaluation of root canal debridement with the endosonic ultrasonic synergistic system, *Oral Surg Oral Med Oral Pathol* 53:527, 1982.

51. Cunningham WT, Martin H, Forrest WR: Evaluation of root canal debridement by the endosonic ultrasonic synergistic system, *Oral Surg Oral Med Oral Pathol* 53:401, 1982.

52. Dakin HD: The antiseptic action of hypochlorite: the ancient history of the "new antiseptic," *Br Med J* 2:809, 1915.

53. Dakin HD: On the use of certain antiseptic substances in treatment of infected wounds, *Br Med J* 2:318, 1915.

54. Dalal MB, Cohil KS: Comparison of silver amalgam, glass ionomer cement and gutta percha as retrofilling materials, an in vivo and an in vitro study, *J Indian Dent Assoc* 55:153, 1983.

55. Dalat DM, Spångberg LSW: Comparison of apical leakage in root canals obturated with various gutta-percha techniques using a dye vacuum tracing method, *J Endod* 20:315, 1994.

56. DeGee AJ, Wu MK, Wesselink PR: Sealing properties of a Ketac-Endo glass ionomer cement and AH26 root canal sealer, *Int Endodont J* 27:239, 1994.

57. Diaz-Arnold AM, Arnold MA, Wilcox LR: Optical detection of hemoglobin in pulpal blood, *J Endod* 22:19, 1996.

58. Diaz-Arnold AM, Wilcox LR, Arnold MA: Optical detection of pulpal blood, *J Endod* 20:164, 1994.

59. Donley DL, Weller RN, Kulild JC, Jurcak JJ: In vitro intracanal temperatures produced by low- and high-temperature thermoplasticized injectable gutta-percha, *J Endod* 17:307, 1991.

60. Ellerbruch ES, Murphy RA: Antimicrobial activity of root canal medicament vapors, *J Endod* 3:189, 1977.

61. Engfelt NO: Die Wirkung der Dakinschon Hypochloritlösong auf gewisse organische Substansen, *Hoppe-Seylers Z Physiol Chem* 121:18, 1922.

62. England MC, West NM, Safavi K, Green DB: Tissue lead levels in dogs with RC-2B root canal fillings, *J Endod* 6:728, 1980.

63. Engström B, Spångberg L: Studies on root canal medicaments. I. Cytotoxic effect of root canal antiseptics, *Acta Odontol Scand* 25:77, 1967.

64. Engström B, Spångberg L: Effect of root canal filling material N2 when used for filling after partial pulpectomy, *Svensk Tandläk T* 62:815, 1969.

65. Engström B, Spångberg L: Toxic and antimicrobial effects of antiseptics in vitro, *Svensk Tandläk T* 62:543, 1969.

66. Eriksson AR, Albrektsson T: Temperature threshold levels for heat-induced bone tissue injury: a vital-microscopic study in the rabbit, *J Prosthet Dent* 50:101, 1983.

67. Eulig HG, Bernhardt H: Die Reaktion verschiedener gewebe auf implantiertes Palavit, Paladon und Gutta-percha, *Dtsch Zahnärztebl* 7:227, 1953.

68. Feldmann G, Nyborg H: Tissue reaction to root filling materials. I. Comparison between gutta-percha and silver amalgam implanted in rabbit, *Odontol Revy* 13:1, 1962.

69. Felt RA, Moser JB, Heuer MA: Flute design of endodontic instruments: its influence on cutting efficiency, *J Endod* 8:253, 1982.

70. Finne K, Nord PG, Persson G, Lennartsson B: Retrograde root filling with amalgam and cavit, *Oral Surg Oral Med Oral Pathol* 43:621, 1977.

71. Fouad AF: The use of electronic apex locators in endodontic therapy, *Int Endodont J* 26:13, 1993.

72. Fouad AF, Krell KV: An in vitro comparison of five root canal length measuring instruments, *J Endod* 15:573, 1989.

73. Fouad AF, Rivera EM, Krell KV: Accuracy of the Endex with variations in canal irrigants and foramen size, *J Endod* 19:63, 1993.

74. Fouad AF et al: A clinical evaluation of five electronic root canal length measuring instruments, *J Endod* 16:446, 1990.

75. Friedman S, Rotstein I, Mahamid A: In vivo efficacy of various retrofills and of CO_2 laser in apical surgery, *Endodont Dent Traumatol* 7:19, 1991.

76. Gazelius B, Olgart L, Edwall B: Restored vitality in luxated teeth assessed by laser Doppler flowmetry, *Endodont Dent Traumatol* 4:265, 1988.

77. Gazelius B, Olgart L, Edwall B, Edwall L: Non-invasive recording of blood flow in human dental pulp, *Endodont Dent Traumatol* 2:219, 1986.

78. Goldberg F: Relation between corroded silver points and endodontic failures, *J Endod* 7:224, 1981.

79. Goldberg F, Abramovich A: Analysis of the effect of EDTAC on the dentinal walls of the root canal, *J Endod* 3:101, 1977.

80. Goldberg F, Spielberg C: The effect of EDTAC and the variation of its working time analyzed with scanning electron microscopy, *Oral Surg Oral Med Oral Pathol* 53:74, 1982.

81. Goldman M et al: New method of irrigation during endodontic treatment, *J Endod* 2:257, 1976.

82. Goldman M et al: The efficacy of several endodontic irrigating solutions: a scanning electron microscopic study: part 2, *J Endod* 8:487, 1982.

83. Goodman A, Schilder H, Aldrich W: The thermomechanical properties of gutta-percha. II. The history and molecular chemistry of gutta-percha, *Oral Surg Oral Med Oral Pathol* 37:954, 1974.

84. Goodman A, Schilder H, Aldrich W: The thermomechanical properties of gutta-percha. Part IV. A thermal profile of the warm gutta-percha packing procedure, *Oral Surg Oral Med Oral Pathol* 51:544, 1981.

85. Grassi MD, Plazek DJ, Michanowicz AE, Chay I-C: Changes in the physical properties of the Ultrafil low-temperature (70°C) thermoplasticized gutta-percha system, *J Endod* 15:517, 1989.

86. Grieve AR, Parkholm JDD: The sealing properties of root filling cements, further studies, *Br Dent J* 135:327, 1973.

87. Grossman LI: Irrigation of root canals, *J Am Dent Assoc* 30:1915, 1943.

88. Grossman LI: Solubility of root canal cements, *J Dent Res* 57:927, 1978.

89. Grossman LI: The effect of pH of rosin on setting time of root canal cements, *J Endod* 8:326, 1982.

90. Gutmann JL, Creel DC, Bowles WH: Evaluation of heat transfer during root canal obturation with thermoplasticized gutta-percha. I. In vitro heat levels during extrusion, *J Endod* 13:378, 1987.

91. Gutmann JL, Rakusin H, Powe R, Bowles WH: Evaluation of heat transfer during root canal obturation with thermoplasticized gutta-percha. II. In vivo response to heat levels generated, *J Endod* 13:441, 1987.

92. Guttuso J: A histopathological study of rat connective tissue responses to endodontic materials, *Oral Surg Oral Med Oral Pathol* 16:713, 1962.

93. Haikel Y, Gasser P, Allemann C: Dynamic fracture of hybrid endodontic hand instruments compared with traditional files, *J Endod* 17:217, 1991.

94. Hand RE, Smith ML, Harrison JW: Analysis of the effect of dilution on the necrotic dissolution property of sodium hypochlorite, *J Endod* 4:60, 1978.

95. Hansen-Bayless J, Davis R: Sealing ability of two intermediate restorative materials in bleached teeth, *Am J Dent* 5:151, 1992.

96. Harris WE: Disintegration of two silver cones, *J Endod* 7:426, 1981.

97. Harrison JW, Baumgartner JC, Zielke DR: Analysis of interappointment pain associated with the combined use of endodontic irrigants and medicaments, *J Endod* 7:272, 1981.

98. Harrison JW, Svec TA, Baumgartner JC: Analysis of clinical toxicity of endodontic irrigants, *J Endod* 4:6, 1978.

99. Hedrick RT, Dove SB, Peters DD, McDavid WD: Radiographic determination of canal length: direct digital radiography versus conventional radiography, *J Endod* 20:320, 1994.

100. Hermann BW: Calciumhydroxyd als Mittel zum Behandel und Füllen von Zahnwurzelkanälen, Würzburg, *Med Diss V* 29:Sept 1920.

101. Hermann BW: Dentin Obliteration der Wurzelkanäle nach Behandlung mit Calcium, *Zahnärztl Rundschau* 39:888, 1930.

102. Hertwig G: Wandständigkeit und durchlässigkeit von wurzelfüllmitteln, *Zahnärztl Praxis* 9:1, 1958.

103. Higginbotham TL: A comparative study of the physical properties of five commonly used root canal sealers, *Oral Surg Oral Med Oral Pathol* 24:89, 1967.

104. Hunter HA: The effect of gutta-percha, silver points and Rickert's root sealer on bone healing, *J Can Dent Assoc* 23:385, 1957.

105. Ingólfsson ÆR, Tronstad L, Hersh E, Riva CE: Effect of probe design on the suitability of laser Doppler flowmetry in vitality testing of human teeth, *Endodont Dent Traumatol* 9:65, 1993.

106. Ingólfsson ÆR, Tronstad L, Riva CE: Reliability of laser Doppler flowmetry in testing vitality of human teeth, *Endodont Dent Traumatol* 10:185, 1994.

107. Jasper EA: Root canal therapy in modern dentistry, *Dent Cosmos* 75:823, 1933.

108. Jerome CE: Warm vertical gutta-percha obturation: a technique update, *J Endod* 20:97, 1994.

109. Kahan RS, Gulabivala K, Snook M, Setchell DJ: Evaluation of a pulse oximeter and customized probe for pulp vitality testing, *J Endod* 22:105, 1996.

110. Kawahara H, Imanishi Y, Oshima H: Biologic evaluation on glass ionomer cement, *J Dent Res* 58:1080, 1979.

111. Kazemi RB, Safavi KE, Spångberg LSW: Dimensional changes of endodontic sealers, *Oral Surg Oral Med Oral Pathol* 76:766, 1993.

112. Kazemi RB, Safavi KE, Spångberg LSW: Assessment of marginal stability and permeability of an interim restorative endodontic material, *Oral Surg Oral Med Oral Pathol* 78:788, 1994.

113. Kazemi RB, Stenman E, Spångberg LSW: The endodontic file is a disposable instrument, *J Endod* 21:451, 1995.

114. Kazemi RB, Stenman E, Spångberg LSW: Machining efficiency and wear resistance of nickel-titanium endodontic files, *Oral Surg Oral Med Oral Pathol Oral Radiol Endod* 81:596, 1996.

115. Keate KC, Wong M: A comparison of endodontic file tip quality, *J Endod* 16:486, 1990.

116. Kehoe JC: Intracanal corrosion of a silver cone producing a localized argyria: scanning electron microscope and energy dispersive x-ray analyzer analyses, *J Endod* 10:199, 1984.

117. Kielt LW, Montgomery S: The effect of Endosonic instrumentation in simulated curved root canals, *J Endod* 13:215, 1987.

118. Kimura JT: A comparative analysis of zinc and nonzinc alloys used in retrograde endodontic surgery. I. Apical seal and tissue reaction, *J Endod* 8:359, 1982.

119. Kimura JT: A comparative analysis of zinc and nonzinc alloys used in retrograde endodontic surgery. II. Optical emmission spectrographic analysis for zinc precipitation, *J Endod* 8:407, 1982.

120. Krupp JD, Brantley WA, Gerstein H: An investigation of the torsional and bending properties of seven brands of endodontic files, *J Endod* 10:372, 1984.

121. Lado EA, Richmond AF, Marks RG: Reliability and validity of a digital pulp tester as a test standard for measuring sensory perception, *J Endod* 14:352, 1988.

122. Langeland K, Guttuso J, Langeland L, Tobon G: Methods in the study of biologic responses to endodontic materials, *Oral Surg Oral Med Oral Pathol* 27:522, 1969.

123. Lauper R, Lutz F, Barbakow F: An in vivo comparison of gradient and absolute impedance electronic apex locators, *J Endod* 22:260, 1996.

124. Lautenschlager EP, Jacobs JJ, Marshall GW, Heuer MA: Brittle and ductile torsional failures of endodontic instruments, *J Endod* 3:175, 1977.

125. Lavelle CLB, Wu C-J: Digital radiographic images will benefit endodontic services, *Endodont Dent Traumatol* 11:253, 1995.

126. Layton CA, Marshall JG, Morgan LA, Baumgartner JC: Evaluation of cracks associated with ultrasonic root-end preparation, *J Endod* 22:157, 1996.

127. Lee D-H, Park B, Saxena A, Serene TP: Enhanced surface hardness by boron implantation in nitinol alloy, *J Endod* 22:543, 1996.

128. Levine M, Rudolph AS: Factors affecting the germicidal efficiency of hypochlorite solutions, *Bull 150 Iowa Exp Sta* 1941.

129. Levy G: Cleaning and shaping the root canal with a Nd:YAG laser beam: a comparative study, *J Endod* 18:123, 1992.

130. Lewis BB, Chestner SB: Formaldehyde in dentistry: a review of mutagenic and carcinigenic potential, *J Am Dent Assoc* 103:429, 1981.

131. Liggett WR, Brady JM, Tsaknis PJ, del Rio CE: Light microscopy, scanning electron microscopy, and microprobe analysis of bone response to zinc and amalgam implants, *Oral Surg Oral Med Oral Pathol* 49:254, 1980.

132. Limkangwalmongkol S et al: A comparative study of the apical leakage of four root canal sealers and laterally condensed gutta-percha, *J Endod* 17:495, 1991.

133. Loushine RJ, Weller RN, Hartwell GR: Stereomicroscopic evaluation of canal shape following hand, sonic, and ultrasonic instrumentation, *J Endod* 15:417, 1989.

134. Margelos J, Verdelis K, Eliades G: Chloroform uptake by gutta-percha and assessment of its concentration in air during the chloroform-dip technique, *J Endod* 22:547, 1996.

135. Marsicovetere ES, Clement DJ, del Rio CE: Morphometric video analysis of the engine-driven nickel-titanium Lightspeed instrument system, *J Endod* 22:231, 1996.

136. Martin LR et al: Histologic response of rat connective tissue to zinc-containing amalgam, *J Endod* 2:25, 1976.

137. Matsuya Y, Matsuya S: Effect of abietic acid and polymethyl methacrylate on the dissolution process of zinc oxide–eugenol cement, *Biomaterials* 15:307, 1994.

138. McComb D, Smith DC: A preliminary scanning electron microscopic study of root canals after endodontic procedures, *J Endod* 1:238, 1975.

139. McComb D, Smith DC, Beagrie GS: The results of in vivo endodontic chemomechanical instrumentation: a scanning electron microscopic study, *J Br Endodont Soc* 9:11, 1976.

140. McDonnell D, Price C: An evaluation of the Sens-A-Ray digital dental imaging system, *Dentomaxillofac Radiol* 22:121, 1993.

141. McElroy DL: Physical properties of root canal filling materials, *J Am Dent Assoc* 50:433, 1955.

142. McKinley IB, Lublow MO: Hazards of laser smoke during endodontic therapy, *J Endod* 20:558, 1994.

143. Messer HH, Chen R-S: The duration of effectiveness of root canal medicaments, *J Endod* 10:240, 1984.

144. Messer HH, Feigal RJ: A comparison of the antibacterial and cytotoxic effects of parachlorophenol, *J Dent Res* 64:818, 1985.

145. Michanowicz A, Czonstkowsky M: Sealing properties of an injection-thermoplasticized low-temperature (70° C) gutta-percha: a preliminary study, *J Endod* 10:563, 1984.

146. Miserendino LJ, Brantley WA, Walia HD, Gerstein H: Cutting efficiency of endodontic hand instruments. IV. Comparison of hybrid and traditional instrument designs, *J Endod* 14:451, 1988.

147. Miserendino LJ, Levy GC, Rizoiu IM: Effects of Nd:YAG laser on the permeability of root canal wall dentin, *J Endod* 21:83, 1995.

148. Miserendino LJ, Miserendino CA, Moser JB, Heuer MA, Osetek EM: Cutting efficiency of endodontic instruments. III. Comparison of sonic and ultrasonic instrument systems, *J Endod* 14:24, 1988.

149. Miserendino LJ, Moser JB, Heuer MA, Osetek EM: Cutting efficiency of endodontic instruments. I. A quantitative comparison of the tip and fluted region, *J Endod* 11:435, 1985.

150. Miserendino LJ, Moser JB, Heuer MA, Osetek EM: Cutting efficiency of endodontic instruments. II. An analysis of the design of the tip, *J Endod* 12:8, 1986.

151. Mitchell DF: The irritational qualities of dental materials, *J Am Dent Assoc* 59:954, 1959.

152. Möller ÅJR: Microbiological examination of root canals and periapical tissues of human teeth, *Odontol Tidskr* 74(special issue):1, 1966.

153. Molyvdas I, Zervas P, Lambrianidis T, Veis A: Periodontal tissue reactions following root canal obturation with an injection-thermoplasticized gutta-percha technique, *Endodont Dent Traumatol* 5:32, 1989.

154. Moshonov J et al: Efficacy of argon laser irradiation in removing intracanal debris, *Oral Surg Oral Med Oral Pathol Oral Radiol Endod* 79:221, 1995.

155. Moshonov J et al: ND:YAG laser irradiationin root canal disinfection, *Endodont Dent Traumatol* 11:220, 1995.

156. Mumford JM, Björn H: Problems in electrical pulp-testing and dental algesimetry, *Int Dent J* 12:161, 1962.

157. Neal RG, Craig RG, Powers JM: Cutting ability of K type endodontic files, *J Endod* 9:52, 1983.

158. Neal RG, Craig RG, Powers JM: Effect of sterilization and irrigants on the cutting ability of stainless steel files, *J Endod* 9:93, 1983.

159. Nelvig P, Wing K, Welander U: Sens-A Ray: a new system for direct digital intraoral radiography, *Oral Surg Oral Med Oral Pathol* 74:818, 1992.

160. Noblett WC et al: Detection of pulpal circulation in vitro by pulse oximetry, *J Endod* 22:1, 1996.

161. Nygaard-Østby B: Chelation in root canal therapy, *Odontol T* 65:3, 1957.

162. Ohara PK, Torabinejad M, Kettering JD: Antibacterial effects of various endodontic irrigants on selected anaerobic bacteria, *Endodont Dent Traumatol* 9:95, 1993.

163. Oliet S, Sorin SM: Effect of aging on the mechanical properties of hand-rolled gutta-percha endodontic cones, *Oral Surg Oral Med Oral Pathol* 43:954, 1977.

164. Omnell K: Electrolytic precipitation of zinc carbonate in the jaw, *Oral Surg Oral Med Oral Pathol* 12:846, 1959.

165. Ørstavik D, Farrants G, Wahl T, Kerekes K: Image analysis of endodontic radiographs: digital subtraction and quantitative densitometry, *Endodont Dent Traumatol* 6:6, 1990.

166. Ørstavik D, Haapasalo M: Disinfection by endodontic irrigants and dressings of experimentally infected dentinal tubules, *Endodont Dent Traumatol* 6:142, 1990.

167. Pascon EA, Spångberg LSW: In vitro cytotoxicity of root canal filling materials. I. Gutta-percha, *J Endod* 16:429, 1990.

168. Pashley EL, Horner JA, Liu M, Pashley DH: Effects of CO_2 laser energy on dentin permeability, *J Endod* 18:257, 1992.

169. Pedicord D, ElDeeb ME, Messer HH: Hand versus ultrasonic instrumentation: its effect on canal shape and instrumentation time, *J Endod* 12:375, 1986.

170. Pissiotis E, Sapounas G, Spångberg LSW: Silver glass ionomer cement as a retrograde filling material: a study in vitro, *J Endod* 17:225, 1991.

171. Powell SE, Simon JHS, Maze B: A comparison of the effect of modified and nonmodified instrument tips on apical canal configuration, *J Endod* 12:293, 1986.

172. Powell SE, Wong PD, Simon JHS: A comparison of the effect of modified and nonmodified instrument tips on apical canal configuration: part II, *J Endod* 14:224, 1988.

173. Pratten DH, McDonald NJ: Comparison of radiographic and electronic working lengths, *J Endod* 22:173, 1996.

174. Ram Z: Effectiveness of root canal irrigation, *Oral Surg Oral Med Oral Pathol* 44:306, 1977.

175. Ramsay DS, Årtun J, Martinen SS: Reliability of pulpal blood-flow measurements utilizing laser Doppler flowmetry, *J Dent Res* 70:1427, 1991.

176. Read RP, Baumgartner JC, Clark SM: Effects of a carbon dioxide laser on human root dentin, *J Endod* 21:4, 1995.

177. Richman MJ: The use of ultrasonics in root canal therapy and root resection, *J Dent Med* 12:12, 1957.

178. Rickoff B et al: Effects of thermal vitality tests on human dental pulp, *J Endod* 14:482, 1988.

179. Roane JB, Sabala CL, Duncanson MG: The "balanced force" concept for instrumentation of curved canals, *J Endod* 11:203, 1985.

180. Rome WJ, Doran JE, Walker WA III: The effectiveness of Gly-Oxide and sodium hypochlorite in preventing smear layer formation, *J Endod* 11:281, 1985.

181. Rutberg M, Spångberg E, Spångberg L: Evaluation of enhanced vascular permeability of endodontic medicaments in vivo, *J Endod* 3:347, 1977.

182. Sabala CL, Powell SE: Sodium hypochlorite injection into periapical tissues, *J Endod* 15:490, 1989.

183. Sabala CL, Roane JB, Southard LZ: Instrumentation of curved canals using a modified tipped instrument: a comparison study, *J Endod* 14:59, 1988.

184. Safavi KE, Nichols FC: Effect of calcium hydroxide on bacterial lipopolysaccharide, *J Endod* 19:76, 1993.

185. Safavi KE, Nichols FC: Alteration of biological properties of bacterial lipopolysaccharide by calcium hydroxide treatment, *J Endod* 20:127, 1994.

186. Safavi KE, Spångberg LSW, Langeland K: Root canal dentinal tubule disinfection, *J Endod* 16:207, 1990.

187. Salzgeber RM, Brilliant JD: An in vivo evaluation of the penetration of an irrigating solution in root canals, *J Endod* 3:394, 1977.

188. Sasano T, Kuriwada S, Sanjo D: Arterial blood pressure regulation of blood flow as determined by laser Doppler, *J Dent Res* 68:791, 1989.

189. Saunders EM: The effect of variation in the thermomechanical compaction techniques upon the quality of the apical seal, *Int Endodont J* 22:163, 1989.

190. Saunders EM: In vivo findings associated with heat generation during thermomechanical compaction of gutta-percha. I. Temperature levels at the external surface of the root, *Int Endodont J* 23:263, 1990.

191. Saunders EM: In vivo findings associated with heat generation during thermomechanical compaction of gutta-percha. II. Histological response to temperature elevation on the external surface of the root, *Int Endodont J* 23:268, 1990.

192. Saunders EM, Saunders WP: Long-term coronal leakage of JS Quick-fill root filling with Sealapex and Apexit sealers, *Endodont Dent Traumatol* 11:181, 1995.

193. Saunders WP, Saunders EM, Gutmann JL: Ultrasonic root-end preparation. II. Microleakage of EBA root-end fillings, *Int Endodont J* 27:325, 1994.

194. Schilder H, Goodman A, Aldrich W: The thermomechanical properties of gutta-percha. I. The compressibility of gutta-percha, *Oral Surg Oral Med Oral Pathol* 37:946, 1974.

195. Schilder H, Goodman A, Aldrich W: The thermomechanical properties of gutta-percha. III. Determination of phase transition temperatures for gutta-percha, *Oral Surg Oral Med Oral Pathol* 38:109, 1974.

196. Schilder H, Goodman A, Aldrich W: The thermomechanical properties of gutta-percha. V. Volume changes in bulk gutta-percha as a function of temperature and its relationship to molecular phase transformation, *Oral Surg Oral Med Oral Pathol* 59:285, 1985.

197. Schmitt W: Die chemischen grundlagenn der erhartenden wurzelfüllungen, *Zahnärztl Welt* 5:560, 1951.

198. Schnettler JM, Wallace JA: Pulse oximetry as a diagnostic tool of pulp vitality, *J Endod* 17:488, 1991.

199. Schroeder A: Mitteilungen über die Abschlussdichtigkeit von Wurzelfüllmaterialien und erster Hinweis auf ein neuartiges Wurzelfüllmittel, *Schweiz Mschr Zahn* 64:921, 1954.

200. Schroeder A: Gewebsverträglichkeit des Wurzelfüllmittels AH 26 *Zahnärz H Welt,* 58:563, 1957.

201. Schroeder A: Zum problem der bacteriendichten Wurzelkanalversorgung, *Zahnärztl Welt Zahnärzt Reform* 58:531, 1957.

202. Seltzer S, Green DB, Weiner N, DeRenzis F: A scanning electron microscope examination of silver cones removed from endodontically treated teeth, *Oral Surg Oral Med Oral Pathol* 33:589, 1972.

203. Senia ES, Marshall FJ, Rosen S: The solvent action of sodium hypochlorite on pulp tissue of extracted teeth, *Oral Surg Oral Med Oral Pathol* 31:96, 1971.

204. Senia ES et al: Rapid sterilization of gutta-percha cones with 5.25% sodium hypochlorite, *J Endod* 1:136, 1975.

205. Seto BG, Nicholls JI, Harrington GW: Torsional properties of twisted and machined endodontic files, *J Endod* 16:355, 1990.

206. Shoji Y: Studies on the mechanism of the mechanical enlargement of root canals, *J Nihon Univ School Dent* 7:71, 1965.

207. Sjögren U, Figdor D, Spångberg L, Sundqvist G: The antimicrobial effect of calcium hydroxide as a short-term intracanal dressing, *Int Endodont J* 24:119, 1991.

208. Sjögren U, Sundqvist G: Bacteriologic evaluation of ultrasonic root canal instrumentation, *Oral Surg Oral Med Oral Pathol* 63:366, 1987.

209. Sjögren U, Sundqvist G, Nair PNR: Tissue reaction to gutta-percha particles of various sizes when implanted subcutaneously in guinea pigs, *Eur J Oral Sci* 103:313, 1995.

210. Smith MA, Steinman HR: An in vitro evaluation of microleakage of two new and two old root canal sealers, *J Endod* 20:18, 1994.

211. Soares I, Goldberg F, Massone EJ, Soares IM: Periapical tissue response to two calcium hydroxide-containing endodontic sealers, *J Endod* 16:166, 1990.

212. Söderberg TA: Effects of zinc oxide, rosin and resin acids and their combinations on bacterial growth and inflammatory cells, Umeå, Sweden, 1990, Umeå University Medical Dissertations No. 280.

213. Soltes EDJ, Zinkel DF: Chemistry of rosin. In Zinkel DF, Russell J, editors: *Naval stores production, chemistry, utilization,* New York, 1989, Pulp Chemical Association, pp 262-331.

214. Sorin SM, Oliet S, Pearlstein F: Rejuvination of aged (brittle) endodontic gutta-percha cones, *J Endod* 5:233, 1979.

215. Spångberg L: Comparison between tissue reactions to gutta-percha and polytetrafluorethylene implanted in the mandible of the rat, *Svensk Tandläk T* 61:705, 1968.

216. Spångberg L: Biological effects of root canal filling materials. II. Effect in vitro of water-soluble components of root canal filling materials on HeLa cells, *Odontol Revy* 20:133, 1969.

217. Spångberg L: Biological effects of root canal filling materials. IV. Effect in vitro of solubilized root canal filling materials on HeLa cells, *Odontol Revy* 20:289, 1969.

218. Spångberg L: Biological effects of root canal filling materials. V. Toxic effect in vitro of root filling materials on HeLa cells and human skin fibroblasts, *Odontol Revy* 20:427, 1969.

219. Spångberg L: Biological effects of root canal filling materials. VI. The inhibitory effect of solubilized root canal filling materials on respiration of HeLa cells, *Odontol T* 77:1, 1969.

220. Spångberg L: Biological effects of root canal filling materials. VII. Reaction of bony tissue to implanted root canal filling material in guinea pigs, *Odontol T* 77:133, 1969.

221. Spångberg L: Biological effects of root canal filling materials: the effect on bone tissue of two formaldehyde-containing root canal filling pastes: N2 and Riebler's paste, *Oral Surg Oral Med Oral Pathol* 38:934, 1974.

222. Spångberg L, Engström B: Studies on root canal medicaments. IV. Antimicrobial effect of root canal medicaments, *Odontol Revy* 19:187, 1968.

223. Spångberg L, Engström B, Langeland K: Biologic effects of dental materials. III. Toxicity and antimicrobial effect of endodontic antiseptics in vitro, *Oral Surg Oral Med Oral Pathol* 36:856, 1973.

224. Spångberg L, Langeland K: Biologic effect of dental materials. I. Toxicity of root canal filling materials on HeLa cells in vitro, *Oral Surg Oral Med Oral Pathol* 35:402, 1973.

225. Spångberg L, Rutberg M, Rydinge E: Biological effects of endodontic antimicrobial agents, *J Endod* 5:166, 1979.

226. Spångberg LSW, Barbosa SV, Lavigne GD: AH26 releases formaldehyde, *J Endod* 19:596, 1993.

227. Stabholz A et al: Sealing of human dentinal tubules by XeCl 308-nm Excimer laser, *J Endod* 19:267, 1993.

228. Staehle HJ, Spiess V, Heinecke A, Müller H-P: Effect of root canal filling materials containing calcium hydroxide and the alkalinity of root dentin, *Endodont Dent Traumatol* 11:163, 1995.

229. Stamos DE, Sadeghi EM, Haasch GC, Gerstein H: An in vitro comparison study to quantitate the debridement ability of hand, sonic, and ultrasonic instrumentation, *J Endod* 13:434, 1987.

230. Stenman E: *Effects of sterilization and endodontic medicaments on mechanical properties of root canal instruments,* Umeå, Sweden, 1977, Ume University Odontological Dissertations No. 8.

231. Stenman E, Spångberg LSW: Machining efficiency of endodontic files: a new methodology, *J Endod* 16:151, 1990.

232. Stenman E, Spångberg LSW: Machining efficiency of endodontic K files and Hedström files, *J Endod* 16:375, 1990.

233. Stenman E, Spångberg LSW: Machining efficiency of Flex-R, K-Flex, Trio-Cut, and S Files, *J Endod* 16:575, 1990.

234. Stenman E, Spångberg L: Root canal instruments are poorly standardized, *J Endod* 19:327, 1993.

235. Sundada I: New method for measuring the length of the root canal, *J Dent Res* 41:375, 1962.

236. Sunzel B: *Interactive effects of zinc, rosin and resin acids on polymorphonuclear leukocytes, gingival fibroblasts and bacteria,* Umeå, Sweden, 1995, Umeå University Odontological Dissertations No. 55.

237. Sunzel B et al: The effect of zinc oxide on *Staphylococcus aureus* and polymorphonuclear cells in a tissue cage model, *Scand J Plast Reconstr Hand Surg* 24:31, 1990.

238. Svec TA, Harrison JW: The effect of effervescence on debridement of the apical regions of root canals in single-rooted teeth, *J Endod* 7:335, 1981.

239. Tagger M: Use of thermo-mechanical compactors as an adjunct to lateral condensation, *Quintessence Int* 15:27, 1984.

240. Tagger M, Tagger E, Kfir A: Release of calcium and hydroxyl ions from set endodontic sealers containing calcium hydroxide, *J Endod* 14:588, 1988.

241. Tani Y, Kawada H: Effects of laser irradiation on dentin. I. Effect on smear layer, *J Dent Mater* 6:127, 1987.

242. Trebitsch H: Über die Verwertung der heilkraft des Silbers, *Zahnäztl Rdsch* 38:1009, 1929.

243. Tronstad L, Barnett F, Flax M: Solubility and biocompatability of calcium hydroxide-containing root canal sealers, *Endodont Dent Traumatol* 4:152, 1988.

244. van der Fehr FR, Nygaard-Østby B: Effect of EDTAC and sulfuric acid on root canal dentine, *Oral Surg Oral Med Oral Pathol* 16:199, 1963.

245. Vessey RA: The effect of filing versus reaming on the shape of the prepared root canal, *Oral Surg Oral Med Oral Pathol* 27:543, 1969.

246. Villalobos RL, Moser JB, Heuer MA: A method to determine the cutting efficiency of root canal instruments in rotary motion, *J Endod* 6:667, 1980.

247. Walia H, Brantley WA, Gerstein H: An initial investigation of the bending and torsional properties of nitinol root canal files, *J Endod* 14:346, 1988.

248. Walker TL, del Rio CE: Histological evaluation of ultrasonic and sonic instrumentation of curved root canals, *J Endod* 15:49, 1989.

249. Walker TL, del Rio CE: Histological evaluation of ultrasonic debridement comparing sodium hypochlorite and water, *J Endod* 17:66, 1991.

250. Webber J, Moser JB, Heuer MA: A method to determine the cutting efficiency of root canal instruments in linear motion, *J Endod* 6:829, 1980.

251. Weine FS, Kelly RF, Lio PS: The effect of preparation procedures on original canal shape and apical foramen shape, *J Endod* 1:255, 1975.

252. Weinreb MM, Meier E: The relative efficiency of EDTA, sulfuric acid, and mechanical instrumentation in the enlargement of root canals, *Oral Surg Oral Med Oral Pathol* 19:247, 1965.

253. Weller RN, Brady JM, Bernier WE: Efficacy of ultrasonic cleaning, *J Endod* 6:740, 1980.

254. Wennberg A, Bergdahl M, Spångberg L: Biologic effect of polyisobutylene on HeLa cells and on subcutaneous tissue in guinea pigs, *Scand J Dent Res* 82:613, 1974.

255. Wennberg A, Ørstavik D: Adhesion of root canal sealers to bovine dentine and gutta-percha, *Int Endodont J* 23:13, 1990.

256. West NM, England MC, Safavi K, Green DB: Levels of lead in blood of dogs with RC-2B root canal fillings, *J Endod* 6:598, 1980.

257. Wong M, Peters DD, Lorton L: Comparison of gutta-percha filling techniques, compaction (mechanical), vertical (warm), and lateral condensation techniques: part I, *J Endod* 7:551, 1981.

258. Wong M, Peters DD, Lorton L, Bernier WE: Comparison of gutta-percha filling techniques: three chloroform-gutta-percha filling techniques: part II, *J Endod* 8:4, 1982.

259. Wong WS, Rosenberg PA, Boylan RJ, Schulman A: A comparison of the apical seals achieved using retrograde amalgam fillings and the Nd:YAG laser, *J Endod* 20:595, 1994.

260. Yahya AS, ElDeeb ME: Effect of sonic versus ultrasonic instrumentation on canal preparation, *J Endod* 15:235, 1989.

261. Yamada RS, Armas A, Goldman M, Sun Lin P: A scanning electron microscopic comparison of a high volume final flush with several irrigating solutions: part III, *J Endod* 9:137, 1983.

262. Yee FS, Krakow A, Gron P: Three-dimensional obturation of the root canal using injection-molded thermoplasticized dental gutta-percha, *J Endod* 3:168, 1977.

263. Zetterqvist L, Anneroth G, Danin J, Roding K: Microleakage of retrograde filling: a comparative investigation between amalgam and glass ionomer cement in vitro, *Int Endodont J* 21:1, 1988.

264. Zetterqvist L, Anneroth G, Nordenram A: Glass ionomer cement as retrograde filling material: an experimental investigation in monkeys, *Int J Oral Maxillofac Surg* 16:459, 1987.

265. Zmener O, Dominquez FV: Tissue response to a glass ionomer used as an endodontic cement, *Oral Surg Oral Med Oral Pathol* 56:198, 1983.

266. Zmener O, Dominquez FV: Corrosion of silver cones in the subcutaneous connective tissue of the rat: a preliminary scanning electron microscope, electron microprobe, and histological study, *J Endod* 11:55, 1985.

Chapter 15

Pulpal Reaction to Caries and Dental Procedures

Syngcuk Kim
Henry O. Trowbridge

At the dental centenary celebration held in Baltimore in 1940, Bodecker commented on the current state of dentistry: "Operative procedures in the reconstruction of teeth have always been governed by engineering principles."[73] Although this is still true today, more than 50 years later, many other basic concepts of restorative dentistry have been changed drastically since then. One fundamental change in dental treatment in the past 40 years has been preservation of dentition and the pulp. Unfortunately, however, greater dental preservation all too often results in damage to the pulp. Of the various forms of dental treatment, operative procedures by far are the most frequent cause of pulpal injury. It is accepted that trauma to the pulp cannot always be avoided, particularly when the tooth requires extensive restoration. Nonetheless, the competent clinician, by recognizing the hazards associated with each step of the restorative process, can often minimize if not prevent trauma and thus preserve the vitality of the tooth.

In the past, pulpal responses to various dental procedures and materials have been discussed almost exclusively from a histologic perspective. Fortunately, active physiologic investigations in the last decade have shed new light on the dynamic changes in the pulp in response to dental procedures and materials. It is the purpose of this chapter to discuss new knowledge together with the old to understand pulpal responses to caries and to various restorative procedures and materials.

DENTAL CARIES

Dental caries is a localized, progressive destruction of tooth structure and the most common cause of pulp disease. It is now generally accepted that for caries to develop, specific bacteria must become established on the tooth surface. Products of bacterial metabolism, notably organic acids and proteolytic enzymes, cause the destruction of enamel and dentin. Bacterial metabolites are also capable of eliciting an inflammatory reaction. Eventually extensive invasion of the dentin results in bacterial infection of the pulp. Basic reactions that tend to protect the pulp against caries involve (1) a decrease in the permeability of the dentin, (2) the formation of new dentin, and (3) inflammatory and immune reactions.

Inward diffusion of toxic substances from carious lesions occurs mainly through the dentinal tubules. Therefore the extent to which toxins permeate the tubules and reach the pulp is of critical importance in determining the extent of pulpal injury. *The most common response to caries is dentin sclerosis.* In this reaction the dentinal tubules become partially or completely filled with mineral deposits consisting of apatite and whitlockite crystals. Researchers[60] reported finding dentin sclerosis at the periphery of carious lesions in 95.4% of 154 teeth examined. Studies using dyes, solvents, and radioactive ions have shown that dentin sclerosis has the effect of decreasing the permeability of dentin, thus shielding the pulp from irritation.[5] Evidence suggests that for sclerosis to occur, vital odontoblast processes must be present within the tubules.[25]

The ability of the pulp to produce reparative dentin beneath a carious lesion is another mechanism for limiting the diffusion of toxic substances to the pulp (see Fig. 11-42). Researchers[60] reported the presence of reparative dentin in 63.6% of teeth with carious lesions and found that it often occurred in combination with dentinal sclerosis. The characteristics of reparative dentin have already been discussed (see Chapter 11). In general, the amount of reparative dentin formed is proportional to the amount of primary dentin destroyed. The rate of carious attack also seems to be an influencing factor, since more dentin is formed in response to slowly progressing chronic caries than to rapidly advancing acute caries. For this reason, carious exposure of the pulp is likely to occur earlier in acute caries than in chronic caries.

Research has shown that along the border zone between primary and reparative dentin, the walls of dentinal tubules are thickened and the tubules are frequently occluded with material resembling peritubular dentin.[53] Thus the border zone appears to be considerably less permeable than ordinary dentin and may serve as a barrier to the ingress of bacteria and their products.

The formation of a dead tract in dentin is yet another reaction that may occur in response to caries. Unlike dentinal sclerosis and the formation of reparative dentin, this response is not considered to be a defense reaction. A dead tract is an area in dentin within which the dentinal tubules are devoid of odontoblast processes. The origin of these tracts in dental caries is uncertain, but most authorities are of the opinion that they are formed as a result of the early death of odontoblasts. Dead tracts are most often observed in young teeth affected by rapidly progressing lesions. Because dentinal tubules of dead tracts are patent, they are highly permeable, and therefore they

Supported in part by NIDR grants DEO-5605 and DEO-0121.

are a potential threat to the integrity of the pulp. Fortunately, the healthy pulp responds to the presence of a dead tract by depositing a layer of reparative dentin over its surface, thus sealing it off.

Dentin is demineralized by organic acids (principally lactic acid) that are products of bacterial fermentation. These acids also play a role in degrading the organic matrix of enamel and dentin. Although very few oral bacteria possess collagenases, the collagenous matrix of dentin can be degraded by bacterial proteases if the collagen is first denatured by acid.

There is some controversy as to when caries first elicits an inflammatory response in the underlying pulp. One study observed an accumulation of chronic inflammatory cells in the pulp beneath enamel caries that had not yet invaded dentin.[10] Another study,[35] however, did not observe pulpal inflammation until the caries had penetrated beyond the enamel. There is general agreement that by the time caries has invaded the dentin, some changes are occurring in the pulp. These changes represent a response to the diffusion of soluble irritants and inflammatory stimuli into the pulp. Such substances include bacterial toxins, bacterial enzymes, antigens, chemotaxins, organic acids, and products of tissue destruction. Substances also pass outward from the pulp to the carious lesion. Researchers reported finding plasma proteins, immunoglobulins, and complement proteins in carious dentin.[41] It is conceivable that some of these factors are capable of inhibiting bacterial activity in the lesion.

Unfortunately, diagnosis of the extent of pulpal inflammation beneath a carious lesion is difficult. Many factors play a role in determining the nature of the caries process, so the individuality of each carious lesion should be recognized. The response of the pulp may vary depending on whether the caries process is progressing rapidly or slowly or is completely inactive (arrested caries). Moreover, caries tends to be an intermittent process with periods of rapid activity alternating with periods of quiescence.[35] The rate of attack may be influenced by any or all of the following:

Age of the host
Composition of the tooth
Nature of the bacterial flora of the lesion
Salivary flow
Buffering capacity of the saliva
Antibacterial substances in the saliva
Oral hygiene
Cariogenicity of the diet and frequency with which acidogenic food is ingested
Caries-inhibiting factors in the diet

Early morphologic evidence of a pulpal reaction to caries is found in the underlying odontoblast layer. Even before the appearance of inflammatory changes in the pulp, there is an overall reduction in the number and size of odontoblast cell bodies.[65] Although odontoblasts are normally tall columnar cells, odontoblasts affected by caries appear flat to cuboidal in shape (Fig. 15-1). Electron microscopic examination of odontoblasts beneath carious lesions has revealed signs of cellular injury in the form of vacuolization, ballooning degeneration of mitochondria, and reduction in the number and size of other cytoplasmic organelles, particularly the endoplasmic reticulum.[34] These findings are in accord with biochemical studies[28] in which a reduction in the metabolic activity of odontoblasts was noted.

Concomitant with changes in the odontoblastic layer, a hy-

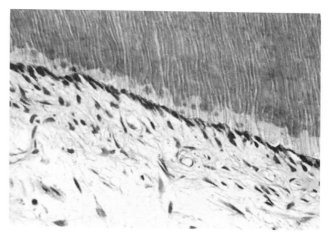

FIG. 15-1 Low cuboidal odontoblasts beneath a carious lesion.

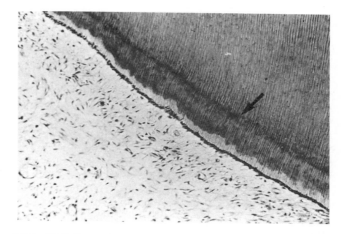

FIG. 15-2 Hyperchromatic line *(arrow)* in dentin beneath a carious lesion. *(From Trowbridge H: J Endod 7:52, 1981.)*

perchromatic line (calciotraumatic response) may develop along the pulpal margin of the dentin (Fig. 15-2). Formation of this line is thought to represent a disturbance in the normal equilibrium of the odontoblasts. It may also delineate the point at which the primary odontoblasts succumbed to the caries process and were replaced by odontoprogenitor cells arising from the cell-rich zone. In either event as new dentin is formed, the hyperchromatic line persists and becomes permanently embedded in the dentin.

Dental caries is a protracted process, and lesions progress over a period of months or years. One investigator found that the average time from the stage of incipient caries to clinically detectable caries in children is 18 ± 6 months. Consequently, it is not surprising that pulpal inflammation evoked by carious lesions begins insidiously as a low-grade, chronic response rather than an acute reaction (Fig. 15-3). The initial inflammatory cell infiltrate consists principally of lymphocytes, plasma cells, and macrophages.[11] Within this infiltrate are immunologically competent cells responding to antigenic substances diffusing into the pulp from the carious lesion.[60] Additionally,

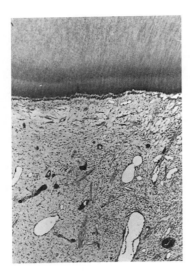

FIG. 15-3 Chronic inflammatory response evoked by a carious lesion in the overlying dentin.

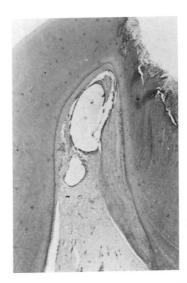

FIG. 15-4 Chronic ulcerative pulpitis.

there is a proliferation of small blood vessels and fibroblasts and the deposition of collagen fibers. This pattern of inflammation is regarded as an inflammatory-reparative process. It is wise to remember that not all injuries result in permanent damage. Should the carious lesion be eliminated or become arrested, connective tissue repair would ensue.

The extent of pulpal inflammation beneath a carious lesion depends on the depth of bacterial invasion and the degree to which dentin permeability has been reduced by dentinal sclerosis and reparative dentin formation. In a study involving 46 carious teeth, investigators found that if the distance between the invading bacteria and the pulp (including the thickness of reparative dentin) averaged 1.1 mm or more, the inflammatory response was negligible.[52] When the lesions reached to within 0.5 mm of the pulp, there was a significant increase in the extent of inflammation; but it was not until the reparative dentin that had formed beneath the lesion was invaded by bacteria that the pulp became acutely inflamed.

As bacteria converge on the pulp, the characteristic features of acute inflammation become manifest. These include vascular and cellular responses in the form of vasodilation, increased vascular permeability, and the accumulation of leukocytes. Neutrophils migrate from blood vessels to the site of injury in response to certain split products of complement that are strongly chemotactic. These products are formed when complement is activated in the presence of antigen-antibody complexes.

Pulpal Abscess

Carious exposure of the pulp results in progressive mobilization of neutrophils and eventually to suppuration, which may be diffuse or localized in the form of an abscess. The exudate associated with this reaction is called pus. Pus is formed when neutrophils release their lysosomal enzymes and the surrounding tissue is digested (a process known as liquefaction necrosis). The digested tissue has a greater osmotic pressure than the surrounding tissue, and this pressure differential is one of the reasons that abscesses are often painful and why drainage provides relief.

Few bacteria are found in an abscess, because bacteria enter-

ing the lesion are promptly destroyed by the antibacterial products of neutrophils. In addition, many bacteria cannot tolerate the low pH resulting from the release of lactic acid from neutrophils. However, as the size of the exposure enlarges and an ever-increasing number of bacteria enter the pulp, the defending forces are overwhelmed. It must be remembered that the pulp has a finite blood supply. Therefore when the demand for inflammatory elements exceeds the ability of the blood to transport them to the site of bacterial penetration, the bacteria become too numerous for the defenders and are able to proliferate without constraint. This ultimately leads to pulp necrosis.

Chronic Ulcerative Pulpitis

In some cases an accumulation of neutrophils may produce surface destruction (ulceration) of the pulp rather than an abscess. This is apt to occur when drainage is established through a pathway of decomposed dentin. The ulcer represents a local excavation of the surface of the pulp resulting from liquefaction necrosis of tissue. Because drainage prevents the buildup of pressure, the lesion tends to remain localized and asymptomatic. The base of the ulcer consists of necrotic debris and a dense accumulation of neutrophils. Granulation tissue infiltrated with chronic inflammatory cells is found within the deeper layers of the lesion. Eventually a space is created between the area of suppuration and the wall of the pulp chamber, giving the lesion the appearance of an ulcer (Fig. 15-4).

Hyperplastic Pulpitis

Hyperplastic pulpitis occurs almost exclusively in primary and immature permanent teeth with open apices. It develops in response to carious exposure of the pulp when the exposure enlarges to form a gaping cavity in the roof of the pulp chamber. This opening provides a pathway for drainage of the inflammatory exudate. Once drainage is established, acute inflammation subsides and chronic inflammatory tissue proliferates through the opening created by the exposure from a "pulp polyp" (Fig. 15-5). Presumably the young pulp does not become necrotic following exposure because its natural defenses and rich supply of blood allow it to resist bacterial in-

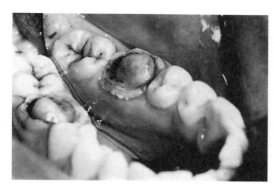

FIG. 15-5 Hyperplastic pulpitis (pulp polyp) in a lower first permanent molar. *(Courtesy Dr. A. Stabholz, Hebrew Univ. School of Dental Medicine, Jerusalem.)*

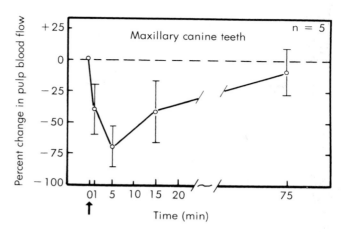

FIG. 15-6 Effects of infiltration anesthesia (2% lidocaine with 1:100,000 epinephrine) on pulpal blood flow in the maxillary canine teeth of dogs. There is a drastic decrease in pulpal blood flow soon after the injection. Arrow indicates the time of injection. Bars depict standard deviation. *(From Kim S: J Dent Res 63[5]:650, 1984.)*

fection. Clinically, the lesion has the appearance of a fleshy mass that may cover most of what remains of the crown of the tooth.

EFFECTS OF LOCAL ANESTHETICS ON THE PULP

The purpose of adding a vasoconstrictor to local anesthetics is to potentiate and prolong the anesthetic effect by reducing blood flow in the area in which the anesthetic is administered. Although this enhances anesthesia, a recent study has shown that an anesthetic such as 2% lidocaine with 1:100,000 epinephrine is capable of significantly decreasing pulpal blood flow.[33] This reduction in blood flow may place the pulp in jeopardy for reasons explained later. Both infiltration and mandibular block injections cause a significant decrease in pulpal blood flow, although the flow reduction lasts a relatively short time (Fig. 15-6). With the ligamental injection, pulpal blood flow ceases completely for about 30 minutes when 2% lidocaine with 1:100,000 epinephrine is used (Fig. 15-7). With a higher concentration of epinephrine the cessation of pulp flow lasts even longer. There is a direct relationship between the length of the flow cessation and the concentration of the vasoconstrictor used.[31] Because the rate of oxygen consumption in the pulp is relatively low, the healthy pulp can probably withstand a period of reduced blood flow. Researchers reported that pulpal blood flow and sensory nerve activity returned to normal levels after 3 hours of total cessation of blood flow.[42] However, a prolonged reduction in oxygen transport could interfere with cellular metabolism and alter the response of the pulp to injury. Irreversible pulpal injury is particularly apt to occur when dental procedures such as full crown preparations are performed immediately following a ligamental injection. At least four documented cases have occurred in which the mandibular anterior teeth were devitalized as a result of crown preparation following ligamental injection.[31] Presumably irreversible pulp damage resulting from tooth preparation is caused by the release of substantial amounts of vasoactive agents, such as substance P, into the extracellular compartment of the underlying pulp.[41] Under normal circumstances these vasoactive substances are quickly removed from the pulp by the blood-

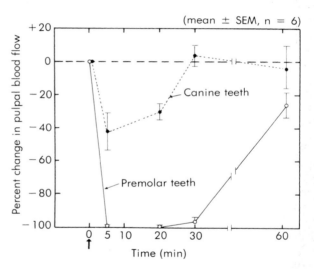

FIG. 15-7 Effects of ligamental injection (2% lidocaine with 1:100,000 epinephrine) on pulpal blood flow in the mandibular canine and premolar teeth of dogs. Injection was given at the mesiodistal sulcus of the premolar teeth. Injection caused total cessation of pulpal blood flow, which lasted about 30 minutes in the premolar teeth. Arrow indicates the time of injection. *(From Kim S: J Endod 12[10]:486, 1986.)*

stream. However, when blood flow is drastically decreased or completely arrested, the removal of vasoactive substance from the pulp is greatly delayed. Accumulation of these substances and other metabolic waste products may thus result in permanent damage to the pulp. One investigator has shown that the concentration of substances diffusing across the dentin into the pulp depends in part on the rate of removal via the pulpal circulation.[43] Thus a significant reduction in blood flow during a restorative procedure could lead to an increase in the concentration of irritants accumulating within the pulp. *Therefore,*

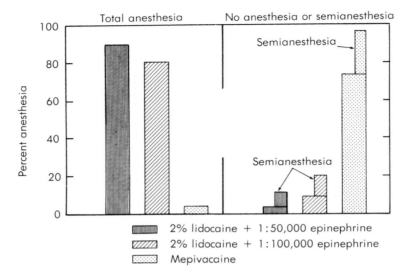

FIG. 15-8 Ligamental injection was effective in obtaining anesthesia in about 90% of cases with 2% lidocaine with 1:50,000 epinephrine and in about 80% of cases with 2% lidocaine with 1:100,000 epinephrine. Injection with mepivacaine (Carbocaine) practically failed to achieve anesthesia. Criterion for total anesthesia is no pain to pulp extirpation and canal instrumentation; semianesthesia is characterized by discomfort as a file approaches the apex.

whenever possible, it is advisable to use vasoconstrictor-free local anesthetics for restorative procedures on vital teeth. Since the addition of epinephrine at a concentration of 1:100,000 to local anesthetics appears to provide adequate vasoconstriction, stronger concentrations should be avoided during routine restorative procedures.

For dental treatments where clinicians need not be concerned about the vitality of the pulp, such as endodontic therapy and extractions, the use of a vasoconstrictor-containing local anesthetic is recommended. When used with an epinephrine-containing anesthetic, the ligamental injection is effective in obtaining anesthesia (Fig. 15-8). Over 80% of the problem teeth were successfully anesthetized with 1:100,000 epinephrine-containing anesthetic. Endodontists have found the ligamental injection to be an important tool to obtain profound anesthesia when treating so-called hot mandibular molars.

CAVITY AND CROWN PREPARATION

"Cooking the pulp in its own juice" is how Bodecker described tooth preparation without proper coolant. As shown in Fig. 15-9, pulpal responses to cavity and crown preparation depend on many factors. These include thermal injury, especially frictional heat; transection of the odontoblastic processes; crown preparation; vibration; desiccation of dentin; pulp exposure; smear layer; remaining dentin thickness; and acid etching.

Thermal Injury

Cutting of dentin with a rotating bur or stone produces a considerable amount of frictional heat. The amount of heat produced is determined by speed of rotation, size and shape of the cutting instrument, length of time the instrument is in contact with the dentin, and amount of pressure exerted on the handpiece. If high temperatures are produced in deep cavities by continuous cutting without proper cooling, the underlying pulp may be severely damaged. According to one investigator,[73] the production of heat within the pulp is the most severe stress that

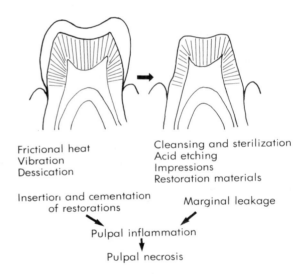

FIG. 15-9 Schematic illustration of factors that might cause pulpal reaction.

restorative procedures impart to the pulp. If damage is extensive and the cell-rich zone of the pulp is destroyed, reparative dentin may not form.[40]

The thermal conductivity of dentin is relatively low. Therefore heat generated during the cutting of a shallow cavity preparation is much less likely to injure the pulp than a deep cavity preparation. One study found that temperatures and stresses developed during dry cutting of dentin were sufficiently high to be detrimental to tooth structure.[13] These investigators found that the greatest potential for damage was within a 1- to 2-mm radius of the dentin being cut.

The importance of the use of water-air spray during cavity preparation has been well established.[61,62] For example, more than 15 years ago it was reported that high-speed cutting with

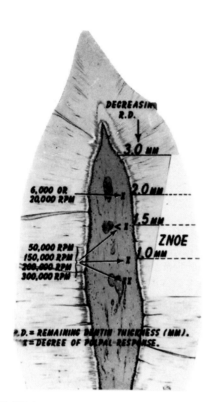

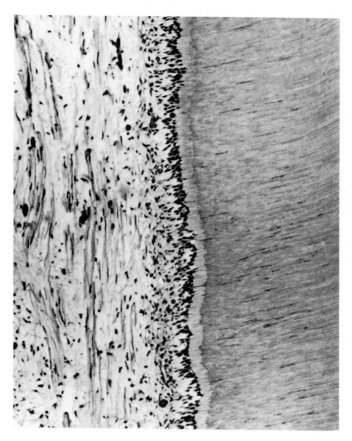

FIG. 15-10 With adequate water-air spray coolant, the same cutting tools, and a comparable remaining dentin thickness, the intensity of the pulpal response with high-speed techniques (decreasing force) is considerably less traumatic than with lower speed techniques (increasing force). *(From Stanley HR, Swerdlow H: J Prosthet Dent 14:365, 1964.)*

FIG. 15-11 Two-day specimen, high-speed with air-water spray. The superficial layers lack infiltrating inflammatory cells. Some odontoblast displacement is present. Pulp architecture is generally intact. *(From Swerdlow H, Stanley HR: J Prosthet Dent 9:121, 1959.)*

an adequate coolant caused cooling of the pulp to a subambient level.[73] Without a coolant the pulpal temperature rose to a critical level, 11° F (−11.6° C) above the ambient temperature. The same is true in the case of slow-speed cutting (11,000 rpm). The reaction of the pulp to cavity preparation with and without a water spray has been studied histologically (Figs. 15-10 to 15-12).[58] When water-air spray was used, there was a negligible response, providing the remaining dentin thickness was greater than 1 mm (Fig. 15-10). However, when the same procedure was performed without using a water spray, severe damage was found underneath the cutting site (Fig. 15-13). The flow was further reduced 1 hour after the completion of the crown preparation, suggesting irreversible damage. In a similar experiment using a water-air spray, only minor changes in pulpal blood flow were observed (Fig. 15-14).

Other researchers[40] investigated the effects of heat on the pulps of anesthetized young premolar teeth scheduled for orthodontic extraction. Class V cavities were prepared in the teeth, leaving an average of 0.5 mm remaining dentin thickness. Subsequently, a constant heat of 302° F (150° C) was applied to the surface of the exposed dentin for 30 seconds. Following this procedure the teeth remained asymptomatic for a month, following which the teeth were extracted. Histologic examination of the pulps revealed varying degrees of pathosis, which

included development of a homogenized collagenous zone along the dentin wall, disappearance of the "cell-rich" zone, and generalized cellular degeneration. Localized abscesses were observed in some of the teeth.

"Blushing" of teeth during or after cavity or crown preparation has been attributed to frictional heat. Characteristically the coronal dentin develops a pinkish hue very soon after the dentin is cut. This pinkish hue represents vascular stasis in the subodontoblastic capillary plexus blood flow. Under favorable conditions this reaction is reversible and the pulp will survive. However, a dark purplish color indicates thrombosis, and this is associated with a poorer prognosis. Histologically, the pulp tissue adjacent to the blushed dentinal surface is engorged with extravasated red blood cells, presumably as a result of the rupture of capillaries in the subodontoblastic plexus.[37] The incidence of dentinal blushing is greatest beneath full crown preparations in teeth that were anesthetized by ligamental injection using 2% lidocaine plus 1:100,000 epinephrine.[31] In such cases the cessation of pulpal blood flow following ligamental injection may be a contributing factor. Tooth preparation may lead to the release of various vasoactive substances such as substance P, and accumulation of such agents as a result of cessation of pulpal blood flow following ligamental injection may cause the tooth to blush.

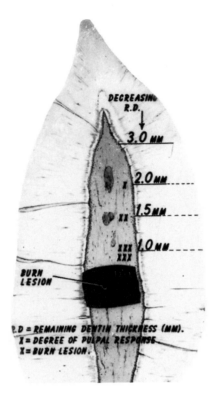

FIG. 15-12 Without adequate water coolant, larger cutting tools (e.g., a No. 37 diamond point) create typical burn lesions within the pulp when the remaining dentin thickness becomes less than 1.5 mm. *(From Stanley HR, Swerdlow H: J Prosthet Dent 14:365, 1964.)*

Transection of the Odontoblastic Processes

The length of the odontoblast process in fully formed teeth is still a matter of controversy. For many years it was believed that the process is confined to the inner third of the dentin. However, recent scanning electron microscopic studies have provided evidence suggesting that many of the processes extend all the way from the odontoblast layer to the dentinoenamel junction.[30] In any event, amputation of the distal segment of odontoblast processes is often a consequence of cavity or crown preparation. Histologic investigation would indicate that amputation of a portion of the process does not invariably lead to death of the odontoblast. We know from numerous cytologic studies involving microsurgery that amputation of a cellular process is quickly followed by repair of the cell membrane. However, it would appear that amputation of the odontoblast process close to the cell body results in irreversible injury.

It is not always possible to determine the exact cause of death when odontoblasts disappear following a restorative procedure, since these cells may be subjected to a variety of insults. Frictional heat, vibration, amputation of processes, displacement as a result of desiccation, exposure to bacterial toxins, and other chemical irritants may each play a role in the demise of odontoblasts.

Investigators[14] studied the effects of class V cavity preparation on rat molar odontoblasts and observed a significant decrease in the amount of rough endoplasmic reticulum and number of mitochondria. There was also a loss of tight junctions between adjacent odontoblasts. Under the conditions of this experiment, these changes were reversible. Tight junctions provide a semipermeable barrier that prevents the passage of macromolecules from the pulp into the predentin. It has been

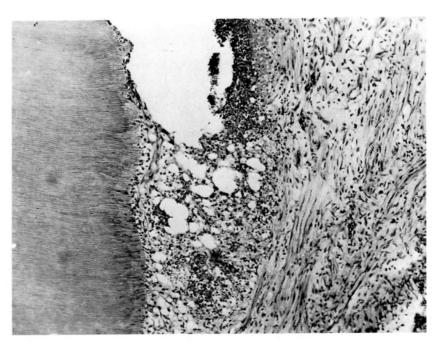

FIG. 15-13 Burn lesion with necrosis and expanding abscess formation in a 10-day specimen. Cavity prepared dry at 20,000 rpm with remaining dentin thickness is 0.23 mm. *(From Swerdlow H, Stanley HR: J Am Dent Assoc 56:317, 1958.)*

shown that cavity preparation disturbs this barrier, thus increasing the permeability of the odontoblast layer.[69] The disruption of tight junctional complexes in the odontoblast layer could increase the potential for entry of toxic substances into the subjacent pulp tissue.

Taylor et al.[63] observed an extensive increase in calcitonin gene-related peptide (CGRP) immunoreactive nerve fibers in the odontoblast layer beneath superficial dentinal cavities in rat molars. It was postulated that this increase represented nerve sprouting. The greatest number of nerve endings was observed at a postoperative interval of 4 days, but within 21 days these fibers had disappeared. The function of nerve sprouting in tissue injury is still unclear.

Crown Preparation

Researchers[16] studied the long-term effects of crown preparation on pulp vitality and found a higher incidence of pulp necrosis associated with full crown preparation (13.3%) as compared with partial veneer restorations (5.1%) and unrestored control teeth (0.5%). The placement of foundations for full crown restorations was associated with an even greater incidence of pulp morbidity (17.7%).

Vibratory Phenomena

Surprisingly little is known about the vibratory agitation that may be produced by high-speed cutting procedures. One study[23] demonstrated violent disturbances in the pulp chambers of teeth beneath the point of application of the bur and at other points remote from the cavity preparation. According to the observations the shock waves produced by vibration were particularly pronounced when the cutting speed was reduced; therefore stalling of the bur by increased digital pressure on the handpiece should be avoided. Obviously this problem deserves further study.

Desiccation of Dentin

When the surface of freshly cut dentin is dried with a jet of air, there is a rapid outward movement of fluid through the den-

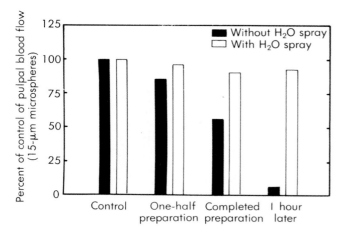

FIG. 15-14 Effects of crown preparation in dogs, with and without water-air spray (at 350,000 rpm), on pulpal blood flow. Tooth preparation without water-air spray caused a substantial decrease in pulpal blood flow, whereas that with water-air spray caused insignificant changes in the flow.

tinal tubules as a result of the activation of capillary forces within.[9] According to the hydrodynamic theory of dentin sensitivity, this movement of fluid results in stimulation of the sensory nerve of the pulp. Fluid movement is also capable of drawing odontoblasts up into the tubules. These "displaced" odontoblasts soon die and disappear as they undergo autolysis. However, desiccation of dentin by cutting procedures or with a blast of air does not injure the pulp.[9] Although one might expect that death of odontoblasts would evoke an inflammatory response, probably too few cells are involved to evoke a significant reaction. Moreover, since death occurs within the dentinal tubules, dentinal fluid would dilute the products of cellular degeneration that might otherwise initiate an inflammatory response. Ultimately, odontoblasts that have been destroyed as a result of desiccation are replaced by new odontoblasts that arise from the cell-rich zone of the pulp, and in 1 to 3 months reparative dentin is formed.

Pulp Exposure

Exposure of the pulp during cavity preparation occurs most often in the process of removing carious dentin. Accidental mechanical exposure may result during the placement of pins or retention points in dentin. In both types of exposure, injury to the pulp primarily appears to be due to bacterial contamination. Investigators demonstrated that surgical exposure of the pulps of germ-free rats was followed by complete healing with no appreciable inflammatory reaction.[27] Another investigator has shown that pulps exposed during the removal of carious dentin become infected by bacteria that are carried into the pulp by dentin chips harboring microorganisms. It is safe to state that carious exposure results in much more bacterial contamination than does mechanical exposure.

Smear Layer

The smear layer is an amorphous, relatively smooth layer of microcrystalline debris whose featureless surface cannot be seen with the naked eye.[44] Although the smear layer may interfere with the adaptation of restorative materials to dentin, it may not be desirable to remove the entire layer, since its removal greatly increases dentin permeability. By removing most of the layer but leaving plugs of grinding debris in the apertures of the dentinal tubules, dentin permeability is not increased, yet the walls of the cavity are relatively clean. Whether or not the smear layer should be removed is a matter of controversy. One view is that microorganisms present in the smear layer may irritate the pulp. Initially few bacteria are present in the smear layer; but if conditions for growth are favorable, these will multiply, particularly if a gap between the restorative material and the dentinal wall permits the ingress of saliva.[8] Brännström believes that most restorative materials do not adhere to the dentinal wall.[8] Consequently, contraction gaps form between such materials and the adjacent tooth structure, and these gaps are invaded by bacteria either from the smear layer or from the oral cavity. As a result, bacterial metabolites diffuse through the dentinal tubules and injure the pulp.

Remaining Dentin Thickness

As discussed in Chapter 11, dentin permeability increases almost logarithmically with increasing cavity depth because of the difference in size and number of dentinal tubules. In short, permeability of the dentin is of great importance in determining the degree of pulpal injury resulting from restorative procedures and materials. Stanley[58] found that the distance between the floor of the cavity preparation and the pulp (i.e., the remaining dentin thickness) greatly influences the pulpal response to restorative procedures and materials. He suggested that a remaining dentin thickness of 2 mm would protect the pulp from the effects of most restorative procedures, provided that all other operative precautions are observed.

Acid Etching

Although acid etching of cavity walls is cleansing, acid etching is specifically designed to enhance the adhesion of restorative materials. In the case of dentin, however, the ability of acid etching to improve long-term adhesion has been questioned. Acid cleansers applied to dentin have been shown to widen the openings of the dentinal tubules, increase dentin permeability, and enhance bacterial penetration of the dentin. One study showed that in deep cavities, pretreatment of the dentin with 50% citric or 50% phosphoric acid for 60 seconds is capable of significantly increasing the response of the pulp to restorative materials.[59] Results of one physiologic investigation have shown that acid etching a small class V cavity having a remaining dentin thickness of 1.5 mm has little effect on pulpal blood flow.[57] Thus direct effect of the acid on the pulpal microvascular vessels appears to be negligible, possibly because of a rapid buffering of the acid by the dentinal fluid. However, it is possible that in very deep cavities acid etching may contribute to pulpal injury.

RESTORATIVE MATERIALS

How do restorative materials evoke a response in the underlying pulp? For many years it was believed that toxic ingredients in the materials were responsible for pulpal injury. However, pulpal injury associated with the use of these materials could not be correlated with their cytotoxic properties. Thus irritating materials such as zinc oxide–eugenol (ZOE) produced a very mild pulpal response when placed in cavities, whereas less toxic materials such as composite resins and amalgam produced a much stronger pulp response. Beside chemical toxicity, some of the properties of materials that might be capable of producing injury include the following:

1. Acidity (hydrogen ion concentration)
2. Absorption of water during setting
3. Heat generated during setting
4. Poor marginal adaptation resulting in bacterial contamination

Investigators[48] found that the pulpal response beneath a material is not associated with the material's hydrogen ion concentration. The acid content in restorative materials is probably neutralized by the dentin and dentinal fluid.[11] As the superficial dentin is demineralized, phosphate ions are liberated, thus producing a buffering effect. However, placement of an acidic material such as zinc phosphate at luting consistency in a deep cavity may have a toxic effect on the pulp, since the diffusion barrier is extremely thin. In a study conducted in our laboratory, zinc phosphate cement of luting consistency placed on a deep (0.5 mm remaining dentin layer) and large class V cavity on canine tooth caused a moderate decrease in pulpal blood flow as measured with the 15 µm microsphere method. After the cement had hardened for about 30 minutes, blood flow had again increased, suggesting that the cement had a temporary

and transitory effect on the pulpal circulation (Fig. 15-15). The changes in pulpal blood flow may have been due to chemical or exothermal effects of the cement. One study[48] found that of all the materials studied, zinc phosphate cement was associated with the greatest temperature rise—an increase of 35.85° F (2.14° C).[48] This amount of temperature increase, however, is not sufficient to produce tissue injury.[73] In a microcirculatory study using hamster cheek pouch, a drop of zinc phosphate liquid caused stasis, followed by hemolysis, resulting in total cessation of blood flow in the vessels that were in contact with the liquid. Thus there seems to be a real possibility of pulpal damage if the pulp is in close contact with the liquid portion of the cement. Absorption of water during the setting of a material can also be ruled out as a cause of pulpal injury. Compared with the removal of fluid from dentin by an airstream during cavity preparation (which produces no inflammatory response in the pulp), absorption of water by a material is insignificant. Researchers[48] found no relationship between the hydrophilic properties of materials and their effect on the pulp.

This brings us to bacterial contamination. It has long been recognized that, in general, dental materials do not adapt to tooth structure well enough to provide a hermetic seal. Thus it has been acknowledged that bacteria may penetrate the gap between the restored material and the cavity wall. Presumably bacteria growing beneath restorations create toxic products that can diffuse through the dentinal tubules and evoke an inflammatory reaction in the underlying pulp. Converging evidence suggests that *products of bacterial metabolism are the major cause of pulpal injury resulting from the insertion of restorations.* Let us briefly review some of that evidence. One inves-

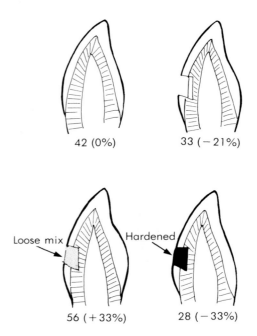

FIG. 15-15 Effects of zinc phosphate cement on pulpal blood flow (ml/min/100 g). Cement of luting consistency was placed in a deep and large class V cavity in the canine teeth of dogs, and pulpal blood flow was measured. A 33% increase was observed initially, but the hardened cement caused a decrease in pulpal blood flow.

tigator showed that material such as composite resins, zinc-phosphate, and silicate cements produced only a localized tissue reaction when placed directly on exposed pulps in germ-free animals.[71] The same procedure in conventional animals resulted in total pulp necrosis. Employing bacterial staining methods, researchers[11] demonstrated that the growth of bacteria under restorations was correlated with the degree of inflammation of the adjacent pulp tissue. They also found that bacteria did not grow when the outer portions of restorations were replaced with ZOE, thus producing a surface seal (Fig. 15-16). When bacterial growth was thus inhibited, pulpal inflammation was negligible. Similar studies[4] showed that colonies of bacteria become established under restorative materials that do not provide an adequate marginal seal. Of the materials tested—Dispersalloy amalgam (Johnson & Johnson Products Co., East Windsor, N.J.), Concise composite resin (3M Co., St. Paul, Minn.), Hygienic gutta-percha (Hygienic Corp., Akron, Ohio), MQ silicate cements (S.S. White Dental Products, Philadelphia, Pa.), and ZOE—only ZOE consistently prevented bacteria from becoming established beneath the restoration. Using ZOE as a surface seal, Cox et al.[15] found that materials such as amalgam, composites, silicate cement, zinc phosphate

cement, and ZOE produced only a thin zone of contact necrosis and no inflammation when placed directly on primate pulps (Fig. 15-17).

In vitro and in vivo studies on marginal adaptation of restorative materials have often yielded conflicting results. Obviously it is difficult to duplicate clinical conditions in the laboratory. Two important factors affecting marginal adaptation are temperature changes and masticatory forces. Nelson et al.[38] were the first to study the opening and closing of the margin of restorations that were subjected to temperature changes. If a material has a different coefficient of thermal expansion than tooth structure, temperature change is likely to produce gaps between the material and the cavity wall. Another investigator[51] demonstrated a marked effect of functional mastication on marginal adaptation of composite restorations. He found gap formation along 71% of the restorations in teeth that were in functional occlusion, whereas leakage occurred in only 28% of teeth with no antagonist.

As yet no permanent filling material has been shown to consistently provide a perfect marginal seal, so leakage and bacterial contamination are always a threat to the integrity of the pulp. Consequently, an adequate cavity liner or cement base should be employed to seal the dentinal tubules before inserting restorative materials. Despite these findings, it must be acknowledged that pulps frequently remain healthy under restorations that leak. Factors that determine whether bacterial growth beneath a restoration will injure the pulp probably include pathogenicity of the microorganisms, permeability of the underlying dentin (i.e., degree of sclerosis, number of tubules, thickness of dentin), and the ability of the irritated pulp to produce reparative dentin.

Since there is convincing evidence that bacterial growth beneath restorations is the primary cause of pulpal injury, the antibacterial properties of filling materials may be of considerable importance. Not all materials have been studied, but there is evidence that ZOE, calcium hydroxide, and polycarboxylate cement have some ability to inhibit bacterial growth. Zinc phosphate cement, the restorative resins, and silicate cements lack antibacterial ingredients, and these materials are most often associated with injury to the pulp.

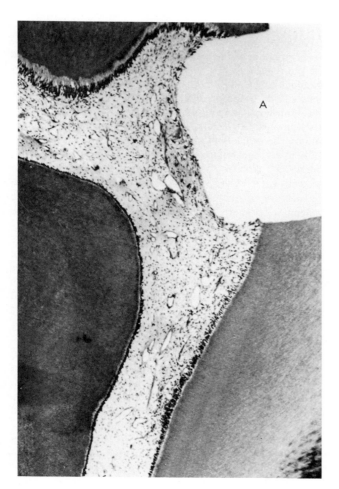

FIG. 15-16 Appearance of pulp 7 days following placement of amalgam restoration *(A)* directly against pulp tissue. Note absence of inflammatory response. *(From Cos CF et al: J Prosthet Dent 57:1, 1987.)*

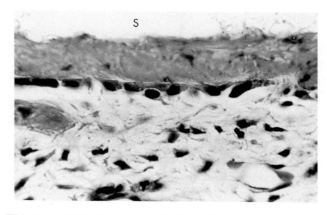

FIG. 15-17 Pulpal response 21 days following placement of silicate cement *(S)* directly against the pulp. Silicate was surface sealed with zinc oxide–eugenol. Note formation of hard tissue and new odontoblasts. *(From Cox CF et al: J Prosthet Dent 57:1, 1987.)*

Zinc Oxide–Eugenol

ZOE is used for a variety of purposes in dentistry. In addition to being a popular temporary filling material, it is used for provisional and permanent cementation of inlays, crowns, and bridges and as a pulp-capping agent and a cement base. Eugenol, a phenol derivative, is known to be toxic, and it is capable of producing thrombosis of blood vessels when applied directly to pulp tissue.[50] It also has anesthetic properties, and is used as an anodyne in relieving the symptoms of painful pulpitis. This presumably results from its ability to block the transmission of action potentials in nerve fibers.[67] Experimentally, ZOE has been shown to suppress nerve excitability in the pulp when applied to the base of a deep cavity.[66] This effect is obtained only when a fairly thin mix of ZOE (e.g., powder-liquid ratio 2:1 w/w) is used. Presumably it is the free eugenol in the cement that is responsible for the anesthetic effect. ZOE has two important properties that explain why it is such an effective base material: (1) it adapts very closely to dentin, thus providing a good marginal seal, and (2) its antibacterial properties inhibit bacterial growth on cavity walls. However, because eugenol injures cells, some authorities question whether ZOE should be used in very deep cavity preparations where there is a risk of pulp exposure.

Zinc Phosphate Cement

One study[24] found that when a liner was omitted, severe pulpal reactions (principally abscess formation) occurred in all teeth in which deep class V cavities were restored with zinc phosphate cement. The pulpal response was attributed to the phosphoric acid contained in the cement. In retrospect, however, it is likely that irritation to the pulp was due primarily to marginal leakage rather than to acidity. Because of its high modulus of elasticity, zinc phosphate is the cement base of choice for amalgam restorations. This results from the fact that it is better able to resist the stresses of mastication than other cements.

Zinc Polycarboxylate Cements

Polycarboxylate cement is well tolerated by the pulp, being roughly equivalent to ZOE cements in this respect.[24] This may be due to its ability to adapt well to dentin. It also has been reported that this cement has bactericidal qualities.[5]

Restorative Resins

The original unfilled resins were associated with severe marginal leakage, caused by dimensional changes that resulted from a high coefficient of thermal expansion. This in turn resulted in marked pulpal injury. The development of sulfinic acid catalyst systems and the nonpressure insertion techniques have improved the performance of resins considerably. The epoxide resins with a benzoyl peroxide catalyst that are 75% filled with glass or quartz (the so-called composite resins) represent another group of resins. These have much more favorable polymerization characteristics and a lower coefficient of thermal expansion than the original unfilled resins. The marginal seal has been further improved by acid etching of beveled enamel and the use of a bonding agent or primer. This reduces the risk of microbial invasion but does not eliminate bacteria that may be present on cavity walls. However, it has been shown that the initial marginal seal tends to deteriorate as the etched composite restoration ages. Furthermore, one study showed that functional mastication is capable of producing gaps that result in increased leakage.[51] Many investigators[11] have shown that unlined composite resins are harmful to the pulp, primarily because of bacterial contamination beneath the restoration. Thus the use of a cavity liner is strongly recommended. Since copal varnish is not compatible with the restorative resins, the use of a polystyrene liner has been advocated.[12] Bases containing calcium hydroxide have also been shown to provide good protection against bacteria.

Glass-Ionomer Cement Restorations

Studies on glass-ionomer cements indicate that they are well tolerated by the pulp.[29] However, researchers[1] have shown that leakage may occur around such fillings, so this material should be used in conjunction with a liner or base. There have been reports of postcementation tooth sensitivity following the use of glass-ionomer cements to cement gold castings, but the cause of this sensitivity has not been determined. It appears that sensitivity is not the result of marginal leakage, because the results of an in vitro leakage study demonstrated that glass-ionomer luting cements provide a good marginal seal.[21]

Dental Amalgam

Dental amalgam, first used for the restoration of carious teeth in the sixteenth century, is still the most popular restorative material in dentistry. Unvarnished amalgam restorations leak severely when they are first inserted, but within a period of 12 weeks a marginal seal develops that resists dye penetration beyond the dentinoenamel junction. Investigators[22] found that pulp responses to unlined amalgams—Sybraloy (Kerr Manufacturing Co., Romulus, Mich.), Dispersalloy (Johnson & Johnson, East Windsor, N.J.), Tytin (S.S. White Dental Products, Philadelphia, Pa.), and Spheraloy (Kerr Manufacturing Co., Romulus, Mich.) consisted of slight to moderate inflammation. The inflammation tended to diminish with time, and within a few weeks reparative dentin was deposited. Other investigators[50] theorized that the high mercury content of amalgam may exert a cytotoxic effect on the pulp, as they found that mercury penetrates into the dentin and pulp beneath an amalgam restoration. They have also reported that rubbing the bottom of the cavity with a calcium hydroxide and water mixture protects the pulp from the irritating effects of amalgam. Bacteria were found beneath unlined amalgams, whereas the pulps of teeth in which a ZOE liner was used exhibited a milder response and no bacteria were present. In vitro bacterial tests indicated that amalgam has no inhibitory effect on bacterial growth.

It is well known that insertion of amalgam restorations may result in postoperative thermal sensitivity, even when amalgam is placed in a shallow cavity. Brännström[7] is of the opinion that such sensitivity results from expansion or contraction of fluid that occupies the gap between the amalgam and the cavity wall. This fluid is in communication with fluid in the subjacent dentinal tubules, so variations in temperature cause axial movement of fluid in the tubules. According to the hydrodynamic theory of dentin sensitivity, this fluid movement would stimulate nerve fibers in the underlying pulp, thus evoking pain.[66] The use of a cavity varnish or base is recommended to seal the dentinal tubules and prevent this form of postoperative discomfort.

Cavity Varnish

The effectiveness of cavity varnish in providing protection for the pulp is highly controversial. One study[18] has called attention to the fact that in vivo surfaces are wet and therefore the application of liners or varnishes may not result in an impervious coating. Even the application of two or three coats of varnish may not prevent gaps from occurring in the lining. Furthermore, other investigators[12] have reported that a double layer of Copalite did not prevent bacterial leakage and growth of bacteria on the cavity walls. Nonetheless, several reports indicate that varnish can act as a barrier to the toxic effects of restorations.[56] One study[39] assessed the ability of several commercial varnishes to decrease microleakage beneath a high-copper spherical alloy restorative material and found Copalite to be the most effective.

EFFECTS OF LASING ON THE PULP-DENTIN COMPLEX

The successful use of various laser systems in medicine has stimulated its application in dentistry. Manufacturers of laser systems make the following claims: lasers can remove caries; modify the dentin surface for stronger bonding; eliminate pits and fissures; and anesthetize and treat hypersensitive teeth. These claims are made for several laser systems with differing wave lengths and energy outputs.[17,49] Two laser systems, the carbon dioxide and Nd:YAG, have demonstrated significant possibilities in clinical dentistry such as those mentioned above. Such results, however, are not the only criteria for evaluating the usefulness and value of lasers in clinical dentistry. Two other requirements are critical for the effectiveness of lasers and the health of the tooth: lasing must provide superior results over traditional procedures, and it must not damage the vital pulp in the process.

Carbon Dioxide Laser

The carbon dioxide laser is well known for cutting soft tissue without bleeding, and thus its usage in soft tissue management in periodontal and oral surgery procedures has been well established. However, its utility in hard tissue management can be contested. Lasing effects on the pulp-dentin complex had not been considered by evaluations of the system, and it has been subsequently shown in several studies that the dentin and the pulp are detrimentally affected by most lasing procedures. For instance, a cat's tooth with a remaining dentin thickness of 1 mm lased at a low energy setting of 2.6 W showed a 50% increase in pulpal blood flow when measured with laser Doppler flowmetry (Fig. 15-18). This indicates a dilation of the blood vessels in response to noxious thermal stimulus. The moderately higher energy of 5 W caused an irreversible flow reduction, indicating damage to the pulp. The most likely cause of the blood flow reduction is an excessive thermal effect.[19] Dentin permeability measured by Pashley's in vitro dentin disk

technique also revealed that permeability increased significantly after lasing. Thus the utility and safety of carbon dioxide laser systems for hard tissues is questionable with the systems currently available.

Nd:YAG Laser

A pulsed Nd:YAG laser with 1.06 mm wavelength has been the most widely tested and used laser system in dentistry with mixed results. White et al.[72] reported that dentin modification by laser increased dentin microhardness, making it more resistant to acid demineralization (i.e., caries). As far as pulp safety is concerned, White et al. also reported that a histologic examination indicated this laser to be safe for the human pulp when used within limited parameters. However, our studies[54] show that the effect of Nd:YAG laser system on the pulp varies greatly depending on the remaining dentin thickness. For instance, using 100 mj/10 pps/10 sec, pulpal blood flow did not change significantly with lasing of the intact enamel. Blood flow increased moderately after lasing of a shallow cavity with a remaining dentin thickness of 1 mm and was irreversibly altered at high energy levels (Fig. 15-19). The pulse per second rate also seems to play an important role. Similarly, when the laser is applied to one area for more than 10 seconds, significant structural damage is caused (Fig. 15-20). When lasing an area just longer than 15 seconds, a crater resulted almost exposing the pulp (Fig. 15-21). These findings suggest that Nd:YAG laser may have certain beneficial effects on the dentin but not on the pulp. Identifying an energy level at a given dentin thickness that provides the desired effects on the dentin for operative dentistry without harming the pulp would be an important step in laser research.

Lasers for Hypersensitive Teeth

Since lasing alters the dentin surface, including blocking of dentin tubules by melted and glazing dentin, some advocate lasing of the hypersensitive dentin as the means of curing the disorder. Pashley's dentin permeability study showed that lasing the dentin surface using carbon dioxide and Nd:YAG systems did not provide sufficient blocking of the dentin tubules. However, our research shows that the Nd:YAG system provides transient anesthesia in cat teeth up to 5 hours as measured with a sensory nerve recording technique. Thus, we feel that successful results obtained in managing hypersensitive teeth using the various laser systems may be due to either permanently damaged sensory nerves or transient anesthesia as observed with the Nd:YAG laser. Our clinical studies indicate that lasing the hypersensitive dentin does not cause pain but desensitizes the tooth only temporarily, with a more severe re-

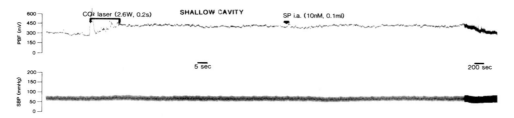

FIG. 15-18 Effect of carbon dioxide lasing on a cat canine pulp blood flow measured with laser Doppler flowmetry. Lasing at 2.6 W/0.2 ms/15 sec caused a 50% flow increase. There was no change in systemic blood pressure or flow response to intraarterial substance P injection, which was used to test vascular reactivity.

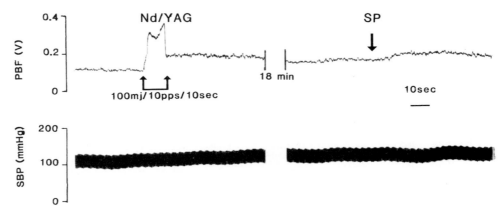

FIG. 15-19 Effect of Nd:YAG lasing on cat canine pulp blood flow measured with laser Doppler flowmetry. Lasing at 100 mj/10 pps/10 sec caused a moderate increase in flow, whereas intraarterial substance P injection caused a slight increase, indicating vascular reactivity after lasing.

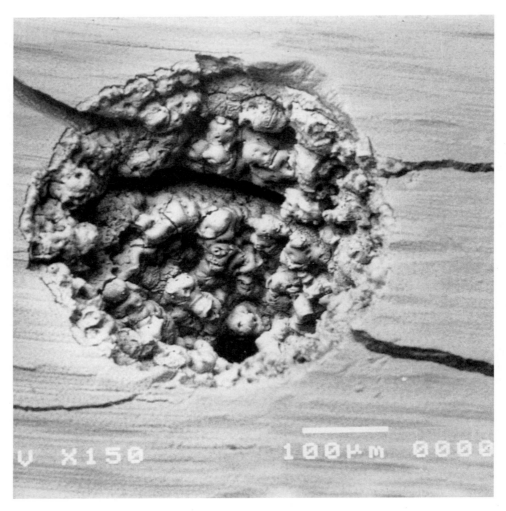

FIG. 15-20 Lasing at 30 mj/10 pps/10 sec at one spot of an extracted human tooth dental surface by Nd:YAG laser. Ablation and melting of the dentin at the irradiated area are found.

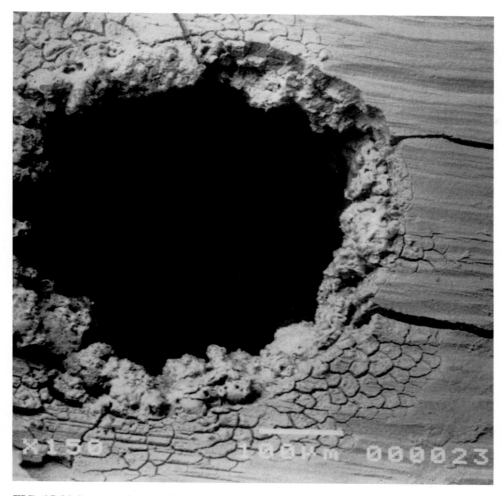

FIG. 15-21 Same tooth as in Fig. 5-20 at the same energy level but at a different site for 30 seconds. Complete removal of the dentin causing a hole connecting to the pulp.

turn of the sensitivity after a short period. Thus, at present the use of lasers for hypersensitive teeth has no biologic basis or benefit.

POSTOPERATIVE SENSITIVITY

Although postoperative discomfort is usually transient, it indicates that the restorative procedure has inflicted trauma on the tooth or the supporting structures. Severe persistent pain almost certainly signifies that pulpal inflammation has resulted in hyperalgesia. Researchers[55] examined 40 patients who had received dental treatment involving insertion of amalgam and composite restorations. They found that 78% of the patients experienced some degree of postoperative discomfort. Sensitivity to cold was the most frequent complaint, whereas sensitivity to heat occurred much less often. Another study[26] found there was a positive correlation between heat sensitivity and pulpal inflammation. The significance of sensitivity to cold has not been fully established. Since the response occurs very soon after stimuli such as ice, cold water, and cold air come into contact with the tooth, it is believed that pain is caused by the stimulation of sensory nerve fibers of the pulp by hydrodynamic forces.[68] Because these fibers have a relatively low excitability threshold, they respond to low-level stimuli that do not necessarily produce tissue injury. However, the presence

of hyperalgesia associated with inflammation produces an exaggerated response to cold. Sensitivity that develops soon after a restoration is placed may also be due to poor marginal adaptation, resulting in leakage of saliva under the filling.

Mechanisms and Management of Hypersensitive Teeth

Tooth sensitivity to various stimuli is a persisting problem that affects as many as one of seven adult dental patients.[20] Although the clinical features of tooth hypersensitivity are well described, the exact causes and their physiologic mechanisms are only beginning to be understood.

Mechanisms

The enamel and cementum covering the dentin, and thus the dentinal nerves, are protective layers. When these protective layers are removed and the dentin tubules are exposed by various means (e.g., scaling, caries, fracture, restorative procedures), the teeth often become hypersensitive. Dentin sensitivity is the result of activation of Aδ type nerve fibers located in the dentinal tubules. Hypersensitivity is characterized as sharp, transient, and well localized. Two mechanisms account for the pain, stimulation of the dentinal *nerves* and dynamics of *exposed dentin*. These two mechanisms are interrelated.

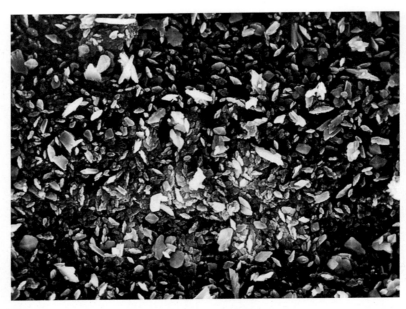

FIG. 15-22 Smear layer treated with 30% dipotassium oxalate for 2 minutes plus 3% monopotassium-monohydrogen oxalate for 2 minutes. Dentin surface is completely covered with calcium oxalate crystals. Original magnification ×1900. *(From Pashley DH, Galloway SE: Arch Oral Biol 30:731, 1985.)*

According to the hydrodynamic theory, dentin sensitivity should be proportional to the hydraulic conductance of dentin. According to Pashley[45] the most important variable related to hydraulic conductance in dentin is the condition of the tubule aperture. Anything, or any agent, that makes the dentin hypoconducting by blocking the aperture alleviates the hypersensitive teeth syndrome.

Another mechanism involves the intradental nerves. Although the nerves themselves are unaffected, the environment surrounding them might be changed so that the normal stimuli, which under normal conditions do not evoke sensation, now evoke the sensation. The causes in the environment may be due to changes in ionic concentration (e.g., excessive sodium or potassium around the nerve terminals in the tubules as the result of pulpal inflammation or exposed dentin).

Hypersensitive teeth and inflamed pulps in many ways present the same symptoms, such as sensitivity to cold, air, and heat. Hypersensitivity due to inflammation of the pulp is the result of excitation of C fibers, which release neuropeptides (e.g., CGRP and substance P) in the pulp. These neuropeptides play a key role in neurogenic inflammation by increasing blood flow and capillary permeability. In the dental pulp in its low-compliance environment the increase in flow and permeability causes a dramatic increase in tissue pressure, which can lower the excitatory threshold level of the intradental nerves, resulting in hypersensitivity.

Agents that block exposed dentinal tubules

As previously discussed, one of the two possible causes of hypersensitive teeth is exposed dentin. To block the exposed tubules would be a simple solution, but finding agents or instruments to do just that has turned out to be not that simple. After many years of experimentation we still do not have an agent or agents that completely block the tubules. Nevertheless, there has been substantial progress in discovering an agent

that blocks dentinal tubules sufficiently to reduce hypersensitivity. Using dentin permeability techniques and scanning electron microscopic examination of the dentin surface, Pashley[45] discovered that oxalate salts are effective agents to block dentinal tubules. Fig. 15-22 shows a dentin surface that was treated with oxalate salts for 2 minutes. When applied to the exposed dentin, potassium oxalate solution forms a microcrystal consisting of calcium oxalate. The calcium oxalate crystals are small enough to block the tubules and thus reduce hydraulic conductance. According to Pashley[45] the oxalate salts reduced dentin permeability by more than 95%. Results of the clinical studies also agree with experimental results.

Agents that reduce intradental nerve excitability

The electrophysiologic method has been used to assess the function of the sensory nerves in response to various potentially useful chemical agents.[32] Sodium, lithium, and aluminum compounds have insignificant effects on reducing sensory nerve activity. Potassium compounds, however, were most effective ingredients for sensory nerve activity reduction. Important potassium compounds were potassium oxalate, potassium nitrate, and potassium bicarbonate. This finding lends credence to the hypothesis that reduction in sensory nerve activity is caused by the increase in potassium concentration around the nerve terminals in the dentinal tubules.

Fig. 15-23 provides the summary diagram illustrating the mechanisms and solutions to these problems. The far left-hand slice represents the sensitive dentin with open tubules. The second slice represents a smear layer covering the exposed dentin surface and occluding the dentinal tubules. However, this smear layer is extremely acid fabrile and is easily removed; therefore it cannot be considered an effective way of managing the problem. The third slice represents other ways of occluding the dentinal tubules. Calcium oxalate is the crystalized product of the chemical reaction between potassium oxalate

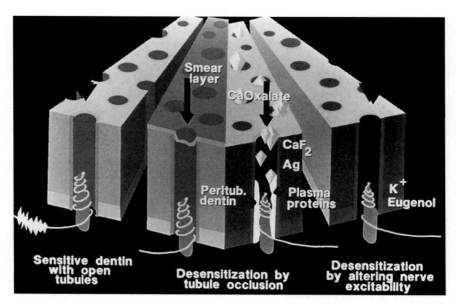

FIG. 15-23 Summary diagram illustrates the mechanisms and solutions to hypersensitivity problems. *(Courtesy Dr. D.H. Pashley, Medical College of Georgia, Augusta, Ga.)*

and dentinal calcium, and is very effective in occluding the tubules. Calcium fluoride and silver nitrate are other agents that showed reasonable effectiveness. Tubular occlusion can also occur from the pulp side, mainly by plasma protein, especially fibrinogen, which is released from blood vessels.[46] The right-hand slice represents desensitization by altering nerve excitability by potassium and possibly by eugenol.

CURRENT THINKING ON THE CAUSE OF PULPAL REACTION TO RESTORATION

In the past, pulp reactions to dental procedures were thought to be due to mechanical insults, such as frictional heat, and generally this is true. The reaction to dental materials, on the other hand, has been attributed to chemical effects, such as acidity of the restorative materials. Although the chemical effects cannot be entirely discounted, especially in a deep cavity where only a very thin layer of dentin remains, in current thinking *pulpal injury is primarily due to microleakage through gaps between the filling material and the walls of the cavity.* It is believed that bacteria growing in these gaps elaborate products that diffuse through the dentinal tubules and irritate the pulp. It must be recognized that *all* permanent filling materials may allow these gaps to form. It is a miracle that all restored teeth do not show some degree of pulpal inflammation. On the other hand, it is not surprising that many teeth that have been restored require endodontic therapy. One study[4] reported that the quantity of bacterial toxins filtered from the base of a class V cavity depends on the type of restorative material used. The greatest amount of leakage occurred with silicate cements, followed by composite resins and amalgam fillings. Little or no leakage occurred when ZOE was used. Even full crown restorations have been found to leak.

It is impossible to examine pulpal reactions without understanding structural and functional properties of the dentin. Pulp reactions begin when irritants make contact with the surface of the dentin. As the dentin's thickness decreases, the danger of pulpal reaction increases dramatically. A simple physiologic law of diffusion states that the rate of diffusion of substances depends on two factors: (1) the concentration gradient of the substances and (2) the surface area available for diffusion. Of importance in determining the extent of pulp reactions is the surface area of dentin available for diffusion. Because the dentinal tubules vary in diameter and density across the thickness of the dentin, the surface area (i.e., product of tubular area and density) available for diffusion varies from one region of the dentin to the other. Table 15-1 demonstrates the available dentin surface for diffusion at various distances from the pulp. For example, the diffusible surface area is 1% of the total dentin surface area at the dentinoenamel junction, whereas it is 22% at the pulp. Thus the harmful effects of an insult increase significantly as the thickness of dentin over the pulp decreases.

The natural defense mechanisms of the tooth should be recognized. In some situations the dentinal tubules may become blocked by hydroxyapatite and other crystals, a condition known as dentinal sclerosis. Another reaction resulting in a decrease in dentin permeability is reparative dentin formation.

The smear layer also influences the permeability of dentin and thus protects the pulp by hindering the diffusion of toxic substances through the tubules.[47] According to one investigation, the smear layer accounts for 86% of the total resistance to flow fluid.[44] Thus acid etching, which removes the smear layer, greatly increases permeability by increasing the diffusible surface area (Fig. 15-24). The question arises of what to do with the smear layer. Should it be removed or left alone? Some authorities are of the opinion that it should be removed, since the smear layer may harbor bacteria. Yet the presence of a smear layer constitutes a physical barrier to bacterial penetration of the dentinal tubules.[36] However, another investigator demonstrated that the presence of the smear layer cannot prevent diffusion of bacterial products, although it effectively blocks actual bacterial invasion.[2] It has been shown that bacterial products reaching the pulp are capable of evoking an inflammatory response.[3] It follows that the best way to solve the problem is to remove the smear layer and replace it with a

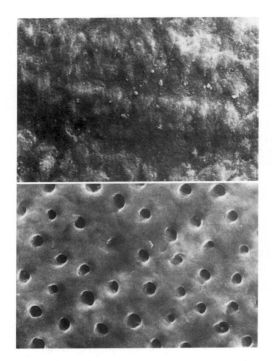

FIG. 15-24 Scanning electron microscopic photomicrographs of smear layer intact and smear layer removed. Notice the patent dentinal tubules. *(Courtesy Dr. D.H. Pashley, Medical College of Georgia, Augusta, Ga.)*

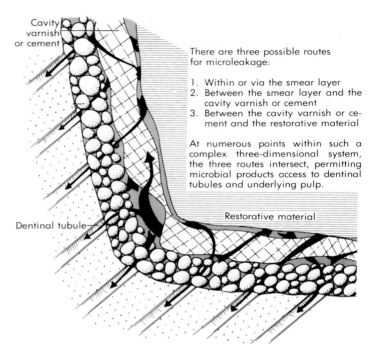

There are three possible routes for microleakage:

1. Within or via the smear layer
2. Between the smear layer and the cavity varnish or cement
3. Between the cavity varnish or cement and the restorative material

At numerous points within such a complex three-dimensional system, the three routes intersect, permitting microbial products access to dentinal tubules and underlying pulp.

FIG. 15-25 Schematic representation of the interface of dentin and restorative material in a typical cavity. Granular constituents of the smear layer have been exaggerated out of their normal proportion for emphasis. Three theoretical routes for microleakage are indicated by arrows. *(Reprinted with permission from Pashley DH et al: Arch Oral Biol 23:391, 1978. Copyright 1978, Pergamon Press, Ltd.)*

Table 15-1. Surface area of dentin available for diffusion at various distances from the pulp

Distance from Pulp	Number of Tubules (million/cm^2)		Tubular Radius (cm $\times$ 10^4)		Area of Surface (Ap) (%)*	
(mm)	Mean	Range	Mean	Range	Mean	Range
	4.5	3.0-5.2	1.25	2.0-3.2	22.1	9-42
0.1-0.5	4.3	2.2-5.9	0.95	1.0-2.3	12.2	2-25
0.6-1.0	3.8	1.6-4.7	0.80	1.0-1.6	7.6	1-9.0
1.1-1.5	3.5	2.1-4.7	0.60	0.9-1.5	4.0	1-8.0
1.6-2.0	3.0	1.2-4.7	0.55	0.8-1.6	2.9	1-9.0
2.1-2.5	2.3	1.1-3.6	0.45	0.6-1.3	1.5	0.3-6
2.6-3.0	2.0	0.7-4.0	0.40	0.5-1.4	1.1	0.1-6
3.1-3.5	1.9	1.0-2.5	0.40	0.5-1.2	1.0	0.2-3

Modified from Garberoglio and Brännström (1976); from Pashley DH: *Operative Dent* 3(suppl):13, 1984.
*$Ap = nr^2$, where n is the number of tubules/cm^2; Ap represents the percentage of the total area of the physical surface available for diffusion.

"sterile, nontoxic" artificial smear layer. Research in the field has yielded some agents that look promising, two of which are potassium oxalate and 5% ferric oxalate.[6]

Since at the present time there is no material that can bond chemically to dentin and thus prevent leakage, the use of a cavity liner to seal dentin is highly recommended. According to one investigator, there are three possible routes for microleakage: (1) within or via the smear layer, (2) between the smear layer and the cavity varnish or cement, and (3) between the cavity varnish or cement and the restorative material (Fig. 15-25).[44]

Compensatory Pulpal Reaction to Outside Insults

Mechanisms exist by which the pulp is able to ward off insults. The ability of the pulp to deposit reparative dentin beneath a restoration is an excellent example. In addition, the vascular system is able to respond to mechanical insults. For example, it has been shown that deep drilling without proper water coolant causes a profound decrease in pulpal blood flow in the area of injury. Blood is shunted away from the area by an abrupt increase in the flow of blood through arteriovenous anastomoses (AVAs) or U-turn loops located in the dental pulp

Pulpal reaction to caries and dental procedures **549**

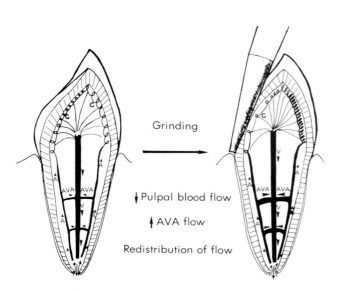

FIG. 15-26 Schematic representation of the changes in pulpal blood flow distribution in response to dry preparation. Notice there is an increase in flow through the arteriovenous anastomoses.

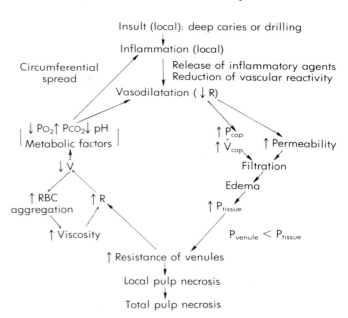

FIG. 15-27 Pathophysiologic mechanism of pulp inflammation and necrosis. This hypothetical mechanism is constructed from the results of many structural and functional investigations.

(Fig. 15-26). It is possible that opening of the previously closed AVAs occurs as pulpal tissue pressure increases to critical levels. The opening of the AVAs is a compensatory mechanism of the pulp to maintain blood flow within physiologically normal limits (see Fig. 15-26).

It should be remembered that the pulp is a very resilient tissue and that it has a great potential for healing. It is only when all compensatory mechanisms fail that the pulp becomes necrotic. Fig. 15-27 depicts the current thinking on the pathophysiologic mechanisms involved in pulp necrosis. Since the pulp is rigidly encased in mineralized tissues, it is protected from most forms of trauma to which the tooth is exposed. Nevertheless, insults such as dental caries and restorative procedures are capable of producing localized inflammatory lesions in the pulp. The tissue adjacent to the inflammatory lesion may show no sign of inflammation, and physiologic analysis may reveal no abnormalities. Thus investigators found that pulpal tissue pressure near a site of localized inflammation was almost normal.[64] This indicates that tissue pressure changes do not spread rapidly. Similar findings have been reported by another researcher.[70] Local insults cause inflammation by triggering the release of various inflammatory mediators and reducing vascular reactivity. These mediators produce vasodilation and decrease the flow resistance in the resistance vessels. Vasodilation and decreased flow resistance cause an increase in both intravascular pressure and blood flow in the capillaries, which in turn precipitate an increase in vascular permeability, favoring filtration of serum proteins and fluid from the vessels. As a result, the tissue becomes edematous. This results in an increase in the tissue pressure. Since the pulp is encased in mineralized tissue, it is in a low-compliance environment. As the tissue pressure increases, it may exceed that of the venules, in which case the venules are compressed, thus producing an increase in flow resistance. This in turn results in a decrease in blood flow,

since the venous drainage is impeded. The sluggish blood flow causes the red blood cells to aggregate, resulting in an elevation of blood viscosity. This vicious cycle leads to even greater problems by producing hypoxia and thus suppressing cellular metabolism in the affected area of the pulp. The stagnation of blood flow not only causes rheologic changes (i.e., red blood cell aggregation and increased blood viscosity), it also causes an increase in carbon dioxide and a decrease in pH levels in the blood. The increase in P_{CO_2} results from impaired removal of waste products from the tissue. These changes in local metabolism lead to vasodilation in the adjacent area and the gradual spread of inflammation. The spread of inflammation is circumferential as was demonstrated in an elegant experiment by Van Hassel.[70] Thus total pulp necrosis is the gradual accumulation of local necroses.

It has been shown that the pulp has tremendous healing potential. This raises the question as to how the pulp recovers from the adverse effects of localized inflammation. Although the exact physiologic mechanisms are not yet known, recent research findings suggest the following. First, as the tissue pressure increases as a result of an increase in blood flow, the AVAs or the U-turn loop vessels open and shunt the blood before it reaches the inflamed region of the coronal pulp. This prevents a further increase in blood flow and tissue pressure. Also the increase in tissue pressure pushes macromolecules back into the bloodstream via the venules in the adjacent healthy region (Fig. 15-28). Once the macromolecules and accompanying fluid leave the extracellular tissue space through the venule, the tissue pressure decreases and normal blood flow is restored.

Prevention

To preserve the integrity of the pulp, the dentist should observe certain precautions while rendering treatment. The fol-

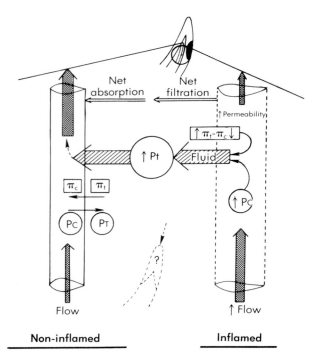

FIG. 15-28 Schematic representation of the compensatory mechanism of the pulp during inflammation. P_C and P_T, hydrostatic pressure of capillary and tissue, respectively; π_c and π_t, osmotic pressure of capillary and tissue, respectively.

lowing is a list of *do's* and *dont's* that should prevent or minimize injury to the pulp:

- Cutting procedures: Use light, intermittent cutting, an efficient cooling system, and high speeds of rotation.
- Avoid desiccating the dentin: Do not overdry the cavity preparation.
- Do not apply irritating chemicals to freshly cut dentin.
- Choose restorative materials carefully, considering the physical and biologic properties of the material.
- Do not use caustic cavity sterilizing agents.
- Assume that all restorative materials will leak: Use a cavity liner or base to seal the openings of exposed dentinal tubules.
- Do not use excessive force when inserting a restoration.
- Employ polishing procedures that do not subject the pulp to excessive heat.
- Establish a patient recall system that ensures periodic evaluation of the status of pulps that have been exposed to injury.

REFERENCES

1. Alperstein KS, Graver HT, Herold RCB: Marginal leakage of glass-ionomer cement restorations, *J Prosthet Dent* 50:803, 1983.
2. Bergenholtz G: Effect of bacterial products on inflammatory reactions in the dental pulp, *Scand J Dent Res* 85:122, 1977.
3. Bergenholtz G, Reit C: Reactions of the dental pulp to microbial provocation of calcium hydroxide treated dentin, *Scand J Dent Res* 88:187, 1980.
4. Bergenholtz G et al: Bacterial leakage around dental restorations: its effect on the dental pulp, *J Oral Pathol* 11:439, 1982.
5. Berggren H: The reaction of the translucent zone to dyes and radio-isotopes, *Acta Odontol Scand* 23:197, 1965.
6. Bowen RL, Cobb EN, Rapson JE: Adhesive bonding of various materials to hard tooth tissues: improvement in bond strength to dentin, *J Dent Res* 61:1070, 1982.
7. Brännström M: A new approach to insulation, *Dent Pract* 19:417, 1969.
8. Brännström M: *Dentin and pulp in restorative dentistry,* London, 1982, Wolfe Medical Publications Ltd.
9. Brännström M: Communication between the oral cavity and the dental pulp associated with restorative treatment, *Operative Dent* 9:57, 1984.
10. Brännström M, Lind PO: Pulpal response to early dental caries, *J Dent Res* 44:1045, 1965.
11. Brännström M, Vojinovic O, Nordenvall KJ: Bacterial and pulpal reactions under silicate cement restorations, *J Prosthet Dent* 41:290, 1979.
12. Brännström M et al: Protective effect of polystyrene liners for composite resin restorations, *J Prosthet Dent* 49:331, 1983.
13. Brown WS, Christensen DO, Lloyd BA: Numerical and experimental evaluation of energy inputs, temperature gradients, and thermal stresses during restorative procedures, *J Am Dent Assoc* 96:451, 1978.
14. Chiego DJ Jr, Wang RF, Avery JK: Ultrastructural changes in odontoblasts and nerve terminals after cavity preparations, *J Dent Res* 68(special issue):1023, 1989 (abstract 1251).
15. Cox CF et al: Biocompatibility of various surface-sealed dental materials against exposed pulps, *J Prosthet Dent* 57:1, 1987.
16. Felton D: Long term effects of crown preparation on pulp vitality, *J Dent Res* 68(special issue):1009, 1989 (abstract 1139).
17. Featherstone J, Nelson D: Laser effects on dental hard tissue, *Adv Dent Res* 1:21-26, 1987.
18. Frank RM: Reactions of dentin and pulp to drugs and restorative materials, *J Dent Res* 54:176, 1975.
19. Friedman S, Liu M, Dörscher-Kim J, Kim S: In-situ testing of CO_2 laser on dental pulp function: the effects on microcirculation, *Lasers Surg Med* 11:325-330, 1991.
20. Graf H, Galasse R: Mobidity, prevalence and intraoral distribution of hypersensitive teeth, *J Dent Res* 162(special issue A):2, 1977.
21. Graver T, Trowbridge H, Alperstein K: Microleakage of castings cemented with glass ionomer cements, *Operative Dent* 15(1):2-9, 1990.
22. Heys DR et al: Histologic and bacterial evaluation of conventional and new copper amalgams, *J Oral Pathol* 8:65, 1979.
23. Holden GP: Some observations on the vibratory phenomena associated with high-speed air turbines and their transmission to living tissue, *Br Dent J* 113:265, 1962.
24. Jendresen M, Trowbridge H: Biologic and physical properties of a zinc polycarboxylate cement, *J Prosthet Dent* 28:264, 1972.
25. Johnson NW, Taylor BR, Berman DS: The response of deciduous dentine to caries studied by correlated light and electron microscopy, *Caries Res* 3:348, 1969.
26. Johnson RH, Daichi SF, Haley JV: Pulpal hyperemia: a correlation of clinical and histological data from 706 teeth, *J Am Dent Assoc* 81:108, 1970.
27. Kakehashi S, Stanley HR, Fitzgerald RJ: The effects of surgical exposures of pulps in germ-free and conventional rats, *Oral Surg* 20:340, 1965.
28. Karkalainen S, LeBell Y: Odontoblast response to caries. In Thylstrup A, Leach SA, Qvist V, editors: *Dentine and dentine reactions in the oral cavity,* Oxford, 1987, IRL Press.
29. Kawahara H, Imanishi Y, Oshima H: Biological evaluation of glass ionomer cement, *J Dent Res* 58:1080, 1979.
30. Kelley KW, Bergenholtz G, Cox CF: The extent of the odontoblast process in rhesus monkeys *(Macaca mulatta)* as observed by scanning electron microscopy, *Arch Oral Biol* 26:893, 1981.
31. Kim S: Ligamental injection: a physiological explanation of its efficacy, *J Endod* 12:486, 1986.
32. Kim S: Hypersensitive teeth: desensitization of pulpal sensory nerves, *J Endod* 12:482, 1986.

33. Kim S et al: Effects of local anesthetics on pulpal blood flow in dogs, *J Dent Res* 63:650, 1984.

34. Magloire H et al: Ultrastructural alterations of human odontoblasts and collagen fibers in the pulpal border zone beneath early caries lesions, *Cell Molec Biol* 27:437, 1981.

35. Massler M: Pulpal reaction to dentinal caries, *J Dent Res* 17:441, 1967.

36. Michelich VJ, Schuster GS, Pashley DH: Bacterial penetration of human dentin in vitro, *J Dent REs* 59:1398, 1980.

37. Mullaney TP, Laswell HR: Iatrogenic blushing of dentin following full crown preparation, *J Prosthet Dent* 22:354, 1969.

38. Nelson RJ, Wolcott RB, Paffenbarger GC: Fluid exchange at the margins of dental restorations, *J Am Dent Assoc* 44:288, 1952.

39. Newman SM: Microleakage of a copal rosin cavity varnish, *J Prosthet Dent* 51:499, 1984.

40. Nyborg H, Brännström M: Pulp reaction to heat, *J Prosthet Dent* 19:605, 1968.

41. Okamura K et al: Dentinal response against carious invasion: localization of antibodies in odontoblastic body and process, *J Dent Res* 59:1368, 1980.

42. Olgart L, Gazalius B: Effects of adrenaline and felypressin (Octapressin) on blood flow and sensory nerve activity on the tooth, *Acta Odontol Scand* 35:69, 1977.

43. Pashley DH: The influence of dentin permeability and pulpal blood flow on pulpal solute concentrations, *J Endod* 5:355, 1979.

44. Pashley DH: Smear layer: physiological consideration, *Operative Dent* 3:13, 1984.

45. Pashley DH: Dentin permeability, dentin sensitivity and treatment through tubule occlusion, *J Endod* 12:465, 1986.

46. Pashley DH, Galloway SE, Stewart F: Effects of fibrinogen in vivo on dentin permeability in the dog, *Arch Oral Biol* 29:725, 1984.

47. Pashley DH, Michelich V, Kehl T: Dentin permeability: effects of smear layer removal, *J Prosthet Dent* 46:531, 1981.

48. Plant CG, Jones DW: The damaging effects of restorative materials. I. Physical and chemical properties, *Br Dent J* 140:373, 1976.

49. Pogrel M, Muff D, Marshall G: Structural changes in dental enamel induced by high energy continuous wave carbon dioxide laser, *Lasers Surg Med* 13:89-96, 1993.

50. Pohto M, Scheinin A: Microscopic observations on living dental pulp. IV. The effects of oil of clove and eugenol on the circulation of the pulp in the rat's lower incisor, *Dent Abstr* 5:405, 1960.

51. Qvist V: The effect of mastication on marginal adaptation of composite restorations in vivo, *J Dent Res* 62:904, 1983.

52. Reeves R, Stanley HR: The relationship of bacterial penetration and pulpal pathosis in carious teeth, *Oral Surg* 22:59, 1966.

53. Scott JN, Weber DF: Microscopy of the junctional region between human coronal primary and secondary dentin, *J Morphol* 154:133, 1977.

54. Shamul J: *Effects of pulsed Nd:YAG laser on pulpal blood flow in cat teeth,* Master of Arts Degree, Oral Biology Thesis, Columbia University, New York, 1992.

55. Silvestri AR, Cohen SN, Wetz JH: Character and frequency of discomfort immediately following restorative procedures, *J Am Dent Assoc* 95:85, 1977.

56. Sneed WD, Hembree JH, Welsh EL: Effectiveness of three varnishes in reducing leakage of a high-copper amalgam, *Operative Dent* 9:32, 1984.

57. Son HG, Kim S, Kim SB: Pulpal blood flow and bonding, *IADR* Abstract for The Hague Meeting, 1986.

58. Stanley HR: Pulpal response. In Cohen S, Burns R, editors: *Pathways of the pulp,* ed 3, St Louis, 1984, Mosby.

59. Stanley HR, Going RE, Chauncey HH: Human pulp response to acid pretreatment of dentin and to composite restoration, *J Am Dent Assoc* 91:817, 1975.

60. Stanley HR et al: The detection and prevalence of reactive and physiologic sclerotic dentin, reparative dentin and dead tracts beneath various types of dental lesions according to tooth surface and age, *J Pathol* 12:257, 1983.

61. Swerdlow H, Stanley HR: Reaction of human dental pulp to cavity preparation. I. Effect of water spray at 20,000 rpm, *J Am Dent Assoc* 56:317, 1958.

62. Swerdlow H, Stanley HR: Reaction of human dental pulp to cavity preparation, *J Prosthet Dent* 9:121, 1959.

63. Taylor PE, Byers MR, Redd PE: Sprouting of CGRP nerve fibers in response to dentin injury in rat molars, *Brain Res* 461:371, 1988.

64. Tönder K, Kvinnsland I: Micropuncture measurement of interstitial tissue pressure in normal and inflamed dental pulp in cats, *J Endod* 9:105, 1983.

65. Trowbridge HO: Pathogenesis of pulpitis resulting from dental caries, *J Endod* 7:52, 1981.

66. Trowbridge HO, Edwall L, Panopoulos P: Effect of zinc oxide–eugenol and calcium hydroxide on intradental nerve activity, *J Endod* 8:403, 1982.

67. Trowbridge H, Scott D, Singer J: Effects of eugenol on nerve excitability, IADR Prog Abstr 56:115, 1977.

68. Trowbridge HO et al: Sensory response to thermal stimulation in human teeth, *J Endod* 6:405, 1980.

69. Turner DF, Marfurt CF, Sattleberg C: Demonstration of physiological barrier between pulpal odontoblasts and its perturbation following routine restorative procedures: horseradish peroxidase tracing study in the rat, *J Dent Res* 68:1261, 1989.

70. Van Hassel HJ: Physiology of the human dental pulp. In Siskin M, editor: *The biology of the human dental pulp,* St Louis, 1973, Mosby.

71. Watts A: Bacterial contamination and toxicity of silicate and zinc phosphate cements, *Br Dent J* 146:7, 1979.

72. White J, Goodis H, Daniel T: Effects of Nd:YAG cases on pulps of extracted teeth, *Lasers Life Sci* 4:191-200, 1991.

73. Zach L: Pulp liability and repair: effect of restorative procedures, *Oral Surg* 33:111, 1972.

PART THREE

RELATED CLINICAL TOPICS

Chapter 16

Traumatic Injuries

Martin Trope
Noah Chivian
Asgeir Sigurdsson

INCIDENCE

Although dental injuries occur at any age, they most commonly affect the permanent teeth at the very active age range of 8 to 12 years old, mostly as a result of bicycle, skateboard, playground, or sports accidents.[18,113,122]

By the time students complete high school it is estimated that as many as one out of three boys and one out of four girls will have suffered a dental injury.[122] This seemingly high incidence of injuries to the permanent teeth is the result of the collective activities of young people throughout their school years. A fourth of the dental injuries in the public schools have been observed to be due to fighting and pushing.[44,54,102] During high school the increased participation of boys and girls in sports increases the risk of injury.

Before the 1960s boys had three times as many injuries as girls. The rapid increase in women's athletics during the 1970s has reduced this ratio, however, to one and one half injuries to boys for each injury to girls.[79,164]

The most vulnerable tooth is the maxillary central incisor, which sustains approximately 80% of dental injuries, followed by the maxillary lateral and the mandibular central and lateral incisors.[78,79,162]

HISTORY AND CLINICAL EXAMINATION

Dental injuries are never convenient for either the patient or the clinician. Consequently, the emergency visit often consists of a distraught patient or parent, or both, meeting a hurried clinician. It is one of the challenges that face clinicians to

---

Revision of this chapter is based in part on original material by Stuart B. Fountain and Joe H. Camp.

control the scene, calm the patient and parents, and take the necessary time to conduct a qualitative evaluation of the patient's injuries. Without such control by the clinician, significant injuries can be easily missed in the haste of the moment.

The medical history (Fig. 1-1) must be completed before all other evaluation and treatment of the patient.

History of the Accident

The *when, how,* and *where* of the accident[14]

When the accident occurred is most important. With the passage of time blood clots begin to form, periodontal ligaments of teeth dry out, saliva contaminates the wound, and all these become factors in making decisions about the sequence of treatment.

Understanding *how* the accident occurred assists the clinician in locating specific injuries. A blow to the lips and anterior teeth could possibly cause crown, root, or bone fractures to the anterior region and is less likely to injure the posterior regions. A blow under the chin or jaw could cause fractures to any tooth in the mouth. A padded blow (e.g., fall against a covered chair arm) could cause a root fracture or tooth displacement, whereas a hard blow (concrete walk) tends to cause coronal fractures.

Where the trauma occurred becomes significant for prognosis. The necessity for prophylactic tetanus toxoid is influenced by the location of the accident. Where the trauma occurred may also be significant because of insurance and possible litigation.

Another important question to ask is whether treatment, of any kind, has been given for this injury by a parent, coach, physician, school nurse, teacher, or ambulance attendant. A normal-appearing tooth may have been replanted or repositioned previously by any of these or by the patient himself, and this influences the prognosis for treatment and sequence of treatment.

Clinical Examination

Chief complaint

Aside from pain and bleeding, there may be a specific complaint that assists in the diagnosis. If the complaint is that the teeth "don't fit together now," the clinician must consider possible displacements or a bone fracture. Pain that occurs *only* when the patient closes the teeth together could indicate crown, root, or bone fractures or displacement.

Neurologic examination

While obtaining the history of the accident and chief complaint, the clinician should observe the patient for neurologic or other medical complications[32] (see Box 16-1). Dental injuries may occur simultaneously with other head and neck injuries. Note should be made of whether the patient is communicating coherently. Does the patient have difficulty focusing or rotating the eyes or breathing?

Can the patient turn the head from side to side? Is there any paresthesia of the lips or tongue? Does the patient complain of ringing in the ears? Have there been persistent headaches, dizziness, drowsiness, or vomiting since the accident? Airway obstruction by dental appliances must be considered.

Before analgesics are prescribed or sedation by inhalation of nitrous oxide or oxygen is used, the clinician must be satisfied that there are no neurologic injuries.[32,83] If there is any question about this, the patient should be referred immediately for appropriate medical treatment.

External examination

Before having the patient open his or her mouth for an intraoral examination, the clinician should first look for external signs of injury. Lacerations of the head and neck are easily detected. However, deviations of normal bone contours must be closely investigated. The temporomandibular joint should be palpated externally while the patient opens and closes the mouth. Does the patient's opening and closing pattern deviate to either side? If so, this could indicate a unilateral mandibular fracture. Similarly, the zygomatic arch, angle, and lower border of the mandible should be bilaterally palpated and note made of any areas of tenderness, swelling, or bruising of the face, cheek, neck, or lips. They could be clues to possible bone fractures.

Intraoral soft tissue examination

One next looks for lacerations of the lips, tongue, cheek, palate, and floor of the mouth. The facial and lingual gingivae and oral mucosae are palpated, with note made of areas of tenderness, swelling, or bruising. The anterior border of the ramus of the mandible is palpated. Any abnormal findings suggest possible tooth or bone injuries, and further radiographic examination of the area is indicated. Lacerations of the lips and tongue must be felt and radiographed for embedded foreign objects.[27,71]

Hard tissue examination

One of the best examinations for evidence of traumatic injuries is simply to look carefully. Each tooth and its supporting structures must be examined with an explorer and periodontal probe. Whether the occlusal plane has been disturbed and whether any teeth are missing must be determined before any thermal or electrical tests are begun.

The examiner looks for gross evidence of injury initially. If several teeth are out of alignment, a bone fracture is the most reasonable explanation. The mandible should be examined for fractures by placing the forefinger on the occlusal plane of the posterior teeth with the thumbs under the mandible and then rocking the mandible from side to side and from an anterior to a posterior direction. A mandibular fracture causes discomfort with these motions, and the grating sound of broken fragments may be heard.[27] Gentle but firm pressure should be used to prevent possible additional trauma to the inferior alveolar nerve and blood vessels.

Also one can try to move the individual teeth with finger

BOX 16-1.
OUTLINE OF INITIAL NEUROLOGIC ASSESSMENT FOR THE PATIENT WITH TRAUMATIC DENTAL INJURIES

Notice unusual communication or motor functions.
Look for normal respiration without obstruction of the airway or danger of aspiration.
Replant avulsed teeth as indicated.
Obtain a medical history and information on the accident.
Determine blood pressure and pulse.
Examine for rhinorrhea or otorrhea.
Evaluate function of the eyes—Is diplopia or nystagmus apparent? Are pupillary activity and movement of the eyes normal?
Evaluate movement of the neck—Is there pain or limitation?
Examine the sensitivity of the surface of the facial skin—Is paresthesia or anesthesia apparent?
Confirm that there is normal vocal function.
Confirm patient's ability to protrude the tongue.
Confirm hearing—Is tinnitus or vertigo apparent?
Evaluate the sense of smell.
Assure follow-up evaluation.

From Croll TP et al: *J Am Dent Assoc* 100:530, 1980.

pressure. Any looseness is indicative of displacement from the alveolar socket. Movement of several teeth together is evidence of an alveolar fracture. Mobility of the crown must be differentiated from the mobility of the tooth. In instances of coronal fractures the crown is mobile, but the tooth remains in position. Occasionally root fractures can be felt by placing a finger on the mucosa over the tooth and moving the crown.

Any freshly fractured cusps or incisal edge fractures should be recorded. Incomplete cusp fractures can be noted by using the tip of a dental explorer as a wedge in the occlusal grooves of the posterior teeth to elicit movement of any cusps. The patient may be asked to bite on a rubber polishing wheel with each tooth in succession to help locate tenderness that could mean an incomplete cusp fracture or displaced tooth.[30]

Each incisal edge and cusp can be gently percussed with the mirror handle to locate incomplete fractures or teeth that have been slightly displaced from the alveolar socket. Accumulation of extravasated fluid and tearing of periodontal fibers around a minimally displaced tooth makes the tooth tender to percussion.

Hemorrhage in the gingival sulcus may indicate a displaced tooth or tooth segment. Any discoloration of the teeth should be noted; viewing from the lingual surface of anterior teeth with a reflected light helps.

Obvious pulp exposures should be noted. Crown fractures with minute pulp exposures can be detected with a cotton pellet soaked in saline and pressed against the area of the suspected exposure.[14] The mechanical pressure of the cotton against an exposure elicits a response. A dry cotton pellet can confuse the diagnosis by dehydrating dentinal tubules in a near exposure, causing pain sensation, and should not be used.

When the visual examination is complete and all abnormal findings are noted, radiographs of the injured areas should be taken. These can be processed while additional tests are being conducted.

Thermal and electrical tests

The reader is referred to Chapter 1 for specific descriptions of pulp tests, but a few general statements in regard to pulp tests on traumatized teeth may be helpful in trying to interpret the results.

For decades controversy has surrounded the validity of thermal and electrical tests on traumatized teeth. Only generalized impressions may be gained from these tests subsequent to a traumatic injury. They are, in reality, sensitivity tests for nerve function and do *not* indicate the presence or absence of blood circulation within the pulp. It is assumed that subsequent to traumatic injury the conduction capability of the nerve endings or sensory receptors is sufficiently deranged to inhibit the nerve impulse from an electrical or thermal stimulus. This makes the traumatized tooth vulnerable to false-negative readings from these tests.

Teeth that give a positive response at the initial examination cannot be assumed to be healthy and continue to give a positive response. Teeth that yield a negative response or no response cannot be assumed to have necrotic pulps, because they may give a positive response later. It has been demonstrated that it may take as long as 9 months for normal blood flow to return to the coronal pulp of a traumatized fully formed tooth. As circulation is restored, the responsiveness to pulp tests returns.[55]

The transition from a negative to a positive response at a subsequent test may be considered a sign of a healthy pulp. The repetitious finding of positive responses may be taken as a sign of a healthy pulp. The transition from a positive to a negative response may be taken as an indication that the pulp is probably undergoing degeneration. The persistence of a negative response would suggest that the pulp has been irreversibly damaged, but even this is not absolute.[22]

In testing teeth for response to cold, the dry ice pencil (carbon dioxide stick described in Chapter 1) test of all teeth in the traumatized area should be performed at the time of the initial examination and carefully recorded to establish a baseline for comparison with subsequent repeated tests in later months. These tests should be repeated at 3 weeks, 3 months, 6 months, 12 months, and yearly intervals following the accident. The purpose of the tests is to establish a trend as to the physiologic status of the pulps of these teeth. Dry ice (which does not drip) gives more accurate responses than does a water ice pencil. The intense cold (172.4° F, −78° C) seems to penetrate the tooth and covering splints or restorations and reach the deeper areas of the tooth.

Radiographic examinations

Radiographs are essential to the thorough examination of traumatized hard tissue. They may reveal root fractures, subgingival crown fractures, tooth displacements, bone fractures, or foreign objects.

However, the fracture line may run in a mesiodistal direction in the tooth and not be evident on the radiograph. Also the fracture line may be diagonal in a faciolingual direction and not obvious on the film. Similarly, a hairline fracture may not be evident on the radiograph at the initial examination but later may become obvious as tissue fluids and mobility spread the broken parts.

In instances of soft tissue laceration it is advisable to radiograph the injured area before suturing to be sure that no foreign objects have been embedded. A soft tissue radiograph with a normal-sized film briefly exposed at a reduced kilovoltage should reveal the presence of many foreign substances, including tooth fragments.

In reviewing the films of traumatized teeth, special attention should be directed to the dimension of the root canal space, the degree of apical closure of the root, the proximity of fractures to the pulp, and the relationship of root fractures to the alveolar crest. Whereas conventional periapical films are generally useful, an occlusal or Panorex film can supplement them when the examiner is looking for bone fractures or the presence of foreign objects.

In summary, the examination of traumatic injuries must be thorough and meticulously recorded. When months or years after the accident the dentist is asked to describe the condition of the patient at the time of the initial examination, the dentist will find a completely documented patient record, including quality radiographs (and photographs, when possible), to be of immense assistance. These records form the basis for the justification of subsequent treatment. In addition, the rapid increase in professional liability claims against dentists further emphasizes the need for complete and accurate patient records (described in greater detail in Chapter 10).

CROWN INFRACTION

Definition: Incomplete fracture or crack of enamel without loss of tooth structure.[14]

Biologic Consequences

Cracks or fractures theoretically are "weak points" through which bacteria and their by-products can travel to challenge the pulp. However, in the vast majority of cases, the pulp, if vital after the initial injury, overcomes the challenge.

Crown infraction rarely occurs alone and can be a sign of a concomitant attachment injury (see Luxation Injuries). The force taken up by the attachment injury leaves only sufficient force to crack (and not fracture) the enamel.

Diagnosis and Clinical Presentation

Crack or craze lines can sometimes be seen with routine examination. However, indirect light or transillumination is of great value for their diagnosis.[14] A fiber-optic or resin-curing light is particularly useful (Fig. 16-1). In fact, indirect light and transillumination should be used routinely when examining all traumatic injuries, since these injuries often occur in teeth adjacent to those that have sustained more serious injuries.

Treatment

Treatment involves establishing a baseline pulp status with routine sensitivity testing.

Follow-Up

Schedule follow-up appointments at 3, 6, and 12 months and yearly thereafter.

Prognosis

Pulpal complications are extremely rare (0.1%).[139]

UNCOMPLICATED CROWN FRACTURE

Definition: Fracture of the enamel only or enamel and dentin without pulp exposure.[14]

Incidence

Uncomplicated crown fracture is very common, accounting for approximately one third of all dental injuries.[139]

Biologic Consequences

If the fracture involves the enamel only, the consequences are minimal and any complications may be due to a concomitant injury to the attachment apparatus. However, if dentin is

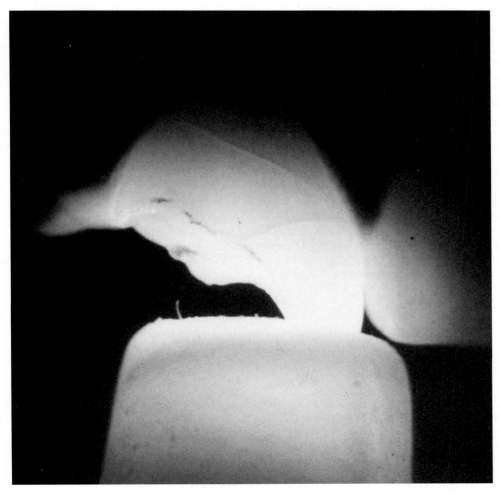

FIG. 16-1 Photograph of traumatized tooth illuminated with a resin-curing light. Enamel infractions are clearly visible.

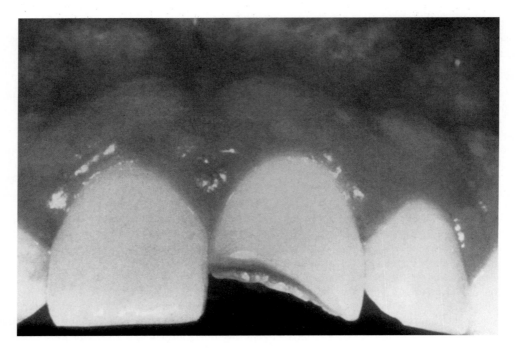

FIG. 16-2 Maxillary central incisor with an uncomplicated crown fracture involving the enamel and dentin.

exposed, a direct pathway exists for noxious stimuli to pass through the dentinal tubules to the pulp. Although the pulp has the potential to successfully defend itself with partial closure of the dentinal tubules and reparative dentin,[28] chronic pulpal inflammation or even necrosis may result.[165] The reaction of the pulp depends on a number of factors including time of treatment, distance of the fracture from the pulp, and the size of the dentinal tubules.[43,125,165]

Diagnosis and Clinical Presentation

Enamel fracture is characterized by a superficial rough edge, which may cause irritation to the tongue or lip. Sensitivity to air or hot or cold liquids is not a complaint.

Similarly enamel/dentin fracture is characterized by a rough edge on the tooth (Fig. 16-2). Sensitivity to air and hot and cold liquids may be a chief complaint. Commonly a lip bruise or laceration is present, since pursing of the lips is automatic when the injury occurs (Fig. 16-3).

Treatment

Enamel fracture only

Smooth the sharp edges and leave if aesthetically acceptable. Use bonded composite resin if necessary for aesthetics.

Enamel/dentin fracture

Treatment should take place as soon as possible.[125] A hard-setting calcium hydroxide base is placed[36] over exposed dentinal tubules to disinfect the fractured dentinal surface and stimulate closure of the tubules, making them less permeable to noxious stimuli[21,105,156] followed by restoration with a bonded resin technique. Controversy exists as to whether dentin bonding can be carried out without an intermediate calcium hydroxide base. It is thought by some authors that

the modern bonding systems seal the cavity sufficiently to protect the pulp. However, while research is abundant as to the increased bond strength with modern dentin bonding systems,[70,81] information is scarce as to whether these bonding systems create a tight enough seal to protect the pulp.[91] It is the authors' opinion that direct dentin bonding (without an intermediate base) should be used on superficial uncomplicated crown fractures only. Direct dentin bonding without a base should be avoided on deep fractures or in young teeth with wide dentinal tubules.

It is essential to account for the fractured tooth fragment. If it can be located and is found intact, it is possible to bond this fragment to the crown with excellent aesthetic results and an acceptable strength[107] (Fig. 16-4, *A* and *B*). If the tooth fragment is not located, a radiograph of the lip should be taken to ensure the fragment has not lodged in the lip. If a lip laceration is present, it must be thoroughly cleansed and sutured. A consult with a plastic surgeon might be prudent is some cases.

Sensitivity testing should be carried out to establish a baseline pulpal status.

Follow-Up

Schedule follow-up as with crown infraction.

Prognosis

The prognosis for uncomplicated crown fracture is extremely good with pulpal complications minimal.[14]

COMPLICATED CROWN FRACTURE

Definition: Crown fractures involving enamel, dentin, and pulp.[14]

Incidence

Complicated crown fractures occur in 2% to 13% of all dental injuries.[94,139]

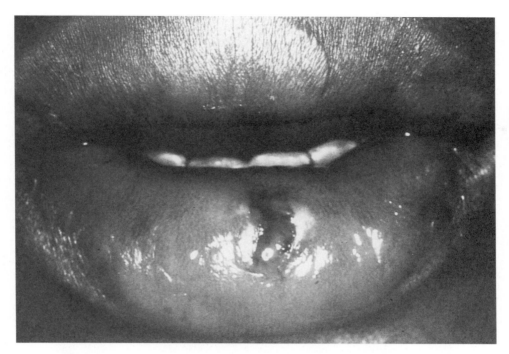

FIG. 16-3 Lip laceration as a result of an injury to the maxillary incisors.

Biologic Consequences

If left untreated, a crown fracture involving the pulp always results in pulp necrosis.[80] However, the manner and time sequence in which the pulp becomes necrotic allows a great deal of potential for successful intervention to maintain pulp vitality. The first reaction after the injury is hemorrhage and local inflammation.[92,135] Subsequent inflammatory changes are usually proliferative but can be destructive. A proliferative reaction is favored in traumatic injuries, since the fractured surface is usually flat, allowing salivary rinsing with little chance of impaction of contaminated debris. Therefore unless impaction of contaminated debris is obvious, it is expected that in the first 24 hours after the injury a proliferative response with inflammation extending not more than 2 mm into the pulp will be present[34,40,66] (Fig. 16-5). In time, the bacterial challenge results in local pulp necrosis and a slow apical spread of the pulpal inflammation.

Treatment

Treatment options are (1) *vital pulp therapy* (comprising pulp capping, partial pulpotomy, and cervical pulpotomy) or (2) *pulpectomy*. Choice of treatment depends on the stage of development of the tooth, time between the accident and treatment, concomitant periodontal injury, and restorative treatment plan.

Stage of development of the tooth

Loss of vitality in an immature tooth can have catastrophic consequences. Root canal treatment on a tooth with a blunderbuss canal is time consuming and difficult. Probably of more importance is the fact that necrosis of an immature tooth leaves it with thin dentinal walls, which are susceptible to fracture both during and after the apexification procedure.[81] Therefore,

every effort must be made to keep the tooth vital at least until the apex and cervical root have completed their development.

Removal of the pulp in a mature tooth is not as significant as in an immature tooth, since a pulpectomy has an extremely high success rate.[59,143] However, it has been shown that vital pulp therapy on a mature tooth performed under optimal conditions can be carried out successfully.[99,160] Therefore this form of therapy can be an option under certain circumstances even though a pulpectomy is the treatment that affords the most predictable success.

In an immature tooth, vital pulp therapy should always be attempted if at all feasible because of the tremendous advantages of maintaining the vital pulp.

Time between the accident and treatment

For 24 hours after a traumatic injury, the initial reaction of the pulp is proliferative with no more than 2-mm depth of pulpal inflammation (see Fig. 16-5). After 24 hours, chances of direct bacterial contamination of the pulp increase and the zone of inflammation progresses apically.[40] Thus as time progresses, the chance of success of maintaining a healthy pulp decreases.

Concomitant periodontal injury

A periodontal injury compromises the nutritional supply of the pulp. This fact is particularly important in mature teeth, where the chance of pulp survival is not as good as for immature teeth.[11,46]

Restorative treatment plan

Unlike an immature tooth where the benefits of maintaining vitality of the pulp are so great, in a mature tooth pulpectomy is a viable treatment option. However, if performed under optimal conditions, vital pulp therapy after traumatic exposures

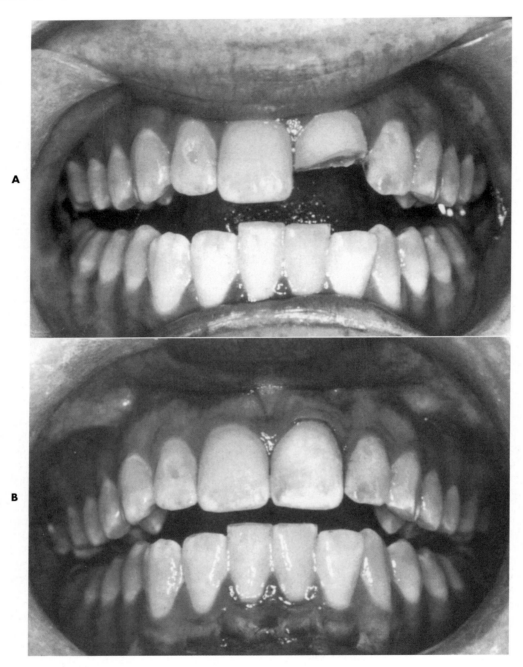

FIG. 16-4 A, Uncomplicated crown fracture of the maxillary central incisor. **B,** Fractured segment is bonded to tooth after placement of a calcium hydroxide base.

can be successful. Thus if the restorative treatment plan is simple and a composite resin restoration will suffice as the permanent restoration, vital pulp therapy should be given serious consideration. However, if a more complex restoration is to be placed (e.g., a crown or bridge abutment), endodontic therapy is recommended.

Vital Pulp Therapy

Requirements for success

Vital pulp therapy has an extremely high success rate if the following requirements are strictly adhered to.

Treatment of a noninflamed pulp. Treatment of a healthy pulp has been shown to be an essential requirement for successful therapy.[149] Vital pulp therapy of the inflamed pulp, on the other hand, affords an inferior success rate.[149]

Therefore the optimal time for treatment is in the first 24 hours when pulp inflammation is superficial. As time increases between the time of injury and therapy, pulp removal must be extended apically to ensure that noninflamed pulp has been reached.

Bacteria-tight seal. In our opinion a bacteria-tight seal is one of the most critical factors for successful treatment. Infection during the healing phase causes failure[31]; however, if the

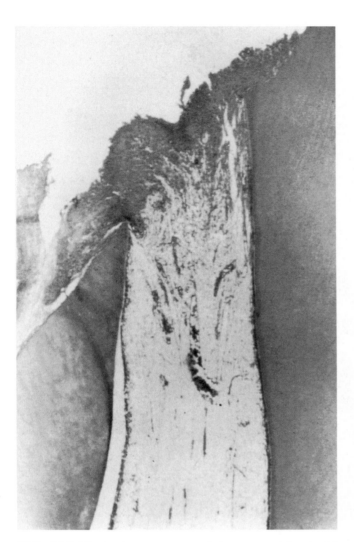

FIG. 16-5 Histologic appearance of the superficial pulp 24 hours after exposure. Proliferative response with inflammation extending 1 to 2 mm into the pulp is seen.

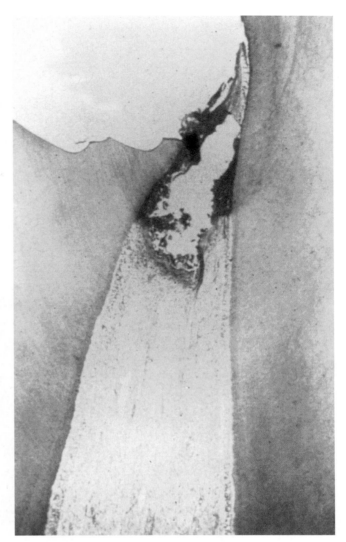

FIG. 16-6 Histologic appearance of the pulp 7 days after dressing with pure calcium hydroxide. Calcium hydroxide has necrosed about 1 to 2 mm of the superficial pulp.

exposed pulp is effectively sealed from bacterial leakage, successful healing of the pulp with a hard tissue barrier occurs independent of the dressing placed on the pulp.[31]

Pulp dressing. Presently calcium hydroxide is the most common dressing used for vital pulp therapy. Its advantages are that it is antibacterial[29,134] and disinfects the superficial pulp. Pure calcium hydroxide necroses about 1.5 mm of pulp tissue,[103] which removes superficial layers of inflamed pulp if present (Fig. 16-6). The high pH of 12.5 of the calcium hydroxide causes a liquefaction necrosis in the most superficial layers of the pulp.[129] The toxicity of the calcium hydroxide appears to be neutralized as the deeper layers of pulp are affected, causing a coagulative necrosis at the junction of the necrotic and vital pulp, resulting in only a mild irritation to the pulp.[129] This mild irritation initiates an inflammatory response and in the absence of bacteria heals with a hard tissue barrier.[129,128] Hard-setting calcium hydroxide does not necrose the superficial layers of pulp but has been shown to initiate healing with a hard tissue barrier also.[141,146]

Vitapex (Neo Dental, Japan), a calcium hydroxide, iodo-form, silicone oil formulation, has been shown to be an effective, antibacterial, hard tissue inducing agent. In its unique syringe format, there is unequaled ease of application into the canal system. Studies have shown Vitapex to be tissue tolerant. The iodoform component is bactericidal, allowing the calcium hydroxide to be more effective. Iodoform also gives a higher degree of radiopacity than other formulations. The silicone vehicle prevents setting of the material, extends shelf life, and allows for ease of manipulation and superior flow characteristics. Vitapex can be used as an antibacterial intracanal medicament for apexification, apexogenesis, treatment of fractures, and internal resorption.

A major disadvantage of calcium hydroxide is that it does not seal the fractured surface. Therefore an additional material must be used to ensure that the pulp is not challenged by bacteria, particularly during the critical healing phase.

Many materials such as zinc oxide–eugenol,[149] tricalcium phosphate,[68] and composite resin[31] have been proposed as medicaments for vital pulp therapy. None to this date have afforded the predictability of calcium hydroxide used in conjunc-

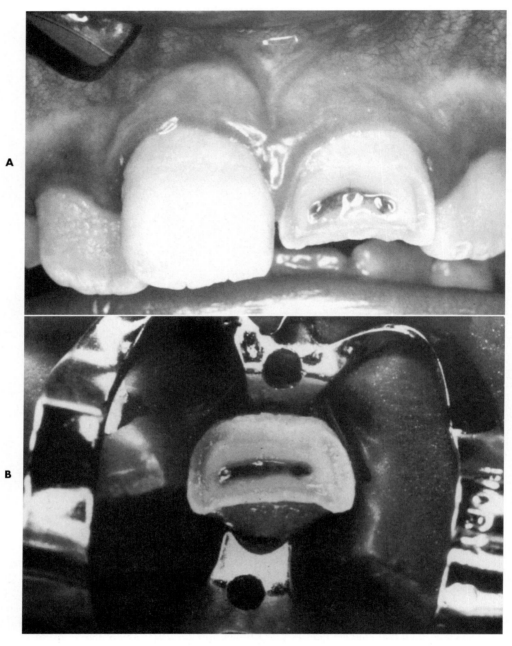

FIG. 16-7 Pulp capping procedure on maxillary central incisor with a complicated crown fracture. **A,** Tooth on presentation to the dentist. **B,** Anesthesia administration, rubber dam placement, and superficial disinfection are performed.

tion with a well-sealed coronal restoration. Mineral trioxide aggregate (MTA), a new material, has been reported to show promise as a pulp capping agent,[119] but as yet the reproducibility of these results and MTA's long-term success have not been tested.

Pulp capping

Pulp capping implies placing the dressing directly onto the pulp exposure.

Indications. Indications for pulp capping are immature permanent tooth, a very recent exposure (<24 hours), and possibly a mature permanent tooth with a simple restorative plan.

Technique. After adequate anesthesia, a rubber dam is placed and the crown and exposed dentinal surface thoroughly rinsed with saline, followed by disinfection with 0.12% chlorhexidine or povidone-iodine (Betadine). Pure calcium hydroxide mixed with sterile saline (or anesthetic solution) is carefully placed over the exposed pulp and dentinal surface. The surrounding enamel is acid etched and bonded with composite resin (Fig. 16-7).

Follow-up. There are two advantages of pulp capping: (1) the final restorative treatment can be completed at the emergency visit; (2) pulp tissue remains coronally, allowing periodic sensitivity testing to be performed. Electrical pulp testing,

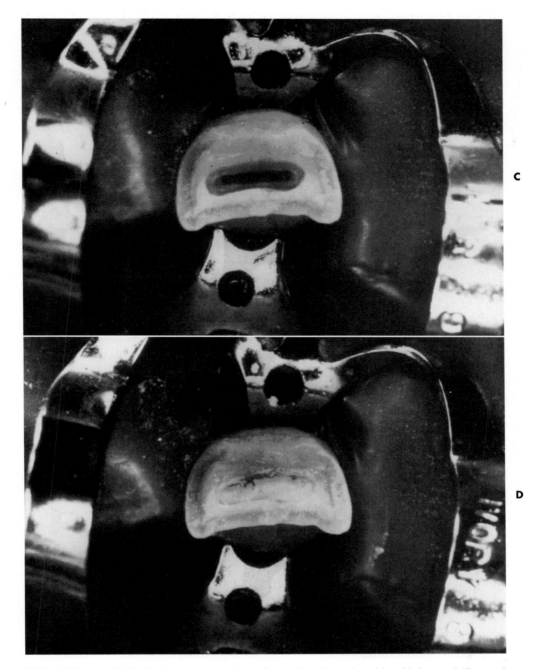

FIG. 16-7, cont'd C, Cavity is prepared 1 to 2 mm into the pulp with a high-speed diamond bur with copious water spray. **D,** Thin layer of calcium hydroxide is placed on the pulp tissue.   *Continued*

thermal testing, and palpation and percussion tests should be carried out at 3 weeks, 3 months, 6 months, and 12 months and every year thereafter. A radiographic examination is extremely important in these cases. A hard tissue barrier can sometimes be visualized as early as 6 weeks after treatment. Also signs of apical periodontitis (an indirect sign of an unhealthy pulp) can be seen as an apical radiolucency. Most importantly, continued root development of the immature root, which was the primary reason for performing the procedure, is checked with this periodic radiographic examination (Fig. 16-8).

Prognosis. The success of the pulp capping procedure relies on the ability of the calcium hydroxide to disinfect the su-

perficial pulp and dentin and to necrose the zone of superficially inflamed pulp. Also the quality of the bacteria-tight seal provided by the enamel-bonded resin restoration is a important factor in successful pulp capping.

Reported prognosis is in the range of 80%.[50,84,123]

Partial pulpotomy

Partial pulpotomy implies the removal of coronal pulp tissue (hopefully) to the level of healthy pulp. This procedure is commonly called the "Cvek pulpotomy."

Indications. Indications for partial pulpotomy are the same as with pulp capping.

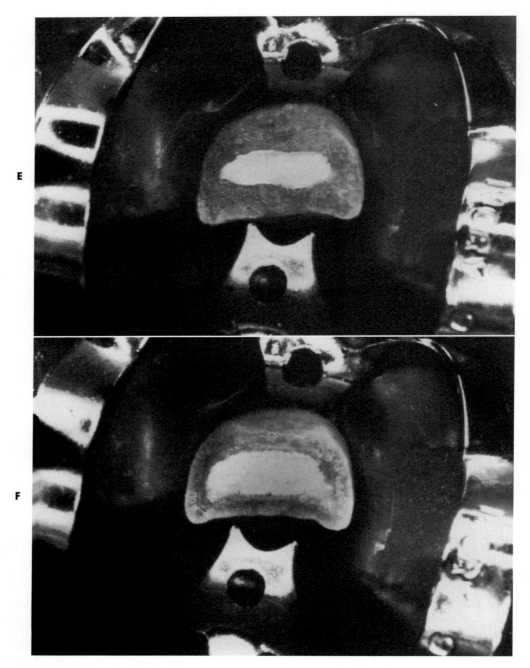

FIG. 16-7, cont'd E, Bacteria-tight seal is created by the placement of a zinc oxide–eugenol temporary restoration into the cavity to the level flush with the fractured dentinal surface. **F,** Calcium hydroxide base is placed to cover the zinc oxide–eugenol and protect the exposed dentin.

When it is predicted that the zone of inflammation in the pulp has extended more than 2 mm apically but has not reached the root pulp (e.g., a traumatic exposure a few days after injury in a large young pulp) partial pulpotomy is indicated. For reasons to be discussed, partial pulpotomy is superior to pulp capping and affords a better prognosis.

Technique. Anesthesia, rubber dam placement, and superficial disinfection are performed as described with pulp capping.

A 1- to 2-mm-deep cavity is prepared into the pulp using a sterile diamond bur of appropriate size with copious water coolant[60] (see Fig. 16-7). A slow-speed bur or spoon excavator should be avoided unless cooling of the high-speed bur is not possible. If bleeding is excessive, the pulp is amputated deeper until only moderate hemorrhage is seen. Excess blood is carefully removed by rinsing with sterile saline or anesthetic solution and dried with a sterile cotton pellet. Care must be taken not to allow a blood clot to develop, as this compromises the prognosis.[34,128] If the pulp is of sufficient size to allow 1- to 2-mm additional pulp necrosis, a thin layer of pure calcium hydroxide is mixed with sterile saline or anesthetic so-

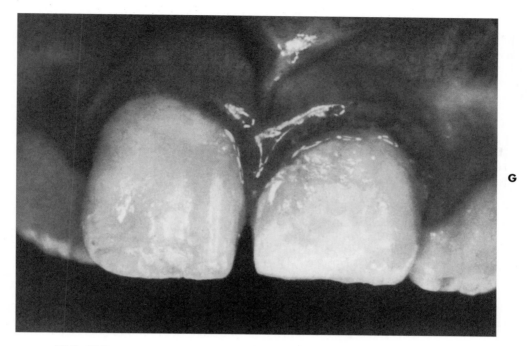

FIG. 16-7, cont'd G, Restoration is completed with bonded composite resin.

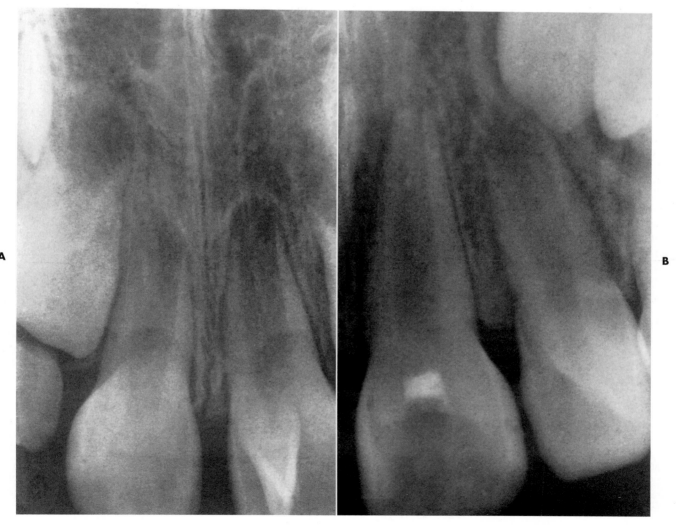

FIG. 16-8 Radiographic follow-up after pulp capping procedure. A, Preoperative. B, Follow-up 1 year later showing continued root development.

lution and carefully placed onto it. If the pulp size does not permit additional loss of pulp tissue, a commercial hard-setting calcium hydroxide can be used.[141] The prepared cavity is filled with a material with the best chance of a bacteria-tight seal (zinc oxide–eugenol or glass-ionomer cement) to a level that is flush with the fractured surface. The material in the pulpal cavity and all exposed dentinal tubules are covered with hard-setting calcium hydroxide, and the enamel is etched and restored with bonded composite resin as in pulp capping.

Follow-up. Schedule follow-up as with pulp capping. Again the emphasis is placed on maintenance of positive sensitivity tests and radiographic evidence of continued root development (see Fig. 16-8).

Prognosis. This method affords many advantages over pulp capping. Superficially inflamed pulp is removed in the preparation of the pulpal cavity. Calcium hydroxide disinfects dentin and pulp and removes additional pulpal inflammation. Most importantly, space is provided for a material that provides a bacteria-tight seal to allow pulpal healing with hard tissue under optimal conditions. Additionally, coronal pulp remains, which allows sensitivity testing to be carried out at the follow-up visits.

Prognosis is extremely good (94% to 96%).[34,51]

Cervical pulpotomy

Cervical pulpotomy involves removal of the entire coronal pulp to a level of the root orifices. This level of pulp amputation is chosen arbitrarily because of its anatomic convenience. Therefore since the inflamed pulp sometimes extends past the canal orifices into the root pulp, many "mistakes" are made, resulting in treatment of an inflamed rather than noninflamed pulp.

Indications. When it is predicted that the pulp is inflamed to the deeper levels of the coronal pulp, cervical pulpotomy is indicated. Traumatic exposures after 72 hours and carious exposures are two examples where cervical pulpotomy may be indicated. Because of the fairly good chance that the dressing will be placed on an inflamed pulp, cervical pulpotomy is contraindicated in mature teeth. However, benefits outweigh risks for this treatment form in the immature tooth with incompletely formed apexes and thin dentinal walls.

Technique. Employ anesthesia, rubber dam placement, and superficial disinfection as with pulp capping and partial pulpotomy. The coronal pulp is removed as in the partial pulpotomy but to the level of the root orifices. Calcium hydroxide dressing, bacteria-tight seal, and coronal restoration are carried out as with partial pulpotomy.[109]

Follow-up. Schedule follow-up as with pulp capping and partial pulpotomy. A major disadvantage of cervical pulpotomy is the fact that sensitivity testing is not possible because of the loss of coronal pulp. Therefore radiographic follow-up is extremely important with this form of treatment to assess for signs of apical periodontitis and to ensure the continuation of root formation.

Prognosis. Since the cervical pulpotomy is performed on pulps that are expected to have deep inflammation and the site of pulp amputation is arbitrary, many more "mistakes" are made, leading to treatment of the inflamed pulp. Consequently, the prognosis, which is in the range of 75%, is poorer for cervical pulpotomy than for partial pulpotomy.[56,61] Because of the inability to evaluate pulp status after cervical pulpotomy, some authors have recommended pulpectomy routinely after the

roots have fully formed (Fig. 16-9). This philosophy is based on the fact that the pulpectomy procedure has a success rate in the range of 95%, whereas if apical periodontitis develops, the prognosis of root canal treatment drops significantly to about 80%.[59,131]

Pulpectomy

Pulpectomy implies removal of the entire pulp to the level of the apical foramen.

Indications

Pulpectomy is indicated in complicated crown fracture of mature teeth (if conditions are not ideal for vital pulp therapy).

Technique

See Chapter 8.

Follow-up

See Chapter 9.

Prognosis

Reported prognosis of pulpectomy of mature teeth is in the range of 90%.[59,143] However, no pulpectomy prognosis study has limited its teeth to those that have undergone a traumatic injury. It is not known if the attachment injury and possible disruption of the apical blood supply that occur in most traumatic injuries affect the prognosis of pulpectomy in these teeth.

Treatment of the Nonvital Pulp

Mature tooth

See Chapters 8 and 9.

Immature tooth: apexification

Indications. Teeth with open apices in which standard instrumentation techniques cannot create an apical stop to facilitate effective obturation of the canal require apexification.

Biologic consequences. A nonvital immature tooth presents a number of difficulties for adequate endodontic therapy. The canal is wider apically than coronally, necessitating the use of a soft gutta-percha technique to mold the gutta-percha to the shape of the apex. Since the apex is extremely wide, no barrier exists to stop this softened gutta-percha from moving into and traumatizing the apical periodontal tissues. Also the lack of apical stop and extrusion of material through the canal might result in a canal that is underfilled and susceptible to leakage. An additional problem in immature teeth with thin dentinal walls is their susceptibility to fracture both during and after treatment.[35,142]

These problems are overcome by stimulating the formation of a hard tissue barrier to allow for optimal obturation of the canal and reinforcing the weakened root against fracture both during and after apexification.[81,93]

Technique

Disinfection of the canal: Since in the vast majority of cases, nonvital teeth are infected,[20,144] the first phase of treatment is to disinfect the root canal system to ensure periapical healing.[29,37,38,80] The canal length is estimated with a parallel preoperative radiograph, and after access to the canals is made, a file is placed to this length. When the length has been confirmed radiographically, *light* filing (because of the thin dentinal walls) is performed with *copious* irrigation with 0.5% sodium hypochlorite.[37,138] An irrigation needle that can passively

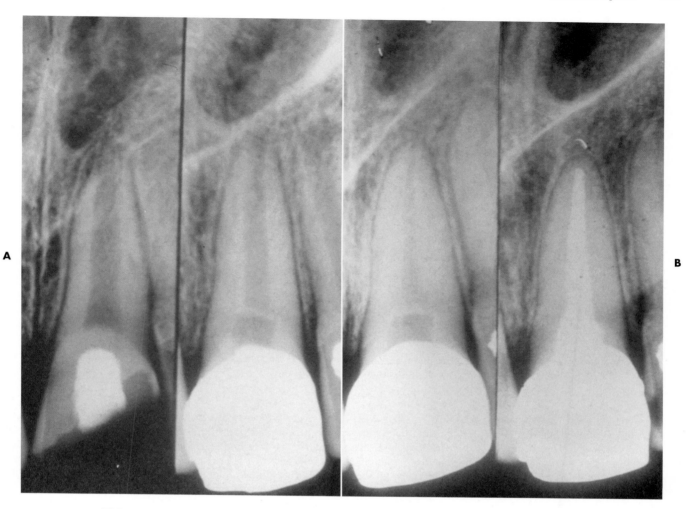

FIG. 16-9 Cervical pulpotomy of an immature maxillary incisor tooth followed by pulpectomy after root formation. **A,** Pulpotomy is initiated *(left)*. Six months later a hard tissue barrier has formed and the root continues to develop *(right)*. **B,** One year later complete root development is complete *(left)*. Pulpectomy followed by permanent root canal therapy is performed *(right)*.

reach close to the apical length is useful in disinfecting the canals of these immature teeth. The canal is dried with paper points, and a soft mix of calcium hydroxide is spun into the canal with a lentulo spiral instrument. The additional disinfecting action of calcium hydroxide is effective for 1 week after its application[134] so that the continuation of treatment can take place any time after 1 week. Further treatment should not be delayed more than 1 month, since the calcium hydroxide could be washed out by tissue fluids through the open apex, leaving the canal susceptible to reinfection.

Stimulation of a hard tissue barrier: The formation of the hard tissue barrier at the apex requires a similar environment to that required for hard tissue formation in vital pulp therapy (i.e., a mild inflammatory stimulus to initiate healing and a bacteria-free environment to ensure that the inflammation is not progressive).

As with vital pulp therapy, calcium hydroxide is presently the medicament of choice for this procedure.[35,67,69]

Pure calcium hydroxide powder is mixed with sterile saline (or anesthetic solution) to a thick (powdery) consistency (Fig.

16-10). Ready-mixed commercial calcium hydroxide can also be used. The calcium hydroxide is packed against the apical soft tissue with a plugger or thick gutta-percha point to initiate hard tissue formation. This step is followed by backfilling with calcium hydroxide to completely obturate the canal, thus ensuring a bacteria-free canal with little chance of reinfection during the 6 to 18 months required for hard tissue formation at the apex. The calcium hydroxide is meticulously removed from the access cavity to the level of the root orifices, and a well-sealing temporary filling is placed in the access cavity. A radiograph is taken; the canal should appear to have become calcified, indicating that the entire canal has been filled with the calcium hydroxide. Because calcium hydroxide washout is evaluated by its relative radiodensity in the canal, it is prudent to use a calcium hydroxide mixture without the addition of a radiopaque substance such as barium sulphate. These additives do not wash out as readily as calcium hydroxide so that if they are present in the canal, evaluation of washout is not possible.

At 3-month intervals a radiograph is taken to evaluate

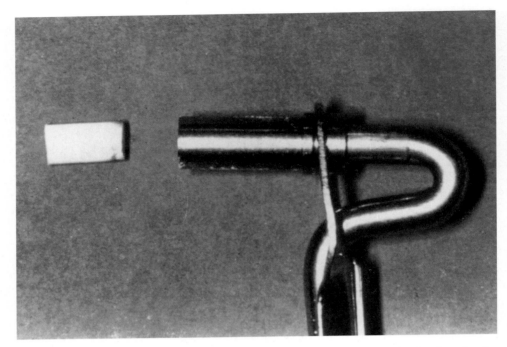

FIG. 16-10 Calcium hydroxide mixed to a thick powdery consistency, allowing it to be deposited in the access cavity with an amalgam carrier.

whether a hard tissue barrier has formed and if the calcium hydroxide has washed out of the canal. If calcium hydroxide washout is seen, it is replaced as previously described. If no washout is evident, it can be left intact for another 3 months. Excessive calcium hydroxide dressing changes should be avoided if at all possible, since the initial toxicity of the material is thought to delay healing.[86]

When completion of a hard tissue barrier is suspected, the calcium hydroxide should be washed out of the canal with sodium hypochlorite and a radiograph taken to evaluate the radiodensity of the apical stop. A file of a size that can easily reach the apex can be used to gently probe for a stop at the apex. When a hard tissue barrier is indicated radiographically and can be probed with an instrument, the canal is ready for obturation.

Obturation of the root canal: Since the apical diameter is larger than the coronal diameter of most of these canals, a softened gutta-percha technique is indicated in these teeth (see Chapter 9). Care must be taken to avoid excessive vertical or lateral force during obturation because of the thin walls of the root. The hard tissue barrier consists of irregularly arranged layers of coagulated soft tissue, calcified tissue, and cementum-like tissue (Fig. 16-11). Included, also, are islands of soft connective tissue, giving the barrier a "Swiss cheese" consistency.[23,39] Because of the irregular nature of the barrier, it is not unusual for cement or softened gutta-percha to be pushed through it into the apical tissues during obturation. Formation of the hard tissue barrier might be some distance short of the radiographic apex because the barrier forms wherever the calcium hydroxide contacts vital tissue. In teeth with wide-open apices vital tissue can survive and proliferate from the periodontal ligament a few millimeters into the root canal. Obturation should be completed to the level of the hard tissue barrier and not forced toward the radiographic apex.

Reinforcement of the thin dentinal walls: The apexification procedure with long-term calcium hydroxide described above has become a predictably successful procedure (see Prognosis).[36,48] However, the thin dentinal walls still present a clinical problem. Should secondary injuries occur, teeth with thin dentinal walls are more susceptible to fractures that render them nonrestorable.[45,145] It has been reported that approximately 30% of these teeth fracture during or after endodontic treatment.[82] Consequently, some clinicians have questioned the advisability of the apexification procedure and have opted for more radical treatment procedures, including extraction[142] followed by extensive restorative procedures such as dental implants. Recent studies have shown that intracoronal acid-etched bonded resins can internally strengthen endodontically treated teeth and increase their resistance to fracture.[121,153]

A new technique has been described to internally strengthen nonvital immature teeth using the Luminex post system. A curing post is used to assist in curing the deeper layers of resin, after which it is removed to allow a channel for calcium hydroxide replenishment and obturation of the canal (Fig. 16-12). In vitro studies have shown the technique to be effective in strengthening these teeth.[81]

Follow-up. Routine recall evaluation should be performed (see Chapter 22) to determine the success in the prevention or treatment of apical periodontitis. Restorative procedures should be assessed to ensure that they in no way promote root fractures.

Prognosis. Periapical healing and the formation of a hard tissue barrier occurs predictably with long-term calcium hydroxide treatment (79% to 96%).[35,82] However, long-term survival is jeopardized by the fracture potential of the thin dentinal walls of these teeth. It is expected that the newer techniques of internally strengthening the teeth described above will increase their long-term survivability.

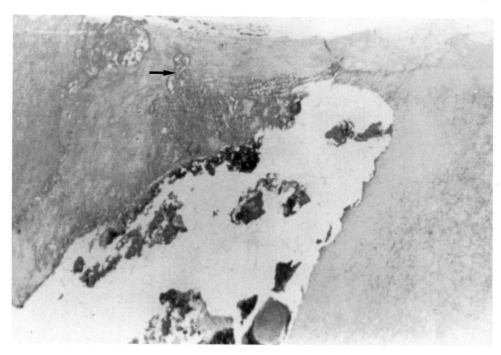

FIG. 16-11 Histologic appearance of hard tissue barrier at the apex of a tooth. It consists of irregularly arranged layers of coagulated soft tissue, calcified tissue, and cementum-like tissue. Included are islands of soft tissue *(arrow)*.

CROWN ROOT FRACTURE

Definition: Crown root fracture involving enamel, dentin, and cementum; pulp may or may not be involved.

Incidence

The incidence of crown root fractures as a direct result of traumatic injuries has been reported to be 5% of all dental injuries.[10]

Biologic Consequences

The biologic consequences of a crown root fracture are identical to an uncomplicated (if the pulp is not exposed) or complicated (if the crown is exposed) crown fracture. In addition, periodontal complications are present because the fracture encroaches on the attachment apparatus. The seriousness of the complication is dependent on the apical extent of the attachment injury.

Diagnosis and Clinical Presentation

Crown root fractures are in most instances due to direct trauma resulting in a chisel-type fracture with a single or multiple fragments below the lingual gingiva[14] (Fig. 16-13). The fragments may be firm, loose, and attached only by the periodontal ligament or lost. Pain on pressure and biting is evident because of the periodontal injury, as is pain to air and hot or cold liquids because of dentin or pulp exposure. Indirect light and transillumination is an effective way of diagnosing crown root fractures.

Treatment

Crown root fractures are treated in the same manner as uncomplicated or complicated crown fractures with additional treatment for the attachment injury.

If a crown root fracture cannot be made into an uncomplicated crown fracture by periodontal (crown lengthening) or orthodontic therapy (root extrusion), or both, the tooth should be extracted because it cannot be properly treated or restored.

After administration of adequate anesthesia, all loose fragments are removed. A periodontal assessment is made as to whether the tooth can be treated periodontally to allow it to be adequately restored. Periodontal therapy could involve a simple removal of tissue with a scalpel, electrosurgical or laser procedure to allow for adequate sealing of the restoration, or forced eruption to extrude the fractured area above the attachment level to allow for adequate restoration (see Coronal Root Fracture).

Follow-Up and Prognosis

Schedule follow-up as with uncomplicated and complicated crown fractures. The quality of the coronal restoration, particularly at the gingival sulcus should be reassessed at each visit, since long-term success is dependent on its quality.[96] Prognosis is similar to that described for uncomplicated or complicated crown fractures.

ROOT FRACTURE

Definition: Fracture of the cementum, dentin, and pulp.

Incidence

Root fractures are relatively infrequent, occurring in less than 3% of all dental injuries.[163] Incompletely formed roots with vital pulps rarely fracture horizontally.[5]

Biologic Consequences

When a root fractures horizontally, the coronal segment is displaced to a varying degree, but generally the apical segment is not displaced. Because the apical pulpal circulation is not

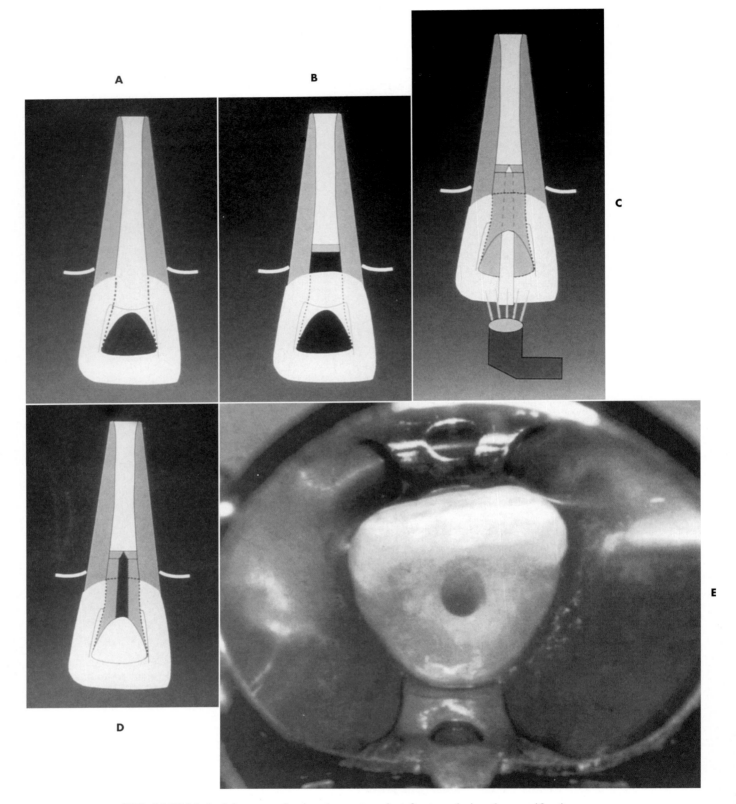

FIG. 16-12 Method for strengthening the root against fracture during the apexification procedure. **A,** Canal is filled with a thick mix of calcium hydroxide. **B,** Calcium hydroxide is removed to below the level of the bone, a thin layer of glass-ionomer cement is placed over it, and a clear Luminex post is seated into the glass-ionomer cement parallel to the long axis of the tooth. The glass ionomer cement is then light cured. **C,** Composite resin is packed into the access cavity, the post is pushed through it to seat into the glass-ionomer cement, and it is cured in the same manner as the glass-ionomer cement. **D,** After the resin is cured, the post is removed leaving a reinforced root and a channel through which medicament changes and obturation can take place. **E,** Clinical picture of the channel, which is sealed with a temporary stopping between medicament changes and is filled with composite resin after obturation. Channel can be widened with a fissure bur to facilitate medicament changes and obturation, after which it is repaired with resin using the same method of curing.

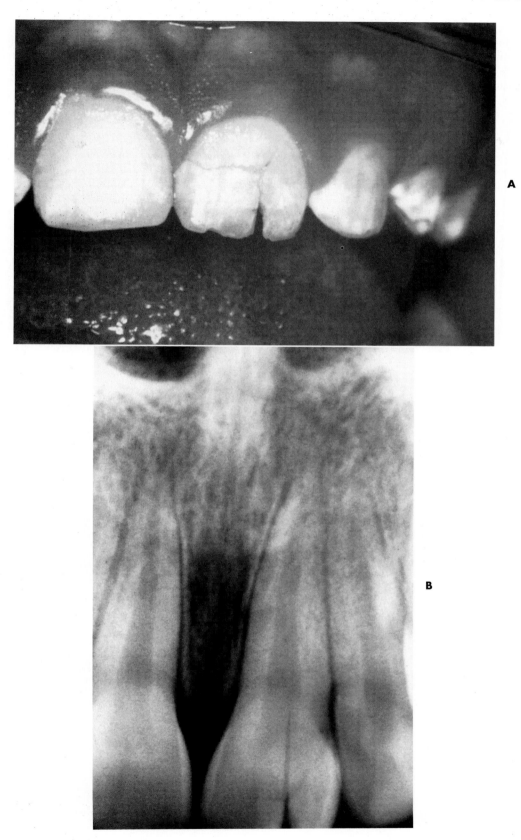

FIG. 16-13 Crown root fracture of maxillary central incisor. **A,** Chisel-type fracture has resulted in multiple fragments, one of which extends below the attachment level. **B,** Radiographic picture of the same tooth.

disrupted, pulp necrosis in the apical segment is extremely rare. Pulp necrosis of the coronal segment results because of coronal segment displacement and occurs in about 25% of cases.[6,7,76]

Rigid stabilization (2 to 4 months) of the segments allows healing and "reattachment" of the fractured segments. The speed of treatment and proximity of the repositioned root segments determine the type of healing that results.

Diagnosis and Clinical Presentation

Clinical presentation is similar to that of luxation injuries (see Luxation Injuries). The extent of displacement of the coronal segment is usually indicative of the location of the fracture and can vary from none, simulating a concussion injury (apical fracture), to severe, simulating an extrusive luxation (cervical fracture).

Radiographic examination for root fractures is extremely important. Since root fractures are usually oblique (facial to palatal) (Fig. 16-14), one periapical radiograph may easily miss its presence. It is imperative to take at least three angled radiographs (45, 90, and 110 degrees) so that at least at one angulation, the x-ray beam passes directly through the fracture line to make it visible on the radiograph (Fig. 16-15).

Treatment

Emergency treatment involves repositioning of the segments in as close proximity as possible and rigidly splinting to adjacent teeth for 2 to 4 months.[120] If a long time has elapsed between the injury and treatment, it is likely not possible to reposition the segments close to their original position, compromising the long-term prognosis of the tooth.

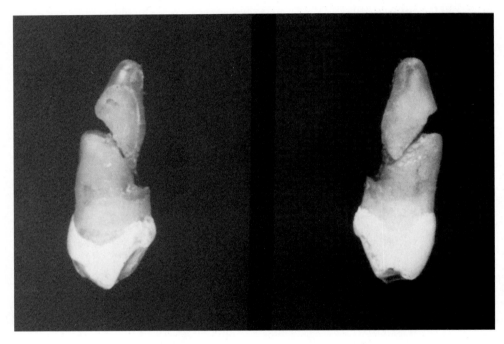

FIG. 16-14 Extracted tooth with an oblique (facial to palatal) root fracture.

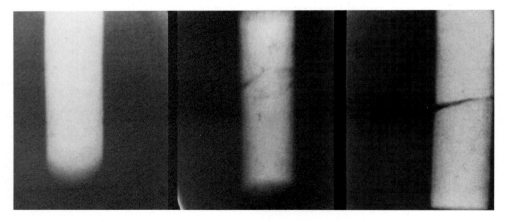

FIG. 16-15 Chalk cut horizontally and radiographed at different angles illustrating the different radiographic pictures that can be obtained. *Left,* At this angle, no "fracture" is seen. *Middle,* The "fracture" appears complicated in nature. *Right,* Only at this angle can the true nature of the fracture can be seen. *(Courtesy Dr. I. B. Bender.)*

Healing Patterns

Andreasen and Hjorting-Hansen[16] have described four types of healing of root fractures.

1. Healing with calcified tissue: Radiographically the fracture line is discernible, but the fragments are in close contact.
2. Healing with interproximal connective tissue: Radiographically the fragments appear separated by a narrow radiolucent line, and the fractured edges appear rounded.
3. Healing with interproximal bone and connective tissue: Radiographically the fragments are separated by a distinct bony ridge (Fig. 16-16, *A*).
4. Interproximal inflammatory tissue without healing: Radiographically a widening of the fracture line or a developing radiolucency corresponding to the fracture line becomes apparent (Fig. 16-16, *B*).

The first three types of healing patterns are considered successful. The teeth are usually asymptomatic and respond positively to sensitivity testing. Coronal yellowing is possible because calcification of the coronal segment is not unusual.[77,163]

The fourth type of healing pattern is typical when the coronal segment loses its vitality. The infective products in the coronal pulp cause an inflammatory response and typical radiolucencies at the fracture line (Figs. 16-16, *B*, and 16-17).[16]

Treatment of Complications

Coronal root fracture

Historically, fractures in the coronal segment were thought to have a poor prognosis, and extraction of the coronal segment was recommended. Research does not support this treatment; in fact if these coronal segments are rigidly splinted, chances of healing do not differ from midroot or apical fractures.[163] However, if the fracture occurs at the level of or coronal to the crest of the alveolar bone, the prognosis is extremely poor.

If reattachment of the fractured segments is not possible, extraction of the coronal segment is indicated. The level of fracture and length of the remaining root are evaluated for restorability. If the apical root segment is long enough, forced eruption of this segment can be carried out to enable a restoration to be fabricated (Fig. 16-18).

Midroot fracture

Pulp necrosis occurs in 25% of root fractures. In the vast majority of cases the necrosis occurs in the coronal segment only, with the apical segment remaining vital. Therefore endodontic treatment is indicated in the coronal root segment only unless periapical pathology is seen in the apical segment. In most cases the pulpal lumen is wide at the apical extent of the coronal seg-

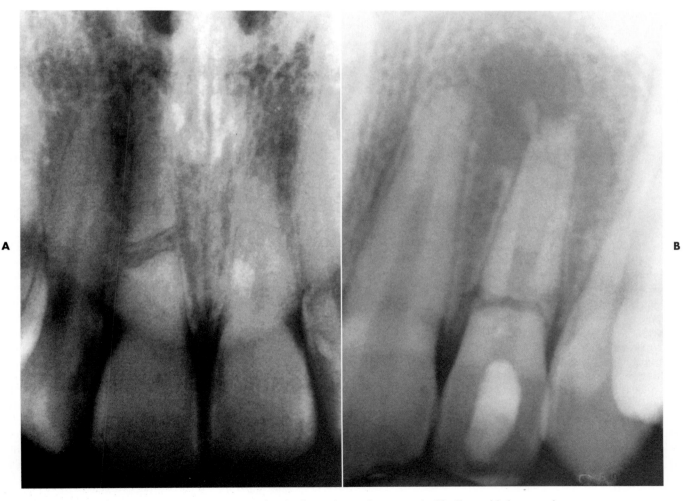

A   **B**

FIG. 16-16 Healing patterns after horizontal root fractures. **A,** Healing with bone and connective tissue. **B,** Interproximal connective tissue without healing.

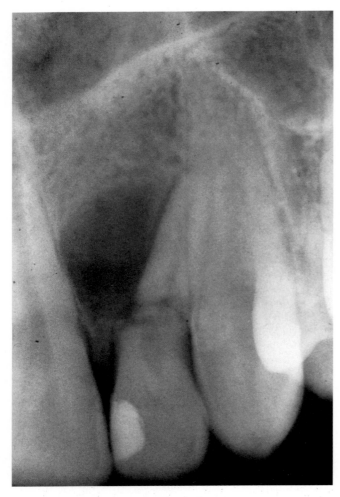

FIG. 16-17 Large radiolucency at the fracture line. Coronal pulp is nonvital, resulting in an inflammatory response at the fracture line.

ment so that long-term calcium hydroxide treatment is indicated (see Immature Tooth: Apexification). The coronal segment is obturated after a hard tissue barrier has formed apically in the coronal segment and periradicular healing has taken place.

In rare cases when both the coronal and apical pulp are necrotic, treatment is more complicated. Endodontic treatment through the fracture is extremely difficult. Endodontic manipulations, medicaments, and filling materials have a detrimental effect on healing of the fracture site (Fig. 16-19). If healing of the fracture has been completed, followed by necrosis of the apical segment, the prognosis is much improved.

In more apical root fractures, necrotic apical segments can be surgically removed. This is a viable treatment if the remaining root is long enough to provide adequate periodontal support. Removal of the apical segment in midroot fractures leaves the coronal segment with a compromised attachment, and endodontic implants have been used to provide additional support to the tooth.

Follow-Up

After the splinting period is completed, follow-up is as with all dental traumatic injuries (i.e., at 3, 6, and 12 months and yearly thereafter).

Prognosis

Factors that influence repair

1. Degree of dislocation and mobility of the coronal fragment are extremely important in determining outcome.[5,77,139,163] Increased dislocation and coronal fragment mobility result in a decreased prognosis.
2. Immature teeth are seldom involved in root fractures, but when they are, the prognosis is good.[73]
3. Prognosis increases with quick treatment, close reduction of the root segments, and rigid splinting for 2 to 4 months.[77,120,139]

Complications are (1) *pulp necrosis,* which can be treated successfully[33,76] by treating the coronal segment with long-term calcium hydroxide and obturation when a hard tissue barrier has formed, and (2) *root canal obliteration,* which is not uncommon if the root segment (coronal or apical) remains vital.

LUXATION INJURIES

Concussion: No displacement, normal mobility, sensitivity to percussion.

Subluxation: Sensitivity to percussion, increased mobility, no displacement.

Lateral Luxation: Displacement labially, lingually, distally, or incisally.

Extrusive Luxation: Displacement in a coronal direction.

Intrusive Luxation: Displacement in an apical direction into the alveolus.

The definitions describe injuries of increasing magnitude in terms of intensity of the injury and subsequent sequelae.

Incidence

Luxation injuries are the most common of all dental injuries, with reported incidences ranging from 30% to 44%.[84,145]

Biologic Consequences

Luxation injuries result in damage to the attachment apparatus (periodontal ligament and cemental layer), the severity of which is dependent on the type of injury sustained (concussion least, intrusion most). The apical neurovascular supply to the pulp is also affected to varying degrees, resulting in an altered or total loss of vitality to the tooth.

Sequelae of attachment damage

Surface resorption. During a luxation injury mechanical damage to the cementum surface occurs, a local inflammatory response, and a localized area of root resorption results. If no further inflammatory stimulus is present, periodontal healing and root surface repair occurs within 14 days.[62] These small resorptive lacunae have been termed *surface resorption* (Fig. 16-20). It is symptomless and in most cases cannot be visualized on routine radiographs.

Dentoalveolar ankylosis and replacement resorption. If the trauma is extensive (e.g., intrusive luxation) with a large area of damage involving more than 20% of the root surface,[87,90] an abnormal attachment can occur after healing. After the initial inflammatory response to remove debris resulting from the injury, a root surface devoid of cementum results.[62,90] Cells in the vicinity of the denuded root now compete to repopulate it.[17] Often cells that are precursors of bone move across from the socket wall and populate the damaged root rather than the slower moving periodontal ligament cells. Bone comes into direct contact with the root without an intermediate attachment

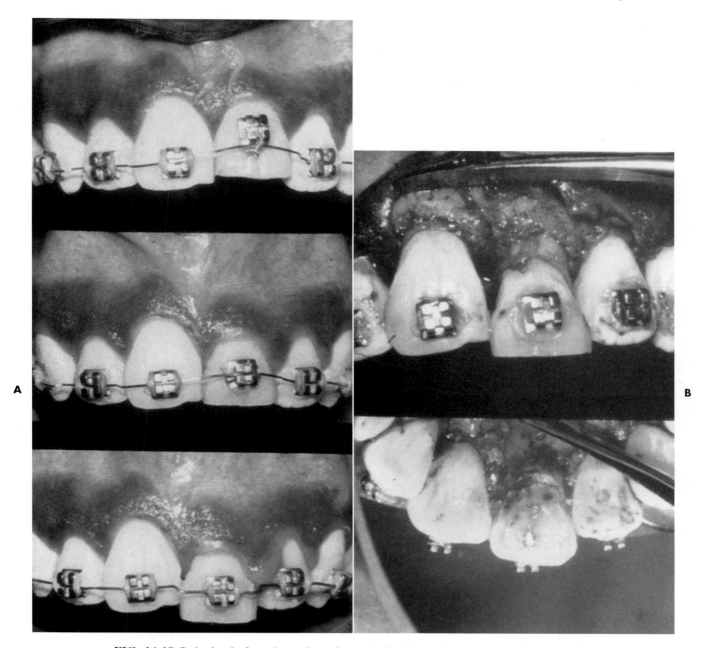

FIG. 16-18 Orthodontic forced eruption of a tooth that has undergone a root fracture at the cervical bone level. **A,** Endodontic treatment is performed. Temporary post is cemented through the crown into the root. Root is erupted approximately 2 mm during a 4-week period. **B,** Flap procedure is performed to ensure that enough tooth structure remains to construct the restoration and to adjust the gingival and bone levels to be compatible with the adjacent teeth.

apparatus. This phenomenon is termed *dentoalveolar anky-losis*.[63] Bone resorbs and reforms physiologically throughout life. The osteoclasts in contact with the root resorb the dentin as though it were bone; in the reforming phase osteoblasts lay down new bone in the area that was previously root, eventually replacing it. This progressive replacement of the root by bone is termed *replacement resorption*.[63] It is characterized histologically by direct contact between bone and dentin without a separating periodontal ligament and cemental layer[14] (Fig. 16-21). Radiographically the distinction between the root and surrounding bone (a traceable lamina dura) is lost, and a

"moth-eaten" appearance results[14,148] (Fig. 16-22). Clinically, lack of mobility of the tooth and a metallic sound to percussion are pathognomonic,[12] as is infraocclusion in the developing dentition. Ultimately the tooth is lost because of loss of root support.

Consequences of apical neurovascular supply damage

Pulp canal obliteration. Pulp canal obliteration is common after luxation injuries. The frequency of pulp canal obliteration appears inversely proportional to that of pulp necrosis. The exact mechanism of pulp canal obliteration is not known. It

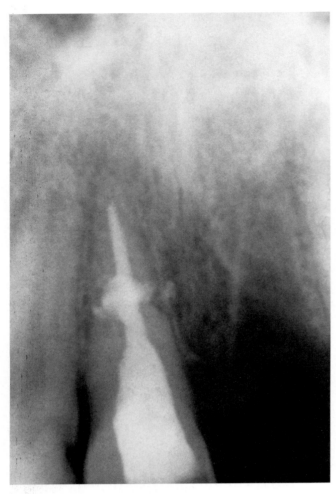

FIG. 16-19 Conservative root canal treatment of the coronal and apical segments. Note the filling material in the fracture line, which compromises the healing response.

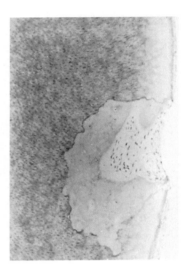

FIG. 16-20 Histologic appearance of surface resorption. Repair of the resorption lacuna with cementum-like tissue is evident. Stain H & E. *(Courtesy Dr. Leif Tronstad.)*

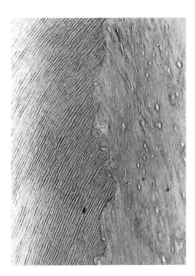

FIG. 16-21 Histologic appearance of dentoalveolar ankylosis with replacement resorption. Note the absence of the periodontal ligament and cemental layer and the direct union of the bone and root.

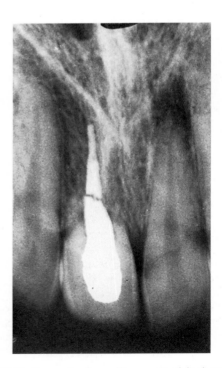

FIG. 16-22 Radiograph of maxillary central incisors with replacement resorption. Note the absence of lamina dura and the moth-eaten appearance of the roots.

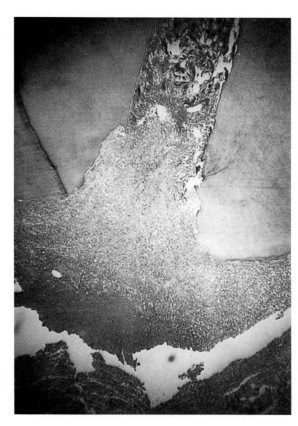

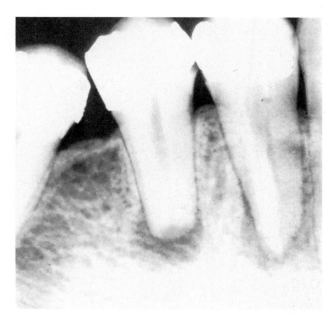

FIG. 16-24 Mandibular premolar with external apical resorption due to apical periodontitis. Pulp of the tooth is necrotic and infected.

FIG. 16-23 Histologic appearance of apical resorption due to an infected root canal. Chronic inflammation is present apically. Resorption of the external and internal aspect of the root can be seen. Stain H & E. *(Courtesy Dr. S. Seltzer.)*

has been theorized that the sympathetic/parasympathetic control of blood flow to the odontoblasts is altered resulting in uncontrolled reparative dentin formation.[5] Another theory is that hemorrhage and blood clot formation in the pulp after injury is a nidus for subsequent calcification if the pulp remains vital.[5] Pulp canal obliteration can usually be diagnosed within the first year after injury.[9] Pulp canal obliteration was found to be more frequent in teeth with open apexes (>0.7 mm radiographically), in teeth with extrusive and lateral luxation injuries, and in teeth that have been rigidly splinted.[9]

Pulp necrosis. The factors most important for the development of pulp necrosis are type of injury (concussion least, intrusion most) and stage of root development (mature apex more than immature apex).[8]

Pulp necrosis can lead to infection of the root canal system with the following consequences.

Apical periodontitis with apical root resorption: Practically all teeth exhibiting apical periodontitis exhibit apical resorption (Fig. 16-23). The resorption can be minor and practically invisible radiographically or can be so extensive that a significant amount of root tip is lost (Fig. 16-24). The cemental layer is a physical barrier that separates the root canal system from the surrounding periodontal attachment. If the cemental layer stays intact after the traumatic injury, it does not allow the passage of toxins through it so that the only communication between the root canal system and the periodontal ligament remains the apical foramen, causing an apical periodontitis with

apical root resorption. It appears that the intense and progressive inflammation confined at the apex overcomes the resistance of the cemental layer to resorption. Apical root resorption is asymptomatic, and symptoms that might lead to its diagnosis are associated with the periapical inflammation. Radiographically it is diagnosed by radiolucencies at the root tip and the adjacent bone. (Pathognomonic of root resorption at all root locations is resorption of the adjacent bone as well.) Treatment is standard root canal treatment (see Chapters 8 and 9) (Fig. 16-25), which has a fairly good success rate.[101,108,114] Apical closure techniques with long-term calcium hydroxide treatment can also be used to ensure a better prognosis for nonsurgical endodontic therapy.[82]

Lateral periodontitis with inflammatory root resorption: After a more serious injury, portions of the cemental covering of the root are damaged and the root's protective (insulating) quality is lost. If the pulp is necrotic and infected, the bacterial toxins can now pass through the dentinal tubules and stimulate an inflammatory response in the corresponding periodontal ligament, resulting in resorption of the root and bone. This process is termed *inflammatory root resorption.*[12,14] The periodontal infiltrate consists of granulation tissue with lymphocytes, plasma cells, and polymorphonuclear leukocytes. The denuded root surface is resorbed by multinucleated giant cells, and this continues until the stimulus (pulp space bacteria) is removed[62] (Fig. 16-26). Radiographically, inflammatory root resorption is observed as progressive radiolucent areas of the root and adjacent bone (Fig. 16-27). When inflammatory root resorption is treated by root canal disinfection, a large area denuded of attachment can result when the inflammation subsides. The competition between cells for the denuded root surface previously described occurs under these circumstances also, possibly resulting in replacement resorption.

It is important to diagnose these resorptive complications, since inflammatory root resorption can be reversed; if ankylosis is present, long-term treatment alternatives must be

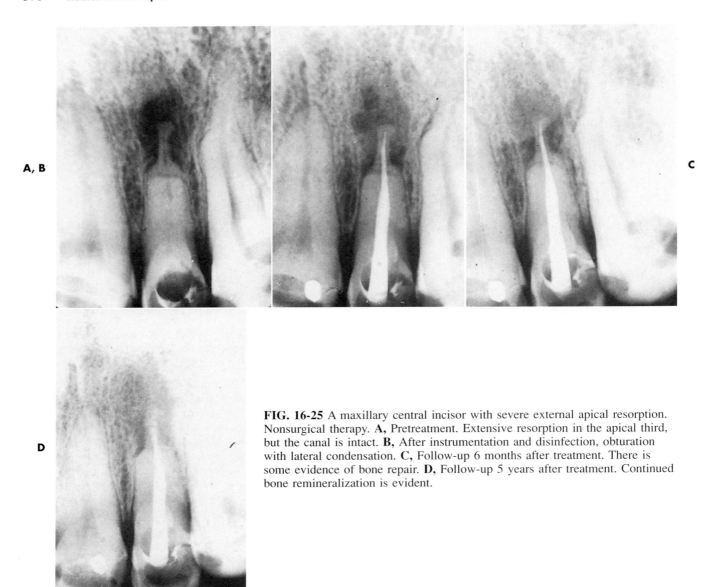

A, B

C

D

FIG. 16-25 A maxillary central incisor with severe external apical resorption. Nonsurgical therapy. **A,** Pretreatment. Extensive resorption in the apical third, but the canal is intact. **B,** After instrumentation and disinfection, obturation with lateral condensation. **C,** Follow-up 6 months after treatment. There is some evidence of bone repair. **D,** Follow-up 5 years after treatment. Continued bone remineralization is evident.

planned. To diagnose these complications it is important to have an understanding of other types of root resorption.

ROOT RESORPTION DEFECTS MIMICKING LATERAL INFLAMMATORY ROOT RESORPTION OF PULPAL ORIGIN

Cervical Root Resorption

Cervical root resorption is a progressive root resorption of inflammatory origin occurring immediately below the epithelial attachment of the tooth (usually but not exclusively the cervical area of the tooth).[14,148,162] It occurs as a delayed reaction after an injury, and its exact pathogenesis is not fully understood. The name *cervical root resorption* implies that the resorption must occur at the cervical area of the tooth. However, the periodontal attachment of teeth is not always at the cervical margin, leading to the same process occurring more apically on the root surface. The anatomic connotation of its name has led to confusion and misdiagnosis of this condition. Be-

cause of this confusion, many attempts have been made to rename this type of external resorption.[19,49,57]

Etiology

Since in its histologic appearance and progressive nature cervical root resorption is identical to other forms of progressive inflammatory root resorption, it appears logical that the pathogenesis would be the same (i.e., an unprotected or altered root surface attracting resorbing cells and an inflammatory response maintained by infection). Cervical root resorption can occur long after orthodontic tooth movement (Fig. 16-28), orthognathic surgery, periodontal treatment, or nonvital bleaching or trauma (Fig. 16-29).[64,148] It is assumed that these procedures are the cause of the denudation or alteration of the root surface immediately below the epithelial attachment of the tooth. *The pulp plays no role in cervical root resorption and is mostly normal in these cases.* Because the source of stimulation (infection) is not the pulp, it has been postulated that bacteria in the sulcus of the tooth stimulate and sustain an in-

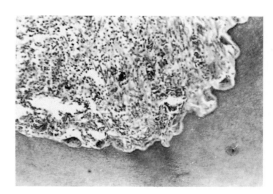

FIG. 16-26 Histologic appearance of inflammatory resorption. Granulomatous tissue in relation to the resorbed root surface. Multinucleated giant cells are present in the areas of active resorption on the root surface. Stain H & E. *(Courtesy Dr. Leif Tronstad.)*

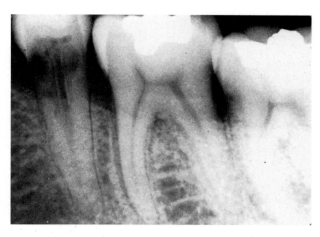

FIG. 16-28 Cervical root resorption on mandibular bicuspid 6 years after completion of orthodontic treatment. Note the mottled appearance of the resorptive defect and the outline of the root canal within the defect.

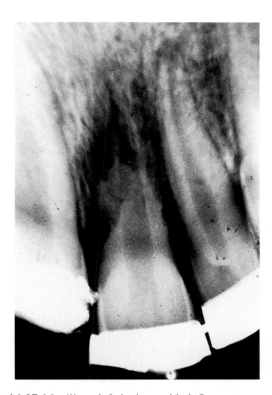

FIG. 16-27 Maxillary left incisor with inflammatory resorption 3 months after replantation without appropriate endodontic treatment. Resorption of the root and bone is apparent. Original root canal can still be traced radiographically.

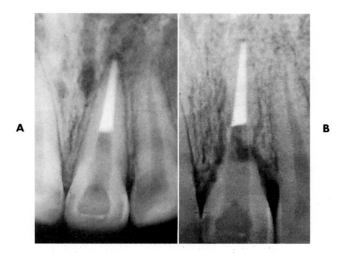

FIG. 16-29 A, Maxillary incisor after completion of root canal therapy and immediate bleaching procedure. **B,** Sixteen-month follow-up showing severe cervical root resorption. *(Courtesy Drs. William Goon and Stephen Cohen.)*

flammatory response in the periodontium at the attachment level of the root.[57,148] The delayed nature (sometimes by many years) of this type of resorption is difficult to explain. It is possible that the inflammatory process does not reach the damaged root surface initially, and that only after years, with eruption of the tooth or periodontal recession, are the chemotactic factors of inflammation close enough to attract resorbing cells to the appropriate root surface. It would seem logical, how-

ever, that if a stimulus were not present immediately after the injury to the root surface, repair would take place and the root surface would no longer be susceptible to resorption. An alternate theory is that the procedures mentioned above cause alteration in the ratio of organic and inorganic cementum,[126] making it relatively more inorganic and less resistant to resorption when challenged by inflammation. Also it has been speculated that the altered root surface registers in the immune system as a different tissue and is attacked as a foreign body.[85] Thus these root surfaces do not possess their original antiresorptive properties on healing and would be susceptible to resorption at all times. When, owing to periodontal recession or tooth eruption, the inflammation in the sulcular gingival area reaches the altered root surface, resorption takes place. Quite clearly, the *pathogenesis of cervical root resorption is not yet fully understood* and further research is required in this area.

Clinical manifestations

Cervical root resorption is asymptomatic and usually is detected only through routine radiographs. As mentioned, the pulp is not involved in this type of resorption, and sensitivity test results would be within normal limits. On occasion if the pulp is exposed by an extensive resorptive defect, abnormal sensitivity to thermal stimuli might be experienced; however, pain to percussion and palpation is not to be expected. The resorption starts on the root surface; but when the predentin is reached, the resorptive process is resisted and the resorption

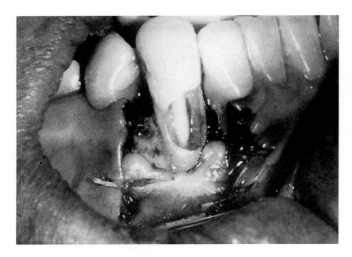

FIG. 16-30 Mandibular canine after removal of granulation tissue of a cervical resorption defect. Note the extensive nature of the defect in the dentin, but the root canal remains intact. *(Courtesy Dr. Henry Rankow.)*

proceeds laterally and in an apical and coronal direction, to envelop the root canal (Fig. 16-30). When cervical root resorption is of long standing, the granulation tissue can be seen undermining the enamel of the crown of the tooth, giving it a pinkish appearance (Fig. 16-31). This "pink spot" has traditionally been used to describe the pathognomonic clinical picture of internal root resorption, resulting in many cervical root resorption cases being misdiagnosed and treated as internal root resorption.

Since as with other inflammatory type of resorptions adjacent bone is resorbed as well as root and in this type of resorption the bone loss is below the epithelial attachment, cervical root resorption is commonly misdiagnosed as an infrabony pocket of periodontal origin. However, when the "pocket" is probed, copious bleeding and a spongelike feeling are observed when the granulation tissue of the resorptive defect is disturbed.

Radiographic appearance

The radiographic appearance of cervical root resorption can be quite variable. If the resorptive process occurs mesially or distally on the root surface, it is common to see a small radiolucent opening into the root. The radiolucency expands coronally and apically in the dentin, and reaches but usually does not perforate the root canal (Fig. 16-32). If the resorptive process is buccal or palatolingual, the radiographic picture is dependent on the extent to which the resorptive process has spread in the dentin. Initially a radiolucency near the attachment level (cervical margin) would be seen. However, if the process is long standing and extensive, the radiolucent area can extend a considerable way in a coronal and apical direction. The resorption site might have a mottled appearance owing to deposition of calcified reparative tissue within the resorptive lesion (see Fig. 16-28).[133] Because the pulp in the root canal

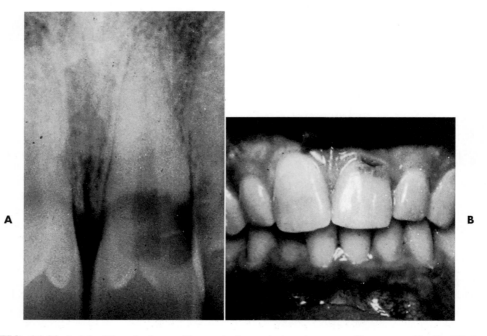

FIG. 16-31 A, Maxillary incisor with cervical root resorption extending coronally. **B,** Clinical appearance shows a pink spot on the labial surface of the tooth, close to the gingival margin.

is not involved in this type of resorption, it is usually possible to clearly distinguish the outline of the canal through the radiolucency of the external resorptive defect (see Figs. 16-28, 16-29, 16-31, and 16-32).

Histologic appearance

The histologic appearance of cervical root resorption is similar to that of other types of inflammatory root resorption (i.e., chronic inflammation and multinucleated resorbing cells). Also it is very common to see histologic evidence of attempts at repair by cementum-like and bonelike material. Union of bone and dentin (replacement resorption) sometimes occurs.

Internal Root Resorption

Internal root resorption is *rare* in permanent teeth. Internal resorption is characterized by an oval-shaped enlargement of the root canal space.[14] External resorption, which is much more common, is often misdiagnosed as internal resorption.

Etiology

Internal root resorption is characterized by resorption of the internal aspect of the root by multinucleated giant cells adjacent to granulation tissue in the pulp (Fig. 16-33). Chronic inflammatory tissue is common in the pulp, but only rarely does it result in resorption. There are different theories on the origin of the pulpal granulation tissue involved in internal resorption. The most logical explanation is that it is pulp tissue that is inflamed owing to an infected coronal pulp space. Communication between the coronal necrotic tissue and the vital pulp is through appropriately oriented dentinal tubules (Fig. 16-34).[147,158] One investigator[140] reported that resorption of the dentin is frequently associated with deposition of hard tissue resembling bone or cementum and not dentin. He postulated that the resorbing tissue is not of pulpal origin but is "metaplastic" tissue derived from the pulpal invasion of macrophage-like cells.[62] Others[159] concluded that the pulp tissue was replaced by periodontium-like connective tissue when internal resorption was present. In addition to the requirement of the presence of granulation tissue, root resorp-

tion takes place only if the odontoblastic layer and predentin are lost or altered.[148,159] Reasons for the loss of predentin adjacent to the granulation tissue are not obvious. Trauma frequently has been suggested as a cause.[42,130] Some[158] report that trauma may be recognized as an initiating factor in internal resorption. They are divided into a transient type and a progressive type, the latter requiring continuous stimulation by infection. Another reason for the loss of predentin might be extreme heat produced when cutting on dentin without an adequate water spray. The heat presumably would destroy the predentin layer; if later the coronal aspect of the pulp became infected, the bacterial products could initiate the typical inflammation in conjunction with resorbing giant cells in the vital pulp adjacent to the denuded root surface. Internal root resorption has been produced experimentally by the application of diathermy.[58]

Clinical manifestations

Internal root resorption is usually asymptomatic and is first recognized clinically through routine radiographs. Pain may be a presenting symptom if perforation of the crown occurs and the metaplastic tissue is exposed to the oral fluids. For internal

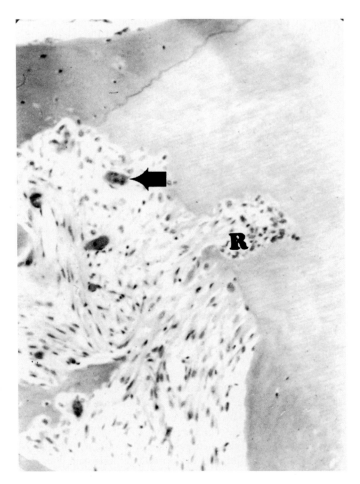

FIG. 16-33 Histologic appearance of internal resorption. Granulation tissue including multinucleated giant cells *(arrow)* is present. Resorptive lacunae *(R)* in dentin. Stain H & E. Original magnification ×100.) *(Courtesy Dr. Harold Stanley.)*

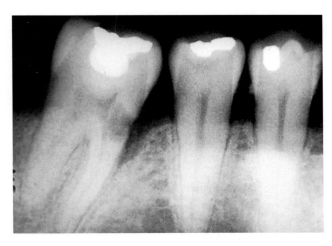

FIG. 16-32 Mandibular molar with cervical resorption on its mesial aspect. Note the small opening into the root, the extensive resorption in the dentin, but the pulp is not exposed. Also a resorptive defect is present in the adjacent bone, appearing radiographically similar to an infrabony pocket.

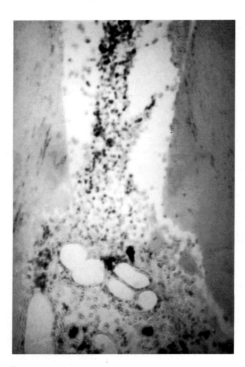

FIG. 16-34 Histologic section of internal resorption stained with Brown and Brenn. Bacteria are seen in the dentinal tubules communicating between the necrotic coronal segment and the apical granulation tissue and resorbing cells. *(Courtesy Dr. Leif Tronstad.)*

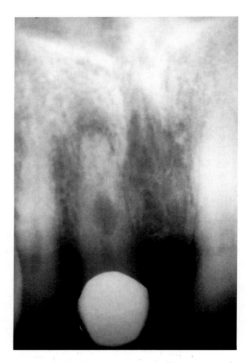

FIG. 16-35 Maxillary incisor with midroot radiolucency typical of internal resorption. Apical radiolucency is also present. Internal resorption must have occurred before the pulp became nonvital.

resorption to be active, at least part of the pulp must be vital, so that a positive response to pulp sensitivity testing is possible. It should be remembered that the coronal portion of the pulp is often necrotic, whereas the apical pulp, which includes the internal resorptive defect, can remain vital. Therefore a negative sensitivity test result does not rule out active internal resorption. It is also possible that the pulp becomes nonvital after a period of active resorption, giving a negative sensitivity test result, radiographic signs of internal resorption, and radiographic signs of apical inflammation (Fig. 16-35). Traditionally the pink tooth has been thought pathognomonic of internal root resorption. The pink color is due to the granulation tissue in the coronal dentin undermining the crown enamel. The pink tooth can also be a feature of cervical root resorption, which must be ruled out before a diagnosis of internal root resorption is made.

Radiographic appearance

Internal root resorption presents radiographically usually as a fairly uniform radiolucent enlargement of the pulp canal (Fig. 16-36). Because the resorption is initiated in the root canal, the resorptive defect includes some part of the root canal space. Therefore the original outline of the root canal is distorted. Only on rare occasions when the internal resorptive defect penetrates the root and impacts the periodontal ligament, does the adjacent bone show radiographic changes.

Histologic appearance

Like that of other inflammatory resorptive defects, the histologic picture of internal resorption is granulation tissue with multinucleated giant cells (see Fig. 16-33). An area of necrotic pulp is found coronal to the granulation tissue. Dentinal tu-

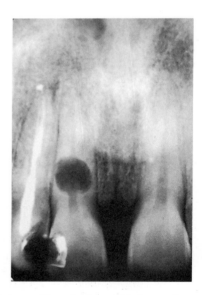

FIG. 16-36 A maxillary incisor with internal root resorption. Uniform enlargement of the pulp space is apparent. Outline of the canal cannot be seen in the resorptive defect.

bules containing microorganisms and communicating between the necrotic zone and the granulation tissue can sometimes be seen (see Fig. 16-34).* Unlike external root resorption, resorption of the adjacent bone does not occur with internal root resorption.

---

*References 148, 150, 151, 154, 157, 158.

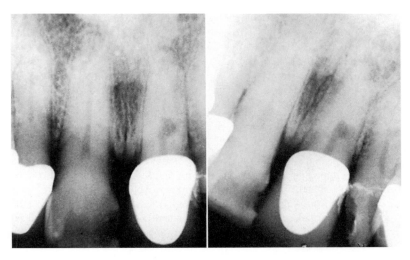

FIG. 16-37 Internal resorption. Radiographs from two different horizontal projections depict the lesion within the confines of the root canal on both views.

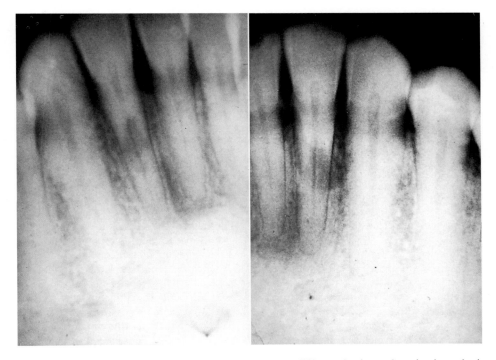

FIG. 16-38 External resorption. Radiographs from two different horizontal projections depict movement of the lesion to outside the confines of the root canal.

Diagnostic Features of External Versus Internal Root Resorption

Sometimes it is very difficult to distinguish external from internal root resorption, so misdiagnosis and incorrect treatment result. The following is a list of typical diagnostic features of each resorptive type.

Radiographic features

Films taken with a change of angulation of x-ray beams should give a fairly good indication of whether a resorptive defect is internal or external. A lesion of internal origin appears close to the canal whatever the angle of the x-ray (Fig. 16-37). On the other hand, a defect on the external aspect of

the root moves away from the canal as the angulation changes (Fig. 16-38). In addition, by using the buccal object rule it is usually possible to distinguish if the external root defect is buccal or linguopalatal.

In internal resorption the outline of the root canal is usually distorted, and the root canal and the radiolucent resorptive defect appear contiguous (see Figs. 16-36 and 16-37). When the defect is external, the root canal outline appears normal and can usually be seen "running through" the radiolucent defect (see Fig. 16-28).

External inflammatory root resorption is always accompanied by resorption of the bone as well (see Figs. 16-24 and 16-27). Therefore radiolucencies are apparent in the root and the adjacent bone. Internal root resorption does not involve the bone, and as a rule the radiolucency is confined to the root (see Figs. 16-35 and 16-36). On rare occasions if the internal defect perforates the root, the bone adjacent to it is resorbed and appears radiolucent on the radiograph.

Vitality testing

External inflammatory resorption in the apical and lateral aspects of the root involves an infected pulp space, so that a negative response to sensitivity tests is required to support the diagnosis. On the other hand, since cervical root resorption does not involve the pulp and the bacteria are thought to originate in the sulcus of the tooth, a normal response to sensitivity testing is usually associated with this type of resorption. Internal root resorption usually occurs in teeth with vital pulps and gives a positive response to sensitivity testing, although in teeth that exhibit internal root resorption it is not too uncommon to register a negative response to sensitivity testing, since often the coronal pulp has been removed or is necrotic and the active resorbing cells are more apical in the canal. Also the pulp might become necrotic after active resorption has taken place (see Fig. 16-35).

Pink spot

With apical and lateral external root resorption, the pulp is nonvital and therefore the granulation tissue that produces the pink spot is not present in these cases. For cervical and internal root resorption the pink spot due to the granulation tissue undermining the enamel is a possible sign.

Summary of Possible Diagnostic Features

Inflammatory root resorption

Apical. Negative pulp sensitivity test, with or without a history of trauma.

Lateral. History of trauma; negative pulp sensitivity test results; lesion "moves" on angled x-ray films; root canal visualized radiographically overlying the defect; bony radiolucency also apparent.

Cervical. History of trauma (often forgotten or not appreciated by the patient); positive pulp sensitivity test results; lesion located at the attachment level of the tooth; lesion "moves" on angled x-ray films; root canal outline is undistorted and can be visualized radiographically; crestal bony defect associated with the lesion; pink spot possible.

Internal. History of trauma, crown preparation, or pulpotomy; positive pulp sensitivity test results likely; lesion may occur at any location along the root canal (not only attachment level); lesion stays associated with the root canal on angled x-ray films; radiolucency contained in the root without an adjacent bony defect; pink spot possible.

The majority of misdiagnoses of resorptive defects are made between cervical and internal root resorptions. The diagnosis should always be confirmed while treatment is proceeding. If root canal therapy is the treatment of choice for an apparent internal root resorption, the bleeding within the canal should cease quickly after pulp extirpation, since the blood supply of the granulation tissue is the apical blood vessels. If bleeding continues during treatment—and particularly if it is still present at the second visit—the source of the blood supply is external, and treatment for external resorption should be carried out. Also on obturation it should be possible to fill the entire canal from within in internal resorption. Failure to achieve this

should make the dentist suspicious of an external lesion. Finally, if the blood supply of an internal resorption defect is removed on pulp extirpation, any continuation of the resorptive process on recall radiographs should alert the dentist to the possibility that an external resorptive defect was misdiagnosed.

DIAGNOSIS OF LUXATION INJURIES AT THE EMERGENCY VISIT

Evaluation

Patients have a history of a recent traumatic injury, a varying degree of displacement of the tooth (based on which the injury is classified), and *pain to percussion.* A thorough history (medical and dental) must be taken and clinical assessment of the teeth must be made with particular emphasis on pain to percussion and mobility. Radiographic assessment (see Root Fracture earlier in this chapter) is extremely important to assess the extent of displacement if present and to assess the presence or absence of a root fracture.

Diagnosis and Emergency Treatment

Concussion

Diagnosis and clinical presentation. Concussion injuries present with no displacement or mobility of the tooth. Pain to percussion is the only presenting feature. A history of the recent traumatic injury, in addition to the pain to percussion, makes the diagnosis possible.

Treatment. Baseline sensitivity tests are performed. A possible root fracture must be ruled out with angled radiographs (see Root Fracture earlier in this chapter). The occlusion must be checked and adjusted if necessary. With concussion injuries as with other luxation injuries it is possible to have a negative response to sensitivity testing and also discoloration of the crown. *Endodontic treatment should not be carried out at this visit because both the sensitivity testing and crown discoloration can be reversible.*[4,5]

Follow-up. Schedule radiographic follow-up for 3 weeks, 3 months, 6 months, 12 months, and yearly.

The major concern in follow-up examinations is the development of pulp necrosis. Sensitivity tests are performed, as are tests for periapical inflammation (i.e., percussion, palpation, and radiographic signs of apical periodontitis). Pulp necrosis has been reported to be discernible within 3 months.[5] Since concussion injuries are relatively minimal injuries in terms of attachment damage, a conservative approach is feasible if sensitivity test results are negative but no signs of apical periodontitis are present.

Subluxation

Diagnosis and clinical presentation. Clinical presentation of subluxation is similar to concussion. In addition, the tooth is slightly mobile and typically has clinical signs of sulcular bleeding (Fig. 16-39).

Treatment. As with concussion.

Follow-up. As with concussion.

Lateral luxation

Diagnosis and clinical presentation. History of a recent traumatic injury. The tooth is displaced laterally (usually the crown to the palatal direction), and sulcular bleeding is usually present. The tooth is usually extremely sensitive to percussion.

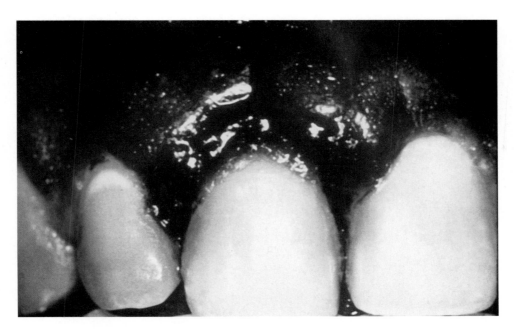

FIG. 16-39 Maxillary central incisor after luxation injury. Sulcular bleeding is an indication that the tooth was displaced in the socket.

Treatment. In most cases of lateral luxation the crown of the tooth is moved palatally and the apex facially (Fig. 16-40). Often the apical root is forced through the labial cortical plate, and the tooth is then frequently locked into its new position and difficult to dislodge. The tooth must be dislodged from the labial cortical plate by moving it coronally and then apically. This is performed as gently as possible by placing coronal and palatal pressure on the apical root with the index finger and labial pressure on the crown with the thumb (see Fig. 16-40). The tooth is thus moved first coronally out of the buccal plate of bone and "snaps back" into its original position. Local anesthetic is usually required for repositioning.

If the tooth is mobile after repositioning, it should be splinted with an acid-etched technique (see Avulsion and Replantation).

Sensitivity testing is of little value at this visit.

Follow-up

Mature tooth: Although pulp survival is possible in a small number of cases,[5] it is our opinion that if at the 3-week follow-up visit sensitivity testing indicates pulp necrosis, endodontic treatment should be performed. Root canal treatment of a noninfected pulp space has an extremely high success rate in a mature tooth[59,143] and in our opinion should be performed rather than risk external root resorption complications.

Immature tooth: Immature teeth present a dilemma. Chances of pulpal vitality (maintenance or revascularization) are fairly good. However, if necrosis and infection do occur, these teeth which have undergone cemental damage because of the traumatic injury are susceptible to inflammatory root resorption and could be lost in a short period of time. Careful follow-up is very important; at the first sign (clinical or radiographic) of apical or periradicular root resorption, endodontic treatment should be initiated (see Avulsion and Replantation). The laser Doppler flowmeter is a promising tool in the diagnosis of revascularization in these young teeth[104] (Fig. 16-41).

Extrusive luxation

Diagnosis and clinical presentation, treatment, and follow-up are essentially the same as with lateral luxations.

Intrusive luxation

Diagnosis and clinical presentation. The tooth may be pushed into its socket, sometimes even giving the appearance that it might have been avulsed (Fig. 16-42). The tooth presents with the clinical presentation of dentoalveolar ankylosis, since it is firm in the socket, gives a metallic sound to the percussion test, and after the injury is in infraocclusion. The obvious difference is the recent traumatic injury. Radiographic evaluation is essential to evaluate the extent and the position of the intruded tooth.

Treatment. Intrusive luxation is probably the most damaging injury that a tooth can sustain. The movement of the tooth into the socket results in extensive attachment damage, with resultant dentoalveolar ankylosis and replacement resorption almost a certainty. In addition, pulp necrosis is extremely common so that inflammatory root resorption will result if timely and adequate endodontic treatment is not performed.

Initial treatment depends on the stage of development of the tooth. Immature teeth usually reerupt spontaneously and establish their original position within a few weeks or months.[74] If reeruption stops before normal occlusion is attained, orthodontic movement should be initiated quickly before the tooth is ankylosed in position (Fig. 16-43). Intruded mature teeth must be repositioned immediately as not to ankylose in the intruded position.[14] If an orthodontic appliance can be attached to the tooth, orthodontic repositioning is favored. If the tooth is severely intruded, surgical access can be made to attach an orthodontic appliance or the tooth can be repositioned by loosening it surgically and immediately repositioning it into alignment with the adjacent teeth.

Endodontic treatment protocols are similar to those for an avulsed tooth (see Avulsion and Replantation).

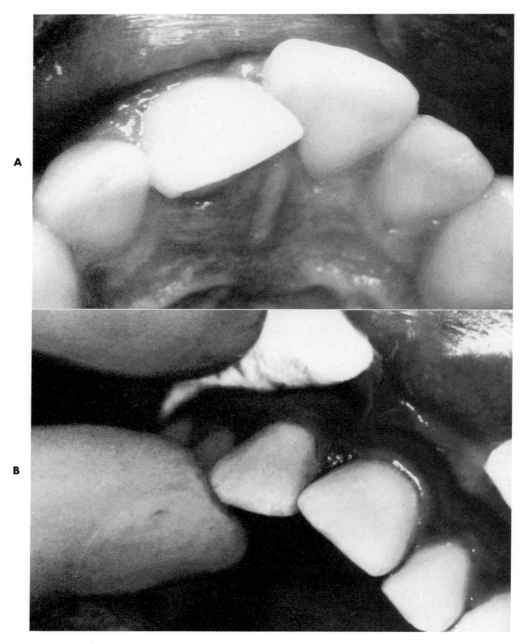

FIG. 16-40 Lateral luxation of maxillary central incisor. **A,** Crown is moved palatally and the root apex facially. **B,** Tooth is moved coronally out of the buccal plate with the index finger and facially with the thumb.

Prognosis of Luxation Injuries

Pulp necrosis

Pulp necrosis is common after luxation injuries. Even a sub-luxation injury that appears to be a minimal injury results in pulp necrosis in the range of 12% to 20% of cases.[95,139] For lateral or extrusive luxations over half of the pulps eventually necrose.[11,75,125,139] Intrusive injuries result in an extremely high incidence of necrosis. Infection of the necrotic pulp takes place after a variable amount of time. Therefore signs of apical periodontitis including pain to percussion can take months or even years.[75]

Pulp canal obliteration

Pulp canal obliteration is a fairly common occurrence in luxated teeth.[11,95,127] Endodontic treatment is *not* routinely indicated in the teeth (see Biologic Consequences).

Root resorption

Root resorption occurs in 5% to 15% of luxation injuries.[95,111,139] Inflammatory root resorption can be treated with a high degree of success with adequate endodontic therapy.[35] However, dentoalveolar ankylosis is irreversible with the methods that are available today so that when it

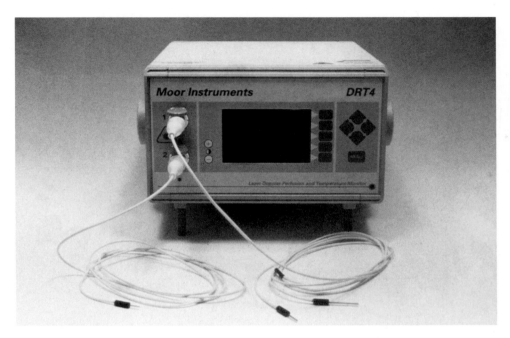

FIG. 16-41 Laser Doppler flowmeter used in the diagnosis of revascularization in luxated and avulsed immature teeth. *(See Mesaros S, Trope M:* Endodont Dent Traumatol *13:1, 24-30, 1997.)*

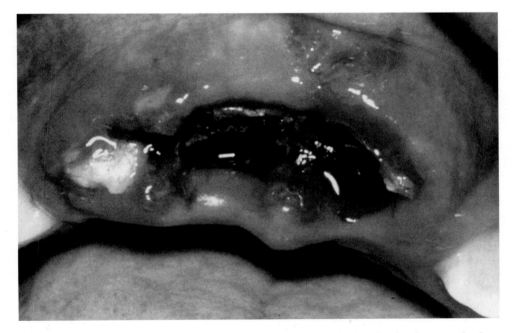

FIG. 16-42 Severely intruded maxillary incisor teeth mistaken as having been avulsed.

occurs, a long-term treatment plan for the ultimate loss of the tooth must be made.

AVULSION AND REPLANTATION

Avulsion (Exarticulation): Complete displacement of the tooth out of the socket.

Incidence

The reported incidence of tooth avulsion ranges from 1% to 16% of all traumatic injuries to the permanent dentition.[47] Like most dental trauma, maxillary central incisors are the most frequently avulsed teeth in the permanent dentition.[47] Sports and automobile accidents are the most frequent causes,[65] and the most frequently involved age group is 7 to 10 years.[15]

Biologic Consequences

The biologic consequences of tooth avulsion are the same as described for tooth luxation. In addition, the drying damage to the periodontal ligament when the tooth is out of the mouth has extremely detrimental effects on healing. Pulp necrosis al-

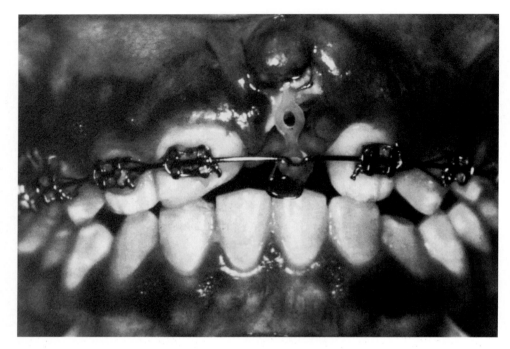

FIG. 16-43 Intruded maxillary incisor is to be orthodontically moved into position soon after the injury. If treatment is delayed, the tooth will be ankylosed in the intruded position.

ways occurs after an avulsion injury, but revascularization can only take place in teeth with immature apexes. Therefore complications after avulsion injuries are common, and treatment must be carried out in a timely and correct fashion to prevent or limit these complications.

Treatment Objectives

Treatment is directed at avoiding or minimizing the effects of the two main complications of the avulsed tooth, namely attachment damage and pulpal infection. Attachment damage as a direct result of the avulsion injury cannot be avoided. However, considerable additional damage can occur to the periodontal membrane in the time that the tooth is out of the mouth (primarily because of drying). Treatment is directed at minimizing this damage so that the fewest possible complications result. When severe additional damage has occurred and replacement resorption is considered certain, steps are taken to slow the resorptive process to maintain the tooth in the mouth for as long as possible. In the open apex tooth, all efforts are made to promote revascularization of the pulp. In the closed apex tooth or in the open apex tooth in which revascularization is unsuccessful, all treatment efforts are made to eliminate potential toxins from the root canal space.

Clinical Management

Management outside the dental office

The damage to the attachment apparatus that occurred during the initial injury is unavoidable. However, all efforts are made to minimize necrosis of the remaining periodontal ligament while the tooth is out of the mouth. Pulpal sequelae are not a concern initially and are dealt with at a later stage of treatment.

The single most important factor in the success of replantation is the *speed* with which the tooth is replanted.[13,14] Of ut-

most importance is the prevention of drying, which causes loss of normal physiologic metabolism and morphology of the periodontal ligament cells.[17,137] Every effort should be made to replant the tooth within the first 15 to 20 minutes.[13,15] This usually requires emergency personnel with experience in this type of injury. Careful instructions to the person at the scene of the accident should be given by the dentist over the phone. A clean tooth with an undamaged root should be replanted as atraumatically as possible. The person should be instructed to hold the tooth by the crown, wash the root gently (but not excessively) in running water or saline, and place it back in the socket as atraumatically as possible. The patient should be brought to the office immediately. If doubt exists that the tooth can be replanted adequately, the tooth should quickly be stored in an appropriate medium until the patient can get to the dental office for replantation. Suggested storage media include the vestibule of the mouth, physiologic saline, milk, and cell culture media in specialized transport containers and water.[72] Water is the least desirable storage medium because the hypotonic environment causes rapid cell lysis.[25] The vestibule of the mouth (saliva) keeps the tooth moist but is not ideal because of incompatible osmolality and pH and the presence of bacteria.[88] However, saliva allows storage for up to 2 hours.[26] Milk is considered the best storage medium for uncomplicated avulsion because it is usually readily available at or near an accident site, it has a pH and osmolarity compatible to vital cells, and it is relatively free of bacteria. Milk effectively maintains the vitality of periodontal ligament cells for 3 hours, which usually allows adequate time for the patient to reach the dentist for replantation.[25] Cell culture media have also been tested as storage media for avulsed teeth and have great potential.[14] However, culture media are seldom available near the site of an accident, rendering their use impractical and of academic interest only.

Recently an avulsed-tooth preserving system (Save-A-

Tooth, 3M-Health Care, St. Paul, Minn.) that contains Hanks Balanced Salt Solution (HBSS) (Biologic Rescue Products, Conshohocken, Pa.), a pH-preserving fluid, and trauma-reducing suspension apparatus has become available and has many potential advantages (Fig. 16-44). This system could be available at schools and contact sport events, in ambulances and hospital emergency rooms, or even in the home. The system makes the use of a variety of storage media practical and enhances the possibility of maintaining the viability of the periodontal ligament cells for an extended time after avulsion. Thus teeth avulsed in serious accidents that relegate replantation to secondary importance might be stored in these devices and replanted after the crisis is over. Media applicable to this type of system extend the storage period significantly as compared with milk.[72,151]

Management in the dental office

Emergency visit. Recognizing that the dental injury might be secondary to a more serious injury is essential. If on examination a serious injury is suspected, immediate referral to the appropriate expert is the first priority. The focus of the emergency visit is the attachment apparatus. The aim is to replant the tooth with the maximal number of periodontal ligament cells that have the potential to regenerate and repair the damaged root surface. Necrotic and irreversibly damaged cells should be removed before replantation if possible. If maintaining the periodontal ligament in a viable state is not possible, steps are taken to alter the root so as to slow the inevitable resorption. The necrotic pulp is not of immediate concern because toxins are usually not present initially in a great enough concentration to elicit an inflammatory response. *Endodontic treatment is not initiated at the emergency visit and is not performed extraorally if any hope exists of the vital periodontal fibers on the root surface reattaching to the attachment apparatus.*

A medical history is extremely important and cannot be overlooked. The possible presence of a more serious trauma than the avulsion must be assessed, and obtaining a full history of the accident is essential. Reconstruction of the accident gives the dentist a good idea of the extent of the injury to the attachment apparatus and the likelihood of damage to other teeth or structures. Information about where the tooth was recovered, dry time, storage media, and mode of transportation of the patient and tooth is essential for formation of the correct treatment choices.

Local anesthesia is usually recommended for conductance of a thorough clinical examination. If the tooth was replanted at the accident site, its positioning in the socket is assessed. If the position is unacceptable, the tooth is gently removed and replanted after the obstruction to correct positioning has been rectified. If the tooth is positioned correctly, splinting, soft tissue management, and adjunctive therapy are the next steps in treatment.

The following clinical steps minimize root resorption when the tooth is not replanted at the accident site.

Diagnosis and treatment planning: The tooth should immediately be placed in an appropriate storage medium while a history of the accident is obtained and the clinical examination is conducted. Hanks Balanced Salt Solution is presently considered the best medium for this purpose. It is commercially available and has a shelf life of 2 years or more. Milk or physiologic saline is also appropriate for storage purposes. The clinical examination should include an examination of the socket

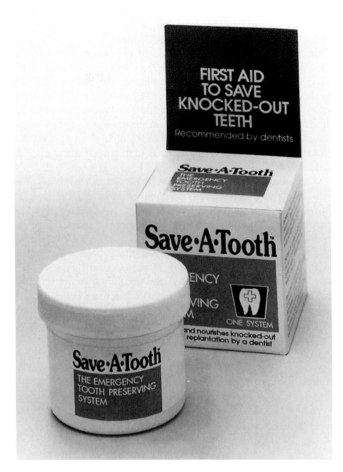

FIG. 16-44 Emergency Tooth Preserving System (Save-A-Tooth, 3M-Health Care, St. Paul, Minn.). Hanks Balanced Salt Solution (Biologic Rescue Products, Conshohocken, Pa.) within the system allows the tooth to be stored for an extended period. Internal net minimizes damage to the periodontal ligament during transportation.

to ascertain if it is intact and suitable for replantation. This is accomplished by palpation facially and palatally. The socket is gently rinsed with saline; when clear of the clot and debris, the socket is examined directly for the presence, absence, or collapse of the socket wall. Palpation of the socket and surrounding apical areas and pressure on surrounding teeth are used to ascertain if an alveolar fracture is present in addition to the avulsion. Movement of a segment of bone and multiple teeth is suggestive of an alveolar fracture. The socket and surrounding areas including the soft tissues should be radiographed.[14] Three vertical angulations are required for diagnosis of the presence of a horizontal root fracture in adjacent teeth. The remaining teeth in both jaws should be examined for crown fractures. Any soft tissue lacerations should be noted. *Sensitivity testing results at the emergency visit are always negative and therefore of limited value and should be delayed until the next visit.*

Preparation of the root

Extraoral dry time less than 20 minutes, closed apex: If the tooth has a closed apex, revitalization is not possible, but because the tooth was dry for less than 20 minutes (replanted or placed in appropriate medium), the chance for periodontal healing is excellent. The root should be rinsed of debris with water or saline and replanted in as gentle a fashion as possible.[14]

Extraoral dry time less than 20 minutes, open apex: In an open apex tooth, revascularization of the pulp and continued root development are possible (Fig. 16-45). In one study[38] revascularization was significantly enhanced by soaking the tooth in doxycycline (1 mg in approximately 10 ml of physiologic saline) for 5 minutes before replantation. The doxycycline inhibits bacteria in the pulpal lumen, thus removing the major obstacle to revascularization.[40,41] As with the tooth with the closed apex, the open apex tooth is then rinsed with water or saline and gently replanted.

Extraoral time 20 to 60 minutes, closed and open apexes: For drying periods of 20 to 60 minutes most authors suggest rinsing the tooth gently and replanting it as soon as possible, accepting that complications are inevitable. Previously an attempt was made to soak the tooth in saline for approximately 30 minutes before replantation with limited success.[100] The theory behind soaking is that dead periodontal ligament cells will wash off the root surface (thus removing a stimulus for inflammation on replantation) and the soaking medium might revitalize cells affected by the extended drying time. A recent study tested newer storage media for soaking of teeth left dry for between 20 and 60 minutes.[115] Although Hanks Balanced Salt Solution was not beneficial for healing after soaking, Via-Span, a liver transplant medium, did decrease the incidence of complications after replantation.[115] Although the results of this study do not yet justify the recommendation to soak such teeth, the newer media show promise that this might be a recommendation in the future.

Extraoral dry time greater than 60 minutes, open and closed apexes: When the root has been dry for 60 minutes or more, all periodontal cells have died[89,137,151] and soaking is ineffective.[100] In these cases the root should be prepared to be as resistant to resorption as possible (attempting to slow the process). These teeth should be soaked in citric acid for 5 minutes to remove all remaining periodontal ligament, in 2% stannous fluoride for 5 minutes, after which they are replanted.[24,132] If the tooth has been dry for more than 60 minutes and no consideration is given to preserving the periodontal ligament, the endodontic treatment could be performed extraorally. In the case of a tooth with a closed apex, no advantage exists to this additional step at the emergency visit. However, in a tooth with an open apex the endodontic treatment, if performed after replantation, involves a long-term apexification procedure. In these cases completing the root canal treatment extraorally, where a seal in the blunderbuss apex is easier to achieve, may be advantageous. When endodontic treatment is performed extraorally, it must be performed aseptically with the utmost care to achieve a root canal system that is free of bacteria.

Preparation of the socket: The socket should be left undisturbed before replantation.[63] Emphasis is placed on removal of obstacles within the socket to facilitate replacement of the tooth into the socket.[151] New evidence suggests that the envi-

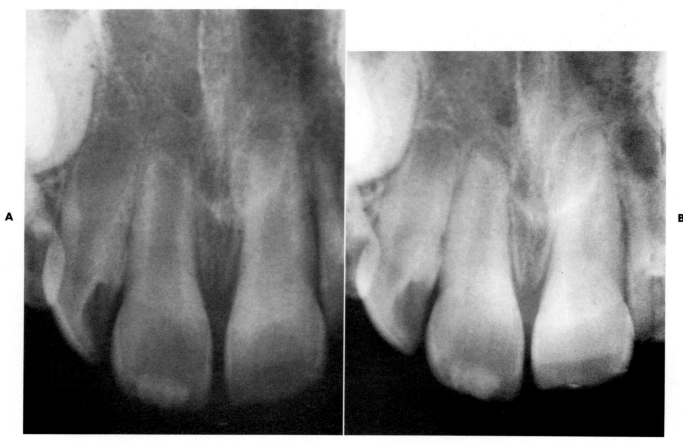

FIG. 16-45 Maxillary incisor with open apex that maintained vitality and continued root development after tooth replantation. **A,** Taken at the time of replantation. **B,** At the 2-year follow-up, the pulp is still vital and the root is fully formed. *(Courtesy Dr. Joe H. Camp.)*

ronment in the socket might change with time, contributing to the prognosis of the replantation.[151,152] These changes have yet to be defined, and no procedures for preparation of the socket can yet be suggested. It should be lightly aspirated if a blood clot is present. If the alveolar bone has collapsed and may prevent replantation or cause it to be traumatic, a blunt instrument should be inserted carefully into the socket in an attempt to reposition the wall.

Splinting: A splinting technique that allows physiologic movement of the tooth during healing and that is in place for a minimal time period results in a decreased incidence of dentoalveolar ankylosis.[3,14] Semirigid (physiologic) fixation for 7

to 10 days is recommended.[3,14] The splint should allow movement of the tooth, should have no memory (so the tooth is not moved during healing), and should not impinge on the gingiva or prevent maintenance of oral hygiene in the area. Many types of splints fulfill these requirements (Fig. 16-46, *A, B,* and *C*). The acid-etched resin and arch wire splint is probably the most commonly used splint for traumatic injuries (Fig. 16-47). A passive wire (size 0.015 to 0.030) is shaped to conform to the facial aspect of the avulsed tooth and one or two teeth on either side. The middle third of the facial surface of the teeth is acid etched, and light-cured composite resin is used to attach the wire to the teeth on either side of the affected tooth. When

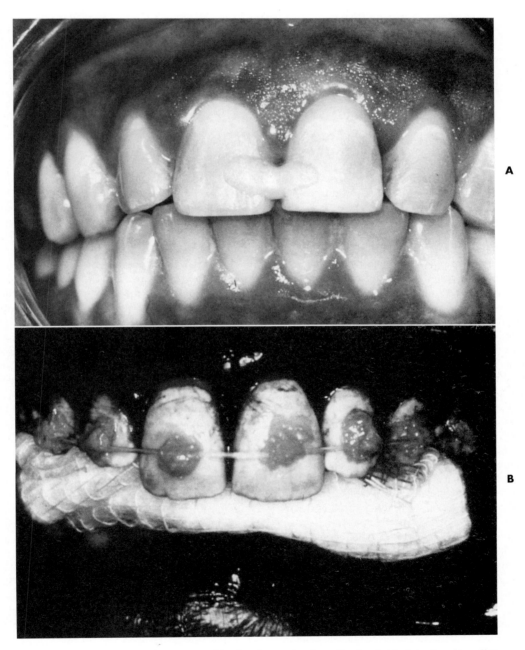

FIG. 16-46 Semirigid splints acceptable for the avulsed tooth. **A,** Acid-etched resin splint between the avulsed tooth and an adjacent tooth. Splint is constructed with resin only and should not extend further than two teeth without wire reinforcement. **B,** Long-span splint constructed with nylon fish line bonded to the teeth with acid-etched resin.

Continued

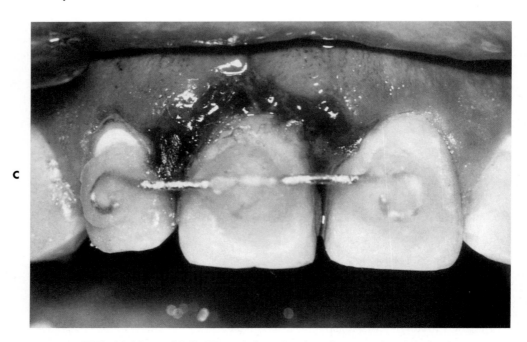

FIG. 16-46, cont'd C, Wire-reinforced resin splint spanning three teeth.

the wire is satisfactorily in place, the patient is asked to bite gently into a bite block (softened pink wax is useful) and gently force the avulsed tooth as far into the socket as possible. The avulsed tooth is then added to the splint with light-cured composite resin (see Fig. 16-47). After the splint is in place, a radiograph should be taken to verify the positioning of the tooth and as a preoperative reference for further treatment and follow-up. When the tooth is in the best possible position, adjusting the bite to ensure that it has not been splinted in a position causing traumatic occlusion is important. One week is sufficient to create periodontal support to maintain the avulsed tooth in position.[14] Therefore the splint should be removed after 7 to 10 days. The only exception is with avulsion in conjunction with alveolar fractures, for which 4 to 8 weeks is the suggested time of splinting.[14]

Management of soft tissues: Soft tissue lacerations of the socket gingiva should be tightly sutured. Lacerations of the lip are fairly common with these types of injuries. The dentist should approach lip lacerations with some caution, and a consultation with a plastic surgeon might be prudent. If these lacerations are sutured, care must be taken to clean the wound thoroughly beforehand because dirt or even minute tooth fragments left in the wound affect healing and the aesthetic result.

Adjunctive therapy: Systemic antibiotics given at the time of replantation and before endodontic treatment are effective in preventing bacterial invasion of the necrotic pulp and therefore subsequent inflammatory resorption.[63] The administration of system antibiotics (penicillin V potassium, 500 mg four times daily or equivalent child dose or alternate antibiotic) is recommended beginning at the emergency visit and continuing until the splint is removed (in 7 to 10 days). The bacterial content of the sulcus also should be controlled during the healing phase. In addition to stressing the need for adequate oral hygiene to the patient, the use of chlorhexidine rinses for 7 to 10 days may be useful. The chlorhexidine rinses assist the patient in maintaining good oral hygiene in the initial stages when the tooth is still painful because of the trauma and the splint is

in place, which makes adequate brushing and flossing difficult. The need for analgesics should be assessed on an individual case basis. The use of pain medication stronger than nonprescription, nonsteroidal antiinflammatory drugs is unusual. *The patient should be sent to a physician for consultation regarding a tetanus booster within 48 hours of the initial visit.*

Second visit. The second visit should take place 7 to 10 days after the emergency visit. At the emergency visit, emphasis was placed on the preservation and healing of the attachment apparatus. The focus of this visit is the prevention or elimination of potential irritants from the root canal space. These irritants, if present, provide the stimulus for the progression of the inflammatory response and bone and root resorption. Also at this visit, the course of systemic antibiotics is completed, the chlorhexidine rinses can be stopped, and the splint is removed.

Endodontic treatment

Tooth with an open apex and less than 60 minutes extraoral dry time: Teeth with open apexes have the potential to revascularize and continue root development, and initial treatment is directed toward reestablishment of the blood supply[136] (see Fig. 16-45). Even when a traumatic injury has not occurred, the assessment of a necrotic pulp in young teeth is difficult with the sensitivity methods currently available.[52,53] The addition of traumatic injury in these immature teeth is an especially difficult diagnostic problem.[110] After trauma, diagnosis of a necrotic pulp is particularly desirable because infection in these teeth is potentially more harmful because of cemental damage accompanying the traumatic injury. Inflammatory root resorption can be extremely rapid in these young teeth because the tubules are wide and allow the irritants to move freely to the external surface of the root.[14]

Patients are recalled every 3 to 4 weeks for sensitivity testing. Recent reports indicate that thermal tests with carbon dioxide snow ($-108.4°$ F, $-78°$ C) or difluordichlormethane ($-58°$ F, $-50°$ C) placed at the incisal edge or pulp horn are the best methods for sensitivity testing, particularly in young

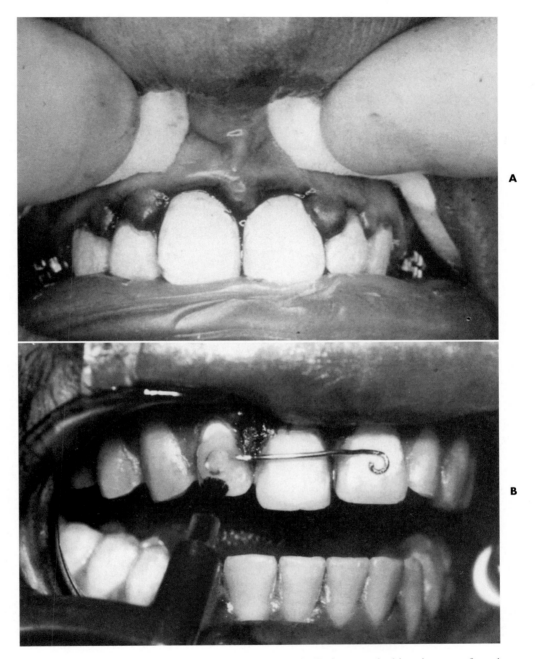

FIG. 16-47 Acid-etched resin and arch wire splint. **A,** Patient gently bites into a softened block of pink wax to assure that the avulsed tooth can be replaced close to its original position. **B,** Passive wire is shaped to conform to the facial aspect of the avulsed tooth, as well as a tooth on either side of it. Middle third of the tooth crown is acid etched, and light-cured composite resin attaches the wire to the adjacent teeth.   *Continued*

permanent teeth[52] (Fig. 16-48). One of these two tests must be included in the sensitivity testing of these traumatized teeth. Radiographic (apical breakdown or signs of lateral root resorption) and clinical (pain to percussion and palpation) signs of pathosis are carefully assessed. At the first sign of pathosis endodontic treatment should be initiated, and after disinfection of the root canal space an apexification procedure should be carried out.

Tooth with an open apex and extraoral dry time of more than 60 minutes: In these teeth the chance of revascularization is extremely poor.[13,154] Therefore no attempt is made to

revitalize these teeth. An apexification procedure is initiated at the second visit if root canal treatment was not performed at the emergency visit. If endodontic treatment was performed at the emergency visit, the second visit is a recall visit to assess initial healing only.

Tooth with a closed apex: No chance exists for revascularization of teeth with a closed apex, and endodontic treatment should be initiated at the second visit at 7 to 10 days after the injury.[14,40] If therapy is initiated at this optimal time, the pulp should be ischemically necrosed without infection or at most only minimal infection.[51,91,155] Therefore endodontic therapy

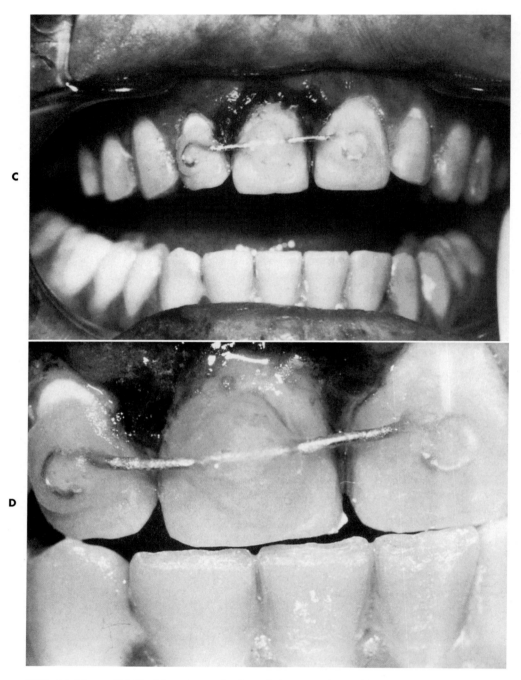

FIG. 16-47, cont'd C, After the avulsed tooth is correctly positioned by the patient again biting into the pink wax, it is added to the splint with light-cured composite resin. **D,** Position of the avulsed tooth and the occlusal adjustment is carefully checked to eliminate the possibility of additional trauma to the tooth during function.

with an effective interappointment antibacterial agent[29] over a relatively short period (7 to 30 days) is sufficient to ensure effective disinfection of the canal.[134] If the dentist is confident of complete patient cooperation, long-term therapy with calcium hydroxide remains an excellent treatment method.[148,155] The advantage of its use is that it allows the dentist to have a temporary obturating material in place until an intact periodontal ligament space is confirmed. Long-term calcium hydroxide treatment should always be used when the injury occurred more than 2 weeks before initiation of the endodontic treat-

ment or if radiographic evidence of resorption is present.[112,155]

The root canal is thoroughly instrumented and irrigated and then filled with a thick (powdery) mix of calcium hydroxide and sterile saline (anesthetic solution is also an acceptable vehicle). The calcium hydroxide is changed every 3 months within a range of 6 to 24 months. The canal is obturated when a radiographically intact periodontal membrane can be demonstrated around the root (Fig. 16-49). Calcium hydroxide is an effective antibacterial agent[29,134] and favorably influences the local environment at the resorption site, theoretically pro-

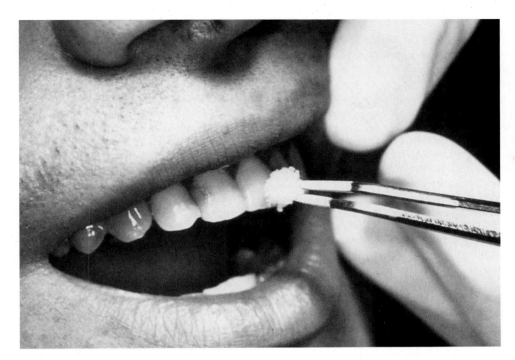

FIG. 16-48 Sensitivity test of previously avulsed tooth. Cotton pellet sprayed with dichlorodifluoromethane (−58° F, −50° C) was placed on the incisal edge of maxillary incisor tooth.

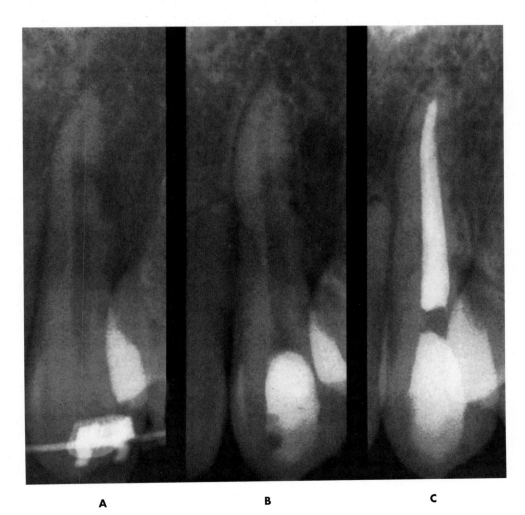

A   B   C

FIG. 16-49 A, Active resorption is seen soon after the tooth was replanted. **B,** After long-term calcium hydroxide treatment the resorptive defects have healed, and an intact lamina dura can be traced around the root. **C,** Tooth is obturated.

moting healing.[150] It also changes the environment in the dentin to a more alkaline pH, which may slow the action of the resorptive cells and promote hard tissue formation.[150] However, the changing of the calcium hydroxide should be kept to a minimum (not more than every 3 months) because it has a necrotizing effect on the cells attempting to repopulate the damaged root surface.[86]

Although calcium hydroxide is considered the drug of choice in the prevention and treatment of inflammatory root resorption, it is not the only medicament recommended in these cases. Some attempts have been made not only to remove the stimulus for the resorbing cells but also to affect them directly. The antibiotic-corticosteroid paste Ledermix is effective in treating inflammatory root resorption by inhibiting the spread of dentinoclasts[117,118] without damaging the periodontal ligament. Its ability to diffuse through human tooth roots has been demonstrated.[1] Its release and diffusion is enhanced when used in combination with calcium hydroxide paste.[2] Calcitonin, a hormone that inhibits osteoclastic bone resorption, also is an effective medication in the treatment of inflammatory root resorption.[116]

Temporary restoration: Effectively sealing the coronal access is essential to prevent infection of the canal between visits. Recommended temporary restorations are reinforced zinc oxide–eugenol cement, acid-etched composite resin, or glass-ionomer cement.[161] The depth of the temporary restoration is critical to its sealability. A depth of at least 4 mm is recommended so that a cotton pellet cannot be placed; the temporary restoration is placed directly onto the calcium hydroxide in the access cavity.[106] Calcium hydroxide should first be removed from the walls of the access cavity because it is soluble and washes out when it comes into contact with saliva, leaving a defective temporary restoration.

After initiation of the root canal treatment, the splint is removed. If time does not permit complete removal of the splint at this visit, the resin tacks are smoothed so as not to irritate the soft tissues and the residual resin is removed at a later appointment.

At this appointment, healing is usually sufficient to perform a detailed clinical examination on the teeth surrounding the avulsed tooth. The sensitivity tests, reaction to percussion and palpation, and periodontal probing measurements should be carefully recorded for reference at follow-up visits.

Obturation visit. The obturation visit occurs 7 to 14 days after the second visit or, in the case of long-term calcium hydroxide therapy, when an intact lamina dura is traced (see Fig. 16-49).

If the endodontic treatment was initiated 7 to 10 days after the avulsion and clinical and radiographic examinations do not indicate pathosis, obturation of the root canal at this visit is acceptable,[154,155] although the use of long-term calcium hydroxide is a proven option for these cases.[148,155] The canal is reinstrumented and irrigated under strict asepsis. After completion of the instrumentation the canal can be obturated by any acceptable technique, with special attention to an aseptic technique and the best possible seal of the obturating material.

Permanent restoration. Much evidence exists that coronal leakage caused by defective temporary and permanent restorations results in a clinically relevant amount of bacterial contamination of the root canal after obturation.[97,124] Therefore the tooth should receive a permanent restoration at or soon after the time of obturation of the root canal. As with the temporary restoration, the depth of restoration is important for its seal, and therefore the deepest restoration possible should be made. A post should be avoided if possible.

Because most avulsions occur in the anterior region of the mouth where aesthetic considerations are important, composite resins with the addition of dentin bonding agents are usually recommended in these cases. They have the additional advantage of internally strengthening the tooth against fracture if another trauma should occur.[70]

Follow-up. Follow-up should continue every 6 months for 5 years and yearly for as long as possible. Follow-up of avulsion cases after completion of the obturation of the canal is extremely important. If replacement resorption is identified (see Fig. 16-22), timely revision of the long-term treatment plan is indicated. In the case of inflammatory root resorption (Fig. 16-50), a new attempt at disinfection of the root canal space by standard retreatment can reverse the process. Teeth adjacent to and surrounding the avulsed tooth or teeth may show pathologic changes long after the initial accident. Therefore these teeth should be tested at recall and the results compared to those collected soon after the accident.

Summary of Treatment of the Avulsed Tooth

Management outside the dental office

Replant immediately after gentle washing if practical

If replantation is not practical, store the tooth in the best medium available.

Storage media in order of preference are Hank's Balanced Salt Solution, milk, saline, and saliva (buccal vestibule).

Water is the least desirable storage medium.

Management in the dental office

Emergency visit

Place tooth in Hank's Balanced Salt Solution while examination is conducted and history is taken.

Prepare socket for gentle repositioning of the tooth.

Prepare the root.

Extraoral dry time less than 20 minutes: Closed apex—replant immediately after gentle washing. Open apex—soak in 1 mg doxycycline in 20 mg saline for 5 minutes.

Extraoral dry time 20 to 60 minutes: Replant.

Extraoral dry time more than 60 minutes: Soak in citric acid, fluoride gel, and replant. Endodontics can be done extraorally.

Semirigid splint for 7 to 10 days. (If alveolar fracture is present, rigid splint for 4 to 8 weeks.) Suture soft tissue lacerations, particularly in the cervical area.

Administer systemic antibiotics (penicillin V potassium if possible).

Chlorhexidine rinses and stringent oral hygiene while the splint is in place (7 to 10 days).

Nonsteroidal antiinflammatory drug analgesics as required.

Second visit after 7 to 10 days

Endodontic treatment

Tooth with open apex and extraoral dry time less than 60 minutes: No endodontic treatment initially. Recall every 3 to 4 weeks to examine for evidence of pathosis. If pathosis is noted, disinfect the pulp space and start apexification procedure.

Tooth with open apex and extraoral dry time more than 60

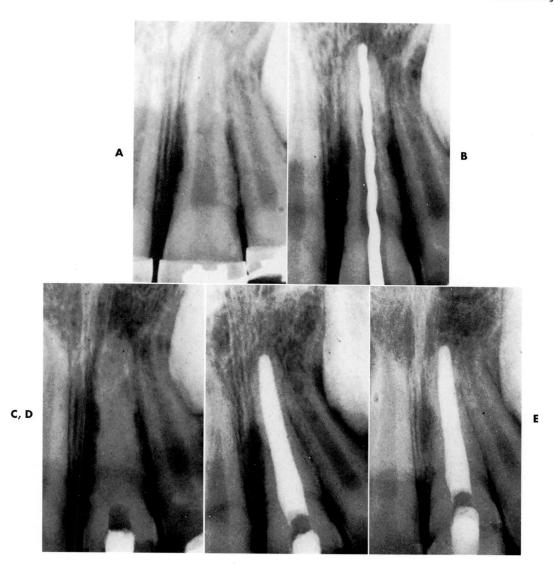

FIG. 16-50 Long-term calcium hydroxide therapy of lateral inflammatory root resorption. **A,** Maxillary central incisor shows radiographic signs of root resorption 1 month after a severe luxation injury. Sensitivity test result is negative. **B,** Root canal therapy is initiated. **C,** Thick mix of calcium hydroxide and anesthetic solution is packed into the canal. **D,** Nine-month recall. Resorption has abated, and there is evidence of bone regeneration. Canal is obturated. **E,** One-year recall. Continued healing is apparent.

minutes: If endodontic treatment was not completed in the emergency visit, start endodontic treatment and follow apexification procedure.

Tooth with closed apex: Endodontic treatment should be initiated after 7 to 10 days. Careful chemomechanical instrumentation under strict asepsis.

Splint removed *at end* of visit.

Obturation visit

If endodontic treatment was initiated 7 to 10 days after the avulsion, obturation can take place after short-term calcium hydroxide treatment.

If endodontic treatment was initiated more than 14 days after the avulsion or inflammatory resorption, long-term calcium hydroxide for 6 to 24 months, obturated when an intact lamina dura is traced.

Temporary restorations: Should be 4 mm deep. Reinforced zinc oxide–eugenol, acid-etched composite resin, glass-ionomer cement.

Permanent restoration: Placed immediately after obturation. Acid-etched resin and dentin bonding agents.

Follow-up

Twice per year for 5 years and yearly for as long as possible.

Late complications are common.

REFERENCES

1. Abbott PV, Heithersay GS, Hume WR: Release and diffusion through human tooth roots in vitro of corticosteroid and tetracycline trace molecules from Ledermix paste, *Endodont Dent Traumatol* 4:55-62, 1988.

2. Abbott PV, Hume WR, Heithersay GS: Effects of combining Leder-mix and calcium hydroxide pastes on the diffusion of corticosteroid and tetracycline through human roots in vitro, *Endodont Dent Traumatol* 5:188-192, 1989.

3. Andersson L, Friskopp J, Blomlof L: Fiber-glass splinting of traumatized teeth, *ASDC J Dent Child* 3:21, 1983.

4. Andreasen FM: Transient apical breakdown and its relation to color and sensibility changes, *Endodont Dent Traumatol* 2:9, 1986.

5. Andreasen FM: *Pulpal healing after tooth luxation and root fractures in the permanent dentition,* Thesis, Denmark, 1995, University of Copenhagen.

6. Andreasen FM, Andreasen JO: Resorption and mineralization processes following root fracture of permanent incisors, *Endodont Dent Traumatol* 4:202, 1988.

7. Andreasen FM, Andreasen JO, Bayer T: Prognosis of root-fractured permanent incisors: prediction of healing modalities, *Endodont Dent Traumatol* 5:11, 1989.

8. Andreasen FM, Vestergaard Pedersen B: Prognosis of luxated permanent teeth: the development of pulp necrosis, *Endodont Dent Traumatol* 1:207, 1985.

9. Andreasen FM et al: The occurrence of pulp canal obliteration after luxation injuries in the permanent dentition, *Endodont Dent Traumatol* 3:103, 1987.

10. Andreasen JO: Etiology and pathogenesis of traumatic dental injuries, *Scand J Dent Res* 78:329, 1970.

11. Andreasen JO: Luxation of permanent teeth due to trauma: a clinical and radiographic follow-up of 189 injured teeth, *Scand J Dent Res* 78:273, 1970.

12. Andreasen JO: Periodontal healing after replantation of traumatically avulsed human teeth: assessment by mobility testing and radiography, *Acta Odontol Scand* 33:325, 1975.

13. Andreasen JO: The effect of extra-alveolar period and storage media upon periodontal and pulpal healing after replantation of mature permanent incisors in monkeys, *Int J Oral Surg* 10:43, 1981.

14. Andreasen JO, Andreasen FM: *Textbook and color atlas of traumatic injuries to the teeth,* ed 3, Copenhagen and St Louis, 1994, Munksgaard and Mosby.

15. Andreasen JO, Hjorting-Hansen E: Replantation of teeth. I. Radiographic and clinical study of 110 human teeth replanted after accidental loss, *Acta Odontol Scand* 24:263, 1966.

16. Andreasen JO, Hjorting-Hansen E: Intra-alveolar root fractures: radiographic and histologic study of 50 cases, *J Oral Surg* 25:414, 1967.

17. Andreasen JO, Kristersson L: The effect of limited drying or removal of the periodontal ligament: periodontal healing after replantation of mature permanent incisors in monkeys, *Acta Odontol Scand* 39:1, 1981.

18. Andreasen JO, Ravn JJ: Epidemiology of traumatic dental injuries to primary and permanent teeth in a Danish population sample, *Int J Oral Surg* 1:235, 1972.

19. Antrim DD, Hicks ML, Altaras DE: Treatment of subosseous resorption: a case report, *J Endod* 8:567, 1982.

20. Bergenholtz G: Microorganisms from necrotic pulp of traumatized teeth, *Odontol Revy* 25:247, 1974.

21. Bergenholtz G, Reit C: Pulp reactions on microbial provocation of calcium hydroxide treated dentin, *Scand J Dent Res* 88:187, 1980.

22. Bhaskar SN, Rappaport HM: Dental vitality tests and pulp status, *J Am Dent Assoc* 86:409, 1973.

23. Binnie WH, Rowe AHR: A histological study of the periapical tissues of incompletely formed pulpless teeth filled with calcium hydroxide, *J Dent Res* 52:1110, 1973.

24. Bjorvatn K, Selvig KA, Klinge B: Effect of tetracycline and SnF_2 on root resorption in replanted incisors in dogs, *Scand J Dent Res* 97:477, 1989.

25. Blomlof L: Milk and saliva as possible storage media for traumatically exarticulated teeth prior to replantation, *Swed Dent J* 8(suppl):1, 1981.

26. Blomlof L et al: Storage of experimentally avulsed teeth in milk prior to replantation, *J Dent Res* 62:912, 1983.

27. Braham RL, Roberts MW, Morris ME: Management of dental trauma in children and adolescents, *J Trauma* 17:857, 1977.

28. Brannstrom M: Observations on exposed dentine and corresponding pulp tissue: a preliminary study with replica and routine histology, *Odontol Revy* 13:253, 1952.

29. Bystrom A, Claesson R, Sundqvist G: The antibacterial effect of camphorated paramonochlorphenol, camphorated phenol and calcium hydroxide in the treatment of infected root canals, *Endodont Dent Traumatol* 1:170, 1985.

30. Cameron CE: The cracked tooth syndrome: additional findings, *J Am Dent Assoc* 93:971, 1976.

31. Cox CF, Keall HJ, Ostro E, Bergenholtz G: Biocompatibility of surface-sealed dental materials against exposed pulps, *J Prosthet Dent* 57:1, 1987.

32. Croll TO et al: Rapid neurologic assessment and initial management for the patient with traumatic dental injuries, *J Am Dent Assoc* 100:530, 1980.

33. Cvek M: Treatment of non-vital permanent incisors with calcium hydroxide. IV. Periodontal healing and closure of the root canal in the coronal fragment of teeth with intra-alveolar fracture and vital apical fragment, *Odontol Revy* 25:239, 1974.

34. Cvek M: A clinical report on partial pulpotomy and capping with calcium hydroxide in permanent incisors with complicated crown fracture, *J Endod* 4:232, 1978.

35. Cvek M: Prognosis of luxated non-vital maxillary incisors treated with calcium hydroxide and filled with guttapercha: a retrospective clinical study, *Endodont Dent Traumatol* 8:45, 1992.

36. Cvek M: Endodontic treatment of traumatized teeth. In Andreasen JO, Andreasen FM, editors: *Textbook and color atlas of traumatic injuries to the teeth,* ed 3, Copenhagen and St Louis, 1994, Munksgaard and Mosby.

37. Cvek M, Hollender L, Nord C-E: Treatment of non-vital permanent incisors with calcium hydroxide. VI. A clinical, microbiological and radiological evaluation of treatment on one sitting of teeth with mature and immature roots, *Odontol Revy* 27:93, 1976.

38. Cvek M, Nord C-E, Hollender L: Antimicrobial effect of root canal debridement in teeth with immature root, *Odontol Revy* 27:1, 1976.

39. Cvek M, Sundstrom B: Treatment of non-vital permanent incisors with calcium hydroxide. V. Histological appearance of roentgenologically demonstrable apical closure of immature roots, *Odontol Revy* 25:379, 1974.

40. Cvek M et al: Pulp reactions to exposure after experimental crown fractures or grinding in adult monkeys, *J Endod* 8:391, 1982.

41. Cvek M et al: Effect of topical application of doxycycline on pulp revascularization and periodontal healing in reimplanted monkey incisors, *Endodont Dent Traumatol* 6:170, 1990.

42. Dargent P: A study of root resorption, *Acta Odontol Stomatol* 117:47, 1977.

43. Darling AI: Response of pulpodentinal complex to injury. In Gorlin RJ, Goldman H, editors: *Thoma's oral pathology,* ed 6, St Louis, 1970, Mosby, p 308.

44. Davis GT, Knott SC: Dental trauma in Australia, *Aust Dent J* 29:217, 1984.

45. Deutsch AS et al: Root fracture during insertion of prefabricated posts related to root size, *J Prosthet Dent* 53:786, 1985.

46. Eklund G, Stalhane I, Hedegard B: A study of traumatized permanent teeth in children aged 7-15. III. A multivariate analysis of post-traumatic complications of subluxated and luxated teeth, *Svensk Tandlak T* 69:179, 1976.

47. Fountain SB, Camp JH: Traumatic injuries. In Cohen S, Burns RC, editors: *Pathways of the pulp,* ed 6, St Louis, 1994, Mosby.

48. Frank AL: Therapy for the divergent pulpless tooth by continued apical formation, *J Am Dent Assoc* 72:87, 1966.

49. Frank AL, Bakland LK: Nonendodontic therapy for supraosseous extracanal invasive resorption, *J Endod* 13:348, 1987.

50. Fuks AB, Bielak S, Chosak A: Clinical and radiographic assessments of direct pulp capping and pulpotomy in young permanent teeth, *Pediatr Dent* 24:244, 1982.

51. Fuks A, Chosak A, Eidelman E: Partial pulpotomy as an alternative treatment for exposed pulps in crown-fractured permanent incisors, *Endodont Dent Traumatol* 3:100-102, 1987.

52. Fulling HJ, Andreasen JO: Influence of maturation status and tooth type of permanent teeth upon electrometric and thermal pulp testing procedures, *Scand J Dent Res* 84:266, 1976.

53. Fuss Z et al: Assessment of reliability of electrical and thermal pulp testing agents, *J Endod* 12:301, 1986.

54. Galea H: An investigation of dental injuries treated in an acute care general hospital, *J Am Dent Assoc* 109:434, 1984.

55. Gazelius B, Olgart L, Edwall B: Restored vitality in luxated teeth assessed by laser Doppler flowmeter, *Endodont Dent Traumatol* 4:265, 1988.

56. Gelbier MJ, Winter GB: Traumatized incisors treated by vital pulpotomy: a retrospective study, *Br Dent J* 164:319, 1988.

57. Gold SI, Hasselgren G: Peripheral inflammatory root resorption, *J Periodontol* 19:523, 1992.

58. Gottlieb B, Orban B: Veranderunngen in Periodontium nach chirurgischer Diathermie, *ZJ Stomatol* 28:1208, 1930.

59. Grahnen H, Hansson L: The prognosis of pulp and root canal therapy: a clinical and radiographic follow-up examination, *Odontol Revy* 12:146, 1961.

60. Granath L-E, Hagman G: Experimental pulpotomy in human bicuspids with reference to cutting technique, *Acta Odontol Scand* 29:155, 1971.

61. Hallet GE, Porteous JR: Fractured incisors treated by vital pulpotomy: a report on 100 consecutive cases, *Br Dent J* 115:279, 1963.

62. Hammarstrom L, Lindskog S: General morphologic aspects of resorption of teeth and alveolar bone, *Int Endodont J* 18:93, 1985.

63. Hammarstrom L et al: Tooth avulsion and replantation: a review, *Endodont Dent Traumatol* 2:1, 1986.

64. Harrington GW, Natkin E: External resorption associated with bleaching of pulpless teeth, *J Endod* 5:344, 1979.

65. Hedegard B, Stalhone I: A study of traumatized permanent teeth in children aged 7-15 years: part I, *Swed Dent J* 66:431, 1973.

66. Heide S, Mjor IA: Pulp reactions to experimental exposures in young permanent teeth, *Int Endodont J* 16:11, 1983.

67. Heithersay GS: Calcium hydroxide in the treatment of pulpless teeth with associated pathology, *J Br Endod Soc* 8:74, 1962.

68. Heller AL et al: Direct pulp capping of permanent teeth in primates using resorbable form of tricalcium phosphate ceramics, *J Endod* 1:95, 1975.

69. Herforth A, Strassburg M: Zur Therapie der chronischapikalen Paradontitis bei traumatisch beschadigten Frontzahnen mit nicht abgeschlossenen Wurzelwachstrum, *Dtsch Zahnartzl Z* 32:453, 1977.

70. Hernandez R, Bader S, Boston D, Trope M: Resistance to fracture of endodontically treated premolars restored with new generation dentin bonding systems, *Int Endodont J* 27:281, 1994.

71. Hill FJ, Picton JF: Fractured incisor fragment in the tongue: a case report, *Pediatr Dent* 3:337, 1981.

72. Hiltz J, Trope M: Vitality of human lip fibroblasts in milk, Hanks Balanced Salt Solution and Viaspan storage media, *Endodont Dent Traumatol* 7:69, 1991.

73. Jacobsen I: Root fractures in permanent anterior teeth with incomplete root formation, *Scand J Dent Res* 84:210, 1976.

74. Jacobsen I: Clinical follow-up study of permanent incisors with intrusive luxation after acute trauma, *J Dent Res* 62:4, 1983.

75. Jacobsen I, Kerekes K: Long-term prognosis of traumatized permanent anterior teeth showing calcific processes in the pulp cavity, *Scand J Dent Res* 85:588, 1977.

76. Jacobsen I, Kerekes K: Diagnosis and treatment of pulp necrosis in permanent anterior teeth with root fracture, *Scand J Dent Res* 88:370, 1980.

77. Jacobsen I, Zachrisson BU: Repair characteristics of root fractures in permanent anterior teeth, *Scand J Dent Res* 83:355, 1975.

78. Jarvinen S: Incisal overject and traumatic injuries to upper permanent incisors: a retrospective study, *Acta Odontol Scand* 36:359, 1978.

79. Jarvinen S: Fractured and avulsed permanent incisors in Finnish children: a retrospective study, *Acta Odontol Scand* 37:47, 1979.

80. Kakehashi S, Stanley HR, Fitzgerald RJ: The effect of surgical exposures on dental pulps in germ-free and conventional laboratory rats, *Oral Surg* 20:340, 1965.

81. Katebzadeh N, Dalton C, Trope M: Strengthening immature teeth during and after apexification, *J Endod* in press.

82. Kerekes K, Heide S, Jacobsen I: Follow-up examination of endodontic treatment in traumatized juvenile incisors, *J Endod* 6:744, 1980.

83. Kopel HM, Johnson R: Examination and neurologic assessment of children with oro-facial trauma, *Endodont Dent Traumatol* 1:155, 1985.

84. Kozlowska I: Pokrycie bezposrednie miazgi preparatem krajowej produccji, *Czas Stomatol* 13:375, 1960.

85. Lado EA, Stanley HR, Weissman MI: Cervical resorption in bleached teeth, *Oral Surg* 55:78, 1983.

86. Lengheden A, Blomlof L, Lindskog S: Effect of delayed calcium hydroxide treatment on periodontal healing in contaminated replanted teeth, *Scand J Dent Res* 99:147, 1991.

87. Lindskog A et al: The role of the necrotic periodontal membrane in cementum resorption and ankylosis, *Endodont Dent Traumatol* 1:96, 1985.

88. Lindskog S, Blomlof L: Influence of osmolality and composition of some storage media on human periodontal ligament cells, *Acta Odontol Scand* 40:435, 1982.

89. Lindskog S, Blomlof L, Hammarstrom L: Repair of periodontal tissues in vivo and in vitro, *J Clin Periodontol* 10:188, 1983.

90. Loe H, Waerhaug J: Experimental replantation of teeth in dogs and monkeys, *Arch Oral Biol* 3:176, 1961.

91. Lundin S-A, Noren JG, Warfvinge J: Marginal bacterial leakage and pulp reactions in class II composite resin restorations in vivo, *Swed Dent J* 14:185, 1990.

92. Luostarinen V, Pohto M, Sheinin A: Dynamics of repair in the pulp, *J Dent Res* 45:519, 1966.

93. Mackie IC, Bentley EM, Worthington HV: The closure of open apexes in nonvital immature incisor teeth, *Br Dent J* 165:169, 1988.

94. Macko DJ et al: A study of fractured anterior teeth in a school population, *J Dent Child* 46:130, 1979.

95. Magnusson B, Holm A: Traumatized permanent teeth in children—a follow-up. I. Pulpal complications and root resorption, *Swed Dent J* 62:61, 1969.

96. Magnusson B, Holm A, Berg H: Traumatized permanent teeth in children—a follow-up. II. The crown fractures, *Swed Dent J* 62:71, 1969.

97. Magura M et al: Human saliva coronal microleakage in obturated canals: an in vitro study, *J Endod* 17:324, 1991.

98. Makkes PG, Thoden van Velzen SK: Cervical external root resorption, *J Dent Res* 3:217, 1975.

99. Masterton JB: The healing of wounds of the dental pulp of man: a clinical and histological study, *Br Dent J* 120:213, 1966.

100. Matsson L et al: Ankylosis of experimentally reimplanted teeth related to extraalveolar period and storage environment, *Pediatr Dent* 4:327, 1982.

101. Maurice CG: Selection of teeth for root canal treatment, *Dent Clin North Am*, 1957, p. 761.

102. Meadow D, Needleman H, Lindner G: Oral trauma in children, *Pediatr Dent* 6:248, 1984.

103. Mejare I, Hasselgren G, Hammarstrom LE: Effect of formaldehyde-containing drugs on human dental pulp evaluated by enzyme histochemical technique, *Scand J Dent Res* 84:29, 1976.

104. Mesaros SV, Trope M: Revascularization of traumatized teeth assessed by laser Doppler flowmetry: case report, *Endodont Dent Traumatol* 13:24, 1997.

105. Mjor IA, Tronstad L: The healing of experimentally induced pulpitis, *Oral Surg* 38:115, 1974.

106. Moller AJR: *Microbiologic examination of root canals and periapical tissues of human teeth,* Thesis, Goteborg, Sweden, 1966, University of Goteborg.

107. Munksgaard EC et al: Enamel-dentin crown fractures bonded with various bonding agents, *Endodont Dent Traumatol* 7:73, 1991.

108. Nichols E: *An investigation into the factors which may influence the prognosis of root canal therapy,* Master's thesis, Faculty of Medicine, 1960, University of London.

109. Nicholls E: Endodontic treatment during root formation, *Int Dent J* 31:49, 1981.

110. Ohman A: Healing and sensitivity to pain in young replanted human teeth: an experimental and histologic study, *Odontol Tidskr* 73:166, 1965.

111. Oikarinen K, Gundlach KKH, Pfeifer G: Late complications of luxation injuries to teeth, *Endodont Dent Traumatol* 3:296, 1987.

112. Olgart L, Brannstrom M, Johnsson G: Invasion of bacteria into dentinal tubules: experiments in vivo and in vitro, *Acta Odontol Scand* 32:61, 1974.

113. O'Mullane DM: Injured permanent incisor teeth: an epidemiological study, *J Irish Dent Assoc* 18:160, 1972.

114. Penick EC: The endodontic management of root resorption, *Oral Surg* 16:344, 1963.

115. Pettiette M et al: Periodontal healing of extracted dog teeth air dried for extended periods and soaked in various media, *Endodont Dent Traumatol* 13:113, 1997.

116. Pierce A, Berg JO, Lindskog S: Calcitonin as an alternative therapy in the treatment of root resorption, *J Endod* 14:459, 1988.

117. Pierce A, Heithersay G, Lindskog S: Evidence for direct inhibition of dentinoclasts by a corticosteroid/antibiotic endodontic paste, *Endodont Dent Traumatol* 4:44, 1988.

118. Pierce A, Lindskog S: The effect of an antibiotic corticosteroid combination on inflammatory root resorption, *J Endod* 14:459, 1988.

119. Pitt Ford TR et al: Using mineral trioxide aggregate as a pulp-capping material, *J Am Dent Assoc* 127:1491, 1996.

120. Rabie G, Barnett F, Tronstad L: Long-term splinting of maxillary incisor with intra-alveolar root fracture, *Endodont Dent Traumatol* 4:99, 1988.

121. Rabie G et al: Strengthening and restoration of immature teeth with an acid-etch resin technique, *Endodont Dent Traumatol* 1:246, 1985.

122. Ravn JJ: Dental injuries in Copenhagen school children, school years 1967-1972, *Community Dent Oral Epidemiol* 2:231, 1974.

123. Ravn JJ: Follow-up study of permanent incisors with complicated crown fractures after acute trauma, *Scand J Dent Res* 90:363, 1982.

124. Ray H, Trope M: Periapical status of endodontically treated teeth in relation to the technical quality of the root filling and the coronal restoration, *Int Endodont J* 28(1):12, 1995.

125. Rock WP et al: The relationship between trauma and pulp death in incisor teeth, *Br Dent J* 136:236, 1974.

126. Rotstein I, Lehr Z, Gedalia I: Effect of bleaching agents on inorganic components of human dentin and cementum, *J Endod* 18:290, 1992.

127. Schindler WG, Gullickson DC: Rationale for the management of calcific metamorphosis secondary to traumatic injuries, *J Endod* 14:408, 1988.

128. Schroder U: Reaction of human dental pulp to experimental pulpotomy and capping with calcium hydroxide (thesis), *Odontol Revy* 24(suppl 25):97, 1973.

129. Schroder U, Granath L-E: Early reaction of intact human teeth to calcium hydroxide following experimental pulpotomy and its significance to the development of hard tissue barrier, *Odontol Revy* 22:379, 1971.

130. Seltzer S: *Endodontology,* Philadelphia, Lea & Febiger, 1988.

131. Seltzer S, Bender IB, Turkenkopf S: Factors affecting successful repair after root canal therapy, *J Am Dent Assoc* 52:651, 1963.

132. Selvig KA, Zander HA: Chemical analysis and microradiography of cementum and dentin from periodontally diseased human teeth, *J Periodontol* 33:303, 1962.

133. Seward GR: Periodontal disease and resorption of teeth, *Br Dent J* 34:443, 1963.

134. Sjogren U, Figdor D, Spangberg L, Sundqvist G: The antimicrobial effect of calcium hydroxide as a short term intracanal dressing, *Int Endodont J* 24:119, 1991.

135. Sheinin A, Pohto M, Luostarinen V: Defence mechanisms of the pulp with special reference to circulation: an experimental study in rats, *Int Dent J* 17:461, 1967.

136. Skoglund A, Tronstad L: Pulpal changes in replanted and autotransplanted immature teeth of dogs, *J Endod* 7:309, 1981.

137. Soder PO et al: Effect of drying on viability of periodontal membrane, *Scand J Dent Res* 85:167, 1977.

138. Spångberg L, Rutberg M, Rydinge E: Biologic effects of endodontic antimicrobial agents, *J Endod* 5:166, 1979.

139. Stalhane I, Hedegard B: Traumatized permanent teeth in children aged 7-15 years: part II, *Swed Dent J* 68:157, 1975.

140. Stanley HR: Diseases of the dental pulp. In Tieck RW, editor: *Oral pathology,* New York, 1965, McGraw Hill.

141. Stanley HR, Lundi T: Dycal therapy for pulp exposures, *Oral Surg* 34:818, 1972.

142. Stormer K, Jacobsen I: Hvor funksjonsdyktige blir rotfylte unge permanente incisiver? Nordisk forening for pedodonti Arsmote, Bergen, Norway 1988.

143. Strinberg LZ: The dependence of the results of pulp therapy on certain factors: an analytic study based on radiographic and clinical follow-up examinations, *Acta Odontol Scand* 14(suppl 21), 1956.

144. Sundqvist G: Ecology of the root canal flora, *J Endod* 18:427, 1992.

145. Trabert KC, Caput AA, Abou-Rass M: Tooth fracture, a comparison of endodontic and restorative treatments, *J Endod* 4:341, 1978.

146. Tronstad L: Reaction of the exposed pulp to Dycal treatment, *Oral Surg* 34:477, 1974.

147. Tronstad L: Pulp reactions in traumatized teeth. In Gutman JL, Harrison JW, editors: *Proceedings of the International Conference on Oral Trauma,* Chicago, 1984, American Association of Endodontists Endowment and Memorial Foundation.

148. Tronstad L: Root resorption: etiology, terminology and clinical manifestations, *Endodont Dent Traumatol* 4:241, 1988.

149. Tronstad L, Mjor IA: Capping of the inflamed pulp, *Oral Surg* 34:477, 1972.

150. Tronstad L et al: pH changes in dental tissues following root canal filling with calcium hydroxide, *J Endod* 7:17, 1981.

151. Trope M, Friedman S: Periodontal healing of replanted dog teeth stored in Viaspan, milk and Hanks Balanced Salt Solution, *Endodont Dent Traumatol* 8:183, 1992.

152. Trope M, Hupp JG, Mesaros SV: The role of the socket in the periodontal healing of replanted dog teeth stored in Viaspan for extended periods, *Endodont Dent Traumatol* 13:171, 1997.

153. Trope M, Maltz DO, Tronstad L: Resistance to fracture of restored endodontically treated teeth, *Endodont Dent Traumatol* 1:108, 1985.

154. Trope M et al: Effect of different endodontic treatment protocols on periodontal repair and root resorption of replanted dog teeth, *J Endod* 18:492, 1992.

155. Trope M et al: Short versus long term Ca(OH)$_2$ treatment of established inflammatory root resorption in replanted dog teeth, *Endodont Dent Traumatol* 11:124, 1995.

156. Warfvinge J, Rozell B, Hedstrom K-G: Effect of calcium hydroxide treated dentin on pulpal responses, *Int Endodont J* 20:183, 1987.

157. Wedenberg C: Evidence for a dentin-derived inhibitor of macrophage spreading, *Scand J Dent Res* 95:381, 1987.

158. Wedenberg C, Lindskog S: Experimental internal resorption in monkey teeth, *Endodont Dent Traumatol* 1:221, 1985.

159. Wedenberg C, Zetterqvist L: Internal resorption in human teeth: a histological, scanning electron microscope and enzyme histochemical study, *J Endod* 13:255, 1987.

160. Weiss M: Pulp capping in older patients, *NY State Dent J* 32:451, 1966.

161. Wilcox LR, Diaz-Arnold A: Coronal microleakage of permanent lingual access restorations in endodontically treated anterior teeth, *Int Endodont J* 23:321, 1990.

162. York AH et al: Dental injuries to 11-13 year old children, *NZ Dent J* 74:218, 1978.

163. Zachrisson BU, Jacobsen I: Long-term prognosis of 66 permanent anterior teeth with root fracture, *Scand J Dent Res* 83:345, 1975.

164. Zadik D, Chosack A, Eidelman E: A survey of traumatized incisors in Jerusalem school children, *J Dent Child* 39:185, 1972.

165. Zadik D et al: The prognosis of traumatized permanent teeth with fracture of enamel and dentin, *Oral Surg* 47:173, 1979.

Chapter 17

Endodontic Pharmacology

Kenneth M. Hargreaves

The effective management of pain is a hallmark of clinical excellence. Pain management is an integral part of the field of endodontics, and the practice of endodontics requires a thorough understanding of pain mechanisms and management.[2] To effectively and efficiently treat pain, the skilled clinician should understand the mechanisms of pain and analgesics and the strategies for the management of pain, including the use of analgesic drugs. Accordingly, this chapter reviews mechanisms of hyperalgesia and the management of odontogenic pain, with an emphasis on endodontic pharmacology. A comprehensive review of pain also includes diagnosis of odontogenic pain (Chapters 1 and 2) and nonodontogenic pain (Chapter 3), neuroanatomy of pulp (Chapter 11), mechanisms of dentinal hypersensitivity (Chapter 11), mediators activated in inflamed pulpal and periradicular tissue (Chapters 12 and 13), and the pharmacology of local anesthetics and anxiolytics (Chapter 19). These topics are reviewed in this chapter.

MECHANISMS OF PAIN

Odontogenic pain is usually caused by either noxious physical stimuli or the release of inflammatory mediators that stimulate receptors located on terminal endings of nociceptive ("pain-detecting") afferent nerve fibers.[33,53,87] Nociceptive fibers are distributed throughout the body and are prevalent in trigeminal nerves innervating tooth pulp and periapical tissue. As described in other chapters, there are two major classes of nociceptors: the C and A delta nerve fibers (Fig. 17-1). In the dental pulp there are at least three to eight times more unmyelinated C fibers as compared to A delta fibers.[10,44,84] Activation of dental pulp nerves by either thermal, mechanical, chemical, or electrical (e.g., electrical dental pulp tester) stimuli results in a nearly pure sensation of pain.[9] Pulpal C fibers are thought to have a predominant role for encoding inflammatory pain arising from dental pulp and periradicular tissue. This hypothesis is supported by the distribution of C fibers in the dental pulp, their responsiveness to inflammatory mediators, and the strikingly similar perceptual qualities (e.g., dull, aching pain) of pain associated with C fiber activation and with pulpitis.[55,65,66]

Following activation, the C and A delta fibers from the orofacial region transmit nociceptive signals primarily via trigeminal nerves to the trigeminal nucleus caudalis located in the medulla.[36,53,77] The nucleus caudalis is an important, but not exclusive, site for processing orofacial nociceptive input.[22,56,76] Blockade of input from C and A delta fibers by the use of long-acting local anesthetics induces profound postoperative analgesia.[17]

The nucleus caudalis has been termed the "medullary dorsal horn," since its anatomic organization is similar to that seen in the spinal dorsal horn. The medullary dorsal horn is not simply a relay station where nociceptive signals are passively transferred to higher brain regions. Rather, the nucleus caudalis plays an important role in processing nociceptive signals, and the output to higher brain regions can be increased (e.g., hyperalgesia), decreased (e.g., analgesia), or misinterpreted (e.g., referred pain) as compared to incoming activity from the relevant C and A delta fibers. For example, during tissue inflammation or following pulpal extirpation, there is a dramatic change in the responsiveness or receptor field size of neurons in the medullary dorsal horn; these and other changes are called dorsal horn plasticity to denote the dramatic alteration in neuronal activity produced by peripheral inflammation.[21,75,76]

The medullary dorsal horn contains at least four major components related to the processing of nociceptive signals: central terminals of afferent fibers, local circuit neurons, projection neurons, and descending neurons. The first component, primary nociceptive afferents (e.g., C and A delta fibers), enter the medullary dorsal horn via the trigeminal tract (Fig. 17-2). The central terminals of these C and A delta fibers end primarily in the outer layers of the medullary dorsal horn. These sensory fibers transmit information by releasing neuropeptides (e.g., substance P or calcitonin gene-related peptide [CGRP]) and amino acids such as glutamate. The administration of receptor antagonists to these neuropeptides or antagonists to glutamate blocks hyperalgesia in animal studies.[21,72] These compounds are likely to serve as prototypes for future classes of analgesic drugs.

Local circuit neurons are a second component of the dorsal horn, and they regulate transmission of nociceptive signals from the primary afferent fibers to projection neurons.[22,53,87] Local circuit neurons are intraneurons whose cell bodies and processes are restricted to the medullary dorsal horn. The third component of the dorsal horn are the projection neurons; the cell bodies of these neurons are within the medullary dorsal horn, and their axons comprise the output system for sending orofacial pain information to more rostral brain regions. A major projection for these axons is the trigeminothalamic tract. This tract crosses to the contralateral side of the medulla and ascends to the thalamus (see Fig. 17-2). From the thalamus, additional neurons relay this information to the cerebral cortex.

Evidence exists that referred pain is due to convergence of afferent input from cutaneous and visceral nociceptors onto the same projection neurons.[78] For example, nociceptors in the maxillary sinus and maxillary molars may stimulate the same neuron located in the nucleus caudalis; this convergence of sensory input probably mediates referred pain.[78] Indeed, about

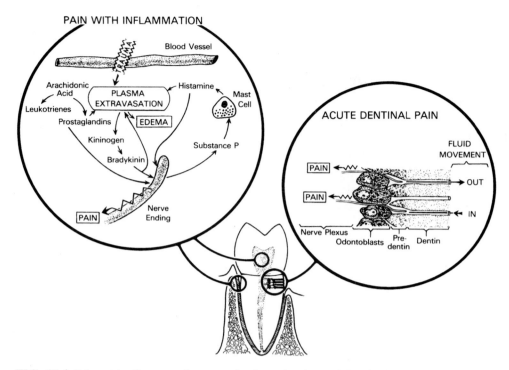

FIG. 17-1 Schematic diagram of two mechanisms for the peripheral stimulation of nociceptive nerve fibers in tooth pulp. *Insert,* Acute dental pain. According to the hydrodynamic theory, stimuli that cause fluid movement in exposed dentinal tubules result in the stimulation of nociceptive nerve fibers. *Insert,* Pain with inflammation. Inflammation is associated with the synthesis or release of mediators including prostaglandins, bradykinin, substance P, and histamine (as well as other mediators not shown). The interrelationships of these inflammatory mediators forms a positive feedback loop allowing inflammation to persist far beyond cessation of the dental procedure. *(From Hargreaves KM, Troullos E, Dionne R:* Dent Clin North Am *31:675-694, 1987.)*

50% of neurons in the nucleus caudalis exhibit convergence of sensory input from cutaneous and visceral structures.[76]

The fourth component of the medullary dorsal horn are the terminal endings of descending neurons (see Fig. 17-2). These terminals act to inhibit the transmission of nociceptive information. An important component of this analgesic system are the endogenous opioid peptides (EOP). The EOPs are a family of peptides that possess many of the properties of exogenous opioids such as morphine and codeine. The EOP family includes the enkephalins, dynorphins, and β-endorphin–related peptides. Importantly, EOPs are found at several levels of the pain suppression system. This fact underlies the analgesic efficacy of endogenous and exogenous opioids, since their administration conceivably activates opioid receptors located at all levels of the neuraxis. The EOPs are probably released during dental procedures, since blockade of the actions of endogenous opioids by administration of the antagonist naloxone can significantly increase the perception of dental pain.[31,37,49]

MECHANISMS OF HYPERALGESIA

The pain system can undergo dramatic changes in response to peripheral inflammation, leading to the development of hyperalgesia.[21,23,50,88] Hyperalgesia can be characterized as spontaneous pain, reduced pain threshold (i.e., allodynia) and increased pain perception to noxious stimuli.[87] Most of us have experienced hyperalgesia; common examples include a sunburn or a thermal injury. A sunburn often induces spontaneous

Table 17-1. Signs of hyperalgesia and endodontic diagnostic tests

Sign of Hyperalgesia	Related Diagnostic Test or Symptom
Spontaneous pain	Spontaneous pain
Reduced pain threshold	Percussion test, palpation test, throbbing pain
Increased response to painful stimuli	Increased response to electric pulp test (EPT or thermal test)

From Hargreaves et al: *Oral Surg Oral Med Oral Pathol* 78:503, 1994.

pain, a reduced pain threshold (e.g., wearing a shirt is painful), and increased pain responsiveness (e.g., increased pain perception occurs when someone slaps sunburned skin). Thus a peripheral injury evokes fundamental changes in the response properties of the pain system.

Hyperalgesia also occurs during inflammation of pulpal or periradicular tissue. Indeed, the outcome of endodontic diagnostic tests and patient symptoms can be used to determine the presence of hyperalgesia (Table 17-1).[9,38] For example, percussion of a tooth with a mirror handle (Chapter 1) tests for one aspect of hyperalgesia: a reduction in the mechanical nociceptive thresholds of neurons innervating the periodontal ligament. Under normal conditions this innocuous stimulation does not elicit pain. However, under conditions of hyperalgesia the mechanical pain threshold is reduced to the point where

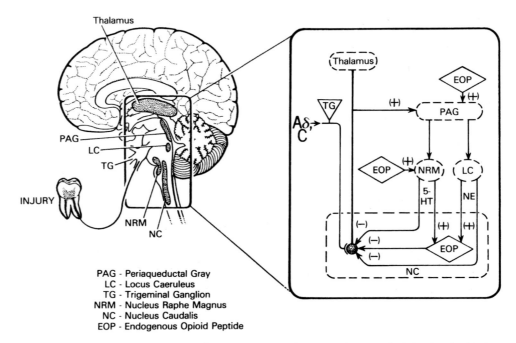

PAG - Periaqueductal Gray
LC - Locus Caeruleus
TG - Trigeminal Ganglion
NRM - Nucleus Raphe Magnus
NC - Nucleus Caudalis
EOP - Endogenous Opioid Peptide

FIG. 17-2 Schematic diagram of the perception and modulation of orofacial pain. Activation of A delta or C nociceptive fibers leads to the entry of a nociceptive signal, which is conveyed across a synapse in the nucleus caudalis of the trigeminal system. Second-order neuron projects to the thalamus; the information is then relayed to the cortex. *Insert,* Endogenous pain suppression system. This insert depicts the functional relationship of several neurotransmitters for the modulation of nociceptive information at the nucleus caudalis (the actual anatomic relationships are more complex). As in the large figure, peripheral activation of A delta or C fibers stimulates the projection neuron in the nucleus caudalis (filled cell body), which relays to the thalamus. This signal is also transmitted to the periaquadactal gray *(PAG),* which receives additional input from other areas not shown. The PAG in turn activates the nucleus raphae magnus *(NRM)* and the locus caeruleus *(LC).* The NRM sends fibers to the first synapse in the nucleus caudalis, where it inhibits the transmission of nociceptive information by the secretion of serotonin *(5-HT)* and other neurotransmitters. In a similar fashion the LC sends fibers to the first synapse, where norepinephrine *(NE)* is released to inhibit transmission. Note that neurons secreting endogenous opioid peptides *(EOP)* are present at all three levels of this system. The "+" sign indicates an excitatory action, whereas the "−" sign denotes an inhibitory action. *(From Hargreaves KM, Troullos E, Dionne R: Dent Clin North Am 31:675-694, 1987.)*

tapping with a mirror handle is now perceived as tender or painful. Similarly, studies in cats have shown that pulpal inflammation lowers the mechanical threshold of pulpal fibers to the level where increases in systolic blood pressure can activate pulpal neurons. The synchrony of firing of pulpal fibers in response to the heartbeat is thought to mediate the "throbbing" pain of pulpitis.[65] Accordingly, mechanisms and management of hyperalgesia are important issues in the field of endodontics.

Hyperalgesia is due to both peripheral and central mechanisms.[21,23,88] Several mechanisms appear to contribute to peripheral hyperalgesia (Table 17-2). It is important to note that dental procedures such as the incision and drainage of an abscess or a pulpectomy may reduce pain by reducing concentrations of mediators and lowering tissue pressure. Many inflammatory mediators found in inflamed pulp or periradicular tissue (Chapters 11 and 12) can either activate or sensitize nociceptors and evoke pain when administered to human volunteers (Table 17-3).[24] Activation of a nociceptor is due to a membrane depolarization sufficient to elicit an action potential, which is then propagated along the neuron to central ter-

Table 17-2. Peripheral mechanisms contributing to hyperalgesia

Mechanism	Reference
Composition and concentration of inflammatory mediators	38, 51
Changes in afferent fiber: activation and sensitization	47, 60, 74
Changes in afferent fiber: sprouting	12
Changes in afferent fiber: proteins	12, 30
Tissue pressure	65, 66
Tissue temperature	62
Sympathetic-primary afferent fiber interactions	43, 50, 69, 85

Modified from Hargreaves et al: *Oral Surg Oral Med Oral Pathol* 78:503, 1994.

minals located in the brain stem trigeminal nuclei. Sensitization of a nociceptor is due to receptor-mediated events leading to spontaneous activity, a decreased threshold for depolarization and prolonged responses (afterdischarges) to suprathreshold stimuli. The actions of peripheral analgesics are based, in part,

Table 17-3. Effect of inflammatory mediators on nociceptive afferent fibers

Mediator	Effect on Nociceptors	Effect on Human Volunteers	Reference
Potassium	Activate	++	45
Protons	Activate	++	54, 80
Serotonin	Activate	++	7, 45
Bradykinin	Activate	+++	7, 45, 51
Histamine	Activate	+	45
Tumor necrosis factor α	Activate	?	85, 92
Prostaglandins	Sensitize	±	8
Leukotrienes	Sensitize	±	8, 55
Nerve growth factor	Sensitize	++	52, 70
Substance P	Sensitize	±	32, 50
Interleukin-1	Sensitize (?)	?	25

Modified from Fields H: *Pain*, New York, 1987, McGraw-Hill, p 32.
+, Positive; ++, very positive; +++, extremely positive; ±, equivalent; ?, unknown.

Table 17-4. Central mechanisms contributing to hyperalgesia

Mechanism	Reference
Increased vesicular release from primary afferent fibers	29
Changes in postsynaptic receptors	27
Changes in second messenger systems	28, 61
Changes in protooncogenes	19
Changes in endogenous opioids	19, 37
Central sensitization	41, 86, 89
Dark neurons	81

Modified from Hargreaves et al: Neuroendocrine and immune responses to injury, degeneration and repair. In Sessle BJ, Dionne RA, and Bryant P, editors: *Temporomandibular disorders and related pain conditions*, Seattle, 1995, IASP Press, pp 273-292.

Table 17-5. Summary of selected nonnarcotic analgesics

Drug	Trade Name	Analgesic Dose Range (mg)	Maximal Dose/Day (mg)
Acetaminophen	Tylenol	325-1000	4000
Aspirin	Many	325-1000	4000
Diclofenac potassium	Cataflam	50-100	150-200
Diflunisal	Dolobid	250-1000	1500
Etodolac	Lodine	200-400	1200
Fenoprofen	Nalfon	200	1200
Flurbiprofen	Ansaid	50-100	200-300
Ibuprofen	Motrin	200-400	2400 (Rx)
Ketoprofen	Orudis	25-75	300 (Rx)
Ketorolac*	Toradol	10 (oral)	40
Naproxen	Naprosyn	250-500	1500
Naproxen sodium	Anaprox	220-550	1650 (Rx)

Modified from Cooper SA: *Postgrad Dent* 2:7, 1995.
*A new package insert for ketorolac tablets contains the instructions that the drug should be used only as a transition from injectable ketorolac and for no more than 5 days.
Rx, Prescription strength.

on the ability of these drugs to reduce nociceptor activation or sensitization by reducing tissue levels of inflammatory mediators. Predictably, drugs that inhibit the actions of these mediators exhibit analgesic activity in models of hyperalgesia.[13,82] Considerable research is being directed to understanding the mechanisms of sensitization of nociceptors in the hope of developing new classes of analgesic drugs.[71]

In addition to activation and sensitization, the peripheral afferent fiber responds to mediators such as nerve growth factor by increasing protein synthesis of substance P and CGRP and by undergoing sprouting of terminal fibers in the inflamed tissue.[12,46] Sprouting increases the density of innervation in inflamed tissue and may contribute to increased pain sensitivity in chronic pulpal or periradicular inflammation.[12] Certain afferent fibers also respond to inflammatory mediators by synthesizing other proteins such as tetrodotoxin (TTX)-insensitive sodium channels. These ion channels are synthesized by a major class of nociceptors and undergo activation by inflammatory mediators.[3,30] Unlike the typical class of TTX-sensitive sodium channels found on sensory neurons, local anesthetics poorly block the TTX-insensitive class of sodium channels. Indeed, it takes four times more lidocaine to block TTX-insensitive channels as it takes to block the typical class of TTX-sensitive ion channels.[73] Given this disparity in lidocaine potency, the synthesis of new types of ion channels on sensory neurons may well contribute to the clinical finding of difficulty in obtaining local anesthesia in certain endodontic pain cases.

In addition to these peripheral mechanisms, several central mechanisms of hyperalgesia have also been proposed (Table 17-4).[21,23,39,88] For example, pulpectomy produces central sensitization as measured both by an expansion of receptive field sizes and an increase in spontaneous activity.[76] In addition, central terminals of afferent fibers continue to exhibit increased release of CGRP even after removal from the animal.[29] Thus even in the absence of peripheral input, central mechanisms of hyperalgesia can persist for some time. Since at least some components of hyperalgesia can persist even without continued sensory input from inflamed tissue, it is not surprising that up to 80% of endodontic patients experiencing pain before treatment continue to report pain after treatment.[58,59] Drugs that block mechanisms of hyperalgesia may well offer new ad-

vances in the control of endodontic pain.[21,28,61] Taken together, it is apparent that the mechanisms of hyperalgesia are clinically significant factors in understanding strategies for diagnosing and managing the patient with endodontic pain.

NONNARCOTIC ANALGESICS

Management of endodontic pain is multifactorial and is directed at reducing the peripheral components of hyperalgesia (see Table 17-2) through combined endodontic procedures and pharmacotherapy. One major class of drugs for managing endodontic pain is the nonnarcotic analgesics, which include both the nonsteroidal antiinflammatory drugs (NSAIDs) and acetaminophen. Although these drugs are classically thought to produce analgesia through peripheral mechanisms, it should be pointed out that the brain is now believed to be an additional site of action.[57]

Numerous NSAIDs are available for management of pain and inflammation (Table 17-5). Unfortunately, there are comparatively few studies, particularly for endodontic pain, that directly compare one NSAID to one another for analgesia and side effect liability. The lack of comprehensive comparative studies in endodontic models means that only general recommendations can be made, and the clinician is encouraged to be

Table 17-6. Summary of selected NSAID-drug interactions

Drug	Possible Effect
Anticoagulants	Increase in prothrombin time or bleeding with anticoagulants (e.g., coumarins)
Angiotensin converting enzyme inhibitors	Reduced antihypertensive effectiveness of captopril (especially indomethacin)
β-Blockers	Reduced antihypertensive effects of β-blockers (e.g., propranolol, atenolol, pindolol)
Cyclosporine	Increased risk of nephrotoxicity
Digoxin	Increase in serum digoxin levels (especially ibuprofen, indomethacin)
Dipyridamole	Increased water retention (especially indomethacin)
Hydantoins	Increased serum levels of phenytoin
Lithium	Increased serum levels of lithium
Loop diuretics	Reduced effectiveness of loop diuretics (e.g., furosemide, bumetanide)
Methotrexate	Increased risk of toxicity (e.g., stomatitis, bone marrow suppression)
Penicillamine	Increased bioavailability (especially indomethacin)
Sympathomimetics	Increased blood pressure (especially indomethacin with phenylpropanolamine)
Thiazide diuretics	Reduced antihypertensive effectiveness

Table 17-7. Analgesic doses of representative opioids

Drug	Dose Equivalent to Codeine 60 mg
Codeine	60
Dihydrocodeine	60
Hydrocodone	10
Meperidine	90
Oxycodone	5-6
Propoxyphene hydrochloride	102
Propoxyphene napsylate	146

Modified from Troullos E, Freeman R, Dionne RA: *Anesth Prog* 33:123, 1986.

Table 17-8. Selected opioid combination analgesic drugs

Formulation*	Trade Name†	Possible Rx
APAP 300 mg and codeine 30 mg	Tylenol with codeine No. 3	2 tablets q4h
APAP 500 mg and hydrocodone 5 mg	Vicodin, Lortab 5/500	1-2 tablets q6h
APAP 325 mg and oxycodone 5 mg	Percocet	1 tablet q6h
APAP 500 mg and oxycodone 5 mg	Tylox	1 tablet q6h
ASA 325 mg and codeine 30 mg	Empirin with codeine No. 3	2 tablets q4h
ASA 325 mg and oxycodone 5 mg	Percodan	1 tablet q6h

*Abbreviations for acetaminophen (APAP) and aspirin (ASA).
†Several generics are available for most formulations.

familiar with several of these drugs. Ibuprofen is generally considered the prototype of NSAID and has a well-documented efficacy and safety profile. Other NSAIDs may offer certain advantages over ibuprofen. For example, etodolac (Lodine) has minimal gastrointestinal irritation, and ketoprofen (Orudis) has been shown in some studies to be somewhat more analgesic than ibuprofen.[4,15] The advantages of NSAIDs include their well-established analgesic efficacy for inflammatory pain. Indeed, many of the NSAIDs listed in Table 17-5 have been shown to be more effective than traditional acetaminophen-opioid combination drugs.[13,17,83]

However, the clinician should be aware of limitations and drug interactions when considering the use of NSAIDs for managing endodontic pain. For example, NSAIDs exhibit an analgesic ceiling that limits the maximal level of analgesia; NSAIDs also induce side effects including those affecting the gastrointestinal (3% to 11% incidence) and central nervous (e.g., dizziness, headache; 1% to 9%) systems. They are contraindicated in patients with ulcers and aspirin hypersensitivity.[14,15,20] Moreover, the NSAIDs have been reported to interact with a number of other drugs (Table 17-6). Acetaminophen-opioid combination drugs represent an alternative to those patients unable to take NSAIDs.[14] Further information is available on the pharmacology and adverse effects of this important class of drugs.[20,26,91]

OPIOID ANALGESICS

Opioids are potent analgesics and are often used in dentistry in combination with acetaminophen or aspirin. Most clinically available opioids activate the μ-opioid receptor. This opioid receptor is located at several important sites in the brain (see Fig. 17-2), and its activation inhibits the transmission of nociceptive signals from the trigeminal nucleus to higher brain regions. However, recent studies indicate that opioids also activate peripheral opioid receptors, and intraligamentary injection of morphine has been shown to significantly reduce pain in endodontic patients.[34,35]

Although opioids are effective as analgesics for moderate to severe pain, their usage is generally limited by their adverse side effect profile. Opioids induce numerous side effects including nausea, emesis, dizziness, drowsiness, and the potential for respiratory depression and constipation. Long-term use of opioids is associated with tolerance and dependence. Since the dose of opioids is limited by their side effect profile, opioids are almost always used in combination drugs for management of dental pain. A combination formulation is preferred, since it permits a lower dose of the opioid to reduce patient side effects (Table 17-7).

Codeine is often considered the prototype opioid for orally available combination drugs. Most studies have found that the 60-mg dose of codeine (the amount in two tablets of Tylenol with codeine No. 3) produces significantly more analgesia than placebo, although it often produces less analgesia than either aspirin 650 mg or acetaminophen 600 mg.[14,15,36] In general, patients taking only 30 mg of codeine report about as much analgesia as those taking a placebo pill.[6,83] Accordingly, Table 17-8 provides doses of other opioids equivalent to the 60-mg dose of codeine.

PAIN MANAGEMENT STRATEGIES

When managing pain in an individual patient, the skilled clinician must customize the treatment plan, balancing the general principles of endodontics, mechanisms of hyperalgesia, and pain management strategies with the particular factors of the individual patient (e.g., medical history, concurrent medications). The following discussion reviews general considerations for pain management strategies.

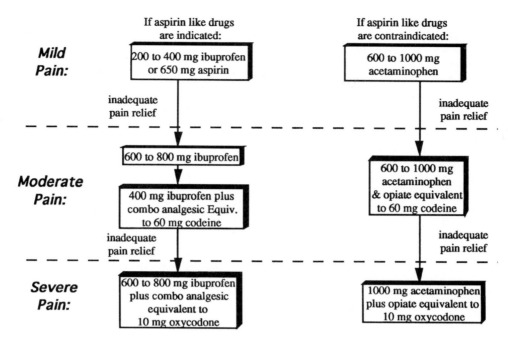

FIG. 17-3 A flexible analgesic strategy.

BOX 17-1.

CONSIDERATIONS FOR EFFECTIVE "THREE-D" PAIN CONTROL

1. Diagnosis
2. Definitive dental treatment
3. Drugs
   a. Pretreat with NSAIDs or acetaminophen when appropriate.
   b. Use long-acting local anesthetics when indicated.
   c. Use a flexible prescription plan.
   d. Prescribe "by the clock" rather than "prn."

Effective management of the patient with endodontic pain starts with the "three Ds": *diagnosis, definitive dental treatment,* and *drugs* (Box 17-1). Comprehensive reviews on diagnosis and definitive dental treatment (e.g., incision and drainage, pulpectomy) are provided in Chapter 2. As described earlier in this chapter, the management of endodontic pain should focus on removal of peripheral mechanisms of hyperalgesia (see Table 17-2). This generally requires treatment that removes or reduces etiologic factors (e.g., bacterial-immunologic factors). For example, both pulpotomy and pulpectomy have been associated with substantial reduction in patient reports of pain as compared to their pretreatment pain levels.[40,68] However, pharmacotherapy is often required to reduce continued nociceptor input (e.g., NSAIDs, local anesthetics) and suppress central hyperalgesia (e.g., opioids).

Pretreatment with an NSAID before a procedure has been demonstrated to produce a significant benefit in many[18,42] but not all studies.[67] The rationale for pretreatment is to block the development of hyperalgesia by reducing the input from pe-

ripheral nociceptors. Interestingly, patients who cannot take NSAIDs may still benefit, since pretreatment with acetaminophen also has been shown to reduce postoperative pain.[64] Patients can be pretreated 30 minutes before the procedure with either an NSAID (e.g., ibuprofen 400 mg or flurbiprofen 100 mg) or with acetaminophen 1000 mg.[42,64]

A second pharmacologic approach for pain management is the use of long-acting local anesthetics. Bupivacaine and etidocaine are two long-acting local anesthetics available for use (Chapter 19). Clinical trials indicate that the long-acting local anesthetics not only provide anesthesia during the procedure, but also significantly delay the onset of posttreatment pain as compared to lidocaine-containing local anesthetics.[16,17] The analgesic benefit of long-acting local anesthetics is observed to a greater extent when administered by block injections as compared to infiltration injections. However, the clinician should also be aware of adverse effects attributed to the long-acting local anesthetics.[5,63]

A third pharmacologic approach is the use of a flexible plan for prescribing analgesics (Fig. 17-3).[1,14,36,83] A flexible prescription plan serves to minimize both patient pain and side effects. With this goal in mind, the strategy is to first achieve a maximally effective dose of the nonnarcotic analgesic (either an NSAID or acetaminophen for patients who cannot take NSAIDs). Second, if the patient is still experiencing pain or if moderate to severe pain is anticipated, the clinician should add an acetaminophen-opioid–containing combination analgesic. In a typical patient the amount of the opioid should be equivalent to codeine 60 mg. Vicoprofen (Knoll Pharmaceutical Co., N.J.) contains both ibuprofen (200 mg) and hydrocodone (7.5 mg) in the same formulation. Even greater analgesia may be possible by combining Vicoprofen with an additional 200 to 400 mg of ibuprofen. An additional strategy to obtain the advantages of both an NSAID and an opioid is to provide alternating treatments.[1,14]

For example, the emergency pain patient could take ibuprofen 400 mg (or an NSAID of choice) at the office. Then the patient could take an acetaminophen-opioid combination 2 hours later (see Table 17-8 for examples). The patient would then take each treatment every 4 hours, taking each drug on an alternating 2-hour schedule. In most cases this treatment need not be continued beyond 24 hours.[1,14] Aspirin-opioid combinations are not, of course, used in this alternating schedule because of potential NSAID-aspirin interactions.

Previous studies have shown that ibuprofen administered concurrently with an acetaminophen-oxycodone combination drug significantly increases patients' reports of analgesia and that patients prefer this combination over acetaminophen-oxycodone alone.[79] Moreover, concurrent administration of acetaminophen and ibuprofen are well tolerated without an apparent increase in side effects or alterations in pharmacokinetics.[48,79,90] Of course, not all patients require concurrent use of NSAIDs with acetaminophen-opioid combinations. Indeed, the basic premise of a flexible prescription plan is that the analgesic prescribed should be matched to the patient's need.

The information and recommendations provided in this chapter were selected to aid the clinician in the management of acute endodontic pain. However, clinical judgment must also take into account other sources of information, including patient history, concurrent medications, nature of the pain, and the treatment plan to provide the best plan for managing the individual pain problem of each patient. Integrating these general principles of pain mechanisms and management with the clinician's assessment of each individual patient provides an effective approach for the successful management of endodontic pain.

REFERENCES

1. American Association of Endodontists: *Endodontics: colleagues for excellence: pain,* Chicago, 1995, The Association.
2. American Association of Endodontists: *1996-97 membership roster,* Chicago, 1996, The Association, p 2.
3. Arbuckle JB, Docherty RJ: Expression of tetrodotoxin-resistant sodium channels in capsaicin-sensitive dorsal root ganglion neurons of adult rats, *Neurosci Lett* 85:70, 1995.
4. Arnold J, Salom I, Berger A: Comparison of gastrointestinal microbleeding associated with use of etodolac, ibuprofen, indomethacin, and naproxen in normal subjects, *Curr Ther Res* 37:730, 1985.
5. Bacsik C, Swift J, Hargreaves KM: Toxic systemic reactions of bupivacaine and etidocaine: review of the literature, *Oral Surg Oral Med Oral Pathol* 79:18, 1995.
6. Beaver W: Mild analgesics: a review of their clinical pharmacology, *Am J Med Sci* 251:576, 1966.
7. Beck P, Handwerker HO: Bradykinin and serotonin effects on various types of cutaneous nerve fibers, *Pflugers Arch* 347:209, 1974.
8. Bisgaard H, Kristensen J: Leukotriene B$_4$ produces hyperalgesia in humans, *Prostaglandins* 30:791, 1985.
9. Brown AC, Beeler WJ, Kloka AC, Fields RW: Spatial summation of pre-pain and pain in human teeth, *Pain* 21:1, 1985.
10. Byers MR: Dental sensory receptors, *Int Rev Neurobiol* 25:39, 1984.
11. Byers MR: Dynamic plasticity of dental sensory nerve structure and cytochemistry, *Arch Oral Biol* 39(suppl):13S, 1994.
12. Byers MR, Taylor P, Khayat B, Kimberly C: Effects of injury and inflammation on pulpal and periapical nerves, *J Endod* 16:78, 1990.
13. Cooper SA: New peripherally acting oral analgesics, *Ann Rev Pharmacol Toxicol* 23:617, 1983.
14. Cooper SA: Treating acute dental pain, *Postgrad Dent* 2:7, 1995.
15. Cooper SA, Berrie R, Cohn P: The analgesic efficacy of ketoprofen compared to ibuprofen and placebo, *Adv Therap* 5:43, 1988.
16. Crout R, Koraido G, Moore PA: A clinical trial of long-acting local anesthetics for periodontal surgery, *Anesth Prog* 37:194, 1990.
17. Dionne RA: Suppression of dental pain by the preoperative administration of flurbiprofen, *Am J Med* 80:41, 1986.
18. Dionne RA et al: Suppression of postoperative pain by preoperative administration of ibuprofen in comparison to placebo, acetaminophen and acetaminophen plus codeine, *J Clin Pharmacol* 23:37, 1983.
19. Draisci G, Iadarola M: Temporal analysis of increases in c-fos, preprodynorphin and preproenkephalin mRNAs in rat spinal cord, *Brain Res Mol Brain Res* 6:31, 1989.
20. *Drug facts and comparisons,* St Louis, 1996, Facts and Comparisons Inc, pp 247-253f.
21. Dubner R, Basbaum AI: Spinal dorsal horn plasticity following tissue or nerve injury. In Wall PD, Melzack R, editors: *Textbook of pain,* ed 3, Edinburgh, 1994, Churchill-Livingstone, pp 225-241.
22. Dubner R, Bennett G: Spinal and trigeminal mechanisms of nociception, *Ann Rev Neurosci* 6:381, 1983.
23. Dubner R, Ruda MA: Activity-dependent neuronal plasticity following tissue injury and inflammation, *Trends Neurosci* 15:96, 1992.
24. Fields H: *Pain,* New York, 1987, McGraw-Hill, p 32.
25. Follenfant R, Nakamura-Craig M, Henderson B, Higgs G: Inhibition by neuropeptides of interleukin-1β-induced, prostaglandin-independent hyperalgesia, *Br J Pharmacol* 98:41, 1989.
26. Gage T, Pickett F: *Mosby's dental drug reference,* St Louis, 1997, Mosby.
27. Galeazza M, Stucky C, Seybold VS: Changes in [125I]h-CGRP binding in rat spinal cord in an experimental model of acute, peripheral inflammation, *Brain Res* 591:198, 1992.
28. Garry MG, Durnett-Richardson J, Hargreaves KM: Carrageenan-induced inflammation alters levels of i-cGMP and i-cAMP in the dorsal horn of the spinal cord, *Brain Res* 646:135, 1994.
29. Garry MG, Hargreaves KM: Enhanced release of immunoreactive CGRP and substance P from spinal dorsal horn slices occurs during carrageenan inflammation, *Brain Res* 582:139, 1992.
30. Gold MS, Reichling DB, Shuster MJ, Levine JD: Hyperalgesic agents increase a tetrodotoxin-resistant Na$^+$ current in nociceptors, *Proc Natl Acad Sci USA* 93:1108, 1996.
31. Gracely R, Dubner R, Wolskee P, Deeter W: Placebo and naloxone can alter post-surgical pain by separate mechanisms, *Nature* 306:264, 1983.
32. Hagermark O, Hokfelt T, Pernow B: Flare and itch produced by substance P in human skin, *J Invest Dermatol* 71:233, 1979.
33. Hargreaves KM, Dubner R: Mechanisms of pain and analgesia. In Dionne RA, Phero J, editors: *Management of pain and anxiety in dental practice,* New York, 1992, Elsevier Press, pp 18-40.
34. Hargreaves KM, Joris J: The peripheral analgesic effects of opioids, *J Am Pain Soc* 2:51, 1993.
35. Hargreaves KM, Keating K, Cathers S, Dionne RA: Analgesic effects of morphine after PDL injection in endodontic patients, *J Dent Res* 70:445, 1991.
36. Hargreaves KM, Troullos E, Dionne RA: Pharmacologic rationale for the treatment of acute pain, *Dent Clin North Am* 31:675, 1987.
37. Hargreaves KM et al: Naloxone, fentanyl and diazepam modify plasma beta-endorphin levels during surgery, *Clin Pharmacol Ther* 40:165, 1986.
38. Hargreaves KM et al: Pharmacology of peripheral neuropeptide and inflammatory mediator release, *Oral Surg Oral Med Oral Pathol* 78:503, 1994.
39. Hargreaves KM et al: Neuroendocrine and immune responses to injury, degeneration and repair. In Sessle BJ, Dionne RA, Bryant P, editors: *Temporomandibular disorders and related pain conditions,* Seattle, 1995, IASP Press, pp 273-292.
40. Hasselgren G, Reit C: Emergency pulpotomy: pain relieving effect with and without the use of sedative dressings, *J Endod* 15:254, 1989.
41. Hylden J, Nahin R, Traub R, Dubner R: Expansion of receptor fields of spinal lamina I projection neurons in rats with unilateral adjuvant-induced inflammation, *Pain* 37:229, 1989.
42. Jackson DL, Moore PA, Hargreaves KM: Preoperative nonsteroidal anti-inflammatory medication for the prevention of postoperative dental pain, *J Am Dent Assoc* 119:641, 1989.

43. Janig W, Kollman W: The involvement of the sympathetic nervous system in pain, *Arzneim Forsch Drug Res* 34:1066, 1984.

44. Johnson D, Harshbarger J, Rymer H: Quantitative assessment of neural development in human premolars, *Anat Rec* 205:421, 1983.

45. Juan H, Lembeck F: Action of peptides and other algesic agents on paravascular pain receptors of the isolated perfused rabbit ear, *Naunyn-Schmeideberg's Arch Pharmacol* 283:151, 1974.

46. Kimberly C, Byers M: Inflammation of rat molar pulp and periodontium causes increased calcitonin gene related peptide and axonal sprouting, *Anat Rec* 222:289, 1988.

47. Kumazawa T, Mizumura K: Thin-fiber receptors responding to mechanical, chemical and thermal stimulation in the skeletal muscle of the dog, *J Physiol* 273:179, 1977.

48. Lanza FL et al: Effect of acetaminophen on human gastric mucosal injury caused by ibuprofen, *Gut* 27:440, 1986.

49. Levine J, Gordon N, Fields H: The mechanism of placebo analgesia, *Lancet* 2:654, 1978.

50. Levine J, Moskowitz M, Basbaum A: The contribution of neurogenic inflammation in experimental arthritis, *J Immunol* 135:843s, 1977.

51. Levine J, Taiwo Y: Inflammatory pain. In Wall PD, Melzack R, editors: *Textbook of pain,* ed 3, Edinburgh, 1994, Churchill-Livingstone, pp 45-56.

52. Lewin GR, Rueff A, Mendell LM: Peripheral and central mechanisms of NGF-induced hyperalgesia, *Eur J Neurosci* 6:1903, 1994.

53. Light AR: The initial processing of pain and its descending control: spinal and trigeminal systems, Basel, 1992, Karger.

54. Lindahl O: Pain: a chemical explanation, *Acta Rheumatol Scand* 8:161, 1962.

55. Madison S, Whitsel EA, Suarez-Roca H, Maixner W: Sensitizing effects of leukotriene B$_4$ on intradental primary afferents, *Pain* 49:99, 1992.

56. Maixner W et al: Responses of monkey medullary dorsal horn neurons during the detection of noxious heat stimuli, *J Neurophysiol* 62:437, 1989.

57. Malmberg A, Yaksh T: Antinociceptive actions of spinal nonsteroidal anti-inflammatory agents on the formalin test in rats, *J Pharmacol Exp Ther* 263:136, 1992.

58. Marshall JG, Liesinger A: Factors associated with endodontic posttreatment pain, *J Endod* 10:584, 1984.

59. Marshall JG, Walton RE: The effect of intramuscular injection of steroid on posttreatment endodontic pain, *J Endod* 19:573, 1993.

60. Martin H et al: Leukotriene and prostaglandin sensitization of cutaneous high-threshold C- and A-delta mechanoreceptors in the hairy skin of rat hindlimbs, *Neuroscience* 22:651, 1987.

61. Meller S, Gebhart G: Nitric oxide (NO) and nociceptive processing in the spinal cord, *Pain* 52:127, 1993.

62. Meyer R, Campbell J: Myelinated nociceptive afferents account for the hyperalgesia that follows a burn to the hand, *Science* 213:1527, 1981.

63. Moore PA: Long-acting local anesthetics: a review of clinical efficacy in dentistry, *Compendium* 11:24, 1990.

64. Moore PA, Werther JR, Seldin EB, Stevens CM: Analgesic regimens for third molar surgery: pharmacologic and behavioral considerations, *J Am Dent Assoc* 113:739, 1986.

65. Narhi M: The characteristics of intradental sensory units and their responses to stimulation, *J Dent Res* 64:564, 1985.

66. Narhi M et al: Role of intradental A and C type nerve fibers in dental pain mechanisms, *Proc Finn Dent Soc* 88(suppl 1):507, 1992.

67. Niv D: Intraoperative treatment of postoperative pain. In Campbell J, editor: *Pain 1996: an updated review,* Seattle, 1996, IASP Press, pp 173-187.

68. Penniston SG, Hargreaves KM: Evaluation of periapical injection of ketorolac for management of endodontic pain, *J Endod* 22:55, 1996.

69. Perl E: Alterations in the responsiveness of cutaneous nociceptors: sensitization by noxious stimuli and the induction of adrenergic responsiveness by nerve injury. In Willis W, editor: *Hyperalgesia and allodynia,* New York, 1992, Raven Press, pp 59-80.

70. Petty BG et al: The effect of systemically administered recombinant human nerve growth factor in healthy human subjects, *Ann Neurol* 36:244, 1994.

71. Rang H, Bevan S, Dray A: Nociceptive peripheral neurons: cellular properties. In Wall PD, Melzack R, editors: *Textbook of pain,* ed 3, Edinburgh, 1994, Churchill-Livingstone, p 57.

72. Ren K, Iadarola MJ, Dubner R: An isobolographic analysis of the effects of N-methyl-D-aspartate and NK$_1$ tachykinin receptor antagonists on inflammatory hyperalgesia in the rat, *Br J Pharmacol* 117:196, 1996.

73. Roy ML, Narahashi T: Differential properties of tetrodotoxin-sensitive and tetrodotoxin-resistant sodium channels in rat dorsal root ganglion neurons, *J Neurosci* 12:2104, 1992.

74. Schaible H, Schmidt R: Discharge characteristics of receptors with fine afferents from normal and inflamed joints: influence of analgesics and prostaglandins, *Agents Actions* 19(suppl):99, 1986.

75. Sessle BJ: Dental deafferentation can lead to the development of chronic pain. In Klineberg I, Sessle BJ, editors: *Oro-facial pain and neuromuscular dysfunction: mechanisms and clinical correlates,* Oxford, 1985, Pergamon Press, p 115.

76. Sessle BJ: Recent developments in pain research: central mechanisms of orofacial pain and its control, *J Endod* 12:435, 1986.

77. Sessle BJ: Neurophysiology of orofacial pain, *Dent Clin North Am* 31:595, 1987.

78. Sessle BJ, Hu JW, Amano N, Zhong G: Convergence of cutaneous, tooth pulp, visceral, neck and muscle afferents onto nociceptive and non-nociceptive neurones in trigeminal subnucleus caudalis (medullary dorsal horn) and its implications for referred pain, *Pain* 27:219, 1986.

79. Stambaugh JE Jr, Drew J: The combination of ibuprofen and oxycodone/acetaminophen in the management of chronic cancer pain, *Clin Pharmacol Ther* 44:665, 1988.

80. Steen KH, Reeh PW, Anton F, Handwerker HO: Protons selectively induce lasting excitation and sensitization to mechanical stimulation of nociceptors in rat skin in vitro, *J Neurosci* 21:86, 1992.

81. Sugimoto T, Bennett G, Kajander K: Transsynaptic degeneration in the superficial dorsal horn after sciatic nerve injury: effects of a chronic constriction injury, transection and strychnine, *Pain* 42:205, 1990.

82. Swift JQ, Garry MG, Roszkowski MT, Hargreaves KM: Effect of flurbiprofen on tissue levels of immunoreactive bradykinin and acute postoperative pain, *J Oral Maxillofac Surg* 51:112, 1993.

83. Troullos E, Freeman R, Dionne RA: The scientific basis for analgesic use in dentistry, *Anesth Prog* 33:123, 1986.

84. Trowbridge H: Review of dental pain: histology and physiology, *J Endod* 12:445, 1986.

85. Wagner R, Myers R: Endoneural injection of TNF-alpha or its second messenger ceramide results in nociceptive behavior in the rat. In *Abstracts 8th World Congress on Pain,* Seattle, 1996, IASP Press, p 353.

86. Wall P, Woolf C: Muscle but not cutaneous C-afferent input produces prolonged increases in the excitability of the flexion reflex in the rat, *J Physiol* 356:443, 1984.

87. Willis W: *The pain system,* Basel, 1985, Karger.

88. Willis W: *Hyperalgesia and allodynia,* New York, 1992, Raven Press.

89. Woolfe C: Evidence for a central component of post-injury pain hypersensitivity, *Nature* 306:686, 1983.

90. Wright CE III, Antal EJ, Gillespie WR, Albert KS: Ibuprofen and acetaminophen kinetics when taken concurrently, *Clin Pharmacol Ther* 34:707, 1983.

91. Wynn R, Meiller T, Crossley H: *Drug information handbook for dentistry 1996-97,* Hudson, Ohio, 1996, Lexi-Comp.

92. Xiao W-H, Wagner R, Myers R, Sorkin L: TNF-alpha applied to the sciatic nerve trunk elicits background firing in nociceptive primary afferent fibers. In *Abstracts 8th World Congress on Pain,* Seattle, 1996, IASP Press, p 354.

Chapter 18

Surgical Endodontics

Gary B. Carr
Scott K. Bentkover

DEFINITION AND SCOPE

Surgical endodontics is the treatment of choice when teeth cannot be treated appropriately by nonsurgical means. The skillful dental surgeon borrows techniques from the periodontist, the oral surgeon, and the restorative dentist and integrates those skills into the art of endodontic surgery. The goal of all endodontic surgery is to remove disease, to prevent it from recurring, and to facilitate healing.

The dental surgeon must have comprehensive knowledge of anatomy and a clear understanding of the biologic principles underlying soft and hard tissue management, including an understanding of surgical wound healing. These requirements have made endodontic surgery a highly disciplined skill.

DIAGNOSIS

Skillful diagnosis in endodontic surgery requires the accurate determination of the reasons for endodontic failure and the dental surgeon's certitude that this failure can be corrected by the appropriate surgical procedure. It is axiomatic that endodontic surgery is not a substitute for careless nonsurgical treatment.[31]

Many root canal systems do not easily lend themselves to surgical therapy. In fact many systems become more difficult to treat when a surgical approach is employed (Fig. 18-1). Once the practitioner is certain that no better result can be achieved by using nonsurgical treatment, the surgical option should be considered.[12,30,63] If the root canal system is properly cleaned, shaped, and obturated, the endodontic failure rate is extremely low, and the need for surgical procedures is minimal.[30,46a] In most cases the surgical approach addresses the inability of the clinician to adequately seal the root canal system three dimensionally. Since research has consistently shown us that incompletely obturated canal systems have a markedly reduced surgical success rate,[31,35] the thoughtful clinician will attempt to three-dimensionally clean, shape, and pack the entire root canal system. Surgery should be the choice only when these attempts have failed (Fig. 18-2).

CONTRAINDICATIONS TO SURGICAL ENDODONTICS

The restorability and the periodontal prognosis of a tooth are important in choosing treatment, but the medical condition of the patient is paramount. Because a surgical entry obviously requires an incision into soft tissue and the removal of bone, the patient must be physically and mentally healthy enough to permit uneventful healing. Thus a thorough medical history (as described in Chapter 1) should be recorded, reviewed, and discussed with the patient to determine if any potential health risks exist.

When doubt arises following an evaluation of the patient's health history, medical consultation with the patient's physician is indicated. All medical concerns and questions should be answered before the surgery. To avert any adverse drug reaction, all medications must be appraised and proper precautions taken. (For appropriate antibiotic prophylactic therapy before surgery, see Chapter 5.)

Few overt medical conditions contraindicate endodontic surgery; however, since apical surgery is an invasive procedure, the dental surgeon should be extremely wary of treating patients with (1) clotting deficiencies or blood dyscrasias, (2) "brittle" diabetes, (3) kidney disease that requires dialysis, or (4) a compromised immune system.

Clotting Deficiencies

Good hemostasis is essential for apical surgery and uneventful healing; therefore careful questioning of the patient regarding potential clotting deficiencies is indicated. The patient's experience with surgery or trauma wounds often reveals details that are unknown, even to the patient or the patient's current attending physician. Do you bruise easily, Ms. Jones? Did you experience bleeding after wisdom teeth extraction? Were there any bleeding complications during pregnancy? These are essential questions to ask. Thus the skilled clinician must be not only a meticulous historian but an adroit detective as well. If any doubt exists, a prothrombin time and bleeding time should be taken before the surgery.

Brittle Diabetes

Patients with brittle diabetes are particularly poor risks for surgery, as they suffer from multisystem organ disease. Since diabetes is essentially a disease of the terminal arterioles, these patients exhibit markedly reduced wound healing capability. Long-term brittle diabetes usually manifests end-stage renal disease, so a serious infection is life threatening. Leukocyte function is severely compromised because of decreased chemotaxis and phagocytosis. Diabetic patients are always prescribed antibiotics and monitored daily until they are out of danger.

Dialysis

Patients receiving dialysis treatments are another high-risk group because they frequently suffer from a multitude of bleeding disorders, viral blood infections (e.g., hepatitis, human immunodeficiency virus [HIV] infection), altered drug metabo-

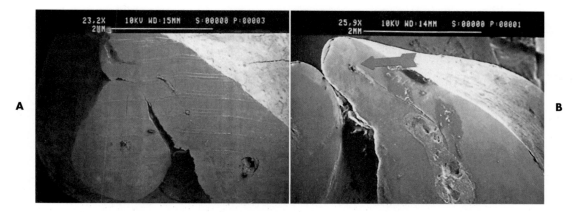

FIG. 18-1 A, Resected root of a maxillary first molar. Note the irregular ramifications between the MB-1 and the MB-2 canals and the difficult retropreparation this would require. **B,** Completed retrofilling material in the mesiobuccal root of a maxillary molar. Note the extreme lingual position of the missed MB-2 canal *(arrow)* and the connecting isthmus.

lism, and impaired wound healing. These patients are managed only after consultation with their nephrologist and after a thorough blood workup is analyzed. Since proteoglycan synthesis and ground substance metabolism are diminished in patients receiving dialysis treatments, delayed or incomplete soft and hard tissue wound repair occurs. All patients receiving dialysis treatments require prophylactic antibiotics because of the presence of arteriovenus shunts and the potential for fatal infective endarteritis.

Compromised Immune System

Immunocompromised patients are also at serious surgical risk. Frequently, these patients take a combination of cytotoxic drugs and corticosteroids and suffer from poor wound healing and susceptibility to infection. Surgical procedures should be avoided if possible.

PRESURGICAL WORKUP

If surgery is necessary, a presurgical workup is in order. The surgeon must first explain to the patient the proposed procedures and all available alternative treatments. A brief explanation, in lay terms, of what is to be done and what the patient can expect postsurgically should be discussed by the dental surgeon. This provides the dental surgeon an opportunity to assess the patient's psychologic status, address concerns, and establish a bond that conveys the doctor's understanding, empathy, and skill. Nothing enhances a surgical result more than a patient's confidence in the dental surgeon.

During the presurgical workup, the dentist must advise patients of any necessary changes in daily activities: drug regimen (i.e., no aspirin 3 days before surgery); the need to begin chlorhexidine rinses 2 days before surgery; the need to arrange for transportation home following surgery; and the need to restrict activities following the procedure (i.e., no smoking or alcohol consumption for 3 days; no vigorous exercise that would dramatically increase blood pressure). These discussions have more impact at the presurgical workup than they would just before the procedure, as they involve changes in lifestyle and scheduling that the patient might not normally anticipate. It contributes to a nonstressful surgical environment if patients know exactly what to expect and what is expected of them.

This professional bonding between doctor and patient often minimizes presurgical anxiety and trepidation.

The clinical presurgical workup should attempt to anticipate all possible complications. Medical history review, blood pressure check, and if necessary consultation with the patient's family physician should be conducted at this time and noted in the chart. It is important to observe the patient's crown contours, pocket depths, alveolar bone topography, zones of attached gingiva and alveolar mucosa, vestibular depth, muscle attachments, root eminences, furcal involvements, and the health and architecture of the interdental papilla. Additional radiographs are exposed if needed to better assess critical anatomic structures that may be endangered by the procedure (e.g., mental or mandibular nerves, the maxillary sinus and floor of the nose). After evaluating these factors, the dentist then outlines the preliminary flap design and enters it into the patient's chart. Time spent in presurgical screening pays dividends by ensuring that the dental surgeon has anticipated and planned for all possibilities.

SURGICAL PROTOCOL AND ANESTHESIA

At the surgical appointment the dental surgeon should again review the procedure with the patient and respond to any additional concerns. Blood pressure is taken, chlorhexidine rinse given, and a nonsteroidal antiinflammatory drug administered preoperatively. Research shows that it is easier to prevent pain than to reduce it after it occurs.[7] Techniques for administering anesthesia are explained in Chapter 19. One of our goals in surgical anesthesia is not only to provide profound anesthesia for the procedure but also to extend this anesthesia for a prolonged period following the surgery. Additionally, the surgeon depends on the anesthesia for its hemostatic effect. Good surgical anesthesia involves a dual-entry technique. The initial injection uses one of the longer acting anesthetics (e.g., bupivacaine, etidocaine). These long-acting anesthetics provide 2 to 4 hours of profound surgical anesthesia and up to 4 to 10 hours of lighter anesthesia. After regional block anesthesia is confirmed, the surgeon administers 2% lidocaine with 1:50,000 epinephrine to achieve good hemostasis. Even in medically compromised patients the *slow* administration *(for a period of 2 minutes)* of 1:50,000 epinephrine poses no systemic risk. It

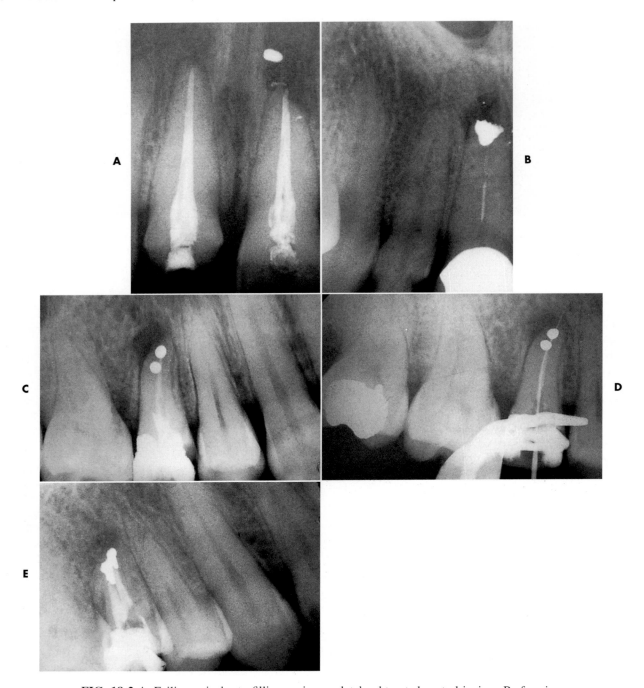

FIG. 18-2 A, Failing apical retrofilling on incompletely obturated central incisor. Performing surgery on such teeth is contraindicated. **B,** Failing apical surgery on incompletely cleaned and obturated central incisor. Appropriate initial therapy is nonsurgical treatment of this tooth. **C** and **D,** Failing apicoectomy on a maxillary premolar. Nonsurgical retreatment reveals a missed lingual canal. Lingual retrofilling has not sealed the apical portal of exit. **E,** Surgical retreatment of the case shown in **C** and **D** with ultrasonic retropreparations placed after the nonsurgical retreatment of both canals.

is only the *rapid* injection of 1:50,000 epinephrine that poses a risk.

The best injection technique to achieve maximal hemostasis involves depositing the solution near the apexes of the root with the needle beveled toward the periostium in the loose connective tissue of the alveolar submucosa.[5,31] Slow (2-minute), multiple injections ensure rapid diffusion without damaging the delicate collagenous bundles that compose the alveolar submu-

cosa (Fig. 18-3). Because the primary blood supply of the gingival tissues emanates from vertically oriented vessels in the alveolar mucosa (Fig. 18-4), enhanced hemostasis is achieved by depositing solution there, *not* by injecting it into the attached gingiva. The attached gingiva consists of dense fibrous connective tissue; its compartmentalized, collagenous nature impedes diffusion of anesthesia. Injections into attached gingiva or worse yet into the papilla to achieve hemostasis are

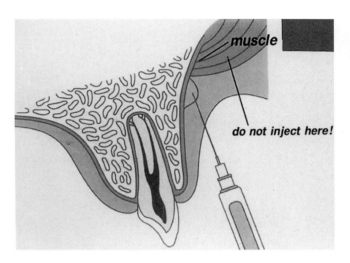

FIG. 18-3 Correct placement of anesthetic is at the apices and not into the muscle attachments.

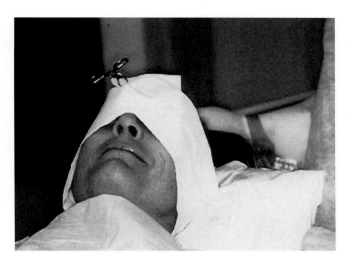

FIG. 18-5 Placement of an eye drape protects the patient's eyes from inadvertent injury and helps shield the patient from the intense light.

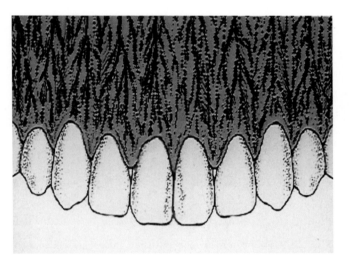

FIG. 18-4 Diagrammatic view of the vertical orientation of blood vessels in the alveolar mucosa and attached gingiva. This orientation means that flaps do not need to be broader at the base and the releasing incisions can be oriented vertically without endangering the vascular supply at the flap corners.

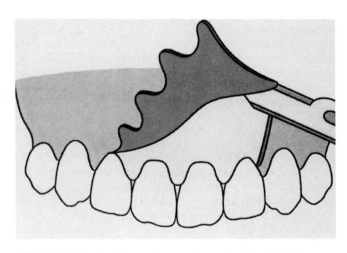

FIG. 18-6 Sulcular triangular or rectangular flap. This flap may have either one or two vertical releasing incisions.

contraindicated and cause unnecessary surgical trauma.[31] Additional injections apical to the root apices into the vestibular tissues are unnecessary.

The hemostatic effect of the epinephrine is produced by its action on α_2-adrenergic receptors on vessels of the terminal microvasculature. Injection into the deeper vestibular tissues or near basal bone, with its muscle attachments, places the solution near tissues that have a much higher concentration of β_2-adrenergic receptors, causing vasodilation. For example, injection of 1:50,000 epinephrine near the buccinator muscle attachment or mentalis muscle attachment results in increased bleeding into the surgical site, compromising surgical visibility.

After profound anesthesia is confirmed, the patient is covered with a gown, the patient's eyes protected by glasses or an eye drape (Fig. 18-5), and the perioral skin cleansed with povidone-iodine (Betadine) or iodine wash to remove skin bac-

teria, cosmetics, and other facial contaminants that can only complicate surgical wound healing. Facial hair (i.e., beards, mustaches) is trimmed at this time if it appears that it could contaminate the surgical field. After the patient is draped, the surgery can begin.

SOFT TISSUE MANAGEMENT IN ENDODONTIC SURGERY

The first surgical trauma is the puncture from the anesthetic needle and injecting the anesthetic. The next trauma is the incision. All flaps for endodontic apical surgery require a horizontal and vertical component. *The horizontal component determines the type of flap.*[28] We recognize the two basic types as *sulcular* and *mucogingival* (Figs. 18-6 and 18-7). The number of vertical releasing incisions determines whether the flap is rectangular or triangular.

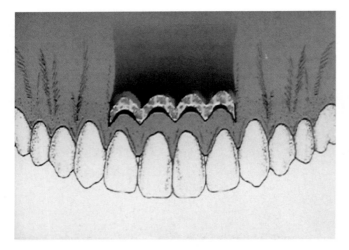

FIG. 18-7 Mucogingival flap with two vertical releasing incisions. Horizontal incision should be at least 2 mm apical to the attachment apparatus.

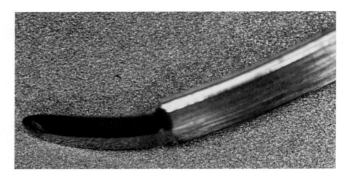

FIG. 18-8 Microsurgical scalpel curved to conform to the cervical convexity of the tooth.

Triangular or Rectangular Flap with Sulcular Incision

A triangular or rectangular flap with sulcular incision provides the best access of all flaps. Of utmost concern when using this design is the health of the gingival tissues. Using the triangular or rectangular flap with a sulcular incision when the gingival tissue is diseased is contraindicated. When sulcular incisions are made in healthy gingiva, every attempt should be made to preserve the integrity of the sulcular epithelium of the gingival crevice and to minimize trauma to the root-attached gingival fibers. Preservation of these soft tissues, especially in the interdental col area, is crucial for obtaining healing by primary intention. If the tissues that comprise the attachment apparatus are handled with skill during incision and elevation, healing by primary intention occurs.[33,34,89]

Vertical releasing incisions are generally made one or two teeth proximal to the involved tooth. This incision should be placed perpendicular to the horizontal sulcular incision, and the two should converge at the mesial or distal line angle of the tooth. Scrupulous care must be taken to place the vertical incision *between* the root eminences and not over the root surface, where the mucosa is thin and therefore difficult to suture. This flap has the advantage of having excellent vascularity because all the supraperiosteal vessels are contained within the flap. Accurate reapproximation is easy to achieve. The disadvantage of this flap is evident; if the attachment apparatus is inflamed or mismanaged during the incision, elevation, or suturing process, healing occurs by secondary intention. Secondary intention healing results in loss of crestal bone, increased pocket depth, and a prolonged healing period. Handled properly, this flap design can preserve the existing epithelial attachment with no loss of marginal gingiva.[33,89] Microsurgical scalpel blades (Figs. 18-8 and 18-9) curved to conform to the cervical contour of the tooth are helpful in preserving the sulcular epithelial lining and minimizing damage to the root-attached gingival fibers, while making the interproximal incision in the col area easier to accomplish.

The elevation of this flap follows the principle of *undermining elevation*.[30,34] Such elevation respects and protects the delicate tissues of the attachment apparatus and preserves

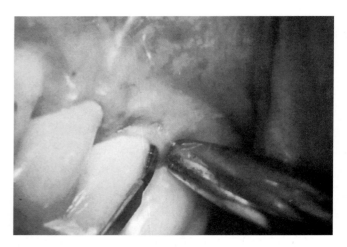

FIG. 18-9 Microsurgical incision using microsurgical scalpel blades permits very accurate and atraumatic incision into the sulcus and interdental papilla area.

its structural integrity so that when they are reapproximated, reattachment begins almost immediately. This elevation technique always begins in the vertical releasing incision, using a sharp Molt or Ruddle 30-degree curette (Fig. 18-10). Periosteum and alveolar mucosa are elevated apical to the attached and marginal gingiva. Then using gentle sharp dissection the dental surgeon frees up the attached gingiva and gently elevates the papilla and marginal gingiva from underneath (Fig. 18-11). This technique avoids the crushing and tearing trauma occasionally associated with traditional methods of flap elevation.[89]

Triangular or Rectangular Flap with Mucogingival Incision

The triangular or rectangular flap with mucogingival incision, referred to as a *Luebke-Ochsenbein flap*, owes its popularity to the fact that the marginal gingiva and attachment apparatus remain undisturbed. If the mucogingival incision is scalloped, reapproximation is simplified (Fig. 18-12). The el-

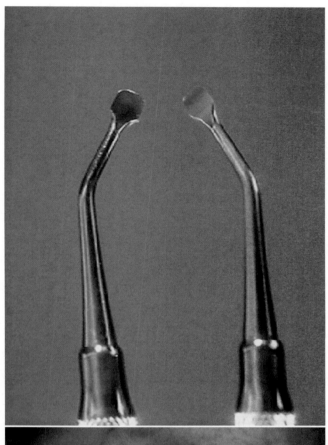

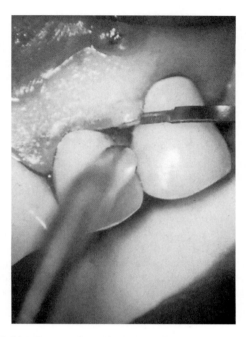

FIG. 18-11 Microsurgical dissection of the interdental col and papilla before elevation. Atraumatic management of this tissue results in primary intention healing. This papilla is elevated from underneath by the Ruddle 30-degree curette. In this technique no crushing or tearing injury is associated with the elevation of the flap.

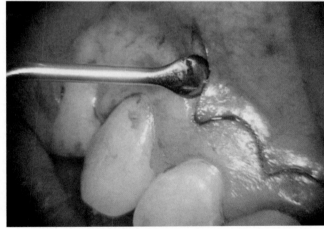

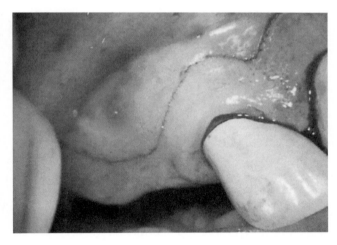

FIG. 18-10 A, Ruddle 30-degree curettes are exceptionally sharp and can be used like a scalpel to perform sharp dissection when elevating the flap. **B,** Correct placement of the Ruddle 30-degree curette. Correct elevation of the flap begins at the releasing incision and elevates the coronal margins of the flap from below.

FIG. 18-12 Scalloped incision permits easy reapproximation of the flapped tissues.

evation of the flap follows the same principles as those for the sulcular flap, beginning at the vertical releasing incision and moving to the coronal margins from an apical direction. This technique protects the wound edges from traumatic crushing and ischemic injury. When reapproximated, the wound edges are ready to heal by primary intention. Since the horizontal incision of this flap severs the major blood supply of the remaining marginal gingiva, the survival of this tissue depends on the

secondary blood supply received from the alveolar bone, which can be highly variable and whose extent, unfortunately, is unknown to the dental surgeon. Another problem one may encounter with this design is flap shrinkage, causing scar formation because of secondary intention healing. This flap design is contraindicated if there is limited attached gingiva or if there are short roots or large periapical lesions, or when the cervical aspect of the root must be examined.

Additional Flap Designs

As the field of endodontic surgery becomes more refined, so too does our understanding of the limitations of other traditional techniques. A wide variety of other flap designs—trapezoidal, gingival, semilunar—are seldom used in endodontic surgery, not only because they offer no additional advantages to those previously discussed, but also because serious disadvantages preclude their use.[31]

Atraumatic Flap Management

Rapid and uneventful healing depends on the dental surgeon's deft, atraumatic handling of the flap throughout surgery and the accurate reapproximation of the wound edges at the conclusion of the procedure. *Most flap injuries result from inadvertent crushing, tearing, or ischemic damage that occurs during incision, elevation, retraction, or suturing.*[89] The surgeon may avoid these multiple injuries if a flap design is developed that is appropriate for the procedure. Microsurgical incisions and undermining elevations reduce the crushing and tearing injury sometimes associated with traditional flap elevation. In cases where the lesion has perforated the buccal cortical bone and has attached itself to the mucoperiosteum, sharp dissection is needed to separate the flap from the lesion (Fig. 18-13).

After the flap has been elevated, the dental surgeon should ensure that minimal tension exists at all perimeters before the osteotomy. If tension exists, one or both releasing incisions may need to be extended.

Once the flap is reflected passively, the retractors are positioned. Because the dental surgeon holds one retractor and the assistant may hold the other retractor, both operators must have unrestricted visibility of the bony architecture and *both* must be certain that the flap is not being impinged. *The most common cause for postsurgical swelling and ecchymosis is inadvertent crushing of the reflected flap by the retractor(s).*[34] Since the dental surgeon's attention is focused on the root end procedure, he or she is frequently unaware of flap impingement until it is too late. This unnecessary trauma can be prevented by preparing two short, shallow grooves in the alveolar bone and letting the retractors rest in the grooves (Fig. 18-14). This technique reduces the visual requirement on the part of the assistant and makes slippage of the retractors over the flap much less likely (Fig. 18-14, *B*).

Dental surgeons who follow this protocol for atraumatic flap management are rewarded with patients who experience remarkable healing rates, even for lengthy surgical procedures.[11]

HARD TISSUE MANAGEMENT

The goal in developing a good flap design is to allow the dental surgeon and the assistant both visual and manual access. Once the flap is atraumatically reflected and both visual and manual access are obtained, the dental surgeon initiates bony access. Like manipulation of the mucoperiosteum, atraumatic surgical manipulation of bone must be deft, skillful, and adroit. Injury to hard tissue in periradicular surgery involves trauma to bone, cementum, and dentin. Of these, dentin is the only tissue that does not repair itself. Bone heals more slowly than cementum and much more slowly than soft tissue, perhaps because the periosteum does not survive the elevation process.[31,34,39] Bone, a very labile organ, sustains mechanical, thermal, and chemical insults during periradicular surgery.

Removal of bone with a rotary bur in an atraumatic manner requires dexterity, patience, and skill. The correct technique requires first positioning a bone-cutting bur (Fig. 18-15) or a No. 4 round bur at high speed (greater than 200,000 rpm), using

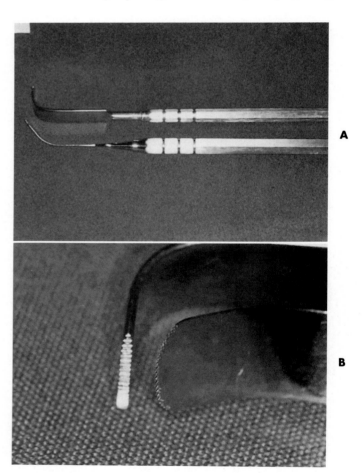

A

B

FIG. 18-14 A and **B,** Carr retractors Nos. 1 and 2 are serrated at their ends to facilitate placement in grooves created in the bone. These notches prevent slippage of the retractor and prevent impingement of soft tissue.

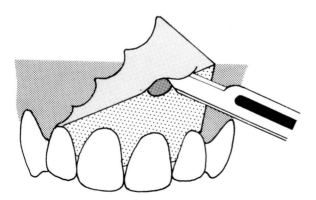

FIG. 18-13 Chronic lesions of long duration occasionally prevent elevation because the granulation tissue perforates through the buccal bone and integrates into the overlying periosteum. Sharp dissection is required to release the lesion from the periosteum.

very light, brushing strokes that minimize mechanical and thermal injury.[10] Because of the danger of air embolism using high-speed handpieces under a flap, handpieces that have no air output at the working end have been devised (Fig. 18-16). These have the added advantage of not spraying surgical debris into the bone and under the flap. Bone burs are designed to minimize clogging and thereby decrease frictional heat buildup. A new bur should be used for every procedure and discarded after use. A copious water spray is important to minimize the generation of heat.

The location of the lesion may not be obvious if the buccal plate has not been perforated by the soft tissue lesion. Presurgical radiographs are helpful for estimating its location, and measurements taken from the radiograph can be transferred to the surgical site. The similar appearance of dentin and bone can further complicate entry; however, dentin is typically slightly yellower and smoother in texture than bone. Once the root outline is observed, cortical bone is removed in an intermittent, brushinglike circular action[74] to allow appropriate visual access to the lesion and root end. When there are few external landmarks, an accurate osteotomy takes skill and judgment. If doubt remains about the location of the root, a piece of sterilized x-ray foil is placed at the entry point and a radiograph is exposed to orient the surgical team. The bony access must be sufficient so that adequate visibility and proper illumination are achieved. Roots that are positioned more lingually require larger bony accesses.

No matter how benign-looking the appearance, tissue from every lesion should be sent for a pathologic examination. Although more than 90% of all lesions are cysts, granulomas, or odontogenic abscesses, a small number are nonodontogenic neoplasms, which may require further medical or dental intervention (Chapter 12).

The dental surgeon should attempt to remove the lesion in toto, using the technique outlined in Fig. 18-17. Whether it is necessary to remove every last remnant of tissue to ensure healing is unclear; in all likelihood, simply disrupting the lining leads to healing if the factors that caused the lesion have been eliminated (Chapter 12). When complete removal of tissue would endanger neurovascular bundles (mental or mandibular nerves) or violate other anatomic structures (floor of the nose, maxillary sinus), aggressive curettement is contraindicated. Research has repeatedly shown that healing proceeds only after the contaminants within the root canal system have been eliminated or sealed from the periapical tissues.[13,27,30] For this reason, apical curettage alone is not considered definitive treatment. Neglecting to rectify the causative factors within the root canal system invites failure.

When operating near vital anatomic structures such as the maxillary sinus or mental or mandibular nerve bundles, conservative osteotomy begins midroot and progresses apically after the surgeon has established landmarks. After achieving suitable bony access and identifying the apex, the dental surgeon curettes and removes the lesion.

APICAL RESECTION (APICOECTOMY)

Once adequate osseous access has been made and the periradicular lesion removed, the dental surgeon is ready to address the cause of the problem: an incompletely cleaned and sealed root canal system. Close scrutiny of the root may reveal more than one possible cause of failure: multiple apical portals of

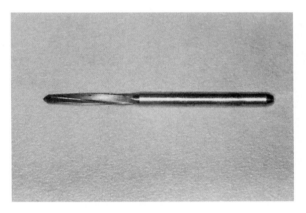

FIG. 18-15 Lindemann bone-cutting bur is designed to reduce clogging and therefore minimize heat buildup.

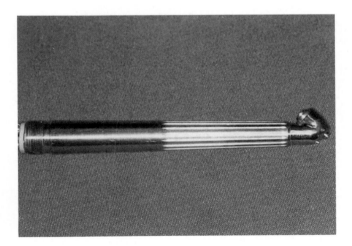

FIG. 18-16 No air exits from the working end of the Impact Air 45 handpiece, reducing the possibility of producing air emphysema or air embolism while operating under the flap.

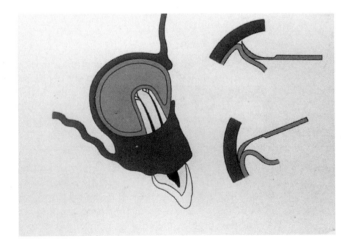

FIG. 18-17 Correct curettement of the soft tissue lesion requires using a sharp spoon in different positions in various locations in the crypt.

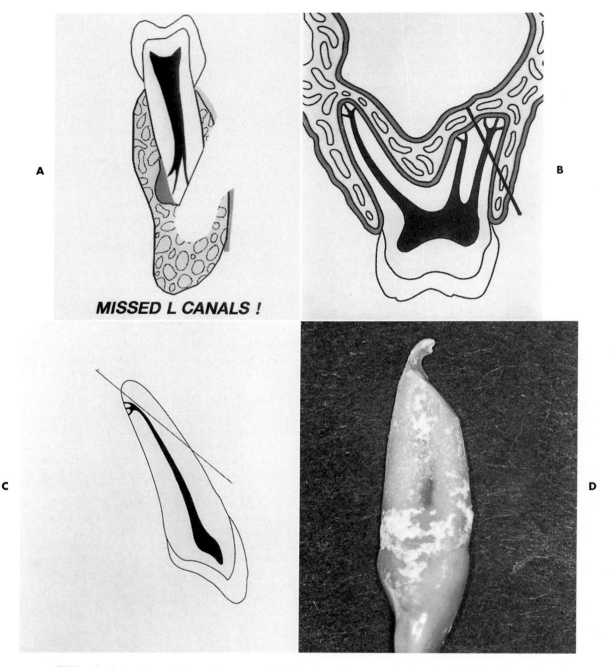

MISSED L CANALS !

FIG. 18-18 A, An acute bevel on a mandibular premolar can entirely miss the lingual canal if the dental surgeon is not aware of the possibility of a second lingual canal. **B,** Acute bevel on a maxillary molar may miss the MB-2 canal or lingual ramifications that are common. **C** and **D,** Failure to completely resect through a maxillary canine may leave the lingual aspect of the root intact or leave the lingual apical ramifications present.

exit, additional roots not seen in the radiograph, extruded filling materials or foreign bodies, apical root fractures, or accessory portals of exit on the lateral root surface. A dental surgeon's knowledge of root canal system anatomy and root morphology is tested every time the surgeon makes an apical examination of a failed root canal. These are opportunities for learning that increase our understanding about endodontic failure.

After root inspection, the dental surgeon forms a three-dimensional mental image of the morphology of the root and

probable internal pulp system anatomy and plans an appropriate resection. For a maxillary anterior tooth close to the labial cortical bone, this apical resection is simple and straightforward. For teeth that are multirooted or multicanaled and lingually inclined, the task is more difficult (Fig. 18-18, *A* and *B*). Because the dental surgeon does not have knowledge about the true buccal or lingual inclination of the root, a resection that appears to cut directly through the root may in fact be an extreme oblique resection (Fig. 18-18, *C*). This is

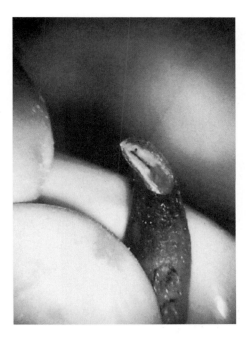

FIG. 18-19 Maxillary premolar with acute bevel demonstrating the additional surface area needed for an adequate retropreparation.

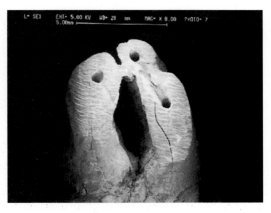

FIG. 18-20 Ultrasonic root end preparations placed very close to the lingual margin of the root because of a very acute bevel.

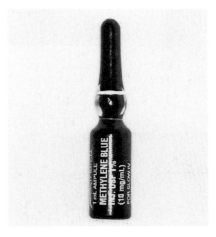

FIG. 18-21 Methylene blue dye can be used to stain vital tissue and can help delineate the pulp and root outline.

especially true in mandibular posterior teeth, where a thick buccal cortex is present, or in mandibular anterior teeth, where roots have a lingual inclination and the surgeon has limited manipulative access due to the mentalis muscle attachment. Failure to cut completely through the root in a buccolingual direction is one of the most common errors in periradicular surgery (Fig. 18-18, *D*). Even when the resection is complete, the bevel is frequently so oblique that the lingual apical ramifications are not eliminated.[11,13] A good rule to follow is this: *Whatever the angle of the bevel, it is almost always greater than it appears to be.* The experienced dental surgeon compensates for this distortion of perspective by reducing the angle of the bevel and positioning it more perpendicular to the longitudinal axis of the root. Another disadvantage of the extreme bevel is that, as the bevel angle increases, the surface area of the cut dentinal tubules likewise increases, and the canal systems, which must be sealed, become elongated in a buccolingual direction (Fig. 18-19). Furthermore, this elongation requires extremely skillful retropreparations close to the lingual aspect of the root (Fig. 18-20).

After the root has been beveled, the cut surface requires close inspection to verify that the root is completely sectioned, the cut smooth, and the bevel angle sufficient enough to provide manual access for the retropreparation.[30]

Frequently the osseous access must be enlarged at this juncture, especially if retropreparations are required in the lingual aspect of the crypt. To clearly identify the complete outline of the root, a small amount of methylene blue dye (Figs. 18-21 and 18-22) can be painted on the root surface (Fig. 18-23). After preliminary inspection is complete and the dental surgeon feels no additional modifications will be needed, the crypt is packed with one of the many surgical dressings available. CollaCote (CaLCITEK, Plainsboro, N. J.; Fig. 18-24) and Avitene (Johnson and Johnson, New Brunswick, N. J.) are particularly

efficacious dressings because they contain collagen, which activates clotting. *The retrofilling procedure must take place in a dry, sterile field, so hemostasis within the crypt is a significant concern.* Adaptic (Johnson & Johnson), Melolite (Smith & Nephew, Memphis, Tenn.) Gelfoam (Upjohn Company, Kalamazoo, Mich.), Surgicel (Johnson & Johnson), and Telfa pads (Kendall Company, Mansfield, Mass; Fig. 18-25) are also useful adjuncts for this packing, as they contain no cotton fibers that could contaminate the field and retard wound healing.[48] Hemostasis within the crypt can also be achieved by using a solution of ferric subsulfate (Fig. 18-26), which has an extremely low pH (0.21) and rapidly causes intravascular coagulation. Since ferric subsulfate is a necrosing agent,[42,43] it must be used judiciously. There are reports that salts of ferric sulfate can remain in tissue, creating a permanent tattoo, and that it should not be used in any cosmetic areas.[1,2] Dermatologic studies have shown that ferric subsulfate can permeate into deeper structures and cause foreign body reactions lasting for weeks.[2] It should therefore be used with extreme caution in areas near vital structures such as the floor of the nose, maxillary sinus, and mental or mandibular nerve bundles. If the dental surgeon finds it necessary to use this hemostatic agent,

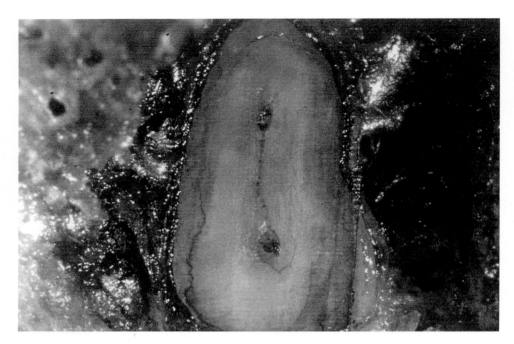

FIG. 18-22 Mesiobuccal root of maxillary molar stained with methylene blue demonstrating vital periodontal ligament and isthmus tissue.

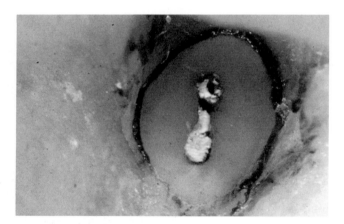

FIG. 18-23 Methylene blue dye stains the periodontal ligament and facilitates identification of the root. It also stains remaining pulp tissue or voids in obturation.

the proper technique is to place a drop on a Telfa pad, remove the excess by squeezing the pad, and then station it against the wall of the crypt for 5 minutes. It is imperative to keep this solution away from the buccal bone, the flap margins, and the periodontal ligament. The cells responsible for initial healing in the periradicular area originate from the periodontal ligament[31,52]; minimizing trauma to these cells is therefore a high priority.

APICAL RETROPREPARATION EXAMINATION

After hemostasis is achieved and the crypt packed, the beveled root end is critically examined with supplemental illumination and magnification,[11] (Plates 18-1 to 18-3). A thorough assessment of the root end should be done with appropriate

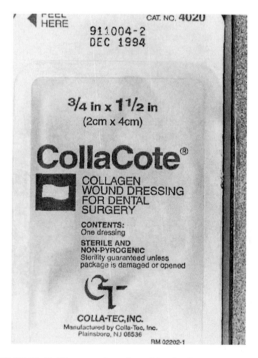

FIG. 18-24 CollaCote can be placed in the bony crypt and promotes hemostasis.

magnification and illumination.[11,13] Perhaps no area of endodontics is in greater need of improvement than in the evaluation of the beveled root end. Since the dental surgeon is confronted with the problem of microscopic leakage, the more detailed the inspection that can be achieved, the more confidence the surgeon can have about the apical seal. The simple act of

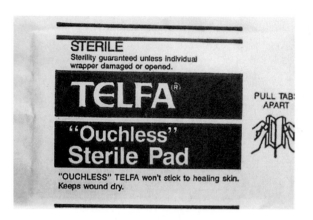

FIG. 18-25 Telfa pads can also be packed into the bony crypt, where they help with hemostasis and prevent contamination by foreign debris.

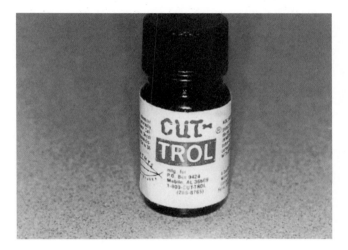

FIG. 18-26 Ferric subsulfate is a powerful hemostatic agent and should be used with caution in the bony crypt.

root resection opens up the entire root canal system, with all its irregularities, to the periapex.

REVIEW OF RETROPREPARATION TECHNIQUE

Retropreparation techniques have historically involved a cursory examination of the root end and an assessment of the adequacy of the root canal filling. Evaluating such seals with the unaided eye is nothing more than a guess. The best assessment of hermetic apical seals requires measurement tolerances on the order of microns, and we do not possess the technology today to confidently evaluate such a seal in a clinical setting. *Until such technology becomes available, prudence dictates that we assume that all beveled root canal fillings are leaking.* Independent scanning electron microscope studies show that the simple act of apical resection disturbs the gutta-percha seal.[72] Therefore the placement of a retrofill is essential unless there are extenuating circumstances.

Even a cursory examination of beveled roots on extracted teeth can reveal to the dental surgeon the infinite variety of pulpal configurations found in nature (Fig. 18-27). Interpreting these configurations in cross section at the time of surgery can be a daunting challenge. The dental surgeon can be con-

fronted with a bewildering array of communicating anastomoses, lateral canals, fracture lines, culs-de-sac, fusion lines, etc. (Fig. 18-28). Additionally, since the root is usually much broader buccolingually than mesiodistally, these confusing arrays are elongated and distorted by the typically angled bevel. Simply understanding what needs to be done to create a seal takes a great deal of skill, judgment, and experience. *The idea that the classic, round, ball bearing type of preparation is adequate is no longer valid because round preparations seldom conform to anatomic structures.* Retropreparations should be oval or slot shaped. Fortunately, the development of ultrasonic retropreparation has helped to standardize these preparations and increased the likelihood that they will be consistently well placed.

Traditional handpiece retropreparation technique uses either miniature contraangle rotary burs or a straight handpiece with limited access. Rarely can a contraangle microhandpiece or a straight handpiece with quarter round bur be placed down the long axis of the root. These preparations are almost always placed obliquely into the root, sometimes even at right angles to the long axis of the pulp canal (Fig. 18-29). Such a misplacement has the major disadvantage of having to rely on the axial wall of the preparation instead of the pulpal floor to effect a seal (Fig. 18-30). Since research has shown that we can expect all nonphysiologic retrofilling materials to undergo some degree of circumferential resorption, the marginal sealing capability will be quickly jeopardized with only minimal resorption.[83]

Retropreparations should accept filling materials that predictably seal off the root canal system from the periradicular tissues. These preparations must fulfill the following requirements:

1. The apical 3 mm of the root is cleaned and shaped.
2. Preparation is parallel to and coincident with the anatomic outline of the pulpal space.
3. Adequate retention form is created.
4. All isthmus tissue is removed.
5. Remaining dentinal walls are not weakened.

In posterior teeth, roots with dual canal systems have multiple anastomoses between them.[57] Once the apex has been removed, the surgeon confronts a much more complex situation. If webbing or interstitial pulp harbors microorganisms or their toxic products, removing these irritants or sealing them off from the periapical tissues is necessary. The endodontic requirements for successful healing are the same for surgical and nonsurgical treatment. Success depends on the cleaning, shaping, and sealing of all portals of exit. Failure to prepare and seal the isthmus areas or any of the anatomic variations present invites failure (Figs. 18-31 and 18-32). The narrow isthmus areas between confluent canal systems can be difficult to see even with a microscope (Fig. 18-33). As a general rule, *all roots with multiple canal systems contain isthmus tissue.*[87] The retropreparation of these narrow isthmus areas presents the dental surgeon with a great challenge. Since the margin of error is less than 1 mm, the surgeon must be especially careful to avoid inadvertent perforation.

For successful retropreparation the dental surgeon must be well versed not only in root canal system anatomy but also in root morphology. The kinds of cases that present for surgery are precisely those in which the anatomy is either aberrant or unusually complex. There are many anatomic studies documenting the infinite variation in tooth morphology and root ca-

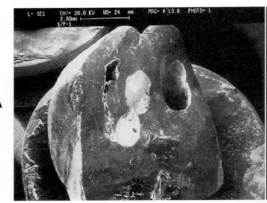
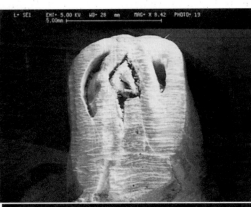

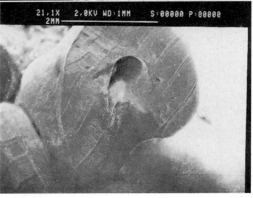

FIG. 18-27 A, Failed apicoectomy shows that the practitioner has mistaken the fusion line between the mesial and distal roots for the MB-2 canal. MB-2 canal and isthmus are completely uninstrumented. **B,** Fused roots can present a confusing picture to the practitioner. Fusion lines and intrafurcal bone can resemble canal spaces. **C,** Incomplete apical retropreparation. Preparation needs to be extended lingually.

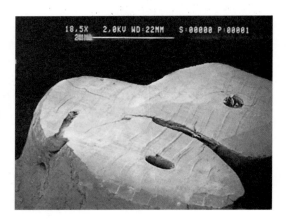

FIG. 18-28 Complex anatomy of maxillary molar shows the need to extend retropreparation to the lingual cementodentinal junction.

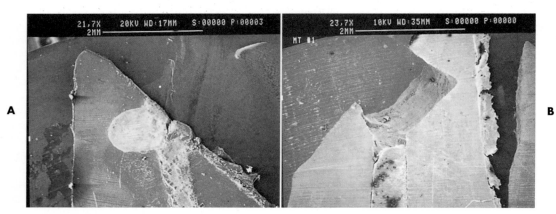

FIG. 18-29 A, Sagittal view of a maxillary lateral incisor shows the oblique placement of the retrofilling material and the probable leakage at the facial margin. **B,** Sagittal view of the retropreparation using a straight handpiece with inverted cone bur. Note the oblique angle of the preparation and the encroachment on the lingual wall of the root.

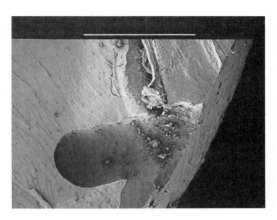

FIG. 18-30 Sectioned longitudinal view demonstrating how the canal is being sealed off by the axial wall of the preparation instead of the pulpal floor of the preparation.

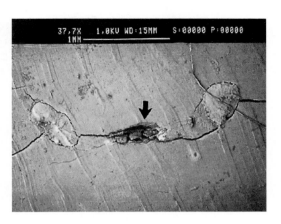

FIG. 18-31 Scanning electron micrograph of a failed apicoectomy with amalgam retrofills in the mesiobuccal and mesiolingual canals and with no instrumentation or filling in the isthmus area connecting the two canals. (Microfractures are artifacts of specimen preparation.)

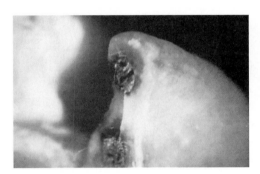

FIG. 18-32 Resected root of the mandibular molar clearly demonstrating the connecting anastomoses between the buccal and lingual canals.

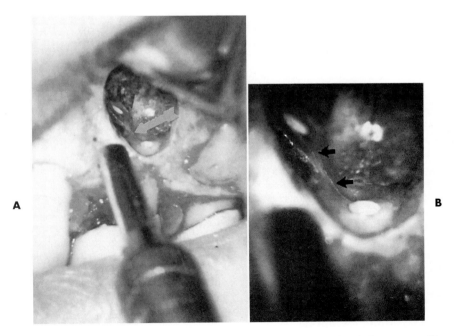

FIG. 18-33 A, Resected root of a maxillary premolar with connecting isthmus area. Even at 6× magnification, the isthmus can be difficult to visualize *(arrow)*. B, Same root seen at 22×. Connecting isthmus is more easily visualized *(arrows)*.

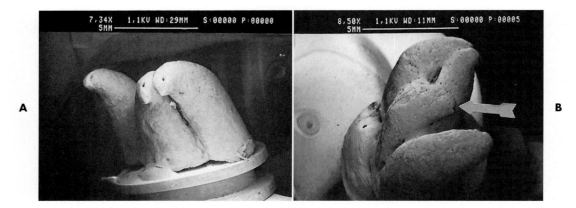

FIG. 18-34 A, Normal-appearing roots of a maxillary molar. **B,** Lingual view reveals hidden MB-2 root *(arrow).*

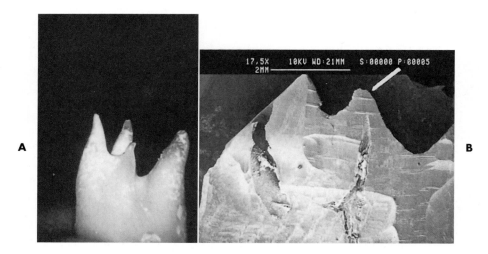

FIG. 18-35 A, MB-2 root of maxillary molar would remain hidden from the dental surgeon even after beveling through the MB-1 root. **B,** Sectioned longitudinal view of ultrasonic root end preparation on the mesiobuccal root with a failure to detect a second MB-2 root *(arrow).*

nal anatomy (Fig. 18-34).[4] Of particular note is the high prevalence of fourth roots on maxillary molars (Fig. 18-35), third roots on mandibular molars, and bifurcated roots on canines and premolars of both arches. The experienced dental surgeon maintains a healthy "anatomic skepticism" at all times.

Another requirement for successful retropreparation is to provide adequate retention form without weakening the root. Silver amalgam, Super EBA, and IRM all require mechanical retention in the form of either undercuts or parallel walls. Creating mechanical undercuts in already very thin dentinal walls is risky, especially in narrow isthmus areas. A parallel preparation avoids hollowing out the delicate root dentin while still providing retention form.

ULTRASONIC RETROPREPARATIONS

Ultrasonic Root End Preparation Technique

Ultrasonic root end preparation technique requires a disciplined, methodical approach. Attempting root end preparations without clear visibility compromises results. Maintaining a dry

crypt is as important as supplementary illumination and magnification.

When the root has been beveled and stained with methylene blue, the outline of the retropreparation is carefully planned after close inspection under magnification (Fig. 18-36). Uncritical or superficial examination of the beveled surface ensures failure (Plates 18-4 and 18-5). A CX-1 Explorer is used to etch, *by hand,* the planned preparation (Figs. 18-37 and 18-38). This preparatory or *tracking groove* simplifies anatomically complex preparation designs, especially when such preparations must be made indirectly using a mirror (Fig. 18-39). After a 0.5-mm to 1-mm-deep tracking groove has been etched by hand, a CT-5, UT-5 or Slim Jim 5 tip is activated with the ultrasonic unit (Fig. 18-40). Using the ultrasonic unit at the *lowest power* and with the lightest possible touch, the tracking groove is gently deepened another 0.5 mm, maintaining complete visibility at all times. This is the only ultrasonic procedure performed dry. Maintaining visibility while following the hand-etched groove is imperative (Fig. 18-41). *The tracking groove enables the ultrasonic tip to glide passively in*

Text continued on p. 627

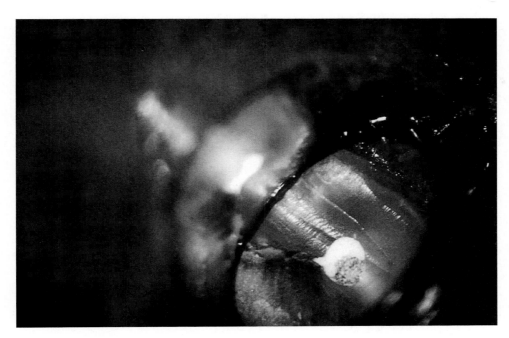

FIG. 18-36 Case showing high-magnification retromirror view of stained buccal and lingual canals with isthmus.

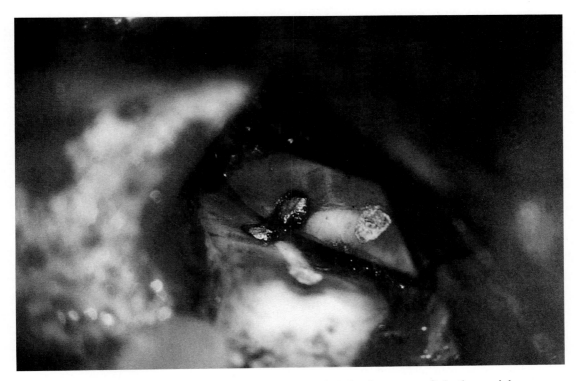

FIG. 18-37 High-magnification retromirror view of failed apicoectomy. Only the mesiobuccal has received a retrofilling. The mesiolingual canal and isthmus area have not been sealed.

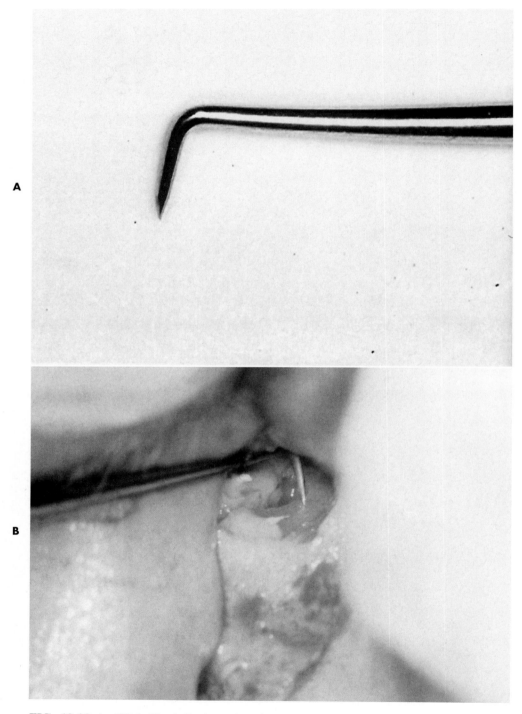

FIG. 18-38 A, CX-1 (Carr) Explorer is manufactured from hardened steel, enabling high stresses to be placed on the tip without causing breakage. This instrument is used to create, *by hand,* a tracking groove. **B,** Creation of a tracking groove from MB-1 to MB-2 using the CX-1.

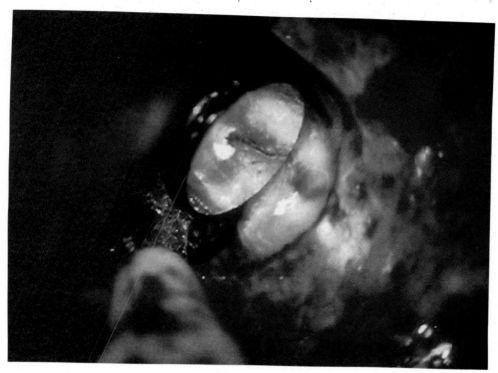

FIG. 18-39 Retromirror view of the tracking groove created with the CX-1 Explorer in the mesiobuccal root of maxillary molar.

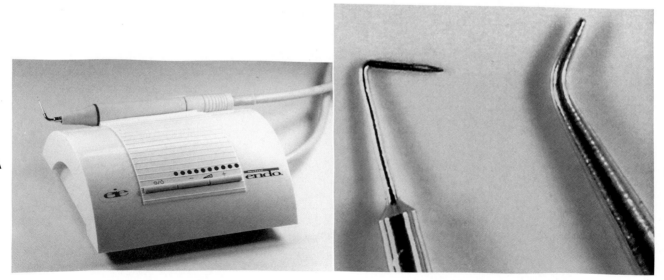

FIG. 18-40 A, EIE/Analytic mini-endo piezoelectrical unit. **B,** Comparison between Slim Jim and CT ultrasonic prepping tip.

Continued

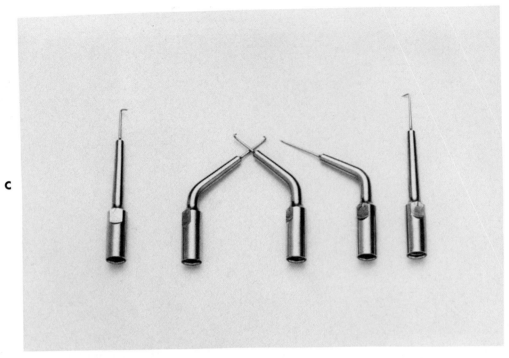

FIG. 18-40, cont'd C, Series of Slim Jim ultrasonic prepping tips.

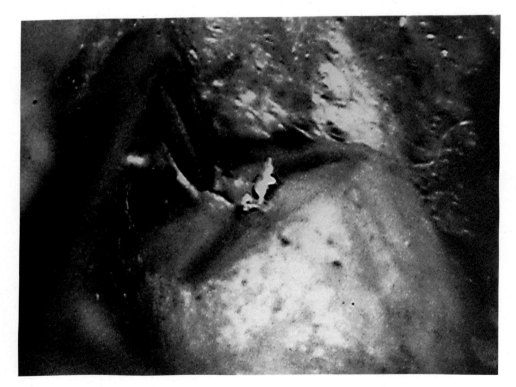

FIG. 18-41 Deepening of the tracking groove by CT-5 ultrasonic tip (dry).

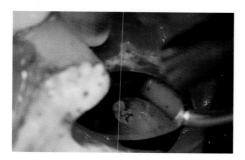

PLATE 18-1 Medium-magnification retromirror view of a beveled root. Notice multiple gutta-percha cones surrounded by sealer.

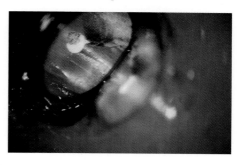

PLATE 18-2 High-magnification retromirror view of MB root maxillary molar. Stained isthmus can clearly be seen, as can dentinal tubules stained with black-pigmented bacteria.

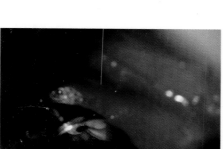

PLATE 18-3 High-magnification retromirror view of stained isthmus.

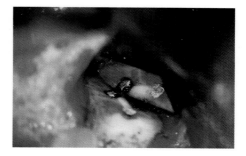

PLATE 18-4 Medium-magnification view of failed retrofilling on maxillary bicuspid. Notice amalgam root end filling in lingual canal and unaddressed isthmus and buccal canal.

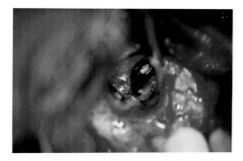

PLATE 18-5 Medium-magnification retroview of failed apicoectomy on MB root of maxillary molar. Notice root end filling in the MB-1 canal and failure to address isthmus and MB-2 canal.

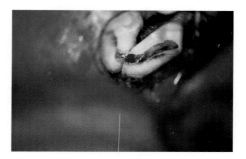

PLATE 18-6 Completed ultrasonic retropreparation of mesial root of a mandibular molar. Notice correct buccolingual extension of preparation with minimal mesiodistal dimensions.

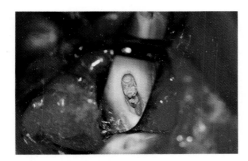

PLATE 18-7 Final ultrasonic root end preparation, maxillary anterior. Examination is improved by completely cleaning and drying preparation prior to viewing.

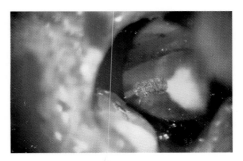

PLATE 18-8 Completed retrofilling, maxillary bicuspid, demonstrating the smoothness of finishing procedures. Notice correct oblong shape of root end filling.

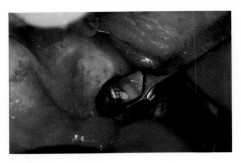

PLATE 18-9 Retromirror view of failed apicoectomy, mandibular bicuspid. Notice placement of amalgam root end filling has not encompassed entire canal area.

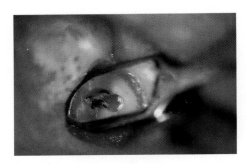

PLATE 18-10 Preliminary ultrasonic root end preparation after removing alloy and gutta-percha of Plate 18-9. Notice the discoloration with possible bacterial contamination on the lingual aspect of ultrasonic preparation.

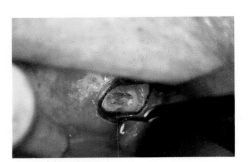

PLATE 18-11 High-magnification retromirror view of completed ultrasonic root end preparation. The preparation has been extended lingually to completely remove bacteria-stained dentin.

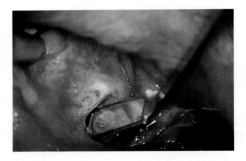

PLATE 18-12 Retromirror view of final root end filling using dentin bonding agent (OptiBond).

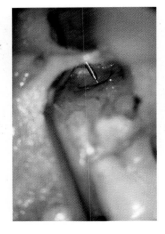

PLATE 18-13 View of ultrasonic preparation of palatal root, maxillary molar, using transsinus (buccal) approach.

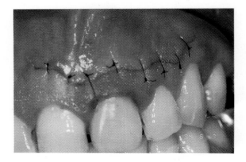

PLATE 18-14 Immediate postoperative view of microsurgical suturing. Notice very close adaptation of flap margins.

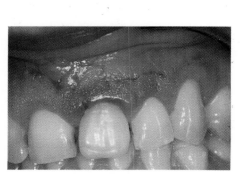

PLATE 18-15 Twenty-four-hour postoperative view of surgical case in Plate 18-13. Excellent healing is evident because of atraumatic flap management techniques.

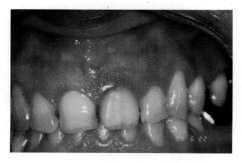

PLATE 18-16 At 2-week recall, soft tissue demonstrates complete absence of scar formation.

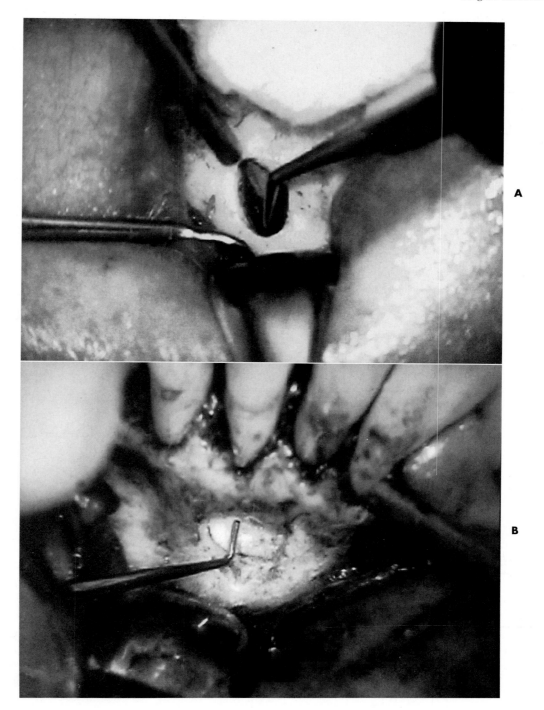

FIG. 18-42 A, CT-3 ultrasonic tip. **B,** CT-1 ultrasonic tip.

the tracking groove without requiring direct vision. Next, an appropriate ultrasonic tip is chosen (that simplifies correct hand placement), the water is turned on, and the preparation is completed by rapidly directing the activated tip back and forth in the tracking groove (Fig. 18-42). The more rapid the movement and the lighter the touch used, the more smooth and uniform the preparation becomes (Fig. 18-43 and Plate 18-6). Ideal retropreparation depth is 3 mm. The steps in this procedure are summarized in Fig. 18-44.

The ultrasonic retropreparation technique was devised to ad-

dress the major shortcomings of conventional rotary bur type of preparations.[11,13] Because of the greatly reduced size of the ultrasonic tip, it is easily placed into the crypt and down the long axis of the root, even in areas that have been traditionally difficult to reach. Ultrasonic units specifically designed for root end preparation are commercially available, as well as a wide variety of tip designs (see Figs. 18-40) that facilitate preparation in all areas of the mouth—even on buccal approaches to palatal roots of maxillary molars (see Plate 18-13).

Comparisons between rotary bur preparations and ultrasonic

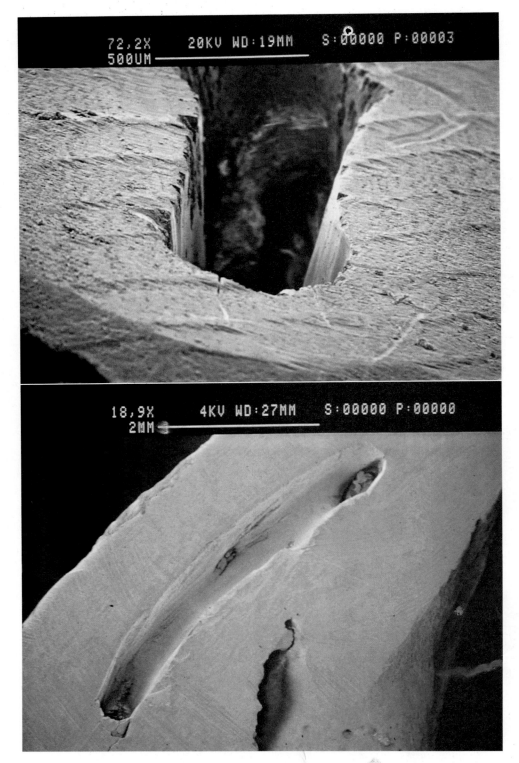

FIG. 18-43 Ultrasonic preparation showing parallel walls and machinelike accuracy of the preparation.

preparations are seen in Fig. 18-45. Particular attention should be paid to the lingual extent of the retropreparations. If the root has been acutely beveled, the preparation frequently encroaches on the lingual wall of the root. By contrast, with ultrasonic root preparation, the required bony access is much smaller than that for rotary bur access, and the preparation can be placed down the longitudinal axis of the canal, preserving precious lingual root structure (Table 18-1).

Ultrasonic retropreparation technique greatly facilitates ideal preparation. Narrow isthmus channels, C-shaped canals, fused

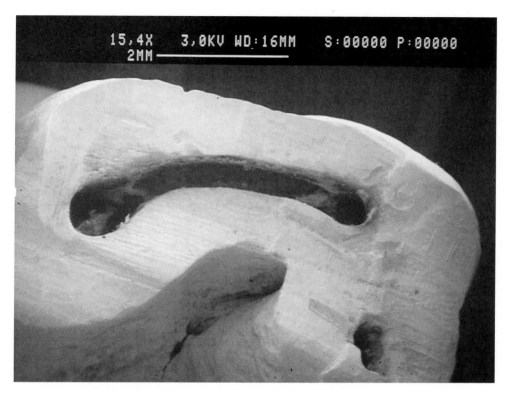

FIG. 18-43, cont'd For legend see opposite page.

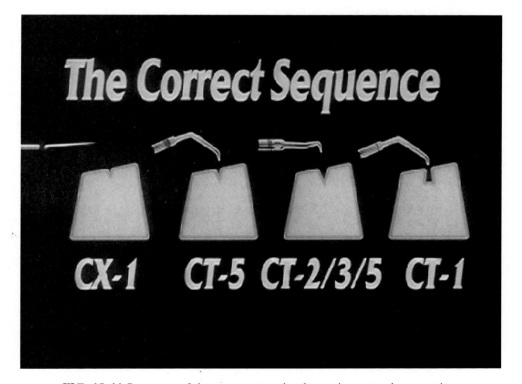

FIG. 18-44 Summary of the correct steps in ultrasonic root end preparation.

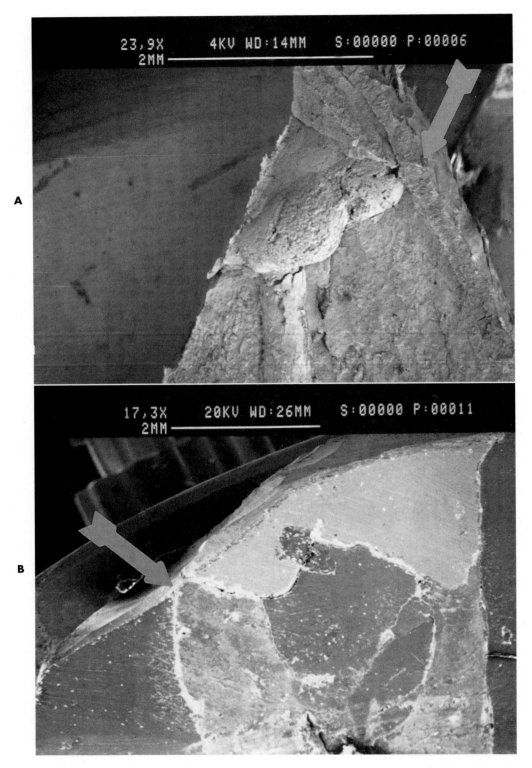

FIG. 18-45 A, Sectioned longitudinal view of the microhandpiece preparation. Note the oblique angle of the preparation and its encroachment on the lingual wall of the root *(arrow).* **B,** Sectioned longitudinal view of amalgam retrofill in mesial root of maxillary molar. Note the oblique orientation of the amalgam retrofill and the failure to seal the buccal margin *(arrow).*

roots with confluent canals, and inaccessible lingual canals can now be not only cleaned and shaped correctly, but also prepared 3 mm down the true axial inclination. *Properly placed ultrasonic root end preparations conform to the true anatomic configuration of the root canal system.*

Table 18-1. Comparison of bevel angles

Perpendicular	Acute
Less root removed	More root removed
Fewer dentinal tubules exposed	More dentinal tubules exposed
Smaller retropreparation needed	Elongated preparation needed
Smaller surface area and marginal perimeter of retrofill	Larger marginal perimeter with increasing chance for marginal leakage
Preparation contained within the root	Risk of lingual perforation
Greater likelihood of cementogenic repair	Greater likelihood of scar formation
Preservation of attachment apparatus on short or lingually inclined roots	Endangerment of attachment apparatus on short or lingually inclined roots

Another advantage of ultrasonic root end preparation is that the resection of the root can be perpendicular to the long axis, therefore eliminating exaggerated bevels and placing the preparation well within the confines of the root, away from the lingual wall. This conserves root structure, decreases the possibility of root perforation, and decreases the surface area and perimeter of the retrofilling material.

Preparations perpendicular to the long axis are important when the roots are short or lingually inclined or when an acute bevel would expose a post placed deep into the root. Acute bevels frequently place the buccal margin of the root section near the marginal gingiva or attachment apparatus. Furthermore, with two-rooted premolars the buccal root often must be reduced well beyond what is desirable to achieve manual access for the lingual root. The ultrasonic root end preparation technique using perpendicular root resections eliminates such excess root removal (Figs. 18-46 and 18-47).

After the ultrasonic preparation is completed, it is cleaned and then examined for completeness. Using a Stropko surgical irrigator (EIE/Analytic, Orange, Calif; Figs. 18-48 and 18-49), the preparation is flushed with either sterile saline or citric acid etchant and dried with a light stream of air. This technique allows for critical scrutiny of the final preparation in a dry field.

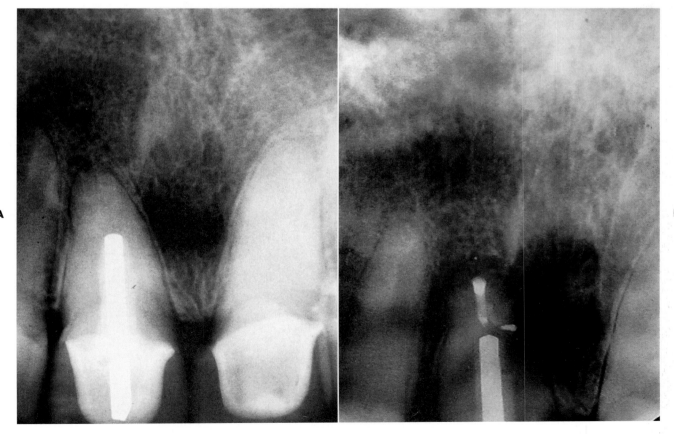

A   B

FIG. 18-46 A, Maxillary central incisor with jacket crown and gold post placed deep into the root. **B,** Ultrasonic retropreparation with retrograde condensation of gutta-percha, which has filled a large lateral canal. Placement of gold foil retrofills in both the apical and lateral portals of exit.

Continued

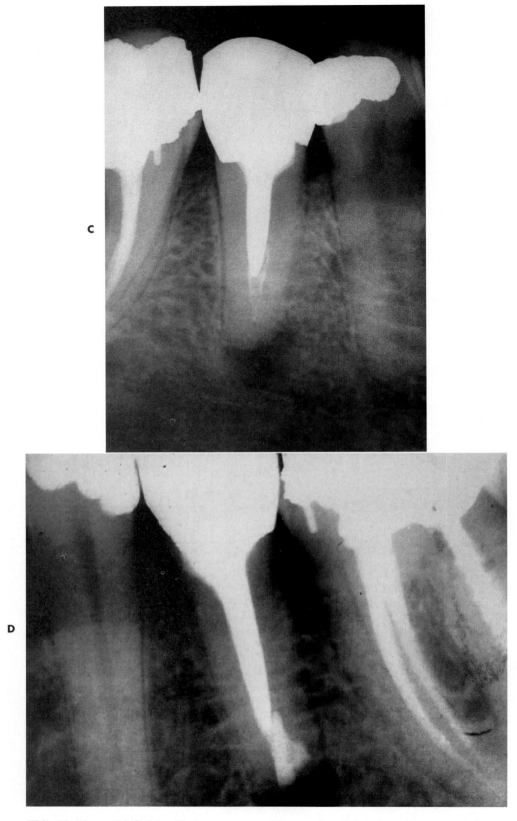

FIG. 18-46, cont'd C, Mandibular premolar with post placed deep into the root with failing endodontic treatment. **D,** Ultrasonic retropreparation with root beveled perpendicular to longitudinal axis and placement of Super EBA up to the level of the post.

The ability to clean and dry the apical preparation and examine it under high magnification is crucial because many deficiencies can be overlooked if the preparation is wet and cluttered with debris (Fig. 18-50 and Plates 18-6 and 18-7). If the dental surgeon is not satisfied with the shape, depth, or extent

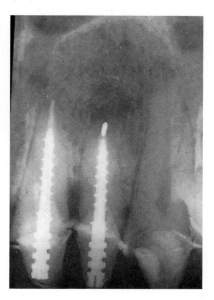

FIG. 18-47 Ultrasonic retropreparation in root with deep post placement. Ability to resect the root perpendicularly to the long axis prevents exposing the post. Conventional bevels would expose the post and compromise the case. *(Courtesy Dr. Keith Kanter.)*

of the retropreparation, modifications are made and the preparation is cleaned, dried, and reexamined (Fig. 18-50, *B*).

ROOT END FILLING MATERIALS

An integral component of periradicular surgery is the placement of a root end filling material. Adequate beveling of the root end exposes a surface that is comprised of dentin with a circumferential covering of cementum and a canal system that *may not be centrally located* and may not contain obturating materials. The root canal system, whether obturated or not invariably contains organic constituents that serve as both a substrate and a reservoir for bacteria and their by-products. It is this central nidus that must be sealed off, since most failures of nonsurgical root canal therapy are due to insufficient debridement.[45] The purpose of a root end filling is to hermetically seal the resected root end, effectively trapping any remaining irritants within the canal system and thereby preventing their egress into the periodontal ligament space. Successful sealing in turn promotes a cementogenic repair of the root end, the most critical step in dentoalveolar wound healing.

An outline of the properties of an ideal root end filling should include many of Grossman's original criteria for a root canal filling material.[29] These criteria can be modified to identify a more physiologic and tissue-specific material for the periradicular environment. An ideal root end filling material should contain the qualities listed in Box 18-1.

The endodontic literature is replete with studies that attempt to identify an ideal root end filling.[49,84,88] Materials that have been studied include amalgam,[91] Cavit,[24] cyanoacrylate, composite resin, desiccated and unmodified zinc oxide–eugenol (ZOE)[88] cement, Diaket sealer, glass-ionomer,[85] gold foil, gutta-percha, Indium, IRM cement, mineral trioxide ag-

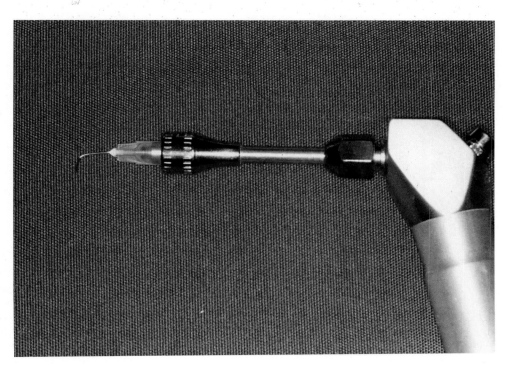

FIG. 18-48 Stropko surgical irrigator connected to triplex syringe is used for irrigating and drying apical retropreparations.

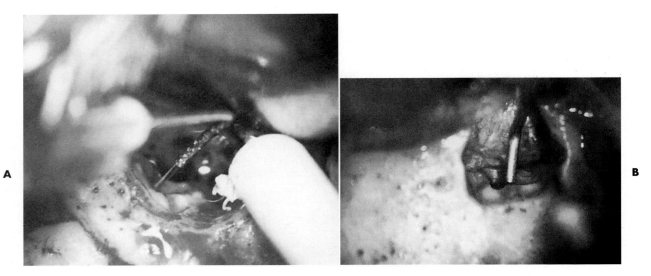

FIG. 18-49 A, Stropko surgical irrigator irrigating an apical retropreparation. **B,** Placement of Stropko surgical irrigator drying an apical retropreparation. This technique is superior to drying with paper points.

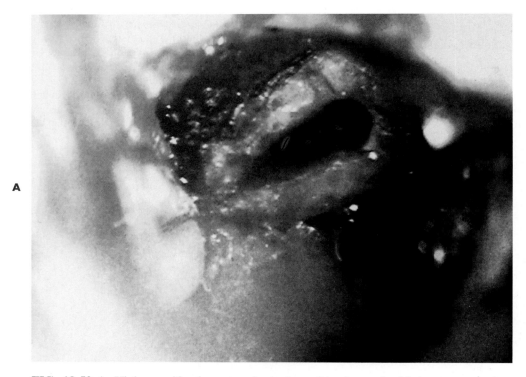

FIG. 18-50 A, High-magnification retromirror view of inadequately dried retropreparation. Note that no detail can be seen.

gregate,[82] polyHEMA,[22,40] polycarboxylate cement, Restodent, Super EBA cement,[78] Titanium screws, Teflon, and zinc phosphate cement. Unfortunately, the ideal material has yet to be developed.

In evaluating dental materials, caution must be used when extrapolating data from benchtop and animal studies to humans. Many techniques exist to evaluate apical leakage, histocompatibility, toxicity, and healing. When leakage studies are considered, it has been proven that the method selected to mea-sure leakage can affect the outcome of the results.[49] Inherent in many of these studies are technical shortcomings that may lead to erroneous findings.[61] Compared with clinical conditions, in vitro dye studies are static and do not reflect the dynamic inter-action between the root canal and periradicular tissues,[79] and they are qualitative, which may not be equatable to clinical suc-cess or failure. Tissue compatibility data also must be viewed skeptically, since, these studies provide conclusions that rarely can be compared to other studies, because of the specificity of

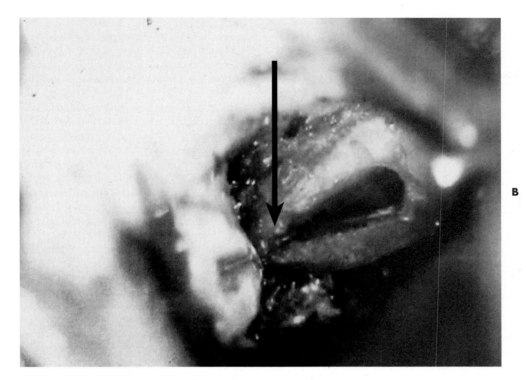

FIG. 18-50, cont'd B, Same view after cleaning and drying with Stropko surgical irrigator. Note the debris *(arrow)* on the axial preparation wall and the inadequate extension of the preparation lingually. "White line" seen on the lingual aspect of the beveled surface indicates where the underextended preparation needs to be completed.

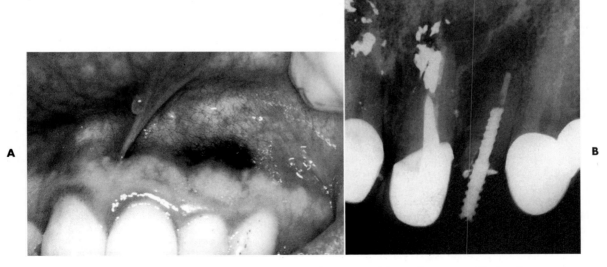

FIG. 18-51 A, Argyria of a maxillary central incisor caused by a silver cone. **B,** Amalgam scatter indicating careless technique.

the cell type and degree of diffusibility.[71,78] In addition, these investigations cannot study the complex interaction between the material and human tissues, and they produce measurements which have little relevance to clinical circumstances.[71,76] Animal model studies can show healing or tissue reaction characteristics that are unique for each specified animal type and may not be transposable to humans.

Clinical usage and retrospective studies include many variables that are difficult to standardize; comparisons between them are nearly impossible.[78] These variables include number of cases, follow-up periods, materials tested, different procedures and techniques used during treatment, different operators, and lack of standardization of evaluation criteria.[78] Finally, a crucial area of concern centers around the statistical analysis and research designs of many studies. Informal audits by statisticians have shown that 39% of published articles contain statistical errors so serious that their conclusions should be considered invalid.[90]

ROOT END FILLING MATERIALS

Amalgam

Historically, numerous materials have been advocated for use as root end fillings, but none have been used as frequently as amalgam. This material satisfies many of the criteria for an ideal Root-end filling material. Amalgam is easy to use and place, adaptable, relatively biocompatible, nonresorbable, bacteriostatic, and radiopaque.

A myriad of studies have been performed evaluating the sealing ability of dental amalgam. Many in vitro studies have shown that the root end amalgam seal is equal to or better than other filling materials,[37,38] whereas additional investigations have indicated that the ability of amalgam to prevent microleakage is quite poor.[70] Numerous conflicting conclusions have been cited as to amalgam type, sealing ability, and presence or absence of moisture or blood contamination.[56] Amalgam cannot create a hermetic seal of the root end preparation, but various compositions attempt to overcome the innate insufficiencies of a metallic restoration. Each formulation behaves slightly different in the highly variable root end environment.[56] Although many studies contradict each other, some tentative conclusions can be drawn. Zinc-free spherical amalgam shows significantly greater leakage than other formulations when used in blood contaminated root end preparations. Zinc and zinc-free alloys seal equally well in a dry environment (when kept dry during the initial set); zinc-containing amalgams will exhibit delayed setting expansion in blood or moisture-laden root end preparations and adversely affect the seal and may contribute to apical dentin fracture. *It is clear that a dry and blood-free field is of paramount importance in the placement of conventional root end fillings.*

Although amalgam shows minimal toxicity, its cementogenic potential is negligible. Amalgam, when used as a retrofilling material, results in fibrous encapsulation.[19] Finally, evidence exists that over time amalgam may not support the properties necessary for clinical success and long-term healing, which is probably indicative of its poor seal (Fig. 18-54).[27]

Additional factors of concern with dental amalgam relate to its electrical and chemical properties. It has been demonstrated that galvanic currents are generated when amalgam contacts other metals (i.e., metallic posts).[3] These currents can promote an increase in corrosion and marginal failure and can lead to the release of metallic precipitates into the periapical tissues.[3] Metallic staining or agyria (Fig. 18-51) can frequently occur in tissues adjacent to the amalgam restoration. This stems from phagocytic uptake of silver and tin with subsequent deposition into the adjacent basement membranes. This may be evidenced by an amalgam stain or tattoo overlaying a previous surgical site, but is not necessarily indicative of postsurgical failure. The staining may be the result of gross amalgam flash during its placement or removal (Fig. 18-51, *B*) or dislodgment of the amalgam subsequent to its placement (Fig. 18-52). Additional causes of agyria are tissue contact with a resected silver point, extensive root end amalgam fillings, or possible leaching from silver composition sealers (Fig. 18-53). Thus accurate control of mercury-containing materials is of critical importance.

Tissue compatibility studies have shown that amalgam exhibits minimal cytotoxicity over time.[24] As with most dental materials it is most cytotoxic in the initial 24-hour period, which in part may be due to the unreacted mercury.[77] Fortunately, the initial cytotoxic effect of amalgam diminishes rapidly through internal mercury bonding over time. The concern of mercury toxicity has become an important area of current controversy. Recent studies have shown that a minimal amount of amalgam alloy is used in the typical root end filling and that mercury release is of little concern.[46] Evidence suggests, however, that varying degrees of cytotoxicity may be elicited from the corrosion products as they form.[54]

Amalgam has many advantages and is considered to be an acceptable material for root end filling. However, initial leakage, secondary corrosion, delayed expansion, lack of adhesion, moisture sensitivity, marginal discrepancies, the need for an undercut in the root end preparation, staining of the hard and soft tissues, and scatter of particles make a convincing argument against its use.

Gutta-Percha

There are several different techniques that use gutta-percha as a root end filling; however, a general consensus cannot be reached as to which one is superior or if they are better than other root end filling methods. Cold-burnished, heat-sealed, resected-but-unaltered, and thermoplasticized techniques have been investigated and compared.[9,72] Varying degrees of adequacy have been demonstrated when the literature compares the sealing ability of gutta-percha to that of amalgam. However, to date most studies show that the resected apical seal of gutta-percha is *inferior* to Super EBA, IRM, glass-ionomer, or

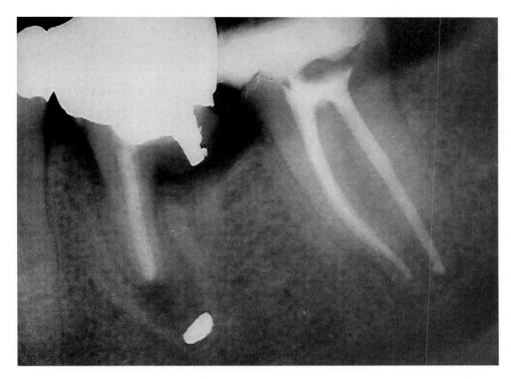

FIG. 18-52 Complete loss of amalgam retrofill subsequent to root resorption.

composite.[23,53] Additionally, in many cases resection of the apical portion of the root may expose canal isthmus, fins, or unfilled or poorly cleansed canal space that is not obvious to the dental surgeon without magnification (Fig. 18-54).

Zinc Oxide–Eugenol Cements

ZOE cements have been used as a root end filling for many years, but until recently amalgam has been the material of choice. Originally, ZOE cements were relied on as a filling material for the apical portion of isolated root canals where surgery was anticipated and only root end resection was to be performed. They were seldom preferred over alloy as a material to fill the root end preparation. Another use was as an insulating material interposed between a root end amalgam and an adjacent post to prevent galvanic currents. Today, the most widely accepted root end filling materials throughout the endodontic community are ZOE cements in the form of Super EBA and IRM. The use of these cements has become more prevalent because of their properties. They are easy to manipulate, have adequate working time, are dimensionally stable, adapt and conform easily to root end preparations, are biocompatible and impervious to tissue fluids, and will not corrode or oxidize. They are unaffected by moisture, bacteriostatic, and radiopaque. They will not discolor the tooth or surrounding tissues and are easily removable, noncarcinogenic, and predictable over time.

Two compositional changes have been made to the ADA type III, class I ZOE formula to increase compressive, tensile, and shear strength and decrease solubility.[15] In one (IRM) polymethyl methacrylate is added to the powder, and in the other (Super EBA) aluminum oxide is added to the powder and ethoxybenzoic acid is added to the liquid. IRM is composed of

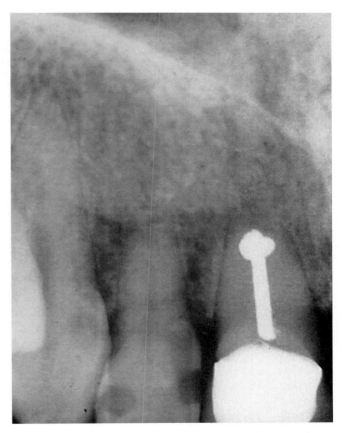

FIG. 18-53 This failing apicoectomy has caused the metallic staining seen in Fig. 18-51, *A*.

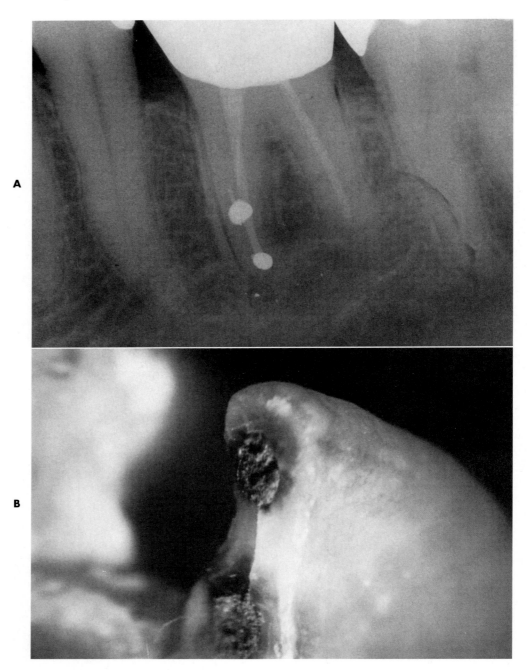

FIG. 18-54 A, Failing apicoectomy mesial root. **B,** Extracted tooth from **A,** showing isthmus. *(Courtesy Dr. R. Burns.)*

80% zinc oxide, 20% polymethyl methacrylate, with the liquid being 99% eugenol and 1% acetic acid. Super EBA is 60% zinc oxide, 34% aluminum oxide, 6% natural resin, with the liquid being 37.5% eugenol and 62.5% ortho-ethoxybenzoic acid (EBA). When the solubility has been measured in buffered phosphate solution, both IRM and Super EBA showed no noticeable signs of disintegration after 6 months.[58] An additional benefit of the ortho-ethoxybenzoic acid is to reduce the amount of the tissue-irritating eugenol in the formula.[8]

Studies have compared the apical leakage of IRM and Super EBA to many frequently used root end filling materials. Statistically, studies have found that there is little difference between the sealing abilities of IRM or Super EBA; many researchers consider them to be equivalent.[8] Some investigations have shown that they seal as well as glass-ionomer or amalgam and cavity varnish initially.[37,70] Most researchers, however, agree that both IRM and Super EBA seal equal to or better than amalgam, glass-ionomer cements, and cold- and hot-burnished gutta-percha.[8,37,38,70]

Tissue compatibility and healing studies have shown mixed results when evaluating ZOE cements. Evidence exists that indicates that Super EBA is less cytotoxic than IRM, suggesting that the decreased eugenol in Super EBA allows it to be less irritating. Intraosseous and subcutaneous implantation studies

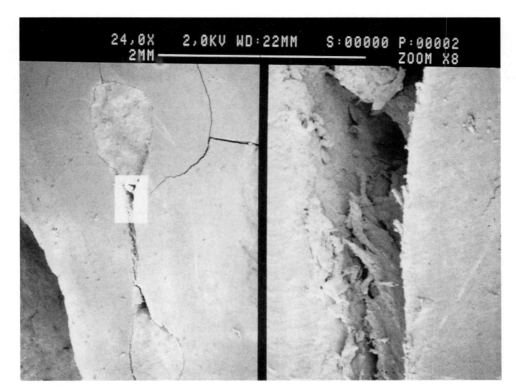

FIG. 18-55 Scanning electron micrography of isthmus area from Fig. 18-54, *A*. Note tissue remnants in isthmus area.

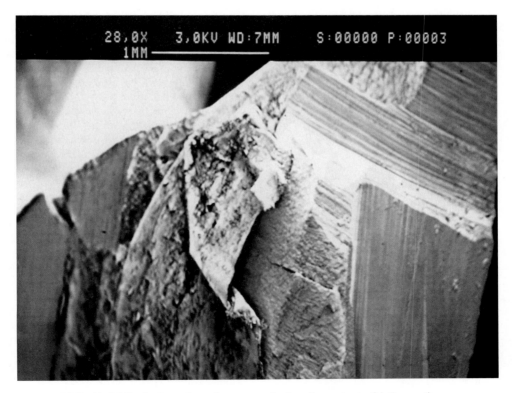

FIG. 18-56 Sagittal section of same tooth showing extent of isthmus tissue.

show initial irritation, but longer term evaluations exhibit that normal bone apposition and fibrous encapsulation occur adjacent to IRM and Super EBA. Clinical evaluation of Super EBA in vivo for 3 years shows collagen fibers impregnating the gaps in the material (Fig. 18-57).[58] Finally, when comparing the healing of periapical tissues following replantation, tissue responses to both IRM and Super EBA were found to be more favorable than that of amalgam.[62]

Mineral Trioxide Aggregate

A new experimental filling material has been advocated for retrofilling. Mineral trioxide aggregate (MTA) is a powder that consists of trioxides combined with other mineral hydrophilic particles, which crystallize in the presence of moisture.[76,77] The principal components of this material are tricalcium silicate, tricalcium aluminate, tricalcium oxide, and silicate oxide.[76] In addition, there are small amounts of other mineral oxides that are responsible for the chemical and physical properties of this aggregate, such as bismuth oxide, which has been added to make the material radiopaque. Hydration of the powder results in a colloidal gel, which solidifies to a hard structure in less than 3 hours.[76,77]

In terms of its usage MTA has several advantageous qualities. First, it is easy to mix and place into the cavity preparation with a small amalgam carrier.[80] Second, because of its hydrophilic nature it is not essential to use in a dry field.[75] Third, it is easy to remove any excess that may accumulate.[80] A possible disadvantage, however, is its long setting time and possible consequent dislodgment or deformation from root end preparations.

In animal studies MTA compares favorably to other filling materials when tested for leakage and biocompatibility. Bacterial and dye leakage studies performed in both dry and blood contaminated root end preparations have indicated that MTA seals better than amalgam, IRM, or Super EBA.[75,79,80] Also when visually evaluating these same materials under scanning electron microscope, MTA had better adaptation to the surrounding dentin of the root end preparation.[81] In addition, tissue cytotoxicity reactions and mutagenicity evaluation results of MTA appear to be excellent and similar to results obtained for amalgam, IRM, and Super EBA.[77]

Tissue compatibility studies of MTA have produced excellent tissue responses, as compared to amalgam in the periapical environment. When placed in a root-end preparation in dogs, MTA elicits less periradicular inflammation and more fibrous encapsulation directly adjacent to the material.[82] Also, the deposition of cementum over the MTA as well as the resected root surface was a frequent finding. Previous electron probe microanalysis data of MTA powder showed that calcium and phosphoros ions are the main ions present in the material.[76] Since they are also the main components in hard tissue, it may be hypothesized that this is one of the qualities that may lead to its biocompatability.[76] Also, MTA has a high pH similar to calcium hydroxide.[76] Thus, it is possible that induction of hard tissue formation may occur following its use, because of its sealing ability,[23,59,62] its high pH, or some unknown property that may activate cementogenesis.[7]

Composite Resins

Composite resin formulations have gained increasing attention because of the less than ideal sealing ability of other root end filling materials. With the advent of "wet bonding" techniques and better hemostasis and crypt control, these materials appear to be a viable option for root end filling.

The primary reason that composites must be emphasized in a differential analysis of root end filling materials available today is because of their excellent sealing abilities. Many researchers have demonstrated that composites with a dentinbonded adhesive (DBA) produce a significantly better seal than amalgam with and without varnish, hot- and cold-burnished guttapercha, resected gutta-percha, Cavit, glass-ionomer, or Durelon cement. Studies have pointed out that a DBA is mandatory, otherwise composite resin alone does not seal better than amalgam or glass-ionomer because of polymerization shrinkage of the filled resin. One study showed that there was no statistically significant difference between composite resin, Teflon, or IRM; however, very little comparison has been performed comparing the sealing ability of resins to ZOE cements. Other studies have shown that composite root end filling in a traditional class I root end preparation may not be necessary and that simply placing a DBA alone or in combination with composite resin directly on the resected root surface may be all that is necessary to obtain an adequate seal.[51,53] Multiple studies also support the placement of root end dentin bonded composite resin in a slightly concave, saucer-shaped preparation on the resected root surface overlaying the canal, which deviates from the conventional ultrasonic root end preparations.[66,67] Finally, many scanning electron microscope studies show that the marginal adaptation of composite resin is superior to Cavit, amalgam, Durelon and zinc phosphate cements, and evidence suggests that this may be correlated with sealing ability.[68]

Long-term healing studies evaluating composite resins also exhibit very favorable results.[65,66,67] Investigations that included patient recalls of up to 9 years for cases treated with Retroplast and Gluma showed complete bone healing over time in a high percentage of cases.[66] This was further emphasized in a previous analysis that revealed significantly higher success rates may be obtained with Retroplast and Gluma as compared to amalgam. In vivo histologic evaluations in both monkeys

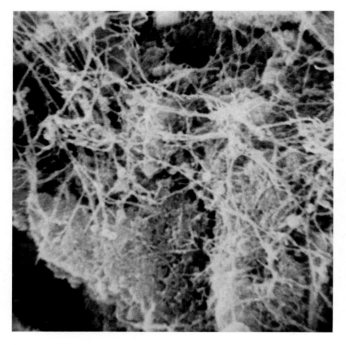

FIG. 18-57 Scanning electron micrograph of collagen fibrils covering surface of Super EBA. *(Courtesy Dr. P. Oynic.)*

and humans comparing the Retroplast and Gluma combination revealed absence of inflammatory cells around the root end filling, with fibroblasts and collagen fibers immediately adjacent.[65] In many cases, cementum deposition with Sharpey's fibers formed in intimate contact with the restoration, indicating that these materials can promote cementogenesis, the most critical step in dentoalveolar wound healing (Fig. 18-58). Additionally, recent evidence exists that suggests that the Geristore and Tenure combination or OptiBond and adhesive may also produce similar favorable results, but further evaluations are necessary[20,21] (Fig. 18-59). Unfortunately, in some cases absence of this complete healing process may be found in conjunction with poor hemostatic control during treatment.[67]

Fifth-generation composite systems support many of the ideal characteristics for root end filling materials. Consequently, resins are considered to be one of the more common options available for root end filling. Unfortunately, many resin materials are not suitable for periradicular use, so care must be exercised in choosing the right material. Other drawbacks include blood or gross moisture sensitivity, additional armamentarium involved in clinical use, and poor biologic and physical properties of older formulations. Fortunately, however, favorable characteristics such as ease of handling, excellent sealing ability, and commendable long-term healing attributes in humans overshadow their weaknesses.

PLACEMENT AND FINISHING OF RETROFILLING MATERIALS

After the retropreparation has been dried and inspected, the retrofilling material is placed. If IRM or Super EBA is used, it is mixed to a claylike consistency, shaped into a narrow cone, and attached to the end of a spoon or Hollenback carver (Fig. 18-60). The material can then be introduced into the surgical site and placed accurately into the retropreparation. It is then compacted using miniature condensers (Fig. 18-61, *A*). The

material is overpacked (Fig. 18-61, *B*) on the root surface and allowed to set. The placement and condensation procedures should occur in a dry field. After the setting is complete, a sharp microsurgical discoid carver can be used to carve away the excess retrofilling material. A 30-fluted composite finishing bur or 8-μm finishing diamond (Fig. 18-62) can be applied to the cut surface to achieve a highly polished surface without fear of ditching either the root surface or the retrofilling material. After finishing, the retrofilling is examined for completeness and marginal integrity (Fig. 18-63 and Plate 18-8). A final radiograph is exposed at this time to confirm the correct placement of the retrofilling (Fig. 18-64).

Every step in this technique is critical for the successful completion of apical surgery. Each of these steps requires not only mastery of technique and a feel for dental materials but also a refinement in the surgeon's visual acuity and an appreciation for the very close tolerances required. Performed on such a miniature scale these skills challenge even the most fastidious dental surgeon. Time spent in perfecting these skills rewards the dental surgeon with a satisfying sense of professional accomplishment (Plates 18-9 to 18-12).

CLOSURE

After final inspection and appropriate radiographs, the crypt packing is removed and the entire surgical site examined for extraneous debris. After irrigation with sterile saline, the wound edges are reapproximated. Time spent in the accurate reapproximation of the wound edges aids in the initiation of primary wound healing.[73] The goal of reapproximation is to enable the wound edges to heal by primary intention. With sulcular incisions the wound edges are located at the attachment apparatus near the cervical aspect of the crown, as well as the papilla and in the interdental col area. If the incision and elevation of these tissues have been atraumatic, primary intention healing should follow.[17] Mucogingival flap margins are

Text continued on p. 647

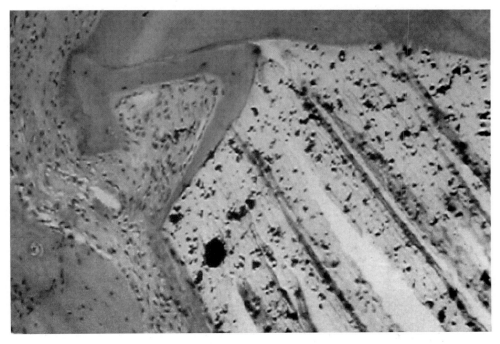

FIG. 18-58 Human histologic section of cementum growth over Retroplast. *(Courtesy Dr. J. Andreason.)*

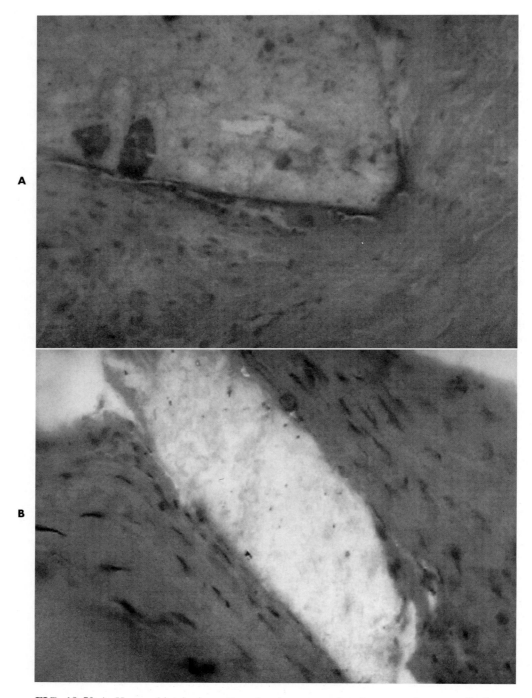

FIG. 18-59 A, Human histologic section showing connective tissue attachment to Geristore. *(Courtesy Dr. M. Dragoo.)* **B,** Tissue-resin interface with OptiBond. Human histology. *(Courtesy Pacific Endodontic Research Foundation.)*

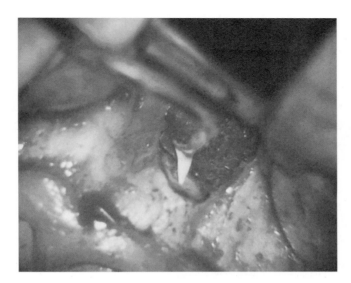

FIG. 18-60 After mixing to a claylike consistency, Super EBA is shaped into a narrow cone and attached to the end of a spoon or Hollenback carver.

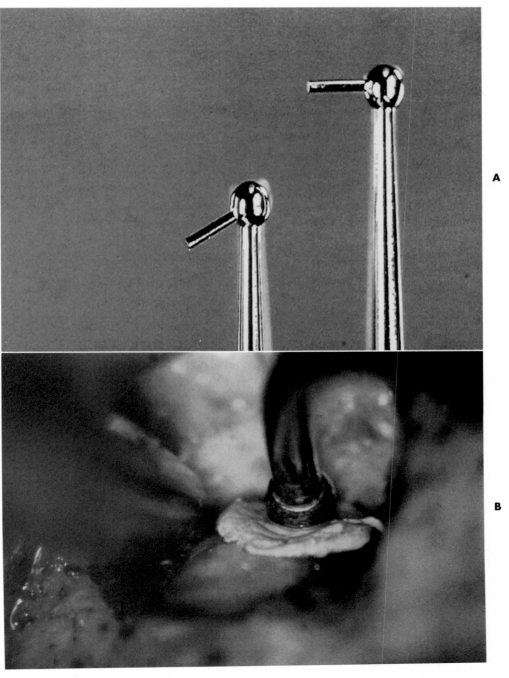

A

B

FIG. 18-61 **A,** Miniature Feinstein condenser. **B,** Miniature ball burnisher.

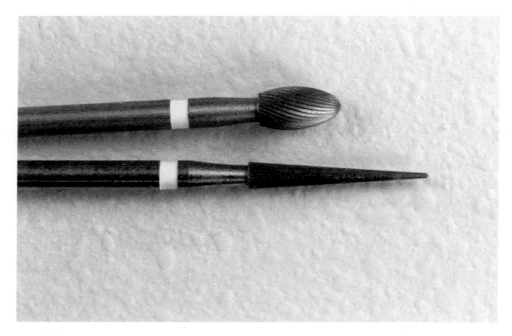

FIG. 18-62 Finishing diamond; finishing bur.

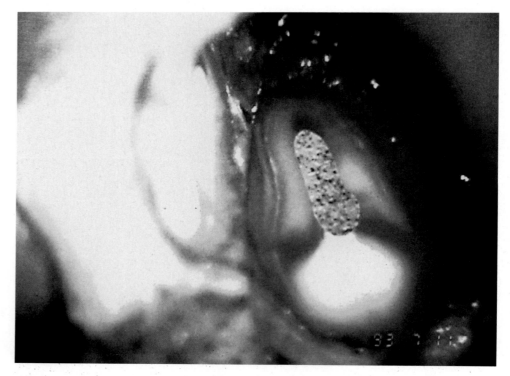

FIG. 18-63 Final inspection of retrofilling after finishing with a composite finishing bur. Smoothness and marginal integrity are checked.

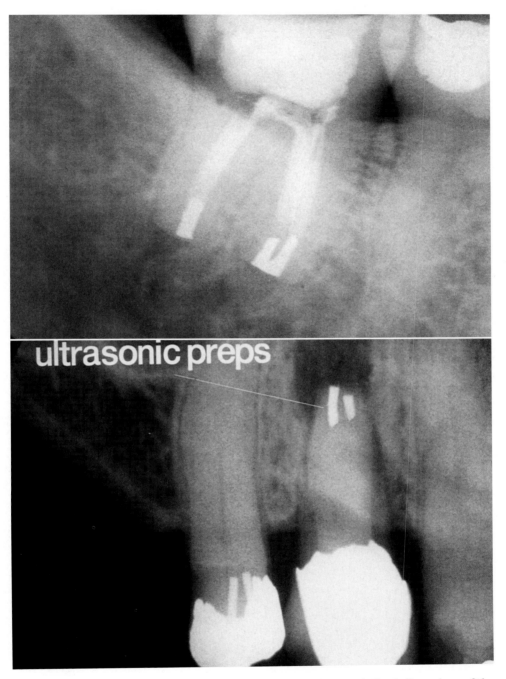

FIG. 18-64 Ultrasonic retropreparations show the conservative mesiodistal dimensions of the retropreparations and their placement parallel to the long axis. *Continued*

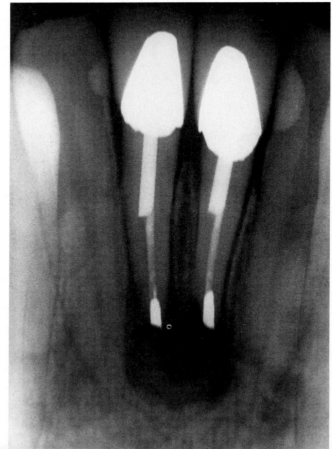

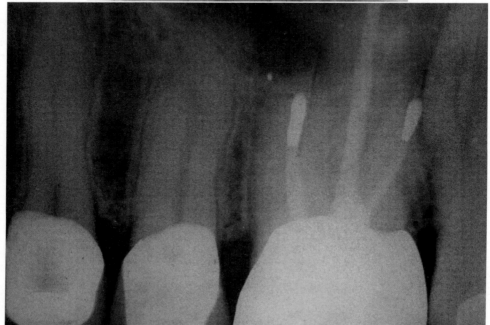

FIG. 18-64, cont'd For legend see preceding page.

easy to approximate if the incisions have been scalloped. After a brief period of compression, the flap is sutured.

The role of sutures is to hold the reapproximated tissues in place during the initial events in wound healing. The thickness of the clot between the opposed edges determines if the tissue heals by primary or secondary intention (Figs. 18-65 and 18-66).[55] For this reason postsurgical compression of the wound site decreases the thickness of the coagulum and allows closer approximation of the wound edges.[31]

The placement of sutures creates another wound. Sutures are longitudinal puncture wounds; they can add significant trauma to the tissues. Sutures are very rapidly colonized by bacteria and can be an impediment to rapid wound healing.[44]

Skillful suturing requires practice and a deft touch. Most flaps reflected during apical surgery can be reapproximated with either interrupted, continuous mattress, continuous blanket, or continuous sling suture designs (Fig. 18-67). Suturing always proceeds from the unattached mucosal surface to the attached mucosal surface. Unnecessary tension on the suture causes the tissue to tear or possibly become ischemic. Vertically releasing incisions rarely require more than one suture, as the releasing incisions are predominantly in alveolar mucosa, which has many elastic fibers. These fibers cannot be approximated once they are cut, no matter how many sutures are used.

Varied suture materials are commercially available, and every dental surgeon quickly develops preferences for one or another. Silk has been favored by many dental surgeons because of its easy handling and low cost, but it is very quickly colonized by bacteria owing to its wicking action and can impede primary intention healing (Fig. 18-68).[44] Nylon suture has working characteristics very similar to those of silk (Fig. 18-69); but it is colonized more slowly and is therefore kinder to tissue. A newly introduced suture (Tevdek EIE/Analytic, Orange, Calif.) (Fig. 18-70, *A*), a polytetraflouroethylene (PTFE) impregnated polyester material, has the advantageous handling characteristics of silk but the bacterial colonization resistance of Gore-tex (Fig. 18-71). Tevdek suture demonstrates dramatic tissue tolerance and is essentially nonirritating. This suture is supplied dual-armed with dissimilar needles at each end, conforming to the dental surgeon's need for different needle sizes to reapproximate the releasing incision and sulcular incision (see Fig. 18-70, *B*). A K-needle combines the sharpness of a side-cutting design while maintaining the atraumatic advantages of a tapered point needle. The removal time for sutures has progressively decreased as our understanding of surgical wound healing has progressed.[25] If no surgical principles have been violated and healing has occurred by primary intention, suture removal is indicated after 48 hours[36,47] (Plates 18-14 to 18-16). With uneventful healing, after 48 hours the suture is performing no function and is simply an irritant.[36] At 72 hours the entire length of suture is typically covered with a bacterial mat that is irritating to the wound site[64] (see Fig. 18-68, *C*).

POSTOPERATIVE CARE

After suturing is complete, the dental surgeon should gently compress the surgical site for 10 to 15 minutes with moist gauze soaked in either chlorhexidine or saline. This procedure reduces clot thickness and achieves hemostasis. Postoperative instructions are given to the patient orally and in writing, and an ice pack is placed over the surgical site with instructions to apply it extraorally for 24 to 48 hours. The ice pack should be applied with light pressure and intermittently, not continuously. Continuous application of ice activates the body's protective mechanisms against frostbite by increasing blood flow to the area, thus increasing swelling.[32] Intermittent postoperative application of ice reduces the vascular rebound phenomenon, reduces postoperative swelling and edema, and acts as an analgesic by interfering with pain fiber transmission. Patients should receive a postsurgical toothbrush with instructions on

Text continued on p. 652

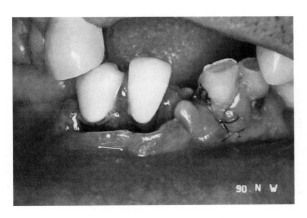

FIG. 18-65 One-week postoperative view demonstrating healing by secondary intention because of poor soft tissue management.

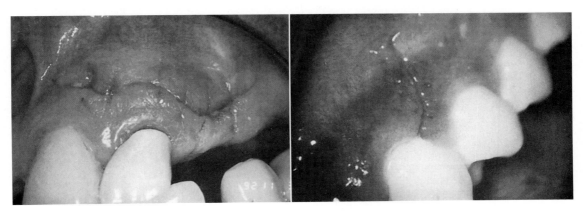

FIG. 18-66 Twenty-four-hour postoperative views demonstrating rapid healing by primary intention following atraumatic flap management.

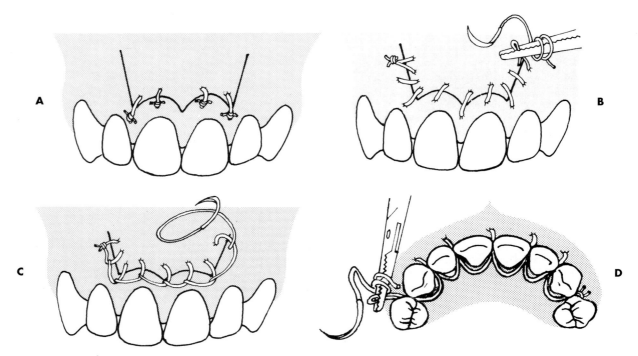

FIG. 18-67 Four suture techniques. **A,** Interrupted. **B,** Continuous mattress. **C,** Continuous blanket. **D,** Continuous sling.

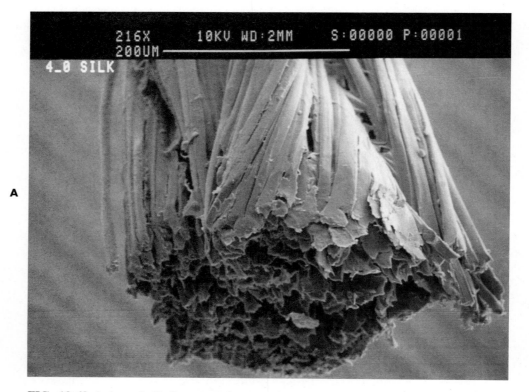

FIG. 18-68 A through **C,** Scanning electron micrographs of silk sutures show its wicking activity. At 48 hours it is completely impregnated with bacterial colonies.

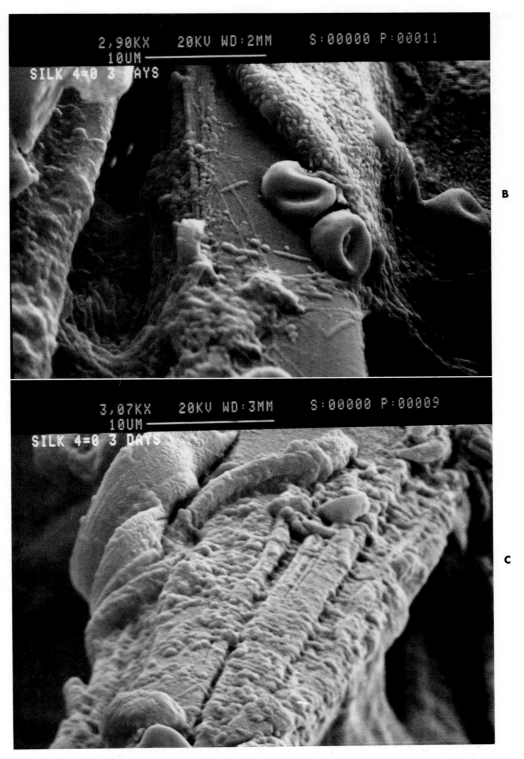

FIG. 18-68, cont'd For legend see opposite page.

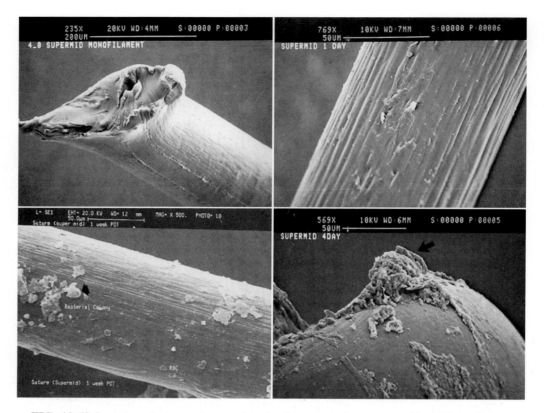

FIG. 18-69 Scanning electron micrographs of nylon suture show minimal bacterial colonization. Bacterial colonization proceeds rapidly after 48 hours.

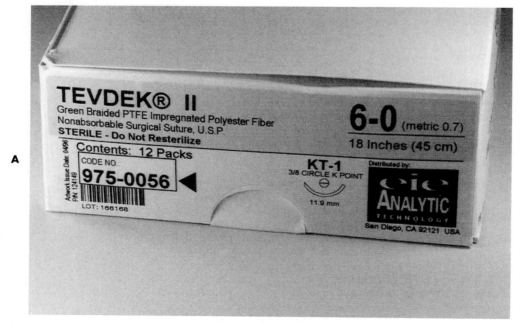

FIG. 18-70 A, Tevdek sutures.

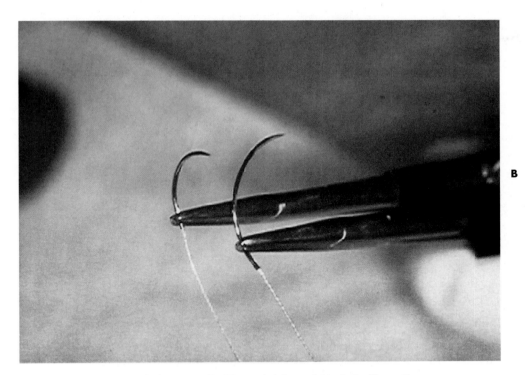

FIG. 18-70, cont'd B, Three eighths and ½ circle K-needle.

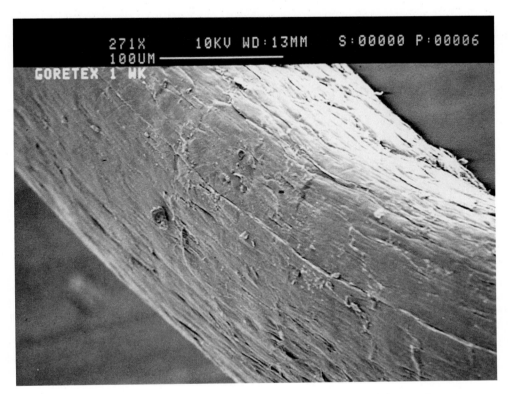

FIG. 18-71 Gore-tex suture with no bacterial colonies after 1 week intraoral exposure.

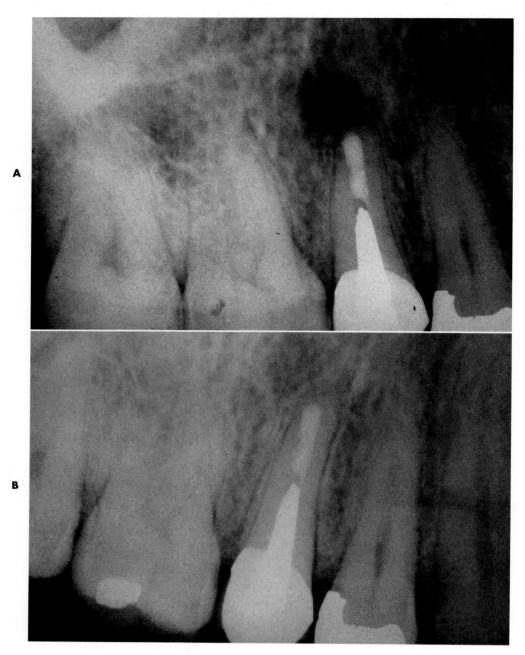

FIG. 18-72 A, Immediate postoperative view shows Super EBA as a retrofilling material. **B,** Two-year recall examination shows resolution of the lesion and apical bone regeneration.

how to use it. This brush reduces plaque buildup without tearing or traumatizing the flap.

All patients should be contacted, preferably by the dental surgeon, that evening, or if the surgery was performed late in the day, the following morning. If this is not possible, the patient should have a way of contacting the dental surgeon by phone should the need arise.

POSTOPERATIVE COMPLICATIONS AND PATIENT MANAGEMENT

Possible postoperative sequelae include bleeding, infection, swelling, discoloration, pain, and delayed healing. Postsurgical bleeding and swelling can be managed by application of pres-

sure with wet gauze or a wet chilled tea bag (which contains tannic acid) for 20 to 30 minutes. If bleeding cannot be controlled by these measures, the patient should be seen by the dental surgeon. If the dental surgeon cannot control the bleeding with pressure techniques, a clotting deficiency should be suspected and the patient accompanied to the hospital for a hematologic workup. Postoperative pain after surgery is usually minimal and is managed appropriately with nonnarcotic analgesics.[19,41,86] Research has consistently shown that nonsteroidal antiinflammatory drugs administered preoperatively are more efficacious than opiate narcotics given after the pain is present.[18,19]

The presurgical administration of antibiotics is not indicated, and research shows that it may actually increase the probability

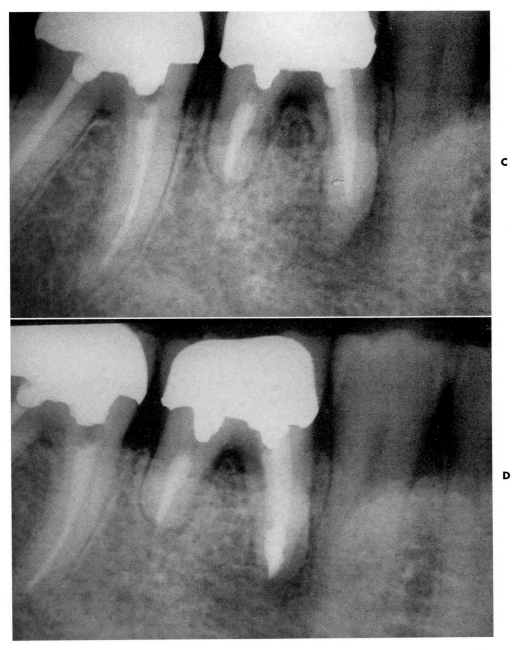

FIG. 18-72, cont'd C, Preoperative radiograph. **D,** Immediate postoperative radiograph with Super EBA retrofill.

Continued

of infection.[59,60] Surprisingly, postoperative infection is rare even though the procedure is performed in a sea of microorganisms. Most postoperative infections develop from either faulty aseptic technique or poor flap reapproximation and closure.[16]

If infection is present, the antibiotic of choice is penicillin V potassium. If the patient is allergic to penicillin, erythromycin or clindamycin can be prescribed.[31] The patient should be monitored daily and the regimen changed if no improvement occurs. The only time antibiotics are routinely prescribed postoperatively, other than for medical reasons, is when during the surgical procedure the maxillary sinus or the floor of the nose has been perforated. These patients should begin taking antibiotics immediately postoperatively and continue for 5 days. These patients should use decongestants while the sinus membrane heals.

Postoperative care involves proper oral hygiene, chlorhexidine mouth rinses for 4 days, liquid food supplements (if needed), and rest. After the suture removal appointment, the patient should be checked again at 10 to 14 days, at which time all swelling and soreness should be gone. At 6 weeks the soft tissue is evaluated again using a periodontal probe to check for a functional attachment.

Yearly recall for at least 2 years is suggested for follow-up care. It is not rare to observe initial osseous healing after 2 years later followed by periapical breakdown.[26]

Successful healing involves the cementogenic repair of the root apex, reestablishment of a functional periodontal ligament, and regeneration of apical alveolar bone (Fig. 18-72). Occasionally we must be satisfied with less than ideal healing, and

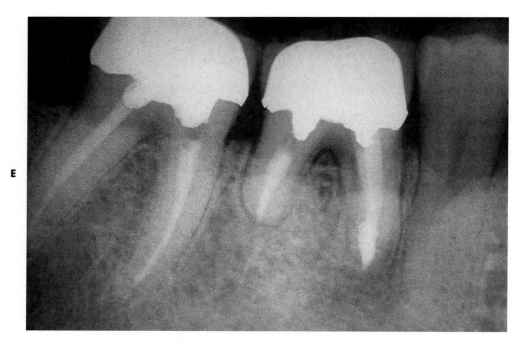

E

FIG. 18-72, cont'd E, At 18-month recall there is good resolution of the lesion.

some surgeries heal with a nonfunctional apical repair (i.e., a scar). Apical scars can be radiographically indistinguishable from recurring disease, and such radiographic lesions should be monitored for changes in size and shape to determine if re-entry is required.

REFERENCES

1. Amazon K, Robinson MJ, Rywlin AM: Ferrugination caused by Monsel's solution: clinical observations and experimentations, *Am J Dermatol* 2:197, 1980.
2. Armstrong RB, Nichols J, Pachance J: Punch biopsy wounds treated with Monsel's solution or collagen matrix: a comparison of healing, *Arch Dermatol* 122:546, 1986.
3. Austin BP, Keating KM, Hohenfeldt PR, Gerstein H: Osseous reactions to bimetallic couples in rat tibias, *Oral Surg* 54:79, 1982.
4. Barber BCW, Parsons KC, Mills PR, Williams GL: Anatomy of root canals. II. Permanent maxillary molars, *Aust Dent J* 19:46, 1974.
5. Bennett CR: *Monheim's local anesthesia and pain control in dental practice,* ed 7, St Louis, 1984, Mosby.
6. Block RM, Bushell A: Retrograde amalgam procedures for mandibular posterior teeth, *J Endod* 8:107, 1982.
7. Bloomquist DS: Pain control in endodontics, *Dent Clin North Am* 23(4):543, 1979.
8. Bondra DL, Hartwell GR, MacPhearson MG, Portell FR: Leakage in vitro with IRM, high copper amalgam, and EBA cement as retrofilling materials, *J Endod* 15:157, 1989.
9. Bramwell JD, Hicks ML: Sealing ability of four retrofilling techniques, *J Endod* 12:95, 1993.
10. Calderwood RG, Hera SS, Davis JR, Waite DE: A comparison of the healing rate of bone after production of defects by various rotary instruments, *J Dent Res* 43:207, 1964.
11. Carr GB: Common errors in periradicular surgery, *Endod Rep* 8:12, 1993.
12. Carr GB: Endodontics at the crossroads, *J Calif Dent Assoc* 24:20, 1996.
13. Carr GB: Ultrasonic root-end preparation, *Dent Clin North Am,* 1997, p. 541.
14. Cox CF, Felton D, Bergenholtz G: Histopathological response of infected cavities treated with Gluma and Scotchbond dentin bonding agents, *Am J Dent* 1:189, 1988.
15. Craig RG: Restorative dental materials, ed 9, St Louis, 1993, Mosby, p 214.
16. Curren JB, Kennet S, Young AR: An assessment of the use of prophylactic antibiotics in third molar surgery, *Int J Oral Surg* 3:1, 1974.
17. Dedolph TII, Clark HB: A histological study of mucoperiosteal flap healing, *J Oral Surg* 16:367, 1958.
18. Dionne RA, Cooper SA: Evaluation of preoperative ibuprofen for postoperative pain after removal of third molars, *Oral Surg* 45:851, 1978.
19. Dionne RA et al: Suppression of postoperative administration of ibuprofen in comparison to placebo, acetaminophen and acetaminophen plus codeine, *J Clin Pharmacol* 23:37, 1983.
20. Dragoo M, Scherer W, Stoll T: Resin-ionomer and hybrid Ionomer cements: I. Comparison of three materials for the treatment of subgingival root lesions, *Int J Periodont Rest Dent* 16:595-601, 1996.
21. Dragoo M, Scherer W, Stoll T: Resin-Ionomer and hybrid Ionomer cements: II. Human clinical and histological wound healing responses in special periodontic lesions, *Int J Periodont Rest Dent* 17:75-87, 1997.
22. Dumsha TC, Sydiskis RJ: Cytotoxicity testing of a dentin bonding system, *Oral Surg* 59:637, 1985.
23. Escobar C, Michaniwicz AE, Czonstowsky M, Miklos FL: A comparative study between injectable low-temperature (700F) gutta-percha and silver amalgam as a retroseal, *Oral Surg* 61:504, 1986.
24. Flanders DH, James GA, Burch B, Dockum N: Comparative histopathologic study of zinc-free amalgam and Cavit in connective tissue of the rat, *J Endod* 1:56, 1975.
25. Forrest L: Current concepts in soft connective tissue wound healing, *Br J Surg* 70:133, 1983.
26. Frank A et al: Clinical and surgical endodontics: concepts in practice, Philadelphia, 1983, JP Lippincott.
27. Frank A et al: Long-term evaluation of surgically placed amalgam fillings, *J Endod* 18:391, 1992.
28. Gerstein H: Surgical endodontics. In Laskin DN, editor: *Oral and maxillofacial surgery, II,* St Louis, 1985, Mosby.

29. Grossman LI, Oliet S, Del Rio C: *Endodontics,* ed 11, Philadelphia, 1988, Lea & Febiger.

30. Gutmann JL: Surgical procedures in endodontic practice. In Levine N, editor: *Current treatment in dental practice,* Philadelphia, 1986, WB Saunders.

31. Gutmann JL, Harrison JW: *Surgical endodontics,* Boston, 1991, Blackwell Scientific Publications.

32. Guyton AC: *Textbook of medical physiology,* ed 7, St Louis, 1986, Mosby.

33. Harrison JW, Jurosky KA: Wound healing in the tissues of the periodontium following periradicular surgery. II. The incisional wound, *J Endod* 17:425, 1991.

34. Harrison JW, Jurosky KA: Wound healing in the tissues of the periodontium following periradicular surgery. II. The dissectional wound, *J Endod* 17:544, 1991.

35. Hartley F et al: The success rate of apicoectomy: a retrospective study of 1,016 cases, *Br Dent J* 129:407, 1970.

36. Hermann JB: Changes in tensile strength and knot security of surgical sutures in vivo, *Arch Surg* 106:707, 1973.

37. Inoue S, Yoshimura M, Tinkle JS, Marshal FJ: A 24-week study of the microleakage of four retrofilling materials using a fluid filtration method, *J Endod* 17:369, 1991.

38. King KT, Anderson RW, Pashley DH, Pantera EA: Longitudinal evaluation of the seal of endodontic retrofillings, *J Endod* 16:307, 1990.

39. Klinsberg J, Butcher EO: Epithelial femar in periodontal repair in the rat, *J Periodontol* 34:315, 1963.

40. Kronman JH: Microbiologic evaluation of poly-HEMA root canal filling material, *Oral Surg* 48:175, 1979.

41. Kusner G et al: A study comparing the effectiveness of ibuprofen (Motrin), Empirin with codeine #3 and Synalgos-DC for relief of postendodontic pain, *J Endod* 10:210, 1984.

42. Lemon RR, Jeansonne BG, Boggs WS: Ferric sulfate hemostasis: effect on osseous wound healing. II. With curettage and irrigation, *J Endod* 19:174, 1993.

43. Lemon RR, Steele PJ, Jeansonne BG: Ferric sulfate hemostasis: effect on osseous wound healing. I. Left in situ for maximum exposure, *J Endod* 19:170, 1993.

44. Lilly GE: Reaction of oral tissues to suture materials, *Oral Surg* 26:128, 1968.

45. Lin L, Skribner J, Shovin F, Langland K: Periapical surgery of mandibular molar teeth: anatomical and surgical considerations, *J Endod* 9:496, 1983.

46. Longos CE, van Cura JE, Alves ME, Nalway C: Blood and urine mercury levels in primates following amalgam retrograde fillings, *J Dent Res* 72:273, 1993 (abstract 1361).

46a. Leubke RG et al: Indications and contradictions for endodontic surgery, *Oral surg.* 7:97, 1964.

47. Mach SD, Krizek TJ: Sutures and suturing: current concepts, *J Oral Surg* 36:710, 1978.

48. Mason RM: Hemostatic mechanisms of microfibuillar collagen. In *Proceedings of a symposium on avitene (MCH),* Ft Worth, 1975, Alcon Laboratories.

49. Matloff IR, Jensen JR, Singer L, Tabibi A: A comparison of methods used in root canal sealability studies, *Oral Surg* 53:203, 1982.

50. Mcarre D, Ellender G: The biocompatibility of restorative materials, *J Dent Res* 69:949, 1990 (abstract 16).

51. McDonald NJ, Dumsha TC: A comparative retrofill leakage study utilizing a dentin bonding material, *J Endod* 13:224, 1987.

52. Melcher AH et al: Cells from bone synthesize cementum-like and bone-like tissue in vitro and may migrate into periodontal ligament in vivo, *J Periodontol Res* 22:246, 1987.

53. Miles DA, Anderson RW, Pashley DH: Evaluation of the bond strengths of dentin bonding agents used to seal resected root apicies, *J Endod* 20:538, 1994.

54. Milleding P, Wennberg A, Hasselgren G: Cytotoxicity of corroded and noncorroded dental silver amalgams, *Scand J Dent Res* 93:76, 1985.

55. Morris ML: Healing of naturally occurring periodontal pockets about vital human teeth, *J Periodontal* 26:285, 1955.

56. Nelson LW, Mahler DB: Factors influencing the sealing behavior of retrograde amalgam fillings, *Oral Surg* 69:356, 1990.

57. Okumura T: Anatomy of the root canal, Trans 7, *Int Dent Congress* 1:170, 1926.

58. Oynick J, Oynick T: A study of a new material for retrograde fillings, *J Endod* 4:203, 1978.

59. Paterson JA, Cardo VA, Stratigos GP: An examination of antibiotic prophylaxis in oral and maxillofacial surgery, *Oral Surg* 28:753, 1970.

60. Pendrill K, Riddy J: The use of prophylactic penicillin in periodontal surgery, *J Periodontol* 51:44, 1980.

61. Peters LB, Harrison JW: A comparison of leakage of filling materials in demineralized and non-demineralized and resected root-ends under vacuum and non-vacuum conditions, *Int Endodont J* 25:273, 1992.

62. Pitt Ford TR, Andreasen JO, Dorn SO, Kariyawasan SP: Effect of Super EBA as a root-end filling on healing after replantation, *J Endod* 21:13, 1995.

63. Reit C, Hirsch J: Surgical endodontic retreatment, *Int Endodont J* 19:107, 1986.

64. Rovee DT, Miller CA: Eipidermal role in the breaking strength of wounds, *Arch Surg* 96:43, 1968.

65. Rud J, Munksgaard EC: Retrograde root filling with dentin-bonded modified resin composite, *J Endod* 22:477, 1996.

66. Rud J, Rud V, Munksgaard EC: Long-term evaluation of retrograde root filling with dentin-bonded resin composite, *J Endod* 22:90, 1996.

67. Rud J et al: Retrograde root filling with composite and a dentin-bonding agent: part 1, *Endodont Dent Traumatol* 7:118, 1991.

68. Shani J, Friedman S, Stabholz A, Abed J: A radionucleic model for evaluating sealibility of retrograde filling materials, *Int J Nucl Med Biol* 11:46, 1984.

69. Siew C et al: Biological safety evaluation of a novel dentine bonding system, *J Dent Res* 63(special issue):313, 1984 (abstract 1277).

70. Smee G et al: A comparative leakage study of P-30 resin bonded ceramic, teflon, amalgam, and IRM as retrofilling seals, *J Endod* 13:117, 1987.

71. Spångberg LSW: The study of biological properties of endodontic biomaterials In Spangberg LSW, editor: *Experimental endodontics,* Boca Raton, Fla, 1990, CRC Press.

72. Tanzilli JP, Raphael D, Moodnik RM: A comparison of the marginal adaptation of retrograde techniques: a scanning electron microscope study, *Oral Surg* 50:74, 1980.

73. Tayler AC, Campbell MM: Reattachment of gingival epithelium to the tooth, *J Periodontol* 43:281, 1972.

74. Telsch P: Development of raised temperatures after osteotomies, *J Maxillofac Surg* 2:141, 1974.

75. Torabinejad M, Higa RK, McKendry DJ, Pitt Ford TR: Dye leakage of four root end filling materials: effects of blood contamination, *J Endod* 20:159, 1994.

76. Torabinejad MT, Hong CU, McDonald F, Pitt Ford TR: Physical and chemical properties of a new root-end filling material, *J Endod* 21:349, 1995.

77. Torabinejad M, Hong CU, Pitt Ford TR, Kettering JD: Cytotoxicity of four root end filling materials, *J Endod* 21:489, 1995.

78. Torabinejad M, Pitt Ford TR: Root end filling materials: a review, *Endodont Dent Traumatol* 12:161, 1996.

79. Torabinejad MT, Rastegar AF, Kettering JD, Pitt Ford RT: Bacterial leakage of mineral trioxide aggregate as a root-end filling material, *J Endod* 21:109, 1995.

80. Torabinejad MT, Watson TF, Pitt Ford TR: Sealing ability of an MTA when used as a root end filling material, *J Endod* 19:591, 1993.

81. Torabinejad MT, Wilder-Smith P, Kettering JD, Pitt Ford TR: Comparative investigation of marginal adaptation of mineral trioxide aggregate and other commonly used root-end filling materials, *J Endod* 21:295, 1995.

82. Torabinejad M et al: Investigation of mineral trioxide aggregate for root-end filling in dogs, *J Endod* 21:603, 1995.

83. Trope M, Lost C, Schmitz HJ, Friedman S: Healing of apical periodontitis in dogs after apicoectomy and retrofilling with various filling materials, *Oral Surg* 81:221, 1996.

84. Vertucci FJ, Beatty RG: Apical leakage associated with retrofilling techniques: a dye study, *J Endod* 12:331, 1986.

85. Vignaroli PA, Anderson RW, Pashley DH: Longitudinal evaluation of the microleakage of dentin bonding agents used to seal resected root apicies, *J Endod* 21:609, 1995.

86. Vogel RI, Gross JI: The effects of nonsteroidal anti-inflammatory analgesics on pain after periodontal surgery, *J Am Dent Assoc* 109:731, 1984.

87. Weller RN, Niemczyk SP, Kim S: Incidence and position of the canal isthmus. I. Mesiobuccal root of the maxillary first molar, *J Endod* 21:380, 1995.

88. Wennberg A, Hasselgren G: Cytotoxicity evaluation of temporary filling materials, *Int Endodont J* 14:121, 1981.

89. Wirthlin MB: The current status of new attachment therapy, *J Periodontol* 52:529, 1981.

90. Yancey JM: Ten rules for reading clinical reports, *Am J Orthod* 109:558, 1996.

91. Yoshimura M, Marshall FJ, Tinkle J: In vitro quantification of the apical sealing ability of retrograde amalgam fillings, *J Endod* 16:9, 1990.

Chapter 19

Management of Pain and Anxiety

Stanley F. Malamed

The problem of managing pain and anxiety in the practice of dentistry is a considerable one. Studies have demonstrated that one of the major reasons why over 50% of adult Americans do not routinely seek dental care is a fear of pain. From interviews with many of these patients it becomes clear that although they may not be in pain when they visit the dentist, a large majority truly believe that they will experience pain at some time during their dental appointment and that the person most likely to be responsible for this discomfort is the dentist.

Not only does the fear of pain minimize visits to the dentist by many patients, usually until they experience excruciating dental pain, but the very pain they are experiencing has been implicated as a significant factor in increasing the incidence of life-threatening medical emergencies arising during dental treatment. This occurs because it becomes clinically more difficult to obtain profound pulpal anesthesia when pain or infection has been present for a significant period of time.

Table 19-1 presents data obtained from 4309 dentists in independent surveys by Fast[12] and Malamed.[23] These dentists reported 30,608 emergency situations arising in their practices over a 10-year period. A wide array of emergencies were reported, from the usually benign (syncope) to the catastrophic (cardiac arrest).

Although specific details of these clinical situations are not available, it can be presumed that as many as 23,105 or 75.5% of the emergencies listed might have been precipitated, in part, by the increased stress (fear or pain) that is so frequently associated with dental treatment. Syncope alone accounted for 50.34% of the reported emergencies. Other potentially "stress-induced" problems include angina pectoris, seizures, acute asthmatic attacks, hyperventilation, cardiac arrest, myocardial infarction, acute pulmonary edema, cerebrovascular accident, acute adrenal insufficiency, and thyroid storm.

That fear and pain are associated with an increased occurrence of emergency situations was further confirmed by Matsuura,[30] who reported that 77.8% of life-threatening systemic complications in the dental office developed either during or immediately following the administration of local anesthesia or during the ensuing dental treatment (Table 19-2). Of those emergencies arising during dental treatment, 38.9% developed during the extraction of teeth and *26.9% occurred during pulpal extirpation,* two procedures where adequate pain control is frequently difficult to obtain (Table 19-3).

In studying which teeth are most difficult to anesthetize, Walton and Abbott[40] found that mandibular molars were implicated in 47% of clinical situations. Malamed,[26] repeating this study at the University of Southern California, found mandibular molars to be "the problem" in 91% of cases of inability to obtain adequate pulpal anesthesia. Table 19-4 compares these two studies.

It appears then that the occurrence of sudden and unexpected pain is able to induce profound stress on the cardiovascular, respiratory, endocrine, and central nervous systems, which may lead in certain situations to potentially significant emergency situations.

The problems of the management of pain and anxiety are closely related. Pain produced by dental treatment can usually be minimized or entirely prevented through thoughtful patient management and the judicious use of the techniques of pain control, especially local anesthesia. Anxiety can also be managed effectively in almost all situations; however, before anxiety can be managed, it must be recognized. Discovery of the cause of a patient's anxiety is the major factor in managing the problem. Once aware of a patient's fears, the dentist has many techniques available with which to care for the patient.

In most areas of dental care the problem of anxiety control is greater than the management of pain. Pain control is almost always manageable through the administration of local anesthetics. Once adequate pain control is achieved, anxiety control is usually more readily achievable. In endodontics, however, more than in any other dental specialty, pain control often proves to be more of a difficult problem than the management of anxiety. Because of this difficulty in providing effective pain control, the patient undergoing endodontic treatment often anticipates the experience with a great deal of apprehension.

The following discussion covers the dual problems of pain control and anxiety control, with special emphasis on the pulpally involved tooth.

PAIN CONTROL

Although achieving adequate pain control for endodontic care is not usually difficult, there are all too many instances when a satisfactory result eludes the dentist. Indeed, in this evolving era of the Internet, many of the queries posted in dental discussion groups deal with exactly this problem: the patient with the "hot" tooth and the dentist's inability to provide satisfactory pain control. The most likely explanation for the greater percentage of anesthetic failures in endodontics than in other areas of dental care lies in the tissue changes that commonly develop in and around pulpally involved teeth.

Local Anesthetics: How They Work

Injectable local anesthetics are acid salts, the weakly alkaline and poorly water-soluble local anesthetic being combined with hydrochloric acid to form the hydrochloride salt (e.g., lidocaine hydrochloride), which is soluble in water and slightly acidic.

Table 19-1. Reported incidence of emergency situations by private practice dentists during a 10-year period[12,23]

	Total
Syncope	15,407
Mild allergic reaction	2,583
Angina pectoris	2,552
Postural hypotension	2,475
Seizures	1,595
Asthmatic attack (bronchospasm)	1,392
Hyperventilation	1,326
"Epinephrine reaction"	913
Insulin shock (hypoglycemia)	890
Cardiac arrest	331
Anaphylactic reaction	304
Myocardial infarction	289
Local anesthetic overdose	204
Acute pulmonary edema (heart failure)	141
Diabetic coma	109
Cerebrovascular accident	68
Adrenal insufficiency	25
Thyroid storm	4

Table 19-2. Time of occurrence of reported systemic complications

Complication	Percentage
Just before treatment	1.5%
During/after local anesthesia	54.9%
During treatment	22.9%
After treatment	15.2%
After leaving dental office	5.5%

Data from Matsuura H: *Anesth Prog* 36:219-228, 1990.

Table 19-3. Type of dental treatment during occurrence of complications

Treatment	Percentage
Tooth extraction	38.9%
Pulp extirpation	26.9%
Unknown	12.3%
Other treatment	9.0%
Preparation	7.3%
Filling	2.3%
Incision	1.7%
Apicoectomy	0.7%
Removal of fillings	0.7%
Alveolar plastics	0.3%

Data from Matsuura H: *Anesth Prog* 36:219-228, 1990.

In solution the local anesthetic exists in two ionic forms: an uncharged anion (RN) and a positively charged cation (RNH⁺). The relative proportions of each ionic form depend on the pH of the anesthetic solution and of the tissue, and on the pK_a of the specific local anesthetic. The pK_a is that pH value at which a solution contains 50% of each ionic form of the local anesthetic.

The pK_a for a given local anesthetic is a constant. pK_as for

Table 19-4. Inability to achieve adequate pulpal anesthesia

	Maxillary		Mandibular	
	Walton and Abbott	Malamed	Walton and Abbott	Malamed
Molars	12%	5%	47%	91%
Premolars	18%	2%	12%	0%
Anteriors	2%	2%	9%	0%

Data from Walton RE, Abbott BJ: *J Am Dent Assoc* 103:571-575, 1981; and Malamed SF: *Handbook of local anesthesia*, ed 4, St Louis, 1997, Mosby.

Table 19-5. Dissociation constants (pK_a) of local anesthetics

Agent	pK_a	Base (RN) at pH 7.4 (%)	Approximate Onset of Action (min)
Mepivacaine	7.6	40	2-4
Etidocaine	7.7	33	2-4
Articaine	7.8	29	2-4
Lidocaine	7.9	25	2-4
Prilocaine	7.9	25	2-4
Bupivacaine	8.1	18	5-8
Tetracaine	8.5	8	10-15
Chloroprocaine	8.7	6	10-15
Procaine	9.1	2	14-18

RN, uncharged molecule.

common local anesthetics are presented in Table 19-5. Since pK_a is a constant, the relative proportion of RN and RNH⁺ ionic forms depends on the pH of the anesthetic solution.

$$RNH^+ \rightleftarrows RN + H^+$$

As the pH of the local anesthetic decreases, H+ ion concentrations increase and the equilibrium shifts toward the charged cationic form. Proportionally more cation is present than free base. Conversely, if the pH of the local anesthetic solution becomes more basic (pH increases), the H+ concentration decreases and a proportionally greater percentage of local anesthetic exists in the RN form.

At the normal tissue pH of approximately 7.4, it can be seen (see Table 19-5) that there exists a greater proportion of local anesthetic cation (RNH⁺). Both ionic forms of the local anesthetic are essential for its anesthetic activity.[35,36]

Several factors are responsible for the ultimate anesthetic profile of a local anesthetic. These include (1) diffusion of the local anesthetic through the lipid-rich nerve sheath (*pK_a and lipid solubility*) and (2) binding of the local anesthetic at the receptor site (*protein binding, nonnervous tissue diffusibility, and intrinsic vasodilator activity*).[10] The lipid-soluble RN ionic form is able to diffuse more readily through the lipoid-rich nerve sheath than does the water-soluble RNH⁺ ionic form. Indeed, clinically local anesthetics with a lower pK_a (more RN ionic forms) possess a more rapid onset of action than do local anesthetics with higher pK_as (see Table 19-5).

The degree of lipid solubility appears to be important in determining the intrinsic potency of a local anesthetic (Table 19-6). Increased lipid solubility permits the anesthetic to penetrate the nerve sheath (which is 90% lipid) more easily.[4] This is re-

Table 19-6. Lipid solubility of local anesthetics

Agent	Approximate Lipid Solubility	Usual Effective Concentration (%)
Procaine	1	2-4
Mepivacaine	1	2-3
Prilocaine	1.5	4
Lidocaine	4	2
Bupivacaine	30	0.5-0.75
Tetracaine	80	0.15
Etidocaine	140	0.5-0.75
Articaine	—	—
Chloroprocaine	—	—

Table 19-7. Protein-binding characteristics and duration of action of local anesthetics

Agent	Approximate Protein Binding	Approximate Duration of Action (min) (Soft Tissue)
Procaine	5	60-90
Prilocaine	55	100-240
Lidocaine	65	90-200
Mepivacaine	75	120-240
Tetracaine	85	180-600
Etidocaine	94	180-600
Bupivacaine	95	180-600
Articaine	95	120-480
Chloroprocaine	—	—

flected clinically as increased potency. Local anesthetics with greater lipid solubility produce more effective conduction blockade at lower concentrations than do less lipid-soluble anesthetics.

Following penetration of the nerve sheath by the RN ions, a reequilibrium occurs between the RN and RNH^+ ionic forms both outside and within the nerve sheath. Within the nerve itself, the RNH^+ ions bind to the (protein) drug receptor site located within the sodium channel. Protein binding of the anesthetic molecule at this receptor site is responsible for (1) suppression of the electrophysiologic events occurring in propagation of a nerve impulse and (2) the duration of anesthetic activity of the drug. Proteins comprise approximately 10% of the nerve membrane. Local anesthetics (e.g., bupivacaine, etidocaine) possessing greater degrees of protein binding (Table 19-7) than others (e.g., procaine) appear to attach more firmly to protein drug receptor sites and are longer acting.

Fig. 19-1 illustrates the sequence of events involved in peripheral nerve block in normal tissues. At a pH of 7.4, an anesthetic with a pK_a of 7.9 reaches equilibrium in the tissues with approximately 75% of its molecules in the RNH^+ ionic form and 25% in the RN ionic form. The RN molecules pass through the barrier to diffusion represented by the lipid nerve sheath more readily than the RNH^+ ionic form. Once the RN ions enter into the nerve, they encounter an intraneural pH of 7.4. The pH of the tissues within the nerve itself remains quite uniform even in the presence of marked changes in the pH of extracellular tissues. The pH of extracellular fluid may therefore differ from the pH within the nerve membrane, and similarly the ratio of RNH^+ to RN at these sites may differ. In

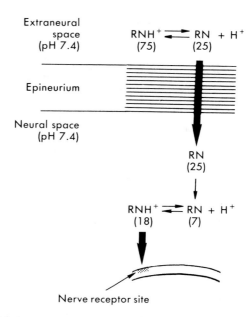

FIG. 19-1 Mode of action of a local anesthetic in normal tissue (pH 7.4). The anesthetic ($pK_a = 7.9$) is deposited in the extraneural tissues. Equilibrium occurs with approximately 75% of the molecules in the charged cationic form and 25% in base form. (Numbers in parentheses represent the proportion of anesthetic cation and base in extracellular and neural compartments.)

this internal environment (pH of 7.4) ionic reequilibration occurs with approximately 75% of the RN reverting to the RNH^+ ionic form, attaching to the drug receptor site within the sodium channel and producing neural blockade.

"Pulpally Involved" Tooth

The problem of inadequate pain control during endodontics can be explained, in part, through changes occurring in periapical tissues. Pulpal and apical pathology (inflammation or infection) decrease tissue pH in the region surrounding the involved tooth below what is normally found. Pus has a pH of approximately 5.5. In the presence of this decreased pH, dissociation of the local anesthetic favors formation of a larger proportion of RNH^+ to RN (Fig. 19-2). Ninety-nine percent of a local anesthetic with a pK_a of 7.9 will be in the RNH^+ ionic form, which is unable to migrate through the neural sheath. The relative absence of RN ions leads to fewer anesthetic molecules entering the nerve sheath and reaching the nerve membrane, where intracellular pH remains 7.4 and reequilibration between RN and RNH^+ can occur. Fewer RNH^+ molecules are present intracellularly, decreasing the likelihood of complete anesthesia developing.

Solutions

One method of obtaining more intense anesthesia in an area of infection would be to deposit a greater volume of anesthetic into the region. A greater number of RN molecules would be liberated, with greater diffusion through the nerve sheath and a somewhat greater likelihood of achieving adequate pain control. Although this procedure is somewhat effective, injection of anesthetics into infected areas is undesirable because of the possibility of the spread of infection into a previously uncontaminated area. Deposition of the anesthetic into an area at a

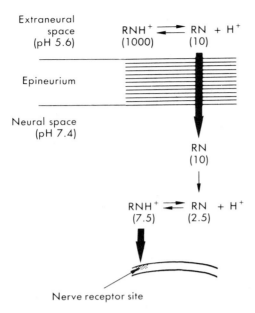

FIG. 19-2 Mode of action of a local anesthetic in an inflamed or infected area. The anesthetic (pK_a = 7.9) is deposited in the extraneural tissues (pH of 5.6). Equilibrium develops with approximately 99% of solution in the cationic form. Fewer anesthetic molecules pass through the epineurium to the neural space. The pH in the neural space is 7.4, and molecules re-equilibrate. However, an insufficient number of molecules may be present, leading to a failure to produce profound clinical anesthesia.

distance from the involved tooth is more likely to provide adequate pain control because of the normal tissue conditions existing there. Regional nerve block anesthesia is therefore a major factor in pain control for pulpally involved teeth.

There are occasions, fortunately rare, when even regional nerve block anesthesia at a distance from the infected tooth fails to provide adequate pain control. Omitting for a moment the most likely cause of this situation (faulty injection technique), Najjar[32] has proposed that inadequate pain control may be due to the fact that morphologic changes (e.g., neurodegenerative changes in the axon or the presence of inflammatory mediators) are developing. He further states that morphologic changes in inflamed nerve, even at a distance from the actual inflammatory site, appear to be a significant barrier for normal electrolyte exchange at membrane level. The net result is reinforcement of a nerve fiber's ability to generate action potentials. Studies[5,37] have demonstrated that inflammation potentiates peripheral nerve excitability.

In addition, when the inflamed tooth is anesthetized, it becomes asymptomatic but, on attempts to gain access to the pulp chamber and canals, becomes exquisitely sensitive to manipulation. Although no entirely satisfactory explanation exists for this circumstance, it may be explainable on the basis of an increase in the rate of stimulation of the nerve endings that occurs with use of the high- or low-speed handpiece. The degree of neural blockade may be adequate for a lower level of stimulation before preparation yet prove inadequate to block completely the rapid flood of impulses arising with the use of the handpiece.

Local Anesthesia: Drugs

Although many drugs are classified as local anesthetics and find use within the health professions, only a handful are currently used in dentistry. In 1980 five local anesthetics were available in dental cartridge form in the United States: *lidocaine, mepivacaine, prilocaine,* and the combination of *procaine* and *propoxycaine.* In the subsequent 17 years increased demand for longer acting local anesthetics led to the introduction, in dental cartridges, of *bupivacaine* (1982 Canada, 1983 United States) and *etidocaine* (1985). In 1983 the thiophene ring–containing amide *articaine* became available in many areas (Europe, United Kingdom, Canada), but not as yet in the United States. Articaine is classified as an intermediate-duration local anesthetic.

With the availability of this increasing number of local anesthetics it is now possible for a dentist to select from a broad spectrum of local anesthetics a drug possessing the specific properties required by the patient for a given dental procedure.

Duration of anesthesia: considerations

The duration of pulpal (hard tissue) and soft tissue (total) anesthesia cited for each drug is an approximation. Factors exist that affect both the depth and the duration of a drug's anesthetic action, either prolonging or (much more commonly) decreasing it. These include the following:

1. Individual variation in response to the drug administered
2. Accuracy in administration of the drug
3. Status of the tissues at the site of drug deposition (vascularity, pH)
4. Anatomic variation
5. Type of injection administered (supraperiosteal ["infiltration"] or nerve block)

The duration of anesthesia (pulpal and soft tissue) is presented as a range (e.g., 40 to 60 minutes). This attempts to take into account the above-mentioned factors that can influence drug action.

Variation in individual response to a drug is quite common and is depicted in the so-called "bell" or normal distribution curve. A majority of patients respond in a predictable manner to a drug's actions (i.e., 40 to 60 minutes). However, some patients (with none of the other factors that influence drug action obviously present) have either a shorter or a longer duration of anesthesia. *This is to be expected and is entirely normal.*

Accuracy in the administration of an injected local anesthetic is a second factor influencing drug action. Although not as significant in certain techniques (i.e., supraperiosteal), accuracy in deposition is a major factor in many nerve blocks in which a considerable thickness of soft tissue must be penetrated to access the nerve to be blocked. The inferior alveolar nerve block is a prime example of a technique in which the duration of anesthesia is greatly influenced by accuracy of injection. Deposition of the anesthetic close to a nerve provides greater depth and duration of anesthetic compared with an anesthetic deposited at a greater distance from the nerve to be blocked.

The *status of the tissues* into which a local anesthetic is deposited influences the observed duration of anesthetic action and is of potentially greater significance in endodontic procedures. The presence of normal healthy tissue at the site of drug deposition is assumed. Inflammation, infection, or pain (acute or chronic) usually decreases the anticipated duration of action. Increased vascularity at an injection site results in a more rapid absorption of the local anesthetic and a decreased duration of anesthesia. This is most notable in areas of infection and inflammation but is also a consideration in "normal" anatomy. For example, the neck of the mandibular condyle, the target for local anesthetic deposition in the Gow-Gates mandibular nerve block, is considerably less vascular than the target area for the inferior alveolar nerve block. The expected duration of anesthesia for any local anesthetic is greater in the less vascular region.

Anatomic variation also influences the duration of clinical anesthesia. If anything, the most notable aspect of "normal" anatomy is the presence of extreme variation (in size and shape of the head, for example) from person to person. The techniques described in this chapter assume a patient in the middle of the bell curve, the so-called "normal responder." Anatomic variations away from this "norm" usually adversely influence the duration of clinical drug action. Although most obvious in the mandible (height of the mandibular foramen, width of the ramus), such variation may also be noted in the maxilla. Supraperiosteal infiltration, usually quite effective in providing pulpal anesthesia for maxillary teeth, provides shorter than expected or inadequate anesthesia where the alveolar bone is more dense than usual. Where the zygomatic arch is lower (primarily in children but occasionally in adults), infiltration anesthesia of the maxillary first and second molars may provide a shorter duration or even fail to provide adequate pulpal anesthesia. In other cases the palatal root of maxillary molars may not be adequately anesthetized, even in the presence of a normal alveolar bony thickness, when that root flares greatly toward the midline of the palate.

Finally, and of potentially great importance, the duration of clinical anesthesia is influenced by the *type of injection administered.* For all the drugs presented, administration of a nerve block provides a longer duration of both pulpal and soft tissue anesthesia than supraperiosteal injection. This assumes that the recommended minimal volume of anesthetic is injected. For example, a duration of 40 minutes may be expected to follow a supraperiosteal injection, whereas a 60-minute duration is to be expected with a nerve block. Less-than-recommended volumes decrease the duration of action. Greater-than-recommended doses do *not* provide increased duration.

Two major classes of injectable local anesthetics, esters and amides, are recognized, distinguished by the type of linkage joining the two ends of the drug. Early local anesthetics, such as cocaine and procaine, were esters, whereas most local anesthetics introduced since 1940 have been amides.

The use of injectable local anesthetics in dentistry is almost exclusively limited to amide type of drugs. In fact no ester is currently being marketed in dental cartridge form in the United States. Given the number of local anesthetic injections administered in dentistry (conservatively estimated at more than 300 million in the United States annually), a drug with minimal risk of allergy is desirable. The risk of allergy to amide anesthetics is significantly less than that with esters. Conversely, the risk of systemic toxicity with amides is somewhat greater than that with esters. However, as toxic reactions are usually dose related, adherence to proper injection techniques—including the use of minimal volumes of anesthetic—minimizes this risk. Amide formulations have also proved more effective than their ester counterparts for achieving intraoral anesthesia. Thus comparison of risk-benefit ratios for local anesthetics used in dentistry greatly favors amide formulations.

BOX 19-1.
EXPECTED DURATION OF PULPAL ANESTHESIA

Short-Duration (<30 Minutes)
Etidocaine 1.5% + epinephrine 1:200,000 (15 minutes via infiltration)
Lidocaine 2% (5-10 minutes)
Mepivacaine 3% (20-40 minutes)
Prilocaine 4% (5-10 minutes via infiltration)

Intermediate-Duration (About 60 Minutes)
Articaine 4% + epinephrine 1:1000,000 and 1:200,000
Lidocaine 2% + epinephrine 1:50,000, 1:100,000
Mepivacaine 2% + levonordefrin 1:20,000
Prilocaine 4% (40-60 minutes via nerve block)
Prilocaine 4% + epinephrine 1:200,000 (60-90 minutes)

Long-Duration (>90 Minutes)
Bupivacaine 0.5% + epinephrine 1:200,000
Etidocaine 1.5% + epinephrine 1:200,000 (via nerve block)

The selection of a local anesthetic for use in a dental procedure is based on the following criteria:
- Duration of the dental procedure
- Requirement for hemostasis
- Requirement for postsurgical pain control
- Contraindication to the selected anesthetic drug or vasoconstrictor

Local anesthetic formulations available in dentistry may be categorized broadly by their expected duration of pulpal anesthesia into short-, intermediate-, and long-acting drugs. Box 19-1 lists local anesthetics, the various combinations in which they are currently available in the United States and Canada, and their expected duration of pulpal anesthesia.

Local Anesthesia: Techniques

Fortunately, many techniques are available to aid the dentist in obtaining clinically adequate pain control during virtually all endodontic procedures, even in the presence of acute or chronic localized tissue changes.

Supraperiosteal injection (local infiltration)

Supraperiosteal anesthesia is described as a technique in which anesthetic is deposited *into* the area of treatment.[25] Small, terminal nerve endings in the area are rendered incapable of transmitting impulses. Infiltration anesthesia is commonly used in maxillary teeth. Because of the ability of the anesthetic solution to diffuse through periosteum and the relatively thin cancellous bone of the maxilla, this technique provides effective pain control in maxillary endodontic procedures when infection is *not* present. Very often, however, when infection *is* present at the onset of an endodontic case and other anesthetic techniques must be relied on initially, infiltration anesthesia may prove effective at subsequent visits, provided cleaning and shaping of the root canals has been accomplished and infection and inflammatory responses are resolved.

Infiltration anesthesia is rarely effective in the adult mandible because of the inability of the anesthetic to penetrate the more dense cortical bone. In pediatric dentistry, however, infiltration anesthesia of the mandible is more successful. As a general rule, infiltration anesthesia in the pediatric mandible is successful when a primary tooth is being treated. Once replaced by a permanent tooth, the success rate of mandibular infiltration anesthesia decreases dramatically. Regional nerve block anesthesia or an accessory technique (periodontal ligament [PDL] or intraosseous [IO] injection) should receive primary consideration for permanent mandibular teeth.

In infiltration anesthesia the target area for deposition of the anesthetic is the apex of the tooth being treated. Only 0.6 ml of anesthetic need be administered for adequate pain control, using a 27-gauge short dental needle. Approximately 3 to 5 minutes are allowed to elapse before starting the procedure (e.g., placement of rubber dam). On rare occasion adequate pulpal anesthesia, even on non-pulpally involved teeth, is not achieved following infiltration. From clinical experience it appears that the most common cause of this is the failure to deposit the anesthetic solution at or above the apex of the tooth. The maxillary canine is most often the culprit, with the maxillary central incisor also frequently involved. Maxillary first and second molars may on rare occasion have buccal root apexes located beneath the thicker bone of the zygoma or may have palatal roots that flare considerably toward the midline. In either case infiltration anesthesia may prove ineffective.

Regional nerve block

In the event that infiltration anesthesia proves ineffective in providing clinically adequate pain control, regional nerve block anesthesia is recommended. Nerve block is defined as a method of achieving regional anesthesia by depositing a suitable local anesthetic close to a main nerve trunk, preventing afferent impulses from traveling centrally beyond that point.[25] Nerve block anesthesia is more likely to be effective when infiltration has failed, since the nerve is being blocked at some distance from the inflamed or infected tissue, where tissue pH and other factors are more nearly normal.

Several nerve blocks are beneficial in dentistry. A brief summary of major intraoral maxillary and mandibular nerve blocks follows.

Maxillary anesthesia. Maxillary nerves that can be anesthetized and are of importance in endodontic procedures are the maxillary (V2), posterior superior alveolar (PSA), anterior superior alveolar (ASA), greater palatine, and nasopalatine nerves.

The *posterior superior alveolar nerve block* provides pulpal anesthesia to the three maxillary molars and their overlying buccal soft tissues and bone. Anesthetic is deposited into the pterygomaxillary space, superior, distal, and medial to the maxillary tuberosity. In 28% of patients the mesiobuccal root of the first molar receives innervation from the middle superior alveolar nerve, in which case a volume of 0.6 ml of anesthetic should be infiltrated high into the buccal fold just anterior to the first maxillary molar.

Posterior superior alveolar nerve block

Teeth anesthetized	Volume of anesthetic (ml)	Recommended needle
1,2,3 or 14,15,16	0.9	25- or 27-gauge short

In addition, palatal infiltration may be required for anesthesia of the palatal soft tissues for placement of the rubber dam clamp.

The *anterior superior alveolar nerve block* is an easy injection to administer, providing anesthesia of the infraorbital, anterior superior alveolar, and the middle superior alveolar nerves in virtually all patients. By depositing local anesthetic outside the infraorbital foramen, anesthesia of the maxillary premolars, anterior teeth, and their overlying buccal soft tissues and bone is obtained. Palatal infiltration may be necessary for placement of a rubber dam clamp. Additionally, the soft tissues of the lower eyelid, lateral portion of the nose, and the upper lip are anesthetized (the infraorbital nerve). An important requirement for successful anterior superior alveolar nerve block is the application of finger pressure over the injection site for a minimum of 2 minutes following deposition of the anesthetic. This converts the infraorbital nerve block (soft tissue only) into the anterior superior alveolar nerve block (teeth, soft tissues, and bone).

Anterior superior alveolar nerve block

Teeth anesthetized	Volume of anesthetic (ml)	Recommended needle
4-8 or 9-13	0.9	25- or 27-gauge long

Palatal anesthesia is frequently required during endodontic procedures and is also needed around the gingival margins of the tooth to be clamped. Deposition of 0.3 ml of anesthetic by infiltration into the palatal gingiva 3 to 5 mm below the gingival margin provides adequate anesthesia. Larger areas of the palate rarely need to be anesthetized for endodontic procedures, but when necessary two nerve blocks are available: the greater palatine and nasopalatine.

The *greater* (or anterior) *palatine nerve block* provides anesthesia to both the palatal hard and soft tissues, ranging from the third molar as far anterior as the medial aspect of the first premolar. At the first premolar soft tissue anesthesia may only be partial because of overlay from the nasopalatine nerve.

Greater (anterior) palatine nerve block

Area anesthetized (soft tissue palatal to teeth numbers)	Volume of anesthetic (ml)	Recommended needle
1-5 or 12-16	0.45	27-gauge long

The *nasopalatine nerves* enter the palate through the incisive foramen, located in the midline just palatal to the central incisors and directly beneath the incisive papilla. They provide sensory innervation to the hard and soft tissues of the premaxilla as far distal as the first premolar, where fibers from the greater palatine nerve may be encountered.

Nasopalatine nerve block

Area anesthetized (soft tissue palatal to teeth numbers)	Volume of anesthetic (ml)	Recommended needle
6-11	0.45 (maximum)	27-gauge long

Because of the density of palatal soft tissues and their firm attachment to bone, especially in the anterior palatal region, palatal injections are considered potentially traumatic, both by patients and dentists. Palatal anesthesia *can* be achieved with a minimum of discomfort if care is taken throughout the procedure to ensure (1) adequate topical anesthesia, (2) adequate pressure anesthesia, (3) slow penetration of tissues, (4) continual slow deposition of anesthetic, and (5) injection of not more than 0.45 ml of solution.

Although rarely necessary, a *maxillary,* or *second division, nerve block* should be considered when other techniques of pain control prove ineffective because of infection accompanied by inflammation. The second division nerve block provides anesthesia of the entire maxillary nerve peripheral to the site of injection: pulps of all maxillary teeth on the side of injection, their overlying buccal soft tissues and bone, palatal hard and soft tissues on the injection side, and the upper lip, cheek, side of the nose, and lower eyelid.

Maxillary nerve block
(high-tuberosity or greater palatine approach)

Teeth anesthetized	Volume of anesthetic (ml)	Recommended needle
1-8 or 9-16	1.8	25-gauge long

Two intraoral approaches are available for the maxillary nerve block.[28,34] The *high-tuberosity approach* follows the same path as the posterior superior alveolar nerve block except that the depth of needle penetration is greater (30mm vs. 16 mm in the p.s.a.). The *greater palatine canal* approach involves entering the greater palatine foramen, usually located palatally between the second and third maxillary molars at the junction of the alveolar process and palatal bone. A 25-gauge long needle is carefully inserted into the foramen to a depth of 30 mm before 1.8 ml of anesthetic is deposited.

Mandibular anesthesia

Inferior alveolar nerve block: Pulpal anesthesia of mandibular teeth is traditionally obtained through the inferior alveolar nerve block (IANB). Additionally, anesthesia of the buccal soft tissues and bone anterior to the mental foramen is provided. If anesthesia of the buccal soft tissues overlying the mandibular molars is needed, the buccal nerve must be blocked. The anterior two third of the lingual nerve is usually blocked along with the inferior alveolar nerve, the floor of the mouth, the mucous membrane and mucoperiosteum on the lingual side of the mandible. A 25-gauge long needle is recommended; following multiple negative aspirations, 1.5 ml of anesthetic is deposited. To block the buccal nerve the same needle (as used for inferior alveolar nerve block) is placed into the buccal fold distal and buccal to the last mandibular molar in the quadrant, and the remaining 0.3 ml of anesthetic deposited.

In the absence of pulpal or periapical pathosis, inferior alveolar nerve block provides clinically adequate anesthesia 85% to 90% of the time. Its rate of success diminishes where periapical disease exists. Because of the density of bone in the adult mandible, infiltration anesthesia is of little value. When inferior alveolar nerve block proves ineffective, fewer alternatives are available. There are, however, other nerve blocks and alternative techniques that may succeed in the mandible.

Inferior alveolar nerve block

Teeth anesthetized	Volume of anesthetic (ml)	Recommended needle
17-24 or 25-32	1.5	25-gauge long

Incisive nerve block: The incisive and mental nerves are terminal branches of the inferior alveolar nerve, arising at the mental foramen. The *mental nerve,* exiting the mental foramen, provides sensory innervation to the skin of the lower lip and chin regions and the mucous membrane lining the lower lip; the *incisive nerve,* remaining within the mandibular canal, provides sensory innervation to the pulps of the premolars, canine, incisors, and the bone anterior to the mental foramen. Pulpal anesthesia of the region served by the incisive nerve should be considered when endodontic treatment is contemplated on premolars or other anterior teeth. Anesthetic is placed *outside* the mental foramen, with finger pressure applied at the injection site for a minimum of 1 minute, preferably 2 minutes, to ensure entry of anesthetic into the mental foramen and mandibular canal.

Incisive nerve block

Teeth anesthetized	Volume of anesthetic (ml)	Recommended needle
20-24 or 25-29	0.6	27-gauge short

Infiltration anesthesia: As mentioned previously, infiltration anesthesia is rarely effective in the adult mandible. The sole exceptions to this are (1) the lateral incisor, where up to 1 ml of anesthetic may be deposited into the mucobuccal fold at the level of the apex of the tooth, and (2) the mandibular molars, where in some patients deposition of 0.9 ml on the *lingual* aspect of the mandible may provide successful anesthesia.

On occasion, adequate pain control is achieved in the mandible except in isolated areas, most often the mesial root of the first molar. Successful pulpal anesthesia of third molars is frequently difficult to achieve because of the multiplicity of accessory innervations that are thought to exist. Indeed, adequate anesthesia is easier to obtain for third molar extraction than for restorative or endodontic procedures.

The mesial root of the mandibular first molar is commonly sensitive to noxious stimuli when all other portions of the same tooth and adjacent structures are insensitive. Although many theories (involving cervical accessory and transverse neck nerves) have been put forward to explain this situation, the mylohyoid nerve (a branch of the posterior division of the mandibular division) appears to be the culprit.[13] The mylohyoid nerve branches off the inferior alveolar nerve well above the inferior alveolar nerve's entry into the mandibular foramen. It passes along the lingual border of the mandible in the mylohyoid groove, sending motor fibers to the anterior belly of the digastric muscle. It has been demonstrated, on occasion, to contain sensory fibers that branch off and enter into the body of the mandible through small foramina on the lingual side of the mandible in the area of the second molar. These fibers presumably pass anteriorly through the body of the mandible to the mesial root of the first molar.

Regardless of the nerve responsible for this phenomenon, the problem of mesial root sensitivity in the inflamed first molar pulp can usually be alleviated with a 27-gauge short needle and 0.6 ml of anesthetic deposited against the lingual side of the mandible at the level of the apex of the mandibular *second* molar. Within 2 to 3 minutes adequate anesthesia should develop. Although usually observed with the first molar, the problem of partial anesthesia can also occur with other teeth. Management consists of depositing 0.6 ml of solution at the apex of the tooth immediately *distal* to the involved tooth, on the lingual of the mandible. PDL or IO anesthesia also resolves this problem.

Mandibular block: Gow-Gates technique: A true mandibular (V3) block injection, one that provides adequate anesthesia of all sensory portions of the mandibular nerve (buccal, inferior alveolar, lingual, mylohyoid), can be obtained through the *Gow-Gates mandibular block.*[15,21] The target area is higher than in the traditional inferior alveolar nerve block technique: the lateral aspect of the neck of the condyle below the insertion of the lateral pterygoid muscle (Fig. 19-3).[15]

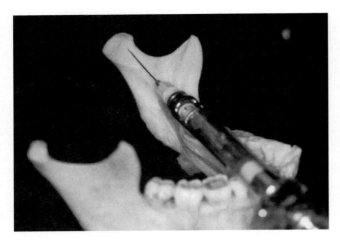

FIG. 19-3 Target area for a Gow-Gates mandibular nerve block: neck of the condyle. *(From Malamed SF:* Handbook of local anesthesia, *ed 4, St Louis, 1997, Mosby.)*

For this reason alone the success rate with the Gow-Gates mandibular block can be expected to be greater than that of the traditional approach *once the dentist learns the technique.* In one study 97.25% of patients receiving the Gow-Gates block did not require supplemental anesthesia.[21] Another advantage is a low positive aspiration rate (1.8%, compared with approximately 10% in inferior alveolar nerve block). A 25-gauge long needle is recommended in the Gow-Gates technique.

Gow-Gates mandibular nerve block

Teeth anesthetized	Volume of anesthetic (ml)	Recommended needle
17-24 or 25-32	1.8-3	25-gauge long

Mandibular block: closed-mouth technique: A new approach to mandibular anesthesia was described in 1977 by Akinosi.[2] This technique, a closed-mouth approach to mandibular anesthesia, is indicated primarily when mandibular opening is limited owing to infection, trauma, or trismus. Significant in endodontics because of the possible presence of edema or infection, the Akinosi-Vazerani technique employs a 25- or 27-gauge long dental needle held in the maxillary buccal fold on the side of injection at the height of the mucogingival junction of the most posterior maxillary tooth. Needle insertion occurs into the soft tissues on the lingual aspect of the mandibular ramus, immediately adjacent to the maxillary tuberosity. The needle is advanced almost parallel to the ramus to a depth of 25 mm (in the average-sized adult) at which point 1.8 ml of anesthetic is deposited following negative aspiration. The primary disadvantage of the closed-mouth mandibular block is the absence of a bony contact to provide a landmark before injection of the anesthetic. However, the closed-mouth mandibular block provides a success rate approaching 80% to 85% (with experience) in a situation (limited or no mandibular opening) in which, in the past, failure was almost guaranteed. Both motor and sensory anesthesia are obtained, allowing the patient to open the jaw, permitting dental treatment to proceed.

Closed-mouth mandibular nerve block

Teeth anesthetized	Volume of anesthetic (ml)	Recommended needle
17-24 or 25-32	1.8	25- or 27-gauge long

Additional local anesthetic procedures

On occasion, the anesthetic techniques previously described fail to produce the required level of pain control. There are several supplemental injection techniques that may be employed to remedy this situation. These include (1) PDL injection, (2) intraseptal injection, (3) intraosseous injection, and (4) intrapulpal injection.

Periodontal ligament injection. The PDL injection, or intraligamentary injection (ILI), is frequently used in restorative dentistry when isolated areas of inadequate anesthesia are present.[40] It may also be used alone to achieve pulpal anesthesia in a single tooth.[22] Although the PDL injection may be used on any tooth, its primary importance lies with mandibular molars, when no nerve block technique has proven to be effective. Advantages to the use of the PDL injection in this way include adequate pulpal anesthesia with a minimal volume of anesthetic (0.2 to 0.4 ml) and the absence of lingual and lower lip anesthesia.

The PDL injection may also prove effective in endodontically involved teeth, where there is no contraindication to its administration. A 27-gauge short or 30-gauge ultrashort needle is firmly placed into the periodontal space between the root of the tooth and the interseptal bone. Although bevel orientation is of little significance in the PDL injection, the author recommends the bevel face the root of the tooth. A volume of 0.2 ml of anesthetic is slowly deposited on *each* root of the tooth. Successful PDL injection anesthesia is indicated by (1) the presence of resistance to anesthetic deposition and (2) ischemia (whitening) of the soft tissues in the immediate area on injection of the anesthetic (Fig. 19-4).

Excessive volumes of anesthetic should not be administered into this confined space.[33] Many devices (e.g., the Peripress) have been marketed to aid in administration of the PDL injection. Although the devices are useful, this author questions their utility because the PDL injection can be administered as successfully with a conventional syringe. The PDL injection is usually quite valuable as an adjunct to nerve block anesthesia in endodontically involved teeth. The most significant contraindication to PDL injection administration is the presence of infection or inflammation in the area of needle insertion. This might prove a significant impediment in endodontics, where periapical infection exists or where periodontal infection is present.

PDL injection

Teeth anesthetized	Volume of anesthetic (ml)	Recommended needle
1 tooth	0.2 per root	27-gauge short

Intraseptal injection. Intraseptal anesthesia, described by Saadoun and Malamed[38] is a variation of the intraosseous technique. A 27-gauge short needle is inserted into the area to be anesthetized (Fig. 19-5). Although not as successful as the IO injection, the intraseptal injection was, until recently, employed more frequently. Because of decreased bone density, intraseptal anesthesia is more successful in younger patients. The needle must be advanced firmly into the cortical plate of bone, the soft tissues having been anesthetized (either by infiltration or topical application) before needle insertion. There must be considerable resistance to drug administration. Ease of administration usually means that the needle is located in soft tissues, not bone. Resistance to injection as the anesthetic is slowly forced under pressure into the cancellous bone is desir-

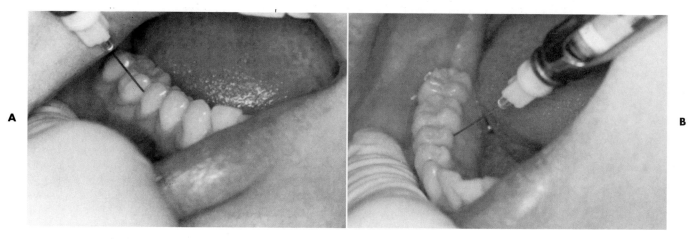

A **B**

FIG. 19-4 If interproximal contacts are tight, the syringe should be directed in from the buccal, **A**, or lingual, **B**, side of the tooth. *(From Malamed SF:* Handbook of local anesthesia, *ed 4, St Louis, 1997, Mosby.)*

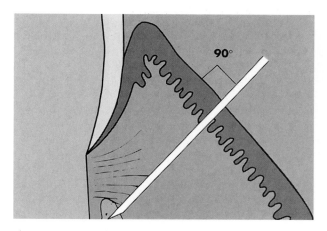

FIG. 19-5 Orientation of the needle for an intraseptal injection. *(From Malamed SF:* Handbook of local anesthesia, *ed 4, St Louis, 1997, Mosby.)*

able. Enough solution must be administered to reach the periapical fibers (approximately 0.3 to 0.5 ml).

Intraseptal injection

Teeth anesthetized	Volume of anesthetic (ml)	Recommended needle
1 tooth	0.3-0.5	27-gauge short

Intraosseous anesthesia. The intraseptal and PDL injections previously described are modifications of true IO anesthesia. In the PDL injection the anesthetic enters the interproximal bone through the periodontal tissues surrounding a tooth, whereas in intraseptal anesthesia the needle is gently embedded into the interproximal bone without use of a bur. Recently IO anesthesia has been repopularized since the introduction of the Stabident Local Anesthesia System (Fairfax Dental, Miami, Fla.). It consists of a perforator, a solid needle that perforates the cortical plate of bone with a conventional slow-speed contraangle handpiece and an 8-mm long, 27-gauge needle that is inserted into this predrilled hole for anesthetic administration (Fig. 19-6). The IO injection can provide anesthesia of a single

tooth or of multiple teeth in a quadrant, dependent on both the site of injection and the volume of anesthetic administered. It is recommended that 0.45 to 0.6 ml of anesthetic be administered when treating one or two teeth. As the injection site is relatively vascular, it is suggested that volumes not exceed those recommended. Additionally, the inclusion of a vasopressor in the anesthetic frequently leads to patient complaints of palpitations. A nonvasopressor-containing anesthetic is preferred.[19]

An advantage of the IO technique is that it is extremely effective in providing pulpal anesthesia in the "hot" mandibular molar. Although no clinical trials have as yet been published that demonstrate this result, clinical experience of many individuals with this technique has provided anecdotal evidence of the IO injection's effectiveness in this difficult clinical situation. When infection is present periapically or periodontally on the tooth to be treated, the PDL and intraseptal injections should not be employed. IO anesthesia can still be administered, the perforation site being moved to the distal of the tooth behind the involved tooth (for example, perforation site distal to the mandibular second molar if the injection site for the involved first molar is unusable because of infection).

Intraosseous injection

Teeth anesthetized	Volume of anesthetic (ml)	Recommended needle
1 or 2 teeth	0.45-0.6	27-gauge short

Intrapulpal injection. When the pulp chamber of a tooth has been exposed while making an access opening or pathologically, the intrapulpal injection may be used to achieve adequate pain control.

A 25- or 27-gauge short needle is inserted into the pulp chamber or specific root canal as needed. Ideally, the needle is firmly wedged into the chamber or canal (Fig. 19-7). On injection, significant resistance is encountered, and the solution must be inserted under pressure. Anesthesia is produced both by the action of the local anesthetic and the applied pressure. There may be a very brief moment of sensitivity as the injection is started; but anesthesia usually occurs immediately thereafter, and instrumentation can proceed painlessly. When a snug fit of the needle is not possible, two procedures are used.

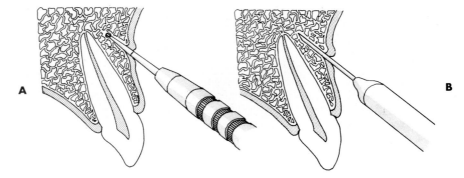

FIG. 19-6 Intraosseous anesthetic is used to obtain adequate pulpal obtundation only when other techniques have failed. Soft tissue over the site has previously been anesthetized through local infiltration. **A,** By means of a small (½ or 1) round bur, a hole is opened in the cortical plate. **B,** A 27-gauge needle is placed in the opening, and anesthetic solution is deposited.

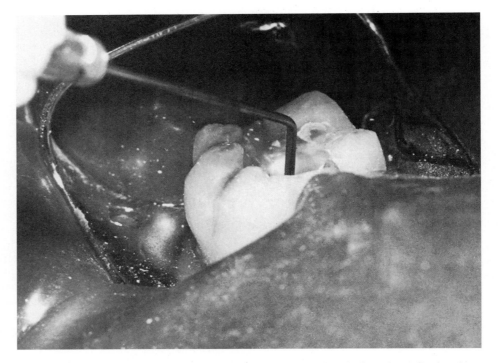

FIG. 19-7 In an intrapulpal injection the needle is inserted directly into the pulp chamber or a specific root canal. Ideally, resistance is met and the solution is expressed under pressure. With the advent of intraligamentary anesthesia, this technique is seldom necessary to employ.

(1) With the needle in the canal, warm base plate gutta-percha is inserted around it. After cooling, injection under pressure may proceed. (2) The anesthetic solution can be deposited into the chamber or canal, with anesthesia being produced by the chemical actions of the solution only. At least 30 seconds should elapse before an attempt is made to proceed with instrumentation. The former technique is preferred whenever possible.[29]

The PDL and intrapulpal injections are the only injections where it may be necessary to bend the local anesthetic needle to gain access to the injection site and to obtain successful anesthesia.

With the reintroduction of IO anesthesia, it has become considerably easier to obtain consistently reliable pulpal anesthesia, even in previously difficult-to-manage situations such as the mandibular molars. The IO technique should become an integral part of the pain control armamentarium of all endodontists and other dentists who frequently treat emergency pain patients.

There are occasions, happily rare, when all of the previously described techniques fail to provide clinically acceptable pain

Intrapulpal injection

Teeth anesthetized	Volume of anesthetic (ml)	Recommended needle
1 tooth	0.2-0.3	25- or 27-gauge short

control, and pulpal anesthesia cannot be attempted until the pulp chamber is exposed. The following sequence of treatment may then be considered:

I. If high-speed instrumentation proves highly traumatic, use of slow-speed high-torque instrumentation is usually less traumatic.

II. Use conscious sedation (which helps to moderate a patient's response to painful stimuli). Inhalation sedation (nitrous oxide and oxygen) or intravenous (IV) sedation, or both, are readily available, safe, and highly effective methods of allaying anxiety and of elevating a patient's pain reaction threshold.

III. When the pulp chamber has been opened, direct intrapulpal anesthesia usually can be administered and proves effective.

IV. If a high level of pain persists and it is still not possible to enter into the pulp chamber, the following sequence should be considered:

A. Place a cotton pellet saturated with local anesthetic loosely onto the pulpal floor of the tooth.

B. Wait 30 seconds.

C. Press the pellet more firmly into the dentinal tubules or the area of pulpal exposure. This area may be initially sensitive but should become insensitive within 2 to 3 minutes.

D. Remove the pellet and continue use of the slow-speed drill until pulpal access is gained, at which time direct injection into the pulp can be performed.

Pain Control: Additional Considerations

In the overwhelming majority of endodontic procedures, if there is difficulty controlling pain at all, this happens only at the first appointment. Once the canals have been located and tissues extirpated, the requirement for pain control becomes minimal. Soft tissue anesthesia may be necessary for rubber dam application; however, if adequate tooth structure exists, even this is unnecessary. Instrumentation with a thoroughly debrided canal seldom requires anesthesia. Overextension of files through the apical foramen may produce a sensitivity that serves as an indicator to the dentist. If the patient overresponds to instrumentation, local infiltration or direct intrapulpal injection can be used.

In the filling of canals, considerable pressure may be exerted during condensation of the filling materials and may produce discomfort or pain. Local infiltration anesthesia should be considered before this procedure is started.

Electronic dental anesthesia

Electronic dental anesthesia (EDA) has received considerable attention since the mid-1980s. EDA devices provide clinical pain control via one or more methods, including the gate control theory of pain,[16] release of endorphins,[6] and release of serotonin.[39] EDA has had some demonstrated clinical success in areas such as restorative, periodontal, and temporomandibular joint treatment. Clark et al.[6] reported no success with EDA in the extirpation of vital pulps. For this reason, EDA is not recommended for endodontic therapy at this time. However, EDA has proven to be an extremely successful technique when used to diminish sensitivity to the administration of local anesthetic injections.

EDA, used as a sole technique in these situations, may prove as effective (or ineffective) as local anesthesia alone. But in combination with local anesthetics (providing chemical anesthesia) and inhalation sedation with nitrous oxide and oxygen (providing an elevation in pain reaction threshold [PRT]), EDA provides both a further elevation of the PRT and an electrical block of pain impulses. These techniques are quite compatible and should be considered in difficult circumstances.

Preoperative and postoperative pain control

The patient suffering from pulpitis most likely has taken oral analgesics for some time before the initial endodontic visit. The dentist should confirm by asking the patient whether he or she is taking medication such as a nonsteroidal antiinflammatory drug (NSAID). A therapeutic blood level should be attained before the initial endodontic visit. Ideally, two oral doses have been taken by this time. The patient should continue to take the NSAID following treatment for a period of time determined by the treating dentist (1 or 2 days, depending on probable posttreatment discomfort). When prescribing analgesic drugs, the dentist should avoid writing "prn pain" in the instructions, for this suggests that the patient is not to take the drug unless he or she is feeling pain, when in fact the goal in managing surgical and postsurgical pain is to prevent it from occurring. Thus it is necessary for the patient to take oral doses on a regular basis (i.e., q4h or qid). When long-acting local anesthetics, such as bupivacaine or etidocaine, are administered in this manner, postendodontic discomfort is minimized.[1]

A telephone call to the patient from the dentist in the early evening following treatment is valuable in minimizing posttreatment complications that may develop early the next morning. It is helpful to determine how the patient is doing, repeat postoperative instructions, and to reaffirm the importance of a patient's continuing to take prescribed medications (i.e., antibiotics and analgesics) as directed. Psychologically, such calls provide a tremendous boost to the patient in the immediate posttreatment period.

Pain control: suggested protocol for the emergency patient

Dentists contacted by a patient who is in acute pain have used the following protocol with considerable success in providing comfortable treatment in an endodontic emergency.

When initially contacted by telephone the dentist determines whether the patient has taken oral analgesic medication. Most often the patient has, but if not, NSAID therapy is started. Preferably the patient has taken two oral doses before the scheduled appointment. Treatment should not be delayed, however, if this cannot be done. The initial goal is to relieve the patient's acute problem, the pain.

On arrival in the office the patient should be seen as soon as possible after completion of the appropriate records (including a health history questionnaire). The dentist identifies the offending tooth and administers the appropriate anesthetic injection technique to provide rapid onset of pain relief. Radiographs can be obtained following successful administration of the local anesthetic. The patient, no longer in pain, can return to the reception area, if necessary, to await definitive treatment. Because the pain cycle has been interrupted, the patient is able to relax, perhaps for the first time in days.

Before the start of definitive endodontic treatment, it is suggested that the patient be reanesthetized, even if the original injection is still effective. All too often the use of a high-speed handpiece evokes even more intense pain than was present when the patient originally entered the office (the "anesthetic window"). Readministration of local anesthetic at this time serves to reinforce the initial block, perhaps by providing additional RN molecules to diffuse into the neuronal tissues.

If the patient still experiences pain in spite of multiple local anesthetic administrations, inhalation sedation should be used. Nitrous oxide at a 35% concentration is equianalgesic to 10 mg morphine or 50 mg meperidine. It does not, in most cases, absolutely eliminate pain, but it does alter the patient's perception of pain, making it more tolerable.

In some few cases, however (most likely in the mandibular molars), adequate pain control may still be unattainable even with the combined use of local anesthesia and inhalation sedation. In such situations use of either IO anesthesia or EDA should be considered. Both IO anesthesia and EDA, have achieved high success rates in these clinical situations. The IO technique is especially recommended in cases of difficult-to-anesthetize mandibular molars.

When the emergency treatment is completed and if the dentist thinks there may be considerable posttreatment pain, the patient should be reanesthetized with a long-acting local anesthetic (etidocaine or bupivacaine), providing that the dosage of local anesthetic thus far has been small enough to permit its administration. This can ensure up to 10 to 12 hours of posttreatment pain relief. The dentist should also reaffirm the importance of continued use of the oral analgesic medication, as directed, even though the patient may still be comfortable. It is easier to keep a patient free of pain than it is to eliminate pain once it recurs.

Again, it is helpful to telephone later the same day to determine how the patient is faring. Minor problems can be managed more easily at this time, and postoperative instructions can be confirmed.

ANXIETY CONTROL

There are many causes of anxiety related to dentistry; most frequently encountered is the fear of pain, and in no specialty of dentistry is the problem of pain control more acute than in endodontics. Because of this many patients are unusually apprehensive when faced with the need for endodontic treatment.

Many adult patients do not openly admit their fears to the doctor. Rather, they sit in the dental chair, undergo dental care, and suffer in silence. Suppression of these anxieties is not always innocuous, as is demonstrated in Tables 19-1 to 19-3. Approximately 75% of the emergency situations reported may have been a result of increased anxiety and dentally related stress.

Children, not having adults' inhibitions about the expression of fear, do not suffer many of the "adult" problems, such as fainting (syncope) and hyperventilation. The child, faced with an unpleasant situation "acts like a child": crying or screaming, perhaps even biting, kicking, or moving about in the dental chair. Significantly, healthy younger children rarely faint or hyperventilate.

The effect of unrecognized and untreated anxiety on medically compromised patients is even more significant. Patients with cardiovascular, respiratory, neurologic, and other metabolic disorders (thyroid disease, diabetes mellitus, adrenal disorders) are considered to be stress intolerant, representing an increased risk during dental care if they become apprehensive or experience pain.

Bennett[3] has stated that the greater the medical risk of the patient, the more important it is to achieve adequate control of both pain and anxiety.

Recognition of Anxiety

Many fearful adult patients do not admit to being apprehensive about their pending dental treatment; therefore the task of exposing their fears becomes a form of detective work—the dentist and members of the office staff seeking clues.

The patient's *prior dental history* can aid in this regard. Fearful patients may exhibit a pattern of cancelled appointments, with any number of excuses for this happening. A dental history of appointments for emergency treatment of painful situations should also be suspect. Once the emergency is alleviated (extraction, pulpal extirpation), the patient does not return until their next episode of dental pain.

On arriving in the dental office, the patient often sits in the reception area and discusses his or her fears of dentistry with other patients or with the office receptionist. The receptionist must be conscious of statements made by patients concerning their attitudes toward dentistry. The receptionist should advise chairside personnel (dental assistant, hygienist, dentist) that "Ms. Jones mentioned to me that she is terrified of 'shots' " or that "she heard that root canal work is very painful." Armed with this knowledge, the dentist and staff are better able to manage this patient's anxieties.

In the dental chair the fearful patient exhibits other clues of anxiety. The dentist must spend some time at each visit speaking with, not to, the patient. This allows the patient to "open up." Many patients complain that doctors (in general) do not allow, or do not seem to want, their patients to talk to them. Anxieties may be expressed at this time. Only a brief period need be devoted to this, but any time thus spent is time well spent.

Touch the patient. The feel of the skin of the apprehensive patient when you shake hands can tell much. Cold, wet palms usually indicate trepidation.

Watch the patient. Apprehensive patients do not stop watching the dentist. They are afraid that they will be "snuck up on" and unpleasantly surprised with a syringe or some other instrument. The patient's posture in the chair is telling. Nonfearful patients look comfortable in the chair, whereas fearful patients appear stiff, unrelaxed, and on the verge of bolting from the chair. Their hands may firmly grip the arm rest of the chair in what is known as the "white knuckle syndrome." They may clutch a handkerchief or shred a paper tissue without even being aware of it.

The forehead and arms of nervous patients may be bathed in perspiration despite effective air-conditioning. Patients may even complain about the warmth of the room.

When these methods of recognizing anxiety in the dental patient are employed, the situation takes on the aspect of a game: Can the dentist detect the patient's anxiety? Will the patient successfully keep his or her fears hidden from the dentist so as not to appear "childish"? Unfortunately, on many occasions the patient wins. Then the dentist, unaware of the patient's fears, proceeds with the dental treatment only to discover that the patient was indeed apprehensive and faints at the sight of the local anesthetic syringe or pushes the dentist's hand away at a critical time during the procedure. Anxiety is obvious at this point, but the ideal time to detect it is *before* dental treatment begins.

The *medical history questionnaire* is a device that may be used to assist in fear recognition before the start of dental treatment. Corah[8] and Gale[14] devised an anxiety questionnaire to help determine the degree of a patient's anxiety. The University of Southern California School of Dentistry has included several of these questions in its medical history questionnaire.[31]

Do you feel very nervous about having dental treatment?

Have you ever had an upsetting experience in the dental office?

Has a dentist ever behaved badly toward you?

Is there anything else about having dental treatment that bothers you? If so, please explain.

These questions permit patients to express their feelings about dentistry, perhaps for the very first time. Many patients who would never verbally admit to anxiety answer these questions honestly.

Management of Anxiety

A variety of techniques for the management of anxiety in dentistry are available. Together these techniques are termed a spectrum of pain and anxiety control (Fig. 19-8). They represent a wide range, from nondrug techniques through general anesthesia. Although general anesthesia has a useful place in this spectrum, its use today is quite limited outside the specialty of oral and maxillofacial surgery (and even within that specialty) and dental anesthesiology. Two reasons for the decreased reliance on general anesthesia as a means of anxiety control have been the introduction and acceptance of the concept of conscious sedation in dentistry and the development in the past two decades of more highly effective drugs for the management of anxiety.

From a practical viewpoint, conscious sedation techniques present relatively safe, reliable, and effective methods of controlling anxiety with little or no added risk to the patient. *Conscious sedation* is defined as "a minimally depressed level of consciousness that retains the patient's ability to independently and continuously maintain an airway and respond appropriately to physical stimulation and verbal command and that is produced by a pharmacological or nonpharmacological method or combination thereof."[9] There are essentially two major types of sedation: *iatrosedation,* techniques that do not necessitate the administration of drugs for the control of anxiety, and *pharmacosedation,* techniques that require drug administration. Iatrosedative techniques include hypnosis, biofeedback, acupuncture, electroanesthesia, and the critically important "chairside manner."

Iatrosedation*

Before discussing pharmacosedation, we must consider nondrug techniques. The techniques of iatrosedation form the building blocks from which all pharmacosedative techniques arise. A relaxed and pleasant dentist-patient relationship favorably influences the action of sedative drugs. Patients who are comfortable with their dentist either require a smaller dose of a given drug to achieve a desired effect or respond more intensely to the usual dose. This is in contrast to patients who are uncomfortable with their dentist. Their greater anxieties or fears cause them, either knowingly or unknowingly, to fight the effect of the drug, the result being poor sedation and an unpleasant experience for both the dentist and the patient.

A determined effort must be made by all members of the dental office staff to help allay the anxieties of the patient.

Pharmacosedation

Although iatrosedation is the starting point for all sedative procedures in the dental office, the level of anxiety present in many patients may prove too great to allow dental care to proceed without pharmacologic intervention. Fortunately, several effective techniques are available to aid in relaxing the apprehensive patient.

The following goals are to be sought whenever pharmacosedation is considered[14]:

The patient's mood must be altered.
The patient must remain conscious.
The patient must be cooperative.
All protective reflexes must remain intact and active.
Vital signs must be stable and within normal limits.
The patient's pain threshold should be elevated.
Amnesia may be present.

---

*This term, introduced by Dr. Nathan Friedman of the University of Southern California School of Dentistry, is defined as "relaxing the patient through the doctor's behavior."

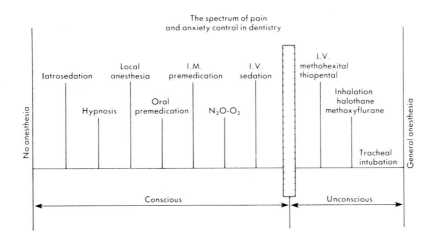

FIG. 19-8 Spectrum of pain and anxiety control in dentistry. Illustration of many of the techniques available in medicine and dentistry for patient management. Vertical bar represents the loss of consciousness. *(From Malamed SF:* Sedation: a guide to patient management, *ed 3, St Louis, 1995, Mosby.)*

There is a second component to ideal sedation that must always be considered:

The level of sedation must never reach beyond the level at which the dentist remains relaxed and capable of completing the dental procedure with uncompromised quality.

Indeed, the quality of the same treatment on that patient should be at least as high as, if not higher than, the quality of the same treatment on that patient without the use of pharmacosedation. Drug administration in dentistry must never become an excuse for inferior quality dentistry.

Oral sedation. The oral route is the most frequently employed technique of pharmacosedation. The oral route offers some definite advantages and possesses some definite disadvantages compared to other techniques.

Advantages	Disadvantages
Practically universally accepted	Slow onset of action (15 to 30 minutes)
Increased safety	Maximal clinical action in about 60 minutes
Adverse reactions less frequent	Long duration of action (3 to 4 hours)
Adverse reactions less severe	Inability to titrate patient to ideal sedation level
	Inability to rapidly increase or decrease sedation level
	Impaired status of patient at conclusion of procedure, requiring escort from office

The disadvantages of oral sedation tend to overshadow its advantages. Because of this the goals of oral sedation should be kept within certain well-defined limits of safety. It is recommended that oral sedation not be employed to achieve deep levels of sedation. Other, more controllable, techniques should be used to achieve these levels. Two recommended uses of the oral route of conscious sedation are (1) 1 hour before going to sleep the evening before a dental appointment if anxiety is severe and (2) 1 hour before scheduled dental treatment to help lessen preoperative anxiety.

Many drugs are available for oral administration. It is strongly recommended that before prescribing any oral sedative to a patient the reader consult a textbook[24] to determine correct dosage, contraindications, precautions, and other important information. In clinical experience the following drugs have proven to be the most effective in reaching the goals just enumerated: benzodiazepines, such as diazepam, oxazepam, triazolam, and flurazepam. The latter two drugs are recommended for hypnosis the evening before scheduled dental treatment, whereas diazepam and oxazepam are recommended for preoperative anxiety management. Oral administration of the parenteral benzodiazepine midazolam has been shown to be effective. An additional advantage to oral midazolam is the occurrence of amnesia (lack of recall of events) in a significant percentage of patients. With the availability of benzodiazepines, the use of oral barbiturates can no longer be recommended. Other benzodiazepines are available for oral administration and prove to be equally effective. Textbooks must be consulted for their doses and other important prescribing information. Table 19-8 lists commonly employed oral antianxi-

Table 19-8. Commonly used oral sedative drugs

Drug Group*	Proprietary Name (U.S.)	Dose† (mg)
Benodiazepines		
Diazepam	Valium	5-10
Flurazepam	Dalmane	15-30
Oxazepam	Serax	15-30
Triazolam	Halcion	0.125-0.25
Chloral hydrate	Noctec, Kessodrate	500-1500
Hydroxyzine	Atarax, Vistaril	50-100

*Please see Chapter 2 and 17 for additional information.
†For a normal, healthy 70-kg man. Patient response to these doses may vary; therefore the reader is advised to consult the drug package insert for specific prescribing information before prescribing any drug.

ety and sedative-hypnotic drugs. Additional information regarding drugs for oral sedation may be found in Chapter 2.

It must be remembered that patients receiving oral sedatives must not be permitted to drive a motor vehicle to or from the dental office.

Oral sedation may be required, especially at the first endodontic appointment, because of the preconceived ideas patients maintain about endodontic care. Proper use of iatrosedation and pain control usually obviate the need for oral sedation at subsequent visits.

Intramuscular sedation. Intramuscular (IM) sedation is infrequently employed in dental practices; however, it remains an effective method of anxiety control in certain situations. Advantages and disadvantages of intramuscular drug administration (compared with the oral route) follow:

Advantages	Disadvantages
More rapid onset of action (10 to 15 minutes)	Inability to titrate to ideal level of sedation
Maximal clinical effect within 30 minutes	Inability to rapidly increase or decrease sedation level
More reliable absorption	Long duration of action (3 to 4 hours)
	Need for an injection
	Impaired status of patient at conclusion of procedure, requiring escort from office

Like the oral route the IM route lacks a degree of control that would be desirable. Therefore the level of sedation sought with IM sedation should remain light to moderate. Only doctors trained in this technique of drug administration and in airway management should consider sedation via the IM route. Indeed 48 states in the United States require the doctor to obtain a parenteral sedation permit to employ IM or IV sedation.

The most effective IM sedative has proven to be the water-soluble benzodiazepine, midazolam (Versed, Hypnovel, Dormicum). Its IM use is frequently associated with the occurrence of amnesia, which is a welcome happenstance, as the patient has a lack of recall of events occurring during the dental procedure.[11,27]

Opioid agonists, such as meperidine (Demerol) are oftentimes used for IM sedation. These drugs are not recommended for use for conscious sedation, the benzodiazepines being significantly more effective in this regard. Respiratory depression and the incidence of nausea and vomiting are increased when opioids are used. Increased vigilance requiring the use of pulse oximetry and automatic vital sign monitors is necessary when IM opioids are used.

IM sedation is not contraindicated in endodontics; however, if an x-ray unit is not readily available chairside, the patient must walk to the x-ray unit, perhaps several times during their appointment. Following IM injection the patient may require assistance in so doing. If an x-ray unit is available chairside, no such problem exists. Patients receiving any IM central nervous system (CNS) depressant must have an adult available to escort them home following their treatment.

Inhalation sedation. Nitrous oxide and oxygen inhalation sedation is a remarkably controllable technique of pharmacosedation employed by approximately 35% of dentists practicing in the United States.[18]

Because of its advantages over other routes of drug administration, inhalation sedation is usually the method of choice when sedation is required.

Advantages	Disadvantages
Rapid onset of action (20 seconds, although 3 to 5 minutes may be required for titration)	Cost and size of equipment
	Requirement for education in proper use of inhalation sedation
Ability to titrate to ideal level of sedation	Potential complications:
Ability to rapidly increase or decrease sedation level	Chronic exposure to low levels of nitrous oxide
Total clinical recovery within 3 to 5 minutes (in virtually all patients)	Abuse potential of nitrous oxide
Ability to discharge most patients without need for adult escort	Sexual phenomena and nitrous oxide (and all other forms of sedation)

Because of the degree of control maintained over inhalation sedation by the dentist, any level of conscious sedation compatible with the dentist's degree of experience can be achieved.

Although nitrous oxide and oxygen inhalation sedation seems to be a nearly perfect technique, as with all drugs there are times when the desired actions do not develop. Approximately 70% of patients receiving nitrous oxide and oxygen are ideally sedated between 30% and 40% nitrous oxide. Fifteen percent require less than 30% nitrous oxide, whereas 15% require in excess of 40%. Of this last 15%, it may be said that some 5% to 10% are unsedatable with any level of nitrous oxide less than 70%. Inhalation sedation units have a number of safety devices incorporated into them whose basic goal is to prevent a patient from ever receiving less than 20% oxygen. Therefore it is probable that approximately 5% of patients receiving inhalation sedation never become adequately sedated. If we add to this other patients who are unable to breathe through their nose and those with a very high anxiety level, it is entirely possible that a failure rate of 10% to 15% could occur with nitrous oxide and oxygen inhalation sedation.

These comments are not meant to denigrate nitrous oxide and oxygen. The purpose in stressing the possibility of failures is to illustrate that no technique of conscious sedation, even inhalation sedation, is universally successful. Failures can

and will occur whenever drugs are administered to patients. The drug administrator must know when to stop the administration. Nitrous oxide does not possess significant analgesic properties, although a degree of soft tissue analgesia does develop in most patients at about 35% nitrous oxide. Local anesthesia must always be administered as it would if inhalation sedation were not being used.

Inhalation sedation is entirely compatible with endodontic treatment. Indeed, use of rubber dam converts most patients into nose breathers, facilitating the administration of nitrous oxide and oxygen. Inhalation sedation with nitrous oxide and oxygen is a highly effective, easy-to-use, and safe technique of pharmacosedation. It is most effective for patients with mild to moderate levels of anxiety. Failures may be noted in unusually apprehensive patients, but for these, other techniques are available (e.g., IM, IV, general anesthesia). Nitrous oxide and oxygen is administered along with the other drugs in these techniques (e.g., IM + nitrous oxide and oxygen; IV + nitrous oxide and oxygen).

In recent years three concerns have arisen relative to use of nitrous oxide and oxygen in dentistry. The first involves the effects of long-term exposure of dental personnel to low levels of nitrous oxide. The use of a scavenger type of device to remove exhaled nitrous oxide from the clinical environment is strongly recommended, despite the continued absence of definitive evidence of danger to dental personnel.[7] A second concern is the abuse of nitrous oxide by dental personnel. This has led to devastating effects, including peripheral sensory nerve deprivation.[20] Nitrous oxide is a potent anesthetic drug, not an innocuous vapor, and must not be abused. A third concern involves the administration of any CNS depressant drug, including nitrous oxide, on a patient of the opposite sex from the doctor. Many cases have been reported in which the dentist was accused of sexual improprieties, sexual misconduct, or rape while the patient received nitrous oxide and oxygen (IV or IM).[17] Most cases have involved nitrous oxide and oxygen, since it is the more commonly employed of these techniques of conscious sedation. Two common threads appear in many of these cases: the patient received high concentrations of nitrous oxide (in excess of 50% to 60%), and the dentist treated the patient without the benefit of a second person (auxiliary) present in the treatment room. Accusations of sexual misconduct or worse may easily be prevented by titrating nitrous oxide to the ideal sedation level and by having an auxiliary, preferably of the same sex as the patient, present in the treatment room at all times.

Intravenous sedation. The goal in the administration of any drug (except obviously, local anesthetics) is to achieve a therapeutic level of that drug in the bloodstream. The delays in onset of action noted with other techniques were due to the slow absorption of drugs from the gastrointestinal tract or from muscle into the blood. The direct administration of a drug into the venous circulation results in a much more rapid onset of action and a greater degree of control than are found with other pharmacosedative techniques.

Only inhalation sedation, in which the inhaled gases rapidly reach the alveoli and capillaries, has an onset of action approaching that of IV sedation. A drop of blood requires between 9 and 30 seconds to travel from the hand to the heart and then to the cerebral circulation. Titration is possible with IV drug administration. The time required to achieve ideal sedation varies with the drug technique: IV diazepam or midazolam may require up to 4 minutes, whereas the Jorgensen technique may require up to 10 minutes. Advantages and disadvantages of IV drug administration are summarized below:

Advantages	Disadvantages
Rapid onset of action (9 to 30 seconds, although several minutes may be required for titration)	Inability to easily lighten level of sedation
Ability to titrate to ideal level of sedation	Inability to reverse the clinical actions of all IV drugs
Ability to rapidly increase sedation level	Potential complications due to rapidity of drug effect mandates increased monitoring (e.g., pulse oximetry, vital signs)
Ability to reverse the clinical actions of many IV drugs	Requirement for education in proper use of inhalation sedation
	Impaired status of patient at conclusion of procedure, requiring escort from office
	Need for venipuncture
	Increase in liability insurance costs

Venipuncture, a learned skill, requires practice and continued repetition if it is to be performed atraumatically. Once venipuncture is accomplished, IV drug administration is quite simple. Because of the degree of control maintained by the dentist the level of sedation sought can vary from light to moderate to deep, entirely dependent on the experience of the dentist and team and the clinical requirements of the patient.

Many techniques of IV sedation are available. Most involve sedative drugs administered alone or in conjunction with opioids. Although many drugs have been successfully used intravenously, several techniques have become more popular, primarily because of their relative simplicity, their effectiveness, and the degree of safety associated with their proper administration. These include the administration of a benzodiazepine, either midazolam or diazepam, or in some cases, both a benzodiazepine and an opioid analgesic.

The use of propofol, a rapid-acting, short-duration nonbarbiturate sedative-hypnotic, or ketamine, a dissociative anesthetic, should not be considered for IV conscious sedation use by dentists not trained in and permitted to use general anesthesia.

Guidelines for teaching IV conscious sedation have been enacted into dental practice acts in 48 states (August, 1997). Most require an intensive didactic (approximately 60 hours) and clinical program (20 patients treated with IV sedation under supervision) and an in-office evaluation program.

IV conscious sedation, particularly with the short-acting benzodiazepines, midazolam and diazepam, or either in combination with an opioid such as meperidine or fentanyl, are ideally suited for endodontic therapy. However, if the x-ray unit is located at a distance from the patient, it may be both difficult and inconvenient to move the patient to the unit. During the early phase of the procedure, immediately following administration of the IV drug(s), the patient may also have difficulty maintaining an open mouth. Bite blocks should be available for use at this time.

Table 19-9 summarizes the recommended levels of sedation for the techniques discussed in this chapter.

Table 19-9. Common routes of sedation in the dental office

Route of Administration	Control		Recommended Safe Sedative Levels
	Titrate	Rapid Reversal	
Oral	No	No	Light only
Intramuscular	No	No	Adults: light, moderate
			Children: light, moderate, deep
Intravenous	Yes	Yes (most drugs)	Children*: light, moderate, deep
			Adults: light, moderate, deep
Inhalation	Yes	Yes	Any level of sedation

From Malamed SF: *Medical emergencies in the dental office*, ed 4, St Louis, 1993, Mosby.
*There is little need for intravenous sedation in normal healthy children. Most children who permit a venipuncture also permit a local anesthetic to be administered intraorally. Intravenous sedation is of great benefit, however, in management of handicapped children or precooperative or uncooperative children.

Combined techniques. On occasion it may be necessary to consider combining several of the techniques just described. Some words of caution are in order.

Quite frequently the patient who requires either inhalation or IV sedation is apprehensive enough to also need oral sedation, either the night before or the day of the dental appointment. There is no contraindication to this practice provided the level of oral sedation is not excessive *and* the inhalation or IV drugs are carefully titrated. Because of the level of oral sedative already in the blood, the requirement for other CNS depressants is usually decreased. If "average" doses of inhalation or IV drugs are used without titration, an overdose is more likely to develop. Titration is an important safety factor. When possible to titrate a drug, it is foolhardy not to.

The combination of inhalation and IV sedation should be avoided by all but the most experienced dentists. Too frequently reports are forthcoming of significant morbidity (and on occasion mortality) resulting from the ill-conceived conjoint use of these two potent techniques. Levels of sedation can vary rapidly; unless constant effective monitoring is maintained, unconsciousness may develop with attendant airway problems before the dentist ever becomes aware of it. Nitrous oxide and oxygen may be employed successfully at the same appointment when a patient requiring IV sedation is apprehensive about venipuncture. Nitrous oxide and oxygen may be used to aid in establishing the IV infusion. Benefits of nitrous oxide and oxygen during venipuncture include (1) a vasodilating effect, (2) anxiety-reducing actions, and (3) some analgesic properties. After the venipuncture is established, the patient should be administered 100% oxygen and returned to the presedative state before any IV drug is administered.

REFERENCES

1. Acute Pain Management Guideline Panel: *Acute pain management: operative or medical procedures and trauma: clinical practice guidelines,* A HCPR Pub No 92-0032, Rockville, Md, 1992, Agency for Health Care Policy and Research, Public Health Service, US Department of Health and Human Resources.
2. Akinosi JO: A new approach to the mandibular nerve block, *Br J Oral Surg* 15:83, 1977.

3. Bennett CR: *Conscious sedation in dental practice,* ed 2, St Louis, 1978, Mosby.

4. Camejo G et al: Characterization of two different membrane fractions isolated from the first stellar nerves of the squid *Dosidicus gigas, Biochim Biophys Acta* 193:247, 1969.

5. Chapman LF, Goodell H, Wolff HG: Tissue vulnerability, inflammation, and the nervous system, Read at American Academy of Neurology, April, 1959.

6. Clark MS et al: An evaluation of the clinical analgesia/anesthesia efficacy on acute pain using high frequency neural modulator in various dental settings, *Oral Surg Oral Med Oral Pathol* 63(4):501, 1987.

7. Cohen F et al: Occupational disease in dentistry and chronic exposure to trace anesthetic gases, *J Am Dent Assoc* 101:21, 1980.

8. Corah N: Development of dental anxiety scale, *J Dent Res* 48:596, 1969.

9. Council on Dental Education, American Dental Association: Guidelines for teaching the comprehensive control of pain and anxiety in dentistry, *J Dent Educ* 36:62, 1972.

10. Covino BJ: Physiology and pharmacology of local anesthetic agents, *Anesth Prog* 28:98, 1981.

11. Dormauer D, Aston R: Update: midazolam maleate, a new water-soluble benzodiazepine, *J Am Dent Assoc* 106:650, 1983.

12. Fast TB, Martin MD, Ellis TM: Emergency preparedness: a survey of dental practitioners, *J Am Dent Assoc* 112:499-501, 1986.

13. Frommer J, Mele FA, Monroe CW: The possible role of the mylohyoid nerve in mandibular posterior tooth sensation, *J Am Dent Assoc* 85:113, 1972.

14. Gale E: Fears of the dental situation, *J Dent Res* 51:964, 1972.

15. Gow-Gates GAE: Mandibular conduction anesthesia: a new technique using extraoral landmarks, *Oral Surg Oral Med Oral Pathol* 36:321, 1973.

16. Hughs J: Identification of two related pentapeptides from the brain with potent opiate antagonist activity, *Nature* 258:577, 1975.

17. Jastak JT, Malamed SF: Nitrous oxide and sexual phenomena, *J Am Dent Assoc* 101:38, 1980.

18. Jones TW, Greenfield W: Position paper of the ADA ad hoc Committee on trace anesthetics as a potential health hazard in dentistry, *J Am Dent Assoc* 95:751, 1977.

19. Leonard M: The efficacy of an intraosseous injection system of delivering local anesthetic, *J Am Dent Assoc* 126(1):81-86, 1995.

20. Malamed SF: The recreational abuse of nitrous oxide by health professionals, *J Calif Dent Assoc* 8:38, 1980.

21. Malamed SF: The Gow-Gates mandibular block: evaluation after 4275 cases, *Oral Surg Oral Med Oral Pathol* 51:463, 1981.

22. Malamed SF: The periodontal ligament injection: an alternative to mandibular block, *Oral Surg Oral Med Oral Pathol* 53:118, 1982.

23. Malamed SF: Managing medical emergencies, *J Am Dent Assoc* 124:40-53, 1993.

24. Malamed SF: *Sedation: a guide to patient management,* ed 3, St Louis, 1995, Mosby.

25. Malamed SF: *Handbook of local anesthesia,* ed 4, St Louis, 1997, Mosby.

26. Malamed SF: Local anesthetics: dentistry's most important drugs, *J Am Dent Assoc* 125:1571-1576, 1994.

27. Malamed SF, Quinn CL, Hatch HG: Pediatric sedation with intramuscular and intravenous midazolam, *Anesth Prog* 36:155, 1989.

28. Malamed SF, Trieger NT: Intraoral maxillary nerve block: an anatomical and clinical study, *Anesth Prog* 30:44, 1983.

29. Malamed SF, Weine F: *Profound pulpal anesthesia,* Chicago, 1988, American Association of Endodontists (audiotape).

30. Matsuura H: Analysis of systemic complications and deaths during dental treatment in Japan, *Anesth Prog* 36:219-228, 1990.

31. McCarthy FM, Pallasch TJ, Gates R: Documenting safe treatment of the medical-risk patient, *J Am Dent Assoc* 119:383, 1989.

32. Najjar TA: Why you can't achieve adequate regional anesthesia in the presence of infection, *Oral Surg* 44:7, 1977.

33. Nelson PW: Injection system, *J Am Dent Assoc* 103:692, 1981 (letter).

34. Poore TE, Carney FMT: Maxillary nerve block: a useful technique, *J Oral Surg* 31:749, 1973.

35. Ritchie JM, Ritchie B, Greengard P: Active structure of local anesthetics, *J Pharmacol Exp Ther* 150:152, 1965.

36. Ritchie JM, Ritchie B, Greengard P: The effect of the nerve sheath on the action of local anesthetics, *J Pharmacol Exp Ther* 150:160, 1965.

37. Rood JP, Pateromichelakis S: Inflammation and peripheral nerve sensitization, *Br J Oral Surg* 19:67, 1981.

38. Saadoun AP, Malamed SF: Intraseptal anesthesia in periodontal surgery, *J Am Dent Assoc* 111:249, 1985.

39. Shanes AM: Electrochemical aspect of physiological and pharmacological action in excitable cells. II. The action potential and excitation, *Pharmacol Rev* 10:165, 1958.

40. Walton RE, Abbott BJ: Periodontal ligament injection: a clinical evaluation, *J Am Dent Assoc* 103:571, 1981.

41. Weisman G: Electronic anesthesia: expanding applications are its future, *Dent Prod Rep* 30(5):88-93, 1996.

Chapter 20

Bleaching Nonvital and Vital Discolored Teeth

Ilan Rotstein

Discoloration of anterior teeth is a cosmetic problem that often requires corrective measures. Although restorative methods such as crowns and laminates are available, discoloration can often be successfully corrected by bleaching.

Bleaching procedures are more conservative than other restorative methods, relatively simple to perform, and less expensive. They can be carried out intracoronally in nonvital teeth or extracoronally in vital teeth. The successful outcome of bleaching depends mainly on the cause of the discoloration, correct diagnosis of the problem, and proper selection of bleaching technique.

CAUSES OF TOOTH DISCOLORATION

Tooth discoloration occurs during or after enamel and dentin formation and may be due to patient-related (natural) or dentist-related (iatrogenic) causes.[48] Patient-related discolorations may be superficial or incorporated into tooth structure. Dentist-related discolorations are usually preventable and should be avoided (Table 20-1).

Patient-Related Causes

Pulp necrosis

Bacterial, mechanical, or chemical irritation to the pulp may result in tissue necrosis and release of tissue disintegration by-products. These compounds may penetrate tubules and discolor the surrounding dentin. The degree of discoloration is directly related to how long the pulp has been necrotic. The longer the discoloration compounds are present in the pulp chamber, the deeper is the penetration into the dentinal tubules and the greater is the discoloration. Such discoloration is usually bleached intracoronally (Plate 20-1, A and B).

Intrapulpal hemorrhage

Intrapulpal hemorrhage and lysis of erythrocytes may follow traumatic injury to a tooth. Blood disintegration products, mainly iron sulfides, are introduced into the tubules and discolor the surrounding dentin. If the pulp becomes necrotic, the discoloration persists and usually becomes more severe with time. If the pulp recovers, the discoloration may be reversed, with the tooth regaining its original shade.

This type of discoloration is also time dependent. Intracoronal bleaching in such cases is usually successful (Plate 20-1, C and D).[32,38]

Dentin hypercalcification

Excessive formation of irregular dentin in the pulp chamber and the canal walls may occur following certain traumatic injuries. In such cases a temporary disruption of blood supply occurs, followed by destruction of odontoblasts. These are replaced by undifferentiated mesenchymal cells that rapidly form irregular dentin on the walls of the pulp lumen. As a result the translucency of the crowns of such teeth gradually decreases and may give rise to a yellowish or yellow-brown discoloration. Extracoronal bleaching should be attempted first. However, sometimes, root canal therapy is required, followed by intracoronal bleaching. Fair aesthetic results are achieved in such teeth.

Age

In elderly patients, color changes in the crown occur physiologically as a result of excessive dentin apposition, thinning of the enamel, and optical changes. Food and beverages also have a cumulative discoloration effect, which becomes more pronounced in the elderly patient because of the inevitable cracking and other changes on the enamel surface of the tooth and in the underlying dentin. In addition, previously applied amalgams and other coronal restorations that become degraded over time cause further discoloration.

Unless tooth structure is badly damaged, bleaching can be successfully applied for many types of discolorations in elderly patients (Plate 20-1, E and F).

Tooth formation defects

Developmental defects. Discoloration may result from developmental defects during enamel and dentin formation.

Defects in enamel formation: Defects in enamel formation are either hypocalcific or hypoplastic. Enamel hypocalcification is a distinct brownish or whitish area, commonly found on the facial aspect of affected crowns. The enamel is well formed with an intact surface. Both the whitish and the brownish spots are amenable to enamel microabrasion techniques, with good results (Plate 20-1, G and H).

Enamel hypoplasia differs from hypocalcification in that the enamel is defective and porous. This condition may be hereditary (as in amelogenesis imperfecta) or a result of environmental factors. In the hereditary type, both deciduous and permanent dentition are involved. Defects caused by environmental factors, such as infections, tumors, or trauma involving one or several teeth, can be detected in both types of dentition. Pre-

Table 20-1. Causes of tooth discoloration

Patient-Related Causes	Dentist-Related Causes
Pulp necrosis	Endodontically related
Intrapulpal hemorrhage	Pulp tissue remnants
Dentin hypercalcification	Intracanal medicaments
Age	Obturating materials
Tooth formation defects	Restoration related
Developmental defects	Amalgams
Drug-related defects	Pins and posts
	Composites

sumably during enamel formation the matrix is altered and does not mineralize properly. The defective enamel is porous and readily discolored by materials in the oral cavity.

Depending on severity and extent of hypoplasia and nature of the discoloration, the enamel surface of such teeth may be bleached with some degree of success.[10] The bleaching effect may not be permanent, with recurring discoloration over time.

Systemic conditions: Various systemic conditions may cause massive lysis of erythrocytes. If this occurs in the pulp at an early age, blood disintegration products may be incorporated into and discolor the forming dentin. One example is the severe discoloration of the primary dentition as a result of erythroblastosis fetalis. This occurs in the fetus or newborn because of Rh incompatibility factors, with resulting massive systemic lysis of erythrocytes. Large amounts of hemosiderin pigment are released, which subsequently penetrate and discolor the forming dentin. Such discoloration is now uncommon and is not amenable to bleaching.

High fever during tooth formation may result in chronologic hypoplasia, a temporary disruption in enamel formation that gives rise to a banding type of surface discoloration. Porphyria, a metabolic disease, may also cause red or brownish discoloration of deciduous and permanent teeth. Thalassemia and sickle cell anemia may cause intrinsic blue, brown, or green discolorations. Amelogenesis imperfecta may result in yellow or brown discolorations. Dentinogenesis imperfecta can cause brownish violet, yellowish, or gray discoloration. These conditions are also not amenable to bleaching and should be corrected by restorative means.

Other staining factors related to systemic conditions are rare and may not be identifiable.

Drug-related defects. Administration or ingestion of certain drugs during the tooth formation period may cause severe discoloration both in enamel and dentin.

Tetracycline: A common cause of discoloration is tetracycline ingestion in children. Tooth shades can be yellow, yellow-brown, brown, dark gray or blue, depending on the type of tetracycline, the dosage, duration of intake, and the patient's age at the time of administration. Discoloration is usually bilateral, affecting multiple teeth in both arches.

Tetracycline discoloration has been classified into three groups according to severity.[20] First-degree discoloration is light yellow, light brown, or light gray and occurs uniformly throughout the crown without banding. Second-degree discoloration is more intense and also without banding. Third-degree discoloration is intense, and the clinical crown exhibits horizontal color banding. This type of discoloration usually predominates in the cervical regions.

The mechanism of tetracycline discoloration is not fully understood. Tetracycline bound to calcium is thought to be incorporated into the hydroxyapatite crystal of both enamel and dentin. However, most of the tetracycline is found in dentin.

Repeated exposure of tetracycline-discolored tooth to ultraviolet radiation can lead to formation of a reddish-purple oxidation by-product that permanently discolors the teeth. In children the anterior teeth often become stained first, and the less exposed posterior teeth are discolored more slowly. In adults natural photobleaching of the anterior teeth is observed, particularly in individuals whose teeth are excessively exposed to sunlight because of maxillary lip insufficiency.

Two approaches have been used to treat tetracycline discoloration: (1) bleaching the external enamel surface (Plate 20-2, *A* through *D*)[3,7] and (2) intracoronal bleaching following intentional root canal therapy.[1,21,49]

Endemic fluorosis: Ingestion of excessive amounts of fluoride during tooth formation may produce a defect in mineralized structures, particularly in the enamel matrix, causing hypoplasia. The severity and degree of subsequent staining generally depends on the degree of hypoplasia and is directly related to the amount of fluoride ingested during odontogenesis.[13] The teeth are not discolored on eruption, but their surface is porous and will gradually absorb colored chemicals present in the oral cavity.

Discoloration is usually bilateral, affecting multiple teeth in both arches. It presents as various degrees of mild, intermittent white spotting, chalky or opaque areas, yellow or brown discoloration, and in severe cases surface pitting of the enamel.

Since the discoloration is in the porous enamel, such teeth are bleached externally. The success of the outcome mainly depends on the degree and duration of the discoloration.

Dentist-Related Causes

Discolorations caused by various dental materials or unsuitable operating techniques should be always avoided. Some of these conditions may be very difficult to correct later by bleaching.

Endodontically related

Pulp tissue remnants. Tissue remaining in the pulp chamber disintegrates gradually and may cause discoloration. Pulp horns must always be included in the access cavity to ensure removal of pulpal remnants and to prevent retention of sealer at a later stage. Intracoronal bleaching in these cases is usually successful.

Intracanal medicaments. Several intracanal medicaments are liable to cause internal staining of the dentin. Phenolics or iodoform-based medicaments sealed in the root canal and chamber are in direct contact with dentin, sometimes for long periods, allowing penetration and oxidization. These compounds have a tendency to discolor the dentin gradually.

Obturating materials. This is the most frequent and severe cause of single tooth discoloration. Incomplete removal of obturating materials from the pulp chamber on completion of treatment often results in dark staining (Plate 20-1, *I* and *J*). This is prevented by removing all materials to a level just below the gingival margin.

Primary offenders are sealer remnants, mainly those containing metallic components.[47] Bleaching prognosis in such cases depends on the type of sealer and duration of discoloration.

Restoration related

The most popular coronal restorations are amalgams and composites. Their modes of tooth discoloration are different.

Amalgams. Amalgams have severe effects on dentin due to dark-colored metallic components that can turn the dentin dark gray. When used to restore lingual access preparation, a developmental groove, or premolar teeth, amalgam may discolor the crown. Such discolorations are difficult to bleach and tend to rediscolor with time.

Sometimes the dark appearance of the crown is due to the amalgam restoration, which can be seen through the tooth structure. In such cases replacement of the amalgam with an aesthetic restoration usually corrects the problem.

Pins and posts. Metal pins and prefabricated posts are sometimes used to reinforce a composite restoration in the anterior dentition. Discoloration from inappropriately placed pins and posts is due to metal that can be seen through the composite or tooth structure. In such cases removal of the metal and replacement of the composite restoration are indicated.

Composites. Microleakage of composites causes staining. Open margins may allow chemicals to enter between the restoration and the tooth structure and discolor the underlying dentin. In addition, composites may become discolored with time, affecting the shade of the crown. These conditions are generally corrected by replacing the old composite restoration with a new well-sealed one.

BLEACHING MATERIALS

Bleaching materials are either oxidizing or reducing agents, but the former are generally used. Many different preparations are available today. Aqueous solutions of various concentrations of hydrogen peroxide, sodium perborate, and carbamide peroxide are commonly used.

Sodium perborate and carbamide peroxide are gradually degraded to release low levels of hydrogen peroxide. Hydrogen peroxide and carbamide peroxide are mainly indicated for extracoronal bleaching, whereas sodium perborate is for intracoronal bleaching.

Hydrogen Peroxide

Various concentrations of hydrogen peroxide are available, but 30% to 35% stabilized aqueous solutions (Superoxol, Perhydrol) are the most common. Silicone dioxide gel forms containing 35% hydrogen peroxide are also available.

Hydrogen peroxide is caustic and burns tissues on contact, releasing toxic free radicals, perhydroxyl anions, or both.

High-concentration solutions of hydrogen peroxide must be handled with care, as they are thermodynamically unstable and may explode unless refrigerated and kept in a dark container.

Sodium Perborate

Sodium perborate is an oxidizing agent available in a powdered form or as various commercial preparations. When fresh, it contains about 95% perborate, corresponding to 9.9% of the available oxygen. Sodium perborate is stable when dry but in the presence of acid, warm air, or water decomposes to form sodium metaborate, hydrogen peroxide, and nascent oxygen.

Various types of sodium perborate preparations are available: monohydrate, trihydrate, and tetrahydrate. They differ in oxygen content, which determines their bleaching efficacy.[50] Commonly used sodium perborate preparations are alkaline,

and their pH depends on the amount of hydrogen peroxide released and the residual sodium metaborate.[30]

Sodium perborate is more easily controlled and safer than concentrated hydrogen peroxide solutions. Therefore sodium perborate should be the material of choice in most intracoronal bleaching procedures.

Carbamide Peroxide

Carbamide peroxide, also known as urea hydrogen peroxide, is available in the concentration range of 3% to 15%. Popular commercial preparations contain about 10% carbamide peroxide with a mean pH of 5 to 6.5. Solutions of 10% carbamide peroxide break down into urea, ammonia, carbon dioxide, and approximately 3.5% hydrogen peroxide.

Bleaching preparations containing carbamide peroxide usually also include glycerin or propylene glycol, sodium stannate, phosphoric or citric acid, and flavor additives. In some preparations, carbopol, a water-soluble polyacrylic acid polymer, is added as a thickening agent. Carbopol also prolongs the release of active peroxide and improves shelf life.

Carbamide peroxide–based preparations have been associated with various degrees of damage to the teeth and surrounding mucosa.[17,39,40,52] They may adversely affect the bond strength of composite resins and their marginal seal.[8,43] Since long-term studies are not yet available, these materials must be used with caution.

BLEACHING MECHANISM

The mechanism of tooth bleaching is unclear. It differs according to the type of discoloration involved and the chemical and physical conditions at the time of the reaction. Bleaching agents, mainly oxidizers, act on the organic structure of the dental hard tissues slowly degrading them into chemical by-products, such as carbon dioxides, which are lighter in color. Inorganic molecules do not usually break down as well. The oxidation-reduction reaction that occurs during bleaching is known as a redox reaction. Generally, the unstable peroxides convert to unstable free radicals. These free radicals may oxidize (remove electrons from) or reduce (add electrons to) other molecules.

Most bleaching procedures use hydrogen peroxide because it is unstable and decomposes into oxygen and water. The mouthguard bleaching technique employs mainly carbamide peroxide as a vehicle for the delivery of lower concentrations of hydrogen peroxide, which require more exposure time. The rate of hydrogen peroxide decomposition during mouthguard bleaching depends on its concentration and the levels of salivary peroxidase. With high levels of hydrogen peroxide, a zero-order reaction occurs so that the time required to clear the hydrogen peroxide is proportional to its concentration. The longer it takes to clear the hydrogen peroxide, the greater the exposure to reactive oxygen species and their adverse effects.

NONVITAL BLEACHING TECHNIQUES

Intracoronal bleaching of nonvital teeth may be successfully carried out at various times, even many years after root canal therapy and discoloration.

The methods most commonly employed to bleach endodontically treated teeth are the walking bleach and the thermocatalytic techniques. The walking bleach technique is preferred since it requires less chair time and is safer and more comfortable for the patient.[27,41]

Walking Bleach

The walking bleach technique should be attempted first in all cases requiring intracoronal bleaching. The walking bleach technique involves the following steps:

1. Familiarize the patient with the possible causes of discoloration, the procedure to be followed, the expected outcome, and the possibility of future rediscoloration.
2. Prepare periapical radiographs to assess the status of periapical tissues and quality of endodontic obturation. End-

---

Table 20-2. Indications and contraindications for nonvital bleaching

Indications	Contraindications
Discolorations of pulp chamber origin	Superficial enamel stains
Dentin stains	Defective enamel formation
Stains not amenable to extracoronal bleaching	Severe dentin loss
	Presence of caries
	Discolored composites

---

odontic failure or questionable obturation should be retreated before bleaching.

3. Assess the quality and shade of any restoration present and replace it if defective. Tooth discoloration frequently is the result of leaking or discolored restorations. In such cases cleaning the pulp chamber and replacing the defective restorations will usually suffice.
4. Evaluate tooth color with a shade guide and if possible take clinical photographs at the beginning of and throughout the procedure; these provide a point of reference for future comparison.
5. Isolate the tooth with a rubber dam. Interproximal wedges and ligatures may also be used for better isolation. If Superoxol is used, protective ointments, such as Orabase or Vaseline, must be applied to the surrounding gingival tissues before dam placement.
6. Remove all restorative material from the access cavity and refine the access. Verify that the pulp horns and other areas potentially containing pulp tissue are properly exposed and clean (Fig. 20-1, *A*). A pulp chamber completely filled with composite presents some clinical difficulties. The shade of the composite resin is often indistinguishable

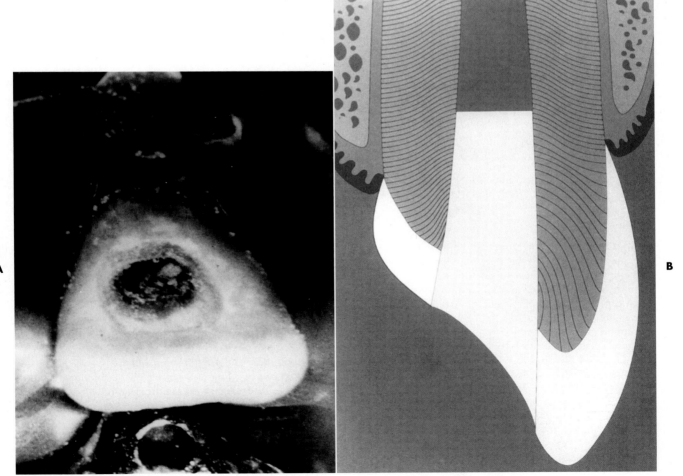

FIG. 20-1 Walking bleach technique. **A,** Coronal restoration is removed, and the access cavity is refined and cleaned. **B,** Root canal obturation has been removed below the level of the gingival margin.

Continued

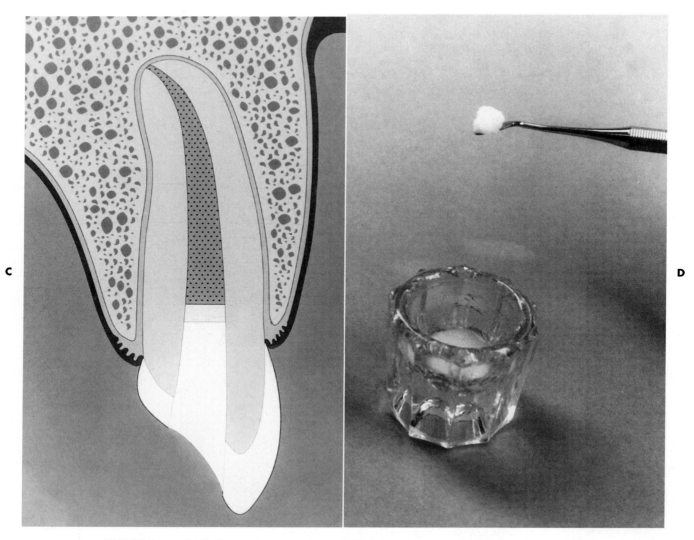

FIG. 20-1, cont'd C, Protective barrier (e.g., IRM) is applied on top of the endodontic obturation. **D,** Walking bleach paste is prepared by mixing sodium perborate and liquid to a thick consistency of wet sand.

from the dentin, and therefore its complete removal from the pulp chamber may be difficult. Removal should be done with care to avoid inadvertent cutting of sound dentin. An ultrasonic device may be used for this purpose. Remember, all the composite must be removed to allow the bleaching agent to penetrate and make contact with the dentin.

7. Remove all materials to a level just below the gingival margin (Fig. 20-1, *B*). Orange solvent, chloroform, or xylol on a cotton pellet may be used to dissolve sealer remnants.

8. Apply a sufficiently thick layer, at least 2 mm of a protective barrier, such as polycarboxylate cement, zinc phosphate cement, glass-ionomer, IRM or Cavit, on the endodontic obturation (Fig. 20-1, *C*). The coronal height of the barrier should protect the dentin tubules and conform to the external epithelial attachment.

9. Prepare the walking bleach paste by mixing sodium perborate and an inert liquid, such as water, saline, or anesthetic solution, to a thick consistency of wet sand (Fig. 20-1, *D*). Although a sodium perborate and 30% hydrogen peroxide mixture bleaches faster, in most cases long-

term results are similar to those with sodium perborate and water, and therefore should not be used routinely.[32,38] Using an amalgam carrier to place the paste, next use a plastic instrument to pack the pulp chamber. Remove the excess liquid by tamping with a cotton pellet (Fig. 20-1, *E*). This also compresses and pushes the paste into all areas of the chamber.

10. Remove the excess bleaching paste from undercuts in the pulp horn and gingival area and apply a thick well-sealed temporary filling (preferably IRM) directly against the paste and into the undercuts. Carefully pack the temporary filling, at least 3 mm thick, to ensure a good seal (Fig. 20-1, *F*).

11. Remove the rubber dam. Inform the patient that the bleaching agent works slowly and that significant lightening may not be evident for several days.

12. Recall the patient approximately 2 weeks later and if necessary repeat the procedure several times.[19] Repeat treatments are similar to the first one.

13. As an optional procedure, if initial bleaching is not satisfactory, strengthen the walking bleach paste by mixing the

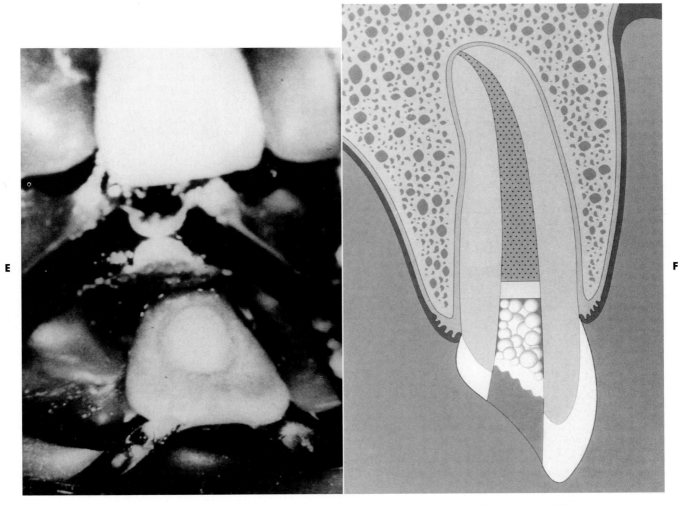

E

F

FIG. 20-1, cont'd E, Pulp chamber is packed with walking bleach paste. **F,** Temporary filling is placed to seal the bleaching paste in the pulp chamber for a few weeks. *(B, C, and* F, *Courtesy Dr. A. Castellucci.)*

sodium perborate with gradually increasing concentrations of hydrogen peroxide (3% to 30%) instead of water. The more potent oxidizers may have an enhanced bleaching effect, but are not used routinely because of the possibility of permeation into the tubules and damage to the cervical periodontium by these more caustic agents.

Thermocatalytic

The thermocatalytic technique involves placement of the oxidizing chemical, generally 30% to 35% hydrogen peroxide, in the pulp chamber (Fig. 20-2) followed by heat application either by electric heating devices (Figs. 20-3 and 20-4) or specially designed lamps (Fig. 20-5).

Potential damage by the thermocatalytic approach is external cervical root resorption caused by irritation to the cementum and periodontal ligament, possibly caused by the oxidizing agent combined with heating.[25,37] Therefore application of a highly concentrated hydrogen peroxide and heat during intracoronal bleaching is questionable.

The thermocatalytic technique does not give more successful long-term results than other methods and is not recommended for most intracoronal bleaching cases.

Ultraviolet Photooxidation

Ultraviolet photooxidation applies ultraviolet light to the labial surface of the tooth to be bleached. A 30% to 35% hydrogen peroxide solution is placed into the pulp chamber on a cotton pellet followed by a 2-minute exposure to ultraviolet light. Supposedly this causes oxygen release, like the thermocatalytic bleaching technique.[24]

There is little clinical experience with this method. It requires more chair time and is probably not more effective than the walking bleach technique.

Intentional Endodontics and Intracoronal Bleaching

Intrinsic tetracycline and other similar stains are incorporated into tooth structure during tooth formation, mostly into the dentin, and therefore are more difficult to treat from the external enamel surface. Intracoronal bleaching of tetracycline-discolored teeth has been shown clinically[1,2] and experimentally[21,49] to lead to significant lightening.

The technique involves standard endodontic therapy followed by an intracoronal walking bleach technique. Preferably only intact teeth without coronal defects, caries, or restorations should be treated. This prevents the need for any additional

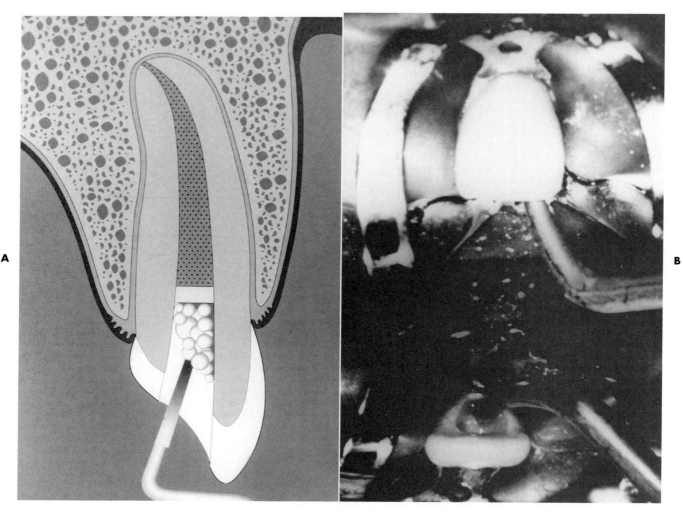

FIG. 20-2 A, Thermocatalytic technique. Oxidizing agent is placed in the pulp chamber and activated with heated tip of the bleaching tool. **B,** Clinical view. (A, *Courtesy Dr. A. Castellucci.*)

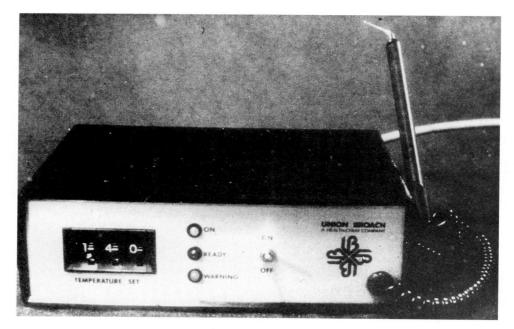

FIG. 20-3 Individual bleaching tool (Union Broach, New York, N.Y.). Heated tip can be used for both external and internal bleaching.

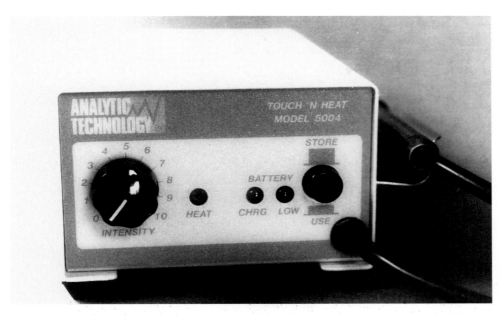

FIG. 20-4 Touch 'n Heat (Analytic Technology, Redmond, Wash.). Specially designed tip can be also used for intracoronal bleaching.

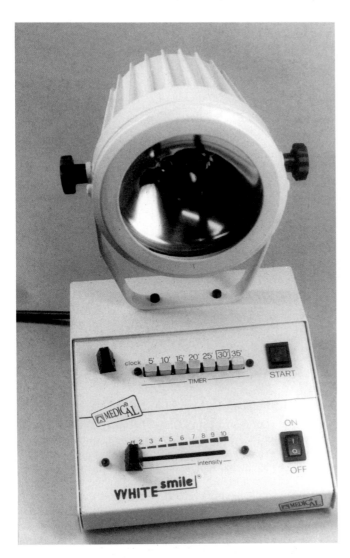

FIG. 20-5 One type of bleaching lamp available. It is usually placed approximately 15 inches from the teeth. Patient's eyes must be protected throughout the bleaching procedure.

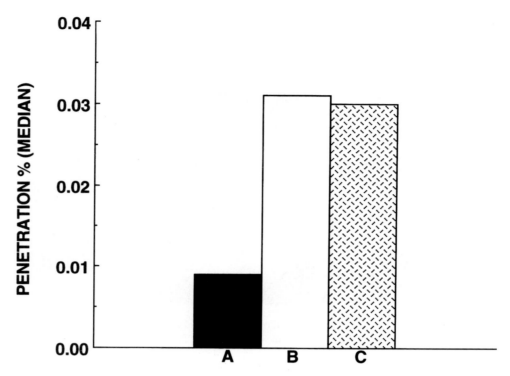

FIG. 20-6 Radicular penetration of hydrogen peroxide following intracoronal thermocatalytic bleaching. Teeth with defects either at the cementoenamel junction *(B)* or midroot *(C)* were significantly more permeable to hydrogen peroxide than those without defects *(A)*. *(From Rotstein et al: J Endod 17:230, 1991.)*

Table 20-3. Clinical reports of external root resorption associated with nonvital bleaching with 30% to 35% hydrogen peroxide

Authors	Published	No. of Cases	Age of Patients (yr)	Previous Trauma		Heat Applied		Barrier Used	
				Yes	No	Yes	No	Yes	No
Harrington and Natkin	*J Endod* 5:344, 1979	7	10-29	7	0	7	0	0	7
Lado et al.	*Oral Surg* 55:78, 1983	1	50	0	1	1	0	0	1
Montgomery	*Oral Surg* 57:203, 1984	1	21	1	0	?		?	
Shearer	*Aust Endod Newslett* 10:16, 1984	1	?	0	1	1	0	0	1
Cvek and Lindvall	*Endodont Dent Traumatol* 1:56, 1985	11	11-26	10	1	11	0	0	11
Latcham	*J Endod* 12:262, 1986	1	8	1	0	0	1	0	1
Goon et al.	*J Endod* 12:414, 1986	1	15	?		0	1	0	1
Friedman et al.	*Endodont Dent Traumatol* 4:23, 1988	4	18-24	0	4	3	1	0	4
Gimlin and Schindler	*J Endod* 16:292, 1990	1	13	1	0	1	0	0	1
Al-Nazhan	*Oral Surg* 72:607, 1991	1	27	0	1	1	0	0	1
Heithersay	*Aust Dent J* 39:82, 1994	4	10-20	4	0	4	0	0	4

restoration, thereby reducing the possibility of coronal fractures and failures. The most discolored tooth should be selected for trial treatment.

The procedure should be carefully explained to the patient, including the possible complications and sequelae. A treatment consent form is recommended. Sacrificing pulp vitality should be considered in terms of the overall psychologic and social needs of the individual patient and the possible complications of other treatment options. The procedure has been shown to be predictable and without significant clinical complications.[1,2]

Complications and adverse effects

External root resorption. Clinical reports (Table 20-3) and histologic studies[25,37] have shown that intracoronal bleaching may induce external root resorption. This is probably caused by the oxidizing agent, particulary 30% to 35% hydrogen peroxide. The mechanism of bleaching-induced damage to the periodontium or cementum has not been fully elucidated. Presumably the irritating chemical diffuses via unprotected dentinal tubules and cementum defects[34] (Fig. 20-6) and causes necrosis of the cementum, inflammation of the periodontal ligament, and fi-

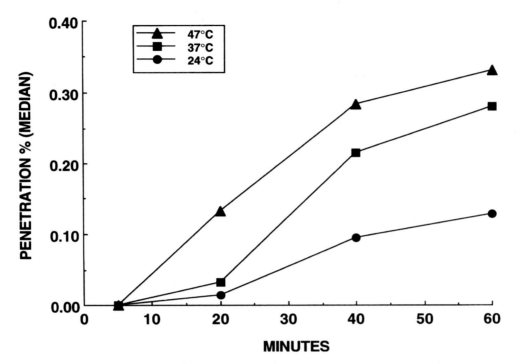

FIG. 20-7 Radicular penetration of hydrogen peroxide following intracoronal bleaching at different temperatures. Elevating the temperature and prolonging the bleaching time increased hydrogen peroxide penetration. *(From Rotstein et al:* Endodont Dent Traumatol *7:196, 1991.)*

nally root resorption. The process may be enhanced if heat is applied[33] (Fig. 20-7) or if bacteria are present.[11,18] Previous traumatic injury and age may act as predisposing factors.[16]

Chemical burns. Thirty percent hydrogen peroxide is caustic and causes chemical burns and sloughing of the gingiva. When such solutions are used, the soft tissues should be always be protected.

Damage to restorations. Bleaching with hydrogen peroxide may affect bonding of composite resins to dental hard tissues.[44] Scanning electron microscopy observations suggest a possible interaction between composite resin and residual peroxide, causing inhibition of polymerization and increase in resin porosity.[45] This presents a clinical problem when immediate aesthetic restoration of the bleached tooth is required. It is therefore recommended that residual hydrogen peroxide is totally eliminated before composite placement.

It has been suggested that immersion of peroxide-treated dental tissues in water at 98.6° F (37° C) for 7 days prevents the reduction in bond strength.[46] Other researchers assessed the efficacy of catalase in removing residual hydrogen peroxide from the pulp chamber of human teeth, as compared to prolonged rinsing in water.[29] Three minutes of catalase treatment effectively removed all the residual hydrogen peroxide.

Suggestions for safer nonvital bleaching

Isolate tooth effectively. Intracoronal bleaching should always be carried out with rubber dam isolation. Interproximal wedges and ligatures may also be used for better protection.

Protect oral mucosa. Protective ointments, such as Orabase or Vaseline, must be applied to the surrounding oral mucosa to prevent chemical burns by caustic oxidizers. Recent reports suggest that catalase applied to oral tissues before hydrogen peroxide treatment totally prevents the associated tissue damage (Plate 20-2, *E* through *H*).[35] The clinical implications of this therapy are currently under investigation.

Verify adequate endodontic obturation. The quality of root canal obturation should always be assessed clinically and radiographically before bleaching. Adequate obturation ensures a better overall prognosis of the treated tooth. It also provides an additional barrier against damage by oxidizers to the periodontal ligament and periapical tissues.

Use protective barriers. Use of protective barriers is essential to prevent leakage of bleaching agents, which may infiltrate between the gutta-percha and root canal walls, reaching the periodontal ligament via dentinal tubules, lateral canals, or the root apex (Fig. 20-8). In none of the clinical reports of postbleaching root resorption was a protective barrier used (see Table 20-3).

Various materials can be used for this purpose. Barrier thickness and its relationship to the cementoenamel junction are most important.[36,42] The ideal barrier should protect the dentinal tubules and conform to the external epithelial attachment.

Avoid acid etching. It has been suggested that acid etching of dentin in the chamber to remove the smear layer and open the tubules would allow better penetration of oxidizer. This procedure has not proven beneficial.[5] The use of caustic chemicals in the chamber is undesirable, as periodontal ligament irritation may result.

Avoid strong oxidizers. Procedures and techniques applying strong oxidizers should be avoided if they are not essential for bleaching. Solutions of 30% to 35% hydrogen peroxide, either alone or in combination with other agents, should not be used routinely for intracoronal bleaching.

Sodium perborate is mild and quite safe, and no additional protection of the soft tissues is usually required. Generally, however, oxidizing agents should not be exposed to more of

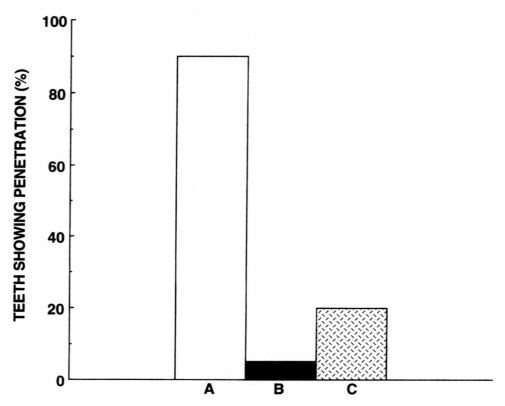

FIG. 20-8 Effect of a protective cement barrier on the radicular penetration of hydrogen peroxide during intracoronal bleaching. Significantly higher penetration was found in teeth without a protective barrier (A). *(From Rotstein et al:* J Endod *18:114, 1992.)*

the pulp space and dentin than absolutely necessary to obtain a satisfactory clinical result.

Avoid heat. Excessive heat may damage the cementum, periodontal ligament dentin, and enamel, especially when combined with strong oxidizers.[25] Although no direct correlation was found between heat applications alone and external cervical root resorption, application of heat should be limited during bleaching procedures.

Recall periodically. Bleached teeth should be frequently examined both clinically and radiographically. Root resorption may occasionally be detected as early as 6 months after bleaching. Early detection improves the prognosis, since corrective therapy may still be applied.

Postbleaching Tooth Restoration

Proper tooth restoration is essential for long-term successful bleaching results. Coronal microleakage of lingual access restorations is a problem,[51] and a leaky restoration may lead to rediscoloration.

There is no ideal method for filling the chamber after tooth bleaching. The pulp chamber and access cavity should be carefully restored with a light-cured acid-etched composite resin, light in shade. The composite material should be placed at a depth that seals the cavity and provides some incisal support. Light curing from the labial surface, rather than the lingual surface, is recommended, since this results in shrinkage of the composite resin toward the axial walls, reducing the rate of microleakage.[22]

Placing white cement under the composite access restora-

tion is recommended. Filling the chamber completely with composite may cause loss of translucency and difficulty in distinguishing between composite and tooth structure during rebleaching.[14]

Residual peroxides from bleaching agents, mainly hydrogen peroxide and carbamide peroxide, may affect the bonding strength of composites.[43,44] Therefore waiting for a few days after bleaching before restoring the tooth with composite resin is recommended. Catalase treatment at the final visit may enhance the removal of residual peroxides from the access cavity; however, this requires further clinical investigation.[29]

Packing calcium hydroxide paste in the pulp chamber for a few weeks before placement of the final restoration to counteract acidity caused by bleaching agents and to prevent resorption has also been suggested; however, this procedure is probably unnecessary and is used mainly with the walking bleach technique.[30,37]

VITAL BLEACHING TECHNIQUES

In vital bleaching techniques, oxidizers are applied to the external enamel surface of teeth with vital pulps. Many techniques have been advocated for extracoronal bleaching of vital teeth. However, the long-term results depend mainly on the nature and location of the discoloration.

Thermobleaching and Photobleaching

The thermobleaching and photobleaching technique basically involves application of 30% to 35% hydrogen peroxide and heat or a combination of heat and light rays to the enamel

Table 20-4. Indications and contraindications for vital thermobleaching and photobleaching

Indications	Contraindications
Light enamel discolorations	Severe dark discolorations
Mild tetracycline stains	Severe enamel loss
Endemic fluorosis stains	Proximity of pulp horns
Age-related discolorations	Hypersensitive teeth
	Presence of caries
	Large/poor coronal restorations

surface. Heat is applied either by electric heating devices (see Fig. 20-3) or heat lamps (see Fig. 20-5). Photobleaching by shortwave ultraviolet light may also be carried out.[24]

With discolored dentin, bleaching agents placed on the enamel do not readily reach the stain. If the stain is on the enamel surface or the enamel is defective and porous, better results are expected. Long-term follow-up studies in humans are limited and have shown partial success only with light yellow stains in young patients. The more prevalent darker stains have generally shown little response to surface bleaching, and the long-term prognosis is poor.

Extracoronal bleaching of vital teeth involves the following steps:

1. Familiarize the patient with the probable causes of discoloration, the procedure to be followed, expected outcome, and the possibility of future rediscoloration.
2. Prepare periapical radiographs to detect the presence of caries, defective restorations, and proximity to pulp horns. Well-sealed small restorations and minimal amounts of exposed incisal dentin are not usually a contraindication for bleaching.
3. Evaluate tooth color with a shade guide and take clinical photographs before and throughout the procedure.
4. Apply a protective ointment to the surrounding gingival tissues and isolate the teeth with a rubber dam and waxed dental floss ligatures. If a heat lamp is used, avoid placing rubber dam metal clamps, as they are subjected to heating and may be painful to the patient.
5. Do not use anesthesia.
6. Position protective sunglasses over the patient's and clinician's eyes.
7. Clean the enamel surface with pumice and water. Avoid prophy pastes containing glycerin or fluoride.
8. Acid etch the darkest or most severely stained areas, as an optional procedure, with buffered phosphoric acid for 5 to 15 seconds and rinse with water for 60 seconds. A gel form of acid provides optimal control. Enamel etching for extracoronal bleaching is controversial and should not be carried out routinely.
9. Place a small amount of 30% to 35% hydrogen peroxide solution into a dappen dish. Apply the hydrogen peroxide liquid on the labial surface of the teeth using a small cotton pellet or a piece of gauze. A bleaching gel containing hydrogen peroxide may be used instead of the aqueous solution.
10. Apply heat with a heating device or a light source. The temperature should be less than the patient can comfortably tolerate, usually between 125° to 140° F (52° to 60° C). Rewet the enamel surface with hydrogen peroxide as

required. If the teeth become too sensitive, discontinue the bleaching procedure immediately. Do not exceed 30 minutes of treatment even if the result is not satisfactory.

11. Remove the heat source and allow the teeth to cool down for at least 5 minutes. Then wash with warm water for 1 minute and remove the rubber dam. Do not rinse with cold water, since the sudden change in temperature may damage the pulp or can be painful to the patient.
12. Dry the teeth and gently polish them with a composite resin polishing cup. Treat all the etched and bleached surfaces with a neutral sodium fluoride gel for 3 to 5 minutes.
13. Inform the patient that cold sensitivity is common, especially during the first 24 hours after treatment. Also instruct the patient to use a fluoride rinse daily for 2 weeks.
14. The patient should return approximately 2 weeks later to evaluate the effectiveness of bleaching. Take clinical photographs with the same shade guide used in the preoperative photographs for comparison purposes. If necessary, repeat the bleaching procedure.

Complications and adverse effects

Postoperative pain. A number of short- and long-term symptoms may occur following extracoronal bleaching of vital teeth. A common immediate postoperative problem is pulpalgia characterized by intermittent shooting pain. It may occur during the bleaching session or later in the day and usually persists for between 24 to 48 hours. The intensity of the pulpalgia is related to the duration and temperature of the bleaching procedure. Shorter bleaching periods and lower temperatures reduce the symptoms.

Long-term sensitivity to cold may also be associated with this procedure. Topical fluoride treatments and desensitizing toothpastes can alleviate these symptoms.

Pulpal damage. Extracoronal bleaching with hydrogen peroxide and heat has been associated with some pulpal damage. Various investigators showed different results, although the majority did not find significant irreversible effects on the pulp.[6,28] Nevertheless, the procedure must be approached and carried out with caution and not performed in the presence of caries, in areas of exposed dentin, or in close proximity to pulp horns. Defective restorations must be replaced before bleaching. Teeth with large coronal restorations should not be bleached.

Dental hard tissue damage. Hydrogen peroxide was shown to cause morphologic and structural changes in enamel, dentin, and cementum in vitro.[31,39,52] A reduction in microhardness was also observed.[23] These changes may cause dental hard tissues to be more susceptible to degradation. More long-term in vivo studies are still required to assess the clinical significance of these changes.

Mucosal damage. Caustic bleaching agents in contact with the oral mucosa may cause peroxide-induced tissue damage (Plate 20-2, *E*). Ulceration and sloughing of the mucosa is caused by oxygen gas bubbles in the tissue (Plate 20-2, *F* and *G*). Generally, the mucosa appears white but does not become necrotic or leave scar tissue. The associated burning sensation is extremely uncomfortable for the patient. Treatment is by extensive water rinses until the whiteness is reduced. In more severe cases a topical anesthetic, limited movements, and good oral hygiene aid healing. Application of protective ointment or catalase (Plate 20-2, *H*) can prevent most of these complications.

Laser-Activated Bleaching

An innovative technique was recently introduced using lasers for bleaching vital teeth. Two types of lasers can be employed: the argon laser, which emits a visible blue light, and a carbon dioxide laser, which emits invisible infrared light. These lasers can be targeted to stain molecules and with the use of a catalyst rapidly decompose hydrogen peroxide to oxygen and water. The catalyst-peroxide combination may be damaging, and therefore exposed soft tissues, eyes, and clothing should be protected.

Combination of both lasers can effectively reduce intrinsic stains in the dentin. The argon laser can be targeted to stain molecules without overheating the pulp. It is easy to use and is best for removal of initial dark stains such as those caused by tetracycline. However, visible blue light becomes less effective as the tooth whitens and there are fewer stain molecules. On the other hand, the carbon dioxide laser interacts directly with the catalyst-peroxide combination and removes the stain regardless of the tooth color.

Laser bleaching is a new technique, and there are currently no long-term studies regarding its benefits or adverse effects.

Mouthguard Bleaching

Mouthguard bleaching is generally used for mild discolorations. It has been basically advocated as a home bleaching technique, with a wide variety of materials, bleaching agents, and frequency and duration of treatment. Numerous products are available, generally either 1.5% to 10% hydrogen peroxide or 10% to 15% carbamide peroxide, which are degraded slowly to release hydrogen peroxide. The carbamide peroxide products are more commonly used.

Because of a lack of consensus concerning treatment techniques the following step-by-step instructions should be used only as a general guideline:

1. Familiarize the patient with the probable causes of discoloration, the procedure to be followed, and the expected outcome.
2. Carry out prophylaxis and assess tooth color with a shade guide. Take clinical photographs before and throughout the procedure.
3. Make an alginate impression of the arch to be treated. Cast the impression and outline the guard in the model. It should completely cover the teeth in the arch; second molars do not need to be covered unless required for retention. Place two layers of die relief on the buccal aspects of the cast teeth to form a small reservoir for the bleaching agent (Fig. 20-9, *A*). Fabricate a vacuum-form soft plastic matrix, approximately 2 mm thick; trim the matrix with crown and bridge scissors to 1 mm past the gingival margins and adjust with an acrylic trimming bur (Fig. 20-9, *B*).
4. Insert the mouthguard to ensure proper fit. Remove the guard and apply the bleaching agent in the space of each tooth to be bleached (Fig. 20-9, *C*). Reinsert the mouthguard over the teeth and remove excess bleaching agent (Fig. 20-9, *D*).
5. Familiarize the patient with the use of the bleaching agent and wearing of the guard. The procedure is usually performed 3 to 4 hours a day and the bleaching agent is replenished every 30 to 60 minutes. Some clinicians recommend wearing the guard during sleep for better long-term aesthetic results; this, however, is of little benefit, since the oxidizer is broken down fairly quickly.

Table 20-5. Indications and contraindications for mouthguard vital bleaching

Indications	Contraindications
Superficial enamel stains	Severe enamel loss
Mild yellow discolorations	Hypersensitive teeth
Brown fluorosis stains	Presence of caries
Age-related discolorations	Defective coronal restorations
	Allergy to bleaching gels
	Bruxism

6. Instruct the patient to brush and rinse the teeth after meals. The guard should not be worn while eating. Inform the patient about thermal sensitivity and minor irritation of soft tissues and to discontinue use of the guard if uncomfortable.
7. Treatment should be for between 4 and 24 weeks. Recall the patient every 2 weeks to monitor stain lightening. Check for tissue irritation, oral lesions, enamel etching, and leaky restorations. If complications occur, stop treatment and reevaluate the feasibility of continuation at a later date. Note that frequently the incisal edges are bleached more readily than the remainder of the crown.

A modification of the technique has also been suggested[9,12] in which the discolored tooth is first treated by enamel microabrasion (described later in the chapter) followed by carbamide peroxide–mouthguard bleaching. This has been said to enhance the aesthetic results of the enamel microabrasion technique.

The long-term aesthetic results of mouthguard bleaching are unknown. However, it appears that rediscoloration is not more frequent than with the other techniques.

To date, no conclusive experimental or clinical studies on the safety of long-term use of the bleaching agents are available. Therefore caution should be exercised in their prescription and application. Of major concern are the products marketed to the public over the counter, often without professional control; their use should be discouraged.

Complications and adverse effects

Systemic effects. Controlled mouthguard bleaching procedures are considered relatively safe with regard to systemic effects.[17] However, some concern has been raised over bleaching gels inadvertently swallowed by the patient. Accidental ingestion of large amounts of these gels may be toxic and cause irritation to the gastric and respiratory mucosa. Bleaching gels containing carbopol, which retards the rate of oxygen release from peroxide, are usually more toxic. Therefore it is advisable to pay specific attention to any adverse systemic effects and to discontinue treatment immediately if they occur.

Dental hard tissue damage. In vitro studies indicate morphologic and chemical changes in enamel, dentin, and cementum associated with some agents used for mouthguard bleaching.[39,40,52] Long-term in vivo studies are still required to determine the clinical significance of these changes.

Tooth sensitivity. Transient tooth sensitivity to cold may occur during or after mouthguard bleaching. In most cases it is mild and ceases on termination of treatment. Treatment for sensitivity consists of removal of the mouthguard for 2 to 3 days, reduction of wearing time, and readjustment of the guard.

Pulpal damage. Long-term effects of mouthguard bleaching on the pulp are still unknown. To date, no correlation was

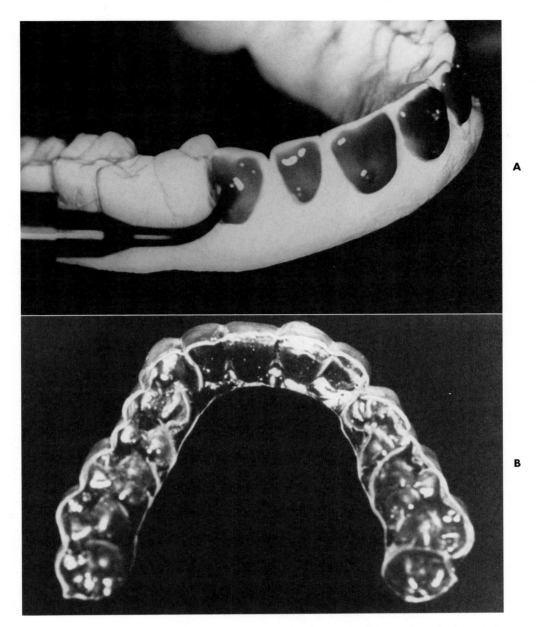

FIG. 20-9 A, Cast model with die relief on the buccal aspects of the teeth to be bleached. **B,** Fabricated vacuum-form soft plastic mouthguard.   *Continued*

found between carbamide peroxide bleaching and irreversible pulpal damage.[17] The pulpalgia associated with tooth hypersensitivity is transient and uneventful.

Mucosal damage. Minor irritations or ulcerations of the oral mucosa were reported to occur during the initial course of treatment. This infrequent occurrence is usually mild and transient. Possible causes are mechanical interference by the mouthguard, chemical irritation by the bleaching active agent, and allergic reaction to gel components. In most cases readjustment and smoothing the borders of the guard will suffice. However, if tissue irritation persists, treatment should be discontinued.

Damage to restorations. Some in vitro studies suggest that damage of bleaching gels to composite resins might be due to softening and cracking of the resin matrix.[8,43] It has been suggested that patients are informed that previously placed com-

posites may require replacement following bleaching. Others reported no significant adverse effects on either surface texture or color of prosthetic restorations.[17] Generally, however, if composite restorations are present in aesthetically critical areas, they may need replacement to improve color matching following successful bleaching.

Occlusal disturbances. Typically, occlusal problems related to the mouthguard may be mechanical or physiologic. From a mechanical point of view the patient may occlude only on the posterior teeth rather than on all teeth simultaneously. Removing posterior teeth from the guard until all the teeth are in contact rectifies this problem. From a physiologic point of view, if the patient experiences pain from the temporomandibular joint, the posterior teeth can be removed from the guard until only the anterior guidance remains. In such cases wearing time should be reduced.

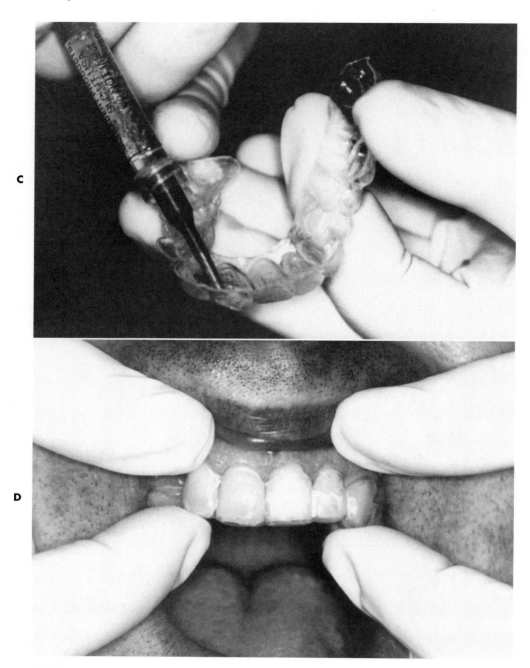

FIG. 20-9, cont'd C, Application of bleaching gel into the spaces of the teeth to be bleached.
D, Insertion of the mouthguard containing bleaching gel.

Enamel Microabrasion

Enamel microabrasion involves removing discolored tooth areas with acid. Two common methods are used to remove stains from the outer tooth surface by stripping the enamel with hydrochloric acid. One combines hydrochloric acid, pumice, and light abrasion (acid-pumice abrasion technique) and the other uses the acid with peroxide and diethyl ether (McInnes technique). The acid-pumice abrasion technique does not actually bleach the stain as in the McInnes technique (which uses hydrogen peroxide) but removes the stain mechanically together with dental hard tissue.

Enamel microabrasion works best on superficial extrinsic stains for which hydrogen peroxide treatment is less success-

ful, such as enamel hypocalcifications (Plate 20-1, *I* and *J*) and endemic fluorosis stains. Although various techniques have been suggested for treating such conditions, the controlled hydrochloric acid-pumice abrasion technique is probably the most effective.[10]

Hydrochloric acid-pumice abrasion

The technique involves the following steps:
1. Photograph the teeth to be treated to serve as a permanent record and as a basis for future comparison.
2. Protect the gingiva and carefully isolate the teeth with a rubber dam and ligatures. Extend the rubber dam over the patient's nostrils.

3. Cover exposed areas of the patient's face and eyes with a towel and protective glasses for added safety from acid spatter.

4. Mix a 36% hydrochloric acid solution with an equal volume of distilled water to make an 18% solution. Always add acid to water. (Adding water to acid can cause splattering.)

5. Add a substantial amount of fine flour of pumice to form a thick paste. In another dappen dish, mix sodium bicarbonate and water to a thick paste for the acid neutralization procedure.

6. Apply the hydrochloric acid and pumice paste to the enamel surface with a piece of wooden tongue blade or crushed orangewood stick end. Simultaneously use a cotton-tipped applicator to absorb any excess solution. Exert firm finger pressure and work the paste into the enamel surface with a swirling motion for 5 to 10 seconds.

7. Rinse the enamel surface thoroughly with water for 10 seconds and evaluate for excessive enamel wear.

8. Wet the tooth with saliva and evaluate for appropriate color change.

9. Reapply the paste until the desired color is achieved. To avoid excessive wear, limit the acid-abrasion applications to a maximum of five attempts.

10. Neutralize with sodium bicarbonate and water and remove the rubber dam. Clean the teeth with a fine fluoride prophylaxis paste and superfine aluminum oxide composite resin polishing disks to smooth the abraded surface. Usually the desired shade is obtained in a single appointment. If not, the stains may be too deep and not amenable to treatment.

The controlled acid-pumice abrasion technique is very effective if an initial lightening effect is achieved.[10] Clinical complications and pulpal effects are minimal.[4,15]

McInnes technique

The McInnes technique is essentially similar to the controlled hydrochloric acid-pumice abrasion technique but uses a solution of 5 parts 30% hydrogen peroxide, 5 parts 36% hydrochloric acid, and 1 part diethyl ether.[26]

The solution is applied directly to the stained areas for 1 to 2 minutes with cotton applicators. While the surface is wet, a fine cuttle disk is run over the stained surfaces for 15 seconds. This is repeated, sometimes in several appointments, until the desired tooth shade is achieved.

REFERENCES

1. Abou-Rass M: The elimination of tetracycline discoloration by intentional endodontics and internal bleaching, *J Endod* 8:101, 1982.

2. Anitua E, Zabalegui B, Gil J, Gascon F: Internal bleaching of severe tetracycline discolorations: four-year clinical evaluation, *Quintessence Int* 21:783, 1990.

3. Arens DE, Rich JJ, Healey HJ: A practical method of bleaching tetracycline-stained teeth, *Oral Surg* 34:812, 1972.

4. Baumgartner JC, Reid DE, Pickett AB: Human pulpal reaction to the modified McInnes bleaching technique, *J Endod* 9:12, 1983.

5. Casey LJ, Schindler WG, Murata SM, Burgess JO: The use of dentinal etching with endodontic bleaching procedures, *J Endod* 15:535, 1989.

6. Cohen SC: Human pulpal response to bleaching procedures on vital teeth, *J Endod* 5:134, 1979.

7. Cohen S, Parkins FM: Bleaching tetracycline-stained vital teeth, *Oral Surg* 29:465, 1970.

8. Crim GA: Post-operative bleaching: effect on microleakage, *Am J Dent* 5:109, 1992.

9. Croll TP: Enamel microabrasion followed by dental bleaching: case reports, *Quintessence Int* 23:317, 1992.

10. Croll TP, Cavanaugh RR: Enamel color modification by controlled hydrochloric acid-pumice abrasion. I. Technique and examples, *Quintessence Int* 17:81, 1986.

11. Cvek M, Lindvall AM: External root resorption following bleaching of pulpless teeth with oxygen peroxide, *Endodont Dent Traumatol* 1:56, 1985.

12. Cvitko E, Swift EJ, Denehy GE: Improved esthetics with a combined bleaching technique: a case report, *Quintessence Int* 23:91, 1992.

13. Driscoll WS et al: Prevalence of dental caries and dental fluorosis in areas with optimal and above-optimal water fluoride concentrations, *J Am Dent Assoc* 107:42, 1983.

14. Freccia WF, Peters DD, Lorton L: An evaluation of various permanent restorative materials' effect on the shade of bleached teeth, *J Endod* 8:265, 1982.

15. Griffen R, Grower M, Ayer W: Effects of solutions used to treat dental fluorosis on permeability of teeth, *J Endod* 3:139, 1977.

16. Harrington G, Natkin E: External resorption associated with bleaching of pulpless teeth, *J Endod* 5:344, 1979.

17. Haywood VB, Heymann HO: Nightguard vital bleaching: how safe is it? *Quintessence Int* 22:515, 1991.

18. Heling I, Parson A, Rotstein I: Effect of bleaching agents on dentin permeability to *Streptococcus faecalis*, *J Endod* 21:540, 1995.

19. Holmstrup G, Palm AM, Lambjerg-Hansen H: Bleaching of discoloured root-filled teeth, *Endodont Dent Traumatol* 4:197, 1988.

20. Jordan RE, Boskman L: Conservative vital bleaching treatment of discolored dentition, *Compend Contin Ed Dent* 5:803, 1984.

21. Lake F, O'Dell N, Walton R: The effect of internal bleaching on tetracycline in dentin, *J Endod* 11:415, 1985.

22. Lemon R: Bleaching and restoring endodontically treated teeth, *Curr Opin Dent* 1:754, 1991.

23. Lewinstein I, Hirschfeld Z, Stabholz A, Rotstein I: Effect of hydrogen peroxide and sodium perborate on the microhardness of human enamel and dentin, *J Endod* 1994; 20:61.

24. Lin LC, Pitts DL, Burgess LW: An investigation into the feasibility of photobleaching tetracycline-stained teeth, *J Endod* 14:293, 1988.

25. Madison S, Walton RE: Cervical root resorption following bleaching of endodontically treated teeth, *J Endod* 16:570, 1990.

26. McInnes JW: Removing brown stain from teeth, *Ariz Dent J* 12:13, 1966.

27. Nutting EB, Poe GS: A new combination for bleaching teeth, *J South Calif Dent Assoc* 31:289, 1963.

28. Robertson WD, Melfi RC: Pulpal response to vital bleaching procedures, *J Endod* 6:645, 1980.

29. Rotstein I: Role of catalase in the elimination of residual hydrogen peroxide following tooth bleaching, *J Endod* 19:567, 1993.

30. Rotstein I, Friedman S: pH variation among materials used for intracoronal bleaching, *J Endod* 17:376, 1991.

31. Rotstein I, Lehr T, Gedalia I: Effect of bleaching agents on inorganic components of human dentin and cementum, *J Endod* 18:290, 1992.

32. Rotstein I, Mor C, Friedman S: Prognosis of intracoronal bleaching with sodium perborate preparations in vitro: 1 year study, *J Endod* 19:10, 1993.

33. Rotstein I, Torek Y, Lewinstein I: Effect of bleaching time and temperature on the radicular penetration of hydrogen peroxide, *Endodont Dent Traumatol* 7:196, 1991.

34. Rotstein I, Torek Y, Misgav R: Effect of cementum defects on radicular penetration of 30% H_2O_2 during intracoronal bleaching, *J Endod* 17:230, 1991.

35. Rotstein I, Wesselink PR, Bab I: Catalase protection against hydrogen peroxide–induced injury in rat oral mucosa, *Oral Surg* 75:744, 1993.

36. Rotstein I, Zyskind D, Lewinstein I, Bamberger N: Effect of different protective base materials on hydrogen peroxide leakage during intracoronal bleaching in vitro, *J Endod* 18:114, 1992.

37. Rotstein I et al: Histological characterization of bleaching-induced external root resorption in dogs, *J Endod* 17:436, 1991.

38. Rotstein I et al: In vitro efficacy of sodium perborate preparations used for intracoronal bleaching of discolored non-vital teeth, *Endodont Dent Traumatol* 7:177, 1991.

39. Rotstein I et al: Histochemical analysis of dental hard tissues following bleaching, *J Endod* 22:23, 1996.

40. Seghi RR, Denry I: Effects of external bleaching on indentation and abrasion characteristics of human enamel in vitro, *J Dent Res* 71:1340, 1992.

41. Spasser HF: A simple bleaching technique using sodium perborate, *NY State Dent J* 27:332, 1961.

42. Steiner DR, West JD: A method to determine the location and shape of an intracoronal bleach barrier, *J Endod* 20:304, 1994.

43. Titley KC, Torneck CD, Ruse ND: The effect of carbamide-peroxide gel on the shear bond strength of a microfil resin to bovine enamel, *J Dent Res* 71:20, 1992.

44. Titley KC, Torneck CD, Ruse ND, Krmec D: Adhesion of a resin composite to bleached and unbleached human enamel, *J Endod* 19:112, 1993.

45. Titley KC et al: Scanning electron microscopy observations on the penetration and structure of resin tags in bleached and unbleached bovine enamel, *J Endod* 17:71, 1991.

46. Torneck CD, Titley KC, Smith DC, Adibfar A: Effect of water leaching on the adhesion of composite resin to bleached and unbleached bovine enamel, *J Endod* 17:156, 1991.

47. van der Burgt TP, Plasschaert AJM: Bleaching of tooth discoloration caused by endodontic sealers, *J Endod* 12:231, 1986.

48. Walton RE: Bleaching procedures for teeth with vital and nonvital pulps. In Levine N: *Current treatment in dental practice,* Philadelphia 1986, WB Saunders, p 202.

49. Walton RE, O'Dell NL, Lake FT: Internal bleaching of tetracycline stained teeth in dogs, *J Endod* 9:416, 1983.

50. Weiger R, Kuhn A, Löst C: In vitro comparison of various types of sodium perborate used for intracoronal bleaching, *J Endod* 20:338, 1994.

51. Wilcox LR, Diaz-Arnold A: Coronal microleakage of permanent lingual access restorations in endodontically treated anterior teeth, *J Endod* 15:584, 1989.

52. Zalkind M, Arwaz JR, Goldman A, Rotstein I: Surface morphology changes in human enamel, dentin and cementum following bleaching: a scanning electron microscopy study, *Endodont Dent Traumatol* 12:82, 1996.

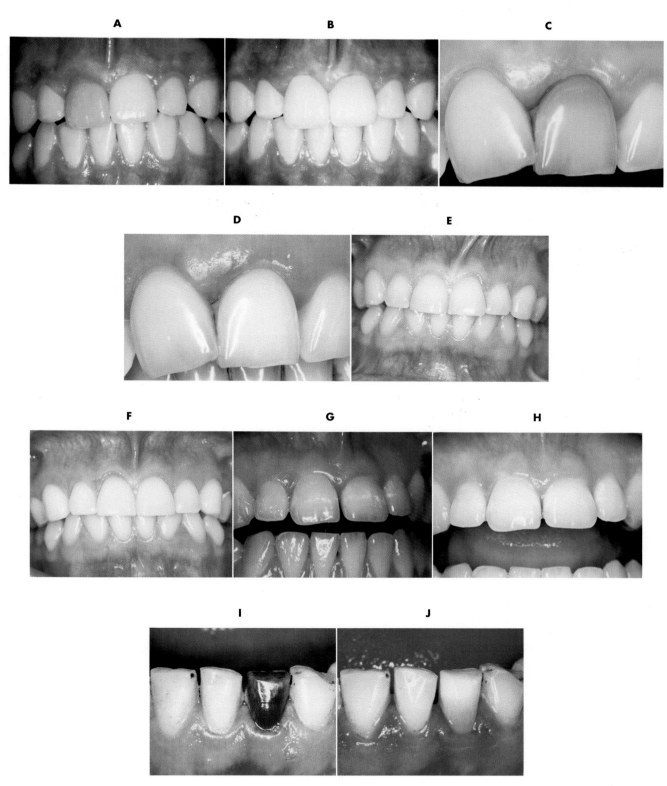

PLATE 20-1 A, Discolored maxillary cental incisor caused by pulp necrosis in a 25-year-old woman. **B,** Following endodontic therapy and two-appointment walking bleach treatment, aesthetic results were markedly improved, thereby preventing the need for prosthetic restoration. **C,** Discolored maxillary central incisor caused by traumatic injury. **D,** Aesthetic results following 3 weeks of walking bleach treatment with sodium perborate and water. **E,** Age-related discoloration of entire dentition. **F,** Improved aesthetic results following 15 days of mouthguard bleaching with carbamide peroxide–based gel. **G,** Enamel hypocalcification with presence of white spot lesions on enamel surface of maxillary anterior dentition. **H,** Aesthetic results following enamel microabrasion treatment. **I,** Discolored mandibular central incisor associated with poor endodontic treatment and coronal restoration. **J,** Aesthetic results following walking bleach treatment with sodium perborate and hydrogen peroxide. (C, D, E, F, G, and H, Courtesy Dr. P. Miara. I and J, Courtesy Dr. M. Amato.)

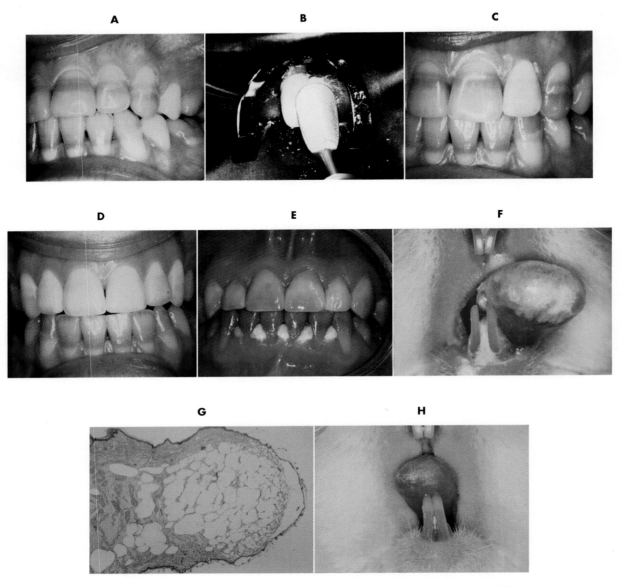

PLATE 20-2 A, Tetracycline discoloration affecting multiple teeth in both arches. **B,** Extra-coronal vital bleaching of a single tooth for assessment of treatment feasibility. **C,** Improved aesthetics of maxillary lateral incisor following vital bleaching with heated solution of hydrogen peroxide. **D,** Immediate postoperative view of bleached maxillary dentition as compared to nontreated mandibular dentition. **E,** Hydrogen peroxide–induced mucosal injury. Clinical appearance of severe gingival burns in a 38-year-old woman. Thermocatalytic vital bleaching was carried out using 30% hydrogen peroxide without effective protection of the gingival tissues. **F,** Rat tongue immediately after experimental application of 30% hydrogen peroxide, showing whitening and marked swelling. **G,** Histologically, large subepithelial vesicles and edematous cisterns are present. **H,** Normal appearance of tongue treated with catalase before hydrogen peroxide application. (**F, G,** and **H,** From Rotstein I et al: *Oral Surg* 75:744, 1993.)

Chapter 21

Restoration of the Endodontically Treated Tooth

Galen W. Wagnild
Kathy I. Mueller

The purpose of this chapter is to discuss the complex endodontic-restorative-periodontal relationship and to describe treatment planning considerations and therapeutic procedures to restore endodontically treated teeth with predictable clinical results.

RESTORATIVE DENTISTRY AND THE VITAL TOOTH

Effect of Restorative Procedures and Materials on the Pulp

The effect of dental restorative techniques and materials on the living pulp has been reported in detail in Chapter 15. Teeth that require extensive restorations suffer pulpal injury from both the dental disease itself and from the treatment procedures used to restore the resultant damage. A number of precautions are listed that can help to reduce the harmful consequences of dental procedures on the pulp. In addition to these, dentin bonding agents can be used to occlude open dentinal tubules and reduce sensitivity.

Risk of postrestorative endodontic complications

Adverse effects on the pulp are an inherent risk of restorative procedures. Despite precautions, pulpal damage from restorative dentistry cannot be entirely eliminated.[2] Intact dentin provides biologic resistance to dental pain and sensitivity, caries, tooth fracture, and pulpal breakdown.[34] As increasing amounts of structural dentin are removed during tooth preparation, the number of exposed dentinal tubules increases dramatically. At the surface of the dentin, or the dentinoenamel junction, dentinal tubules range between 15,000 and 20,000/mm². At the pulpal surface, the number of dentinal tubules increases threefold to 45,000 to 60,000/mm² and the tubule diameter increases. Therefore deep preparations expose a large number of wide dentinal tubules to trauma, dental materials, and bacterial products. Dentin permeability is greatest on thin axial surfaces, particularly mesial surfaces. These surfaces are often extensively reduced during preparation for full veneer crowns, and especially for fixed partial dentures involving mesially tipped abutments. Pulpal irritation becomes significant when the dentin thickness is reduced to 0.3 mm.[41]

The process of tooth preparation and restoration is irritating to the pulp, and the injury can occasionally be irreversible. Dental procedures are considered to be responsible for those endodontic complications that develop in restored teeth for no

other known reason. Abutment teeth have a higher risk of developing subsequent pulpal necrosis than vital teeth restored with single crowns, undoubtably because of the increased preparation required for parallelism. In a study of endodontic complications in restored teeth, approximately 0.3% of crowned teeth and 4% of abutment teeth became endodontically involved, when no caries, fracture, or other etiologic factors were present. When known etiologic factors were also present, pulpal necrosis significantly increased. The combined effect of dental procedures and recurrent dental disease nearly quadrupled the rate of endodontic involvement for abutment teeth and increased the rate for teeth with single crowns by more than tenfold.[3]

Endodontic involvement increases in proportion to the degree of dental destruction and the complexity of the restoration. Teeth treated with a buildup and a full veneer crown became necrotic roughly 30 times more frequently than unrestored teeth.[17] In complex cases requiring periodontal-prosthetic reconstruction, twice as many teeth with advanced periodontal disease developed endodontic complications compared to teeth with moderate periodontal disease.[19] This reflects a complicated interplay between multiple disease processes, more extensive tooth preparation, and the cumulative effects of previous dental breakdown and restoration.

Pulpal degeneration also increases with time following the insertion of the restorations. The pulpal insult initiated by the preparation and restoration procedures can continue undetected for many years. Among restored teeth that became endodontically involved for no known reason, 12% deteriorated in the first 3 years after the restorative treatment. The necrosis rate tripled by year 7 and increased to 50% of the restored teeth by year 12.[3]

The clear risks of endodontic involvement in teeth that require restorations mandate a careful prerestorative evaluation, particularly as the case size and complexity increases. Endodontic intervention should be planned and integrated into a logical treatment sequence before any therapy is started. Both the patient and the clinician must be aware of the interdisciplinary nature of this approach.

Indications for prerestorative endodontic therapy

The evaluation of teeth to be restored should include the following endodontic considerations: (1) the health of the root canal system, (2) the impact of planned restorative procedures

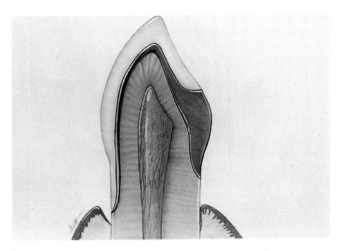

FIG. 21-1 Attachment loss often results in elongated clinical crowns. Restorative procedures require additional dentin removal from the axial walls and may be detrimental to pulpal vitality.

on the pulp, and (3) the magnitude of the restorative effort. Instances in which restorative requirements significantly decrease predictability of pulpal health should be managed with preventive endodontics.

Restorative Procedures and the Pulp

Prophylactic endodontics

Teeth to be restored are candidates for prophylactic endodontic therapy when restorative procedures requiring significant dentin removal are likely to endanger pulpal integrity. For example, vital teeth with minimal remaining tooth structure often require auxiliary retention for restorations. Retentive grooves, boxes, and pins are placed at the expense of the dentin; this can ultimately compromise vitality. Judicious endodontic therapy can be crucial to the success of the restoration when substantial tooth structure is missing. A tooth that has lost pivotal coronal dentin to caries, fracture, or old restorations may remain vital but exhibit insufficient supragingival tooth structure for retention of a new restoration. In this case the root canal system may be considered an extension of the restorative zone and the tooth devitalized to allow placement of a dowel-core-crown restoration.

Substantial tooth preparation is common in cases with missing or malposed teeth, and this can jeopardize pulpal health. Preparation of nonparallel abutment teeth for fixed restorations entails extensive dentin removal from axial walls, which can encroach on the pulp. Intracoronal attachments are also used to solve problems of missing or malposed teeth. However, the additional preparation needed for placement of the attachment within the confines of the crown can result in irreversible pulpal injury.

Periodontally involved teeth are at risk for pulpal involvement when crown margins are placed considerably apical to the cementoenamel junction (Fig. 21-1). The narrow circumference of the root dictates increased dentin removal to prepare tapered axial walls. The remaining layer of tooth structure overlying the pulp may be too thin to protect against irreversible degeneration from the combined effects of the

tooth preparation process and potentially irritating restorative materials.

Prerestorative endodontic therapy is also prescribed before restoration of periodontally involved vital teeth when root amputation or hemisection is planned to salvage portions of guarded teeth. Similarly, teeth with significant periodontal bone loss can be endodontically treated and the roots retained to provide needed support for an overdenture.

Major occlusal correction of vital teeth may also dictate endodontic treatment before crown placement. Decreasing the occlusal height of a hypererupted tooth to restore a proper occlusal plane may necessitate devitalizing the tooth. Similarly, correction of an unfavorable crown-root ratio is accomplished by decreasing the clinical crown height through substantial coronal reduction. Prophylactic endodontics should be considered to avoid access preparation through the crown at a later date.

Endodontic therapy should be planned in advance for teeth with fragile pulpal systems that require a cast restoration. Treatment of chronic pulpitis is more efficient and effective when the tooth is endodontically treated before placement of a crown or bridge retainer. The dental history of a tooth must be considered before crown preparation. Teeth that have undergone multiple episodes of dental disease or trauma and multiple dental procedures have an increased risk for subsequent pulpal breakdown. Vital teeth should be treated endodontically first if they have a guarded pulpal prognosis and would be difficult to treat endodontically after completion of the planned restoration.

Magnitude of the restorative treatment. As the size and complexity of the restorative effort increase, the need for prerestorative endodontics simultaneously increases. The hazards associated with retroactive treatment are serious and dangerous risks. Endodontic access through an existing restoration can remove a significant portion of the underlying dentin core and vertical walls of the underlying preparation. This can disrupt the cement seal integrity and compromise retention and resistance of the restoration. Loss of cement seal and ensuing leakage at the crown margins can result in severe caries of the dentin core inside the crown. Core caries of a nonvital tooth is difficult to detect with radiographs or symptoms until the damage is severe (Fig. 21-2). Extensive caries extending into the root may require periodontal crown lengthening surgery to expose the carious dentin for repair. Root caries is sometimes not restorable, resulting in a need for extraction and possible loss of a multitooth fixed restoration. Creation of an access opening through an all-ceramic or a porcelain-fused-to-metal crown also structurally weakens the restoration. Simply perforating the glazed porcelain surface reduces porcelain strength significantly. Perforation of the occlusal porcelain and the metal coping can weaken the porcelain bond strength enough to cause separation of the porcelain veneer from the metal substructure. Clearly, although it is possible to perform endodontic procedures after restorations are complete, postrestorative endodontics should be avoided whenever possible.

In more compromised dentitions, occlusal requirements may alter the normal relationship of root anatomy to clinical crown in the restored dentition. The disorientation of crown morphology and underlying root form can lead to difficulty in endodontic access and result in excessive removal of coronal tooth structure. In the severe case this disorientation can contribute to a mechanical perforation of the root (Fig. 21-3). These clinical realities may not greatly impact a treatment plan for the

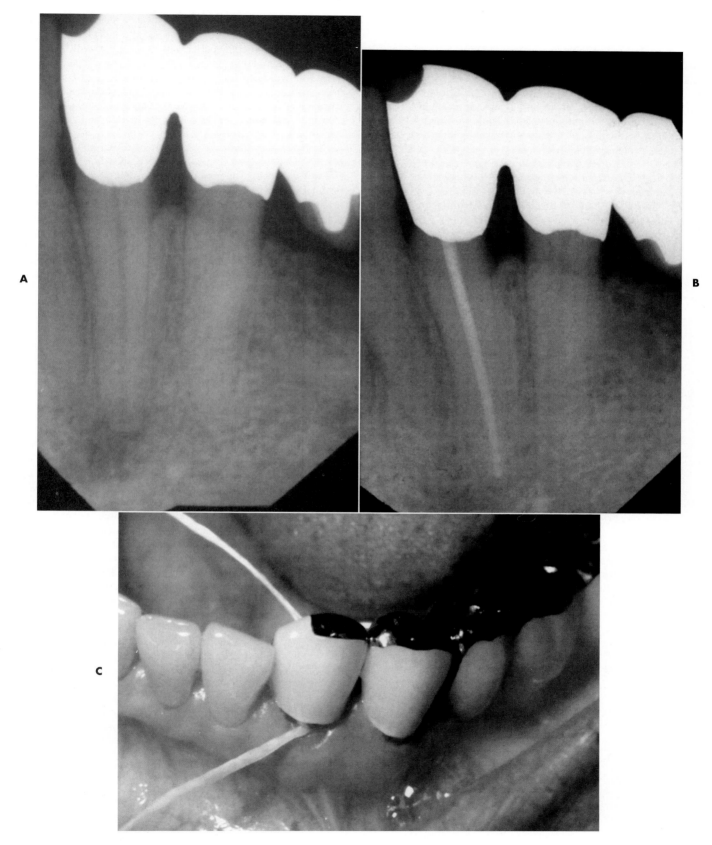

FIG. 21-2 A, Existing fixed partial denture with periapical lesion. **B,** After endodontic therapy. **C,** Rapid loss of cement seal with resultant carious destruction of anterior abutment. *(Courtesy Dr. George Gara.)*

tooth requiring a single crown but may cause rapid destruction of the larger, more fragile, more complex restoration. These cases require prerestorative endodontic evaluation and the definitive treatment of strategic teeth with questionable pulpal prognosis.

Pretreatment evaluation. Before initiation of restorative therapy the tooth must be thoroughly evaluated to ensure success of all ultimate treatment goals. The tooth should be examined individually and in the context of its contribution to the overall treatment plan. Adjacent teeth, opposing teeth, and patient desires for treatment should be considered. This survey includes endodontic, periodontal, restorative, and aesthetic evaluations.

Endodontic evaluation: In addition to identification of nonvital teeth and the endodontic evaluation of vital teeth described above, the prerestorative examination should include an inspection of the quality of existing endodontic treatment. New restorations, particularly complex restorations, should not

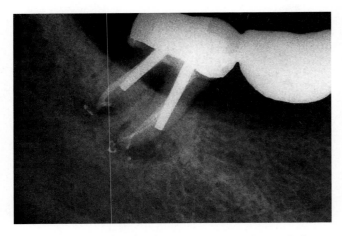

FIG. 21-3 Root anatomy dictates dowel location and dimension. Occlusal surface anatomy of this molar was used to project root location. Long axis dislocation of the restored crown and the root can result in dramatic clinical errors.

be placed on abutment teeth with a questionable endodontic prognosis. Endodontic retreatment may be indicated for teeth that exhibit radiographic periapical pathology or clinical symptoms of inflammation (see Chapter 24). Restorations that require a dowel need a dowel space, which is prepared by removal of gutta-percha from the canal. Canals obturated with a silver cone or other inappropriate filling materials should be identified and endodontically retreated before the start of restorative therapy.

Periodontal evaluation: Maintenance of periodontal health is critical to the long-term success of endodontically treated and restored teeth. The periodontal condition of the tooth must be determined before initiation of endodontic therapy. In addition to a conventional periodontal examination the effect of the planned restoration on the attachment apparatus must be considered. Many teeth suffer from significant structural defects that jeopardize coronal reconstruction. Extensive caries, tooth fracture, previous restorations, perforations, and external resorption can destroy tooth structure at the level of the periodontal attachment. An attempt to place restorative margins on solid tooth structure beyond these defects further invades the biologic attachment zone. Violation of the biologic width is an invitation to failure of the clinical results (Fig. 21-4). A mutilated tooth in which restorative treatment would compromise the junctional epithelium or connective tissue attachment levels should be scheduled for periodontal crown lengthening surgery or orthodontic extrusion, in addition to endodontic and restorative procedures.

Restorative evaluation: A restorative examination of the tooth should be performed before initiation of any definitive therapy. It is essential to determine if the tooth is restorable before endodontic treatment is performed. The strategic importance of a tooth should be determined before a final plan is formulated. Mutilated teeth may not warrant extensive treatment if adjacent healthy teeth are available as abutments; extraction of an extensively damaged tooth may be indicated. Conversely, the distal-most tooth in a quadrant can be critical to avoid a distal extension removable partial denture and may merit extensive reconstructive efforts. Similarly, the success of a large restoration may depend on the availability of an intermediate abutment or strategic tooth within a sextant.

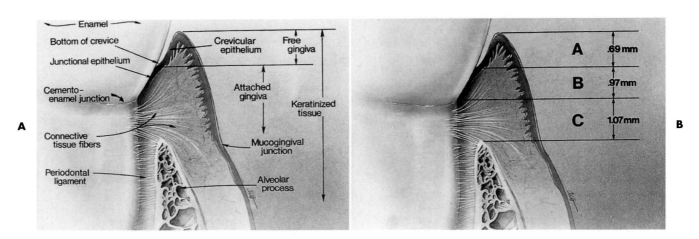

FIG. 21-4 A, Anatomy of the healthy attachment apparatus. **B,** Defective tooth structures necessitating margin placement into zones B and C are indications for crown lengthening surgery or orthodontic extrusion. These zones contain the junctional epithelium and the connective tissue attachments.

In addition to the strategic position the reliability of the tooth after restoration should be considered before inclusion in a final treatment plan. The tooth to be retained must be able to withstand the functional forces placed on it after reconstruction. Large amounts of missing tooth structure can be replaced with a cast restoration, a core, and possibly a dowel. However, a critical amount of solid coronal dentin is required, and this must be encased in a metal coping for structural integrity of the restored tooth. This ferrule has been shown to significantly reduce the incidence of fracture in the root canal–treated tooth.[49] If sufficient solid tooth structure to accommodate a restoration with a ferrule is not available, the tooth should first be treated periodontally, orthodontically, or extracted.

Aesthetic evaluation: Potential aesthetic complications should be investigated before initiation of endodontic therapy. Thin gingiva may transmit a shadow of dark root color through the tissue. Metal, carbon, or amalgam dowels placed in the canal can result in unacceptable gingival discoloration from the underlying root. The translucency of all-ceramic crowns must be considered in the selection of dowel and buildup materials; zirconium and other translucent dowels are recent additions to the aesthetic armamentarium. Similarly, tooth-colored, rather than opaque, composite core material should be selected for the aesthetic case. An aesthetic tooth that does not need a crown after endodontic treatment requires critical control of endodontic filling materials in the coronal third of the canal and the pulp chamber (Fig. 21-5). The color and translucency of most uncrowned teeth are adversely affected by opaque substances. Similarly, discoloration from gutta-percha can be visible in the coronal aspect of an endodontically treated tooth and should be limited to an apical level in the root. Endodontic and restorative materials in these aesthetically critical cases must be selected to provide the best health service with the minimum of aesthetic compromise.

The total evaluation of clinical problems should be completed before any definitive therapy is started. When endodontic treatment is initiated by an acute pulpitis, treatment should be restricted to emergency care. After stabilization, the clinician should return and complete the entire evaluation before continuing treatment. Accurate assimilation of endodontic, periodontal, restorative, and aesthetic variables contributes to a rational, successful treatment outcome. There are instances in which endodontic therapy could succeed but failure would occur in other disciplines of dentistry. These conditions should be detected and treated with an interdisciplinary approach to maximize success. In the extreme case, extraction may be indicated for teeth where endodontics could succeed but completion of the total treatment plan is impossible because of periodontal or restorative deficiencies that cannot be corrected. These cases must be identified in the planning stage, and replacement of the condemned teeth must then be included in the overall treatment plan.

RESTORATIVE DENTISTRY AND THE NONVITAL TOOTH

Effects of Endodontics on the Tooth

Changes in endodontically treated teeth

The disease processes and restorative procedures that create the need for endodontic therapy affect much more than the pulp vitality. The tooth structure that remains after endodontic treatment has been undermined and weakened by the previous epi-sodes of caries, fracture, tooth preparation, and restoration. Endodontic manipulation further removes important intracoronal and intraradicular dentin. Finally, the endodontic treatment changes the actual composition of the remaining tooth structure. The combined result of these changes is the common clinical finding of increased fracture susceptibility and decreased translucency in nonvital teeth. As restorations for endodontically treated teeth are designed to compensate for these changes, it is important to understand the effects of endodontics on the tooth and the significance of each factor. The major changes in the endodontically treated tooth include (1) loss of tooth structure, (2) altered physical characteristics, and (3) altered aesthetic characteristics of the residual tooth.

Loss of tooth structure. The decreased strength seen in endodontically treated teeth is primarily caused by the loss of coronal tooth structure and is not a direct result of the endodontic treatment. Endodontic procedures have been shown to reduce tooth stiffness by only 5%, whereas a mesioocclusodistal (MOD) preparation reduces stiffness by 60%.[43] Endodontic access into the pulp chamber destroys the structural integrity provided by the coronal dentin of the pulpal roof and allows greater flexing of the tooth under function.[25] In cases with significantly reduced remaining tooth structure, normal functional forces may fracture undermined cusps or fracture the tooth in the area of the smallest circumference, frequently at the cementoenamel junction. The decreased volume of tooth structure from the combined effect of prior dental procedures create a significant potential for fracture of the endodontically treated tooth.

Altered physical characteristics. The tooth structure remaining after endodontic therapy also exhibits irreversibly altered physical properties. Changes in collagen cross-linking and dehydration of the dentin result in a 14% reduction in strength and toughness of endodontically treated molars. Maxillary teeth are stronger than mandibular teeth, and mandibular incisors are the weakest.[25] The combined loss of structural integrity, loss of moisture, and loss of dentin toughness compromises endodontically treated teeth and necessitates special care in the restoration of pulpless teeth.

Altered aesthetic characteristics. Aesthetic changes also occur in endodontically treated teeth. Biochemically altered dentin modifies light refraction through the tooth and modifies its appearance. The darkening of nonvital anterior teeth is well known. Inadequate endodontic cleaning and shaping of the coronal area also contributes to this discoloration by staining the dentin from degradation of vital tissue left in the pulp horns. Medicaments used in dental treatment and remnants of root canal filling material can affect the appearance of endodontically treated teeth. Endodontic treatment and restoration of teeth in the aesthetic zone require careful control of procedures and materials to retain a translucent, natural appearance.

Treatment planning for restoration of nonvital teeth

All the changes that accompany root canal therapy influence the selection of restorative procedures for endodontically treated teeth. Tooth structure loss can range from very minimal access preparations in intact teeth to very extensive damage that endangers the longevity of the tooth itself. A wide array of restorative materials and techniques are available to address problems presented by nonvital teeth at every point along this damage scale.

Restorative treatment decisions depend on the amount of remaining tooth structure, the functional demands that will be

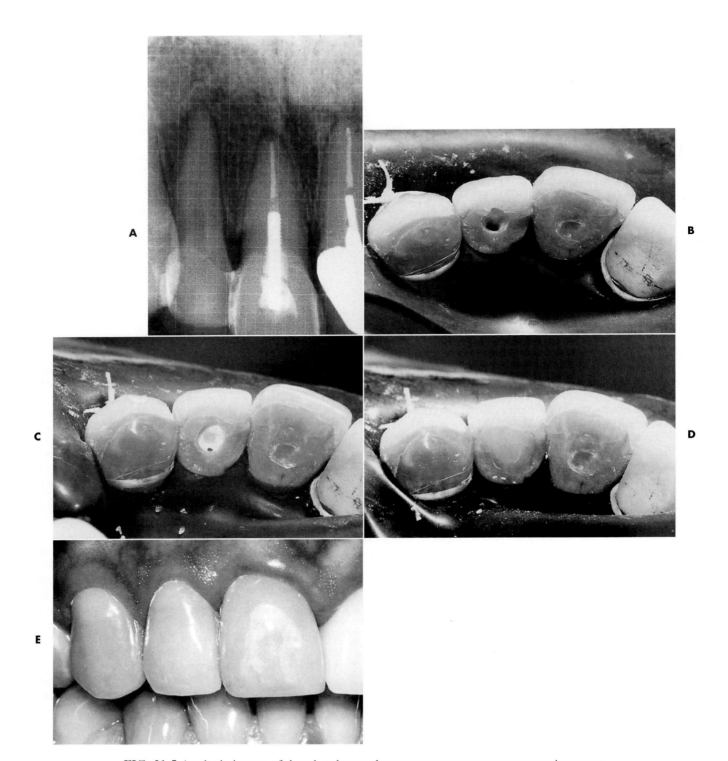

FIG. 21-5 Aesthetic impact of dowel and core placement on contemporary restorations must be understood. **A,** Trauma necessitated restorative and endodontic therapy in the anterior maxilla. Lateral incisor subsequently became nonvital. **B,** Conservative access is made, leaving the porcelain veneer intact. **C,** Pulp chamber and coronal orifice of canal are filled with glass-ionomer cement. **D,** Bonded resin restoration placed in the access opening. **E,** Anterior aesthetics of the veneer are unaltered by the restorative materials selected.

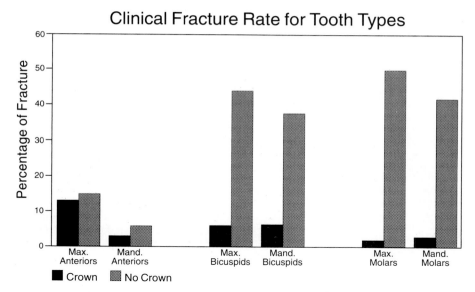

Clinical Fracture Rate for Tooth Types

(y-axis: Percentage of Fracture)

Categories: Max. Anteriors, Mand. Anteriors, Max. Bicuspids, Mand. Bicuspids, Max. Molars, Mand. Molars

■ Crown   ▨ No Crown

FIG. 21-6 Fracture of nonvital teeth increases in the posterior dentition when a coronal coverage restoration is not used.[52]

placed on the tooth, and the need for the tooth as an abutment in a larger restoration. Posterior teeth carry greater occlusal forces than anterior teeth, and restorations must be planned to protect posterior teeth against fracture (Fig. 21-6). The horizontal and torquing forces endured by abutments for fixed or removable partial dentures dictate more extensive protective and retentive features in the restoration. Teeth with minimal remaining tooth structure have an increased risk for fracture, provide decreased retention for the restoration, and are in jeopardy for invasion of the periodontal attachment.

As the remaining tooth structure decreases and functional forces increase, greater restorative control is needed. Extensively damaged or missing tooth structure fundamentally alters the use of restorative procedures and the need for adjunctive treatment from the other specialties. Misunderstanding or misuse of integrated therapy can lead to an ever-shortening cycle of treatment, breakdown, and retreatment.

Basic Components Used in Restoration of the Nonvital Tooth

Restorations for endodontically treated teeth are designed to replace the missing tooth structure and to protect the remaining tooth structure from fracture. The final restoration will include some combination of (1) dowel, (2) core, and (3) coronal restoration. The selection of the individual components for the restoration depends on whether the nonvital tooth is an anterior or posterior tooth and whether significant coronal tooth structure is missing. Not every endodontically treated tooth needs a crown or a dowel. Some teeth need all three components, and some need only an access seal for the coronal restoration.[36] It is critically important to understand the clinical indications for each component, for overuse or underuse of dowels and crowns can increase the risk of unrestorable fracture. The purpose of each component, restoration design guidelines, and clinical procedures are described in the following sections.

Intact anterior teeth. Nonvital anterior teeth that have not lost tooth structure beyond the endodontic access preparation are at minimal risk for fracture and do not require a crown,

core, or dowel. Restorative treatment is limited to sealing of the access cavity.

Extensively damaged teeth. When a nonvital anterior or posterior tooth has lost significant tooth structure, a cast coronal restoration is required. An intermediary restoration, the dowel and core, is used to support and retain the crown. The final configuration of the restored tooth includes four parts (Fig. 21-7):

1. Residual tooth structure and periodontal attachment apparatus
2. Dowel material, located within the root
3. Core material, located in the coronal area of the tooth
4. Definitive coronal restoration

The dowel and core function together. The core replaces lost coronal tooth structure and provides retention for the crown. The dowel provides retention for the restorative material of the core and must be designed to minimize the potential for root fracture from functional forces. The crown restores function and aesthetics and protects the remaining root and coronal structure from fracture. The specific design of each dowel and core is determined by the relative clinical need for each of these functions.[7] The major design classifications are discussed in relation to their ability to satisfy these requirements.

Dowel (post) (Fig. 21-7)

The dowel is a post or other rigid restorative material placed in the radicular portion of a nonvital tooth. It functions primarily to aid retention of the restoration and secondarily to distribute forces along the length of the root. The dowel thus has a retentive role and does not strengthen a tooth. Instead, the tooth is weakened if dentin is sacrificed to facilitate larger dowel placement. This is an important distinction, as significant damage can result from misplaced efforts to fortify roots with large dowels (Fig. 21-8). The foremost function of the dowel is to provide retention for the core and coronal restoration and to do so without increasing the risk of root fracture.

Retentive role of the dowel. When a tooth has suffered significant coronal damage, insufficient sound tooth structure

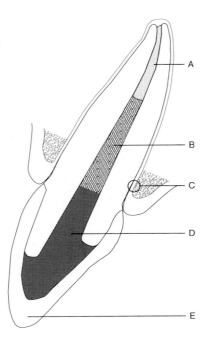

FIG. 21-7 Final configuration of the restored, endodontically treated tooth. Apical endodontic seal is preserved with 3 to 5 mm of gutta-percha *(A)*. Dowel *(B)* is the restorative material within the root. Core *(D)* replaces missing coronal tooth structure and retains the final coronal restoration *(E)*. Restorative and endodontic therapy must preserve the residual root and its attachment mechanism *(C)*.

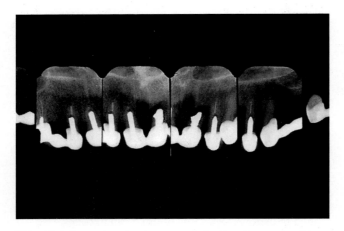

FIG. 21-8 Excessive dentin removal for the placement of large dowels results in weakened tooth structure.

is left above the periodontal attachment to secure a restoration. The dowel within the residual root extends apically to anchor the materials used to support the crown. The root and dowel collectively can be considered an extension of the restorative zone.

For the dowel to function in this retentive role, there must be clinically adequate retention between both the dowel and root and between the dowel and core. Dowel design, cementing media, core material, and functional load effect the ability of dowels to be retained within the root and simultaneously to anchor the core. It is important, however, to differentiate be-

tween clinically adequate and excessive retention. Retention between the dowel and the root that is greater than necessary is not desirable and can lead to failure from untreatable root fracture rather than from loss of the restoration. Cementation technology is rapidly changing clinical concepts regarding dowel retention. Basic dowel design guidelines will change with the continued development of improved adhesive dental agents.

Nonthreatening role of the dowel. Occlusal forces are transferred through the core to the dowel and ultimately along the length of the root. The dowel must be designed in such a way that it serves its retentive function without endangering the root or coronal integrity. The remaining dentin and dowel together must have adequate rigidity to withstand the functional loads sustained by the tooth without deformation. Distortion of the dowel under function results ultimately in the failure of the dowel, remaining tooth structure, and the restoration.

The dowel must remain in the root for a successful restoration, but must not damage the root in attempts to achieve maximal retention. Dowels should be retained by cementation to the dentin walls of the root; active engagement of the dowel space by screw threads is contraindicated. Maximal retention but a maximal incidence of fracture is found with screw type of dowels.[6,18] The risk of root fracture is significant and partially dependent on dowel length and surface configurations. In a clinical evaluation of dowels and cores beneath existing crowns, 10% of all failures were due to root fracture.[21] In an earlier clinical study, 40% of self-threaded dowels failed by angular and vertical root fracture, whereas almost 98% of cemented, parallel-sided dowels were successful.[51]

Dowel design. The nonthreatening and retentive capacity of the dowel depends on the appropriate combination of mechanical design features. The relevant variables are the dowel (1) length, (2) taper, (3) diameter, (4) surface configuration, and (5) cement type. Dowels are designed to take best advantage of each of these qualities; thus no single approach or single system for the intermediary dowel and core restoration is sufficient for all cases. The following discussion of dowel variables is derived from research based on the use of metal dowels with nondentin bonded cements. Acceptable dowel design guidelines for length, taper, diameter, and surface configuration change with increased understanding of these variables as they relate to dentin bonding technology. Additionally, the proliferation of nonmetallic dowel materials further modifies existing dowel guidelines.

Dowel classifications. The two major categories of dowels consist of preformed dowel systems (Fig. 21-9) and custom cast dowels (Fig. 21-10). The proprietary preformed dowel systems include various sizes of premade dowels. The traditional dowel material is metal, but the preformed dowel classification has been expanded to include numerous nonmetal dowel structures. Matching instrumentation is used to form a dowel space within the root (Fig. 21-11). The corresponding, preformed dowel is secured to the root by cement, and a core is formed from a variety of restorative materials. A custom cast dowel system uses a casting procedure to fabricate a one-piece metal dowel and core, which has no interface between the dowel and the core. By using instrumentation that is paired with castable plastic patterns (Fig. 21-12), the dowel space is shaped to standardized dimensions and may incorporate some customizing of the final dowel shape to that of the canal. A custom resin dowel and core pattern is produced, invested, and cast in a crown and

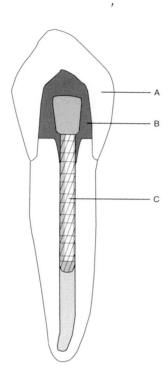

FIG. 21-9 Preformed dowel and core restoration. Preformed metal dowel *(C)* is cemented into the prepared dowel space. Core material *(B)* is retained by the dowel, by bonding to the tooth structure by undercuts in the pulp chamber and occasionally by auxiliary retentive pins, grooves, or boxes. Coronal restoration *(A)* provides the ferrule and restores aesthetics and function.

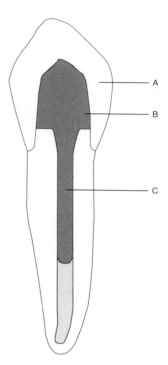

FIG. 21-10 Cast dowel and core restoration. Dowel and the core *(B)* are cast of the same material and cemented to the tooth as a single unit. Coronal restoration *(A)* provides the ferrule and restores aesthetics and function.

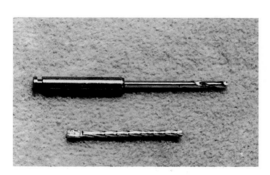

FIG. 21-11 Instrumentation used for fabrication of a preformed dowel. Drill refines the dowel space after initial gutta-percha removal. Corresponding preformed metal dowel should seat easily without active engagement of the dentin walls. *(Courtesy Para Post System, Whaledent International, Mahwah, N.J.)*

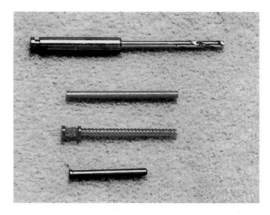

FIG. 21-12 Instrumentation used for fabrication of a cast dowel. *From top,* Drill refines the dowel space after initial gutta-percha removal. Color-coded plastic impression dowel and plastic burnout dowel are used for the indirect technique; plastic burnout dowel only is used for the direct cast dowel. Corresponding aluminum dowel is used to retain a provisional restoration. *(Courtesy Para Post System, Whaledent International, Mahwah, N.J.)*

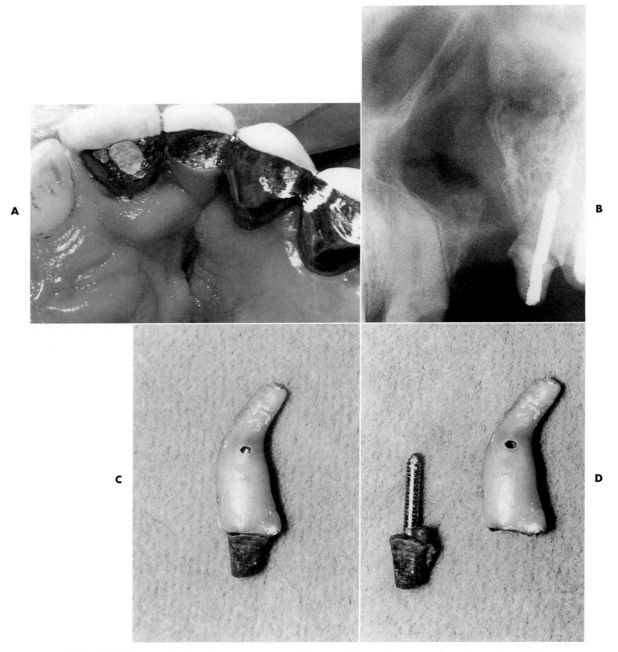

FIG. 21-13 Substantial tooth structure (a minimum of 1 mm) must surround the dowel for strength. **A,** Persistent symptoms in the treated canine adjacent to the cleft were diagnosed as a root perforation. **B,** Radiograph appears to demonstrate an intact root surface. **C,** Extracted tooth reveals the dowel visible through the perforation. **D,** Dowel and core separation from the root verify that the perforation occurred at the apex of the dowel.

bridge alloy. The final cast dowel and core are cemented to the residual tooth structure at a subsequent appointment.

Alternative custom dowel techniques are sometimes used, but they generally require increased fabrication time and are often technique sensitive. These include two-part dowel and core restorations for nonparallel roots, totally custom-tapered dowels, and other highly individualized approaches to clinical problems.

Dowel length. Dowel retention is proportional to dowel length; increasing the dowel length increases the retention. The dowel length selected for a given root depends on a number of factors. Generally stated, the dowel should be long enough to satisfy clinical requirements without jeopardizing the root integrity. The standard parameters for dowel length in a tooth with normal periodontal support range between (1) two thirds the length of the canal, (2) an amount equal to the coronal length of the tooth, and (3) half the length of root supported by bone. These guidelines are reasonable and useful clinical tools.[21] The final length of the dowel in the periodontally healthy tooth is limited by two major variables, the root morphology and the need for sufficient apical seal in the root canal system.

Root morphology plays a great role in the determination of dowel length. The total root length is the most obvious factor in dowel length design. Equally important are root taper, root curvature, and cross-sectional root form. Clear and nondistorted radiographs reveal root length, taper, and curvature. The root should have more than 1 mm of tooth structure remaining circumferentially around the apical end of the dowel to avoid perforation and resist fracture (Fig. 21-13). This concept dictates a shorter dowel in a tapered root so that the apical extent of the dowel does not impinge on converging root walls. A longer dowel can safely be placed in a parallel-sided root of equal length. Root curvature reduces dowel length in a similar manner; the greater the curve of the root and the more coronally located the curve, the shorter will be the dowel. Cross-sectional root form cannot be determined by conventional radiographs, as root concavities are not readily visible in a two-dimensional film. Thorough knowledge of root morphology for each tooth is mandatory for dowel placement. Furcations, both faciolingual and mesiodistal, along with developmental depressions are present in predictable locations in the dentition (Fig. 21-14). Maxillary first molars have deep concavities on the furcal surface of 94% of the mesiobuccal roots, 31% of distobuccal roots, and 17% of palatal roots. Mandibular first molars have root concavities on the furcal surface of 100% of mesial roots and 99% of distal roots.[4] Maxillary first premolars have deep mesial concavities and slender roots with minimal dentin walls. Endodontically treated teeth with these root concavities require alteration of the length and placement of dowel materials to eliminate thin dentinal walls or outright root perforations.[25]

The need to maintain adequate obturation is the second major factor limiting dowel length. Retaining the last 3 to 5 mm of filling material at the apex is sufficient for the endodontic seal.[22] A dowel placed closer to the apex than this distance, even when surrounded by adequate tooth structure, risks failure of the seal and thus of the restorative effort (Fig. 21-15). Alveolar bone height also influences dowel length. Occlusal forces generate the least risk to the remaining tooth structure and surrounding bone when a dowel extends apical to the alveolar crest. Short dowels transfer forces to the unsupported root extending above the alveolus and can cause root fracture.

When dowels are indicated, they should be placed in roots that are husky, straight, and long. Root anatomy of multirooted teeth is most suitable in the palatal roots of maxillary molars, palatal roots of maxillary premolars, and distal roots of mandibular molars.

Dowel shape. Placement of a parallel-sided dowel within the canal improves both the retention and the force distribution of the dowel. Parallel-sided dowels are more retentive than tapered dowels and distribute functional loads to the root passively. Parallel dowels are indicated for the majority of cases. Tapered dowels act like a wedge to exert significant lateral forces on the tooth structure. These forces may ultimately result in a vertical root fracture. Tapered dowel form has been generally reserved for the significantly tapered canal system where use of a parallel-sided dowel would necessitate rigorous alteration of the radicular dentin walls. Tapered canals with thin, fragile walls may be reinforced internally with composite resin, cured by light-transmitting dowels. The design of the crown is critical to protect teeth with thin dentin walls against root fracture.

As root canals are not parallel in shape, some preparation of the canal is required for a parallel-sided dowel. The taper of the canal system dictates the amount of tooth structure to be removed for dowel placement. Instrumentation of the radicular dentin walls during dowel space preparation should be very conservative. Severe alteration of a tapered canal system to accept a parallel dowel defies the concept of preservation of tooth structure. This means that conservative parallel dowels in funnel-shaped canals do not contact the coronal aspect of the canal wall and are surrounded by layer of cement. It is not necessary to have intimate tooth-to-dowel contact in all areas of the restoration (Fig. 21-16). To the contrary, tapered dowels that are closely adapted to the internal shape of the root canal are more likely to result in extensive root fracture than parallel-sided dowels.[49]

Dowel diameter. The dowel must be of a sufficient diameter to resist functional forces. The dowel-to-root dynamics are not improved by increasing the diameter beyond that point. A larger diameter gives little or no improvement in the dowel-to-root retention but significantly reduces the resistance of the tooth to fracture (Fig. 21-17). The preservation of dentin in the radicular areas takes precedence over the larger diameter dowel.

Dowel surface configuration. The surface of a dowel can be smooth or serrated. Serrated surfaces provide mechanical undercuts for cement and significantly increase retention of parallel dowels over that of smooth surfaces, when cemented with traditional, nonadhesive cements. Serrations can be horizontal with a single vertical vent channel, or patterned with flutes or diamond shapes, such that the serrations from a series of vents reduce hydraulic forces generated during cementation.

The mechanical features that contribute the greatest retention with traditional cements are increased length, parallel sides, and a serrated surface of the dowel. The mechanical features that contribute most to the ability of the dowel to resist forces are an increased length, parallel sides, and moderate diameter of the dowel. The most important aspect of fracture prevention, however, is not the dowel design but the final crown. The majority of early dowel and force studies were performed on unrestored teeth. The differences in fracture rate between various dowel designs disappeared when crowns were placed.[20]

Dowel materials. Materials used in dowel construction must be able to withstand functional stresses, must resist corrosion, and must not be harmful to the patient. Traditional dowel materials include alloys of gold, stainless steel, titanium, and dental amalgam. Newer, nonmetallic dowel materials may mimic the physical and aesthetic characteristics of dentin.

Desirable properties: The dentition in function is subject to intermittent forces, loaded in multiple directions, which must be considered when selecting materials to reconstruct teeth after endodontic therapy. Important physical requirements for dowels include adequate stiffness, high yield strength, and favorable fatigue properties. Insufficient stiffness results in stress concentration as the dowel repeatedly deforms and springs back under function. This stress concentration can ultimately cause fracture and failure of the tooth or restoration. Of the newer nonmetallic structures, dowels of carbon fiber material have demonstrated significantly lower tooth fracture occurrence in vitro when compared to metal dowels.[30] The stiffness of the dowel also plays a role in the maintenance of marginal integrity of the coronal restoration by protecting fragile restorative margins from high functional loads. This can cause failure of the restorative material at the crown margin or degradation of the cement, resulting in caries at or under the margin.

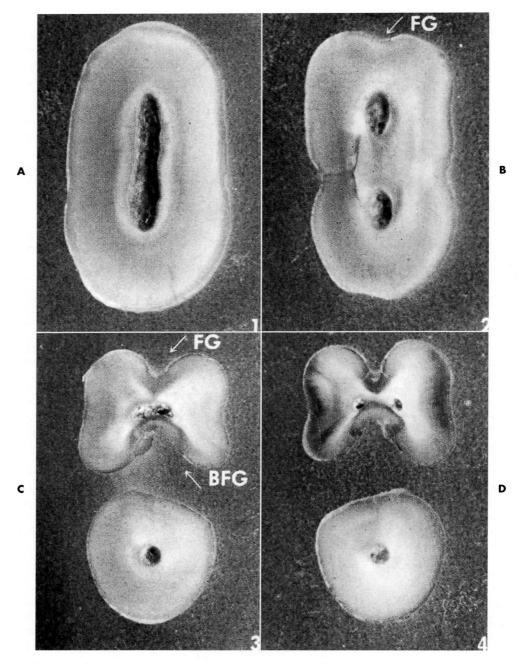

FIG. 21-14 Root anatomy has significant influence over dowel placement. **A,** Cross section of a maxillary first premolar at the cementoenamel junction; the buccal surface faces the top of the section. **B,** Two millimeters apical to the cementoenamel junction, root irregularities and developmental depressions become apparent. **C,** Four millimeters apical to the cemento-enamel junction, the root has separated into buccal *(top)* and palatal roots and developmental grooves have deepened. **D,** Six millimeters apical to the cementoenamel junction, the buccal root continues to demonstrate more accentuated depressions. Placement of a dowel in the buc-cal root risks perforation into the furcation of this tooth. Palatal root is a better choice for dowel placement. *(From Gher ME, Vernino AR:* Int J Periodont Rest Dent *1(5):52-63, 1981.)*

Low yield strength materials bend and transfer stresses to the restoration. Deformation of the dowel endangers the remaining tooth structure, core material, crown, and cement. Similarly, dowels possessing unfavorable fatigue properties are subject to premature failure when exposed to the repetitive characteristics of oral function. This metal fatigue manifests as a fracture of the dowel and may lead to fracture of the tooth.

Dowel materials should be selected that are inert or highly resistant to the corrosive effects of oral fluids. The most significant corrosion occurs in stainless steel dowels that have been invested, heated, and allowed to cool when a custom core is cast onto a preformed metal dowel.[50] Corrosion is not an issue with entirely custom cast dowel and cores, as these are fabricated completely from nonreactive gold alloys. Preformed systems traditionally use dowels made of stainless steel alloys containing nickel and chrome. The preformed dowels exhibit high strength and ease of use for reconstructing the endodontically treated tooth. Recent concern about the potential for sensitivity and allergy production by nickel alloys has been raised. Biocompatible titanium or nonmetallic preformed dowels have less allergenic potential than stainless steel alloys. These non-stainless steel dowels, however, are significantly less radiopaque than the nickel-chrome alloys. The radiopacity of titanium dowels is similar to gutta-percha.[24] These dowels are difficult to distinguish in radiographs with densely condensed, gutta-percha filled canals (Fig. 21-18).

In summary, conventional dowels should be passive and cemented into place. The residual dentin should undergo minimal alteration to accept the dowel. Length and diameter should be the minimal dimensions needed to withstand functional loading. Dowels should be parallel walled with a serrated surface. They should be fabricated from materials that exhibit physical properties for long-term success and materials that will not corrode. The dowel should be an extension into the conservatively shaped root canal system, not an intrusion into the radicular dentin. The goal of dowel design is clinically sufficient retention of the dowel and maximal fracture resistance of the root, not the converse (Fig. 21-16).

Core (see Fig. 21-7)

The core consists of restorative material placed in the coronal area of a tooth. This material replaces carious, fractured, or otherwise missing coronal structure and retains the final crown.

The core is anchored to the tooth by extending into the coronal aspect of the canal or through the endodontic dowel. The

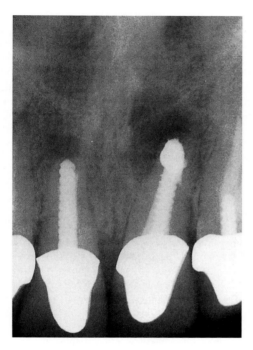

FIG. 21-15 Long, large diameter dowels obliterate the apical seal and cause endodontic failure of two central incisors. Three to five millimeters of intact endodontic seal must be retained at the apex.

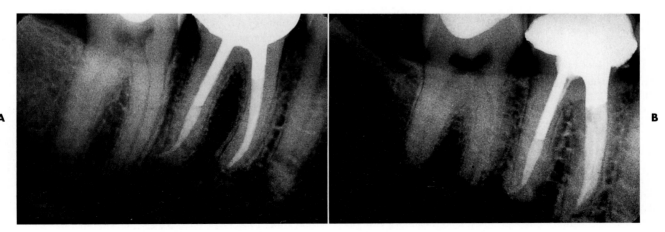

FIG. 21-16 Components of a successful restoration can be seen in these two radiographs of the same tooth. **A,** Gutta-percha seal is intact. Minimal dowel space instrumentation allows the dowel to be an extension of the canal system in the distal root. Cementing medium is evident in the larger, coronal opening of the distal canal. **B,** Mesial roots contain alloy condensed into the first 2 to 4 mm of the canal. Coronal restoration provides protection, function, and if needed aesthetics. *(Courtesy Dr. Frank Casanova.)*

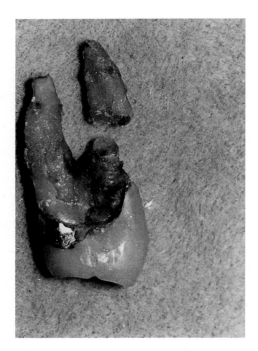

FIG. 21-17 Large dowel diameter in the buccal root resulted in a functional fracture of this premolar. Coronal to the fracture, the dowel can be seen through the thinned root surface. Excessive radicular dentin removal weakened the tooth.

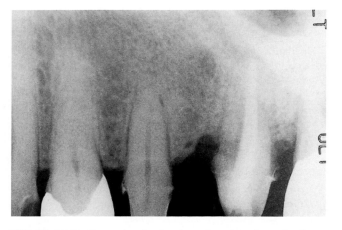

FIG. 21-18 Radiograph of a titanium dowel in the palatal root of the maxillary first molar. This material is more difficult to detect on radiographs than stainless steel or cast dowels.

attachment between tooth, dowel, and core is mechanical or chemical, as the core and dowel are usually fabricated from different materials.

The remaining tooth structure can also be altered to augment retention of the core or to provide resistance to core rotation under function. Pins, grooves, and channels can be placed in the dentin in a position remote from the dowel space and keyways. However, these modifications increase the core retention and resistance to rotation at the expense of tooth structure. In most cases the irregular nature of the residual coronal tooth structure and the normal morphology of the pulp chamber and canal orifices eliminate the need for these tooth

alterations. Using restorative materials that bond to tooth structure enhances retention and resistance without the need to remove valuable dentin. Therefore if additional retentive or antirotation form for the core is deemed necessary, dentin removal should be kept to a minimum.

Desirable physical characteristics of a core include (1) high compressive strength, (2) dimensional stability, (3) ease of manipulation, (4) short setting time, and (5) an ability to bond to both tooth and dowel. Contemporary cores include cast metal, amalgam, composite resin, and glass-ionomer materials.[9,13]

Cast metal core (Fig. 21-10). A cast dowel and core are a traditional and proven method to restore endodontically treated teeth. The core is an integral extension of the dowel, and the cast core does not depend on mechanical means for retention to the dowel. This construction avoids dislodgment of the core and crown from the dowel and root when minimal tooth structure remains. Noble metals are noncorrosive, and ceramometal alloys exhibit increased stiffness for decreased dentin deformation. The cast dowel and core can provide antirotation features with eccentric preparations in the dentin, retentive pins, or a cervical collar at the base of the core.[28] These antirotation features also increase core and crown retention. The cast dowel and core are indicated in small anterior and premolar teeth, as well as teeth with major coronal destruction. In addition, they may be used when functional forces on a tooth put the dowel-to-core retention at risk.

The disadvantages of the cast dowel and core system, however, are considerable. The financial cost of providing this service is high, as two appointments are needed to complete the cast dowel and core. The laboratory expense may be significant, and the laboratory phase is technique sensitive. Casting a large core in contact with a small diameter dowel pattern can result in porosity at the dowel-core interface. Fracture of the metal at this interface under function results in the failure of the restoration. Attempts to circumvent this problem by casting a core to a proprietary stainless steel preformed dowel are contraindicated. The heating and casting procedures necessary in the laboratory degrade the physical characteristics of the stainless steel. Final qualities of this dowel-core restoration are not sufficiently strong or inert to withstand clinical forces over time.

Amalgam core. Dental amalgam is a traditional core buildup material with a long history of clinical success. Amalgam is a strong, economical material that is easy to use. It is very stable to thermal and functional stresses and therefore transmits minimal stress to the residual tooth structure, cement, and crown margins. When used with dentin bonding agents, the seal at the tooth-alloy junction can be improved by incorporating a layer of a resin that chemically bonds to both dentin and metal.[14,47] The resultant low microleakage discourages recurrent caries and coronal-apical endodontic contamination. High compressive strength, high tensile strength, and high modulus of elasticity are attributes of dental amalgam and are ideal for a core material.

Amalgam is easily manipulated and can have a rapid setting time. Placement of a fast-setting, high-copper alloy core permits final crown preparation at the initial operative appointment, although the early strength is low. Amalgam cores are highly retentive when used with a preformed dowel in posterior teeth; they require more force to dislodge than cast dowel and cores. This is largely due to high mechanical retention of amalgam to tooth and dowel undercuts.[37] Additional retention and antirotation can be procured with auxiliary pins, irregular dentin preparation, and dentin bonding agents. Bonded amalgam exhibits moderate retention to dentin and has been shown to increase the strength of restored teeth.[9,11,15,47]

A significant disadvantage of amalgam cores is the potential for corrosion and subsequent discoloration of the gingiva or remaining dentin. This core material can be used in almost all teeth where sufficient bulk of amalgam for strength is possible. Amalgam dowels should be avoided in teeth with high aesthetic value and in patients with known metal allergies. Use of amalgam is declining worldwide because of legislative, safety, and environmental issues. However, the nature and significance of any adverse effects from dental amalgam remains controversial.[46]

Composite resin core. A third core material is composite resin, which exhibits favorable ease of manipulation and very rapid set. Preparation for the final restoration is readily accomplished during the core placement session. Additional retention and antirotation mechanisms are also easily achieved with auxiliary pins, dentin preparations, or dentin bonding materials.

Composite resin properties pertaining to microleakage and retention to tooth structure are dependent on the intermediary bonding agent, as composite resin alone has no capability of self-bonding to tooth structure. Research reports from different generations of composite and bonding systems are not directly comparable, as earlier studies preceded the development of dentin bonding agents. These earlier systems exhibit several undesirable properties that limit their use as a core material. Polymerization shrinkage and contraction away from the tooth structure of nondentin-bonded, light-cured composite resin can result in core or tooth marginal opening, microcracks, and microleakage. Composite resin has no anticariogenic properties, and these openings are potential avenues of extensive invasion for oral fluids following a break in the cement seal or marginal integrity of the crown. Microleakage exceeds that of amalgam, glass-ionomer, or glass-ionomer resin. Composite resin is dimensionally unstable in wet conditions, regardless of dentin bonding agents. Loss of a provisional crown can result in moisture-mediated expansion of the core, which can cause marginal openings from incomplete seating of a new crown. High expansion can also affect the cement seal of the final crown.[1] Dentin bonding agents improve the physical characteristics and reduce microleakage of the composite resin core and tooth junction. However, no bonding agent entirely eliminates microleakage.[56] Therefore as with all buildup materials for decimated teeth, more than 2 mm of sound tooth structure should remain at the margin for optimal composite resin core function.

Composite resin has undergone significant development and improvement in physical characteristics and bond strengths. Improved mechanical properties from increased filler content, decreased filler size, and dual or chemical cure formulations contribute to composite resin's suitability for core fabrication. The physical characteristics of composite resin will continue to evolve, along with adhesive dental technologies. These advances will dictate that composite resin will be among the most widely used core materials in clinical practice.[27,42]

Glass-ionomer core. High-viscosity glass-ionomer and glass-ionomer–silver core materials are adhesive, and are useful for small buildups or to fill undercuts in prepared teeth. The major benefit of glass-ionomer materials is an anticariogenic quality resulting from the presence of fluoride in the chemical composition. Microleakage of glass-ionomer is low, less than that of composite resin or glass-ionomer resin.[16]

The physical characteristics of glass-ionomer materials limit their application to specific clinical conditions. Glass-ionomer is soluble and sensitive to moisture. Adhesive failure can result from contamination of the tooth surface with cutting debris, saliva, blood, or protein. Glass-ionomer cores have low strength and are brittle because of low fracture toughness, which contraindicates the use of glass-ionomer buildups in thin anterior teeth or to replace unsupported cusps. Glass-ionomer cores also exhibit low retention to preformed dowels.[37] Glass-ionomer can be used for small buildups under single crowns, but is not strong enough for an abutment tooth core. It is indicated in posterior teeth where (1) a bulk of core material is possible, (2) significant sound dentin remains, (3) additional retention is available with pins or dentin preparations, (4) moisture control is assured, and (5) caries control is indicated.

Glass-ionomer resin core: Glass-ionomer resin materials are a combination of glass-ionomer and composite resin technologies and exhibit properties of both parent materials. The precise properties of fluoride release, thermal expansion, and bond to dentin depend on the proportion of glass-ionomer and composite resin in a specific brand of glass-ionomer resin buildup material. Glass-ionomer resin exhibits moderate strength, greater than glass-ionomer and less than composite resin. As a core material, it is adequate for moderate-sized buildups. Solubility of glass-ionomer resin is between that of glass-ionomer and composite resins. Fluoride release is equal to glass-ionomer and far more than composite resin. The bond to dentin is closer to that of a dentin-bonded composite resin and significantly higher than traditional glass-ionomer. Glass-ionomer resin is nearly insoluble and exhibits minimal microleakage.[5,8]

Dowel and core selection. Successful restoration of the endodontically treated tooth requires careful planning and meticulous instrumentation. Many of the dowel and core systems use common procedures, which are presented together in this chapter. Understanding the general technique of the major dowel and core subgroups allows the clinician to easily adapt to the specifics of a proprietary system in that group. It is not the object of this chapter to be an exhaustive compilation of available dowel systems. Many factors affect the selection of a particular dowel and core system for tooth restoration. Two variables that have major influence on this decision are the amounts of remaining tooth structure and the functional stresses anticipated for the tooth. When a coronal restoration is indicated, the amount of tooth structure remaining after final preparation has the greatest importance in determining the design of the intermediary dowel and core. Tooth structure that appears adequate before the crown preparation may be grossly unsatisfactory after occlusal and axial reductions. Therefore the initial crown preparation is first completed and the bulk and position of the prepared tooth structure is evaluated before dowel and core selection. Selection and placement of a specific dowel and core system before tooth preparation can create significant restorative problems and greatly compromise the final restoration.

The second major consideration in designing dowel and core restorations is the functional requirement of the tooth. Abutment teeth for removable partial dentures are subject to greater stress and fracture more frequently than abutment teeth for fixed partial dentures or individual teeth within the dental arch. Consequently, endodontically treated abutment teeth for removable partial dentures require a dowel to distribute forces, as well as a core and crown. Fixed partial denture abutments and individual teeth can use pin-retained cores or coronal-radicular alloys without dowels, when residual tooth structure volume permits.

Improper selection of the dowel and core system may result in clinical failure. Significant functional forces and minimal remaining tooth structure concentrate stress at the core to the dowel-tooth interface. Fracture of the core material from the dowel and the tooth can occur. The crown, with the core inside, separates from the dowel and root complex. A new core and crown may be fabricated if the existing dowel is satisfactory and increased retention is achieved with the added core material. If the existing dowel is unsatisfactory, a delicate removal procedure is indicated. Persistent vibration with an ultrasonic cleaning device degrades the cement and allows withdrawal of the dowel. Extreme care must be used to protect the remaining tooth structure, as additional dentin loss will compound the restorative problem. Forced removal of the dowel from the root is contraindicated and may result in fracture of the root and loss of the tooth.

Coronal restoration

The final component of the endodontic reconstruction is the coronal restoration (see Fig. 21-7). All coronal restorations reestablish function and isolate the dentin and endodontic filling materials from microleakage. They may also restore aesthetics. Cast crowns are coronal restorations that fulfill all these requirements and also distribute functional forces and protect the tooth against fracture.

As described earlier, the physical characteristics of the endodontically treated tooth differ from the vital tooth. Previous concern over the loss of dentinal resiliency assumed that all endodontically treated teeth became brittle and required a cast crown. Currently the fundamental issue for fracture potential is the missing tooth structure and loss of architectural integrity of the remaining tooth. This view has altered the clinical criteria for placement of a coronal restoration. Depending on the tooth type and the degree of tooth structure decimated by previous disease, repair, and iatrogenic misadventures, the coronal restoration can range from a simple access seal to a crown replacing essentially all the coronal tooth structure.

As a general rule, all endodontically treated posterior teeth and those anterior teeth that are structurally damaged should be restored with a crown. Crowns prevent a significant number of fractures in posterior teeth but do not similarly protect anterior teeth (see Fig. 21-6). In a large clinical study the fracture rate for uncrowned premolars and molars was double that for those restored with crowns. The success rate for maxillary molars dropped from 97.8% for those with crowns to 50% for those without crowns. Anterior teeth are less at risk for fracture than posterior teeth and showed no further improvement when restored with a crown. Maxillary anterior teeth exhibited a success rate of 87.5% for crowned teeth and 85.4% for uncrowned teeth. Therefore endodontically treated anterior teeth do not require a crown or dowel unless extensive tooth structure is missing and integrity, function, and aesthetics must be restored. The coronal restoration for endodontically treated intact anterior teeth consists of sealing the lingual access cavity. Posterior teeth need coronal coverage to protect against fracture from occlusal forces, regardless of the amount of remaining tooth structure.

Crown preparation for endodontically treated teeth is identical to that of vital teeth when substantial tooth structure remains. Once restored with a crown, the underlying sound tooth structure provides greater resistance to fracture than any dowel type or design. Natural tooth structure should be carefully preserved during all phases of dowel space and crown preparation.[23] The crown preparation design for extensively damaged nonvital teeth is critical. The minimal remaining tooth structure must be used effectively so that the crown can restore function without harm to remaining roots or to the periodontal attachment. The residual tooth between the core and the gingival sulcus must be structurally sound and a minimum of 2 mm in height for the crown ferrule and margin. As caries, fracture, and other endodontic precedents can decimate the tooth to the tissue level, this amount of unaffected tooth structure is often not available and adjunctive procedures are indicated to first obtain the necessary length.

The final coronal restoration provides added security to the tooth by consolidating the remaining cusps and prepared tooth structure and by creating a ferrule effect (Fig. 21-19). The ferrule is a band of metal or ceramic material that encircles the external aspect of the residual tooth, similar to the metal bands around a barrel or a shovel handle. It is formed by the walls of the crown (Fig. 21-20) or cast telescopic coping (Fig. 21-21) encasing the gingival 1 to 2 mm of the axial walls of the preparation above the crown margin. A properly executed ferrule significantly reduces the incidence of fracture in the nonvital tooth by reinforcing the tooth at its external surface and dissipating force, which concentrates at the narrowest circum-

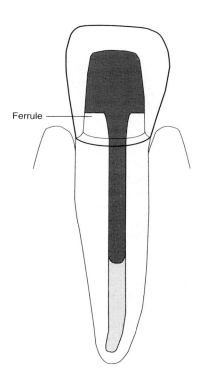

Ferrule

FIG. 21-19 Ferrule is an encircling band of metal, usually provided by the coronal restoration. It greatly increases the resistance of a tooth to fracture. Ferrule should (1) be a minimum of 1 to 2 mm in height, (2) have parallel axial walls, (3) totally encircle the tooth, (4) end on sound tooth structure, and (5) not invade the attachment apparatus of the tooth.

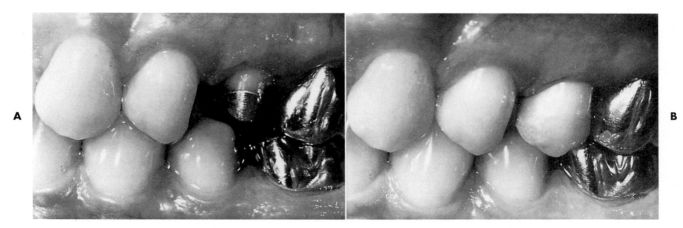

FIG. 21-20 Ferrule effect is provided by the coronal restoration. **A,** Second premolar with a preformed dowel and alloy core. **B,** Coping of the porcelain and metal crown supplies the ferrule. This encirclement significantly increases the fracture resistance of the tooth.

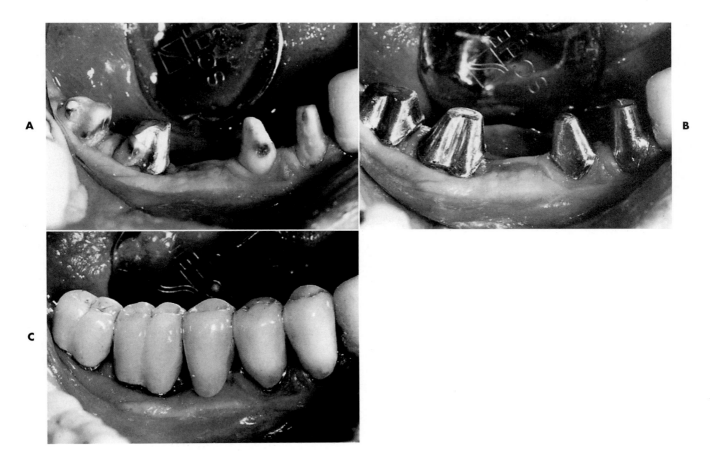

FIG. 21-21 Ferrule is produced by the primary coping. **A,** Second premolar and second molar both contain dowel and core restorations. **B,** Primary copings are seated. They encircle the tooth structure and provide the ferrule. **C,** Superstructure prosthesis is cemented. Superstructure does not add to the ferrule in this case.

ference of the tooth. The ferrule also resists lateral forces from tapered dowels and leverage from the crown in function and increases the retention and resistance of the restoration. Crown preparations with a 1-mm coronal extension of dentin above the margin exhibit double the fracture resistance when compared to preparations with the core terminating on a flat surface immediately above the margin.[38,49]

To be successful, the ferrule must encircle a vertical wall of sound tooth structure above the margin and must not terminate on restorative material. The crown and crown preparation together must meet five requirements: (1) a minimum of 1 to 2 mm of dentin axial wall height is required; (2) the axial walls must be parallel; (3) the metal must totally encircle the tooth; (4) the metal must be on solid tooth structure; and (5) the metal must not invade the attachment apparatus.

A tooth with remaining structure that is insufficient to construct a ferrule as described above should be evaluated for periodontal crown lengthening surgery or orthodontic extrusion to gain access to additional root surface.[33] The lack of a sufficient ferrule in the final restoration forces the core and the dowel to accept high functional stresses, often resulting in fracture caused by material failure (Fig. 21-22).

The true extent of caries or other damage in a broken-down tooth can be difficult to determine before tooth preparation. Placement of a provisional restoration or a temporary crown allows total evaluation of the tooth and supporting structures before committing the patient to definitive endodontics. As discussed above in Pretreatment Evaluation, structural, occlusal, and periodontal findings may condemn a tooth to extraction even though endodontic therapy can be successful. It is prudent to discover these facts before the canals are treated.

Provisional restorations. Once the decision to retain a tooth is made, crown preparation and provisional restoration in advance of endodontic treatment can assist the endodontic endeavor. Removal of this temporary crown at the endodontic appointment allows structural evaluation of the remaining coronal dentin and facilitates access entry to the chamber. When the procedure is completed, the provisional restoration is recemented and the function, aesthetics, and protective qualities of the tooth are returned.

The provisional crown may also aid in rubber dam isolation. Left in place during root canal therapy, the provisional crown provides normal axial contours to the tooth and allows engagement of the rubber dam clamp. Access is then attained through the occlusal or lingual surface of the provisional restoration. A temporary material is used when the operative appointment for endodontics is complete.

Finally, preendodontic preparation and provisionalization may assist in the differential diagnosis. Proper diagnosis can be difficult when multiple clinical problems are present on the same tooth or on adjacent teeth. Clarification of the true etiologic origin is aided by the removal of potential symptomatic variables, including caries, defective restorations, and cracked cusps. Decisions about the restorability of the tooth can be made and the tooth returned to temporary aesthetics and function before scheduling definitive endodontic treatment or extraction of the tooth.

Provisional crown fabrication techniques. Provisional crowns are fabricated using conventional fixed prosthodontic techniques and cementation procedures. Due to its superior strength and color stability, methyl methacrylate acrylic resins or composite-based materials should be used when crowns are

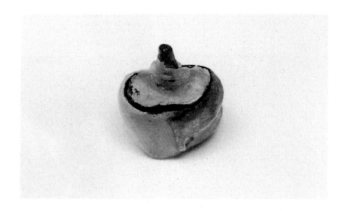

FIG. 21-22 Failed restoration with inadequate ferrule. Level of the core material is coincident with the restorative margin; functional forces were not resisted by adequate axial walls of sound tooth structure.

required to function over extended periods of time. These are stable materials, which allow various dental supportive therapies to be completed in an organized and controlled fashion without provisional restoration maintenance problems. Temporary crowns formed from ethyl methacrylate resins or cement-filled aluminum crown shells cannot be expected to provide the needed time and control to finish a prescribed treatment sequence.

After endodontic treatment a provisional crown with an attached temporary dowel can restore aesthetics and function to the tooth with limited supragingival tooth structure until definitive restoration is possible (Fig. 21-23). Many proprietary dowel systems include temporary dowels for fabrication of dowel-retained provisional crowns. An appropriate temporary dowel is selected to fit the prepared dowel space. The dowel is seated and sized to fit within the confines of a crown shell or of the existing provisional crown. Slight internal relief in the crown allows resin material to attach to both the crown and the dowel. Undercuts within the tooth are blocked out or removed at the dowel-tooth interface. The tooth structure is lightly lubricated, and a small amount of the resin is placed in the relief area of the provisional crown. The crown is seated over the tooth and dowel and held in position until the resin is set and attached to the temporary dowel. Occlusion and marginal adaptation of an existing provisional crown are not altered by this procedure. The combined crown and dowel are then cemented into place with a temporary cementing medium.

Provisional crowns for endodontically treated teeth must be used with extreme caution. A partial loss of cement seal does not provoke symptoms in the tooth and may go undetected for some time. This leakage can lead to severe carious invasion and result in the loss of the tooth. This is especially true when the combination provisional crown and temporary dowel are used. The lack of tooth structure necessitating this combination predisposes the cement seal to breakdown and places these teeth at risk. In addition to caries formation, leakage of the post-obturation temporary restoration can jeopardize success of the endodontic treatment. Coronal to apical degradation of the root canal sealer can occur when the endodontically completed canal system is contaminated by oral fluids. This loss of seal and resultant reentry of bacteria into the canal system necessitates endodontic retreatment. The timely placement of the final

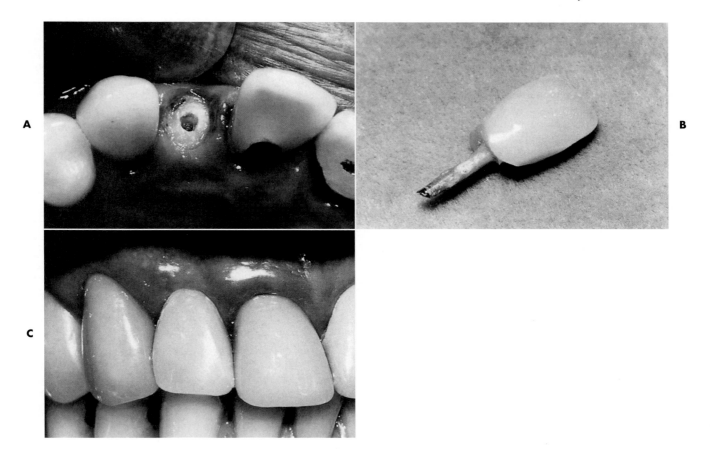

FIG. 21-23 Provisional crowns may be retained by temporary dowels until definitive therapy can be provided. **A,** Lateral incisor fractured below the level of the free gingival margin. **B,** Endodontic therapy was completed and a provisional crown fabricated with an aluminum dowel. **C,** Provisional restoration in place. This procedure allowed time for orthodontic extrusion of the root. Final dowel, core, and coronal restoration were placed after sufficient tooth structure was present above the periodontal attachment.

dowel and core and coronal restoration in the endodontically treated tooth is critical to therapeutic success.

Dowel and core fabrication techniques. There are numerous techniques for the fabrication and placement of the dowel and core restoration. Most of these share the initial steps, including gutta-percha removal and initial preparation of the dowel space. The procedures for each subgroup (preformed passive dowels and cast dowels) then diverge. The preformed systems use common procedures for attachment of the core, a step which is unnecessary for cast dowel and core systems.

The first step for all types of dowel and core restorations is the removal of the gutta-percha from the dowel space. The amount of gutta-percha to be removed is dictated by the desired dowel length, the bone height, and the root morphology, as discussed earlier. The procedure is generally best accomplished by the clinician providing the endodontic service, as that person has clear knowledge of the canal system size and form. Removal of the filling material to form the dowel space should be completed in a passive manner so as not to disturb the apical seal. A hot root canal plugger or electronic heating device can be safely used to remove gutta-percha.[26] It is important to heat the instrument hot enough to sear and remove the gutta-percha. An instrument that is too cool melts the filling into a sticky mass, which can dislodge the entire canal filling when the instrument is withdrawn. Extreme care must be taken with the heated instruments so that the patient is not injured.

Rotary instrumentation for gutta-percha removal is also available. However, rotation instruments carry the risk of straying from the canal and cutting radicular dentin (see Fig. 21-3). This weakens the root structure and could result in lateral root perforation, particularly in the area of root flutings or concavities. If mechanical rotation is deemed necessary, instruments such as Peeso reamers or Gates-Glidden burs are indicated. They are designed to center themselves within the confines of the gutta-percha filling. However, occasional deviation into the dentin walls or dislodgment of the apical seal can occur.

The use of chemicals for gutta-percha removal should be discouraged. Containment of the chemical within the canal and total control to the desired depth is very difficult. The result of chemical removal may be leakage in the lateral canal complex or in the apical areas.

The initial dowel space preparation procedure is similar for most dowel and core systems. The space cleared of gutta-percha has the form of the canal after cleaning and shaping and must be refined to the correct dimension and shape for the dowel space. All the proprietary systems are supplied with a series of drills to prepare the internal surface of the canal. The drills gradually increase the size of the canal, remove natural undercuts, and shape the canal to correspond with the provided dowel or dowel pattern. The drills are sized to match preformed dowels, preformed impression dowels, or preformed plastic dowel forms. The goal at the refinement step is to establish a proper dowel space with a minimum of dentin wall alteration. Intimate contact of the dowel and dentin surfaces is not indicated for the passive dowel systems; adequate depth and proper cementation provide sufficient retention for these restorations. The drills provided for the internal refinement should be used with great caution. It is often possible to achieve proper form in the dowel space by rotation of these drills with finger force only. Correct depth can be measured by a periodontal probe or other small measuring device. The distance from a coronal landmark to the apical gutta-percha is recorded. This measurement is transferred to the smallest drill for use in the canal; drills of progressively larger size are used until the apical 2 or 3 mm of dentin are engaged during rotation. Rotation with a dental handpiece is dangerous as deviation from the cleared canal is easy and hazardous. In addition, power-driven instrumentation risks unnecessary enlargement of the canals and could damage the apical endodontic seal. The dowel space is now ready for the final clinical procedure, the actual dowel and core construction.

Cast dowel and core fabrication technique: Cast dowel and core restorations can be fabricated with either direct or indirect techniques. These procedures differ only in the means by which the dowel and core pattern is generated. Both use instrumentation and materials from the same proprietary systems (see Fig. 21-12). In the direct technique a castable dowel and core pattern is fabricated directly on the prepared tooth in the patient's mouth. The indirect technique uses an impression and stone die of the tooth for the pattern fabrication. The pattern from either the direct or indirect technique is then invested and cast with gold or other crown and bridge alloy.

When the direct technique is used, the final dowel and core pattern is fabricated during the first appointment. After the initial crown preparation and dowel space refinement, a preformed plastic dowel pattern that corresponds to the last drill size used is selected. This plastic rod is seated completely in the dowel space. The pattern should not bind on the internal walls of the root. If the passive fit is not present, a second pattern should be tried or the canal refined again. Passivity is important. After the dowel pattern is fit, any necessary antirotation pins or dentin preparations are added, ensuring that they are parallel to the path of withdrawal. Undercuts should be eliminated by blocking out with glass-ionomer cement or alloy rather than removing valuable dentin. The tooth is lubricated lightly, and the plastic dowel is seated. Self-curing acrylic resin or wax is added to the tooth to create a core attached to the dowel pattern. The final core shape is completed in the patient's mouth by carving wax or preparing the hardened resin with a dental handpiece using copious water flow. The prepared pattern is removed from the tooth, the dowel orifice is protected with a cotton pledget, and the provisional crown is cemented. If a dowel-retained provisional crown is used, no cement should be placed on the temporary dowel or in the canal (Fig. 21-24).

When the indirect technique is used, a final impression of the prepared tooth and prepared dowel space is made during the first appointment. The final pattern is then fabricated on a die made from this impression. The crown margins need not be accurately reproduced at this stage, unless a more complex telescopic dowel and core are planned. Again, proprietary systems provide matched drills, impression dowels, and laboratory casting patterns of various diameters. As a first clinical step, an impression dowel is selected and fit to the refined dowel space. This impression dowel must seat easily in the prepared dowel space. Adhesive is applied to the coronal portion of the impression dowel and a final impression is made using conventional crown and bridge materials. The impression captures the form of the coronal tooth structure and picks up the dowel impression dowel. The block out of undercuts need not be done in the patient's mouth at this time. The provisional crown is cemented in place and the patient dismissed. A dental cast is fabricated with a die that precisely reproduces the prepared dowel space and the residual coronal tooth structure. In the laboratory, undercuts are removed by block out on the cast. A preformed plastic dowel pattern is fit into the die dowel space and wax added to form the core. The final core shape is carved in the wax and the dowel and core pattern removed from the cast. Patterns generated from both the direct and the indirect techniques are invested and cast in the same way. The final cast custom dowel and core are now ready for the patient's second appointment.

After removal of the provisional crown and temporary cement, the casting is carefully seated in the dowel space. It should slide easily into place without binding and without the need for pressure. This is a passive dental restoration. Obstructions to easy seating should be detected by a silicone paste or paint type of disclosing medium and removed. This process is repeated until the casting seats completely and easily in the preparation. It is important to note that total marginal integrity between the casting and the tooth is not mandatory, except as an indication of complete seating. This is an internal restoration; the entire cast dowel and core along with the tooth structure of the ferrule will be encapsulated by the coping of the final restoration. The final crown must have marginal integrity. The dowel and core restoration is now ready for cementation (see Cementation later in this chapter).

Preformed dowel and core fabrication technique: Preformed dowel and core combinations are the restoration of choice for most clinical situations. They make up the vast majority of intermediary restorations placed in dental practices today. Although there are many variations, most of these systems contain preformed dowels corresponding to the instrumentation used in refining the dowel space (see Fig. 21-11). Once the dowel space preparation is complete, the matching dowel is easily selected by a numbering or color system. This dowel is placed in the finished dowel space and should slide easily to the apical extension of the preparation. There should be no binding and no force necessary to place this dowel. Resistance to seating should be removed by refining the dowel space; the preformed dowel should not be altered to fit the tooth as any grinding on the apical area alters the dowel to root dynamics. Total seating is assessed by measuring the length of the dowel space from a fixed coronal landmark with a periodontal probe. This distance is transferred to the preformed dowel to confirm total embedment. Complete seating may also be confirmed by radiograph. After achieving a passive fit within the root, the excess dowel material must be shortened to an appropriate length. This must be completed before the dowel is cemented into the dowel space. Trimming the dowel after final cementation causes vibration and risks degradation of the cement, decreased retention, and possible

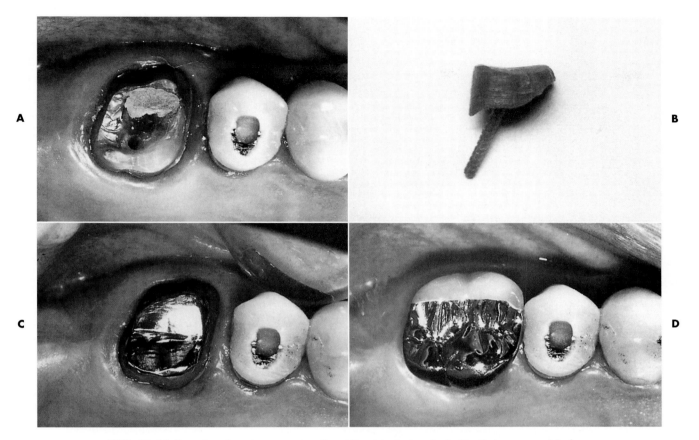

FIG. 21-24 Cast dowel and core restoration (direct technique). **A,** Tooth is prepared before the final selection of a dowel and core system. Buccal canal undercuts are blocked out to form a path of withdrawal for the pattern without additional dentin removal. Plastic burnout dowel is fit to the refined dowel space in the palatal root, and resin is added to form the core portion of the pattern. **B,** One-piece pattern is removed from the tooth and cast. **C,** Cast dowel and core are cemented in the preparation. **D,** Final coronal restoration is fabricated.

microleakage into the canal space. The dowel should be short of the internal occlusal surface of the final coronal restoration but must be long enough to retain the core. The dowel is now ready for cementation (Fig. 21-25) (see Cementation later in this chapter).

Core fabrication technique: After the dowel is luted to the root, any necessary retentive and antirotation mechanisms are added. A minimal number of additional retentive devices should be used, as these pins, grooves, and other dentin preparations remove tooth structure. Often the undercut nature of the remaining pulp chamber, the irregularities of the residual coronal tooth structure, and the angle at which the dowel exits the tooth are adequate to ensure core retention. These features, along with normal irregular cervical root anatomy, provide adequate antirotation to most restorations. The core material is then placed around the dowel, into the remaining pulp chamber and built up to form the coronal area. A suitable matrix may be necessary. Manufacturers' instructions should be followed for mixing and placement of each of the core materials. Isolation from moisture contamination is vital during the core formation. Amalgam alloys, composite resins, glass-ionomer, glass-ionomer resin, and dentin bonding agents require a dry field to obtain optimal physical characteristics. After the core material is set, it can be prepared for the final coronal restora-

tion. The dowel and any additional retentive devices used should not extend to the surface of the core when this preparation is completed. The tooth is now ready for the final coronal restoration.

Coronal-radicular restoration technique (Fig. 21-26). An alternative to the traditional dowel and core for posterior teeth is the direct coronal-radicular restoration. This restoration consists of a core that replaces coronal tooth structure and extends 2 to 4 mm into the coronal portion of the canals. The core is retained by a combination of the divergence of the canals in a multirooted tooth, the natural undercuts in the pulp chamber, adhesion with dentin bonding agents, and retentive channels or preparations in the dentin.

The coronal-radicular core uses conventional restorative materials, including amalgam, composite resin, or glass-ionomer resin. The ease of manipulation and a rapid set of these core materials are advantages. The buildup can be placed and prepared for a final coronal restoration in one visit. A single, homogeneous material is used for the entire restoration, as opposed to the dual phases of a conventional preformed dowel and core. The coronal-radicular core is indicated for posterior teeth that have large pulp chambers and multiple canals for retention. The retention of coronal-radicular alloy buildups in molars is equal to that of pin-retained amalgam cores.[31] The

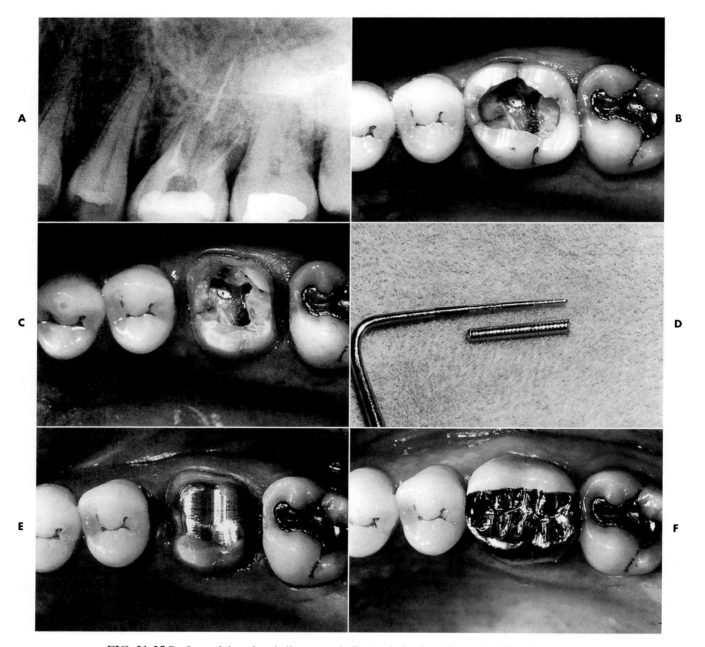

FIG. 21-25 Preformed dowel and alloy core. **A,** Postendodontic radiograph with a dowel space prepared in the palatal root. **B,** Occlusal view before preparation. Dowel and core system has not yet been selected. **C,** Final coronal preparation with sufficient tooth structure for a preformed dowel and alloy core. **D,** Dowel is cut to size before cementation; a periodontal probe is used to measure from a fixed coronal landmark to the base of the dowel space. **E,** Final preparation with the core in place. **F,** Final coronal restoration.

physical characteristics of alloy and composite resins allow this restoration to function well when up to 50% of the coronal tooth structure has been lost. Greater amounts of tooth structure must be present if glass-ionomer is used because of its low tensile strength. Because no dowel is present to distribute functional forces to the apical tooth structure, this restoration should be used cautiously in teeth that are abutments for large restorations generating high functional loads.

The technique for a coronal-radicular buildup of the nonvital tooth is straightforward. Because this restoration requires no dowel and because the restorative material is not rigid when placed, exact refinement of the coronal segment of the canals is not critical. The removal of 2 to 4 mm of gutta-percha from these canals is sufficient for preparation; no dentin need be altered. Undercuts and irregularities found in the canal walls are actually advantages, as they increase retention of the restoration. Restorative materials should be bonded to the available tooth structure to increase retention, decrease microleakage, and increase fracture resistance of the tooth. The tooth is now ready for the final coronal restoration.

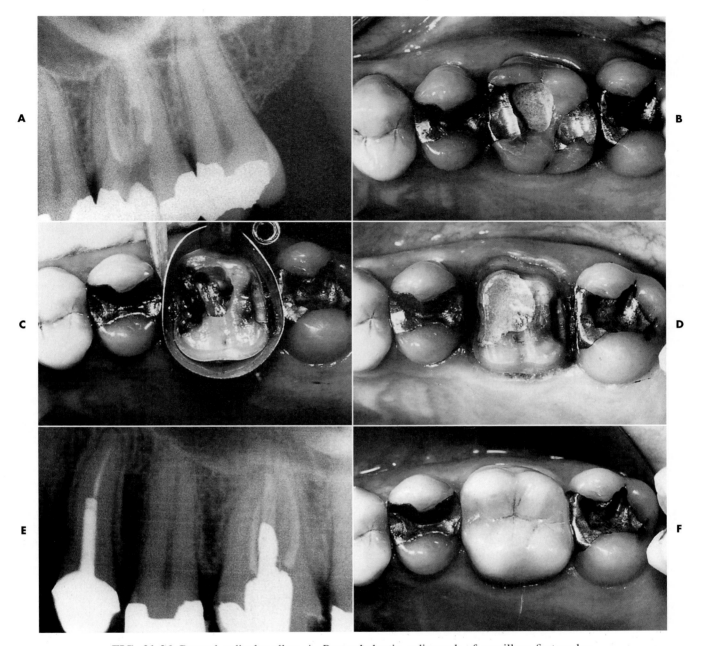

FIG. 21-26 Coronal-radicular alloy. **A,** Postendodontic radiograph of maxillary first molar. **B,** Occlusal view before preparation. Dowel and core system has not yet been selected. **C,** Final coronal preparation with sufficient tooth structure for a bonded coronal-radicular alloy. Matrix is used when condensing the alloy. **D,** Final preparation with core in place. **E,** Radiograph before final restoration. **F,** Final coronal restoration.

Cementation: Dowel and core cementation materials have changed markedly in recent years. The ability to bond to dentin has significantly expanded the options available to the restorative dentist and have altered every phase of dowel and core restoration. Dowels can be cemented with zinc phosphate, glass-ionomer, glass-ionomer resin, or resin cements. Use of a cement that bonds to the tooth structure and the dowel and core material offers obvious advantages.

Nonadhesive cements: Zinc phosphate cement is a traditional dental luting agent with a long and satisfactory clinical history. It provides retention through interlocking of small mechanical undercuts in the tooth structure and restorative materials. The retention is sufficient for well-designed dowels, cores, and coronal restorations but does not equal that of the chemically adhesive resin cements. This level of adequate but not excessive retention can be advantageous in the event of trauma or dowel removal, as loosening occurs by cement failure rather than by root fracture. The inability to chemically bond to residual tooth structure is also a disadvantage. Zinc phosphate cement retains the restoration but does not increase the resistance to fracture by direct bond to the tooth and does not inhibit marginal leakage by the same method. Zinc phosphate cement has no anticariogenic properties.[32]

Adhesive cements: Adhesive cements bond to dentin within the root and residual tooth, as well as to most dowel and core materials.[35] Traditional glass-ionomer cement is fluoride releasing and anticariogenic, a major advantage. However, it is moisture sensitive, soluble, and slow setting. Glass-ionomer cement is not indicated in areas where moisture control is compromised.

Glass-ionomer resin cements combine the qualities of glass-ionomer and resin groups, resulting in a cement that is superior to either.[10,12,48,55] Glass-ionomer resin cement exhibits moderate retention, high strength, low or no solubility, high fluoride release, and favorable ease of use. Removal of excess cement is accomplished before the cement has set completely. Partially set cement is readily removed, whereas removal of completely set cement is very difficult. Moderate retention is preferable to maximal retention for most cases, as restorations and dowels may require removal at a later time. Restorative retreatment is more difficult and risky when restorations are placed with excessively retentive cements.

Resin cement can result in maximal possible retention but makes subsequent dowel removal risky. Bond strength achievable with a specific resin cement can be very high. Parallel dowels set with a cement are equal in retention to active or screw type of dowels, without the inherent risk from screw threads in dentin. This cement-mediated maximal retention is not risk free, however, as 80% of the roots fractured when dowels were dislodged by force.[53,54] Conversely, adhesive cements may help the tooth resist fracture, as the dentin wall, cementing medium, and dowel become an integrated unit.[29] The retention of the core is also enhanced by these cements. Core materials of amalgam, composite resin, or glass-ionomer can be bonded to the dentin, to the dowel, and to most cements used to lute the dowel.[39] Resin cement does not have anticariogenic properties, although the adhesive bond inhibits fluid microleakage between the tooth and the restoration. Reduced microleakage and cement insolubility are major advantages over traditional, nonadhesive cements to diminish recurrent caries around a restoration and to minimize coronal-apical contamination of the root canal system. However, these cements can be difficult to use and to remove excess set cement from furcations and other periodontally sensitive areas.

The general cementation procedure for insertion of dowel and core restorations is very similar, regardless of cement type. Once mixed, the cement is delivered to the dowel space with a lentulo spiral to ensure that all walls are coated. At the same time the dowel or dowel and core are coated with a thin layer of cement; retention is greatest when both the dowel and canal are coated, rather than either one alone.[44] The restoration should slide slowly and easily into place with light finger pressure. Most preformed dowels include a vent that allows dissipation of hydraulic back pressure during the cementation process. Excess cement must escape coronally, as the dowel nearly fills the dowel space. Significant pressure generation in nonvented cases may cause the root to crack during cementation.[40] Biting pressure to seat the restoration is not necessary. Tapping with a mallet or other instrument is absolutely contraindicated. Once the restoration is fully seated, it should remain untouched until the cement has set passively. The excess cement is removed, and the dowel and core portion of the restoration is complete.

Compromised teeth. Restoration of endodontically treated teeth becomes more complex as the teeth or supporting structures become increasingly diseased. The compromises created by extensive loss of tooth structure alter the restorative procedures and affect the longevity of the tooth and the prosthesis. Mechanical requirements for structural integrity of the restoration and biologic requirements for the periodontal attachment apparatus often conflict. The narrow band of tooth structure that remains after severe breakdown is needed by both the restoration for a ferrule and by the tissue for periodontal health. Adjunctive dental procedures from other specialties may be needed before endodontic restoration of the severely damaged tooth.

Endodontic treatment can also become a form of adjunctive therapy to facilitate treatment of periodontally compromised teeth. Portions of teeth that otherwise may be candidates for extraction can sometimes be retained with hemisection or root amputation procedures. Periodontally guarded anterior teeth can be shortened and roots used as overdenture abutments. Adjunctive or supportive endodontic treatment is needed for these periodontal procedures. Dowel, core, and coronal restorations must also be designed for the new shape and function of the altered, endodontic teeth. Lastly, the compromised tooth may not be a candidate for rehabilitation. In some circumstances, endodontic, restorative, and periodontal therapy do not add predictably to the prognosis of a tooth or teeth. Inclusion of implant dentistry into treatment planning options makes heroic attempts to salvage some compromised teeth unnecessary.

Posterior dentition: Teeth with diminished periodontal support may require integrated periodontal, endodontic, and restorative treatment.[45] Moderate to severe attachment loss results in a significant alteration of crown-root ratio. The complexity caused by diminished periodontal attachment is increased with multirooted teeth. The furcation involvement is common in the posterior dentition. Additionally, the loss of supporting tissues and periodontal therapy used to correct these problems often compromise restorative options.

Coronal preparation for both a path of withdrawal and reduction of the horizontal furcation invasion usually results in severe diminution of tooth structure. Establishment of a satisfactory taper for these teeth requires aggressive tooth preparation. The axial walls begin on the root surface, which has a smaller circumference than the cementoenamel junction. The axial walls of the prepared tooth must converge throughout the elongated clinical crown. This dentin removal brings the operative procedure, as well as the final restoration, in close proximity to the root canal system. The problem is exacerbated in the multirooted tooth when restorative procedures attempt to diminish furcation invasions. Teeth that exhibit attachment loss apical to the root trunk have horizontal defects into the furcation area. Tooth preparation to minimize this dimension requires removal of significant tooth structure coronal to the furcation. The resultant "fluted" preparation is seen throughout the full length of the axial wall (Fig. 21-27). This procedure decreases the horizontal dimension of the furcation invasion but also increases pulpal morbidity. As discussed in Pretreatment Evaluation earlier in this chapter, preventive endodontics is indicated in cases with a strong suspicion of future pulpal involvement. The probability of pulpal degeneration in these teeth is statistically high.

When prerestorative root canal therapy is indicated for elongated, periodontally involved teeth, it is extremely important to retain as much radicular dentin as possible. These teeth are subject to fracture because of increased leverage caused by

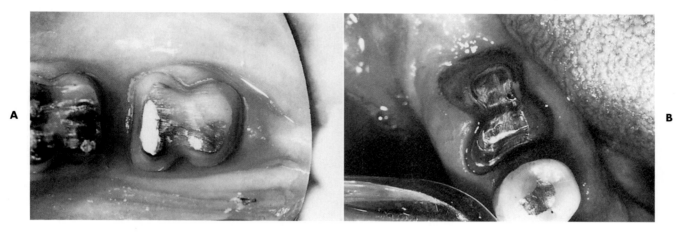

FIG. 21-27 Tooth preparation advantageous to the periodontium can prove deleterious to the pulp. **A,** Dentin reduction to decrease furcation invasions brings the preparation and restoration in close proximity to the pulp chamber. **B,** Increased osseous destruction in the furcation results in exaggerated preparation designs.

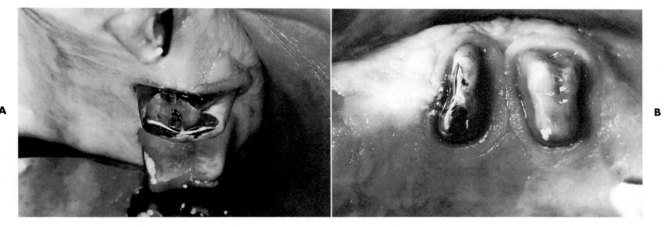

FIG. 21-28 Sectioned maxillary first molar with a preformed dowel and alloy core in place. **A,** Mesial view shows the core after removal of the mesiobuccal root. Alloy obliterates the pulp chamber and is separated from the attachment by the thin chamber floor. **B,** Root morphology and degree of periodontal attachment loss dictate margin geometry. Ultimate tooth reduction and preparation form converge from this level.

greater crown length and the smaller diameter of root structure at the alveolar crest. Dowel placement may be needed for retention of the core. However, conventional dowel guidelines do not apply in the restoration of the severely periodontally compromised tooth. The dowel is rarely as long as the clinical crown and often does not reach to the alveolar crest. Narrowing root morphology further limits the apical extension. The apical end of the dowel should not be at the level of the alveolar crest but should terminate above or below the alveolus. The bony crest and dowel terminus are both stress concentrators, and coincident placement increases fracture potential.

Root amputation or tooth sectioning may be included in periodontal treatment of the multirooted tooth. The restorative strategy is significantly modified by this procedure. When the margin of the preparation is placed in the gingival crevice, all convexity on the axial wall must be removed. The root structure just coronal to the attachment level dictates the geometry of the restorative finish line. As the axial walls converge from

the margin area, this outline form is retained. Thus the morphology of the remaining root structure at the attachment level dictates the preparation design in the amputated or sectioned tooth (Figs. 21-28 and 21-29). Concern for long-term structural integrity of the tooth is always heightened by this finding. Predictably, studies of these teeth reveal the major cause of failure over time is root fracture, followed by recurrent periodontal disease, endodontic failure, caries, or loss of cement seal. As with periodontally sound teeth, the endodontic, periodontal, and initial restorative preparation should be completed before the selection of a dowel and core system. Maintenance of dentin is again the primary goal. Anatomy of the remaining roots indicates the best location for dowel placement. Long, straight, round roots of larger diameter should be selected for the dowel site. Adequate ferrule and exquisite control of occlusion are critical for longevity of these teeth.

Anterior dentition: The same caution in restoration of the periodontally compromised posterior dentition is present in the

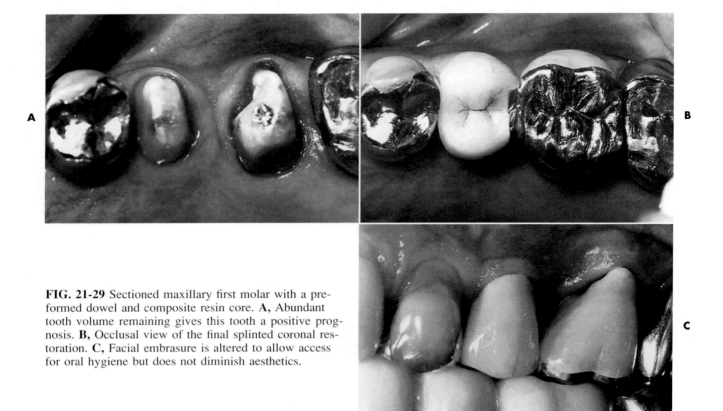

FIG. 21-29 Sectioned maxillary first molar with a pre-formed dowel and composite resin core. **A,** Abundant tooth volume remaining gives this tooth a positive prognosis. **B,** Occlusal view of the final splinted coronal restoration. **C,** Facial embrasure is altered to allow access for oral hygiene but does not diminish aesthetics.

anterior sextants. Single root formation is an anatomic advantage in this area, as the furcation is eliminated. However, aesthetic demands are a compounding issue. Margin location coronal to the free gingiva or minimal axial tooth reduction can lessen pulpal embarrassment in the posterior preparation. Heightened aesthetic demands in the anterior dentition may not allow these compromises. Margin placement in the gingival crevice and full-depth facial reduction for veneering material may be aesthetic requirements. The anterior sextant may also require connection to some or all of the posterior dentition. Paralleling these abutments usually mandates added dentin removal in the anterior segment. The cumulative effects of these insults on the anterior teeth may require preventive root canal therapy.

Anterior teeth with significant periodontal attachment loss may be retained as overdenture abutments. This option is available but less frequently used in the posterior areas. Guidelines for tooth selection and techniques for restoration of these teeth have been fully documented. Of importance here is the relationship between endodontics and restorative dentistry. The majority of these overdenture teeth function to support a removable prosthesis. Denture retention and lateral stability are minimal requisites. As such, functional forces to these abutments are directed mainly through the long axis of the tooth. Stress dissipation to the residual root through the use of a dowel is not required. These teeth may need only a restoration in the access opening to restore tooth contour and to seal the canal system. A preparation depth of approximately 3 mm is sufficient to retain the restoration and protect the canal system. Coverage of the entire dome-shaped overdenture abut-

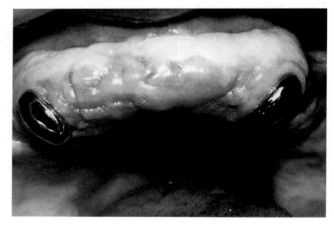

FIG. 21-30 Conventional overdenture teeth do not require dowels for stress distribution. Endodontic therapy is completed to allow reduction of the crown-root ratio. This case has cast gold copings for root coverage. In cases with sound tooth structure and low caries potential, bonded amalgam in the coronal segment of the canal is sufficient restoration.

ment is occasionally indicated for caries control and restoration (Fig. 21-30). A dowel may be used in such a case to retain the coronal restoration; again force dissipation is minimal, and the dowel length can be shortened. Only when the overdenture abutment is used for active retention of the prosthesis should guidelines for full-length dowels be followed. In addition to supplying support in a tissue-ward direction, these abutments also provide lateral stability and retain the prosthesis. Dowel placement distributes the functional load to the residual root and retains the precision attachment.

REFERENCES

1. Abou-Rass M: Post and core restorations of endodontically treated teeth, *Curr Opin Dent* 2:99, 1992.
2. Barnett F: Pulpal response to restorative procedures and materials, *Curr Opin Dent* 2:93, 1992.
3. Bergenholtz G, Nyman S: Endodontic complications following periodontal and prosthetic treatment of patients with advanced periodontal disease, *J Periodontol* 55:63, 1984.
4. Bower RC: Furcation morphology relative to periodontal treatment, *J Periodontol* 50:366, 1979.
5. Burgess J, Norling B, Summitt J: Resin-ionomer restorative materials: the new generation, *J Esthet Dent* 6:192, 1994.
6. Burns DA, Drause WR, Douglas HB, Burns DR: Stress distribution surrounding endodontic posts, *J Prosthet Dent* 64:412, 1990.
7. Christensen G: Post & core—state of the art—'92, *Clin Res Assoc Newsletter* 16:1, 1992.
8. Christensen G: Glass ionomer-resin: state of art, *Clin Res Assoc* 17:1, 1993.
9. Christensen G: Should teeth be built up for crowns? *J Am Dent Assoc* 124:93, 1993.
10. Christensen G: A promising new category of dental cements, *J Am Dent Assoc* 126:781, 1995.
11. Christensen G: Bonding amalgam update—1995, *Clin Res Assoc* 19:1, 1995.
12. Christensen G: Glass ionomer-resin cements, *Clin Res Assoc* 19:1, 1995.
13. Christensen G: When to use fillers, build-ups or post and cores, *J Am Dent Assoc* 127:1397, 1996.
14. Cooley RL: Dentinal bond strengths and microleakage of a 4-META adhesive to amalgam and composite resin, *Quintessence Int* 22:979, 1991.
15. Covey DA, Moon PC: Shear bond strength of dental amalgam bonded to dentin, *Am J Dent* 4:19, 1991.
16. Erickson R, Glasspoole EA: Bonding to tooth structure: a comparison of glass-ionomer and composite-resin systems, *J Esthet Dent* 6:192, 1994.
17. Felton D: Long term effects of crown preparation on pulp vitality, *J Dent Res* 68(special issue):1009, 1989 (abstract 1139).
18. Felton DA, Webb EL, Kanoy BE, Dugoni J: Threaded endodontic dowels: effect of post design on incidence of root fracture, *J Prosthet Dent* 65:179, 1991.
19. Ferrara A: Personal communication, January 1993.
20. Gelfand M, Golman M, Sunderman EJ: Effect of complete veneer crowns on the compressive strength of endodontically treated posterior teeth, *J Prosthet Dent* 52:635, 1984.
21. Goodacre CJ, Spolnik KJ: The prosthodontic management of endodontically treated teeth: a literature review. I. Success and failure data, treatment concepts, *J Prosthodont* 3:243, 1994.
22. Goodacre CJ, Spolnik KJ: The prosthodontic management of endodontically treated teeth: a literature review. II. Maintaining the apical seal, *J Prosthodont* 4:51, 1995.
23. Goodacre CJ, Spolnik KJ: The prosthodontic management of endodontically treated teeth: a literature review. III. Tooth preparation considerations, *J Prosthodont* 4:122, 1995.
24. Goss JM, Wright WJ, Bowles WF: Radiographic appearance of titanium alloy prefabricated posts cemented with different luting materials, *J Prosthet Dent* 67:632, 1992.
25. Gutmann JL: The dentin-root complex: anatomic and biologic considerations in restoring endodontically treated teeth, *J Prosthet Dent* 67:458, 1992.
26. Haddix JE, Mattison GD, Shulman CA, Pink FE: Post preparation techniques and their effect on the apical seal, *J Prosthet Dent* 64:515, 1990.

27. Hakajima M et al: Tensile bond strength and SEM evaluation of caries-affected dentin using dentin adhesives, *J Dent Res* 74:1679, 1995.
28. Hemmings KW, King PA, Setchell DJ: Resistance to torsional forces of various post and core designs, *J Prosthet Dent* 66:325, 1991.
29. Hussey DL: Resin retained posts, possible strengthening effects on dentine, *J Dent Res* 68(special issue): 1989 (abstract S54).
30. Isodore F, Odman P, Brondum K: Intermittent loading of teeth restored using prefabricated carbon fiber posts, *Int J Pros* 9:131, 1996.
31. Kane JJ, Burgess JO, Summitt J: Fracture resistance of amalgam coronal-radicular restorations, *J Prosthet Dent* 63:607, 1990.
32. Kydd WL et al: Marginal leakage of cast gold crowns luted with zinc phosphate cement: an in vitro study, *J Prosthet Dent* 75:9, 1996.
33. Lenchner NH: Restoring endodontically treated teeth: ferrule effect and biologic width, *Pract Periodont Aesth Dent* 1:19, 1989.
34. Marshall GW: Dentin: microstructure and characterization, *Quintessence Int* 24:606, 1993.
35. McComb D: Adhesive luting cements: classes, criteria, and usage, *Compend Contin Educ Dent* 17:759, 1996.
36. McDonald AV, King PA, Setchell DJ: An in vitro study to compare impact fracture resistance of intact root-treated teeth, *Int Endodont J* 23:304, 1990.
37. Millstein PL, Ho J, Nathanson D: Retention between a serrated steel dowel and different core materials, *J Prosthet Dent* 65:480, 1991.
38. Milot P, Stein RS: Root fracture in endodontically treated teeth related to post selection and crown design, *J Prosthet Dent* 68:428, 1992.
39. Nathanson D, Ashayeri N: New aspects of restoring the endodontically treated tooth, *Alpha Omegan* 83:76, 1990.
40. Obermayr G, Walton RE, Leary JM, Krell KV: Vertical root fracture and relative deformation during obturation and post cementation, *J Prosthet Dent* 66:181, 1991.
41. Pashley DH: Clinical correlations of dentin structure and function, *J Prosthet Dent* 66:777, 1991.
42. Pashley DH et al: Adhesion testing of dentin bonding agents: a review, *Dent Mater* 11:117, 1995.
43. Reeh ES, Messer HH, Douglas WH: Reduction in tooth stiffness as a result of endodontic and restorative procedures, *J Endod* 15:512, 1989.
44. Reel DC, Hinton T, Riggs G, Mitchell RJ: Effect of cementation method on the retention of anatomic cast post and cores, *J* 62:162, 1989.
45. Rosenberg MM, Kay HB, Keough BE, Holt RL: *Periodontal and prosthetic management for advanced cases,* Chicago, 1988, Quintessence Publishing.
46. Saxe SR et al: Dental amalgam and cognitive function in older women: findings from the nun study, *J Am Dent Assoc* 126:1495, 1995.
47. Scherer W et al: Bonding amalgam to tooth structure: a scanning electron microscope study, *J Esthet Dent* 4:199, 1992.
48. Sidhu SK, Watson TF: Resin-modified glass ionomer materials: a status report for the *American Journal of Dentistry, Am J Dent* 8:59, 1995.
49. Sorensen JA, Engelman MJ: Ferrule design and fracture resistance of endodontically treated teeth, *J Prosthet Dent* 63:529, 1990.
50. Sorensen JA, Engleman MJ, Daher T, Caputo AA: Altered corrosion resistance from casting to stainless steel posts, *J Prosthet Dent* 63:630, 1990.
51. Sorensen JA, Martinoff JT: Clinically significant factors in dowel design, *J Prosthet Dent* 52:28, 1984.
52. Sorensen JA, Martinoff JT: Endodontically treated teeth as abutments, *J Prosthet Dent* 53:631, 1985.
53. Standlee JP, Caputo AA: Endodontic dowel retention with resinous cements, *J Prosthet Dent* 68:913, 1992.
54. Standlee JP, Caputo AA: The retentive and stress distributing properties of split threaded endodontic dowels, *J Prosthet Dent* 68:436, 1992.
55. Thakur A, Johnston WM: Fluoride release of resin-based luting cements, *J Dent Res* 75:68, 1996 (abstract).
56. van Meerbeek B, Vanherle G, Lambrechts P, Braem M: Dentin and enamel bonding agents, *Curr Opin Dent* 2:117, 1992.

Chapter 22

Pediatric Endodontic Treatment

Joe H. Camp

Despite water fluoridation and emphasis on the prevention of caries, premature loss of primary and young permanent teeth continues to be common. The total prevention of caries is the ultimate goal of dentistry; but meanwhile, procedures must be used to preserve the primary and young permanent teeth ravaged by caries. This chapter deals with preservation of the primary and young permanent teeth that are pulpally involved. The objective of pulpal therapy is conservation of the tooth in a healthy state functioning as an integral component of the dentition.

Preservation of arch space is one of the primary objectives of pediatric dentistry. Premature loss of primary teeth may cause aberration of the arch length, resulting in mesial drift of the permanent teeth and consequent malocclusion. Whenever possible, the pulpally involved tooth should be maintained in the dental arch—provided, of course, that it can be restored to function, free of disease.

Other objectives of preserving primary teeth are to enhance aesthetics and mastication, prevent aberrant tongue habits, aid in speech, and prevent the psychologic effects associated with tooth loss. Premature loss of the maxillary incisors before age 3 has been shown to cause speech impairment that may persist in later years.[149]

Loss of pulpal vitality in the young permanent tooth creates special problems. Since the pulp is necessary for the formation of dentin, if the pulp is lost before root length is completed the tooth will have a poor crown-root ratio. Pulpal necrosis before the completion of dentin deposition within the root leaves a thin root more prone to fracture in the event of trauma. This situation also creates special problems in endodontic treatment, since endodontic techniques are usually not adequate to obturate the large blunderbuss canals. Additional procedures of apexification or apical surgery often become necessary to maintain the pulpless immature permanent tooth; the prognosis for permanent retention of the tooth is poorer than for the completely formed tooth.

In this chapter emphasis is on maintenance of pulpal vitality in the primary and young permanent teeth whenever possible to avoid many of the problems discussed elsewhere in this book.

Successful pulpal therapy in the primary dentition requires a thorough understanding of primary pulp morphology, root formation, and the special problems associated with resorption of primary tooth roots. Differences in the morphology of the primary and permanent pulps, in root formation, and in pri-

mary root resorption are covered later in this chapter. The reader is referred to Chapter 11 for a complete description of pulp and dentin formation.

DIFFERENCES IN PRIMARY AND PERMANENT TOOTH MORPHOLOGY (Fig. 22-1)

According to Finn[40] and Wheeler[198] the basic differences between the primary and the permanent teeth are these:

1. Primary teeth are smaller in all dimensions than the corresponding permanent teeth.
2. Primary crowns are wider in the mesial to distal dimension in comparison to their crown length than are permanent crowns.
3. Primary teeth have narrower and longer roots in comparison to crown length and width than do permanent teeth.
4. The facial and lingual cervical thirds of the crowns of anterior primary teeth are much more prominent than those of permanent teeth.
5. Primary teeth are markedly more constricted at the dentino-enamel junction than are permanent teeth.
6. The facial and lingual surfaces of primary molars converge occlusally so that the occlusal surface is much narrower in the facio-lingual than the cervical width.
7. The roots of primary molars are comparatively more slender and longer than the roots of permanent molars.
8. The roots of primary molars flare out nearer the cervix and more at the apex than do the roots of permanent molars.
9. The enamel is thinner, about 1 mm, on primary teeth than on permanent teeth, and it has a more consistent depth.
10. The thickness of the dentin between the pulp chambers and the enamel in primary teeth is less than in permanent teeth.
11. The pulp chambers in primary teeth are comparatively larger than in permanent teeth.
12. The pulp horns, especially the mesial horns, are higher in primary molars than in permanent molars.

A detailed discussion of the anatomy of the individual primary root canals is presented later in this chapter.

Diagnosis

Before the initiation of restorative procedures on a tooth, a thorough clinical and radiographic examination must be concluded. The case history and any pertinent medical history must be thoroughly reviewed. Comprehensive coverage of diagnosis is to be found in Chapter 1, and the reader is referred to that chapter for a more in-depth discussion.

The author wishes to thank Dr. Ronald B. Mack for his contribution in revising this chapter.

Good periapical and bite-wing radiographs are essential to complete the diagnosis. Examination of the soft and hard tissues for any apparent pathosis is a routine part of the examination.

In the event that pulp therapy is required, the preoperative diagnosis is of utmost importance and should dictate the type of treatment to be carried out. If the pulpal status is not determined before operative procedures are begun and pulp therapy becomes necessary during the treatment, an adequate diagnosis may be impossible.

There are no reliable clinical diagnostic tools for accurately evaluating the status of the pulp that has become inflamed. An accurate determination of the extent of inflammation within the pulp cannot be made short of histologic examination.[173] Diagnosis of pulpal health in the exposed pulp of children is difficult, and the correlation between clinical symptoms and histopathologic conditions is poor.[109]

Although the diagnostic tests are admittedly poor for evaluating the degree of inflammation within the primary and young permanent pulp, they must always be performed to obtain as much information as possible to aid in the diagnosis before treatment is rendered. The recommended diagnostic tests for use in primary and young permanent teeth are discussed next.

Radiographs

Current radiographs are essential to examining for caries and periapical changes. Interpretation of radiographs is complicated in children by physiologic root resorption of primary teeth and by incompletely formed roots of permanent teeth. If one is not familiar with diagnosing radiographs of children or does not have radiographs of good quality, these normally occurring circumstances can easily lead to misinterpretation of normal anatomy for pathologic changes.

The radiograph does not always demonstrate periapical pathosis, nor can the proximity of caries to the pulp always be accurately determined. What may appear as an intact barrier of secondary dentin overlying the pulp may actually be a perforated mass of irregularly calcified and carious dentin overlying a pulp with extensive inflammation.[109]

The presence of calcified masses within the pulp is important to making a diagnosis of pulpal status (Fig. 22-2). Mild, chronic irritation to the pulp stimulates secondary dentin formation. When the irritation is acute and of rapid onset, the defense mechanism may not have a chance to lay down secondary dentin. When the disease process reaches the pulp, the pulp may form calcified masses away from the exposure site. These calcified masses are always associated with advanced pulpal degeneration in the pulp chamber and inflammation of the pulp tissue in the canals.[109]

Pathologic changes in the periapical tissues surrounding primary molars are most often apparent in the bifurcation or trifurcation areas rather than at the apexes, as in permanent teeth (Figs. 22-2 and 22-3, *A*). Pathologic bone and root resorption is indicative of advanced pulpal degeneration that has spread into the periapical tissues. The pulpal tissue may remain vital even with such advanced degenerative changes.

Internal resorption occurs frequently in the primary dentition following pulpal involvement. It is always associated with ex-

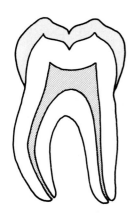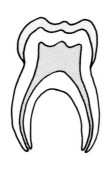

FIG. 22-1 Cross section of primary and permanent molars.

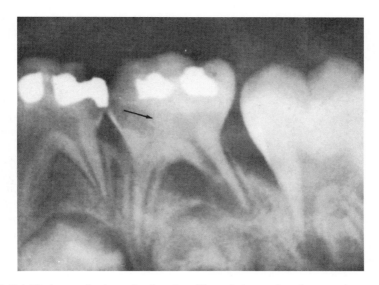

FIG. 22-2 Calcified mass in the pulp chamber. There is internal and external root resorption. Calcified mass *(arrow)* is an attempt to block a massive carious lesion. Because of resorption, this tooth should be extracted. Note the bone loss in the bifurcation area.

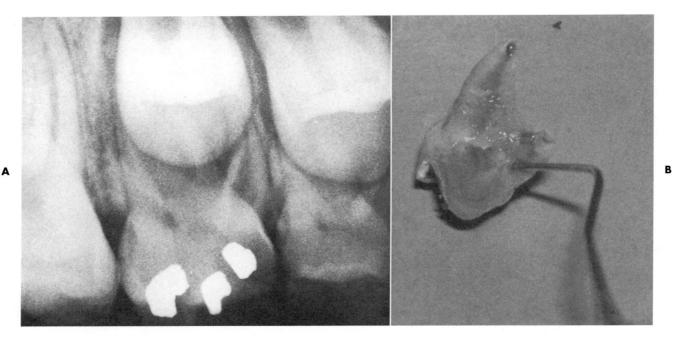

FIG. 22-3 Internal resorption caused by inflammation from carious pulp exposure. **A,** Note the bone loss in the trifurcation and the internal resorption in the mesial root. **B,** Extracted tooth. Note the perforation of internal resorption. Probe is extended through the resorption defect.

tensive inflammation[59] and usually occurs in the molar root canals adjacent to the bifurcation or trifurcation area. Because of the thinness of primary molar roots, once the internal resorption has become advanced enough to be seen radiographically, there is usually a perforation of the root by the resorption (Fig. 22-3, *B*). After the occurrence of perforation of the primary tooth root by internal resorption, all forms of pulpal therapy are contraindicated. The treatment of choice is extraction.

Pulp tests

The electrical pulp tester is of little value in the primary dentition or in young permanent teeth with incompletely developed apexes. Although the tester may indicate vitality, it will not give reliable data as to the extent of inflammation within the pulp. Many children with perfectly normal teeth do not respond to the electrical pulp tester even at the higher settings. Added to these factors is the unreliability of the response in the young child because of apprehension, fear, or management problems.

Thermal tests are also generally unreliable in the primary dentition for determining pulpal status.

Percussion and mobility

Teeth with extensive pulpal inflammation usually exhibit tenderness to percussion; however, this test is not very reliable in primary teeth of young children because of the psychologic aspects involved.

Tooth mobility is also not a reliable test of pulpal pathosis in primary teeth. During phases of active physiologic root resorption, primary teeth with normal pulps may have varying degrees of mobility. Furthermore, teeth with varying degrees of pulpal inflammation may have very little mobility.

Pulpal exposures and hemorrhage

It has been reported that the size of the exposure, the appearance of the pulp, and the amount of hemorrhage are important factors in diagnosing the extent of inflammation in a cariously exposed pulp. A true carious exposure is always accompanied by pulpal inflammation (see Chapter 15).[109,173] The pinpoint carious exposure may have pulpal inflammation varying from minimal to extensive to complete necrosis. However, the massive exposure always has widespread inflammation or necrosis and is not candidate for any form of vital pulp therapy. Excessive hemorrhage at an exposure site or during pulp amputation is evidence of extensive inflammation. These teeth should be considered candidates for pulpectomy or extraction.

History of pain

A history of spontaneous toothache is usually associated with extensive degenerative changes in the pulp of a primary tooth[59]; nevertheless, absence of pain cannot be used to judge pulpal status, since varying degrees of degeneration or even complete necrosis of the pulp are seen without any history of pain.

Guthrie et al.[59] attempted to use the first drop of hemorrhage from an exposed pulp site as a diagnostic aid for determining the extent of degeneration within the pulp. A white blood cell differential count (hemogram) was made for each of 53 teeth included in the study. A detailed history, including percussion, electrical pulp test, thermal tests, mobility, and history of pain, was obtained. The teeth were extracted and histologically examined. On correlation of the histologic findings with the hemogram and a detailed history, it was determined that percussion, electrical and thermal pulp tests, and mobility were *unreliable* in establishing the degree of pulpal inflammation.

The hemogram did not give reliable evidence of pulpal degeneration, even though teeth with advanced degeneration of the pulp involving the root canals did have an elevated neutrophil count. A consistent finding of the study, however, was advanced degeneration of pulpal tissue in teeth with a history of spontaneous toothache.

Primary teeth with a history of spontaneous, unprovoked toothache should not be considered for any form of pulp therapy short of pulpectomy or extraction.

INDIRECT PULP THERAPY

Indirect pulp therapy is a technique for avoiding pulp exposure in the treatment of teeth with deep carious lesions in which there exists no clinical evidence of pulpal degeneration or periapical disease. The procedure allows the tooth to use the natural protective mechanisms of the pulp against caries. It is based on the theory that a zone of affected demineralized dentin exists between the outer infected layer of dentin and the pulp. When the infected dentin is removed, *the affected dentin can remineralize and the odontoblasts form reparative dentin,* thus avoiding a pulp exposure.[25]

Disagreement exists as to whether the deep layers of the carious dentin are infected. Several studies[86,92] showed deep carious lesions to be infected, whereas another[50] reported an area of softened and discolored dentin far in advance of bacterial contamination in acute caries. Still others[164,200] found that most organisms had been removed after the removal of the softened dentin, although the incidence of bacterial contamination was higher in primary teeth than in permanent teeth; however, some dentinal tubules still contained small numbers of bacteria.

Kopel[90] summarized the results of various studies of the carious process and identified three distinct layers in active caries: necrotic soft dentin not painful to stimulation and grossly infected with bacteria, firm but softened dentin painful to stimulation but containing fewer bacteria, and slightly discolored hard sound dentin containing few bacteria and painful to stimulation.

In indirect pulp therapy the outer layers of carious dentin are removed. Thus most of the bacteria are eliminated from the lesion. When the lesion is sealed, the substrate on which the bacteria act to produce acid is also removed. Exposure of the pulp occurs when the carious process advances faster than the reparative mechanism of the pulp. With the arrest of the carious process, the reparative mechanism is able to lay down additional dentin and avoid a pulp exposure.

Although carious dentin left in the tooth probably contains some bacteria, the number of organisms can be greatly diminished when this layer is covered with zinc oxide–eugenol (ZOE) or calcium hydroxide.[37,86]

The reparative and recuperative powers of the dental pulp have long been recognized in dentistry. In the mideighteenth century Pierre Fauchard advised that all caries in deeply carious sensitive teeth should not be removed because of the danger of pulp exposure.[90] The principles of indirect pulp therapy were recognized as early as 1850. Early investigators[61,73,201] proposed leaving a layer of partially softened dentin to avoid exposure of the pulp and suggested that recalcification of areas of soft decalcified dentin could occur when the softened dentin was sealed under a filling. All these early investigators attributed their success to proper selection of cases. The techniques

suggested were only for teeth without a history of pain or teeth in which slight inflammation was suspected. Although the techniques were empiric, the treatment was judged successful.

Dimaggio and Hawes[29,30] selected primary and permanent teeth that were free of clinical signs of pulpal degeneration and periapical pathosis and that appeared radiographically to have a pulp exposure if all the decay were removed. On removal of all decay, pulp exposure occurred in 75% of the teeth. In another group of teeth judged clinically to be the same as the first group, the authors achieved 99% success in avoiding pulp exposures with indirect pulp therapy. Reporting on an expanded number of teeth observed from 2 weeks to 4 years, their success rate remained at 97% for the indirect pulp therapy technique.[63]

Indirect pulp therapy has proved to be a very successful technique when cases are properly selected. Reports[85,128,186] show successes ranging from 74% to 99%. Differences in case selection, length of study, and type of investigation are responsible for the variations in success. Frankl's report[43] of pulp therapy in pediatric dentistry provides a complete review of the literature on indirect pulp therapy.

Indirect Pulp Therapy Technique

Indirect pulp therapy is used when pulpal inflammation has been judged to be minimal and complete removal of caries would probably cause a pulp exposure (Fig. 22-4, *A*). Careful diagnosis of the pulpal status is completed before the treatment is initiated. Any tooth judged to have widespread inflammation or evidence of periapical pathosis should receive endodontic therapy or be extracted.

The tooth is anesthetized and isolated with a rubber dam. All the caries except that immediately overlying the pulp is removed. Care must be taken to eliminate all the caries at the dentinoenamel junction. Because of its closeness to the surface, caries left in this area will likely cause failure. If there is communication of the caries with the oral cavity, the carious process will continue, resulting in failure.

Care must also be taken in removing the caries to avoid exposure of the pulp. A large round bur is best to remove the caries. The use of spoon excavators when approaching the pulp may cause an exposure by removal of a large segment of decay. Nevertheless, if used judiciously, a spoon excavator is not contraindicated for removing caries near the dentinoenamel junction. All undermined enamel is not removed, for it will help retain the temporary filling.

After all caries except that just overlying the pulp has been removed, a sedative filling of either ZOE or calcium hydroxide is placed over the remaining carious dentin and areas of deep excavation. The tooth may then be sealed with ZOE or amalgam (Fig. 22-4, *B* and *C*).

If the remaining tooth structure is insufficient to retain the temporary filling, a stainless steel band or temporary crown must be adapted to the tooth to maintain the dressing within the tooth (Fig. 22-5). If the dressing is lost and the remaining caries reexposed to the oral fluids, the desired effects cannot be achieved and a failure will occur.

If this preliminary caries removal is successful, the inflammation will be resolved and deposition of reparative dentin beneath the caries will allow subsequent eradication of the remaining caries without pulpal exposure.

The sedative dressing to be used in indirect pulp therapy may be either calcium hydroxide or ZOE. Studies have shown

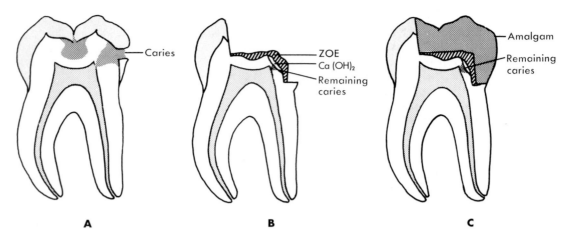

FIG. 22-4 Indirect pulp therapy. **A,** Pulp would probably be exposed if all caries is removed. **B,** All decay is eliminated except that just overlying the pulp. Calcium hydroxide–zinc oxide–eugenol is placed over the remaining caries and deep carious excavation. (Calcium hydroxide may be deleted and only ZOE placed.) **C,** Tooth is sealed with amalgam.

both materials to be effective, and no compelling evidence has been presented that calcium hydroxide is superior to ZOE.[34,85]

The treated tooth is reentered in 6 to 8 weeks, and the remaining caries is extirpated. The rate of reparative dentin deposition has been shown to average 1.4 μm/day following cavity preparations in dentin of human teeth. The rate of reparative dentin formation decreases markedly after 48 days.[170] Dentin is laid down fastest during the first month following indirect pulp therapy, and the rate then diminishes steadily with time. Pulpal floor depth reportedly has little effect on the amount of reparative dentin formed.[186] By contrast, another report[157] has stated that dentin formation is accelerated by thin dentin, that more dentin formation occurs with longer treatment times, and that greater dentin formation is observed in primary than in permanent teeth.

If the initial treatment is successful, when the tooth is reentered, the caries appears to be arrested. The color changes from a deep red rose to light gray or light brown. The texture changes from spongy and wet to hard, and the caries appears dehydrated. *Practically all bacteria are destroyed under ZOE and calcium hydroxide dressing sealed in deep carious lesions.*[4,86]

Following removal of the remaining caries, the tooth may be permanently restored. The usual procedure of pulpal protection with adequate bases is, of course, mandatory before placement of permanent restorations.

DIRECT PULP CAPPING AND PULPOTOMY

Direct pulp capping and pulpotomy involve the application of a medicament or dressing to the exposed pulp in an attempt to preserve its vitality. Pulpotomy differs from pulp capping only in that a portion of the remaining pulp is removed before application of the medicament. These procedures have been employed for carious, mechanical, and traumatic exposures of the pulp—with reported high incidence of success as judged radiographically and by the absence of clinical signs and symptoms. Histologic examinations, however, have shown chronic inflammation under many carious pulp caps and diminished success rates.

Orban[129] described the histopathology of the pulp and concluded that the cells of the pulp were the same as those of loose connective tissue. He believed these cells could differentiate and healing could occur in the dental pulp. In subsequent years much experimentation has taken place, with advocates both for and against pulp-capping and pulpotomy procedures.

Although disagreement exists concerning pulp capping and pulpotomy as permanent procedures in mature secondary teeth, it is universally accepted that vital technique must be employed in teeth with incompletely formed roots with exposed pulps. Once root formation has been completed, routine endodontic treatment may be performed.

Cvek[19,21,22] has reported that pulp capping and partial pulpotomy with calcium hydroxide on *traumatically exposed pulps* are successful 96% of the time. He found that the time between the accident and treatment was not critical as long as the superficially inflamed pulp tissue was removed before capping. The size of the exposure had no bearing on success or failure. The study included both mature teeth and teeth with incompletely formed roots. Continued calcification of the pulp following pulp capping was not a consistent finding; and when it occurred, it was usually within the first year. These findings have been substantiated by subsequent studies.[47,66,88]

In a technique termed *partial pulpotomy,* young posterior teeth with deep carious exposures were subjected to removal of 1 to 3 mm of the exposed pulp. The exposure site was covered with calcium hydroxide and the tooth sealed with IRM and a permanent restoration. In cases with no clinical or radiographic signs of pathology a success rate of 91% was reported.[110] Twenty-nine of 31 cases were successful when followed 24 to 140 months. The same study reported four of six cases with temporary pain and radiographic signs of minor periapical involvement responding successfully. Since loss of the pulp in teeth with immature apexes is so devastating, it seems advisable to attempt the partial pulpotomy procedure. If failure occurs, apexification can always be performed.

Because of the normal aging of the dental pulp, chances of successful pulp capping diminish with age. Increases in fibrous and calcific deposits and a reduction in pulpal volume may be observed in older pulps. With age the fibroblast proliferation observed in the teeth of young animals is significantly reduced.[160]

Teeth with calcifications of the pulp chamber and root canals

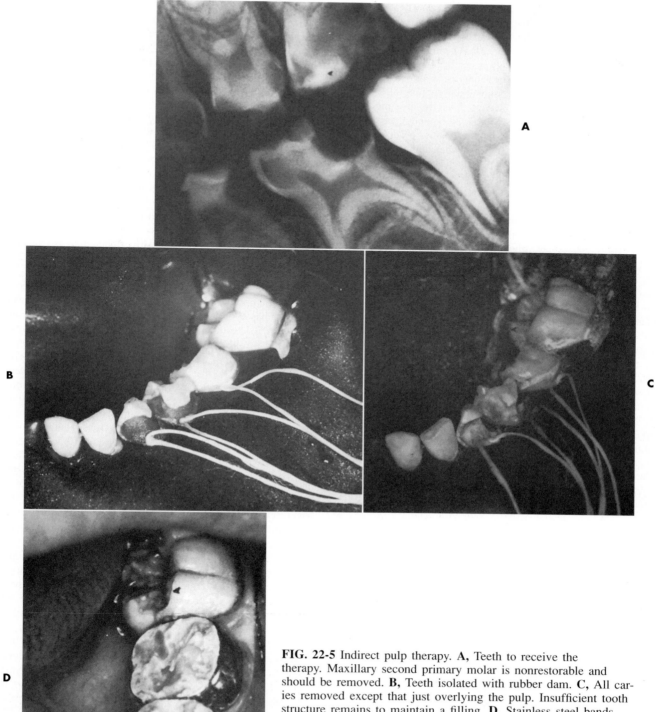

FIG. 22-5 Indirect pulp therapy. **A,** Teeth to receive the therapy. Maxillary second primary molar is nonrestorable and should be removed. **B,** Teeth isolated with rubber dam. **C,** All caries removed except that just overlying the pulp. Insufficient tooth structure remains to maintain a filling. **D,** Stainless steel bands placed for retention of zinc oxide–eugenol temporary fillings.

are not candidates for pulp-capping procedures. These calcifications are indicative of previous inflammatory responses or trauma and render the pulp less responsive to vital therapy.[20]

Agreement generally exists concerning pulp caps in young permanent teeth with blunderbuss apexes, but there is disagreement as to whether mature permanent teeth should be pulp capped after a carious pulp exposure. Pulp capping after carious pulp exposure is widely accepted as the treatment of choice. Many clinicians believe that to obtain good results teeth must be carefully selected; pulp capping should be done only in the absence of a history of pain and when there is little or no bleeding at the exposure site.[109] However, other clinicians recommend extirpation of all cariously exposed pulps except those with incompletely formed apexes, the rationale being that although there may be no pain, enough toxic products remain in the pulp to maintain the inflammation.[93]

These long-standing inflammations with circulatory disturbances are frequently accompanied by apposition and resorption of the canal walls and calcification in the pulp. The inflammation, calcification, apposition, and resorption may thrive under pulp caps, regardless of which material is used as the pulp-capping agent. In teeth with blunderbuss apices, some clinicians recommend pulp extirpation and filling of the canals after a pulp cap as soon as the apical foramen has closed because continued calcification may eventually render the canals unnegotiable.[93]

Few disagree that the ideal treatment for all carious pulp exposures on mature permanent teeth should be pulpal extirpation and endodontic treatment. It is unrealistic, however, to believe that this can be achieved in all cases. Extirpating the pulp is economically unfeasible in many cases and is time consuming and difficult to accomplish in certain teeth. If vital pulp therapy fails, one usually still has the option of endodontic treatment.

Agreement exists that exposed caries on primary teeth should *not* be pulp capped. *Pulp-capping procedures in primary teeth should be reserved for teeth with mechanical exposures.* The pulpotomy procedure for primary teeth (see below) has been shown to be much more successful than pulp capping, and the time requirements for performing the procedures are similar. Therefore *it is recommended that carious pulp exposures on primary teeth not be pulp capped.*[172,173]

According to Seltzer and Bender[160] pulp capping should be discouraged for carious pulp exposures, since microorganisms and inflammation are invariably associated. Macroscopic examination of such exposures is difficult, and areas of liquefaction necrosis may be overlooked. Because of accelerated aging processes in carious teeth and teeth having undergone operative procedures, they are poorer candidates for pulp caps than noncarious teeth; because of diminished blood supply, periodontally involved teeth are poor risks for pulp capping.

There is general agreement[25,109,160] that the larger the area of carious exposure the poorer the prognosis for pulp capping. With a larger exposure more pulpal tissue is inflamed, and there is greater chance for contamination by microorganisms. With larger exposures there is also greater damage from crushing of tissues and hemorrhage, causing a more severe inflammation. However, when exposure occurs as a result of traumatic or mechanical injury to a healthy pulp, the size of the exposure does not influence healing.[19,134]

Location of the pulp exposures is an important consideration in the prognosis. If the exposure occurs on the axial wall of the pulp, with pulp tissue coronal to the exposure site, this tissue may be deprived of its blood supply and undergo necrosis, causing a failure. Then a pulpotomy or pulpectomy should be performed rather than a pulp cap.[168]

If pulp capping or pulpotomy is to be done, care must be exercised in removal of caries or dentin over the exposure site to keep to a minimum the pushing of dentin chips into the remaining pulp tissue. Decreased success has been shown when dentin fragments are forced into the underlying pulp tissue.[79] Inflammatory reaction and formation of dentin matrix are stimulated around these dentin chips.[112] In addition, microorganisms may be forced into the tissue. The resulting inflammatory reaction can be so severe as to cause failure.

Experiments on germ-free animals have shown the importance of microorganisms in the healing of exposed pulp tissues; injured pulp tissue contaminated by microorganisms did not heal, whereas tissue in germ-free animals did heal regardless of the severity of the exposure.[78,133] Pulp procedures should always be carried out with rubber dam isolation and aseptic conditions to prevent introduction of microorganisms into the pulp tissue.

Marginal seal over the pulp-capping or pulpotomy procedure is of prime importance. In deep cavities without pulp exposure, Kanka[80] has hypothesized that pulpal inflammation is a consequence of bacterial microleakage rather than acid etching of dentin. In a follow-up study[199] it was shown that healing following acid etching was better with composite resin adhesives than with controls of ZOE or silicate cement when placed in deep dentinal preparations. Leakage of bacteria in the controls was associated with severe pulpal inflammation. Thus it was concluded that bacterial leakage rather than acid etching impairs pulpal healing in deep dentinal cavities. Healing and the formation of secondary dentin are inherent properties of the pulp. If allowed to do so, the pulp, like any connective tissue, will heal itself. Healing following pulp amputation has been shown to be essentially the same as initial calcification events that occur in other normal and diseased calcified tissues.[64] Factors promoting healing are conditions of the pulp at the time of amputation, removal of irritants, and proper postoperative care such as proper sealing of the margins.

After mechanical exposure of the pulp, an acute inflammation occurs at the exposure site. Blood vessels dilate, edema occurs, and polymorphonuclear leukocytes accumulate at the injury site. If the initial tissue damage is too severe, the pulp becomes chronically inflamed, with eventual necrosis of the pulp. It has been shown, however, that repair can occur after pulp exposure. Mechanical exposures have a much better prognosis than do carious exposures because of the lack of previous inflammation and infection associated with the carious exposures. Repair depends on the amount of tissue destruction, the presence of hemorrhage, the patient's age, the resistance of the host, and other factors involved in connective tissue repair.[160]

After pulpal injury, reparative dentin is formed as part of the repair process. Although formation of a dentin bridge has been used as one of the criteria for judging successful pulp capping or pulpotomy procedures, bridge formation can occur in teeth with irreversible inflammation. Moreover, successful pulp capping has been reported without the presence of a reparative dentin bridge over the exposure site.[158,194]

Pulp-Capping Agents

Many materials and drugs have been employed as pulp-capping agents. Camp's[14] report provides a complete review of the literature on pulp-capping agents. Materials, medicaments, antiseptics, antiinflammatory agents, antibiotics, and enzymes have been used as pulp-capping agents; but *calcium hydroxide is generally accepted as the material of choice for pulp capping.*[20,109,160]

Before 1930, when Hermann[67] introduced calcium hydroxide as a successful pulp-capping agent, pulp therapy had consisted of devitalization with arsenic and other fixative agents. Hermann demonstrated the formation of secondary dentin over the amputation sites of vital pulps capped with calcium hydroxide.

In 1938 Teuscher and Zander[183] introduced calcium hydroxide in the United States; they histologically confirmed complete dentinal bridging with healthy radicular pulp under calcium hydroxide dressings. Further reports[55,204] firmly established calcium hydroxide as the pulp-capping agent of choice. After these early works many studies have reported various forms of calcium hydroxide used, with success rates ranging from 30% to 98%.[43] The dissimilar success rates are attributed to many factors, including selection of teeth, criteria for success and failure, differences in responses among different animals, length of study, area of pulp to which the medicament was applied (coronally or cervically), and the type of calcium hydroxide employed.

When calcium hydroxide is applied directly to pulp tissue, there is necrosis of the adjacent pulp tissue and an inflammation of the contiguous tissue. Dentin bridge formation occurs at the junction of the necrotic tissue and the vital inflamed tissue. Although calcium hydroxide works effectively, the exact mechanism is not understood. Compounds of similar alkalinity (pH of 11) cause liquefaction necrosis when applied to pulp tissue. Calcium hydroxide maintains a local state of alkalinity that is necessary for bone or dentin formation. Beneath the region of coagulation necrosis, cells of the underlying pulp tissue differentiate into odontoblasts and elaborate dentin matrix.[160]

Occasionally in spite of successful bridge formation, the pulp remains chronically inflamed or becomes necrotic. Internal resorption may occur following pulp exposure and capping with calcium hydroxide. In other cases complete dentin mineralization of the remaining pulp tissue occludes the canals to the extent that they cannot be penetrated for endodontic therapy if necessary. For these reasons pulpal extirpation and canal filling have been recommended as soon as root formation is completed after the use of calcium hydroxide[93,160] (Fig. 22-6). However, in view of the low incidence of this occurrence, it does not seem to be routinely justified unless necessary for restorative purposes.

It was postulated[204] that calcium would diffuse from a calcium hydroxide dressing into the pulp and participate in the formation of reparative dentin. Experiments with radioactive ions, however, have shown that calcium ions from the calcium hydroxide do *not* enter into the formation of new dentin. Radioactive calcium ions injected intravenously were identified in the dentin bridge. Thus it was established that *the calcium for the dentin bridge comes from the bloodstream.*[6,137,159] The action of calcium hydroxide to form a dentin bridge appears to be a result of the low-grade irritation in the underlying pulpal tissue following application. This theory was supported by the demonstration of successful dentin bridging after application of calcium hydroxide for short periods of time, followed by removal of the material.[23]

Different forms of calcium hydroxide have produced marked differences when applied to a pulp exposure.[136,180,188]

Commercially available compounds of calcium hydroxide in modified forms are known to be less alkaline and thus less

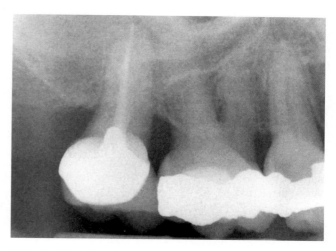

FIG. 22-6 Calcification of pulp chambers and root canals after calcium hydroxide pulp capping. Pulp chamber is completely obliterated, and the root canals are partially obliterated. Because of calcification after the pulp capping, the root canals are extremely difficult to locate and negotiate.

caustic on the pulp. The reactions to Dycal, Prisma VLC Dycal, Life, and Nu-Cap have been shown to be similar.[168,169,180] The chemically altered tissue created by application of these compounds is resorbed first, and the bridge is then formed in contact with the capping material.[187,188] With calcium hydroxide powder (or Pulpdent) the bridge forms at the junction of the chemically altered tissue and the remaining subjacent vital pulp tissue. The altered tissue degenerates and disappears, leaving a void between the capping material and the dentin bridge. This is the reason a bridge can be seen better radiographically with calcium hydroxide powder or Pulpdent than with the other commercial compounds. The quality of the dentin bridging was equally good with either material.

The ideal treatment for all carious exposures, except those in teeth with incompletely formed roots, might be pulp extirpation and root canal filling; nevertheless, there are still indications for direct pulp capping. Economics, time, and difficulty of achieving root canal filling in certain teeth are a few of the reasons one may choose pulp capping over another form of pulp therapy. *The pulp capping material of choice at the present time remains calcium hydroxide.* If pulp capping is considered, one must consider all the factors discussed in this section to determine the prognosis of each case. In the event of failure of direct pulp capping, there is usually the option of endodontic therapy.

Pulp capping should *not* be considered for primary carious pulp exposures or for permanent teeth with a history of spontaneous toothache, radiographic evidence of pulpal or periapical pathosis, calcifications of the pulp chamber or root canals, excessive hemorrhage at the exposure site, or exposures with purulent or serous exudates.

PULPOTOMY

The pulpotomy procedure involves removing pulp tissue that has inflammatory or degenerative changes, leaving intact the remaining vital tissue, which is then covered with a pulp-capping agent to promote healing at the amputation site or an agent to cause fixation of the underlying tissue. The only difference between pulpotomy and pulp capping is that in pulpotomy additional tissue is removed from the exposed pulp. Traditionally, the term "pulpotomy" has implied removal of pulp tissue to the cervical line. However, the depth to which tissue is removed is determined by clinical judgment. All tissue judged to be inflamed should be removed to place the dressing on healthy, uninflamed pulp tissue. Better results are obtained if the amputation level is shallow because of better visualization of the working area. In multirooted teeth the procedure may be simplified by removing tissue to the orifices of the root canals.

The difficulties of assessing the extent of inflammation in cariously exposed pulps have been previously discussed. However, several studies[22,65,66] have shown that inflammation is confined to the surface 2 to 3 mm of the pulp when traumatically exposed and left untreated for up to 168 hours. In experimental animals the results were the same whether the crowns were fractured or ground off. Direct invasion of vital pulp tissue by bacteria did not occur, even though the pulps were left exposed to the saliva. Under the same circumstances with cavity preparations into the teeth that left areas to impact food, debris, and bacteria in contact with the pulp, the inflammation ranged from 1 to 9 mm with abscess and pus formation.[22,65] The same results have been obtained in permanent teeth with incompletely formed roots, as well as those with mature ones. Pulpotomy procedures for primary teeth are discussed later in this chapter.

Calcium Hydroxide Pulpotomy on Young Permanent Teeth

Despite the fact that vital pulp-capping and pulpotomy procedures for cariously exposed pulps in teeth with developed apexes remain controversial, it is universally accepted that vital techniques be employed in those teeth with incompletely developed apexes. Although many materials and drugs have been used as pulp-capping agents (described earlier), the application of calcium hydroxide to stimulate dentin bridge formation in accidentally or cariously exposed pulps of young permanent teeth continues to be the treatment of choice.

The indirect pulp therapy technique should be used whenever possible with deep carious lesions to avoid exposure of the pulp (see p. 721). Every attempt should be made to maintain the vitality of these immature teeth until their full root development has been completed. Loss of vitality before root completion leaves a weak root more prone to fracture. Loss of vitality before completion of root length may leave a poor crown-root ratio and a tooth more susceptible to periodontal breakdown because of excessive mobility. If necessary, the remaining pulp tissue can be extirpated and conventional endodontic therapy completed when root formation has been accomplished.

Endodontic treatment is greatly complicated in teeth with necrotic pulps and open apexes. Although apexification procedures have been perfected for these teeth, the treatment is extensive and costly for the patient and the resulting root structure is weaker than in teeth with fully developed roots. If the calcium hydroxide pulpotomy is not successful, the apexification procedure or surgical endodontics may still be performed.

Technique

After the diagnosis is completed, the tooth is anesthetized. If possible, pulpal procedures should always be performed under rubber dam isolation and aseptic conditions to prevent further introduction of microorganisms into the pulp tissues. Care must be taken when placing the rubber dam on a traumatized tooth. If any loosening of the tooth has occurred, the rubber dam clamps must be applied to adjacent uninjured teeth. If this is impossible because of lack of adjacent teeth or partially erupted ones that cannot be clamped, careful isolation with cotton rolls and constant aspiration by the dental assistant may be used to maintain a dry field (Fig. 22-7).

In traumatically exposed pulps, only tissue judged to be inflamed is removed. Cvek[19] has shown that with pulp exposures resulting from traumatic injuries, regardless of the size of the exposure or the amount of lapsed time, pulpal changes are characterized by a proliferative response with inflammation extending only a few millimeters into the pulp. When this hyperplastic inflamed tissue is removed, healthy pulp tissue is encountered.[19] In teeth with carious exposure of the pulp, it may be necessary to remove pulp tissue to a greater depth to reach uninflamed tissue.

The instrument of choice for tissue removal in the pulpotomy procedure is an abrasive diamond bur, using high speed and adequate water cooling. This technique has been shown to create the least damage to the underlying tissue.[56] Care must be exercised to ensure removal of all filaments of the pulp tissue coronal to the amputation site; otherwise, hemorrhage will be impossible to control. Following pulpal amputation, the preparation is thoroughly washed with physiologic saline or sterile water to remove all debris. The water is removed by vacuum and cotton pellets. Air should not be blown on the exposed pulp, since it will cause desiccation and tissue damage.

Hemorrhage is controlled by slightly moistened cotton pellets (wetted and blotted almost dry) placed against the stumps of the pulp. Completely dry cotton pellets should not be used, since fibers of the dry cotton will be incorporated into the clot and, when removed, will cause hemorrhage. Dry cotton pellets are placed over the moist pellets, and slight pressure is exerted on the mass to control the hemorrhage. Hemorrhage should be controlled in this manner within several minutes (Fig. 22-7, C). It may be necessary to change the pellets to control all hemorrhage. If hemorrhage continues, one must carefully check to be sure that all filaments of the pulp coronal to the amputation site were removed and that the site is clean.

If hemorrhage cannot be controlled, amputation should be performed at a more apical level. Should it become necessary to extend into the root canals, a small endodontic spoon or round abrasive diamond bur may be used to remove the tissue on anterior teeth with single canals (Fig. 22-8). On posterior teeth the use of endodontic files or reamers may be necessary if tissue is being amputated within the canals. *Obviously, extension of the amputation site is carried into the root canals only in teeth with blunderbuss apexes.*

On teeth with blunderbuss apexes, if tissue removal has been extended several millimeters into the root canals and hemorrhage continues, a compromise treatment should be considered. The hemorrhage is controlled with chemicals such as aluminum chloride or other hemostatic agents. Once the hemorrhage is controlled, calcium hydroxide is placed in the canal against the pulp stump and the tooth is sealed. These compromised teeth must be closely monitored for development of pathologic conditions. If necrosis of the remaining pulp tissue occurs, apexification procedures are instituted. If vitality is maintained, further root development with dystrophic calcification usually

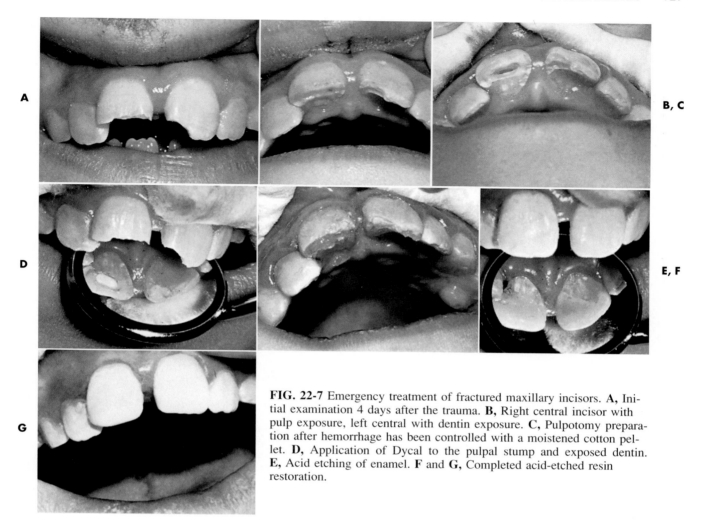

FIG. 22-7 Emergency treatment of fractured maxillary incisors. **A,** Initial examination 4 days after the trauma. **B,** Right central incisor with pulp exposure, left central with dentin exposure. **C,** Pulpotomy preparation after hemorrhage has been controlled with a moistened cotton pellet. **D,** Application of Dycal to the pulpal stump and exposed dentin. **E,** Acid etching of enamel. **F** and **G,** Completed acid-etched resin restoration.

occurs. In these compromised cases, once the apex has formed, the tooth is reentered and conventional endodontic therapy is completed with gutta-percha obliteration.

In the normal pulpotomy procedure, once the hemorrhage has been controlled, a dressing of calcium hydroxide is placed over the amputation site (see Fig. 22-7, *D*). If the pulpal amputation extends into the tooth only a few millimeters, the use of a hard-setting material (e.g., Dycal or Life) is usually easiest. However, for deeper amputation, calcium hydroxide powder carried to the tooth in an amalgam carrier is the easiest method of application. The amalgam carrier is tightly packed with powder; then all but one fourth to one third of the pellet is expressed from the carrier and discarded. The remaining calcium hydroxide in the carrier is then expressed into the preparation site. The pellet of calcium hydroxide powder is carefully teased against the pulp stump with a rounded-end plastic instrument. The entire pulp stump must be covered with a thin layer of calcium hydroxide. Care must be taken not to pack the calcium hydroxide into the pulp tissue, as this causes greater inflammation and increases the chances of failure, or if pulpotomy is successful, there is increased calcification of the remaining pulp tissues around the particles of calcium hydroxide.[189]

Pulpdent (calcium hydroxide in a methylcellulose base) may also be used for the pulpotomy procedure. If commercial preparations of calcium hydroxide are used, care must be taken to avoid trapping air bubbles when applying the material.

After the calcium hydroxide has been applied to the pulp stumps, a creamy mix of ZOE or other cement base must be flowed over the calcium hydroxide and allowed to set completely. When a composite resin restoration is to be used, eugenol compounds must be avoided, since these interfere with a setting reaction of the composite. In these cases a second layer of Dycal or Life is placed. After setting, the cement base layer should be thick enough to allow for condensation of a permanent restoration to effectively seal the tooth.

A permanent type of restoration should always be placed in the tooth to ensure the retention of the calcium hydroxide cement base dressing. Unless a crown is necessary, amalgam is the material of choice for posterior teeth, and an etched composite restoration (see Fig. 22-7, *E* through *G*) is preferred for anterior teeth.

Follow-up after pulp capping and pulpotomy

After pulp capping and pulpotomy, the patient should be recalled periodically for 2 to 4 years to determine success. Although the normal vitality tests such as electrical and thermal sensitivity are reliable after pulp capping, they are usually not helpful in the pulpotomized tooth. Although histologic success

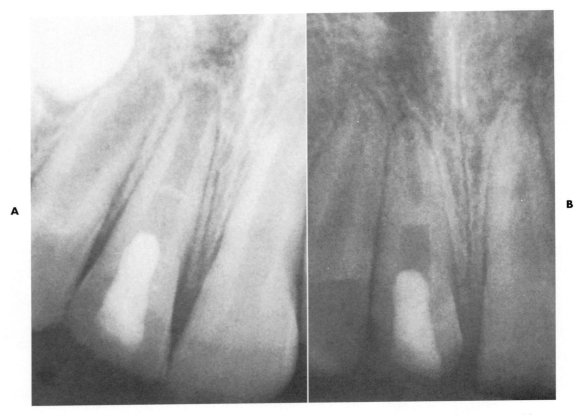

FIG. 22-8 Deep calcium hydroxide pulpotomy. **A,** Central incisor with an immature apex 10 weeks after a traumatic exposure of the pulp and a calcium hydroxide pulpotomy. Note the dentin bridge. **B,** Three years after pulpotomy. Note the thickening of the dentin bridge and the completion of root development. Tooth remained asymptomatic. No further endodontic treatment is indicated at this time.

cannot be determined, clinical success is judged by the absence of any clinical or radiographic signs of pathosis, the verification of a dentin bridge both radiographically and clinically, and the presence of continued root development in teeth with incompletely formed roots.

Controversy exists as to whether the pulp should be reentered after the completion of root development in the pulpotomized tooth. Some researchers[93,160] believe that pulp capping and pulpotomy procedures invariably lead to progressive calcification of the root canals. After successful root development, they advocate extirpation of the remaining pulp tissue and endodontic treatment. They recommend endodontic therapy because of the high incidence of continued calcification, which would render the canals nonnegotiable at some future time when endodontic therapy might be required because of disease. However, it has been my experience and the experience of others[21,47,66] that with good case selection, if a gentle technique is used in removing pulp tissue, care is taken to avoid contamination of the pulp with bacteria and dentin chips, and the dressing of calcium hydroxide is not packed into the underlying pulp tissue, progressive calcification of the pulp is an infrequent sequela of pulpotomy (Fig. 22-9).

In a follow-up study of clinically successful pulpotomies previously reported,[19] researchers[21] removed the pulps 1 to 5 years later for restorative reasons and found histologically normal pulps. They concluded that changes seen in the pulps do not represent sufficient histologic evidence to support routine pulpectomy after pulpotomy in accidentally fractured teeth with pulp exposures. Thus the routine reentry to remove the pulp and place a root canal filling after completion of root development is contraindicated unless dictated by restorative considerations such as the necessity for retentive post placement. Nevertheless, canal calcification, internal resorption, and pulp necrosis are potential sequelae of pulp-capping and pulpotomy procedures. Although unlikely, they are possible, and the patient should be clearly informed.

In posterior teeth, where surgical endodontics is difficult, if continued calcification of the canal is observed following root closure, reentry of the tooth for endodontic therapy is recommended. In anterior teeth, if calcification of the canal has made conventional endodontics impossible, surgical endodontics may be performed with relative ease. Therefore in anterior teeth, routine endodontic therapy following completion of root development is contraindicated unless clinical signs and symptoms of pathosis are present or unless such therapy is necessary for restorative procedures (placement of a post for retention of a crown because of missing tooth structure; Fig. 22-10).

Formocresol Pulpotomy on Young Permanent Teeth

Because of the reported clinical and histologic success with the formocresol pulpotomy on primary teeth, there has been much interest in this technique on young permanent teeth. Evi-

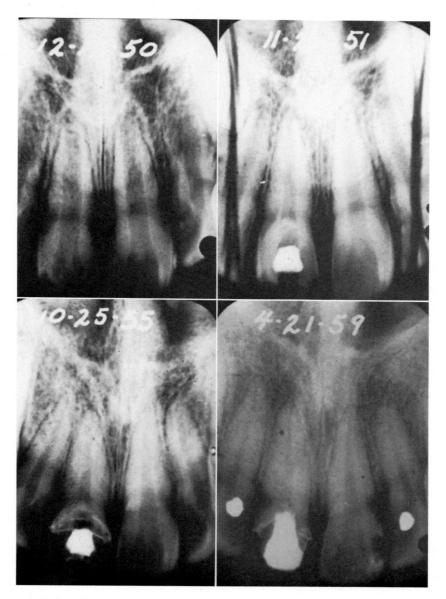

FIG. 22-9 Calcium hydroxide pulpotomy on a permanent incisor with an immature (or blunderbuss) apex. Traumatic exposure of the pulp of the central incisor was treated with a calcium hydroxide pulpotomy. The tooth at 1 year, 5 years, and 8½ years after pulpotomy remained asymptomatic. Root formation was completed, and the root canal appears to be a similar size to that of the adjacent incisor. *(Courtesy Dr. Ralph McDonald.)*

dence of continued apical development following formocresol pulpotomy procedures on young permanent teeth with incompletely developed apexes has been reported.[39,117,155,192] Several authors have reported better results with diluted formocresol. However, they reported a high incidence of internal resorption, which increased in severity with longer periods of time.[46,135]

The formocresol procedure has appeal because there is a lack of calcification of the remaining pulp tissue, as may be seen with calcium hydroxide pulpotomy. After root completion the tooth can easily be reentered, the pulp extirpated, and routine endodontic therapy performed. Contrary to these findings, one group of researchers[5] has shown calcification of the canals by continuous apposition of dentin on the lateral walls

with equal frequency whether using calcium hydroxide or formocresol. The only common denominator to this reaction was the presence of dentin chips that had accidentally been pushed into the radicular pulp tissue.

A retrospective study using clinical and radiographic criteria reported successful results; however, there was a high degree of root canal obliteration by calcification, which might preclude future root canal treatment.[182]

Other studies[83,116] have shown complete replacement of the pulp tissue with granulation tissue and the formation of osteodentin along the walls of the canals in permanent teeth following formocresol pulpotomies. The reaction was described as a healing rather than a destructive process, but persistent chronic inflammation was noted.

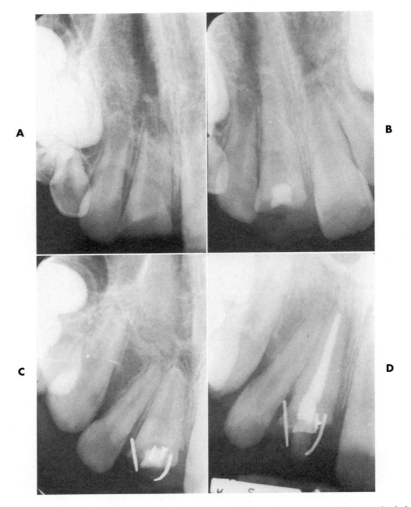

FIG. 22-10 Apexogenesis following calcium hydroxide pulpotomy. **A,** Traumatic injury has exposed the pulp in the maxillary central incisor before formation of the root was completed. **B,** Two months after calcium hydroxide pulpotomy, a dentin bridge has formed. **C,** Two and a half years after the pulpotomy, the root has completed its development. Note the lack of further pulpal calcification and a misplaced pin for retention of a temporary composite restoration. **D,** Root canal treatment has been completed so that the tooth may be permanently restored with a post and core and crown.

Although this treatment has been reported to be partly successful, it cannot be routinely recommended until further research showing the technique to be successful has been completed.

Formocresol pulpotomy procedures have been reported as temporary treatments on permanent teeth with necrotic pulps. Clinical success after 3 years has been reported.[185] The formocresol pulpotomy was performed rather than extraction when routine endodontic therapy could not be completed because of financial considerations. Complete endodontic treatment was advocated at a later date, with the formocresol pulpotomy used only as a *temporary* treatment.

PULPOTOMY ON PRIMARY TEETH

The 1996 American Academy of Pediatric Dentistry Guidelines[58] for pulp therapy for primary and young permanent teeth describes the pulpotomy procedure in primary teeth as the amputation of the affected or infected coronal portion of the den-

tal pulp, preserving the vitality and function of all or part of the remaining radicular pulp. Evidence of success in therapy includes (1) vitality of the majority of the radicular pulp, (2) no prolonged adverse clinical signs or symptoms such as prolonged sensitivity, pain, or swelling, (3) no radiographic evidence of internal resorption or abnormal canal calcification, (4) no breakdown of periradicular tissue, and (5) no harm to succedaneous teeth.

Many pharmacotherapeutic agents have been employed to achieve the above criteria. Formocresol has been the most popular agent mainly because of its ease in use and excellent clinical success. Yet despite its good clinical results, formocresol has come under close scrutiny because of concerns regarding the systemic distribution of this agent and its potential for toxicity, allergenicity, carcinogenicity, and mutagenicity. Other medicaments such as glutaraldehyde, calcium hydroxide, collagen, and ferric sulfate have been suggested as possible replacements. However, varying success rates and concerns regarding the safety of these materials make it clear that additional research on the use of these and other pharmaco-therapeutic agents is required.

Nonpharmacologic hemostatic techniques have been recommended including electrosurgery[103,138,153,161,162] and laser therapy.[163] Research on both of these techniques is sparse. However, electrosurgical pulpotomy is currently being taught in several dental schools and continues to grow in popularity among clinicians.

The formocresol, glutaraldehyde, and electrosurgical pulpotomy techniques are discussed further in this section. Ranly[142] provides a thorough review of pulpotomy agents and discusses new modalities for possible future use.

Formocresol Pulpotomy on Primary Teeth

The use of formocresol in dentistry has become a controversial issue since reports of wide distribution of the medicament following systemic injection[119] and the demonstration of an immune response to formocresol-fixed autologous tissue implanted in connective tissues or injected into root canals.[11,184] However, the formocresol pulpotomy continues to be one treatment of choice for primary teeth with vital carious exposures of the pulp in which inflammation or degeneration are judged to be confined to the coronal pulp. The last reported worldwide survey of dental schools in 1987[7] showed a majority of pediatric dentistry departments and practicing pediatric dentists advocated the formocresol pulpotomy technique. Currently it is still widely taught and used in clinical practice. The current formocresol pulpotomy technique is a modification of that reported by Sweet in 1930.[179]

Histologic studies[105,107] have demonstrated the effects of formocresol on pulps of primary and permanent human teeth. Formocresol-saturated cotton pellets caused the surface of the pulp to become fibrous and acidophilic within a few minutes. After exposure to the formocresol for a period of 7 to 14 days, three distinct zones became evident: (1) a broad acidophilic zone of fixation, (2) a broad pale-staining zone with diminished cellular and fiber definition (atrophy), and (3) a broad zone of inflammatory cells concentrated at the pale-staining zone junction and diffusing apically into normal pulp tissue. There was no evidence of an attempt to wall off the inflammatory zone by fibrous tissue or calcific barrier. After 60 days to 1 year, the pulp was progressively fixed and the entire pulp ultimately became fibrous.

Subsequent investigations[35] showed that the effect of formocresol on the pulp varied depending on the length of time the drug was in contact with the tissue. After 5 minutes there was a surface fixation blending into normal pulp tissue apically. Formocresol sealed in contact with the pulp for 3 days caused calcific degeneration, and the technique was termed vital or nonvital, according to the length of time of the application. As a part of this report, the clinical data from Sweet's files were compiled and showed a 97% success rate.

The ingrowth of fibroblasts in tissue underlying formocresol-pulpotomized noncarious human primary canines has been reported.[27] At 16 weeks the entire pulp had degenerated and was being replaced with granulation tissue. Mild inflammation in addition to some calcific degeneration was noted.

Doyle et al.[31] compared calcium hydroxide and formocresol pulpotomies on mechanically exposed, healthy, primary dental pulps. A formocresol pellet was sealed in place 4 to 7 days, and the histologic study was conducted from 4 to 388 days. Of the 18 teeth in the calcium hydroxide group, only 50% were judged histologically to be successful; of the 14 teeth treated with formocresol, 92% were histologically successful. Radiographically the success rates were 64% and 93%, whereas the clinical success rates were 71% and 100% (calcium hydroxide versus formocresol pulpotomy). The authors were able to identify vital tissue in the apical third of the root canals after treatment with formocresol pulpotomies.

Studies of the effect of adding formocresol to the ZOE filling over the 5-minute formocresol-pulpotomized primary tooth[192] have shown no appreciable differences between cases in which formocresol was included in the cement and those in which it was not; and histologic investigations[167,192] have reported no significant differences between two-appointment and one-appointment (5-minute) formocresol pulpotomies.

Accumulation of formocresol has been demonstrated in the pulp, dentin, periodontal ligament, and bone surrounding the apexes of pulpotomized teeth.[49,118] Formaldehyde was shown to be the component of formocresol that interacts with the protein portion of cells. The addition of cresol to formaldehyde appears to potentiate the effect of formaldehyde on protein.[124] In a study using human pulp fibroblast cultures, formaldehyde was shown to be the major component of formocresol that caused cytotoxic effects and to be 40 times more toxic than cresol.[75]

Application of radioactive formocresol to amputated pulp sites has been shown to result in immediate absorption of the material. The systemic absorption was limited to about 1% of the applied dose, regardless of the amount of time the drug was applied. It was shown that formocresol compromised the microcirculation, causing vessel thrombosis, which limited further systemic accumulation.[118]

Animal experiments[11,184] have demonstrated that in vivo formocresol-fixed autologous tissue produced an immune response when implanted into connective tissues or injected into root canals. The tissue became antigenically altered by formocresol and activated a specific cell-mediated lymphocyte response.

Other studies have demonstrated no evidence of this response in nonpresensitized animals,[166] and presensitized animals showed only a weak allergic potential.[191] This is in agreement with researchers[28] who have shown that formaldehyde demonstrated a low level of antigenicity in rabbits and as such would be an acceptable pulp medicament in regard to immunoreactive potential. Other investigators[98] studied lymphocyte transformation induced by formocresol-treated and untreated extracts of homologous pulp tissue in children with varying past experience with formocresol pulpotomies. Significant transformation responses were noted in over half the children, but they were unrelated to a clinical history of formocresol pulpotomy. Sensitization to pulp-related antigens was a common finding in the study. The authors concluded that formocresol pulpotomy does not induce significant immunologic sensitization to extracted antigens of homologous pulp or to pulp antigen altered by treatment with formocresol and therefore does not support other animal studies in which intense immunization schedules were used.[98] Clinical use of formocresol for many years without reports of allergic reaction has quite obviously substantiated this finding.

Concerns regarding the systemic effects of formocresol have also led to investigations concerning its possible embryotoxic and teratogenic effects.[44] In a study using injections of 25% and

50% formocresol into chick embryos, significant increases were noted in mortality, structural defects, and retarded development.

After systemic administration of formocresol in experimental animals, formocresol is distributed throughout the body. Metabolism and excretion of a portion of the absorbed formocresol occur in the kidneys and lungs. The remaining drug is bound to tissue predominantly in the kidneys, liver, and lungs. When administered systemically in large doses, acute toxic effects (including cardiovascular changes, plasma and urinary enzyme changes, and histologic evidence of cellular injury to the vital organs) were noted. The degree of tissue injury appeared to be dose related, with some of the changes being reversible in the early stages. The authors[119] were careful to point out that the administered doses were far in excess of those used clinically in humans and should not be extrapolated to clinical dental practice. In another study the same authors emphasized that the quantities of formaldehyde absorbed systemically via the pulpotomy route were small and did not contraindicate the use of formocresol.[132]

A subsequent study[120] in which 16 pulpotomies (5-minute application of full-strength formocresol) were performed on a dog displayed early tissue injury to the kidneys and liver; however, cellular recovery could be expected, since there was no evidence of the onset of an inflammatory reaction. In animals subjected to only one to four pulpotomies, there was no injury to the kidneys or liver. The heart and lungs of all the animals were normal. The authors pointed out that 16 pulpotomies expose a small dog to a much higher systemic level of formocresol than would several pulpotomies in a human. They further concluded that no clinical implications regarding the toxicity of absorbed formocresol should be drawn from this study. Other investigators[51] have shown that the effect of formocresol on pulp tissue is controlled by the quantity that diffuses into the tissue, and the quantity can be controlled by the length of time of application, the concentration used, the method of application, or a combination of all these factors.

With the use of isotope-labeled 19% formaldehyde, the presence of the drug was demonstrated in the lung, liver, kidney, muscle, serum, urine, and carbon dioxide following a 5-minute application of the drug to pulpotomy sites. The concentrations achieved in the tissues were equivalent to those found following an infusion of 30% of the amount placed in the pulp chamber.[141]

Another study using ^{14}C-labeled formocresol showed that 12% of the material used in a 5-minute full-strength pulpotomy was recovered after 36 hours, chiefly from the teeth, plasma, urine, and also from the liver, kidneys, lungs, heart, and spleen.[62]

Implantation of undiluted formocresol-fixed tissue in animals causes necrosis of the surrounding connective tissues,[12] and dilution of the formocresol decreases the tissue irritation potential.[53] Investigations using one-fifth concentration formocresol for pulpotomies have noted little difference as related to the initial effects on tissue fixation; however, earlier recovery of enzyme activity was apparent with the diluted formocresol than with the undiluted. Postoperative complications were reduced, and there was an improvement in the rate of recovery from the cytotoxic effects for formocresol when diluted.[99,100,177] It has been reported clinically that the same success is achieved with the diluted formocresol as with the undiluted.[45,113,114] *Therefore it is recommended that one-fifth concentration formocresol be used for pulpotomy procedures, since it is as effective as and less damaging than the traditional preparation.*

One-fifth concentration formocresol is prepared in the following manner. The dilute solution is prepared by mixing three parts glycerin with one part distilled water. One part formocresol is then thoroughly mixed with four parts diluent.

A histologic study on teeth with induced pulpal and periapical pathosis[84] showed no resolution of inflammation or periapical pathosis after a 5-minute pulpotomy procedure. Canals with vital tissue exhibited more internal resorption than was reported by other researchers, and more apical resorption was seen in teeth with periapical and furcal involvement than was seen in teeth with vital pulps. Ingrowth of tissue was not observed in canals with necrotic tissue. Also noted was the lack of evidence of formocresol fixation of either apical or furcal lesions. Despite extensive inflammatory reactions around the apexes of primary teeth close to the permanent tooth germs, no ill effects were observed on any tooth germs from the formocresol. Formocresol fixation was confined within the canals in all instances. Since the authors[84] concluded that the formocresol pulpotomy is an unacceptable procedure for teeth with pulpal and periapical pathosis, this study points out the importance of confining formocresol pulpotomies to primary teeth containing vital tissue in the root canals. Clinically, these results have also been substantiated.[182]

The fear of damage to the succedaneous tooth has been offered as an argument against formocresol pulpotomy on primary teeth. Studies have shown conflicting findings, ranging from the same incidence of enamel defects in treated and untreated contralateral teeth[115,152] to an increase in defects and positional alterations of the underlying permanent tooth.[111] It should be pointed out that studies of this nature are follow-up studies long after treatment, without knowledge of the existing status of the pulp before pulpotomy. Nor has anyone devised a study to ascertain the effects of the condition that necessitated the pulpotomy procedure. If the strict criteria outlined in this section are followed, the incidence of defects to the permanent teeth does not increase after formocresol pulpotomy.

Studies have shown that the exfoliation time of primary molars following formocresol pulpotomy is not affected.[115,190]

Indications and contraindications

The formocresol pulpotomy is indicated for pulp exposure on primary teeth in which the inflammation or infection is judged to be confined to the coronal pulp. If inflammation has spread into the tissues within the root canals, the tooth should be considered a candidate for pulpectomy and root canal filling or extraction. The contraindications for formocresol pulpotomy on a primary tooth are (1) a nonrestorable tooth, (2) a tooth nearing exfoliation or with no bone overlying the permanent tooth crown, (3) a history of spontaneous toothache, (4) evidence of periapical or furcal pathology, (5) a pulp that does not hemorrhage, (6) inability to control hemorrhage following a coronal pulp amputation, (7) a pulp with serous or purulent drainage, and (8) the presence of a fistula.

Technique (Fig. 22-11)

The formocresol pulpotomy is used on primary teeth whose roots are judged to be free of inflammation and infection. Compromise on this principle leads to a diminished success rate and possible damage to the succedaneous tooth. Therefore the importance of a proper diagnosis cannot be overstressed.

After the diagnosis has been completed, the primary tooth is anesthetized and isolated with a rubber dam. All caries is

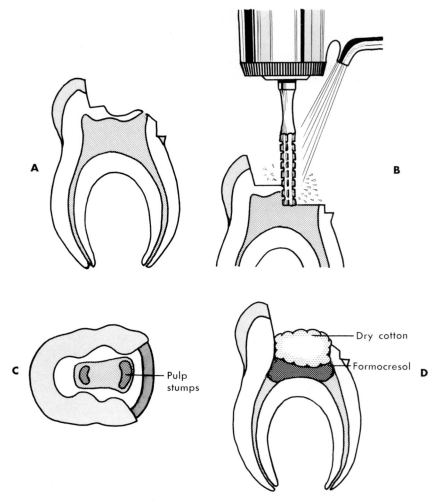

FIG. 22-11 Formocresol pulpotomy. **A,** Carious pulp exposure in the primary tooth. **B,** Removal of the roof of the pulp chamber. **C,** Pulp stumps after hemorrhage controlled. **D,** Formocresol application for 5 minutes. After fixation of the pulp stumps, a base zinc oxide–eugenol is applied and the tooth is permanently restored.

removed. The entire roof of the pulp chamber is cut away with a high-speed bur and copious water spray. All the coronal pulp is removed with a bur or spoon excavator. Care must be exercised to extirpate all filaments of the coronal pulp. If any filaments remain in the pulp chamber, hemorrhage will be impossible to control. The pulp chamber is thoroughly washed with water to remove all debris. The water is removed by vacuum and cotton pellets.

Hemorrhage is controlled by slightly moistened cotton pellets (wetted and blotted almost dry) placed against the stumps of the pulp at the openings of the root canals. Completely dry cotton pellets should not be used, since fibers of the cotton will be incorporated into the clot and, when removed, will cause hemorrhage. Dry cotton pellets are placed over the moist pellets, and pressure is exerted on the mass to control the hemorrhage. Hemorrhage should be controlled in this manner within several minutes. It may be necessary to change the pellets to control all hemorrhage. If hemorrhage occurs, carefully check to be sure that all filaments of the pulp were removed from the pulp chamber and that the amputation site is clean.

If hemorrhage cannot be controlled within 5 minutes, the pulp tissue within the canals is probably inflamed and the tooth is not a candidate for a formocresol pulpotomy. The clinician should then proceed with pulpectomy, or the tooth should be extracted.

When the hemorrhage has been controlled, one-fifth dilution formocresol on a cotton pellet is placed in direct contact with the pulp stumps. Fixation does not occur unless the formocresol is in contact with the stumps. The cotton pellet is blotted to remove excess formocresol after saturation and before the tooth is entered. Formocresol is caustic and creates a severe tissue burn if allowed to contact the gingiva.

The formocresol is left in contact with the pulp stumps for 5 minutes. When it is removed, the tissue appears brown and no hemorrhage should be present. If an area of the pulp was not contacting the medication, the procedure must be repeated for that tissue. Small cotton pellets for applying the medication usually work best, since they allow closer approximation of the material to the pulp.

A cement base of ZOE is placed over the pulp stumps and allowed to set. The tooth may then be restored permanently. The restoration of choice is a stainless steel crown for primary

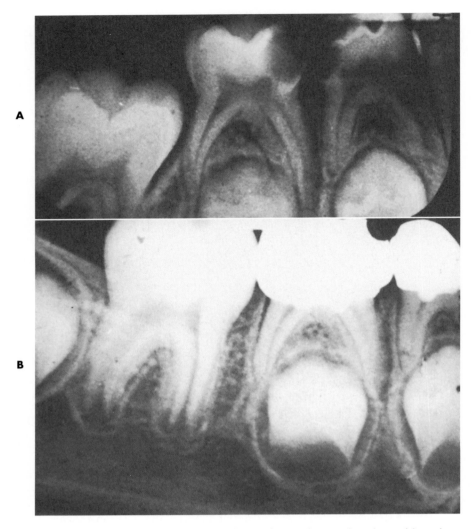

FIG. 22-12 Formocresol pulpotomy. **A,** Primary first and second molars with carious pulp exposures. **B,** Eighteen months after formocresol pulpotomy. Note the eruption of the permanent first molar.

molars. On anterior primary teeth a composite tooth-colored restoration is the treatment of choice unless the tooth is so badly broken down that it requires a crown.

With the formocresol, no dentin bridge formation occurs as with the calcium hydroxide pulpotomy (Fig. 22-12).

Failure of a formocresol pulpotomy is usually detected radiographically (Fig. 22-13). The first signs of failure are often internal resorption of the root adjacent to the area where the formocresol was applied. This may be accompanied by external resorption, especially as the failure progresses. In the primary molars a radiolucency develops in the bifurcation or trifurcation area. In the anterior teeth a radiolucency may develop at the apexes or lateral to the roots. With more destruction the tooth becomes excessively mobile. A fistula usually develops. It is rare for pain to occur with the failure of a formocresol pulpotomy. Consequently, unless patients receive follow-up checks after a formocresol pulpotomy, failure may be undetected. When the tooth loosens and is eventually exfoliated, the parents and child may consider the circumstances normal.

The development of cystic lesions following pulp therapy in primary molars has been reported.[156] An amorphous, eosi-

nophilic material shown to contain phenolic groupings similar to those present in medicaments was found in the lesions. Other researchers[122] have observed furcal lesions in untreated pulpally involved primary molars containing granulomatous tissue with stratified squamous epithelium, suggesting the potential for cyst formation. In a subsequent study involving failed pulpotomized primary molars, most specimens were diagnosed as furcation cysts.[123] These findings point out the importance of follow-up to endodontic treatment on primary teeth.

Glutaraldehyde Pulpotomy

A body of evidence has accumulated that has led some investigators to suggest that glutaraldehyde should replace formocresol as the medicament of choice for chemical pulpotomy procedures on primary teeth. Numerous studies[28,181,195] have shown that the application of 2% to 4% aqueous glutaraldehyde produces rapid surface fixation of the underlying pulpal tissue, although its depth of penetration is limited. Unlike the varied response to formocresol, a large percentage of the underlying pulp tissue remains vital and is free of inflammation. A narrow zone of eosinophilic-stained and compressed fixed

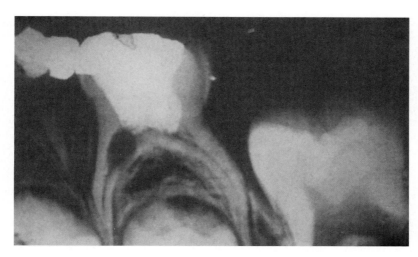

FIG. 22-13 Formocresol pulpotomy failure. Note the internal resorption in the mesial root and the radiolucency in the bifurcation.

tissue is found directly beneath the area of application, which blends into vital normal-appearing tissue apically. With time, the glutaraldehyde-fixed zone is replaced through macrophagic action with dense collagenous tissue; thus the entire root canal tissue is vital.[91]

Glutaraldehyde is absorbed from vital pulpotomy sites but, unlike formocresol, which is absorbed and distributed throughout the body within minutes of placement,[132] glutaraldehyde does not perfuse the pulp tissue to the apex and demonstrates less systemic distribution immediately after application.[26,96,196] Autoradiographs of isotope-labeled glutaraldehyde show that the drug is limited largely to the pulp space, with little evidence of escape outside the tooth following pulpotomy.[121] No differences have been reported in the incidence of enamel defects on succedaneous teeth with the use of formocresol- or glutaraldehyde-based pulpotomy techniques.[1]

Also unlike formaldehyde, which is mostly tissue bound with only a small fraction being metabolized, glutaraldehyde exhibits very low tissue binding and is readily metabolized. Glutaraldehyde is metabolized mostly in the kidney and lungs but is also found in liver, heart, and muscle tissues.[81,121] Glutaraldehyde is eliminated primarily in urine and expired in gases; 90% of the drug is gone within 3 days.[146]

Virtually no toxic effects have been shown following glutaraldehyde administration either via pulpotomy or systemic application. Large doses (up to 500 times the amount applied in a pulpotomy procedure) caused little toxic effect.[146] Cytotoxicity studies in human pulp fibroblasts showed 2.5% glutaraldehyde to be 15 to 20 times less toxic than formocresol or 19% formaldehyde.[75]

Isotope methods have shown that much of the glutaraldehyde distributed systemically is neutralized by oxidation to carbon dioxide, excretion by the kidney, and binding to plasma proteins.[145] It has also been shown that glutaraldehyde is not incorporated in the nuclear portion of fractionated liver cells, and it is felt to have little potential for chromosomal interference or mutagenicity.[143]

The concentrations of glutaraldehyde and formocresol that are necessary for adequate antimicrobial effect without excessive cytotoxic results have also been reported. A concentration of not less than 3.125% glutaraldehyde is recommended for adequate antimicrobial effect. At this concentration, less cytotoxic effect is exerted on surrounding tissues than by formocresol.[70] It has also been noted that the longer time required for tissue fixation by glutaraldehyde may make its cytotoxicity in clinical applications closer to that of formocresol than was previously reported.[178]

Although glutaraldehyde has been shown to produce antigenic products in much the same manner as formocresol,[148] it has a relatively low antigenicity[147] as compared with formocresol. Unfortunately, purified solutions of glutaraldehyde have been shown to be unstable.[140]

The indications, contraindications, and technique for the glutaraldehyde pulpotomy are the same as for the formocresol pulpotomy, except that glutaraldehyde is substituted for formocresol. Unfortunately, neither the optimal concentration of glutaraldehyde nor the amount of time of application has been conclusively established.

Investigators[52,97,144] have reported the effects of various concentrations and lengths of application of glutaraldehyde. Application of the glutaraldehyde through incorporation in ZOE led to a high failure rate, thus contraindicating this route of administration.[52] Buffering glutaraldehyde, increasing its concentration, and applying it for longer periods enhance the degree of fixation. Only stronger solutions increase the depth of fixation.[97,144] Increased fixation gives greater resistance to removal and replacement of the fixed tissue. Weak concentrations and short application times lead to more severe inflammatory responses in the underlying pulp tissue and to eventual failure.[97]

Their research has led Ranly et al.[144] to recommend 4% buffered glutaraldehyde with a 4-minute application time or 8% for 2 minutes.

In a 24-month follow-up of pulpotomies performed with 2% glutaraldehyde, the failure rate rose to 18% after 2 years, and the authors could not justify its use over formocresol.[48] Other authors have examined the evidence with regard to toxicity, mutagenicity, and systemic distribution and do not recommend the substitution of glutaraldehyde for formocresol in pulpotomy technique.[38] The majority of training institutions continue to teach the formocresol technique, and a large majority of practicing pediatric dentists employ formocresol.[7]

Given comparable success rates and the undesirable effects of formocresol and glutaraldehyde, it has been suggested to substitute the pulpectomy technique for the pulpotomy in primary teeth.[203]

Electrosurgical Pulpotomy

Although electrocoagulation on the pulps of teeth was reported in 1957,[95] it was a decade later that Mack[102] became the first U.S. dentist routinely to perform electrosurgical pulpotomies. Oringer[131] also strongly advocated this technique in his 1975 text on electrosurgery. Several clinical studies[153,162] have produced results comparable to those found with the use of formocresol. Conflicting results have been reported from histologic studies ranging from comparable results to formocresol pulpotomy[161] to pathologic root resorption with periapical and furcal involvement.[165] A retrospective human study by Mack and Dean[103] in 1993 showed a success rate of 99% for primary molars undergoing electrosurgical pulpotomies. Compared to a formocresol pulpotomy study of similar design, the success rate of the electrosurgery technique was shown to be significantly higher. A more recent clinical study[138] showed success rates of 95% and 87% respectively for electrosurgical and formocresol pulpotomies.

The steps in the electrosurgical pulpotomy technique (Fig. 22-14) are basically the same as those for the formocresol technique through the removal of the coronal pulp tissue. Large sterile cotton pellets are placed in contact with the pulp and pressure applied to obtain hemostasis. The Hyfrecator Plus 7-797 (Birtcher Medical Systems, Irvine, Calif.) is set at 40% power (high at 12 W), and the 705A dental electrode is used to deliver the electrical arc. Lowering of the intensity of the overhead dental light allows better visualization of the electrical arc. The cotton pellets are quickly removed, and the electrode is placed 1 to 2 mm above the pulpal stump (Fig. 22-14, D). The electrical arc is allowed to bridge the gap to the pulpal stump for 1 second, followed by a cooldown period of 5 seconds. Heat and electrical transfer are thus minimized by keeping the electrode as far away from the pulpal stump and tooth structure as possible while still allowing electrical arcing to occur. If necessary this procedure may be repeated up to a maximum of three times. The procedure is then repeated for the next pulpal stump. When the procedure is properly performed, the pulpal stumps appear dry and completely blackened (Fig. 22-14, E). The chamber is filled with ZOE placed directly against the pulpal stumps. Research[41] has shown no difference between ZOE or calcium hydroxide as the dressing. The tooth should then be restored with a stainless steel crown (Fig. 22-14, G).

PULPECTOMY IN PRIMARY TEETH

Primary Root Canal Anatomy

To complete endodontic treatment on primary teeth successfully, the clinician must have a thorough knowledge of the anatomy of the primary root canal systems and the variations that normally exist in these systems. To understand some of the variations in the primary root canal systems requires an understanding of root formation.

Root Formation

According to Orban[130] development of the roots begins after enamel and dentin formation has reached the future cemen-

toenamel junction. The epithelial dental organ forms Hertwig's epithelial root sheath, which initiates formation and molds the shape of the roots. Hertwig's sheath takes the form of one or more epithelial tubes (depending on the number of roots of the tooth, one tube for each root). During root formation the apical foramen of each root has a wide opening limited by the epithelial diaphragm. The dentinal walls taper apically, and the shape of the pulp canal is like a wide-open tube. Each root contains one canal at this time, and the number of canals is the same as the number of roots (Fig. 22-15, A). When root length is established, the sheath disappears but dentin deposition continues internally within the roots.

Differentiation of a root into separate canals, as in the mesial root of the mandibular molars, occurs by continued deposition of dentin; this narrows the isthmus between the walls of the canals and continues until there is formation of dentin islands within the root canal and eventual division of the root into separate canals. During the process, communications exist between the canals as an isthmus, then as fins connecting the canals (Fig. 22-15, B). The reader is referred to Chapter 11 for a complete description of pulp and dentin formation.

As growth proceeds, the root canal is narrowed by continued deposition of dentin and the pulp tissue is compressed. Additional deposition of dentin and cementum closes the apex of the tooth and creates the apical convergence of the root canals common to the completely formed tooth (Fig. 22-15, C).

Root length is not completed until 1 to 4 years after a tooth erupts into the oral cavity. In the primary teeth the root length is completed in a shorter period of time than in the permanent tooth because of the shorter length of the primary roots.

The root-to-crown length of the primary teeth is greater than that of the permanent teeth. The primary roots are narrower than the permanent roots. The roots of the primary molars diverge more than those of the permanent teeth. This feature allows more room for the development of the crown of the succeeding premolar[198] (see Fig. 22-1).

The primary tooth is unique insofar as resorption of the roots begins soon after formation of the root length has been completed. At this time the form and shape of the root canals roughly correspond to the form and shape of the external anatomy of the teeth. Root resorption and the deposition of additional dentin within the root canal system, however, significantly change the number, size, and shape of the root canals within the primary tooth.

It should be noted that most of the variations within the root canals of primary teeth are in the faciolingual plane and that dental radiographs do not show this plane but show the mesiodistal plane. Therefore when we view radiographs of primary teeth, many of the variations that are present are not visible.

Primary anterior teeth

The form and shape of the root canals of the primary anterior teeth (Figs. 22-16 and 22-17) resemble the form and shape of the roots of the teeth. The permanent tooth bud lies lingual and apical to the primary anterior tooth. Owing to the position of the permanent tooth bud, resorption of the primary incisors and canines is initiated on the lingual surface in the apical third of the roots (see Fig. 22-16, A).

Maxillary incisors. The root canals of the primary maxillary central and lateral incisors are almost round but somewhat compressed. Normally these teeth have one canal without bi-

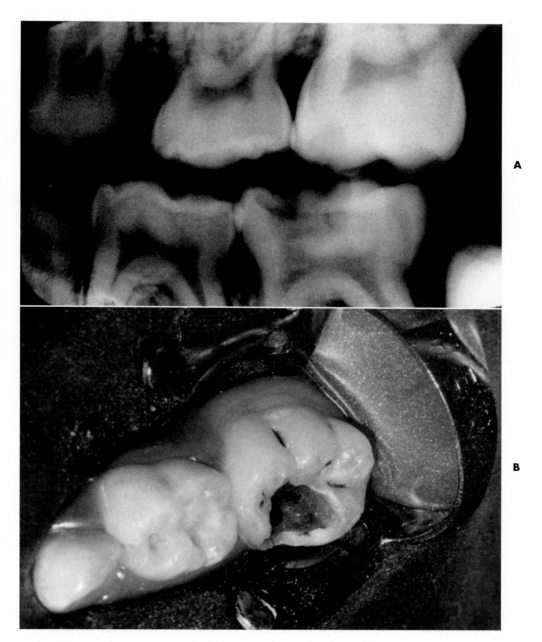

FIG. 22-14 Electrosurgical pulpotomy on a mandibular right second primary molar. **A,** Pre-operative radiograph showing caries into the pulp. **B,** Tooth isolated with the rubber dam.

Continued

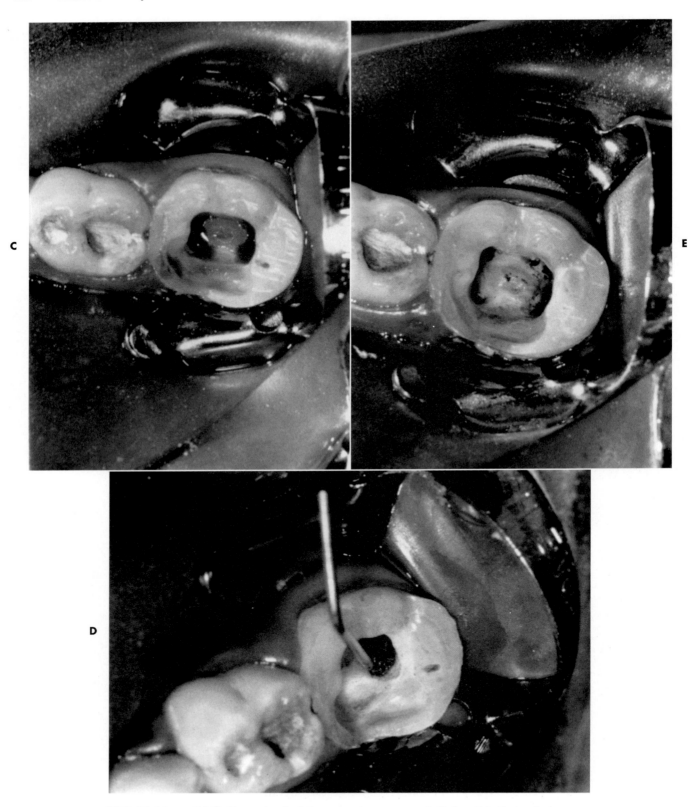

FIG. 22-14, cont'd C, Coronal pulpal tissue has been removed. Before this the occlusion was reduced and occlusal amalgams placed in the first primary molar. **D,** The 705A dental electrode in the Hyfrecator Plus 7-797 is activated over each pulpal stump for 1 second. **E,** Pulpal stumps appear dry and completely blackened following the electrosurgery pulpotomy.

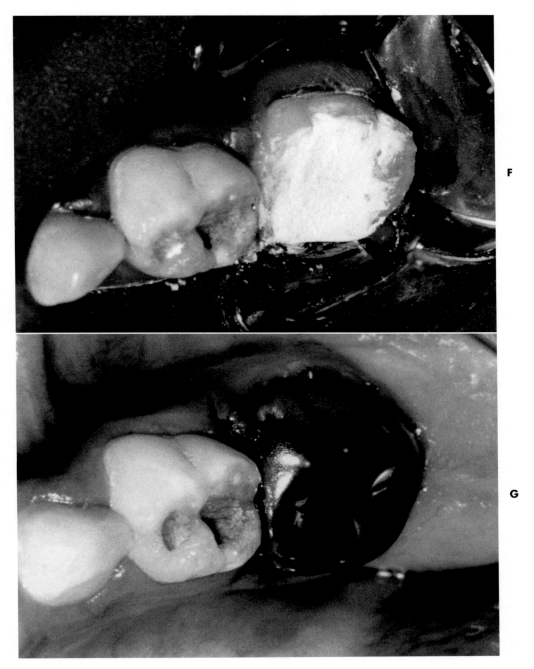

FIG. 22-14, cont'd F, Pulp chamber is filled with zinc oxide–eugenol placed directly against the pulpal stumps. **G,** Tooth is restored with a stainless steel crown.

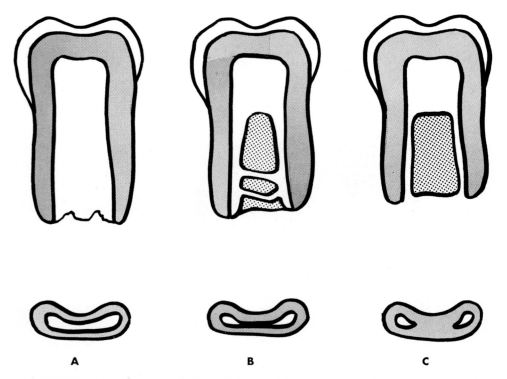

FIG. 22-15 Faciolingual cross section of the mesial root of a mandibular primary molar. **A,** Formation of the root at the time the root length is completed and only one canal is present. **B,** Differentiation of the root into separate canals by the continued deposition of dentin *(shaded areas).* Small fins and connecting branches are present between the two canals. **C,** Canals are completely divided, and root resorption has begun.

furcations. Apical ramifications or accessory canals and lateral canals are rare but do occur[205] (see Fig. 22-16).

Mandibular incisors. The root canals of the primary mandibular central and lateral incisors are flattened on the mesial and distal surfaces and sometimes grooved, pointing to an eventual division into two canals. The presence of two canals is seen less than 10% of the time. Occasionally lateral or accessory canals are observed.[205]

Maxillary and mandibular canines. The root canals of the maxillary and mandibular canines correspond to the exterior root shape, a rounded triangular shape with the base toward the facial surface. Sometimes the lumen of the root canal is compressed in the mesiodistal direction. The canines have the simplest root canal systems of all the primary teeth and offer few problems when being treated endodontically. Bifurcation of the canal does not normally occur. Lateral canals and accessory canals are rare[205] (see Fig. 22-17).

Primary molars

The primary molars (Fig. 22-18) normally have the same number of roots and position of the roots as the corresponding permanent molars. The maxillary molars have three roots, two facial and one palatal; the mandibular have two roots, mesial and distal. The roots of the primary molars are long and slender compared with crown length and width, and they diverge to allow for permanent tooth bud formation.

When full length of the roots of the primary molars have just been completed, only one root canal is present in each of the roots. The continued deposition of dentin internally may divide the root into two or more canals. During this process, communications exist between the canals and may remain in the fully developed primary tooth as isthmuses or fins connecting the canals (see Fig. 22-15, *B*).

The deposition of secondary dentin in primary teeth has been reported.[10,69,74] After root formation the basic morphologic pattern of the root canals may change, producing variations and alterations in the number and size of the root canals caused by the deposition of secondary dentin. This deposition begins at about the time root resorption begins. Variations in form are more pronounced in teeth that show evidence of root resorption.[69]

The most variation in the morphology of the root canals is found in the mesial roots of both maxillary and mandibular primary molars. This variation originates in the apical region as a thinning of the narrow isthmus between the facial and lingual extremities of the apical pulp canals. Subsequent deposition of secondary dentin may produce a complete separation of the root canal into two or more individual canals. Many fine connecting branches or lateral fibrils form a connecting network between the facial and lingual aspects of the root canals.

The variations found in the mesial roots of the primary molars are also found in the distal and lingual roots but to a lesser degree. Accessory canals, lateral canals, and apical ramifications of the pulp are common in primary molars—occurring in 10% to 20%.[69,205]

In the primary molars, resorption usually begins on the inner surfaces of the roots next to the interradicular septum. The effects of resorption on canal anatomy and root canal filling on the primary teeth are discussed in detail later in this chapter.

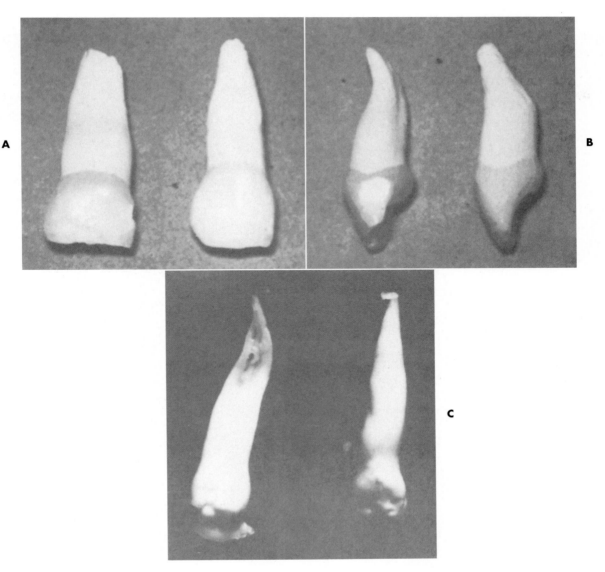

FIG. 22-16 Primary central incisors and silicone models of the pulp canals. **A,** Facial surfaces. **B,** Beginning resorption of the roots on the apical third of the lingual surfaces. **C,** Models. The pulp canals were injected with silicone and the tooth structure decalcified away, leaving a model of the root canal systems. Note the division of the canal on the left.

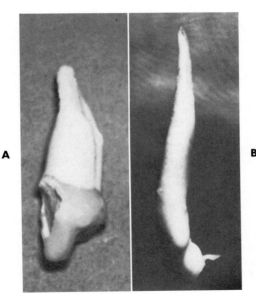

FIG. 22-17 Maxillary primary canine and silicone model of the root canal. **A,** Mesial surface. **B,** Model of the root canal.

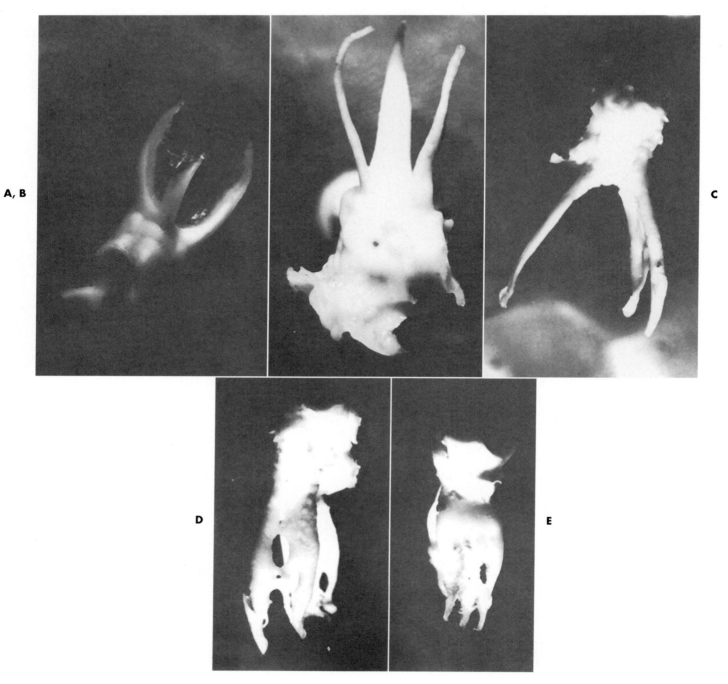

FIG. 22-18 Silicone models of the root canal systems of primary molars. **A,** Maxillary first molar. Note the fused distal and palatal roots. Note the thin fin connecting the roots. **B,** Maxillary second molar, facial surface. **C,** Mandibular first molar, facial view. **D,** Same tooth from the mesial surface. Note the connecting fibrils between the facial and lingual canals. **E,** Mandibular second molar, distal view. Three canals are present.

Maxillary first primary molar. The maxillary first primary molar has from two to four canals that roughly correspond to the exterior root form with much variation. The palatal root is often round; it is often longer than the two facial roots. Bifurcation of the mesiofacial root into two canals occurs in approximately 75% of maxillary first primary molars.[69,205]

Fusion of the palatal and distofacial roots occurs in approximately one third of the maxillary primary first molars. In most of these teeth, two separate canals are present with a very narrow isthmus connecting. Islands of dentin may exist between the canals, with many connecting branches and fibrils (Fig. 22-18, *A*).

Maxillary second primary molar. The maxillary primary molar has two to five canals roughly corresponding to the exterior root shape. The mesial-facial root usually bifurcates or contains two distinct canals. This occurs in approximately 85% to 95% of maxillary second primary molars[69,205] (Fig. 22-18, *B*).

Fusion of the palatal and distofacial roots may occurs. These fused roots may have a common canal, two distinct canals, or two canals with a narrow connecting isthmus of dentin islands between them and many connecting branches or fibrils.

Mandibular first primary molar. The mandibular first primary molar usually has three canals roughly corresponding to the external root anatomy but may have two to four canals. It is reported that approximately 75% of the mesial roots contain two canals, whereas only 25% of the distal roots contain more than one canal[69,205] (Fig. 22-18, C and D).

Mandibular second primary molar. The mandibular second primary molar may have two to five canals but usually has three. The mesial root has two canals approximately 85% of the time, whereas the distal root contains more than one canal only 25% of the time[69,205] (Fig. 22-18, E).

ROLE OF RESORPTION ON CANAL ANATOMY AND APICAL FORAMINA

In the newly completed roots of the primary teeth the apical foramina are located near the anatomic apexes of the roots. After the deposition of additional dentin and cementum, there are multiple apical ramifications of the pulp as it exits the root, just as in the mature permanent tooth.

Because of the position of the permanent tooth bud, physiologic resorption of the roots of the primary incisors and canines is initiated on the lingual surfaces in the apical third of the roots. In the primary molars, resorption usually begins on the inner surfaces of the roots near the interradicular septum.

As resorption progresses, the apical foramen may not correspond to the anatomic apex of the root but be coronal to it. Therefore radiographic establishment of the root canal length may be erroneous. Resorption may extend through the roots and into the root canals, creating additional communications with the periapical tissues other than through the apical foramina or lateral and accessory canals (Fig. 22-19). This has been shown to occur at all levels of the root.[150]

Permanent Tooth Bud

The effects of primary endodontic therapy on the developing permanent tooth bud should be of paramount concern to the clinician.

Manipulation through the apex of the primary tooth is contraindicated, since the permanent tooth bud lies immediately adjacent to the apex of the primary tooth. Overextension of root canal instruments and filling materials must be avoided. If signs of resorption are visible radiographically, it is advisable to establish the working length of endodontic instruments 2 or 3 mm short of the radiographic apex. The use of the radiographic paralleling technique with a long cone for maximal accuracy when measuring canal lengths is recommended.

Anesthesia is usually necessary for pulp extirpation and enlargement of the canals but is rarely needed when primary teeth are filled at a subsequent appointment. The response of the patient can sometimes be used as a guide to the approach to the apex and as a check to the length of the canal that was previously established radiographically. Hemorrhage after pulp removal indicates overextension into the periapical tissues.

The filling material used to obliterate the root canals on primary teeth must be absorbable so it can be absorbed as the tooth resorbs and so it offers no resistance or deflection to the eruption of the permanent tooth. *Materials such as gutta-percha or silver points are contraindicated as primary root canal fillers.*

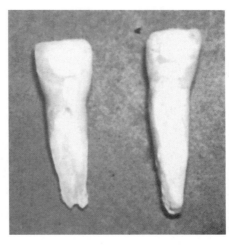

FIG. 22-19 These two primary mandibular incisors have lingual and apical resorption. Note that the left incisor has the apical foramen just beneath the cervical line, whereas the right one has its apical foramen at the apex of the root.

Pulpectomy

Pulpectomy and root canal filling procedures on primary teeth have been the subject of much controversy. Fear of damage to developing permanent tooth buds and a belief that the tortuous root canals of primary teeth could not be adequately negotiated, cleaned, shaped, and filled have led to the needless sacrifice of many pulpally involved primary teeth.

Much has been written regarding potential damage to the developing permanent tooth bud from root canal fillings. While magnifying these dangers, many authors have advocated extraction of pulpally involved primary teeth and placement of space maintainers. However, there is no better space maintainer than the primary tooth. Also nothing has been written concerning the damage of space maintainers on existing teeth in the mouth. For many space maintainers that are placed, adequate follow-up is not achieved because of the carelessness of either the patient or the clinician. Decalcification and rampant caries are frequent sequelae of loosened bands retained for extended periods of time. Poor oral hygiene around space maintainers contributes to increased decay and gingival problems. Deflection of erupting permanent teeth because of prolonged retention of space maintainers is sometimes encountered. Loss of space maintainers with resulting space loss can occur if the patient delays returning for treatment. These are a few of the problems that may be avoided by retention of the pulpally involved primary tooth when possible.

It has been reported[72] that although severe hypoplasia and disturbances in root development do not intensify, minor hypoplasia is increased in succedaneous teeth after root canal treatment of the primary precursors. Others[16] have reported the same amount of defects on the untreated side and concluded that there are no effects from primary pulpectomy on the succedaneous teeth. Enamel defects increased as the amount of preoperative primary root resorption increased. It was summarized that defects result from the infection existing before the pulpectomy and not the procedure itself. It should be pointed out that all such studies are retrospective, involving erupted permanent teeth, and as such cannot ascertain the causes of defects.

Economics has been advanced as an argument against endodontic treatment of primary teeth, but it is not a reasonable argument when compared with the cost of space maintainers, including the required follow-up treatment. In fact endodontic treatment is probably the less expensive of the two alternatives when the entire treatment sequence is considered.

Success of endodontic treatment on primary teeth is judged by the same criteria that are used for permanent teeth. The treated primary tooth must remain firmly attached in function without pain or infection. Radiographic signs of furcal and periapical infection should be resolved, with a normal periodontal attachment. The primary tooth should resorb normally and in no way interfere with the formation or eruption of the permanent tooth.

Success rates ranging from 75% to 96% have been reported.[2,71,94,203] The usual means of studying root canal filling on primary teeth have been clinical and radiographic. There exists a great need for histologic study in this area.

Early reports of endodontic treatment on primary teeth usually involved devitalization with arsenic in vital teeth and the use of creosote, formocresol, or paraformaldehyde pastes in nonvital teeth. The canals were filled with a variety of materials, usually consisting of zinc oxide and numerous additives.[33,54,76,171]

The first well-documented scientific report of endodontic procedures on primary teeth was published by Rabinowitch in 1953.[139] A 13-year study of 1363 cases of partially or totally nonvital primary molars was reported. Only seven cases were failures. Most patients were followed for 1 or 2 years clinically and radiographically. Fillings of ZOE and silver nitrate were placed only after a negative culture result was obtained for each tooth. Periapically involved teeth required an average of 7.7 visits to complete treatment; teeth with no periapical involvement required an average of 5.5 visits. Rabinowitch listed internal resorption and gross pathologic external resorption as contraindications to primary root canal fillings.

Another well-documented study reported a success rate of 95% in both vital and infected teeth using a filling material of thymol, cresol, iodoform, and zinc oxide.[2]

The reader is referred to Bennett[8] for a review of the techniques of partial and total pulpectomy.

In a well-controlled clinical study of primary root canals using Oxpara paste as the filling material,[94] five preexisting factors were reported to render the prognosis less favorable: perforation of the furcation, excessive external resorption of roots, internal resorption, extensive bone loss, and periodontal involvement of the furcation. When teeth with these factors were eliminated, a clinical success rate of 96% was achieved. When all symptoms of residual infection were resolved before filling of the canals, the success rate improved. No radiographic evidence of damage to the permanent teeth was noted.

After reviewing the literature on root canal fillings on primary teeth, one is impressed with the lack of histologic material in this area. There exists a great need for further research on the subject.

Contraindications for Primary Root Canal Fillings

Except for the following situations, all primary teeth with pulpal involvement that has spread beyond the coronal pulp are candidates for root canal fillings whether they are vital or nonvital:

1. A nonrestorable tooth
2. Radiographically visible internal resorption in the roots

3. Teeth with mechanical or carious perforations of the floor of the pulp chamber
4. Excessive pathologic root resorption involving more than one third of the root
5. Excessive pathologic loss of bone support with loss of the normal periodontal attachment
6. The presence of a dentigerous or follicular cyst

Internal resorption usually begins just inside the root canals near the furcation area. Because of the thinness of the roots of the primary teeth, once internal resorption has become visible radiographically, there is invariably a perforation of the root by the resorption (see Fig. 22-3). The short furcal surface area of the primary teeth leads to rapid communication between the inflammatory process and the oral cavity through the periodontal attachment. The end result is loss of the periodontal attachment of the tooth and ultimately further resorption and loss of the tooth.

Mechanical or carious perforations of the floor of the pulp chamber fail for the same reasons.

It has been shown that root length is the most reliable criterion of root integrity, and at least 4 mm of root length is necessary for the primary tooth to be treatable.[150]

ACCESS OPENINGS FOR PULPECTOMY ON PRIMARY TEETH

Anterior Teeth

Access openings for endodontic treatment on primary or permanent anterior teeth have traditionally been through the lingual surface. This continues to be the surface of choice except for the maxillary primary incisors. Because of problems associated with the discoloration of endodontically treated primary incisors, it has been recommended to use a facial approach followed by an acid-etched composite restoration to improve aesthetics (Fig. 22-20).[104] Bleaching techniques that are quite successful in permanent teeth are unsuccessful in primary teeth.

Many maxillary primary incisors requiring pulpectomy have discoloration caused by the escape of hemosiderin pigments into the dentinal tubules following a previous traumatic injury. Subsequent to pulpectomy and root canal filling, most primary incisors discolor.

The anatomy of the maxillary primary incisors is such that access may successfully be made from the facial surface. The only variation to the opening is more extension to the incisal edge than with the normal lingual access to give as straight an approach as possible into the root canal.

The root canal is filled with ZOE (see below), then the ZOE is carefully removed to near the cervical line. A liner of Dycal or Life is placed over the ZOE to serve as a barrier between the composite resin and the root canal filling. The liner is extended over the darkly stained lingual dentin to serve as an opaquer. The access opening and entire facial surface are acid etched and restored with composite resin (Fig. 22-20).

Unlike posterior primary teeth, anterior primary teeth have one single canal without ramifications and lateral or accessory canals. Therefore primary anterior root canals may be filled immediately after cleaning, provided the canal can be dried.

Posterior Teeth

Access openings into the posterior primary root canals are essentially the same as those for the permanent teeth. (Chapter 7 contains a detailed description of access openings.) Impor-

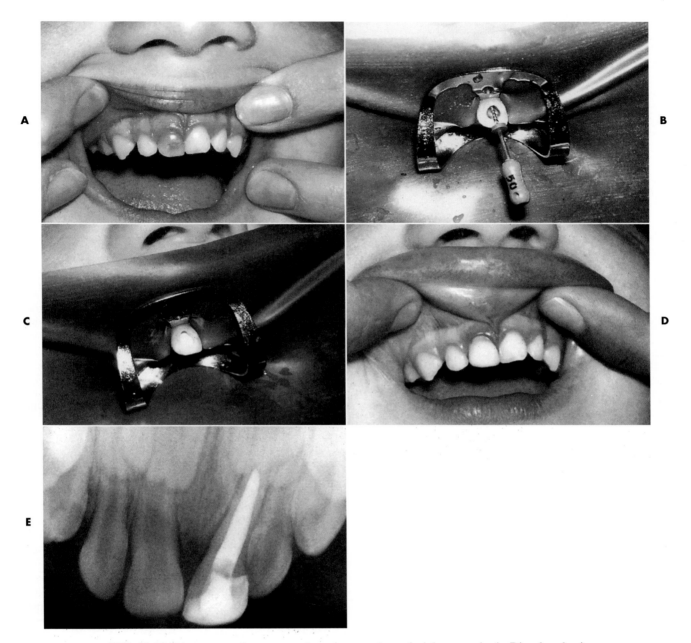

FIG. 22-20 Primary anterior root canal treatment using a facial approach. **A,** Discolored primary central incisor with a necrotic pulp. **B,** Tooth during root canal cleansing. **C,** Root canal filling with zinc oxide–eugenol has been completed. ZOE was removed to the cervical line and a Dycal liner was placed over the dentin. Tooth has been acid etched. **D,** Composite resin has been bonded over the facial surface to achieve aesthetics. **E,** Postoperative radiograph showing the completed procedures.

tant differences between the primary and permanent teeth are the length of the crowns, the bulbous shape of the crowns, and the very thin dentinal walls of the pulpal floors and roots. The depth necessary to penetrate into the pulpal chamber is quite less than that in the permanent teeth. Likewise, the distance from the occlusal surface to the pulpal floor of the pulp chamber is much less than in permanent teeth. In the primary molars, care must be taken not to grind on the pulpal floor, since perforation is likely (Fig. 22-21).

When the roof of the pulp chamber is perforated and the

pulp chamber identified, the entire roof should be removed with the bur. Since the crowns of the primary teeth are more bulbous, less extension toward the exterior of the tooth is necessary to uncover the openings of the root canals than in permanent teeth.

As in permanent endodontic therapy, canal cleaning and shaping is one of the most important phases of primary root canal treatment. The main objective of the chemical-mechanical preparation of the primary tooth is debridement of the canals. Although an apical taper is desirable, it is not nec-

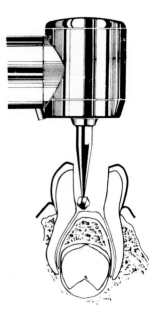

FIG. 22-21 Access opening in primary molar. No. 4 round bur has been used to remove the root of the pulp chamber and the dentin ledges over the canal orifices. Note the minimal length of the bur needed to penetrate to the pulpal floor. Caution must be exercised to avoid perforation of the pulpal floor. *(From Goerig AC, Camp JH: Pediatr Dent 5:33, 1983.)*

essary to have an exact shape to the canals, since the filling is with an absorbable paste rather than gutta-percha. As with any endodontic procedure, use of the rubber dam is mandatory.

A preliminary working length is determined by measurement of a radiograph taken with a paralleling technique. The working length is then determined from a radiograph with an endodontic file in the canal. The use of apex locators may be unreliable as root resorption may create lateral openings into the periodontal tissues at any level.[150] To prevent overextension through the apical foramen, it is advisable that the working length be shortened 2 to 3 mm short of the radiographic length, especially in teeth exhibiting signs of apical root resorption.

Following establishment of the working length, the canal is cleaned and shaped basically as described in Chapter 8. Because of the thin walls of the roots, sonic and ultrasonic cleaning devices should not be used to prepare the canals of primary teeth. Also the use of Gates-Glidden or Peeso drills is contraindicated because of the danger of perforation or stripping of the roots.

Because of their greater flexibility nickel-titanium instruments are recommended rather than stainless steel. Either hand or rotary techniques are ideal for primary teeth. If stainless steel files are used, the instruments must be gently curved to help negotiate the canals. Shaping of the canals proceeds in much the same manner as is done to receive a gutta-percha filling. Care must be taken not to perforate the thin roots during cleaning and shaping procedures. The canals are enlarged several sizes past the first file that fits snugly in the canal, with a minimal size of 30 to 35.

Since many of the pulpal ramifications cannot be reached mechanically, copious irrigation during cleaning and shaping must be maintained (Chapter 8). Debridement of the primary root canal is more often accomplished by chemical means than by mechanical means.[90] This statement should not be misinterpreted as a deemphasis of the importance of thorough debridement and disinfection of the canal. The use of sodium hypochlorite to digest organic debris and RC-Prep to produce effervescence must play an important part in removal of tissue from the inaccessible areas of the root canal system.

After canal debridement the canals are again copiously flushed with sodium hypochlorite and are then dried with sterile paper points; a pellet of cotton is barely moistened with camphorated parachlorophenol (CMCP) and sealed into the pulp chamber with a temporary cement.

At a subsequent appointment the rubber dam is placed and the canals reentered. As long as the patient is free of all signs and symptoms of inflammation, the canals are again irrigated with sodium hypochlorite and dried before filling. If signs or symptoms of inflammation are present, the canals are recleaned and remedicated and the filling procedure delayed until a later time.

Filling of the Primary Root Canals

The filling material for primary root canals must be absorbable so that it absorbs as the roots resorb and does not interfere with the eruption of the permanent tooth. Most reports in the U.S. literature have advocated the use of ZOE as the filler, whereas other parts of the world have used iodoform paste[71] (KRI paste, Pharmachemic AG, Zurich, Switzerland) or ZOE. The antibacterial activity of KRI paste has been shown to be less than ZOE, whereas its cytotoxicity in direct and indirect contact with cells is equal to and greater respectively than ZOE. *The filling material of choice is ZOE without a catalyst.* The lack of a catalyst is necessary to allow adequate working time for filling the canals. The use of gutta-percha or silver points as primary root canal fillers is contraindicated.

The filling of the primary tooth is usually performed without a local anesthetic. This is preferable if possible so the patient's response can be used to indicate approach to the apical foramen. It is, however, sometimes necessary to anesthetize the gingiva with a drop of anesthetic solution to place the rubber dam clamp without pain.

The ZOE is mixed to a thick consistency and is carried into the pulp chamber with a plastic instrument or on a lentulo spiral. The material may be packed into the canals with pluggers or the lentulo spiral. A cotton pellet held in cotton pliers and acting as a piston within the pulp chambers is quite effective in forcing the ZOE into the canals. The endodontic pressure syringe[9,57] is also effective for placing the ZOE in the root canals. In a study of apical seal and quality of filling evaluated radiographically, no statistically significant differences were determined when the canal was filled with the lentulo spiral, pressure syringe, or incrementally with a plugger.[24]

Regardless of the method used to fill the canals, care should be taken to prevent extrusion of the material into the periapical tissues. It is reported that a significantly greater failure rate occurs with overfilling of ZOE than with filling just to the apex or slightly underfilling.[16,71] The adequacy of the obturation is checked by radiographs (Figs. 22-22 through 22-24).

In the event a small amount of the ZOE is inadvertently forced through the apical foramen, it is left alone, since the material is absorbable. It has been reported that defects on succedaneous teeth have no relationship to length of the ZOE filling.[16]

When the canals are satisfactorily obturated, a fast-setting

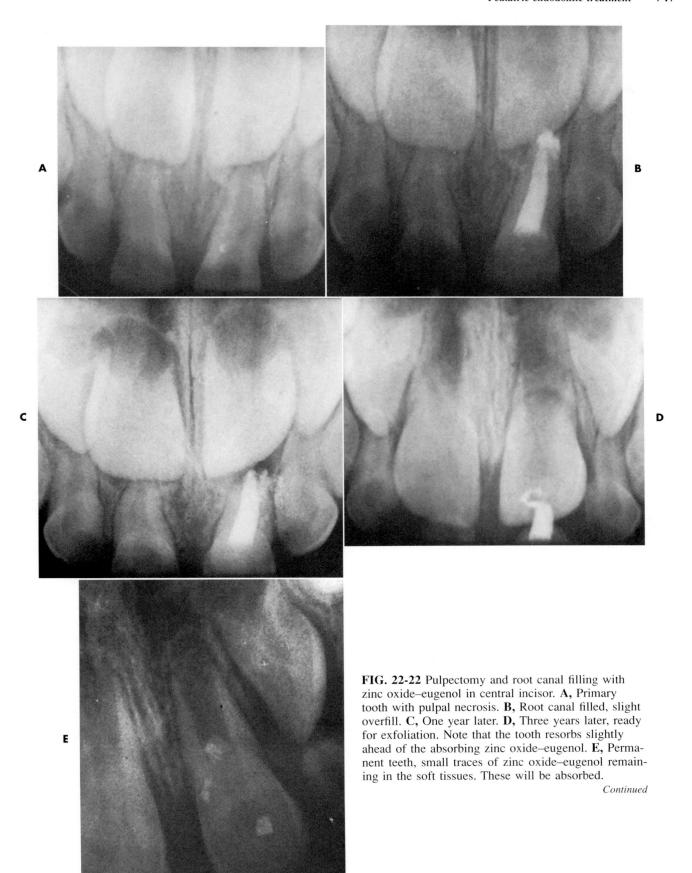

FIG. 22-22 Pulpectomy and root canal filling with zinc oxide–eugenol in central incisor. **A,** Primary tooth with pulpal necrosis. **B,** Root canal filled, slight overfill. **C,** One year later. **D,** Three years later, ready for exfoliation. Note that the tooth resorbs slightly ahead of the absorbing zinc oxide–eugenol. **E,** Permanent teeth, small traces of zinc oxide–eugenol remaining in the soft tissues. These will be absorbed.

Continued

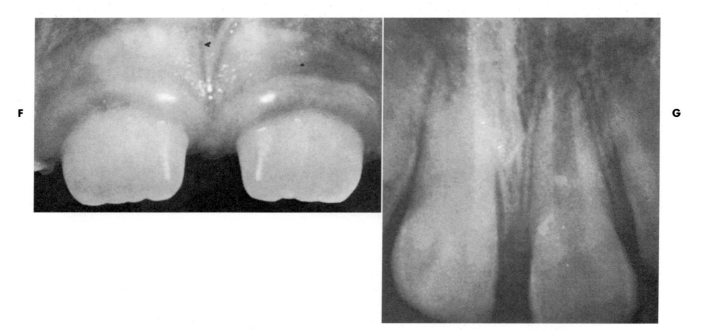

FIG. 22-22, cont'd F, Permanent central incisors newly erupted. Note that no defects are present on the crown even though there was a slight overfill of the primary root canal filling. **G,** Five years after pulpectomy and root canal filling. Note the normal apical closure and the almost total absorption of the zinc oxide–eugenol remnants.

temporary cement is placed in the pulp chamber to seal over the ZOE canal filling. The tooth may then be restored permanently.

In the primary molars it is advisable to place a stainless steel crown as the permanent restoration to prevent possible fracture of the tooth.

When the succedaneous permanent tooth is missing and the retained primary tooth becomes pulpally involved, the canals are filled with gutta-percha following pulpectomy. Since eruption of the permanent tooth is not a factor in these cases, gutta-percha is substituted for ZOE as the filling material of choice (Fig. 22-25).

Follow-up after Primary Pulpectomy

As previously stated, the rate of success following primary pulpectomy is high. However, these teeth should be periodically recalled to check for success of the treatment and to intercept any problem associated with a failure. While resorbing normally without interference with the eruption of the permanent tooth, the primary tooth should remain asymptomatic, firm in the alveolus, and free of pathosis. If evidence of pathosis is detected, extraction and conventional space maintenance are recommended.

It has been pointed out[16,174] that pulpally treated primary teeth may occasionally present a problem of overretention. One study[16] reported 20% incidence of crossbites or palatal eruption of permanent incisors following pulpectomy on primary incisors. In the posterior teeth extraction was required in 22% of cases because of ectopic eruption of the premolars or difficulty in exfoliation of the treated primary molar.[16] After normal physiologic resorption of the roots reaches the pulp chamber, the large amount of ZOE present may impair the absorption and lead to prolonged retention of the crown. Treatment usually consists of simply removing the crown and allowing the permanent tooth to complete its eruption.

Retention of ZOE in the tissues is a common sequela to primary pulpectomy. One long-term study reported that after loss of the tooth 50% of cases had retained ZOE. Teeth filled short of the apices had significantly less retained filler. In time most showed complete absorption or reducing amounts. Retention of filler was not related to success and caused no pathology.[154] Therefore no attempt is made to remove retained filler from the tissues (see Figs. 22-22, *E* and *G* and 22-23, *D* and *E*).

APEXIFICATION

A thorough knowledge of normal root formation is necessary to help one understand the processes involved in treating the pulpless permanent tooth with a wide-open immature apex.

Endodontic management of the pulpless permanent tooth with a wide-open blunderbuss apex has long presented a challenge to dentistry. Before the introduction of apical closure techniques, the usual approach to this problem was surgical. Although the surgical approach was successful, the mechanical and psychologic aspects offered many contraindications. In the pulpless tooth with an incompletely formed apex, the thin fragile dentinal walls made it difficult to achieve an apical seal. When a portion of the root was removed to obtain a seal, the crown-root ratio was poor. Since this situation was usually present in the child patient, a less traumatic approach was desirable.

Many techniques have been advocated to manage the pulpless permanent tooth with an incompletely developed apex. The canals are cleaned and filled with a temporary paste to stimulate the formation of calcified tissue at the apex. The temporary paste is later removed after radiographic evidence of apical closure has been obtained, and a permanent filling of gutta-percha is placed in the canal. The term *apexification* is used to describe this procedure.[175]

Many materials have been reported to successfully stimulate

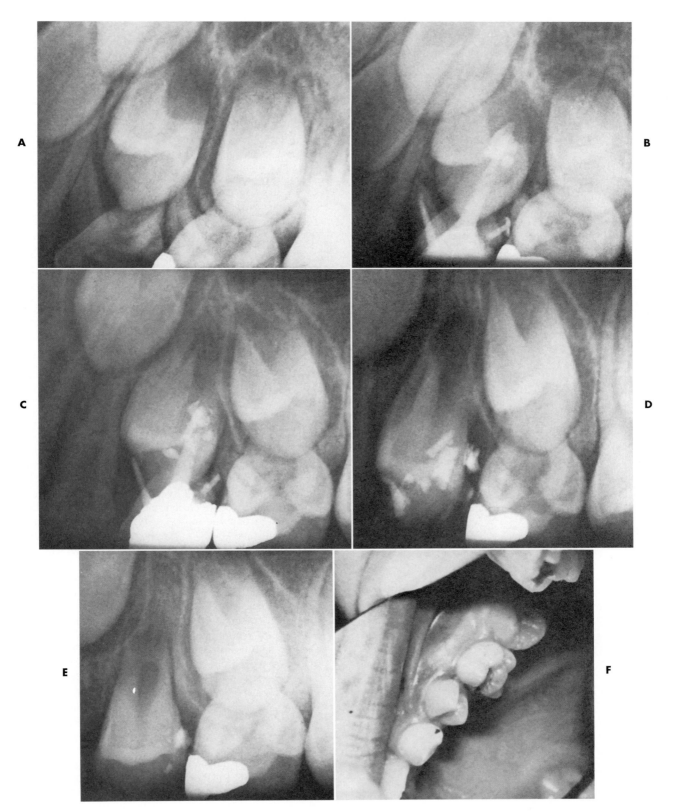

FIG. 22-23 Pulpectomy and root canal filling with zinc oxide–eugenol in a maxillary posterior tooth. **A,** Carious exposure of a primary first molar. **B,** Root canals filled with zinc oxide–eugenol. **C,** One year later. **D,** Two and one half years later. Tooth is ready to exfoliate. **E,** Erupted permanent premolar. Note the slight amount of zinc oxide–eugenol retained in the soft tissue. Zinc oxide–eugenol will undergo absorption. **F,** Note the permanent crown, free of defects.

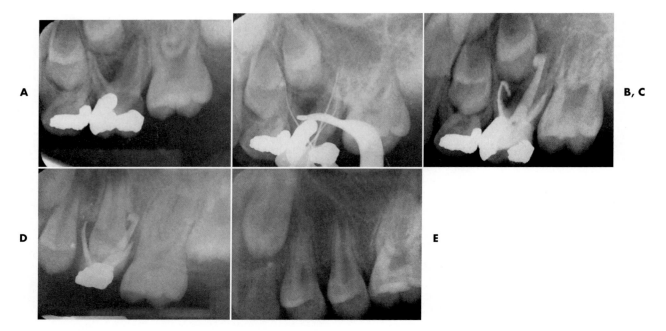

FIG. 22-24 Pulpectomy and root canal filling with ZOE in a maxillary primary second molar. A, Carious pulp exposure with a chronic abscess. Note the furcal and periapical radiolucencies. B, Instruments in place establishing the working length. C, Root canal filled with zinc oxide–eugenol. D, Four and one half years following root canal treatment. Tooth is near exfoliation. E, One year later. Premolar is fully erupted and all traces of the zinc oxide–eugenol have been resorbed.

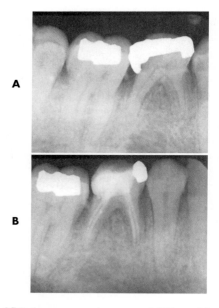

FIG. 22-25 Pulpectomy and root canal filling with gutta-percha in a retained mandibular primary second molar with with no succedaneous permanent tooth. A, Carious exposure of pulp. B, Because the permanent premolar is absent, the root canals of the primary tooth were filled with gutta-percha rather than zinc oxide–eugenol.

apexification. The use of calcium hydroxide for apexification in the pulpless tooth was first reported by Kaiser in 1964.[77] The technique was popularized by the work of Frank.[42] Since that time, calcium hydroxide alone or in combination with other drugs has become the most widely accepted material to promote apexification.

The calcium hydroxide powder has been mixed with CMCP, metacresyl acetate, Cresanol (a mixture of CMCP and metacresyl acetate), physiologic saline, Ringer's solution, distilled water, and anesthetic solution. Although some of these materials appear to enhance the action of the calcium hydroxide better than others, all have been reported to stimulate apexification. Most reports in the U.S. literature[13,60,176] have advocated mixing the calcium hydroxide with CMCP or Cresanol, whereas reports from other parts of the world[18,108] show the same success using distilled water or physiologic saline as the vehicle with which the calcium hydroxide is mixed. The addition of barium sulfate to calcium hydroxide to enhance radiopacity has been shown to produce apexification. The recommended ratio of barium sulfate is one part added to eight parts calcium hydroxide.[193]

In the teeth of humans and primates, tricalcium phosphate promotes apexification similar to that found with calcium hydroxide.[89,151] The material has also been packed into the apical 2 mm of the canal to act as a barrier against which gutta-percha is condensed.[17] The treatment was achieved in one appointment. Using radiographic assessment, the authors reported successful apexification comparable to that achieved in multiple appointments with calcium hydroxide.[17] Calcium hydroxide has also been used successfully as an apical barrier against which to pack gutta-percha.

Collagen–calcium phosphate gel has been reported to produce apexification faster than calcium hydroxide in animals and humans. Various forms of hard and soft tissues were shown revitalizing pulpless root canals within 12 weeks. Formation of cementum, bone, and reparative dentin was noted within the connective tissue ingrowths; a normal periodontal ligament and the absence of ankylosis was also noted. The gel appears to function as an absorbable matrix, supporting hard tissue growth into the debrided root canals.[125-127] In contrast to this, however, another investigator[15] showed that collagen–calcium phosphate gel inhibits the reparative process, with extensive destruction of periapical tissues and no evidence of apexification. Despite the fact that this area of research shows promise for the future, at present it must be considered experimental.

Numerous other materials to promote apexification have been studied with mixed results. Webber[193] and Camp[14] provide expanded data on these materials. Although apexification occurs with many materials, it has been reported even without the presence of canal filling material after removal of the necrotic pulp tissue.[36] The most important factors in achieving apexification seem to be thorough debridement of the root canal (to remove all necrotic pulp tissue) and sealing of the tooth (to prevent the ingress of bacteria and substrate). Apexification does not occur when the apex of the tooth penetrates the cortical plate. To be successful, the apex must be completely within the confines of the cortical plates.

Although highly successful, apexification should be the treatment of last resort in a tooth with an incompletely formed root. Attention should be focused on the maintenance of vitality in these teeth so that as much root length and dentin formation as possible can occur in the root. Indirect pulp therapy and vital pulp-capping and pulpotomy techniques have proved to be successful, aided by the tremendous blood supply present with the open apex. These procedures should be the treatment of choice if there is the possibility of success with any of them. When the tooth with an incompletely formed apex becomes pulpless or periapical disease has developed, apexification is the preferred treatment.

Apexification has been reported in an adult following failed conventional endodontic treatment and apicoectomy performed in childhood.[197] It has also been achieved during active orthodontic treatment.[3]

Determination of the extent of apical closure is many times difficult to ascertain. Radiographic interpretation of apical closure is often misleading. It must always be remembered that the dental radiograph is a two-dimensional picture of a three-dimensional object. Under normal conditions the dental radiograph shows the mesiodistal plane of the tooth rather than the faciolingual plane. The faciolingual aspect of the root canal, however, is usually the last to become convergent apically as the root develops. Therefore it is possible to have a dental radiograph showing an apically convergent root canal while in the faciolingual plane the root canal is divergent (Fig. 22-26).

In teeth with vital tissue remaining in the root canal, techniques to maintain the vitality, rather than pulpectomy, should be used until complete root formation has occurred.

Technique

Diagnosis of pulpal necrosis in the tooth with an incompletely formed apex is sometimes difficult unless a frank exposure of the pulp chamber exists.

The usual cause of endodontic involvement in a tooth with an incompletely developed root is trauma. A detailed history, as well as documentation for insurance and dental-legal reasons, of any injury is of prime importance from both a diagnostic and a treatment point of view.

Radiographic diagnosis of disease is complicated in these teeth because of the normal radiolucency occurring at the apex as the root matures. Comparison of root formation with that in contralateral teeth should always be considered.

The electrical pulp tester usually does not provide meaningful data in teeth with incompletely formed roots. Thermal tests are more reliable for ascertaining vitality but may be complicated by the reliability of the response in the young child.

The presence of acute or chronic pain, percussion sensitivity, mobility, and any discoloration of the crown should be considered in the diagnosis.

In the tooth without a pulp exposure—if any doubt persists after all the foregoing tests have been completed—take a watch-and-wait approach before entering the tooth endodontically to be certain that conclusive evidence of pulpal necrosis exists. If dentin exposure is present, the tooth must be restored in such a manner as to prevent any further pulpal irritation.

In the apexification technique the canal is cleaned and sanitized in the routine endodontic manner. (See Chapter 8 for an in-depth discussion of this technique.) As in any endodontic procedure, the use of the rubber dam is mandatory.

The access opening is made as usual but may require some extension, especially in the anterior teeth, to accommodate the larger-sized instruments necessary to clean the root canals.

The length of the canal is established radiographically, and the canal is cleaned as thoroughly as possible. Frequent irrigation with sodium hypochlorite helps remove debris from the canal. Since the coronal half of the root canal is of smaller diameter than the apical half, root canal instruments that are smaller than the canal space must be used. Thus while mechanically cleaning and shaping the canal, lean the instruments toward each surface of the tooth to contact all surfaces of the root because the canal diverges apically. Sonic and ultrasonic devices are extremely helpful in debriding the canal.

After thorough debridement the canal is dried and just *barely* medicated with CMCP or some other suitable intracanal medicament. The canal is then sealed with a temporary cement.

If symptoms persist or any signs of infection are present at a subsequent appointment or if the canal cannot be dried, the debridement phase is repeated and the canal is medicated with a slurry of calcium hydroxide paste and sealed.

When the tooth is free of signs and symptoms of infection, the canal is dried and filled with a stiff mix of calcium hydroxide and CMCP. The filling procedure is usually performed without the use of local anesthetic. This is preferable if possible so that the patient's response can be used to indicate the approach to the apical foramen.

The material should be spatulated as little as possible, since spatulation decreases the working time and may cause the material to set into a semihard mass before the filling procedure is completed. If this happens, the canal may contain voids and should be recleaned; the filling procedure is then repeated.

The paste may be carried into the canal with an amalgam carrier, lentulo spiral, disposable syringe, or endodontic pressure syringe. Pluggers are helpful for packing the material to the apex. The addition of some dry calcium hydroxide powder within the canal by means of an amalgam carrier aids in condensing the paste of the apex. The canal should ideally be com-

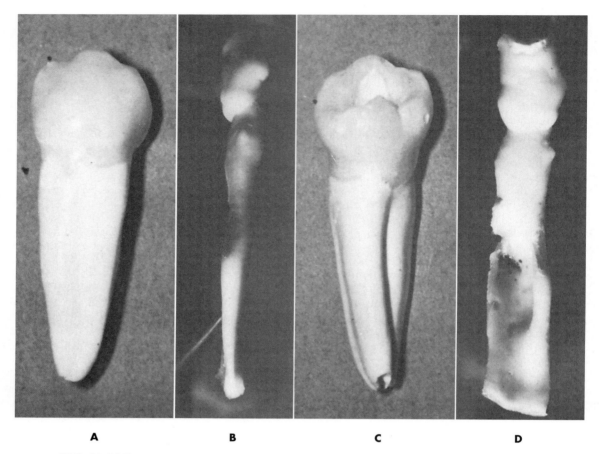

FIG. 22-26 Extracted mandibular premolar and silicone model of the root system. **A,** Facial view. **B,** Model from the facial surface. Note that the root canal diverges apically, which would correspond to the radiographic view of the tooth in the mouth. **C,** Lingual view. **D,** Model from the proximal view, apically divergent canal. With further development the root canal system will divide into two canals.

pletely filled with the paste but should not be overfilled. The response of the patient is used as a guide in approaching the apex; however, because of differences in patient response, this method is not wholly reliable. Radiographic checks of the depth of the filling are essential to verify an adequate filling. The addition of small amounts of barium sulfate to the paste aids in radiographic interpretation without altering the response of the material.

Commercial pastes of calcium hydroxide (Calasept, Pulp-dent, Hypo-cal, and Calyxl) may be used to fill the canals. In this technique, the paste is placed in the canal via the sterile needle supplied with the paste. The liquid portion of the paste is then absorbed with paper points placed into the canal. Injection and absorption of the liquid are repeated until filling of the canal is achieved. Condensation of the dried paste with pluggers is necessary to completely obliterate the canal space.

It has been reported that successful apexification can occur with an overfill of material; in fact it has been reported that an overfill is preferable to an underfill.[13] In the event of an over-fill, the material (being absorbable) is not removed from the apical tissues. The presence of an overfill rarely causes post-operative pain.

After the canal is filled, the access opening must be sealed with a permanent filling material. If the outer seal is defective, the calcium hydroxide paste is lost and recontamination of the canal results. For this reason a temporary type of cement should never be used to seal the tooth after the filling proce-dure. Composite resin or silicate cement is recommended for anterior teeth and amalgam for posterior teeth.

Periodic Recall

The usual time required to achieve apexification is 6 to 24 months (average 1 year $\pm$ 7 months).[87] Factors that lead to increased time are the presence of a radiolucent lesion, inter-appointment symptoms, and loss of the external seal with re-infection of the canal. During this time the patient is recalled at 3-month intervals for monitoring of the tooth.

If any signs or symptoms of reinfection or pathology occur during this phase of treatment, the canal is recleaned and re-filled with the calcium hydroxide paste. The patient is recalled until radiographic evidence of apexification has become appar-ent. Then the tooth is reentered and clinical verification of apexification is made by the failure of a small instrument to penetrate through the apex after removal of the calcium hy-droxide paste. If apexification is incomplete, the canal is re-packed with the calcium hydroxide paste, and the periodic re-call continues (Fig. 22-27).

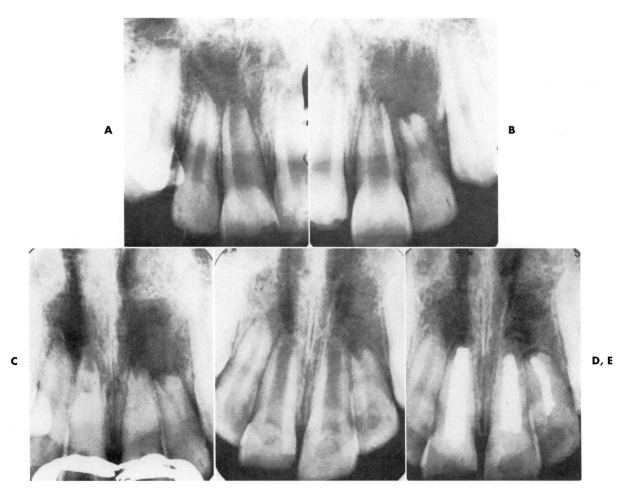

FIG. 22-27 Apexification in three permanent incisors, using calcium hydroxide–camphorated parachlorophenol filling material. **A** and **B,** Open apexes of the three incisors with periapical pathosis. Note the calcification that has occurred in the lateral incisor before pulpal necrosis. **C,** Calcium hydroxide–camphorated parachlorophenol filling placed in two teeth. Note the void in the left incisor requiring further filling. **D,** Radiographic appearance of apexification a year later. **E,** Permanent root canal filling of gutta-percha after apexification.

Histology of Apexification

The calcified material that forms over the apical foramen has been histologically identified as an osteoid (bonelike) or cementoid (cementum-like) material by investigators who have done apexification following periapical involvement of the treated teeth.[13,60,175] The formation of osteodentin after the placement of calcium hydroxide paste immediately on conclusion of a vital pulpectomy has also been reported.[32]

Histologic studies consistently report the absence of Hertwig's epithelial root sheath. Normal root formation usually does not occur following apexification. Instead, there appears to be a differentiation of adjacent connective tissue cells into specialized cells; there is also deposition of calcified tissue adjacent to the filling material. The calcified material is continuous with the lateral root surfaces. The closure of the apex may be partial or complete but consistently has minute communications with the periapical tissues (Fig. 22-28). For this reason apexification must always be followed by filling of the canal with a permanent root canal filling of gutta-percha.

Various types of apical closure have been reported in clinical studies of apexification. In view of the histologic evidence of subsequent studies, it would appear that these types of apical closure simply relate to the level to which the filling material was placed within or beyond the apical foramen.

Many of the failures of apexification have been shown histologically to arise from the difficulty of adequately cleaning and sanitizing the wide-open canals. The tooth with an apically divergent root canal is much more difficult to clean thoroughly than is the mature tooth, which becomes increasingly smaller as the apex is approached.

Although the formation of calcified tissue was noted in the presence of mild inflammation,[13] the results were consistently better in specimens that were free of inflammation. It is recommended therefore that the cleaning and filling procedure be done at separate appointments rather than in a single appointment. Likewise, ideally all signs and symptoms of infection and inflammation should be absent before the calcium hydroxide paste is placed.

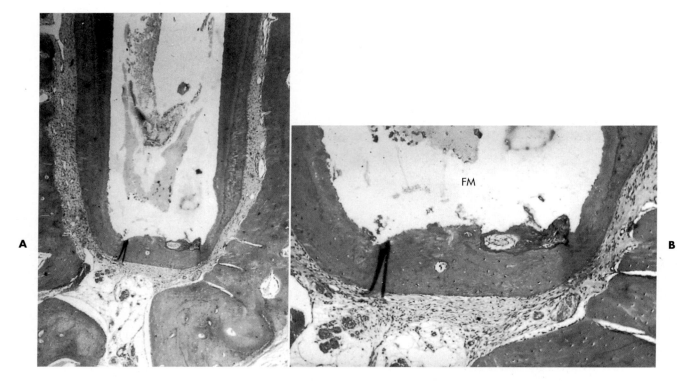

FIG. 22-28 Histologic sections of a dog's tooth after apexification. **A,** Cementum-like calcified tissue is closing the wide-open apical foramen. Note the presence of debris within the canal because of inadequate cleaning of the canal before filling. **B,** Higher magnification showing cellular detail. Periodontal ligament *(P)* is free of inflammation. Filling material *(FM),* calcium hydroxide–camphorated parachlorophenol, was lost during processing. Note the presence of tissue communication through the calcified tissue. Stain H & E.

Obturation with Gutta-Percha

After verification of successful apexification, the canal is thoroughly cleaned, care being taken not to damage the calcific barrier at the apex. The canal is then obturated with gutta-percha in the usual manner. Because of the large size of the canal, it may be necessary to prepare a customized gutta-percha point as described in Chapter 9. Although the apexification procedure is highly successful, the root of such a tooth is weak and prone to fracture with subsequent injuries. Therefore apexification should be a treatment of last resort after all attempts at vital therapy have failed.

Restoration Following Apexification

Because of the thin dentinal walls there is a high percentage of root fractures in teeth following apexification. Restoration of the immature tooth following obturation with gutta-percha must be designed to strengthen the tooth as much as possible. The use of newer dentinal bonding techniques has been shown to strengthen endodontically treated teeth to levels close to that of intact teeth.[68,82]

Placement of an autocuring composite is difficult because of the short working time. Light-curing composites allow sufficient time for proper placement in the canal but have the disadvantage of incomplete polymerization in the deeper depths of the canal because of limited transmission of light through the material. Clear plastic posts, the Luminex System (Dentatus USA, New York, N.Y.), have been developed to allow light

transmission throughout the canal, curing the entire mass of composite.

Following obturation, the gutta-percha is removed to a depth of 3 to 4 mm below the cervical line. A Luminex post is selected. The dentin is acid etched, and a dentin bonding agent applied to the internal surfaces of the canal. Light-curing composite is placed in the canal, and care is taken not to trap bubbles. The Luminex post is placed to the depth of the preparation and the composite cured by transmitting light through the post. Following curing, the plastic post may be removed and a corresponding metal post cemented, which will further increase strength.[82]

REFERENCES

1. Alacam A: Long-term effects of primary teeth pulpotomies with formocresol, glutaraldehyde–calcium hydroxide and glutaraldehyde–zinc oxide–eugenol on succedaneous teeth, *J Pedodont* 13:307, 1989.
2. Andrew P: The treatment of infected pulps in deciduous teeth, *Br Dent J* 98:122, 1955.
3. Anthony DR: Apexification during active orthodontic movement, *J Endod* 12:419, 1986.
4. Aponte AJ, Hartsook JT, Crowley MC: Indirect pulp capping success verified, *J Dent Child* 33:164, 1966.
5. Armstrong RL et al: Comparison of Dycal and formocresol pulpotomies in young permanent teeth in monkeys, *Oral Surg* 48:160, 1979.
6. Attala MN, Noujaim AA: Role of calcium hydroxide in the formation of reparative dentin, *J Can Dent Assoc* 35:267, 1969.

7. Avram DC, Pulver F: Pulpotomy medicaments for vital primary teeth: surveys to determine use and attitudes in pediatric dental practice and in dental schools throughout the world, *J Dent Child* 56:426, 1989.

8. Bennett CG: Pulpal management of deciduous teeth, *Pract Dent Monogr*, p 1, May-June, 1965.

9. Berk II, Krakow AA: Endodontic treatment in primary teeth. In Goldman HM et al, editors: *Current therapy in dentistry,* vol 5, St Louis, 1974, Mosby.

10. Bevelander G, Benzer D: Morphology and incidence in secondary dentin in human teeth, *J Am Dent Assoc* 30:1079, 1943.

11. Block RM et al: Cell-mediated immune response to dog pulp tissue altered by formocresol within the root canal, *J Endod* 3:424, 1977.

12. Brian JD et al: Reaction of rat connective tissue to unfixed and formaldehyde-fixed autogenous implants enclosed in tubes, *J Endod* 6:628, 1980.

13. Camp JH: *Continued apical development of pulpless permanent teeth following endodontic therapy,* master's thesis, Bloomington, 1968, Indiana University School of Dentistry.

14. Camp JH: Pediatric endodontic treatment. In Cohen S, Burns RC, editors: *Pathways of the pulp,* ed 6, St Louis, 1994, Mosby.

15. Citrome GP, Kaminski EJ, Heuer MA: A comparative study of tooth apexification in the dog, *J Endod* 5:290, 1979.

16. Coll JA, Sadrian R: Predicting pulpectomy success and its relationship to exfoliation and succedaneous dentition, *Pediatr Dent* 18:57, 1996.

17. Coviello J, Brilliant JD: A preliminary clinical study of the use of tricalcium phosphate as an apical barrier, *J Endod* 5:6, 1979.

18. Cvek M: Treatment of non-vital permanent incisors with calcium hydroxide, *Odontol Rev* 23:27, 1972.

19. Cvek M: A clinical report on partial pulpotomy and capping with calcium hydroxide in permanent incisors with complicated crown fractures, *J Endod* 4:232, 1978.

20. Cvek M: Endodontic treatment of traumatized teeth. In Andreasen JO: *Traumatic injuries of the teeth,* ed 2, Philadelphia, 1981, WB Saunders.

21. Cvek M, Lundberg M: Histological appearance of pulps after exposure by a crown fracture, partial pulpotomy, and clinical diagnosis of healing, *J Endod* 9:8, 1983.

22. Cvek M et al: Pulp reactions to exposure after experimental crown fracture or grinding in adult monkey, *J Endod* 8:391, 1982.

23. Cvek M et al: Hard tissue barrier formation in pulpotomized monkey teeth capped with cyanoacrylate or calcium hydroxide for 10 and 60 minutes, *J Dent Res* 66:1166, 1987.

24. Dandashi MB et al: An in vitro comparison of three endodontic techniques for primary incisors, *Pediatr Dent* 15:254, 1993.

25. Dannenberg JL: Pedodontic-endodontics, *Dent Clin North Am* 18:367, 1974.

26. Davis MJ, Myers R, Switkes MD: Glutaraldehyde: an alternative to formocresol for vital pulp therapy, *J Dent Child* 49:176, 1982.

27. Dietz D: *A histological study of the effects of formocresol on normal primary pulpal tissue,* master's thesis, Seattle, 1961, School of Dentistry, University of Washington.

28. Dilley GJ, Courts FJ: Immunological response to four pulpal medicaments, *Pediatr Dent* 3:179, 1981.

29. Dimaggio JJ, Hawes RR: Evaluation of direct and indirect pulp capping, *J Dent Res* 40:24, 1962 (abstract).

30. Dimaggio JJ, Hawes RR: Continued evaluation of direct and indirect pulp capping, *J Dent Res* 41:38, 1963 (abstract).

31. Doyle WA, McDonald RE, Mitchell DF: Formocresol versus calcium hydroxide in pulpotomy, *J Dent Child* 29:86, 1962.

32. Dylewski JJ: Apical closure of non-vital teeth, *Oral Surg* 32:82, 1971.

33. Easlick KA: Operative procedures in management of deciduous molars, *Int J Orthod* 20:585, 1934.

34. Ehrenreich DW: A comparison of the effects of zinc oxide and eugenol and calcium hydroxide on carious dentin in human primary molars, *J Dent Child* 35:451, 1968.

35. Emmerson C et al: Pulpal changes following formocresol applications on rat molars and human primary teeth, *J South Calif Dent Assoc* 27:309, 1959.

36. England MC, Best E: Noninduced apical closure in immature roots of dogs' teeth, *J Endod* 3:411, 1977.

37. Fairbourn DR, Charbeneau GT, Loesche WJ: Effect of improved Dycal and I.R.M. on bacteria in deep carious lesions, *J Am Dent Assoc* 100:547, 1980.

38. Feigal RJ, Messer HH: A critical look at glutaraldehyde, *Pediatr Dent* 12:69, 1990.

39. Feltman EM: *A comparison of the formocresol pulpotomy techniques and Dycal pulpotomy technique in young permanent teeth,* master's thesis, Bloomington, 1972, School of Dentistry, Indiana University.

40. Finn SB: Morphology of the primary teeth. In Finn SB et al, editors: *Clinical pedodontics,* ed 3, Philadelphia, 1967, WB Saunders.

41. Fishman SA et al: Success of electrofulguration pulpotomies covered by zinc oxide and eugenol, *Pediatr Dent* 18:385, 1996.

42. Frank AL: Therapy for the divergent pulpless tooth by continued apical formation, *J Am Dent Assoc* 72:87, 1966.

43. Frankl SN: Pulp therapy in pedodontics, *Oral Surg* 34:293, 1972.

44. Friedberg BH, Gartner LP: Embryotoxicity and teratogenicity of formocresol on developing chick embryos, *J Endod* 16:434, 1990.

45. Fuks AB, Bimstein EC: Clinical evaluation of diluted formocresol pulpotomies in primary teeth of school children, *Pediatr Dent* 3:321, 1981.

46. Fuks AB, Bimstein E, Bruchimn A: Radiographic and histologic evaluation of the effect of two concentrations of formocresol on pulpotomized primary and young permanent teeth in monkeys, *Pediatr Dent* 5:9, 1983.

47. Fuks AB et al: Partial pulpotomy as a treatment alternative for exposed pulps in crown-fractured permanent incisors, *Endodont Dent Traumatol* 3:100, 1987.

48. Fuks AB et al: Assessment of a 2 percent buffered glutaraldehyde solution in pulpotomized primary teeth of school children, *J Dent Child* 57:371, 1990.

49. Fulton R, Ranly DM: An autoradiographic study of formocresol pulpotomies in rat molars using ^{3}H-formaldehyde, *J Endod* 5:71, 1979.

50. Fusayama T, Okuse K, Hosoda H: Relationship between hardness, discoloration and microbial invasion in carious dentin, *J Dent Res* 45:1033, 1966.

51. Garcia-Godoy F, Novakovic DP, Carvajal IN: Pulpal response to different application times of formocresol, *J Pedodont* 6:176, 1982.

52. Garcia-Godoy F, Ranly D: Clinical evaluation of pulpotomies with ZOE as the vehicle for glutaraldehyde, *Pediatr Dent* 9:144, 1987.

53. Gazi HA, Nayak RG, Bhat KS: Tissue-irritation potential of dilute formocresol, *Oral Surg* 51:74, 1981.

54. Gerlach E: Root canal therapeutics in deciduous teeth, *Dent Surv* 8:63, 1932.

55. Glass RL, Zander HA: Pulp healing, *J Dent Res* 28:97, 1949.

56. Granath LE, Hagman G: Experimental pulpotomy in human bicuspids with reference to cutting technique, *Acta Odontol Scand* 29:155, 1971.

57. Greenberg M: Filling root canals of deciduous teeth by an injection technique, *Dent Dig* 67:574, 1964.

58. Guidelines for pulp therapy for primary and young permanent teeth: *American Academy of Pediatric Dentistry Reference Manual, Pediatr Dent* 18:44, 1996.

59. Guthrie TJ, McDonald RE, Mitchell DF: Dental hemogram, *J Dent Res* 44:678, 1965.

60. Ham JW, Patterson SS, Mitchell DF: Induced apical closure of immature pulpless teeth in monkeys, *Oral Surg* 33:438, 1972.

61. Harris CA: *The principles and practice of dental surgery,* ed 4, Philadelphia, 1850, Lindsay & Blakiston.

62. Hata G et al: Systemic distribution of ^{14}C-labeled formaldehyde applied in the root canal following pulpectomy, *J Endod* 15:539, 1989.

63. Hawes RR, Dimaggio JJ, Sayegh F: Evaluation of direct and indirect pulp capping, *J Dent Res* 43:808, 1964 (abstract).

64. Hayashi Y: Ultrastructure of initial calcification in wound healing following pulpotomy, *J Oral Pathol* 11:174, 1982.

65. Heide S: Pulp reactions to exposure for 4, 24 and 168 hours, *J Dent Res* 59:1910, 1980.

66. Heide S, Kerekes K: Delayed partial pulpotomy in permanent incisors of monkeys, *Int Endodont J* 19:78, 1986.

67. Hermann BW: Dentinobliteran der Wurzelkanale nach der Behandlung mit Kalzium, *Zahaertzl Rund* 39:888, 1930.

68. Hernandez R, Bader S, Boston D, Trope M: Resistance to fracture of endodontically treated premolars restored with new generation dentin bonding systems, *Int Endodont J* 27:281, 1994.

69. Hibbard ED, Ireland RL: Morphology of the root canals of the primary molar teeth, *J Dent Child* 24:250, 1957.

70. Hill S et al: Comparison of antimicrobial and cytotoxic effects of glutaraldehyde and formocresol, *Oral Surg Oral Med Oral Pathol* 71:89, 1991.

71. Holan G, Fuks AB: A comparison of pulpectomies using ZOE and KRI paste in primary molars: a retrospective study, *Pediatr Dent* 15:403, 1993.

72. Holan G, Topf J, Fuks AB: Effect of root canal infection and treatment of traumatized primary incisors on their permanent successors, *Endodont Dent Traumatol* 8:12, 1992.

73. Inglis OE: Can recalcification of dentin occur? A proposition, *Pacific Dent Gaz* 8:763, 1900.

74. Ireland RL: Secondary dentin formation in deciduous teeth, *J Am Dent Assoc* 28:1626, 1941.

75. Jeng HW, Feigal RJ, Messer HH: Comparison of the cytotoxicity of formocresol, formaldehyde, cresol, and glutaraldehyde using human pulp fibroblast cultures, *Pediatr Dent* 9:295, 1987.

76. Jordon ME: *Operative dentistry for children*, New York, 1925, Dental Items of Interest Publishing Co.

77. Kaiser JH: Management of wide-open canals with calcium hydroxide. Paper presented at the meeting of the American Association of Endodontics, Washington, DC, April 17, 1964. Cited by Steiner JC, Dow PR, Cathey GM: Inducing root end closure of nonvital permanent teeth, *J Dent Child* 35:47, 1968.

78. Kakehashi S, Stanley HR, Fitzgerald RT: The effects of surgical exposures of dental pulps in germ-free and conventional laboratory rats, *Oral Surg* 20:340, 1965.

79. Kalnins V, Frisbie HE: Effect of dentin fragments on the healing of the exposed pulp, *Arch Oral Biol* 2:96, 1960.

80. Kanka J III: An alternative hypothesis to the cause of pulpal inflammation in teeth treated with phosphoric acid on the dentin, *Quintessence Int* 21:83, 1990.

81. Karp WB, Korb P, Pashley D: The oxidation of glutaraldehyde by rat tissues, *Pediatr Dent* 9:301, 1987.

82. Katebzadeh N, Dalton BC, Trope M: Strengthening immature teeth during and after apexification, *J Endod* 1997, in press.

83. Kelley MA, Bugg JL, Skjonsby HS: Histologic evaluation of formocresol and oxpara pulpotomies in rhesus monkeys, *J Am Dent Assoc* 86:123, 1973.

84. Kennedy DB et al: Formocresol pulpotomy in teeth of dogs with induced pulpal and periapical pathosis, *J Dent Child* 40:44, 1973.

85. Kerkhove BC et al: A clinical and television densitometric evaluation of the indirect pulp capping technique, *J Dent Child* 34:192, 1967.

86. King JB, Crawford JJ, Lindahl RL: Indirect pulp capping: a bacteriologic study of deep carious dentine in human teeth, *Oral Surg* 20:663, 1965.

87. Kleier DJ, Barr ES: A study of endodontically apexified teeth, *Endodont Dent Traumatol* 7:112, 1991.

88. Klein H et al: Partial pulpotomy following complicated crown fracture in permanent incisors: a clinical and radiographic study, *J Pedodont* 9:142, 1985.

89. Koenigs JF et al: Induced apical closure of permanent teeth in adult primates using a resorbable form of tricalcium phosphate ceramic, *J Endod* 1:102, 1975.

90. Kopel HM: Pediatric endodontics. In Ingle JI, Beveridge EE, editors: *Endodontics*, ed 2, Philadelphia, 1976, Lea & Febiger.

91. Kopel HM et al: The effects of glutaraldehyde on primary pulp tissue following coronal amputation: an in vivo histologic study, *J Dent Child* 47:425, 1980.

92. Langeland K: Management of the inflamed pulp associated with deep carious lesion, *J Endod* 7:169, 1981.

93. Langeland K et al: Human pulp changes of iatrogenic origin, *Oral Surg* 32:943, 1971.

94. Laurence RP: *A method of root canal therapy for primary teeth*, master's thesis, Atlanta, Ga, 1966, School of Dentistry, Emory University.

95. Laws AJ: Pulpotomy by electro-coagulation, *New Zealand Dent J* 53:68, 1957.

96. Lekka M, Hume WR, Wolinsky LE: Comparison between formaldehyde and glutaraldehyde diffusion through the root tissues of pulpotomy-treated teeth, *J Pedodont* 8:185, 1984.

97. Lloyd JM, Seale NS, Wilson CFG: The effects of various concentrations and lengths of application of glutaraldehyde on monkey pulp tissue, *Pediatr Dent* 10:115, 1988.

98. Longwill DG, Marshall FJ, Creamer HR: Reactivity of human lymphocytes to pulp antigens, *J Endod* 8:27, 1982.

99. Loos PJ, Han SS: An enzyme histochemical study of the effect of various concentrations of formocresol on connective tissues, *Oral Surg* 31:571, 1971.

100. Loos PJ, Straffon LH, Han SS: Biological effects of formocresol, *J Dent Child* 40:193, 1973.

101. Lui JL: Depth of composite polymerization within simulated root canals using light-transmitting posts, *Oper Dent* 19:165, 1994.

102. Mack ES: Personal communication, 1967.

103. Mack RB, Dean JA: Electrosurgical pulpotomy: a retrospective human study, *ASDC J Dent Child* 60:107, 1993.

104. Mack RB, Halterman CW: Labial pulpectomy access followed by esthetic composite resin restoration for nonvital maxillary deciduous incisors, *J Am Dent Assoc* 100:374, 1980.

105. Mansukhani N: *Pulpal reactions to formocresol*, master's thesis, Urbana, 1959, College of Dentistry, University of Illinois.

106. Mass E, Zilberman U: Clinical and radiographic evaluation of partial pulpotomy in carious exposures of permanent molars, *Pediatr Dent* 15:257, 1993.

107. Massler M, Mansukhani H: Effects of formocresol on the dental pulp, *J Dent Child* 26:277, 1959.

108. Matsumiya S, Susuki A, Takuma S: *Atlas of clinical pathology*, vol 1, Tokyo, 1962, Tokyo Dental College Press.

109. McDonald RE, Avery DR: Treatment of deep caries, vital pulp exposure, and pulpless teeth in children. In McDonald RE, Avery DR, editors: *Dentistry for the child and adolescent*, ed 3, St Louis, 1978, Mosby.

110. Mejare I, Cvek M: Partial pulpotomy in young permanent teeth with deep carious lesions, *Endodont Dent Traumatol* 9:238, 1993.

111. Messer LB, Cline JT, Korf NW: Long-term effects of primary molar pulpotomies on succedaneous bicuspids, *J Dent Res* 59:116, 1980.

112. Mjör IA, Dahl E, Cox CF: Healing of pulp exposures: an ultrastructural study, *J Oral Pathol Med* 20:496, 1991.

113. Morawa AP et al: Clinical studies of human primary teeth following dilute formocresol pulpotomies, *J Dent Res* 53:269, 1974, (abstract).

114. Morawa AP et al: Clinical evaluation of pulpotomies using dilute formocresol, *J Dent Child* 42:360, 1975.

115. Mulder GR, van Amerongen WE, Vingerling PA: Consequences of endodontic treatment of primary teeth. II. A clinical investigation into the influence of formocresol pulpotomy on the permanent successor, *J Dent Child* 54:35, 1987.

116. Mūniz MA, Keszler A, Dominiguez FV: The formocresol technique in young permanent teeth, *Oral Surg* 55:611, 1983.

117. Myers DR: *Effects of formocresol on pulps of cariously exposed permanent molars*, master's thesis, 1972, College of Dentistry, University of Tennessee.

118. Myers DR et al: Distribution of ^{14}C-formaldehyde after pulpotomy with formocresol, *J Am Dent Assoc* 96:805, 1978.

119. Myers DR et al: Acute toxicity of high doses of systemically administered formocresol in dogs, *Pediatr Dent* 3:37, 1981.

120. Myers DR et al: Tissue changes induced by the absorption of formocresol from pulpotomy sites in dogs, *Pediatr Dent* 5:6, 1983.

121. Myers DR et al: Systemic absorption of ^{14}C-glutaraldehyde from glutaraldehyde-treated pulpotomy sites, *Pediatr Dent* 8:134, 1986.

122. Myers DR et al: Histopathology of furcation lesions associated with pulp degeneration in primary molars, *Pediatr Dent* 9:279, 1987.

123. Myers DR et al: Histopathology of radiolucent furcation lesions associated with pulpotomy-treated primary molars, *Pediatr Dent* 10:291, 1988.

124. Nelson JR et al: Biochemical effects of tissue fixatives on bovine pulp, *J Endod* 5:139, 1979.

125. Nevins AJ et al: Revitalization of pulpless open apex teeth in rhesus monkeys, using collagen–calcium phosphate gel, *J Endod* 2:159, 1976.

126. Nevins A et al: Hard tissue induction into pulpless open-apex teeth using collagen-calcium phosphate gel, *J Endod* 3:431, 1977.

127. Nevins A et al: Induction of hard tissue into pulpless open-apex teeth using collagen-calcium phosphate gel, *J Endod* 4:76, 1978.

128. Nirschl RF, Avery DR: Evaluation of new pulp capping agent in indirect pulp therapy, *J Dent Child* 50:25, 1983.

129. Orban B: Contribution to the histology of the dental pulp and periodontal membrane with special reference to the cells of defense of these tissues, *J Am Dent Assoc* 16:965, 1929.

130. Orban BJ, editor: *Oral histology and embryology,* ed 4, St Louis, 1957, Mosby.

131. Oringer MJ: *Electrosurgery in dentistry,* ed 2, Philadelphia, 1975, WB Saunders.

132. Pashley EL et al: Systemic distribution of ^{14}C-formaldehyde from formocresol-treated pulpotomy sites, *J Dent Res* 59:603, 1980.

133. Paterson RC, Watts A: Further studies on the exposed germ-free dental pulp, *Int Endod J* 20:112, 1987.

134. Pereira JC, Stanley HR: Pulp capping: influence of the exposure site on pulp healing—histologic and radiographic study in dogs' pulp, *J Endod* 7:213, 1981.

135. Peron LC, Burkes EJ, Gregory WB: Vital pulpotomy utilizing variable concentrations of paraformaldehyde in rhesus monkeys, *J Dent Res* 55:B129, 1976 (abstract 269).

136. Phancuf RA, Frankl SN, Ruben M: A comparative histological evaluation of three calcium hydroxide preparations on the human primary dental pulp, *J Dent Child* 35:61, 1968.

137. Pisanti S, Sciaky I: Origin of calcium in the repair wall after pulp exposure in the dog, *J Dent Res* 43:641, 1964.

138. Rabbach VP et al: Comparison of the effectiveness of electrosurgery versus formocresol in the pulpotomy procedure for primary teeth: a prospective human study, in press.

139. Rabinowitch BZ: Pulp management in primary teeth, *Oral Surg* 6:542, 1953.

140. Ranley DM: Glutaraldehyde purity and stability: implications for preparation, storage, and use as a pulpotomy agent, *Pediatr Dent* 6:83, 1984.

141. Ranley DM: Assessment of the systemic distribution and toxicity of formaldehyde following pulpotomy treatment. I, *J Dent Child* 52:431, 1985.

142. Ranley DM: Pulpotomy therapy in primary teeth: new modalities for old rationals, *Pediatr Dent* 16:403, 1994.

143. Ranley DM, Lazzari EP: A biochemical study of two biofunctional reagents as alternatives to formocresol, *J Dent Res* 62:1054, 1983.

144. Ranley DM, Garcia-Godoy F, Horn D: Time, concentration, and pH parameters for the use of glutaraldehyde as a pulpotomy agent: an in vivo study, *Pediatr Dent* 9:199, 1987.

145. Ranley DM, Horn D, Hubbard GB: Assessment of the systemic distribution and toxicity of glutaraldehyde as a pulpotomy agent, *Pediatr Dent* 11:8, 1989.

146. Ranley DM, Horn D, Zislis T: The effect of alternatives to formocresol on antigenicity of protein, *J Dent Res* 64:1225, 1985.

147. Ranley DM, Amstutz L, Horn D: Subcellular localization of glutaraldehyde, *Endodont Dent Traumatol* 6:251, 1990.

148. Ranley DM, Horn D: Distribution, metabolism, and excretion of (^{14}C) glutaraldehyde, *J Endod* 16:135, 1990.

149. Rickman GA, Elbadrawy HE: Effect of premature loss of primary incisors on speech, *Pediatr Dent* 7:119, 1985.

150. Rimondini L, Baroni C: Morphologic criteria for root canal treatment of primary molars undergoing resorption, *Endodont Dent Traumatol* 11:136, 1995.

151. Roberts SC Jr, Brilliant JD: Tricalcium phosphate as an adjunct to apical closure in pulpless permanent teeth, *J Endod* 1:263, 1975.

152. Rølling I, Poulsen S: Formocresol pulpotomy of primary teeth and occurrence of enamel defects on the permanent successors, *Acta Odontol Scand* 36:243, 1978.

153. Ruemping DR, Morton TH Jr, Anderson MW: Electrosurgical pulpotomy in primates—a comparison with formocresol pulpotomy, *Pediatr Dent* 5:14, 1983.

154. Sadrian R, Coll JA: A long-term follow-up on the retention of zinc oxide eugenol filler after primary tooth pulpectomy, *Pediatr Dent* 15:249, 1993.

155. Sanchez ZMC: *Effects of formocresol on pulp-capped and pulpotomized permanent teeth of rhesus monkeys,* master's thesis, Ann Arbor, 1971, University of Michigan.

156. Savage NW et al: An histological study of cystic lesions following pulp therapy in deciduous molars, *J Oral Pathol* 15:209, 1986.

157. Sayegh FS: Qualitative and quantitative evaluation of new dentin in pulp capped teeth, *J Dent Child* 35:7, 1968.

158. Sayegh FS: The dentinal bridge in pulp-involved teeth. I, *Oral Surg* 28:579, 1969.

159. Sciaky I, Pisanti S: Localization of calcium placed over amputated pulps in dogs' teeth, *J Dent Res* 39:1128, 1960.

160. Seltzer S, Bender IB: Pulp capping and pulpotomy. In Seltzer S, Bender IB, editors: *The dental pulp, biologic considerations in dental procedures,* ed 2, Philadelphia, 1975, JB Lippincott.

161. Shaw DW et al: Electrosurgical pulpotomy—a 6-month study in primates, *J Endod* 13:500, 1987.

162. Sheller B, Morton TH Jr: Electrosurgical pulpotomy: a pilot study in humans, *J Endod* 13:69, 1987.

163. Shoji S, Nakamura M, Horiuchi H: Histopathological changes in dental pulps irradiated by CO_2 laser: a preliminary report on laser pulpotomy, *J Endod* 11:379, 1985.

164. Shovelton DS: A study of deep carious dentin, *Int Dent J* 18:392, 1968.

165. Shulman ER, Melver FT, Burkes EJ Jr: Comparison of electrosurgery and formocresol as pulpotomy techniques in monkey primary teeth, *Pediatr Dent* 9:189, 1987.

166. Simon M, van Mullem PJ, Lamers AC: Formocresol: no allergic effect after root canal disinfection in non-presensitized guinea pigs, *J Endod* 8:269, 1982.

167. Spedding RH: The one-appointment formocresol pulpotomy for primary teeth, *J Tenn Dent Assoc* 48:263, 1968.

168. Stanley HR, Lundy T: Dycal therapy for pulp exposure, *Oral Surg* 34:818, 1972.

169. Stanley HR, Pameijer CH: Pulp capping with a new visible-light–curing calcium hydroxide composition (Prisma VLC Dycal), *Oper Dent* 10:156, 1985.

170. Stanley HR, White CL, McCray L: The rate of tertiary (reparative) dentine formation in the human tooth, *Oral Surg* 21:180, 1966.

171. Stanton WG: The non-vital deciduous tooth, *Int J Orthod* 21:181, 1935.

172. Starkey PE: Methods of preserving primary teeth which have exposed pulps, *J Dent Child* 30:219, 1963.

173. Starkey PE: Management of deep caries of pulpally involved teeth in children. In Goldman HM et al, editors: *Current therapy in dentistry,* vol 3, St Louis, 1968, Mosby.

174. Starkey PE: Treatment of pulpally involved primary molars. In McDonald RE et al, editors: *Current therapy in dentistry,* vol 7, St Louis, 1980, Mosby.

175. Steiner JC, Dow PR, Cathey GM: Inducing root end closure of nonvital permanent teeth, *J Dent Child* 35:47, 1968.

176. Steiner JC, Van Hassel HJ: Experimental root apexification in primates, *Oral Surg* 31:409, 1971.

177. Straffon LH, Han SS: Effects of varying concentrations of formocresol on RNA synthesis of connective tissue in sponge implants, *Oral Surg* 29:915, 1970.

178. Sun HW, Feigal RJ, Messer HH: Cytotoxicity of glutaraldehyde and formaldehyde in relation to time of exposure and concentration, *Pediatr Dent* 12:303, 1990.

179. Sweet CA: Procedure for the treatment of exposed and pulpless deciduous teeth, *J Am Dent Assoc* 17:1150, 1930.

180. Tagger M, Tagger E: Pulp capping in monkeys with Reolite and Life, two calcium hydroxide bases with different pH, *J Endod* 11:394, 1985.

181. Tagger E, Tagger M, Sarnat H: Pulpal reaction for glutaraldehyde and paraformaldehyde pulpotomy dressings in monkey primary teeth, *Endodont Dent Traumatol* 2:237, 1986.

182. Teplitsky PE: Formocresol pulpotomies on posterior permanent teeth, *J Can Dent Assoc* 50:623, 1984.

183. Teuscher GW, Zander HA: A preliminary report on pulpotomy, *Northwest Univ Dent Res Grad Q Bull* 39:4, 1938.

184. Thoden van Velzen SK, Feltkamp-Vroom TM: Immunologic consequences of formaldehyde fixation of autologous tissue implants, *J Endod* 3:179, 1977.

185. Trask PA: Formocresol pulpotomy on (young) permanent teeth, *J Am Dent Assoc* 85:1316, 1972.

186. Traubman L: *A critical clinical and television radiographic evaluation of indirect pulp capping,* master's thesis, Bloomington, 1967, Indiana University School of Dentistry.

187. Tronstad L: Reaction of the exposed pulp to Dycal treatment, *Oral Surg* 38:945, 1974.

188. Turner C, Courts FJ, Stanley HR: A histological comparison of direct pulp capping agents in primary canines, *J Dent Child* 54:423, 1987.

189. Tziafas D, Molyvdas I: The tissue reaction after capping of dog teeth with calcium hydroxide experimentally crammed into the pulp space, *Oral Surg Oral Med Oral Pathol* 65:604, 1988.

190. van Amerongen WE, Mulder GR, Vingerling PA: Consequences of endodontic treatment in primary teeth. I. A clinical and radiographic investigation into the influence of the formocresol pulpotomy on the life-span of primary molars, *J Dent Child* 53:364, 1986.

191. van Mullen PJ, Simon M, Lamers AC: Formocresol: a root canal disinfectant provoking allergic skin reactions in presensitized guinea pigs, *J Endod* 9:25, 1983.

192. Venham LL: *Pulpal responses to variations in the formocresol pulpotomy technique: a histologic study,* master's thesis, Columbus, 1967, College of Dentistry, Ohio State University.

193. Webber RT: Apexogenesis versus apexification, *Dent Clin North Am* 28:669, 1984.

194. Weiss MB, Bjorvatn K: Pulp capping in deciduous and newly erupted permanent teeth of monkeys, *Oral Surg* 29:769, 1970.

195. Wemes JC et al: Histologic evaluation of the effect of formocresol and glutaraldehyde on the periapical tissues after endodontic treatment, *Oral Surg* 54:329, 1982.

196. Wemes JC et al: Diffusion of carbon-14-labeled formocresol and glutaraldehyde in tooth structures, *Oral Surg* 54:341, 1982.

197. West NM, Lieb RJ: Biologic root-end closure on a traumatized and surgically resected maxillary central incisor: an alternative method of treatment, *Endodont Dent Traumatol* 1:146, 1985.

198. Wheeler RC: *A textbook of dental anatomy and physiology,* ed 4, Philadelphia, 1965, WB Saunders.

199. White KC et al: Pulpal response to adhesive resin systems applied to acid-etched vital dentin: damp versus dry primer application, *Quintessence Int* 25:259, 1994.

200. Whitehead FI, MacGregor AB, Marsland EA: The relationship of bacterial invasions of softening of the dentin in permanent and deciduous teeth, *Br Dent J* 108:261, 1960.

201. Williams JL: The non-removal of softened dentine before filling, *Int Dent J* 20:210, 1899.

202. Wright KJ, Barbosa SV, Araki K, Spangberg LSW: In vitro antimicrobial and cytotoxic effects of KRI 1 paste and zinc oxide–eugenol used in primary tooth pulpectomies, *Pediatr Dent* 16:102, 1994.

203. Yacobi R et al: Evolving primary pulp therapy techniques, *J Am Dent Assoc* 122:83, 1991.

204. Zander HA: Reaction of the pulp to calcium hydroxide, *J Dent Res* 18:373, 1939.

205. Zurcher E: *The anatomy of the root canals of the teeth of the deciduous dentition and of the first permanent molars,* New York, 1925, William Wood & Co.

Chapter 23

Geriatric Endodontics

Carl W. Newton
Cecil E. Brown, Jr.

Dental service requirements are determined by four demographic and epidemiologic factors: the population at risk, the incidence and prevalence of dental diseases, the accepted standards of care, and the perceived need and expectations toward dental health by the public.[10] As a result of the aging of the population, all these factors are changing.

According to the U.S. Census Bureau, the number of persons aged 65 and older is expected to reach 35,000,000 by the year 2000 (Fig. 23-1), approximately 13% of the U.S. population.[44] The bureau also reported that 9% of those in the 65-and-over age group are 85 years or older. This figure will grow steadily to almost 17% by 2010. For census purposes the geriatric population is generally divided into two groups, those 65 to 80 and those 80 and older.

The Social Security Administration (Fig. 23-2) shows the percentage distribution of the U.S. population by age from 1985 to 2020.[36] The oldest (85+) segment of the population will grow most rapidly before 2000.[25] The group aged 65 to 74 years will increase most rapidly between the year 2000 and 2020, as the post–World War II baby-boom generation enters the older adult category.

Increased longevity of the dentition with expanding fields of advanced restorative procedures and implantology lend support that dentistry will see a substantial growth in the number of older adult patients. Until 1983 persons aged 65 and older made an average of 1.5 dental visits annually, a lower utilization rate than that of any other age group.[46] Between 1983 and 1986 a 29% increase in visits by those 65 years and older was noted by the National Health Survey.[45] According to this survey, older adults currently make more visits per year, on average, than those in the "all ages combined" category. In the future, general dentists will routinely serve a growing number of older persons, who will account for one third to two thirds of their workload.[21]

Dental services, including root canal procedures, for the older adult population of the future are anticipated to be of two general types: (1) services for relatively healthy older adults who are functionally independent, and (2) services for older adult patients with complex conditions and problems who are functionally dependent.[25] The latter group will require care from dentists who have advanced training in geriatric dentistry. This age group is being targeted in dental education programs and advanced training through improved curriculum, research, and publications on aging. The National Institute on Aging stated that all dental professionals should receive education concerning treatment of the elderly as part of basic professional education.[25]

The purpose of this chapter is to discuss the effect of aging on the diagnosis of pulpal and periapical disease and successful root canal treatment. The quality of life for older patients can be significantly improved and reflected in their oral health and functions.

A simple pleasure in life is being able to eat what one wishes, and with age the simplest pleasures may become even more important, as does the need for proper diet and nourishment. Every tooth may be strategic, and old age is no time to be forced to replace sound teeth with removable appliances or dentures. Consultation with older adult patients should help them overcome what may be a very limited knowledge of root canal treatment and lack of appreciation for regular dental care. Well-meaning friends and spouses who contend that their dentures are as good or better than their natural teeth may have had a lifetime of poor dental experiences or have forgotten what it is like to enjoy natural dentition.

Negative social attitudes toward older adults tend to carry over into their care. Older adult patients are in danger of being dismissed as hopeless or not worth the effort. At times, we are too eager to consider the probability of benefit for the investment (treatment and cost). Sometimes we tend to shy away from providing care for seniors because of the perceived difficulty of certain treatment procedures or because of complicated medical conditions. We also, at times, consider older adult patients less able to pay for treatment because of their age and appearance. However, the vast majority of older adults engage in normal activity and can recognize and afford the value of good dentistry.[4]

It should be considered that most of our older adult patients have had active, productive lives and they are very interested in maintaining their dignity and do not consider themselves a bad investment. As with any age group, older patients must be considered as individuals. This may prove difficult in the face of the tendency of many health care professionals to assign any person older than 65 to the classification *geriatric* and to stereotype patients (e.g., confusion, dementia, poor treatment response). Each older adult patient comes with unique psychologic and social life history, with a set of values, needs, and resources unlike those of any other patient the provider will see. Most seniors are more concerned with maintaining control of their lives than being old.[31]

Since the primary function of teeth is mastication, it is presumed that loss of teeth leads to detrimental food changes and reduction in health.[15] However, this may not be the driving force when seniors are seeking treatment. Social issues many times are the motivation for a senior to visit our office. After

Population 65 Years and Older (Millions)

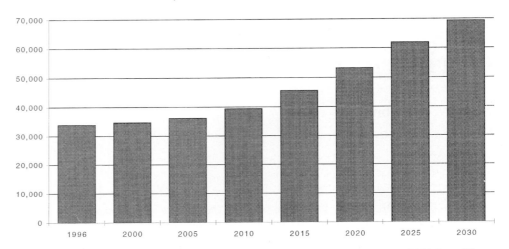

FIG. 23-1 Projections of U.S. population 65 years and older from 1996 to 2030 in millions.

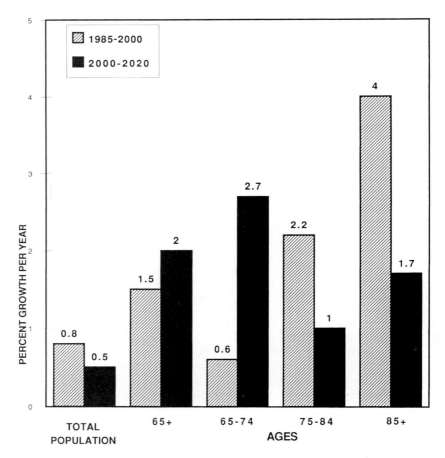

FIG. 23-2 Percentage growth rate and distribution of the U.S. population by age from 1985 to 2020.

suggesting to a 93-year-old man that he have a mandibular anterior tooth extracted, an author was told, "I can't, Doctor. You see, I go dancing every Saturday night, and I need that tooth. I can't look like that." Dentists should not presume that they know what is best for senior patients or what they can afford

without the patient's full awareness. The needs, expectations, desires, and demands of older people may exceed those of any age group, and the gratitude shown by older adult patients is among the most satisfying of professional experiences.

The desire for root canal treatment among aging patients has increased considerably in recent years. Older adult patients are aware that treatment can be performed comfortably and that age is *not* a factor in predicting success.[2,40,42] Obtaining informed consent also requires that root canal treatment should be offered as a favorable alternative to the trauma of extraction and the cost of replacement. The distribution of specialists and the improved endodontic training of all dentists have broadened the availability of most endodontic procedures to everyone, regardless of age. Expanded dental insurance benefits for retirees and a heightened awareness of the benefits of saving teeth have encouraged many older adult patients to seek endodontia rather than extraction.[14]

This chapter compares the typical geriatric patient's endodontic needs with those of the general population. Pulp changes attributed to age are discussed in Chapter 11; their effects on clinical treatment are also discussed in this chapter.

MEDICAL HISTORY

A medical history should be taken before the patient is brought into the treatment room, and a standardized form (see p. 2) should be used to identify any disease or therapy that would alter treatment or its outcome. Some older patients may need assistance in filling out the forms and may not be fully aware of their conditions or history. Some patients may withhold their date of birth to conceal their age for reasons of vanity or even fear of ageism. Vision deficits caused by outdated glasses or cataracts can adversely affect a patient's ability to read the typically small print on many history forms. Consultation with family, guardian, or physician may be necessary to complete the history, but the dentist is ultimately responsible for the treatment.

An updated history, including information on compliance with any prescribed treatment and sensitivity to medications, must be obtained at each visit and reviewed. In general, older adults use more drugs than younger patients, and most of these medications are potentially important to the dentist.[22] *The Physicians' Desk Reference* should be consulted and any precaution or side effect of medication noted.

Although geriatric patients are usually knowledgeable about their medical history, some may not understand the implications of their medical conditions in relation to dentistry or may be reluctant to let the clinician into their confidence. Their perceptions of their illnesses may not be accurate, so any clue to a patient's conditions should be investigated.

Symptoms of undiagnosed illnesses may present the dentist with a screening opportunity that can disclose a condition that might otherwise go untreated or lead to an emergency. Management of medical emergencies in the dental office is best directed toward prevention rather than treatment.

Few families are without at least one member whose life has been extended as a result of medical progress. A great number have had diseases or disabilities controlled with therapies that may alter the clinician's case selection. Root canal treatment is certainly far less traumatic in the extremes of age or health than is extraction.

Chief Complaint

Most patients who are experiencing dental pain have a pulpal or periapical problem that requires root canal treatment or extraction. Dental needs are often manifested initially in the form of a complaint, which usually contains the information necessary to make a diagnosis. The diagnostic process is directed toward determining whether pulpal or periapical disease is present, whether palliative or root canal therapy is indicated, the vitality of the pulp, and which tooth is the source (see Chapter 1).

The clinician should, without leading, allow the patient to explain the problem in his or her own way. This gives the examiner an opportunity to observe the patient's level of dental knowledge and ability to communicate. Visual and auditory handicaps may become evident at this time.

Patiently encouraging the patient to talk about problems may lead into areas of only peripheral interest to the dentist, but it establishes a needed rapport and demonstrates sincere interest. A patient may exhibit some feelings of distrust if there is a history of failed treatments or if there are well-meaning denture-wearing friends or relatives who claim normal function and are now free of the need for dental treatment. The effect of the "focal infection" theory is still evident when other aches and pains cannot be adequately explained and loss of teeth is accepted as inevitable. The best patients are those who have already had successful endodontic treatment.

Most geriatric patients do not complain readily about signs or symptoms of pulpal and periapical disease and may consider them to be minor compared to other health concerns and discomfort. A disease process usually arises as an acute problem in children, but assumes a more chronic or less dramatic form in the older adult. The *mere presence* of teeth indicates proper maintenance or resistance to disease. A lifetime of experiencing pains puts a different perspective on interpreting dental pain.

Pain associated with vital pulps (that which is caused by heat, cold, or sweets; or referred pain) seems to be reduced with age, and the severity of symptoms diminish. Heat sensitivity that occurs as the only symptom suggests a reduced pulp volume such as that occurring in the older pulps.[16] Pulpal healing capacity is also reduced, and necrosis may occur quickly following microbial invasion, again with reduced symptoms.

Although complaints are fewer, they are usually more conclusive evidence of disease. The complaint should isolate the problem sufficiently to allow the clinician to take a periapical radiograph before proceeding. Studying radiographs before an examination can prejudice rather than focus attention; accordingly, they should be reviewed *after* the clinical examination has been completed.

DENTAL HISTORY

Search the patient's records and explore his or her memories to determine the history of the involved teeth or surrounding area. The history may be as obvious as a recent pulp exposure and restoration, or as subtle as a routine crown preparation 15 or 20 years ago. Any history of pain before or after treatments may establish the beginning of a degenerative process. Subclinical injuries caused by repeated episodes of decay and its treatment may accumulate and approach a clinically significant threshold that can be later exceeded following additional routine procedures. Multiple restorations on the same tooth are common (Fig. 23-3).

Recording information at the time of treatment may seem to be unnecessary busy work, but it could prove to be helpful in identifying the source of a complaint or disease many years later. A patient's recall of dental treatments is usually limited to a few years, but the presence of certain materials or appliances such as silver points can sometimes date a procedure.

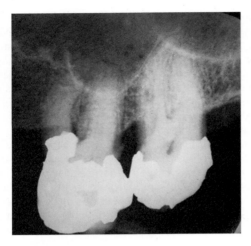

FIG. 23-3 Multiple restorations on this 74-year-old patient suggest repeated episodes of caries and restorative procedures whose pulpal effects can accumulate in the form of subclinical inflammation and calcification.

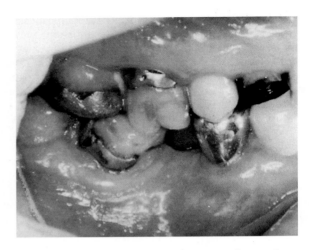

FIG. 23-4 Missing teeth and the subsequent tilt, rotation, and supereruption of adjacent and opposing teeth contribute to reduced functional ability and increased susceptibility to caries and periodontal disease.

Aging patients' dental histories are rarely complete and may indicate treatment by several dentists and at different locations. They likely have outlived at least one dentist and been forced to establish a relationship with a new, younger dentist that may find dental needs that require an updated treatment plan.

Subjective Symptoms

The examiner can pursue responses to questions about the patient's complaint, the stimulus or irritant that causes pain, the nature of the pain, and its relationship to the stimulus or irritant. This information is most useful in determining whether the source is pulpal disease, whether inflammation or infection has extended to the apical tissues, and its reversibility and can thus suggest what types of tests are necessary to confirm findings or suspicions. For further information the reader is referred to Chapter 1.

It is important to remember that pulpal symptoms are usually chronic in older adult patients, and other sources of orofacial pain should be ruled out when pain is not soon localized. Much of the information to be obtained from the complaint, history, and description of subjective symptoms can be gathered in a screening interview by the clinician's assistant or over the phone by the receptionist. The need for treatment can be established and can provide a focus for the examination.

Objective Signs

The intraoral and extraoral clinical examination provides valuable first-hand information about disease and previous treatment. The overall oral condition should not be overlooked while centering on the patient's complaint, and all abnormal conditions should be recorded and investigated. Exposures to etiologic factors that contribute to oral cancers accumulate with age, and many systemic diseases may initially manifest prodromal oral signs or symptoms.

Missing teeth contribute to reduced functional ability (Fig. 23-4). The resultant loss of chewing efficiency leads to a higher-carbohydrate diet of softer and more cariogenic foods. Increased sugar intake to compensate for loss of taste[13,24] and

xerostomia[3] are also factors in the renewed susceptibility to decay.

Gingival recession, which creates sensitivity and is hard to control, exposes cementum and dentin that are less resistant to decay. A clinical study of 600 patients older than age 60 showed that 70% had root caries and 100% had some degree of gingival recession.[47] The removal of root caries is irritating to the pulp and often results in pulp exposures or reparative dentin formation that affect the negotiation of the canal should root canal treatment later be needed (Fig. 23-5). Asymptomatic pulp exposures on one root surface of a multirooted tooth can result in the uncommon clinical situation of the presence of both vital and nonvital pulp tissue in the same tooth. Interproximal root caries is difficult to restore, and restoration failure as a result of continued decay is common (Fig. 23-6). Although the microbiology of diseases is not substantially different in different age groups, the altered host response during aging may modify the progression of these diseases.[43]

Attrition (Fig. 23-7), abrasion, and erosion (Fig. 23-8) also expose dentin through a slower process that allows the pulp to respond with dentinal sclerosis and reparative dentin.[38] Secondary dentin formation occurs throughout life and may eventually result in almost complete pulp obliteration. In maxillary anterior teeth the secondary dentin is formed on the lingual wall of the pulp chamber[29]; in molar teeth the greatest deposition occurs on the floor of the chamber.[7] Although this pulp may appear to recede, small pulpal remnants can remain or leave a less calcific tract that may lead to a pulp exposure.

In general, canal and chamber volume are inversely proportional to age: as age increases, canal size decreases (Fig. 23-9). Reparative dentin resulting from restorative procedures, trauma, attrition, and recurrent caries also contributes to diminution of canal and chamber size. In addition, the cementodentinal junction moves farther from the radiographic apex with continued cementum deposition (Fig. 23-10).[18] The thickness of young apical cementum[33] is 100 to 200 μm and increases with age to two or three times that thickness.[51]

The calcification process associated with aging appears clinically to be of a more linear type than that which occurs in a

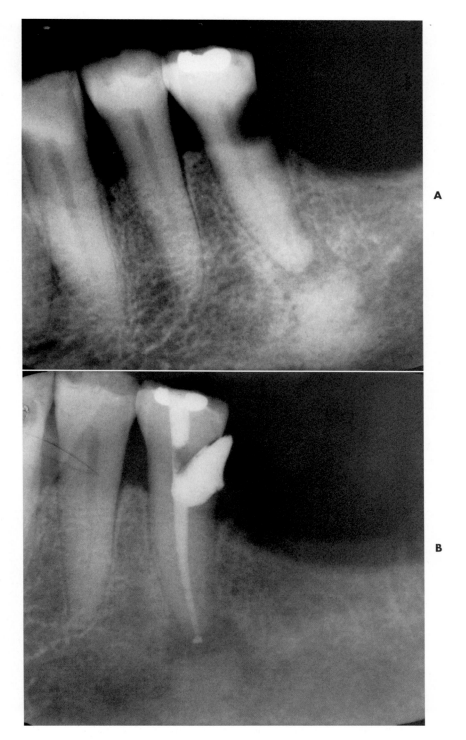

FIG. 23-5 Gingival recession exposes cementum and dentin, which are less resistant to decay. Root caries (**A**) often results in pulp exposures (**B**) that require endodontic treatment.

younger tooth in response to caries, pulpotomy, or trauma (Fig. 23-11). Dentinal tubules become more occluded with advancing age, decreasing tubular permeability.[23] Lateral and accessory canals can calcify, thus decreasing their clinical significance.

The compensating bite produced by missing and tilted teeth or attrition can cause temporomandibular joint dysfunction (less common in the elderly) or loss of vertical dimension. Any

limitation in opening reduces available working time and the space needed for instrumentation.

The presence of multiple restorations indicates a history of repeated insults and an accumulation of irritants. Marginal leakage and microbial contamination of cavity walls is a major cause of pulpal injury.[8] Violating principles of cavity design combines with the loss of resiliency that results from a

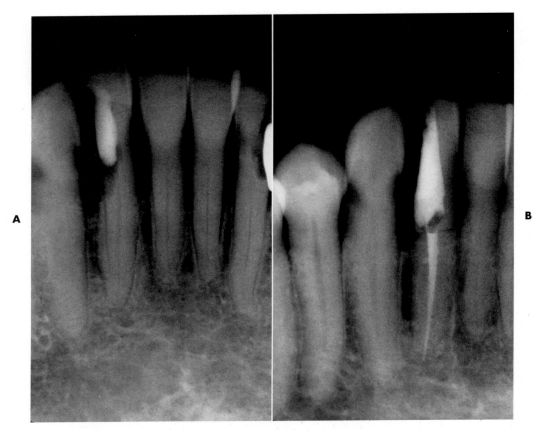

FIG. 23-6 A, Interproximal root decay is hard to restore and creates a very difficult isolation problem if endodontic treatment is indicated **(B).**

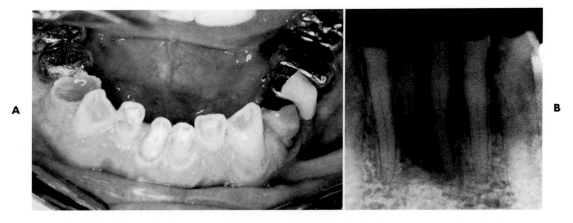

FIG. 23-7 A, Attrition exposes dentin through a slow process that allows the pulp to respond with reparative dentin, but pulp exposure eventually becomes clinically evident **(B).**

reduced organic component to the dentin to increase susceptibility to cracks and cuspal fractures. In any further restorative procedures on such teeth, the clinician should consider the effect on the pulp and the effect on accessing and negotiating canals through such restorations if root canal therapy is indicated later.

Many cracks or craze lines (see Fig. 23-8) may be evident as a result of staining, but they do not indicate dentin penetra-

tion or pulp exposure. Pulp exposures caused by cracks are less likely to present acute problems in older patients and often penetrate the sulcus to create a periodontal defect, as well as a periapical one. If incomplete cracks are not detected early, the prognosis for cracked teeth in older patients is questionable.

Periodontal disease may be the principal problem for dentate seniors.[11] The relationship between pulpal and periodontal disease can be expected to be more significant with age.

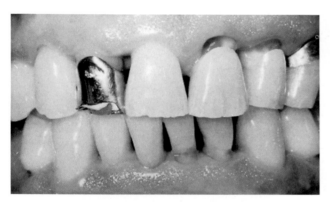

FIG. 23-8 Gingival recession also exposes cementum and dentin that are less resistant to abrasion and erosion, which can expose pulp or require restorative procedures that could result in pulp irritation.

Retention of teeth alone demonstrates some resistance to periodontal disease. The increase in disease prevalence is largely attributable to an increase in the proportional size of the population who have retained their teeth.[20] The periodontal tissues must be considered a pathway for sinus tracts (Fig. 23-12). Narrow, bony-walled pockets associated with nonvital pulps are usually sinus tracts, but they can be resistant to root canal therapy alone when with time they become chronic periodontal pockets. Periodontal treatment itself can produce root sensitivity, disease, and pulp death.[19] In developing a successful treatment plan it is important to determine the effects on the pulp of periodontal disease and its treatment. The mere increase in incidence and severity of periodontal disease with age increases the need for combined therapy. The chronic nature of pulp disease demonstrated with sinus tracts can often be manifested in a periodontal pocket. Root canal treatment is commonly indicated before root amputations are performed. With age, the size and number of apical and accessory foramen are actually reduced as pathways of communication,[32] as is the permeability of dentinal tubules.

Examination of sinus tracts should include tracing with gutta-percha cones to establish the tracts' origin. Sinus tracts may have long clinical histories and usually indicate the presence of chronic periapical inflammation. Their disappearance after treatment is an excellent indicator of healing. The presence of a sinus tract reduces the risk of interappointment or postoperative pain, although drainage may follow canal debridement or filling.

Pulp testing

Information collected from the patient's complaint and history and from the examination may be adequate to establish pulp vitality and should direct the clinician toward the techniques that are most useful in determining which tooth or teeth are the object of the complaint.

Slow and gentle testing should be done to determine pulp and periapical status and whether palliative or definitive therapy is indicated. Vitality responses must correlate with clinical and radiographic findings and be interpreted as a supplement in developing clinical judgment. Techniques for clinical pulp-testing procedures are discussed in Chapter 1.

Transilluminating[30] and staining have been advocated as

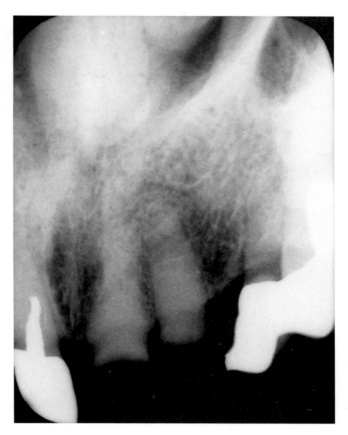

FIG. 23-9 In general, canal and chamber volume are inversely proportional to age: as age increases, canal size decreases. These maxillary incisors illustrate reduced canal and chamber volume in an older patient.

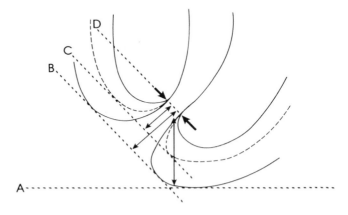

FIG. 23-10 The cementodentinal junction at *D* is the smallest diameter of the root canal system, and treatment at this point produces the smallest wound and greatest resistance to condensation during filling procedures. With continued cementum deposition throughout life, the distance from the anatomic apex increases (from *C* to *B*), as does the distance from the radiographic apex, *A*.

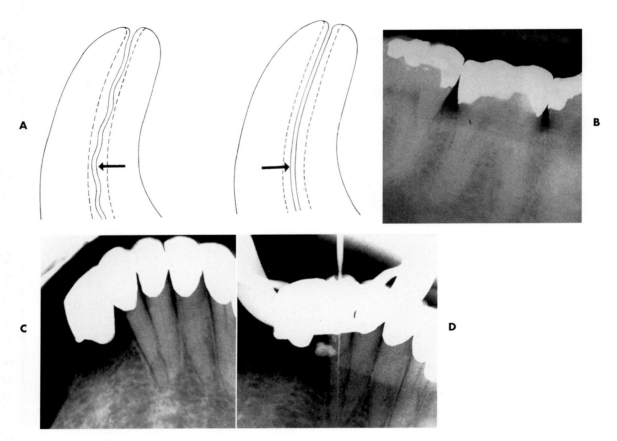

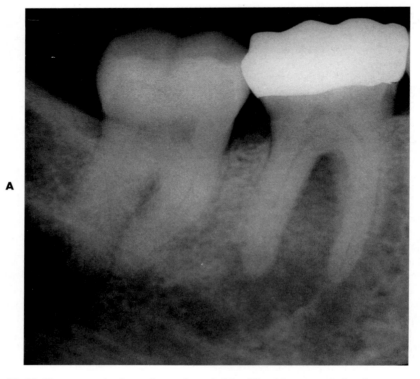

FIG. 23-11 A, Calcification process in aging appears clinically to be linear *(right)* and probably more easily negotiated than the irregular calcification diagrammatically illustrated *(left)* that occurs in a younger tooth. **B,** Treatment of this mandibular molar, with mesial canals calcified because of a pulp cap 15 years earlier, presents a much more difficult negotiation than **C** and **D,** the mandibular incisor in a 79-year-old patient.

FIG. 23-12 Sinus tract in the sulcus of tooth No. 30 with a nonvital pulp may appear as periodontal disease **(A).**

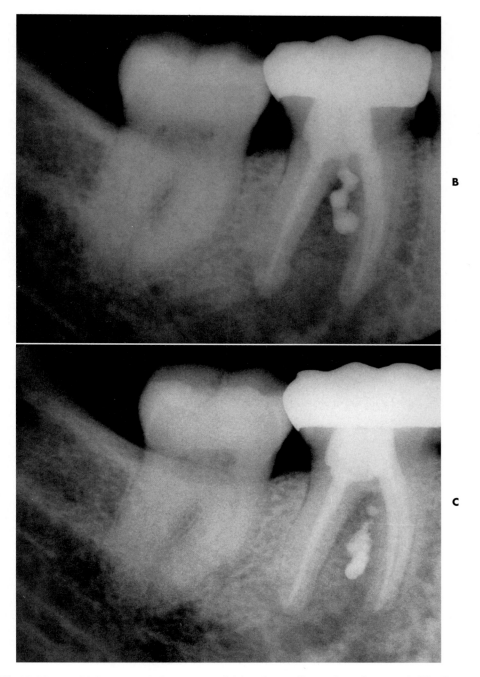

FIG. 23-12, cont'd Root canal therapy was initiated revealing a furcation canal **(B).** Complete healing may occur without further treatment **(C).**

means to detect cracks, but the presence of cracks is of little significance in the absence of complaints because most older teeth, especially molars, demonstrate some cracks. Vertically cracked teeth should always be considered when pulpal or periapical disease is observed and little or no cause for pulpal irritation can be observed clinically or radiographically. The high magnification available with microscopes during access opening and canal exploration now permits visualization of the extent of cracks in determining prognosis. Cracks that are de-

tected while the pulp is still vital can offer a reasonable prognosis if immediately restored with full cuspal coverage. The chronic nature of any periapical pathology caused by vertically cracked teeth indicates that it is long-standing, and the prognosis is questionable even when pocket depths appear normal. Periodontal pockets associated with cracks indicate a hopeless prognosis.

The reduced neural and vascular component of aged pulps,[6] the overall reduced pulp volume, and the change in character of

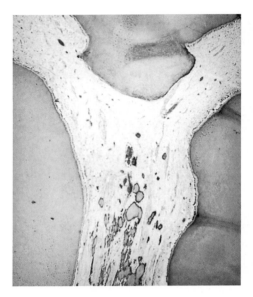

FIG. 23-13 There is a gradual decrease in the cellularity of older pulp tissue, and the odontoblasts decrease in size and number and may disappear altogether in certain areas, particularly on the pulpal floor in multirooted teeth.

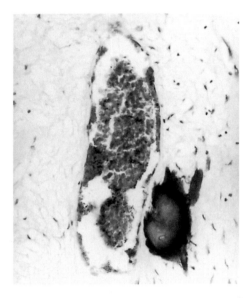

FIG. 23-14 Fibrosis appears to occur along the pathways of degenerated vessels and may serve as foci for pulpal calcification.

the ground substance[37] create an environment that responds differently to both stimuli and irritants than that of younger pulps (Fig. 23-13).

There are fewer nerve branches in older pulps. This may be due to retrogressive changes resulting from mineralization of the nerve and nerve sheath (Fig. 23-14).[5] Consequently, the response to stimuli may be weaker than in the more highly innervated younger pulp.

There is no correlation between the degree of response to electrical pulp testing and the degree of inflammation. The presence or absence of response is of limited value and must be correlated with other tests, examination findings, and radiographs. Extensive restorations, pulp recession, and excessive calcifications are limitations in both performing and interpreting results of electrical and thermal pulp testing. Attachments that reduce the amount of surface contact necessary to conduct the electrical stimulus are available from Analytic Technology, and bridging the tip to a small area of tooth structure with an explorer has been suggested.[27] Use of even this small electrical stimulus in patients with pacemakers[48] is not recommended; any such risk would outweigh the benefit. The same caution holds true for electrosurgical units.

A test cavity is generally less useful as the test of last resort because of reduced dentin innervation. Vital pulps can sometimes be exposed and even negotiated with a file with minimal pain (Fig. 23-15); then the root canal treatment becomes part of the diagnostic procedure. Test cavities should be used only when other findings are suggestive but not conclusive.

Diffuse pain of vague origin is also uncommon in older pulps and limits the need for selective anesthesia. Pulpal disease is progressive and produces diagnostic signs or symptoms in a relatively short time. Nonodontogenic sources should be considered when etiologic factors associated with pulpal disease are not readily identified or when acute pain does not localize within a short time.

Discoloration of single teeth may indicate pulp death, but

this is a less likely cause of discoloration with advanced age. Dentin thickness is greater and the tubules are less permeable to blood or breakdown products from the pulp. Dentin deposition produces a yellow, opaque color that would indicate progressive calcification in a younger pulp but is common in older teeth.

Radiographs

Indications for and techniques of taking radiographs do not differ much among adult age groups, although several physiologic, anatomic changes can significantly affect their interpretation. Film placement may be adversely affected by tori but can be assisted by the apical position of muscle attachments that increase the depth of the vestibule. Older patients may be less capable of assisting in film placement, and holders that secure the position should be considered. The presence of tori, exostoses, and denser bone (Fig. 23-16) may require increased exposure times for proper diagnostic contrast. The subjective nature of interpretation can be reduced with correct processing, proper illumination, and magnification.

The periapical area must be included in the diagnostic radiograph, which should be studied from the crown toward the apex. Angled radiographs should be ordered only after the original diagnostic radiograph suggests that more information is needed for diagnosis or to determine the degree of difficulty of treatment. Radiovisiography may be more useful than conventional radiography in detecting early bone changes.[50]

In older patients, pulp recession is accelerated by reparative dentin and complicated by pulp stones and dystrophic calcification. Deep proximal or root decay and restorations may cause calcification between the observable chamber and root canal.

The depth of the chamber should be measured from the occlusal surface and its mesiodistal position noted. Receding pulp horns apparent on a radiograph may remain microscopically much higher. Deep restorations or extensive occlusal crown reduction may produce pulp exposures that were not expected.

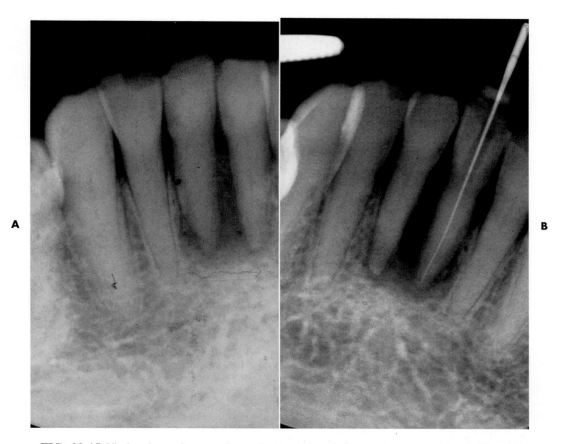

FIG. 23-15 Vital pulp testing was inconclusive (**A**) and the canal was negotiated (**B**) with little discomfort even though this was primarily periodontal disease.

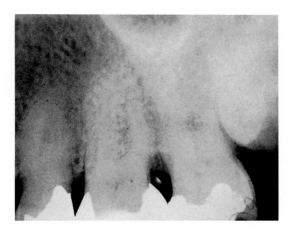

FIG. 23-16 Dense bone may indicate the need for increased exposure times to improve contrast needed to see the canal and root anatomy.

The axial inclinations of crowns may not correlate with the clinical observation when tilted teeth have been crowned or become abutments for fixed or removable appliances. Access to the root canals is the most limiting condition in root canal treatment of older patients.

Canals should be examined for their number, size, shape, and curvature. Comparisons to adjacent teeth should be made. Small canals are the rule in older patients. A midroot disap-pearance of a detectable canal may indicate bifurcation rather than calcification. Canals calcify evenly throughout their length unless an irritant (decay, restoration, cervical abrasion) has separated the chamber from the root canal. Retrograde fillings during apicoectomies, more common during retreatment of older patients, indicate missed canals and roots as a common cause of failure.[1]

The lamina dura should be examined in its entirety and ana-tomic landmarks distinguished from periapical radiolucencies and radiopacities. The incidence of some odontogenic and non-odontogenic cysts and tumors characteristically increases with age, and this should be considered when vitality tests do not correlate with radiographic findings. The incidence of osteo-sclerosis and condensing osteitis, however, decreases with age.

Resorption associated with chronic apical periodontitis may significantly alter the shape of the apex and the anatomy of the foramen through inflammatory osteoclastic activity (Fig. 23-17).[9] The narrowest point in the canal may be difficult to determine; it is positioned farther from the radiographic apex because of continued cementum deposition.

A continued normal rate of cementum formation may be demonstrated by a canal or foramen that appears to end or exit short of the radiographic apex, and hypercementosis (Fig. 23-18) may completely obscure the apical anatomy.

DIAGNOSIS AND TREATMENT PLAN

A clinical classification that accurately reflects the histologic status of the pulp and periapical tissues is not possible and not

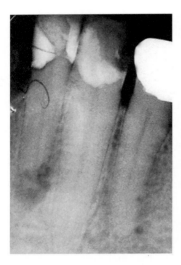

FIG. 23-17 Resorption associated with chronic apical periodontitis may alter the shape and the position of the foramen through osteoclastic activity. Narrowest point in the canal lies farther from the radiographic apex.

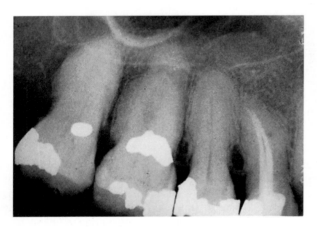

FIG. 23-18 Hypercementosis may completely obscure the apical anatomy and result in a constriction farther from the radiographic apex.

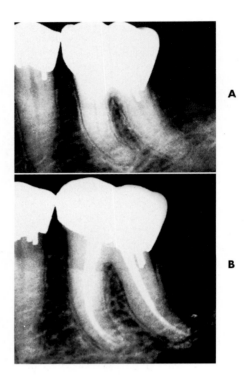

FIG. 23-19 A, Mandibular molar diagnosed with irreversible pulpitis in an 87-year-old patient who traveled 50 miles one way and was treated in one visit. **B,** Crown access restored at the same visit. Comfort of the patient was monitored, and treatment was tolerated very well even though total chair time was 2 hours.

necessary beyond determining whether root canal treatment is indicated. A clinical judgment can be made, based on the patient's complaint, history, signs, symptoms, testing, and radiographs, as to the vitality of the pulp and the presence or absence of periapical pathology. This classification has not been shown to be a factor in predicting success, interappointment or postoperative pain, or the number of visits necessary to complete treatment when the objectives of cleansing, shaping, and filling are clearly understood and consistently met. Of great clinical significance in treatment procedures is the assessment of pulp status to determine the depth of anesthesia necessary to perform the treatment comfortably.

One-appointment procedures offer obvious advantages to older adult patients (Fig. 23-19). The length of a dental appointment does not usually cause inconvenience, as may more numerous appointments, especially if a patient must rely on another person for transportation or needs physical assistance to get into the office or operatory.

Root canal treatment as a restorative expediency on teeth with normal pulps must be considered when cusps have fractured or when supraerupted or malaligned teeth, intracoronal attachments, guide planes for partial abutments, rest seats, or overdentures require significant tooth reduction (Fig. 23-20). Predicting future need for root canal treatment and a clinician's ability to perform treatment later is even more important, because the risk of losing the restoration during later access preparation increases with the thickness of the restoration and the reduction in canal size (Fig. 23-21). Because of a reduced blood supply, pulp cappings are not as successful in older teeth as in younger ones and therefore are not recommended. Any risk to the patient's future health and the effect that health may have on his or her ability to withstand future procedures should also be considered. Endodontic surgery at a later time is not as viable an alternative as for a younger patient.

Consultation and Consent

Good communication should be established and maintained with all patients, regardless of whether they are visual or hearing impaired or are fully responsible for making treatment decisions.

Relatives or trusted friends should be included in consultations if their judgment is valued by the patient or needed for consent. Procedures should be explained so that they are completely comprehensible and opportunities provided for questions and discussions. "Patient-friendly" pamphlets are available from the American Association of Endodontists to thoroughly explain and illustrate most endodontic procedures.

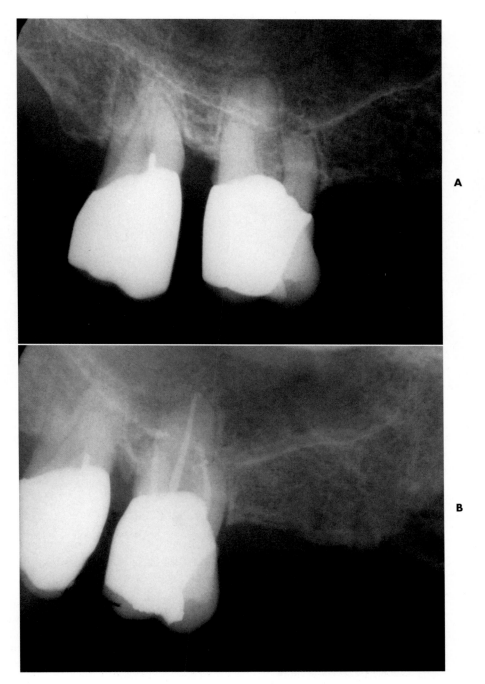

FIG. 23-20 A, Valuable maxillary first and second molar abutments in an 85-year-old patient. **B,** Later need for endodontic therapy was made very challenging because of access difficulties.

Obtaining signed consent to outlined treatment is encouraged and may be especially useful if the patient is forgetful.

Determining the patient's desires is as important as determining his or her needs and is required in obtaining informed consent. Priorities in treating pain and infection to properly and anesthetically restore teeth to health and function should be unaffected by age (Fig. 23-22). A patient's limited life expectancy

should not appreciably alter treatment plans and surely is no excuse for extractions or poor root canal treatment. It is important that each geriatric patient be well informed of risks and alternatives.

Acceptance of the eventual loss of teeth has been replaced by an understanding of the psychologic and functional importance of maintaining dentition. Older adult patients whose lives

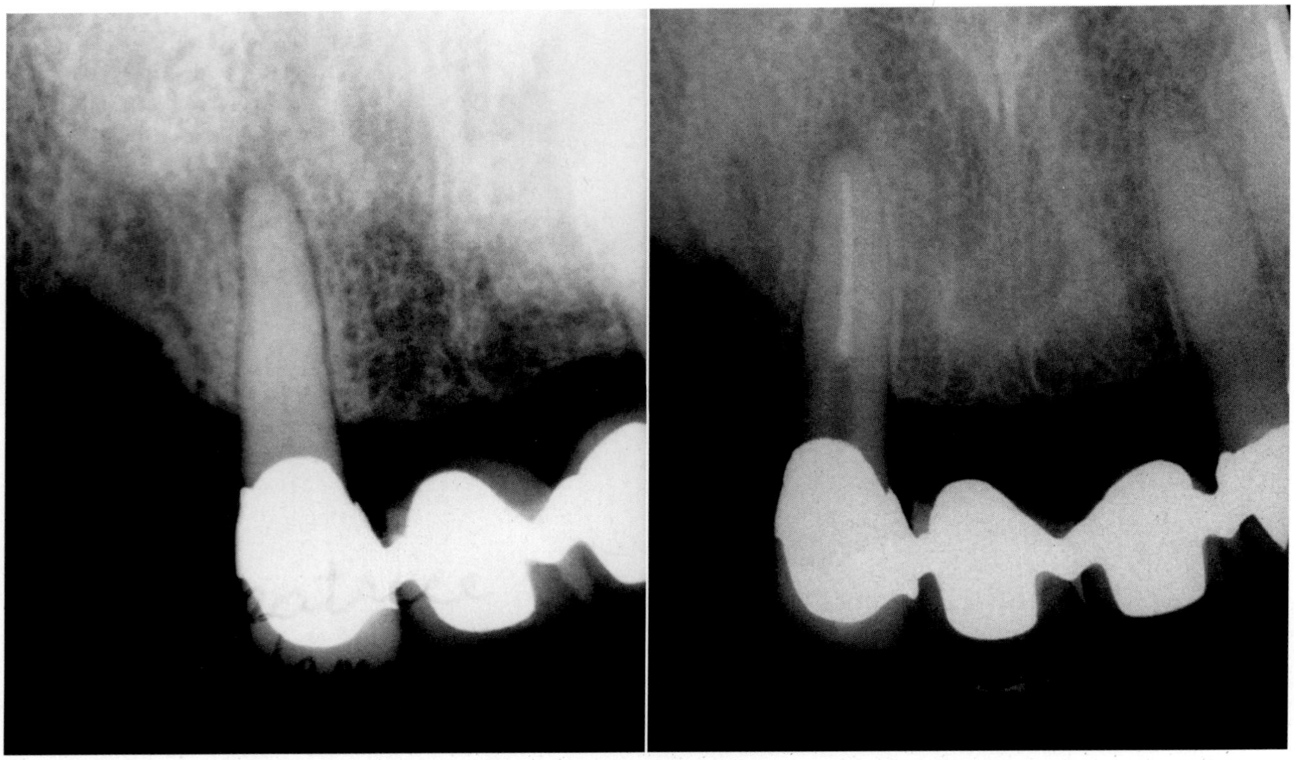

A

B

FIG. 23-21 **A,** Intracoronal attachments, guide planes, and rest seats for partial abutments require significant tooth reduction and a bulk of metal that makes endodontic treatment more likely and difficult. **B,** Successful treatment and preservation of the restoration when the canal is small are challenges to the most skilled clinician.

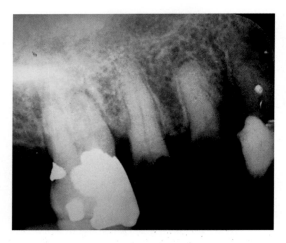

FIG. 23-22 This 84-year-old patient was pleased to find that all these teeth could be saved with root canal procedures and crown and was eager to make the investment in time and money in spite of her limited life expectancy. Her concern focused on why these procedures had not been recommended by her previous dentist, whom she visited regularly.

have been changed for the worse by a previous surgical procedure may readily recognize the implications of the loss of teeth.

The capability of the clinician and the availability of endodontic specialists should also be considered. The obligation to offer root canal treatment as an alternative to extraction may exceed a clinician's ability to perform the procedure efficiently or successfully, and referral may be indicated.

Obtaining informed consent before dental procedures usually is not a problem. However, medically compromised or cognitively impaired patients may make it difficult to acquire valid informed consent. Neuropsychiatric impairment may result in gross manifestations and indicate a reduced level of competency. Physicians or mental health experts should be consulted as needed, and no elective procedures performed until valid consent is established. Fortunately, acute pulpal and periapical episodes in which immediate treatment is indicated for pain or infection are less common than the low-grade signs and symptoms of chronic disease.

TREATMENT

The vast majority of geriatric patients who need and demand endodontic therapy are not institutionalized and are ambulatory. Institutionalized and nonambulatory patients require clinicians trained in those environments and facilities designed for access to dental health care. Such access is a benefit required in most institutions, but alternatives to root canal therapy may be the only services available. Extended health care facilities are now required to have dentists on staff before Medicare certification can be obtained. The dental office building, including both the interior design and the exterior approach, must be able to accommodate people with any handicapping condition.[26] Access for those who use ambulation aids such as canes, walkers, and wheelchairs should include comfort and safety in the parking lot, reception room, operatory, and rest room.

A physical and mental evaluation of the patient should determine the ideal time of day and length of time necessary to schedule treatment. A patient's daily personal, eating, and resting habits should be considered, as well as any medication schedule. Morning appointments are preferable for some older patients, and their comfort, which varies with the procedure indicated, dictates the length of the appointment. Some patients prefer late morning or early afternoon visits, to allow "morning stiffness" to dissipate.[12] They are more likely to tolerate long appointments better than most, although chair positioning and comfort may be more important for older adults than for younger patients. Patients should be offered assistance into the operatory and into or out of the chair. Chair adjustments should be made slowly and the ideal position established and used if possible. Pillows should be offered, as well as assistance in positioning them comfortably. Every effort should be made to accommodate the ideal position, even at some expense to the clinician's comfort or access. The patient's eyes should be shielded from the intensity of the clinician's light. If the temperature selected for the comfort of the office staff is too cool for the patient, a blanket should be available. As much work as possible should be performed at each visit and a rest room break offered at intervals as the patient's needs indicate. Jaw fatigue is readily recognizable and may be the most limiting factor in a long procedure, requiring periods of rest; however, once such fatigue is evident, the procedure should be terminated as soon as possible. Bite blocks are useful in comfortably maintaining freeway space and reducing jaw fatigue.

Retired persons may rely on rides from friends or relatives or public transportation to get to the dental office and are very often early for appointments, but they are usually in no hurry once they arrive. Enough time should be scheduled to allow some social exchange, and a sincere personal interest should be demonstrated before proceeding. Allow patients to initiate handshakes, which may be very uncomfortable to arthritic joints. From a behavioral and management standpoint, geriatric patients are among the most cooperative, available, and appreciative.

Medically compromised patients among older adults are at no more risk of complications than those in any other age group, and the chronicity of their diseases can alert the clinician to necessary precautions. It should again be recognized that for older people root canal therapy is far less traumatic than extraction.

The need for anesthesia is determined by the pulp vitality status and the cervical positioning of the rubber dam clamp. Older adult patients more readily accept treatment without anesthesia and sometimes even must be convinced that anesthesia is necessary for root canal treatment if their routine operative procedures have been performed without it. Teeth with

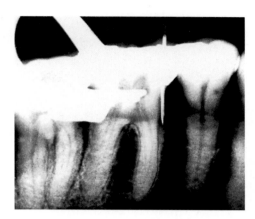

FIG. 23-23 Reduced width of the periodontal ligament makes needle placement for supplementary intraligamentary injections more difficult. Smaller needles may penetrate farther but bend more easily and may stick into root structure. Small amounts of anesthetic should be deposited slowly and under pressure with this technique.

necrotic pulps occasionally may be treated without anesthesia, if possible, to allow the patient's response to instrumentation through the apical foramen to determine file length or need for adjustment; this reduces the risk of overinstrumentation and inoculation of canal contents into the periapical tissue. Older patients demonstrate less anxiety about dental treatment in general and may have previous experience with root canal treatment.

The cutting of dentin does not produce the same level of response in an older patient for the same reason that a test cavity is not as revealing during examination. The number of low-threshold, high–conduction velocity nerve endings in dentin are reduced or absent and do not extend as far into the dentin, and the dentinal tubules are more calcified.[6,37] A painful response may not be encountered until actual pulp exposure has occurred.

Anatomic landmarks that are used as guides to needle placement during block and infiltration injections are usually more distinguishable in older patients. Anesthetics should be deposited very slowly and skeletal muscle avoided if epinephrine is the vasoconstrictor. The effects of epinephrine should be considered when selecting anesthetics for routine endodontic procedures.

The reduced width of the periodontal ligament[17] makes needle placement for supplementary intraligamentary injections more difficult (Fig. 23-23). Placing an anesthetic under pressure produces an intraosseous anesthesia that extends to the apex and to adjacent teeth, but it also distributes small amounts of solution systemically.[35] Smaller amounts of anesthetic should be deposited during intraosseous injections, and the depth of anesthesia should be checked before repeating. Like intrapulpal anesthesia, intraosseous anesthesia is not prolonged; therefore the pulp tissue must be removed within 20 minutes.

The reduced volume of the pulp chamber makes intrapulpal anesthesia difficult in single-rooted teeth and almost impossible in multirooted teeth. Initial pulp exposures are also hard to identify. Wedging a small needle into each canal to produce the necessary pressure for anesthesia is the method of last resort (Fig. 23-24). Every effort should be made to produce pro-

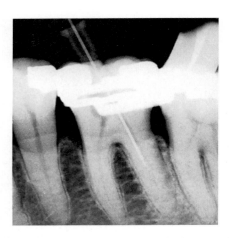

FIG. 23-24 Intraligamentary anesthesia is far superior to intrapulpal anesthesia, which is the method of last resort, and actual penetration into the canal may be necessary to generate sufficient pressure to produce profound anesthesia. Canal contents should be removed immediately because this is not a long-lasting anesthesia.

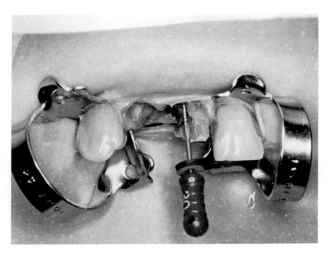

FIG. 23-25 Multiple tooth isolation techniques protect the patient from instruments but do not provide the fluid-tight environment preferred for the safe use of sodium hypochlorite.

found anesthesia. Patients should be encouraged to report any unpleasant sensation, and a prompt response should be made to any complaint. Patients should never be expected to tolerate pulpal pain.

Isolation

Single-tooth rubber dam isolation should be used whenever possible. Badly broken-down teeth may not provide an adequate purchase point for the rubber dam clamp, and alternate rubber dam isolation methods should be considered (see Chapter 5). Multiple-tooth isolation may be used if adjacent teeth can be clamped and saliva output is low or a well-placed saliva ejector can be tolerated (Fig. 23-25). A petroleum-based lubricant for the lips and gingiva reduces chafing from saliva or perspiration beneath the rubber dam. Reduction in salivary flow and gag reflex reduces the need for a saliva ejector.

Canals should be identified and their access maintained if restorative procedures are indicated for isolation. The clinician should not attempt isolation and access in a tooth with questionable marginal integrity of its restorations. Fluid-tight isolation cannot be compromised when sodium hypochlorite is used as an irrigant. Difficult-to-isolate defects produced by root decay (see Fig. 23-6) present a good indication, in initial preparation, for the use of sonic handpieces that use flow-through water as an irrigant.

The many merits of single-visit root canal procedures described in Chapter 4 should again be considered when isolation is compromised. The few minor benefits of multiple-visit treatment are further reduced if an interappointment seal is difficult to obtain.

Access

Adequate access and identification of canal orifices are probably the most difficult parts of root canal treatment on aged teeth. Although the effects of aging and multiple restorations may reduce the volume and coronal extent of the chamber or canal orifice, its buccolingual and mesiodistal positions remain the same and can be predicted from radiographs and clinical examination. Canal position, root curvature, and axial inclinations of roots and crowns should be considered during the examination (Fig. 23-26). The effects of access on existing restorations and the possible need for actual removal of the restoration should be discussed with the patient before proceeding. Coronal tooth structure or restorations should be sacrificed when they compromise access for preparation or filling (Fig. 23-27). The reader is referred to Chapter 7 for more details on proper access openings.

Magnification in the range of ×2.5 to ×4.5 (e.g., Designs for Vision) has become a common tool and can be designed to fit the clinician's most comfortable working distance. The growing acceptance and availability of endodontic microscopes offers clear magnification of ×25 or greater and has obvious advantages in treating smaller geriatric canals.

Pain, bleeding, disorientation of the probing instruments, or an unfamiliar feel to the canal may indicate a perforation (Fig. 23-28). The size of the perforation and the extent of contamination determine the success of repair (which should be done immediately) and do not necessarily indicate failure (Fig. 23-29). Supererupted teeth can be easily perforated (Fig. 23-30) if the reduced distance to the furcation is not noted.

A lengthy, unproductive search for canals is fatiguing and frustrating to both the clinician and the patient. Scheduling a second attempt at this procedure is often productive. Personal clinical experiences and judgment determine when the search for the canals must be terminated and referral or alternatives to nonsurgical root canal treatment considered (Fig. 23-31).

Modifications to enhance access vary from widening the axial walls to increasing visibility or light to complete removal of the crown. Alterations may be indicated after canal penetration to the apex if tooth structure interferes with instrumentation or filling procedures.

Very few canals of older teeth, even maxillary anterior teeth, have adequate diameter to allow the safe and effective use of broaches. Older pulps may give a clinical appearance that re-

Text continued on p. 778

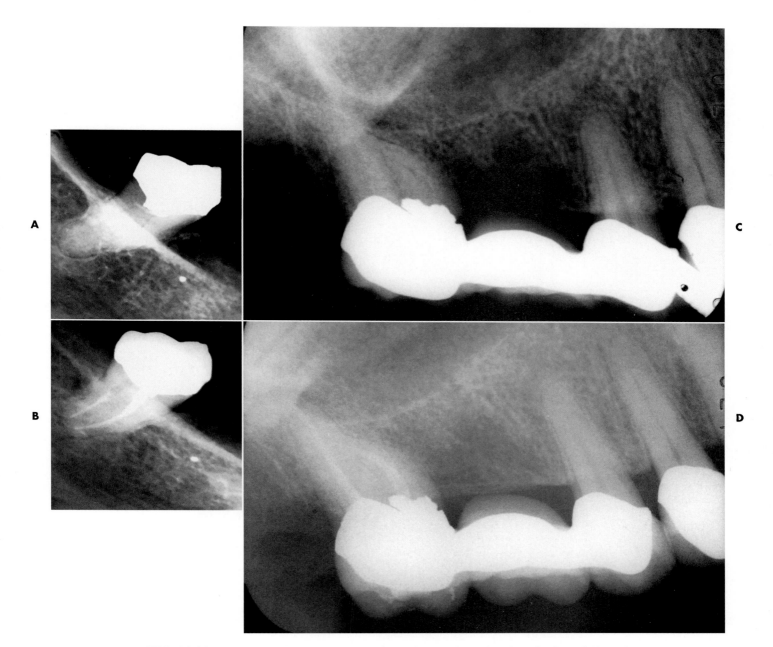

FIG. 23-26 A, This mandibular third molar in a 78-year-old patient has tilted mesially and has been restored with a full crown, upright to allow a path of insertion for a removable partial denture. **B,** Successful root canal treatment is the primary objective; retaining the crown, when possible, also represents significant savings to the patient. This crown will be replaced; a post space has been prepared. **C,** This maxillary third molar on the same patient is tilted mesially and rotated, making access (**D**) the most difficult part of this treatment.

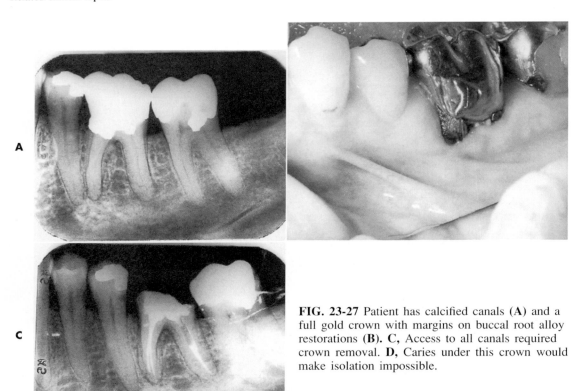

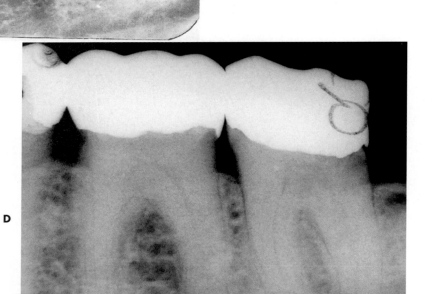

FIG. 23-27 Patient has calcified canals (**A**) and a full gold crown with margins on buccal root alloy restorations (**B**). **C,** Access to all canals required crown removal. **D,** Caries under this crown would make isolation impossible.

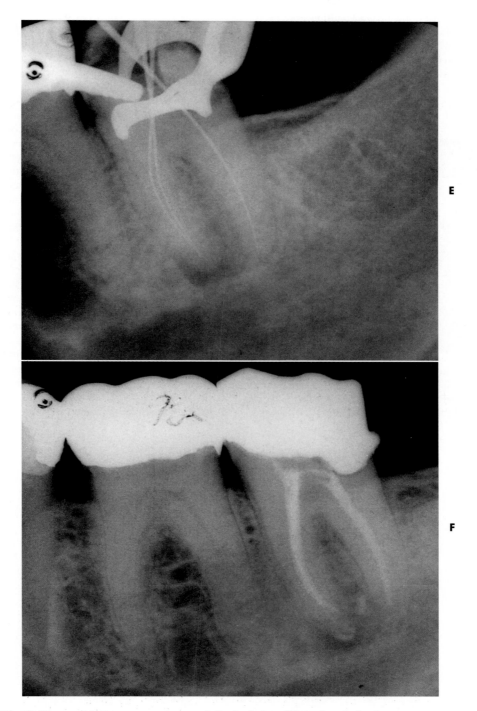

FIG. 23-27, cont'd Crown was removed for isolation (**E**) and endodontic treatment completed in one visit (**F**).

flects their calcified, atrophic state with the stiffened, fibrous consistency of a wet toothpick. Any broached canals should be thoroughly instrumented at the same appointment.

Preparation

The calcified appearance of the canals resulting from the aging process presents a much different clinical situation than that of a younger pulp in which trauma, pulpotomy, decay, or restorative procedures have induced premature canal obliteration. Unless further complicated by reparative dentin formation, this calcification appears to be much more concentric and linear.

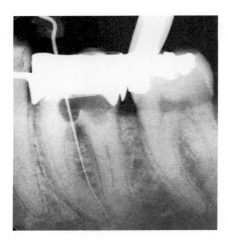

FIG. 23-28 Pain, bleeding, or disorientation of the probing instrument may indicate a perforation and should be immediately investigated radiographically. Repair is possible when the opening is pinpointed and the periodontal tissues are still normal.

This allows easier penetration of canals, once they are found. An older tooth is more likely to have a history of earlier treatments, with a combination of calcifications present. For a description of cleaning and shaping root canals, the reader is referred to Chapter 8.

The length of the canal from the actual anatomic foramen to the cementodentinal junction increases with the deposition of cementum throughout life.[18] The advantage of this situation in the treatment of teeth with vital pulps is countered by the presence of necrotic, infected debris in this longer canal when periapical pathosis is already present. The actual cementodentinal junction width or most apical extent of the dentin remains constant with age.[39]

Flaring of the canal should be performed as early in the procedure as possible to provide for a reservoir of irrigation solution and to reduce the stress on metal instruments that occurs when they bind with the canal walls. Thorough and frequent irrigation should be performed to remove the debris that could block access. Files with a triangular or square cross section may penetrate into the walls with greater force than the fracture resistance of small files when used with a reaming action and result in instrument fatigue and fracture. The benefits of instruments with no rake angle and a crown-down technique should be considered.

Since this cementodentinal junction is the narrowest constriction of the canal, it is the ideal place to terminate the canal preparation. This point may vary from 0.5 to 2.5 mm from the radiographic apex and be difficult to determine clinically. Calcified canals reduce the clinician's tactile sense in identifying the constriction clinically, and reduced periapical sensitivity in older patients reduces the patient's response that would indicate penetration of the foramen. Increased incidence of hypercementosis, in which the constriction is even farther from the apex, makes penetration into the cemental canal almost impossible.

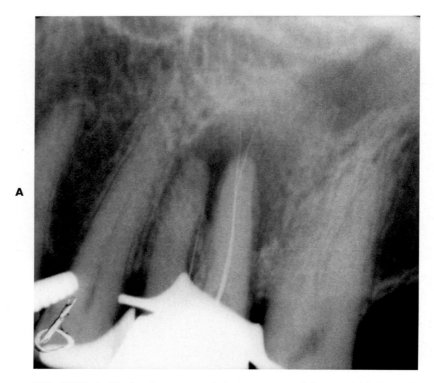

FIG. 23-29 A, Perforation occurred during access of these calcified canals.

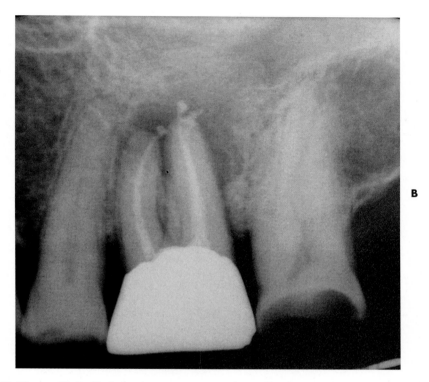

FIG. 23-29, cont'd B, Endodontic treatment was immediately completed after the perforation repair.

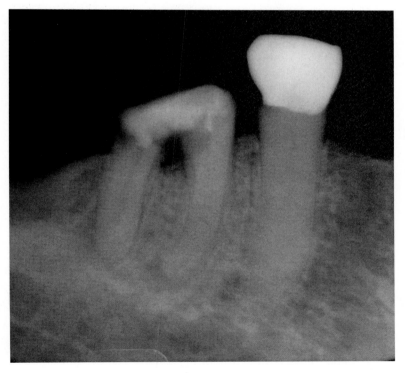

FIG. 23-30 Supraerupted mandibular first molar that was perforated during access.

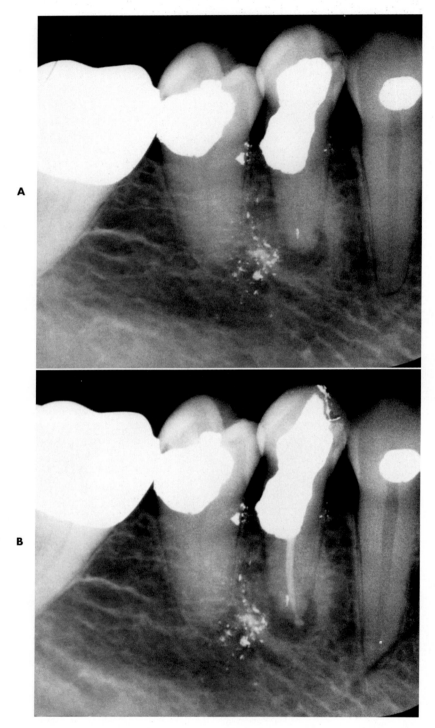

FIG. 23-31 A, Midtreatment referral of a mandibular first premolar only after perforation and repair with amalgam. **B,** Canal was still detectable with enhanced vision technique and treatment completed.

Achieving and maintaining apical patency is more difficult. Apical root resorption associated with periapical pathosis further changes the shape, size, and position of the constriction.

The frequency and intensity of discomfort following instrumentation has not been shown to be related to the amount of preparation, the type of interappointment medication or temporary filling, pulp or periapical status, whether the root canal filling is completed at the same appointment, tooth number, or age.[40] The more constricted dentinocemental junction permits a much smaller pulp wound and resists penetration with even the initial small files. Patency is difficult to establish and maintain. Dentin debris creates a matrix early in the preparations[49] and further reduces the risk of overinstrumentation or the forcing of debris into the periapical tissues,[28] which could cause an acute apical periodontitis or abscess. Further access to periapical tissues through the canal is likewise limited.

Obturation

For the older adult patient the prudent clinician selects gutta-percha filling techniques that do not require unusually large midroot tapers and do not generate pressure in this area, which could result in root fracture. The reader is referred to Chapter 9 for the most appropriate technique to use to seal the canal.

The role of the dentinal plug and its effect on the apical seal and success has been discussed. The likelihood of plug formation increases when the apex is constricted or when a file length is established at a distance from the radiographic apex and canals are calcified. These characteristics are all common in older teeth. The plug may create its own seal, contribute to a solid matrix for producing a condensed gutta-percha seal, and reduce the effects of overinstrumentation and filling.[28]

Coronal seal plays an important role in maintaining the apically sealed environment and has significant impact on long-term success.[41] Even a root-filled tooth should not have its canals exposed to the oral environment. Permanent restorative procedures should be scheduled as soon as possible and intermediate restorative materials selected and properly placed to maintain a seal until then. Glass-ionomer cements are of value for this purpose when mechanical retention is not ensured with the preparation.

Success and Failure

Repair of periapical tissues following endodontic treatment in older patients is determined by most of the same local and systemic factors that govern the process in all patients. With vital pulps, periapical tissues are normal and can be maintained with an aseptic technique, confining preparation and filling procedures to the canal space. Infected, nonvital pulps with periapical pathology must have this process altered in favor of the host tissue, and repair is determined by the ability of this tissue to respond. Factors that influence repair have their greatest effect on the prognosis of endodontic therapy when periapical pathology is present.

With aging, arteriosclerotic changes of blood vessels increase and the viscosity of connective tissue is altered, making repair more difficult. The rate of bone formation and normal resorption decreases with age, and the aging of bone results in greater porosity and decreased mineralization of the formed bone. A 6-month recall period to evaluate repair radiographically may not be adequate; it may take as long as 2 years to produce the healing that would occur at 6 months in an adolescent (Fig. 23-32).

Studies that suggest a difference in success between age groups must note the smaller numbers usually in this older treatment group and the local factors that make treatment difficult. Overlooked canals are a more common cause of failure in older patients (Fig. 23-33), which explains the increased clinical indications for retrograde fillings when surgical treatment is attempted.[1] Heat sensitivity as an isolated symptom may indicate a missed canal. For further information on assessing failures and possible retreatment, the reader is referred to Chapter 24.

ENDODONTIC SURGERY

Considerations and indications for endodontic surgery are not much affected by age. The need for establishment of drainage and relief of pain are not common indications for surgery. Anatomic complications of the root canal system such as small (Fig. 23-34) or completely calcified canals (Fig. 23-35), nonnegotiable root curvatures, extensive apical root resorption, and pulp stones occur with greater frequency in older patients. Perforation during access, losing length during instrumentation, ledging, and instrument separation are iatrogenic treatment complications associated with treatment of calcified canals.

Medical considerations may require consultation but do not contraindicate surgical treatment when extraction is the alternative (Fig. 23-36). In most instances surgical treatment may be performed less traumatically than an extraction, which may also result in the need for surgical access to complete root removal. A thorough medical history and evaluation should reveal the need for any special considerations, such as prophylactic antibiotic premedication, sedation, hospitalization, or more detailed evaluation.

Local considerations in treatment of older patients include an increase in the incidence of fenestrated or dehisced roots and exostoses (Fig. 23-37). The thickness of overlying soft and bony tissue is usually reduced, and apically positioned muscle attachments extend the depth of the vestibule. Smaller amounts of anesthetic and vasoconstrictor are needed for profound anesthesia. Tissue is less resilient, and resistance to reflection appears to be diminished. The oral cavity is usually more accessible with the teeth closed together because the lips can more easily be stretched. The apex can actually be more surgically accessible in older patients. Ability to gain such access varies with the skill of the surgeon; however, some areas are unreachable by even the most experienced.

The position of anatomic features such as the sinus, floor of the nose, and neurovascular bundles remains the same, but their relationship to surrounding structures may change when teeth have been lost. The need may arise to combine endodontic and periodontic flap procedures, and every effort should be made to complete these procedures in one sitting.

When apicoectomy is to be performed, the surgeon must consider whether the root that will be left is long enough and thick enough for the tooth to continue to remain functional and stable. This factor is especially important when the tooth will be used as an abutment. Detailed surgical procedures are presented in Chapter 18.

Ecchymosis is a more common postoperative finding in older adult patients and may appear to be extreme. The patient should be reassured that this condition is normal and that normal color may take as long as 2 weeks to return. The blue discoloration will change to brown and yellow before it disappears. Immediate application of an ice pack following surgery

Text continued on p. 786

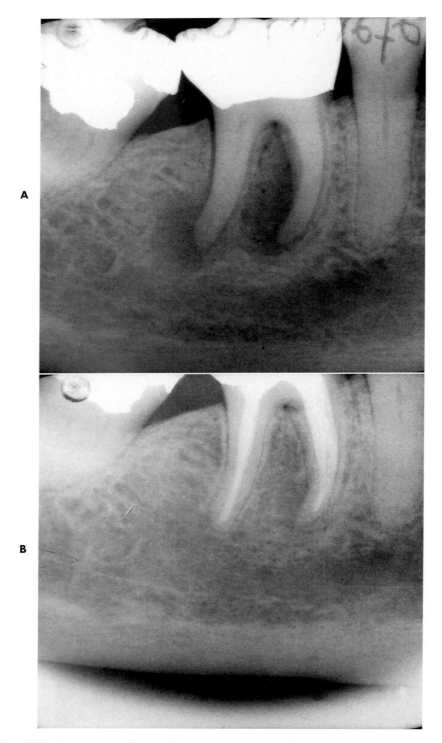

FIG. 23-32 A, Long-standing periapical radiolucency with a draining sinus tract indicated the need for endodontic treatment on this crowned mandibular first molar of an 82-year-old patient. **B,** One-year recall examination shows remineralization.

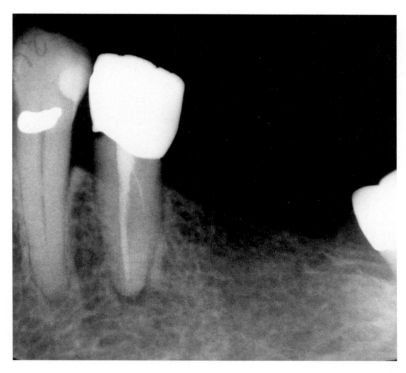

FIG. 23-33 Overlooked canals are a more common cause of failure in older patients than in younger patients, which explains increased clinical indications for retrograde fillings when surgical treatment is performed.

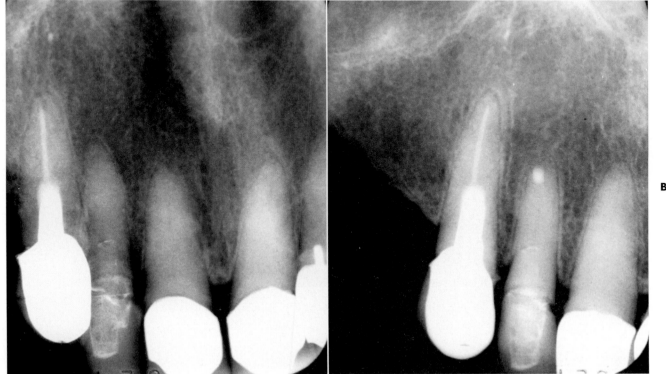

FIG. 23-34 A, Even though a small canal is detectable on the radiograph, it appears that an earlier unsuccessful attempt has been made to find it. **B,** It was decided that the risk of damage to a satisfactory restoration justified surgical treatment for this patient.

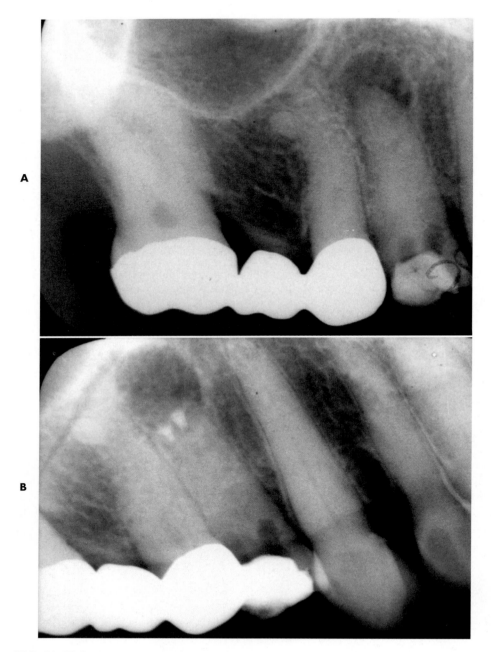

FIG. 23-35 A, Completely calcified canals were nonnegotiable. **B,** Surgical access was the only alternative.

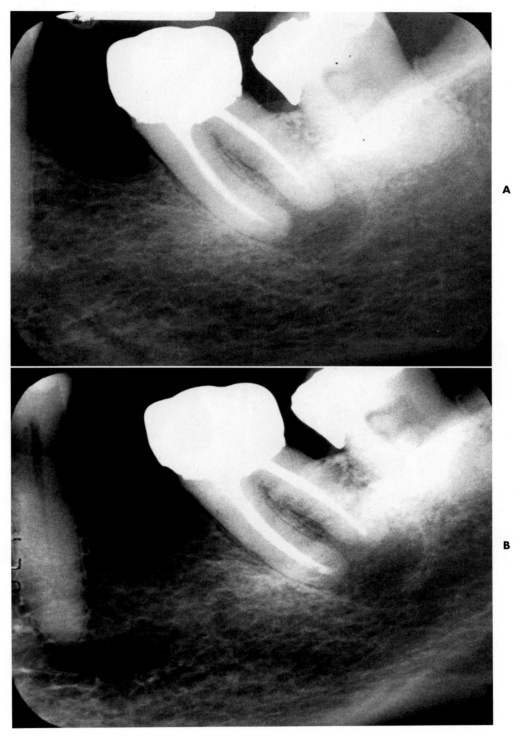

FIG. 23-36 A, Unsuccessful and symptomatic treatment on a mandibular second molar of a 78-year-old patient was surgically treated **(B)** with less trauma than the extraction alternative.

Continued

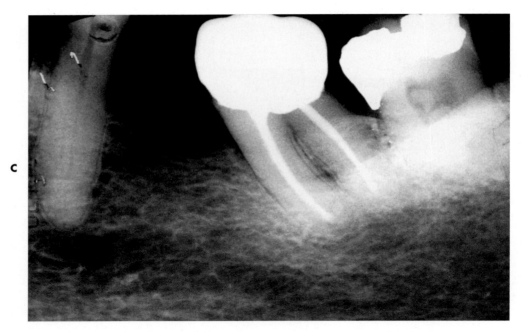

FIG. 23-36, cont'd C, Complete healing at 1 year apparently unaffected by age.

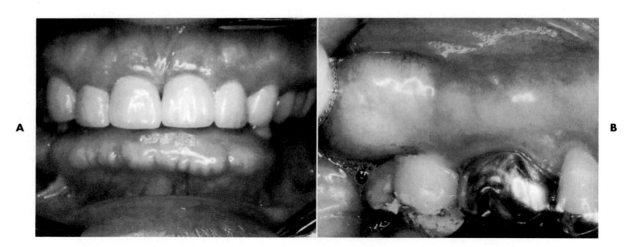

FIG. 23-37 Exostoses, as illustrated in this mandibular anterior (**A**) and maxillary molar (**B**) covered with thin tissue that can easily be torn during flap reflection, as well as the more obvious heavy bone and its effect on surgical access.

reduces bleeding and initiates coagulation to reduce the extent of ecchymosis, and later application of heat helps to dissipate the discoloration.

RESTORATION

Root canal treatment saves roots, and restorative procedures save crowns. Combined, these procedures are returning more teeth to form and function than was thought possible just a few decades ago. General considerations and procedures for postendodontic restoration are detailed in Chapter 21. Special consideration must be given to post design, especially when small posts are used in abutment teeth; root fracture is common in older adults when much taper is used. Post failure or

fracture occurs when small diameter parallel posts are used (Fig. 23-38). Posts are not usually needed when root canal treatment is performed through an existing crown that will continue to be used (Fig. 23-39).

The value of the tooth, its restorability, its periodontal health, and the patient's wishes should be part of the evaluation preceding endodontic therapy. The restorability of older teeth can be affected when root decay has limited access to sound margins or reduced the integrity of remaining tooth structure (Fig. 23-40). There can also be insufficient vertical and horizontal space when opposing or adjacent teeth are missing. Patient desires to save appliances can sometimes be fulfilled with creative attempts that just might outlive them (Fig. 23-41).

Text continued on p. 790

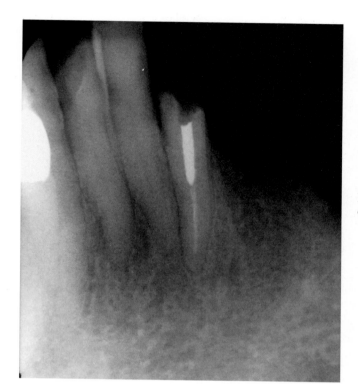

FIG. 23-38 This fracture of a cast post presents a very difficult challenge to remove.

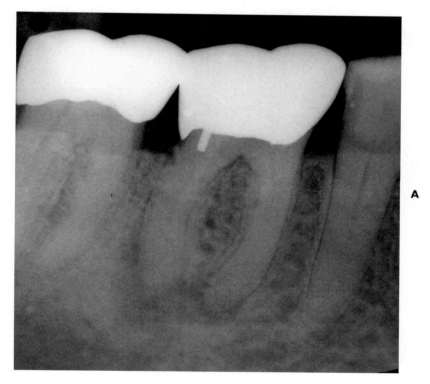

A

FIG. 23-39 A, Intact margins permitted the continued use of this crown and the access was restored with an amalgam-bond core (B).

Continued

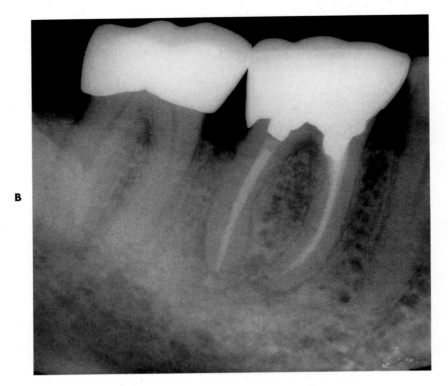

FIG. 23-39, cont'd For legend see previous page.

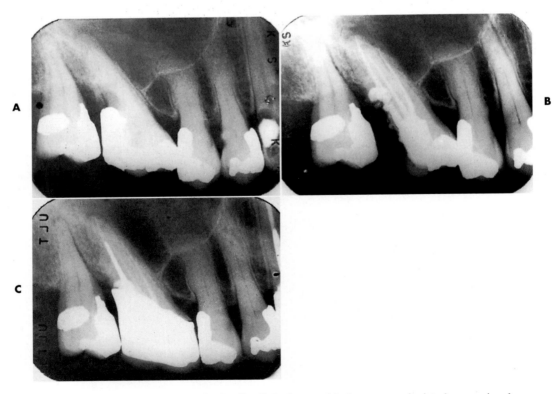

FIG. 23-40 A, This older adult, fragile diabetic, an elderly woman, insisted on saving her tooth in spite of extensive root caries on the palatal root. Root canal treatment was performed **(B),** and healing followed restoration **(C).**

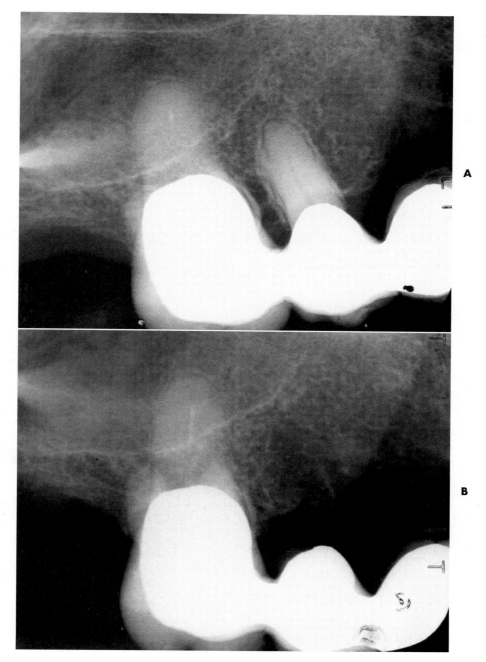

FIG. 23-41 A, Unrestorable caries contraindicated endodontic therapy on this second premolar abutment. **B,** Root was surgically extracted from beneath the bridge, which was still functional at this 3-year recall period.

In conclusion, it can be seen that geriatric endodontics will gain a more significant role in complete dental care as our aging population recognizes that a complete dentition, and not complete dentures, is a part of their destiny.

REFERENCES

1. Allen RK, Newton CW, Brown CE Jr: A statistical analysis of surgical and nonsurgical endodontic retreatment cases, *J Endod* 15:261, 1989.
2. Barbakow FH, Cleaton-Jones P, Friedman D: An evaluation of 566 cases of root canal therapy in general dental practice: postoperative observations, *J Endod* 6:485, 1980.
3. Baum BJ: Evaluation of stimulated parotid saliva flow rate in different age groups, *J Dent Res* 60:1292, 1981.
4. Berkey DB et al: The old-old dental patient, *J Am Dent Assoc* 127:321, 1996.
5. Bernick S: Effect of aging on the nerve supply to human teeth, *J Dent Res* 46:694-699, 1967.
6. Bernick S, Nedelman C: Effect of aging on the human pulp, *J Endod* 3:88, 1975.
7. Bhaskar H: *Orban's oral histology and embryology,* ed 5, St Louis, 1962, Mosby.
8. Browne RM, Tobias RS: Microbial microleakage and pulpal inflammation: a review, *Endodont Dent Traumatol* 2:177, 1986.
9. Delzangles B: Scanning electron microscopic study of apical and intracanal resorption, *J Endod* 14:281, 1989.
10. Douglas CW, Furino A: Balancing dental service requirements and supplies: epidemiologic and demographic evidence, *J Am Dent Assoc* 121(5):587, 1990.
11. Douglas CW, Gammon MD, Orr RB: Oral health status in the U.S.: prevalence of inflammatory periodontal disease, *J Dent Educ* 49:365, 1985.
12. Ettinger R, Beck T, Glenn R: Eliminating office architectural barriers to dental care of the elderly and handicapped, *J Am Dent Assoc* 98(3):398, 1979.
13. Frank ME, Hettinger TP, Mott AK: The sense of taste: neurobiology, aging, and medication effects, *Crit Rev Oral Biol Med* 3(4):371, 1992.
14. Ingle JI: Geriatric endodontics, *AO* 79:47, 1986.
15. Joshipura KJ, Willett WC, Douglass CW: The impact of edentulousness on food and nutrient intake, *J Am Dent Assoc* 127:459, 1996.
16. Kier DM et al: Thermally induced pulpalgia in endodontically treated teeth, *J Endod* 17:38, 1991.
17. Klein A: Systematic investigations of the thickness of the periodontal ligament, *Ztschr Stomatol* 26:417, 1928.
18. Kuttler Y: Microscopic investigation of root apexes, *J Am Dent Assoc* 50:544, 1955.
19. Lowman JV, Burke RS, Pelleu GB: Patent accessory canals: incidence in molar furcation region, *Oral Surg* 36:580, 1973.
20. MacNeil RC: The geriatric patient: a periodontal perspective, *J Ind Dent Assoc* 70:24, 1991.
21. Meskin LH: Economic impact of dental service utilization by older patients, *J Am Dent Assoc* 120:665, 1990.
22. Miller CS: Documenting medication use in adult dental patients: 1987-1991, *J Am Dent Assoc* 123:41, 1992.
23. Miller WA, Massler M: Permeability and staining of active and arrested lesions in dentine, *Br Dent J* 112:187, 1962.
24. Moeller TM: Sensory changes in the elderly, *Dent Clin North Am* 33:29, 1989.
25. National Institute on Aging: *Personnel for health needs of the elderly through year 2020: report to Congress,* Washington, DC, 1987, US Government Printing Office, 1, 14.
26. Palmer C: New federal law will ban discrimination, *ADA News* 21(11):1-2, 1990.
27. Pantera EA, Anderson RW, Pantera CT: Use of dental instruments for bridging during electric pulp testing, *J Endod* 18:37, 1992.
28. Patterson SM et al: The effect of an apical dentin plug in root canal preparation, *J Endod* 14:1, 1988.
29. Philippas GG, Applebaum E: Age changes in the permanent upper canine teeth, *J Dent Res* 47:411, 1968.
30. Polson AM: Periodontal destruction associated with vertical root fracture, *J Periodontol* 48:27, 1977.
31. Rossman I: *Clinical geriatrics,* ed 3, Philadelphia, 1986, JB Lippincott.
32. Rubach WC, Mitchell DF: Periodontal disease, accessory canals and pulp pathosis, *J Periodontol* 36:34, 1965.
33. Selvig KF: The fine structure of human cementum, *Acta Odontol Scand* 23:423, 1965.
34. Shafer WG, Hine MK, Levy BM: *A textbook of oral pathology,* ed 3, Philadelphia, 1974, WB Saunders.
35. Smith GN, Walton RE: Periodontal ligament injections: distribution of injected solutions, *Oral Surg* 55:232, 1983.
36. Social Security Administration, 1985.
37. Stanley HR, Ranney RR: Age changes in the human dental pulp. I. The quantity of collagen, *Oral Surg* 15:1396, 1962.
38. Stanley HR et al: The detection and prevalence of reactive and physiologic sclerotic dentin, reparative dentin and dead tracts beneath various types of dental lesions according to tooth surface and age, *J Oral Pathol* 12:257, 1983.
39. Stein TJ, Corcoran JF: Anatomy of the root apex and its histologic changes with age, *Oral Surg Oral Pathol Oral Med* 69:238, 1990.
40. Strindberg L: The dependence of the result of pulp therapy on certain factors: an analytic study based on radiographic and clinical follow-up examinations, *Acta Odontol Scand* 14(suppl 21): 1956.
41. Swanson K, Madison S: An evaluation of coronal microleakage in endodontically treated teeth. I. Time periods, *J Endod* 13:56, 1987.
42. Swartz DB, Skidmore AK, Griffin JA: Twenty years of endodontic success and failure, *J Endod* 9:198, 1983.
43. Tenovuo J: Oral defense factors in the elderly, *Endodont Dent Traumatol* 8:93, 1992.
44. US Census Bureau: *US population projections: US Census Bureau,* Washington, DC, 1996, US Government Printing Office.
45. US Department of Health and Human Services: *Personnel for health needs of the elderly through year 2020: September 1987 report to Congress,* Bethesda, Md, 1987, US Public Health Service, NIH Publication No 87-2950.
46. US Department of Health and Human Services: *Use of dental services and dental health, United States: 1986,* Washington, DC, 1988, US Government Printing Office, Publication No 88-1593 (National Health Survey; series 10; No 165.)
47. Wallace MC, Retief DH, Bradley EL: Prevalence of root caries in a population of older adults, *Geriodontics* 4:84, 1988.
48. Woodly L, Woodworth J, Dobbs JL: A preliminary evaluation of the effect of electric pulp testers on dogs with artificial pacemakers, *J Am Dent Assoc* 89:1099, 1974.
49. Yee RDS et al: The effect of canal preparation on the formation and leakage characteristics of the apical dentin plug, *J Endod* 10:308, 1984.
50. Yokota ET, Miles DA, Newton CW, Brown CE: Interpretation of periapical lesions using Radiovisiography, *J Endod* 20:490, 1994.
51. Zander H, Hurzeler B: Continuous cementum apposition, *J Dent Res* 37:1035, 1958.

Chapter 24

Retreatment

Gary B. Carr

RETREATMENT: DEFINITION

Endodontic retreatment has traditionally been referred to as an attempt to rectify unsatisfactorily completed treatment. The current *American Association of Endodontists Glossary of Contemporary Terminology for Endodontics*[1] defines retreatment as:

A procedure to remove root canal filling materials from the tooth and again clean, shape, and obturate the canals; usually accomplished because the original treatment appears inadequate or has failed or because the root canal has been contaminated by prolonged exposure to the intraoral environment.

The limitation of this definition is that it describes only one kind of retreatment (i.e., the kind that requires removal of filling materials) and ignores many other kinds of retreatments that are comonly performed. For example, Fig. 24-1 shows a case referred for completion. The referring doctor spent hours searching for the canal and, at the demand of the patient, the case was finally referred to an endodontist. The endodontist had to locate the canal, despite the destruction of all anatomic landmarks, and repair a buccal perforation made by the first dentist. This is certainly retreatment, although it has nothing to do with removing canal filling materials.

Fig. 24-2 shows prior apical surgery. The retreatment of the case consisted of nonsurgical cleaning, shaping, and obturating of the canals. This too is retreatment, although, again, no filling materials were removed from the canals. Fig. 24-3 shows a completed case with a missed MB-2 canal. The canal was nonsurgically retreated, but no filling materials were removed in the process. Fig. 24-4 shows a previously attempted treatment, many years earlier, on a calcified canal. Microscopic retreatment of the case resulted in locating and treating the canal. Here too no filling materials were removed from the root in completing this case. The AAE's *Glossary of Contemporary Technology for Endodontics* is correct, but with the conditions outlined above the definition could be expanded.

New Definition of Retreatment

A definition of retreatment that would include all possibilities means several additional factors must be considered. The first consideration is *whether the prior treatment has complicated or added to the difficulty of the subsequent treatment.* A patient who has had several teeth opened and has received multiple antibiotic and narcotic analgesic regimens—with no relief—is more difficult to treat than the patient who was properly diagnosed initially. The retreating dentist now must not only reconstruct the initial presenting signs and symptoms but must factor in the complications caused by careless diagnosis or inappropriate treatment.

For example, a patient who is suffering from myofacial pain syndrome (MFP) and has temporomandibular dysfunction (TMD) while complaining of acute pain in the maxillary quadrant presents a difficult diagnostic dilemma. If three endodontic treatments are started on teeth Nos. 12, 13, and 14 in an unsuccessful attempt to alleviate the pain, the primary source of the pain may be impossible to determine if the initial doctor's testing procedures were incomplete. This case must also be considered a retreatment because the prior treatment has complicated the diagnosis and the time needed to manage the case has greatly increased because of the original improper diagnosis.

Therefore what is needed is an updated definition of retreatment that includes a classification of prior treatment but does not include procedures performed for simple pain control (such as pulpotomy or pulpectomy). The following definition is offered as an alternative that more closely reflects the actual clinical practice of retreatment:

Endodontic retreatment is a procedure performed on a tooth that has received prior attempted definitive treatment resulting in a condition requiring further endodontic treatment to achieve a successful result.

Objective of Retreatment

The objective of retreatment is to *perform endodontic therapy in order to return the treated tooth to function and comfort and to allow the supporting structures to repair completely.*

Classifications of Retreatment

Teeth requiring retreatment may be classified as follows:
1. Discontinued treatment by prior dentist
2. Incomplete treatment
3. Complete but inadequate treatment
4. Complete and *apparently* adequate treatment, but with a questionable long-term prognosis

ENDODONTIC FAILURE

Endodontic retreatment predominantly addresses endodontic failure or probable endodontic failure. Evaluating endodontic failure is complicated and resists simple analysis. Table 24-1 summarizes the major studies on endodontic failure over the last two decades. It would appear that the failure rate for endodontic treatment varies between 5% and 34%, depending on the study. Such a huge discrepancy illustrates the significant problems involved with determining the actual success rate for a procedure that has so many variables that cannot be well controlled.

Much scientific evidence suggests that the success/failure ratio is *not* appreciably affected by age, sex, ethnicity, tooth type,

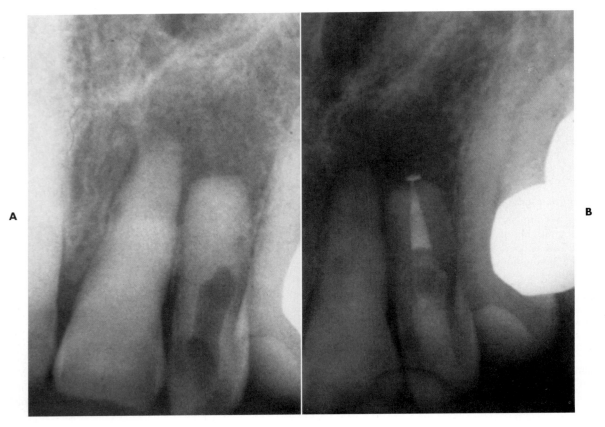

FIG. 24-1 A, Initial attempt to locate calcified canal using round burs. **B,** Retreatment using microscopic techniques.

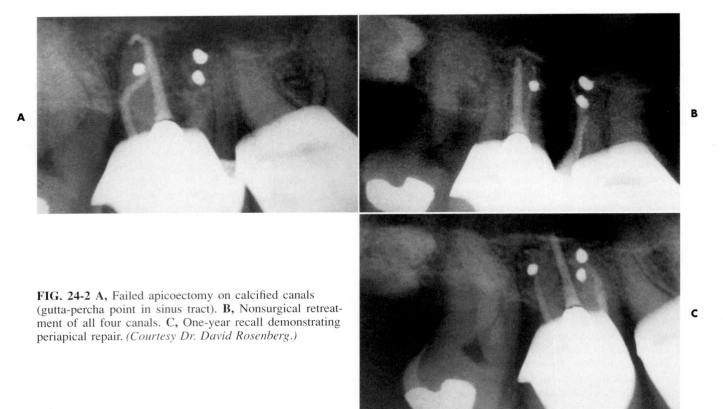

FIG. 24-2 A, Failed apicoectomy on calcified canals (gutta-percha point in sinus tract). **B,** Nonsurgical retreatment of all four canals. **C,** One-year recall demonstrating periapical repair. *(Courtesy Dr. David Rosenberg.)*

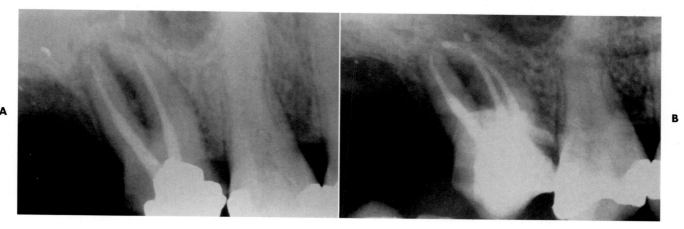

FIG. 24-3 A, Failing treatment of maxillary molar with palatal root amputation. **B,** Retreatment of mesial root with two canals allows remineralization.

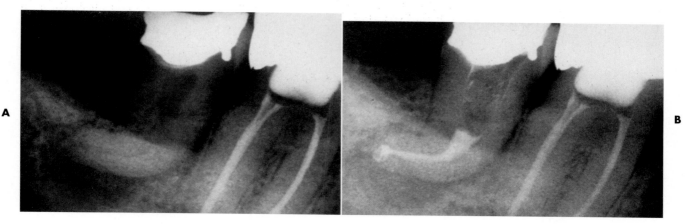

FIG. 24-4 A, Failure to find canal leads to discontinued treatment. **B,** Successful completion using a microscope. *(Courtesy Dr. David Rosenberg.)*

size of lesion, location of lesion, or number of treatment sessions (Table 24-2), but *is* affected greatly by the operator's skill.[44,45] The essential question is this: *What is the success rate of endodontic therapy if the root canal system is completely cleaned, shaped, and obturated?* The answer to this question is that the success rate is very close to 100%.[45,57,56] Endodontic disease *is* a bacterial infection originating in the pulp and progressing apically to the periapical region.[29,36,43] The theory that lesions of endodontic origin form adjacent to the portals of exit in avascular root canal systems is one of the linchpins of modern endodontic practice.[57] That these lesions do not form in the absence of bacteria creates a disease model of relative simplicity. *In the absence of bacteria, periapical lesions do not form.* Cleansing infected root canal systems in their entirety results in the elimination of all pulpally originating periapical disease.[16,29,44] Fig. 24-5 shows a series of scanning electron micrographs demonstrating the bacterial contamination of a lateral canal, which has led to endodontic failure and periapical pathology.

However, there are also examples of apparently completely debrided canal systems that do not respond successfully to treatment and hence must either undergo a surgical procedure or ex-

traction. Whether these failures are due to persistent infection in the periapex following skillful completion of the endodontic therapy or due to a concomitant infection of the periradicular cementum because of an immunologic defect or syndrome is unknown and is the focus of current research.[16,45,75]

Common Errors in the Diagnosis of Endodontic Failure

Conclusions drawn from a careful history and thorough examination should be discussed with the patient and recorded. Before retreatment, pain of nonodontogenic origin should be ruled out. MFP, TMD, vascular headache syndromes, neurogenic pain, CNS pathology, herpetic or other viral infection, and psychosomatic pain must be included in the differential diagnosis.[2,4,24] Nonodontogenic pain is discussed in Chapter 3.

Odontogenic pain may be of nonendodontic origin. For example, endodontically treated teeth subjected to occlusal trauma may remain persistently tender; retreatment does not address the true cause of this tenderness.[35,51] Similarly, periodontally involved teeth may remain sensitive after successful endodontic therapy, especially to percussion and palpation; therefore careful periodontal probings and recording are abso-

Table 24-1 Characteristics of reports on endodontic success and failure

Year	Authors	No. of Cases (Teeth)	Operator	Follow-up Period (yr)	Reported Treatments Results (%)			Factors Studied That Related to Results	Remarks
					Success	Uncertain	Failure		
1956	Strindberg	529	Author	4	87	2	11	a,b,c,d,f,g,i,k,q,s,t*	
1961	Grahnen & Hansson	763	Students	4-5	81	—	19	a,b,c,e,h,i	
1963	Seltzer et al.	2921	Authors	0.5	80	—	20	a,b,d,l,m	
1963	Zeldow & Ingle	42	Faculty	2	83.3	—	16.7	l	Nonvital teeth only, with positive cultures before obturation
1964	Bender et al.	706	Authors	2	82	—	18	a,b,g,l,m	
1964	Grossman et al.	432	Students	1-5	90	1	9	a,d,f,j	Success rate represents the mean value between nonvital and vital teeth
1965	Ingle	1229	Students and practitioners	2	91.5	—	8.5	c,d,e,v	
1969	Storms	158	Students	1	81	14	5	a,b,d,f,h,i,l,p,q	
1970	Harty et al.	1139	Faculty and students	0.5	90	—	10	b,d,f,n	Anterior teeth only; post-graduate student patients
1970	Heling & Tamse	213	Students	1-5	70	—	30	a,b,	
1974	Selden	1571	Author	0.5	94	—	6	a,c,g	
1976	Adenubi & Rule	870	Hospital staff	5-7	88.2	4.8	7	a,b,e,f,g,h,j,k,n	Anterior teeth only; all patients younger than 16 yr
1978	Jokinen et al.	1304	Students	2-7	53	13	34	a,b,c,d,e,g,h,j,p	"Number of cases" represents number of roots
1979	Kerekes & Tronstad	501	Students	3-5	91	4	5	a,c,d,f,g,i,o,u	
1980	Barbakow et al.	566	Practitioners	1 and up	87.4	5.7	6.9	a,b,c,d,i	
1983	Morse et al.	220	Author	0.5-3	94.5	—	5.5	a,b,c,h	Results analyzed per 458 canals also
1983	Oliet	338	Author	1.5 and up	89	—	11	a,b,c,d,e,o	153 teeth treated in single visits
1983	Swartz et al.	1007	Students	1 and up	87.8	—	12.2	a,b,c,d,e,k,p	Single visit only
1986	Pekruhn	925	Author	1	94.8	—	5.2	a,c,r	
1989	Petersson et al.	3383	Practitioners	—	74	—	26	b,f	Results based on radiographic survey only
1993	Smith et al.	821	Faculty and students	5 and up	84.3	—	15.71	a,b,c,d,e,f,g,k	Results based on radiographic survey only
1993	De Cleen et al.	97	Practitioners	—	60.8	—	39.2	b,f	Results based on radiographic survey only
1995	Ray et al.	1010	Practitioners	1 and up	61.1	—	38.93	a,b,f,p	Results based on radiographic survey only

*The factors are presented in descending order of frequency at which they were investigated in the reviewed studies.

Table 24-2 Biologic and therapeutic factors reported to potentially influence endodontic success or failure

Code	Factor
a	Apical pathosis
b	Extension of filling material
c	Tooth type (anterior teeth, premolars, and molars)
d	Age
e	Sex
f	Obturation quality
g	Observation period
h	Tooth type (maxillary or mandibular)
i	Pulp vitality
j	Type of intracanal medication
k	Type of filling material
l	Bacterial status of root canal before obturation
m	Obturation technique
n	Procedural periapical disturbances
o	Number of treatment sessions
p	Postoperative restoration
q	Patient's general health status
r	Preoperative pain
s	Postoperative pain
t	Apical resorption
u	Length of endodontic session

lutely imperative before initiating any endodontic therapy. Teeth that present vertical or oblique crown or root fracture remain tender to percussion and may never become asymptomatic.[17,49,53] *A decision to retreat must be based on having a confidence regarding the cause of the failure and a belief that retreatment can successfully correct the deficiency.*

REVOLUTION IN RETREATMENT TECHNIQUES

Retreatment techniques have undergone a renaissance recently. The use of the operating microscope has revolutionized our approach to failing endodontic cases and also greatly expanded our proficiency in treating prior inadequate endodontic therapy. The use of the operating microscope has enabled us to not only dismantle sophisticated restorative dentistry but has expanded our capabilities in finding calcified or occluded canals, removing separated instruments or silver cones, and repairing perforations. Sophisticated use of the operating microscope permits the clinician to enjoy visual mastery previously not attainable and to employ techniques and procedures on a microscopic scale that have hitherto not been possible.[12,13,68]

The rapid growth of microscopic techniques has led to the development of a dedicated armamentarium specifically designed for such an approach. Fig. 24-6 shows an example of several instruments used in microperforation repairs. Note their small size and unusual shapes.

The following discussion reviews how these new techniques are used in retreatment.

Tooth Disassembly Techniques

Retreatment of endodontic cases frequently requires the removal of fixed restorations to adequately gain access. The anatomic landmarks present in the unrestored dentition are invaluable guides to the clinician. Rotated teeth, labially or lingually inclined teeth, malformed teeth, and teeth tipped mesially or distally are conditions that can be obscure to the clinician because of the presence of restorations. The removal of these restorations greatly facilitates visibility and orientation. Nothing is more disconcerting to the clinician than perforating through the side of a tooth or through the furcation because the clinician did not realize the tooth was tipped or rotated. Furthermore, it is much easier to view and evaluate subgingival caries when all restorative materials are removed, as illustrated in Chapter 5.

Crown Removal Techniques

Crowns that have long, parallel preparations and have been cemented with dentin bonding agents may be almost impossible to remove without sectioning the crown. Crowns with good marginal integrity are also more difficult to remove, as are crowns that are splinted or double- or triple-abutted.

If it is important to preserve the existing restoration, several techniques are available. The crown remover shown in Figs. 24-7 and 24-8 incorporates hardened rubber plugs attached to the jaws of a specially configured hemostat that can engage the crown with sufficient force to remove most crowns cemented with temporary cements or loose crowns cemented with permanent cement. This instrument is particularly helpful in removing temporarily cemented porcelain restorations because the rubber beaks do not damage the porcelain. This device is also very useful in removing heat-cured, provisional splints, as these restorations can have significant retention caused by multiple parallel abutments.

Another helpful device is the Crown-O-Matic shown in Fig. 24-9. This device imparts a sudden, controlled vertical component of force directed in an axial direction that frequently is sufficient to break cement bonds. The hooked end of the device is placed under a margin to gain purchase on the crown. Unfortunately, this action can damage the margin of the crown or fracture the porcelain. The Crown-O-Matic is especially effective in removing three-unit bridges, as it can hook under the pontic area and direct an axial component of force sufficient to remove most bridges.

The Richwil crown remover is another nondestructive way to remove permanently cemented restorations. The Richwil material is heated in a container of hot water and then placed over the occlusal surface of the crown and closely adapted circumferentially around the crown with finger pressure (Figs. 24-10 and 24-11). The patient is then asked to bite down into the softened material until the opposing tooth occludes with the crown to be removed. After allowing the material to cool, the patient is instructed to open his mouth, causing the crown to dislodge because of the exceptional adhesive characteristics of the Richwil material.

If the crown does not need to be salvaged, there are several devices that can quickly and nontraumatically remove well-retained restorations. The EIE crown splitter (Fig. 24-12) is a hand instrument that uses a gradual spreading action of two extensions that engage a predrilled vertical slot in the crown. With one push of the plunger, these extensions impart a powerful, lateral component of force sufficient to separate the metal segments so that mechanical retention on the tooth is lost (Fig. 24-13). This method of removal is especially useful when removing semiprecious or nonprecious crowns.

An orthodontic band remover (Fig. 24-14) is also an efficient way to remove crowns. A pilot hole is drilled through the center of the occlusal table until dentin is reached. The

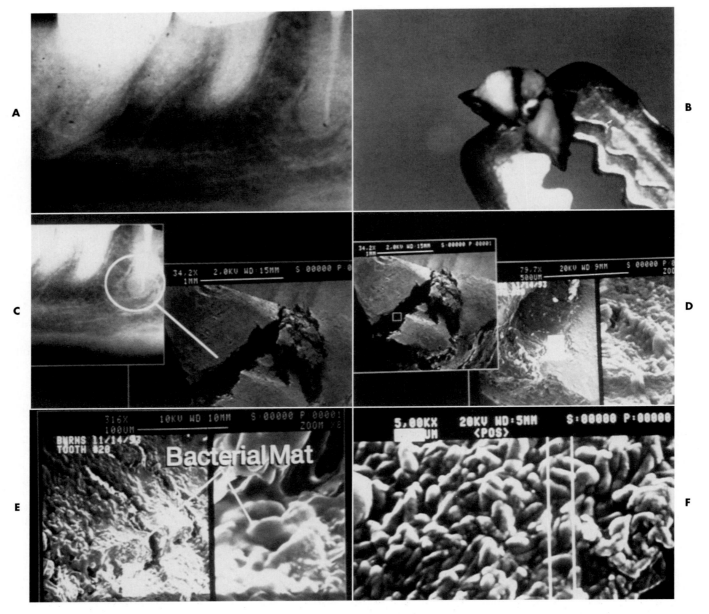

FIG. 24-5 A, Failed endodontic treatment in a mandibular second premolar. **B,** Resected. **C,** Scanning electron micrograph showing unfilled apical canal. **D,** Higher magnification of canal. **E,** Higher magnification view of bacterial mat on canal wall. **F,** Individual rod bacteria at periphery of canal wall. *(Courtesy Pacific Endodontic Research Foundation.)*

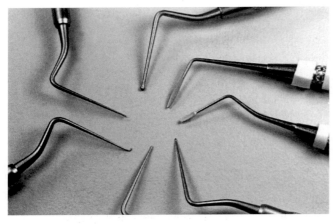

FIG. 24-6 Sharp and West series of perforation repair instruments. *(EIE/Analytic, Orange, Calif.)*

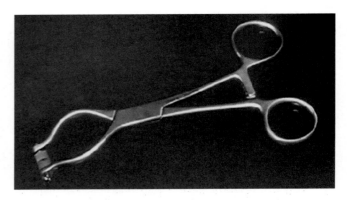

FIG. 24-7 Crown remover.

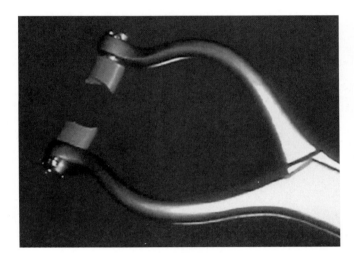

FIG. 24-8 Crown remover beaks.

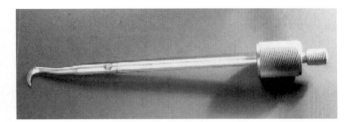

FIG. 24-9 Crown-O-Matic.

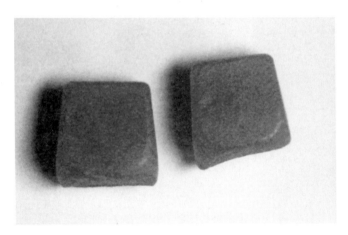

FIG. 24-10 Richwil crown and bridge remover by Almore.

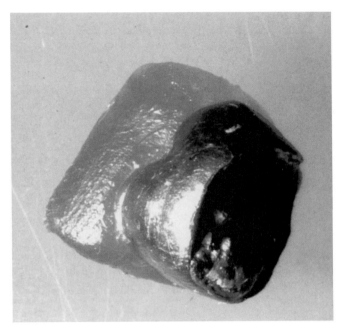

FIG. 24-11 Removal of crown using Richwil material.

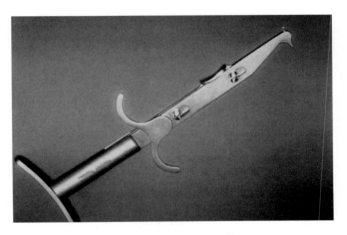

FIG. 24-12 EIE crown splitter.

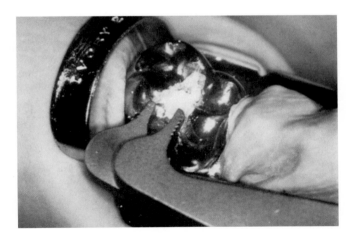

FIG. 24-13 EIE crown splitter activated.

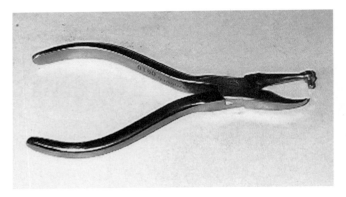

FIG. 24-14 Orthodontic band remover.

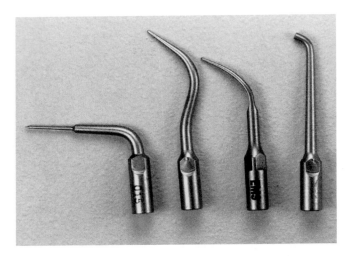

FIG. 24-17 Ultrasonic tips designed to vibrate bridge abutments.

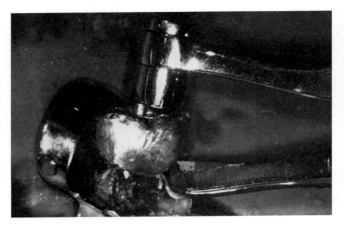

FIG. 24-15 Band remover in use.

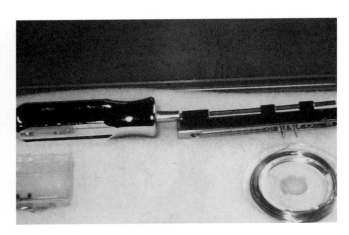

FIG. 24-18 Higa bridge remover.

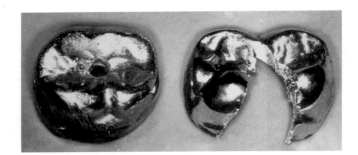

FIG. 24-16 Two methods for removing crowns.

piston-shaped head of the plier is placed into the pilot hole, and the jaw of the plier is placed under a margin or directed under the gingival height of contour of the crown. As the plier is closed, vertical pressure is applied to the crown, breaking the cement bond and dislodging the crown (Fig. 24-15).

Fig. 24-16 presents two methods commonly used for the removal of crowns.

Bridge Removal Techniques

The procedure for removal of a bridge is similar to that for crown removal, but the procedure carries more risk because it is more difficult to determine the exact path of insertion and withdrawal. When multiple abutments are involved, especially with fragile mandibular anterior teeth, even a minor force applied off-angle to the path of withdrawal can cause the teeth to fracture horizontally. For this reason it is advisable to loosen the cement bond on at least one abutment, and preferably two, before applying a force. Ultrasonic manufacturers provide special inserts specifically designed to vibrate bridge abutments (Fig. 24-17). These ultrasonic attachments are effective with conventional cements but appear to be ineffective with resin cements or dentin-bonded cements.

If the cement bonds cannot be broken on one or more abutments, the Higa bridge remover (Fig. 24-18) is capable of removing a well-cemented bridge with little risk of abutment damage. Pilot holes are prepared in the two abutment teeth, and the Higa pistons are placed in the pilot holes until they contact dentin (Fig. 24-19, *A* through *C*). Orthodontic wire is then placed under and around the appropriate pontic and in-

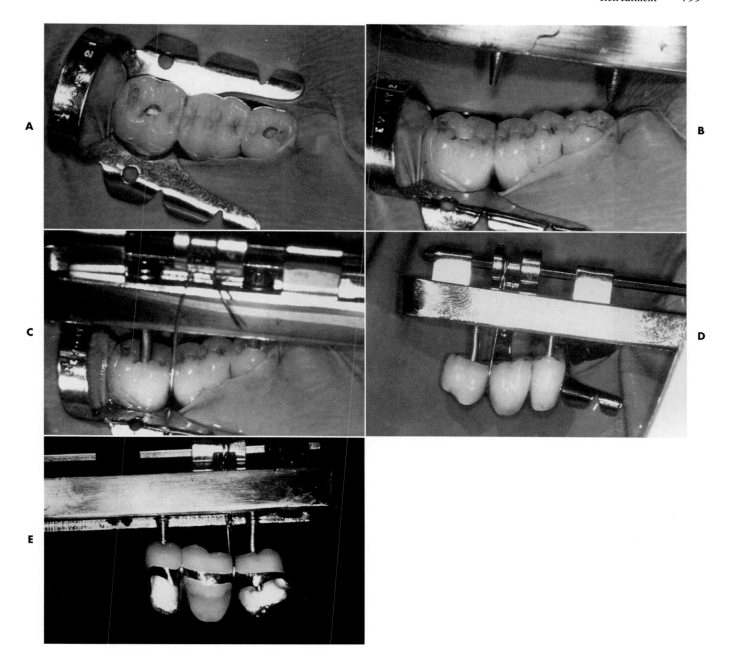

FIG. 24-19 A, Pilot holes prepared. **B,** Higa pistons inserted. **C,** Orthodontic wire engaged. **D,** Bridge removal. **E,** Nondestructive removal.

serted through a take-up reel in the device. The hand crank is then turned, rotating the take-up reel and cinches up the wire. This intraoral wench gradually hoists the bridge through steadily increasing vectors of force as the reel is rotated (Fig. 24-19, *C*). This device can be used for both metal and porcelain bridges and is completely nondestructive to the margins of the restorations (Fig. 24-19, *D* and *E*).

Post and Core Removal Techniques

The safe removal of posts and cores is one of the most important techniques in retreatment. The archaic method of drilling out the post and core with a carbide bur and high-speed handpiece is risky and requires both guesswork and luck. De-

signing a strategy for post and core removal requires a knowledge and understanding of the cementing medium, the composition and characteristics of the post, and the composition of the core material. For example, screw type of posts cemented with zinc oxyphosphate require a different approach than parallel posts cemented with dentin-bonded resin cement. What follows is a summary of the various strategies available.

Ultrasonic vibration

Many posts can be loosened and then removed by sonic or ultrasonic vibration transmitted to the post or core material by tips specifically designed for this purpose. Ultrasonic vibration appears to be more effective than sonic vibration for breaking

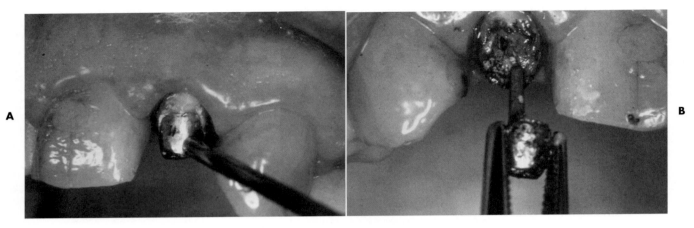

FIG. 24-20 A, Vibrator tip in place. **B,** Removal of post and core.

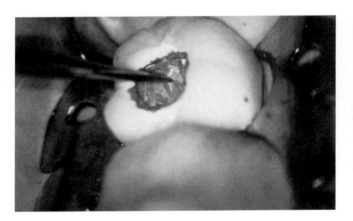

FIG. 24-21 CT-4 ultrasonic tip troughing around composite buildup material.

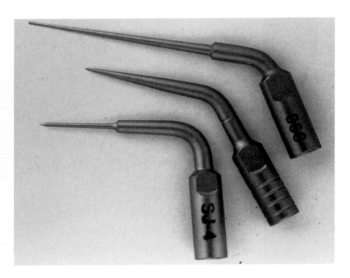

FIG. 24-23 Troughing instruments.

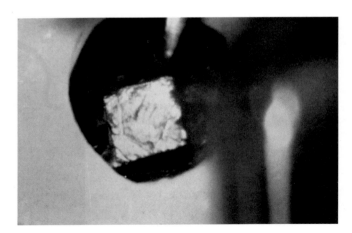

FIG. 24-22 Troughing procedure—undermining the post.

cement bonds.[9] The technique requires intimate contact of the vibrator tip to the metal of the post as shown in Fig. 24-20. The cement bond may break at the metal-cement interface or at the dentin-cement interface. Precautions include using coolant water to avoid heat buildup during the vibrating period and taking care to avoid fracturing delicate roots.

Root fracture is another cause for concern when vibrating posts ultrasonically. Although the incidence of root fracture appears to be low, the kinetic energy transmitted to the post is certainly within the range to exceed the tensile strength of dentin (12,000 psi), and caution must be exercised, especially when the remaining dentinal wall thickness is 2 mm or less.

Removing posts cemented with dentin-bonded cements can be challenging. If the post cannot be loosened with the standard vibration technique described above, another approach is to use an ultrasonic tip (Fig. 24-21) to trough around the post, removing the resin cement at the base of the post and essentially undermining its support and increasing the available reciprocal range of vibration (Figs. 24-22 and 24-23). This troughing procedure must be performed under high magnifi-

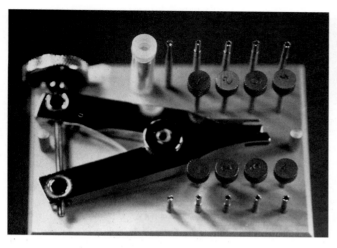

FIG. 24-24 Gonon post removal kit.

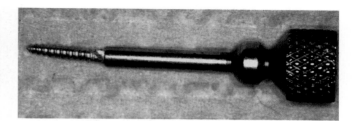

FIG. 24-26 Extractor device.

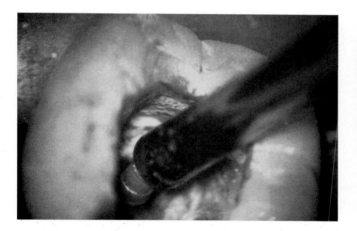

FIG. 24-25 Tubular tap.

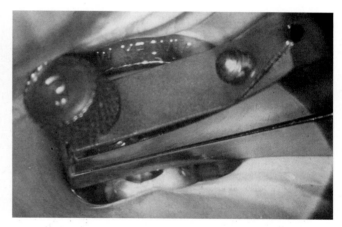

FIG. 24-27 Extractor engaged by removal device.

cation because the fine tips used in the troughing are easily damaged if they contact metal. The clinician circles the post with the tip, removing the cementing medium while *avoiding* contact with the post. The assistant, looking through the co-observer scope, uses a Stropko irrigator to keep the operative site free of debris so that the clinician's view is never hindered. This procedure is performed without water, thus enabling the clinician to maintain complete visibility throughout the entire troughing procedure. After the post has been undermined, the vibrator tip is used again to loosen the post.

Gonon post removal instrument

Another very effective method for atraumatically removing post and cores is by using the Gonon post remover (Fig. 24-24). This device contains a series of incrementally sized trephine burs made of drill-rod steel that has been heat treated to a very high Brinell hardness. This hardened steel enables these trephine burs to cut into and shape most posts made of surgical stainless steel. After choosing a trephine closest in size to the post, the trephine bur engages the post and prepares it like a tap and die. After threading the post with the trephine, a female-threaded cannula, called a tubular tap, engages the post and is screwed onto the post tightly (Fig. 24-25). This cannula

is also made of hardened drill-rod steel and has a fitting at its extremity that allows it to be attached to an extractor device that incrementally expands its jaws and pulls the post out gradually (Fig. 24-26). This device can remove even deeply seated posts placed with resin cements (Fig. 24-27).[46] It is especially useful in removing posts from teeth with ceramic restorations, as the extractor forces are cushioned and dissipated by a silicone washer. After the post is removed, the post hole is cleaned by ultrasonics with a CT-4 tip.

RISK ASSESSMENT IN RETREATMENT: RISK-BENEFIT CONSIDERATIONS

Nonsurgical retreatment is one alternative among several options. If the patient is asymptomatic but a pathologic condition is present, a judgment must be made to simply observe or treat. The decision to observe, although attractive to the asymptomatic patient, must be tempered by the consideration that failing, asymptomatic endodontics has a high incidence of inopportune flare-ups; delayed treatment frequently makes the eventual retreatment more problematic.[66,67] If treatment is chosen, the options are nonsurgical retreatment, surgical treatment, a combination of both, or extraction. Factors such as oral hygiene, age, remaining dentition, patient motivation, probability of success,

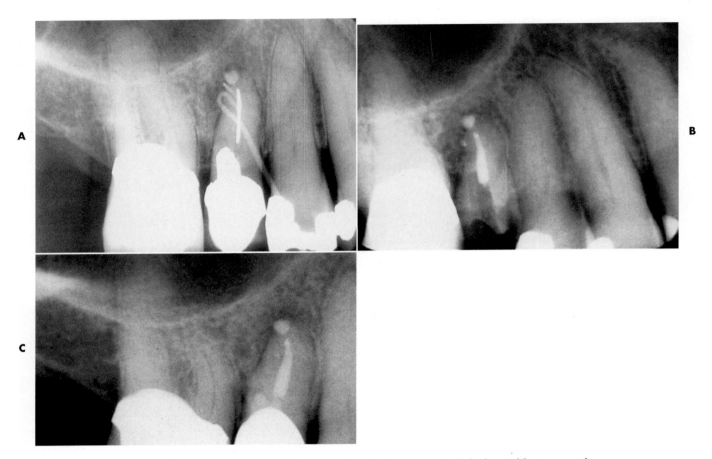

FIG. 24-28 A, Surgical retreatment of tooth No. 13. Note lateral root lesion (with gutta-percha point tracking in sinus tract). **B,** Nonsurgical retreatment. Warm, well-compacted gutta-percha replaced the silver point. **C,** One-year recall shows healing. *(Courtesy Dr. David Rosenberg.)*

and cost must be weighed in making a decision. The decision about which option to choose must be made by the patient *and* the clinician. The clinician should emphasize to the patient that the *most* expensive endodontic treatment is that which must be repeatedly redone.[19] Occasionally a surgical approach is attempted in retreating a failed case, but only later is it discovered that nonsurgical retreatment is the only approach that can salvage the case (Fig. 24-28). As discussed in Chapter 18, surgical treatment frequently fails to comprehensively address the singular cause of the failure (Fig. 24-29). *It is wise to retreat nonsurgically before any attempted surgical correction, unless there are extenuating circumstances.*

Treatment planning for teeth that have undergone inadequate endodontic therapy that is *not* failing with no evident pathology presents a dilemma for the clinician. Predicting whether a poorly completed case will fail at some time in the future is highly speculative. For example, as shown in Fig. 24-30, the patient was to have a full-mouth reconstruction over previously endodontically treated teeth. The endodontic treatment is failing only on tooth No. 25. However, should teeth Nos. 24 and 26 fail in the future, the entire reconstruction could be at risk. In this particular case the better decision is to retreat the questionable teeth, because of potential complications in the future.

We dentists have a conundrum when restoring asymptomatic teeth with silver points or paste fills. The exact pathogenesis of these delayed failures is unknown.[16,60,71] However, in

all likelihood, certain restorative procedures contribute to increased coronal leakage, which leads to canal contamination and subsequent failure. *Observing questionable endodontic therapy that appears to be successful is considered acceptable treatment but is not advised if the treated tooth is to receive a new restoration or is to be included as a critical abutment in a comprehensive reconstruction.*

RETREATMENT OF DISCONTINUED CARE BY PRIOR DENTIST

There are many reasons why endodontic treatment can be interrupted and not completed. When the prior clinicians can be contacted, their treatment records can be invaluable. In cases where there were personality conflicts with the initial treating doctor or failure of pain control, simply establishing a trusting rapport with the patient may avoid potential problems. Clinicians should be cautious about treating patients who have been treated by multiple clinicians, with no resolution of symptoms. Clear and honest communication with the patient and detailed testing and record keeping can avert misunderstanding and lead to successful resolution of the patient's problem..

If the discontinued treatment is due to a recalcitrant patient or one who seeks care only when in pain, clear guidelines must be set at the first visit. The patient should be made aware in writing that failure to follow the treatment regimen places the patient at great risk (with possible loss of the tooth and significant

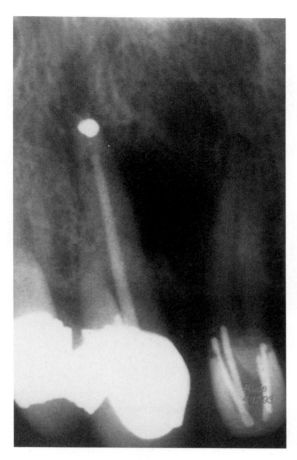

FIG. 24-29 Inappropriate surgery on case with a lateral root lesion. Correct treatment is nonsurgical retreatment.

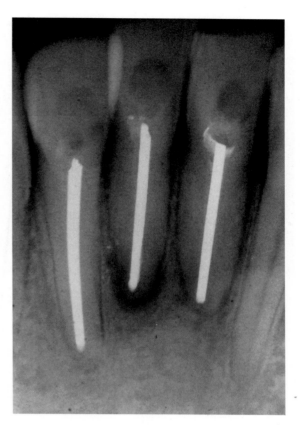

FIG. 24-30 Teeth Nos. 24, 25, and 26 have silver point treatment. Only No. 25 is failing. Should all be retreated?

pain and swelling), and that the offered treatment is conditional on following directions and keeping scheduled appointments.

If the prior treating dentist cannot be contacted and behavioral difficulties are not the reason for the discontinued treatment, one must assume there was some procedural difficulty causing the discontinued treatment. Continuation of care must address whatever that procedural difficulty may have been. For example, if treatment was stopped because of limited access caused by the patient's inability to open the mouth adequately, the patient's ability to open the mouth either must be compensated for (by bending files or using a hemostat instead of fingers) or otherwise resolved. For example, patients with limited mouth opening because of muscle trismus can be helped by physical therapy and home exercises, which can increase their range of motion significantly. Ethyl chloride spray, applied to the temporalis and masseter muscles during treatment, blocks pain impulses and prevents the incremental closing these patients frequently experience during long appointments. Preoperative muscle relaxants or minor tranquilizers can also aid the anxious patient who experiences trouble opening the mouth. Finally, intravenous sedation or general anesthesia is an acceptable approach for the patient who cannot be helped by other means. Whatever course is taken, the competent retreatment of discontinued therapy must address and solve the particular problem that was the initial reason for the interruption in treatment.

Treatment is most frequently discontinued because of diffi-

culties with the tooth itself. The most common reason is calcification of the pulp chamber or canals. Fortunately, with the advent of the operating microscope, calcified canals can be located, even in the apical thirds of roots. The calcified material that is formed is irregular and globular and lacks the symmetry and organization of secondary or tertiary dentin. The optical refractance of calcified pulp is different enough from secondary dentin that the trained eye can detect the dissimilarity between these substances, even in the apical one third of a canal (Fig. 24-31).[12,68]

The microscopic approach has enabled the routine retreatment of previously untreatable calcified canals and has dramatically lessened the need for a surgical approach to these cases. *The clinician should never determine the untreatability of a tooth based on radiographic evidence alone, or on the prior dentist's conviction that the canals were not negotiable* (Fig. 24-32). The technique for removing calcified pulp relies both on the visual skills of the clinician (being able to distinguish dentin from calcified pulp) and the skillful use of specialized instruments that have been designed specifically for the purpose of removing calcified pulp or other coronal obstructions. Fig. 24-33 shows the family of specialized ultrasonic instruments, each having its own function for different stages of pulp removal. These instruments have completely replaced the need for bur type of removal of the calcified material. They can discreetly and definitively remove calcified pulp without gouging the root and subjecting it to unnecessary

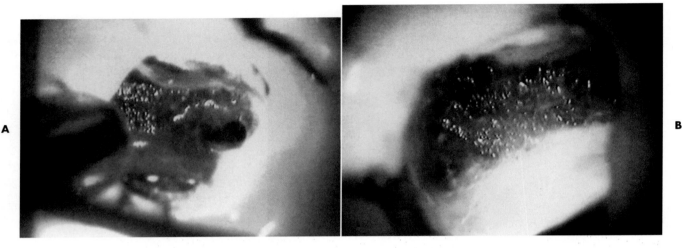

FIG. 24-31 **A,** Texture and color difference (between calcified pulp and secondary dentin) can be clearly detected. **B,** Subcoronal transillumination demonstrates "globular" appearance of calcified pulp.

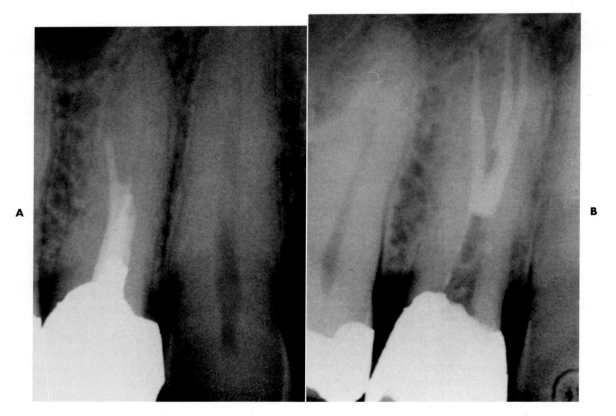

FIG. 24-32 **A,** Prior treatment discontinued due to calcified canals. **B,** Microscopic retreatment. *(Courtesy Dr. David Rosenberg.)*

weakening. The larger tips are used for rapid and gross removal of chamber calcifications, and increasingly smaller tips are used as one proceeds apically. The smaller the tip, the less aggressive the cutting action.

The role of the assistant at the microscope is crucial for this procedure to be completed efficiently. As the clinician is dusting away the calcified pulp ultrasonically, the assistant is using the Stropko irrigator to continually sweep away dental and pulpal debris formed by the ultrasonic activity. This teamwork approach enables the clinician to work without interruption and renders complete visual control even in areas previously thought impossible to view (Fig. 24-34). Accessory fiber-optic wands placed adjacent to the soft tissue (at the level of the root) are capable of transilluminating the root sufficiently to obtain enough intracanal illumination to work confidently (Fig. 24-35 and Plate 24-3).

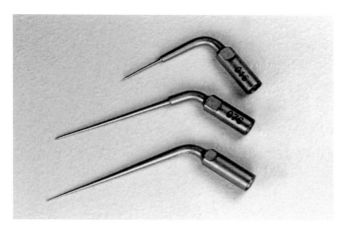

FIG. 24-33 Selection of EIE/Analytic's ultrasonic tips for removal of coronal/midroot and apical obstructions.

RETREATMENT OF INCOMPLETE ENDODONTIC THERAPY

No clinician deliberately fails to instrument a canal. Canals are missed because they are not seen. Canals are not seen either because calcifications are present coronal to the visible part of the canal, or the canal orifice is located in an anomalous location, or the access opening is too small to thoroughly inspect the pulpal floor in its entirety. Fig. 24-36 and Plates 24-4 to 24-7 demonstrate one such example of a failing root canal treatment caused by an untreated canal.

Commonly missed canals include the MB2/MB3 of maxillary molars, L canals of maxillary premolars, L canals of mandibular central and lateral incisors, second or third canals in mandibular premolars, second or third D canals in mandibular molars, and third MB canals in mandibular molars (Fig. 24-37). The clinician, however, must maintain constant anatomic skepticism because anomalous canals can be found in *any* tooth (Fig. 24-38).[20,72,73]

There are many new techniques for locating difficult-to-find canals. They are summarized as follows:

1. Radiographic methods
2. Transillumination methods
3. Troughing methods: Using the "white line test"
4. Staining methods
5. Bubble tests

Radiographic Methods

In retreating a case the first consideration by the clinician is a missed canal.[7,25,69,70] Off-angled radiographs are particularly useful in developing an accurate conceptual image of the tooth. Extreme mesial and distal views can reveal hitherto unsuspected anatomy (Fig. 24-39). Occlusal radiographs are beneficial, especially when pathology is present. The buccal object rule is employed to great benefit (Chapter 5) when multiple canal systems are present in broad mesiodistal roots (Fig. 24-40).[32]

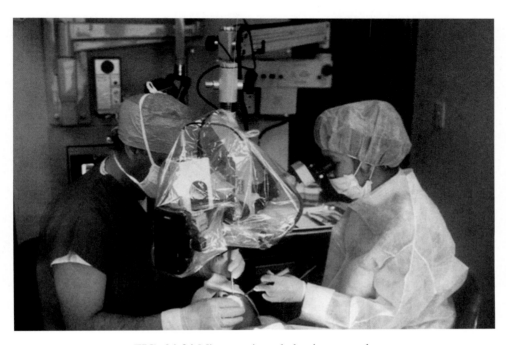

FIG. 24-34 Microscopic endodontic approach.

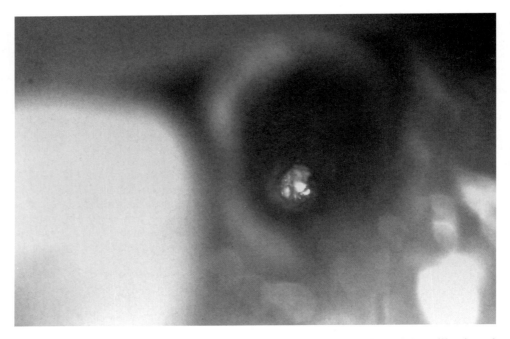

FIG. 24-35 High magnification view of silver point in apical third of canal (transilluminated by fiber optic wand).

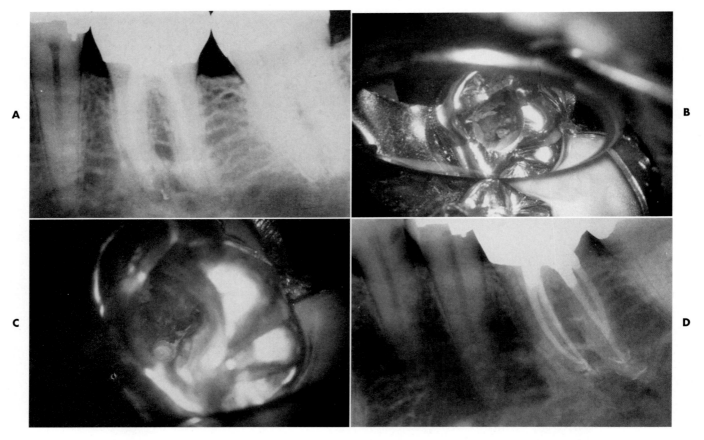

FIG. 24-36 A, Failing endodontic therapy. **B,** Initial access revealing calcified pulp not removed. **C,** After ultrasonic removal of calcified pulp. **D,** Final retreatment.

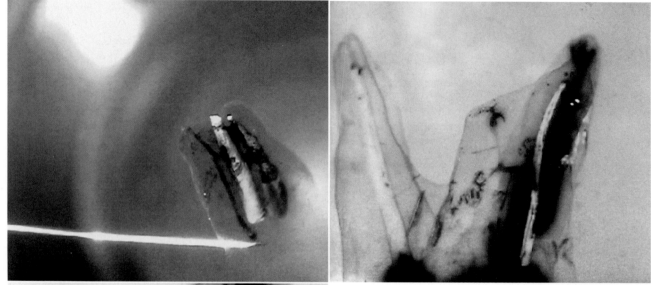

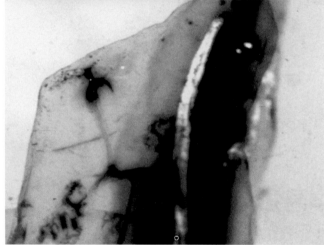

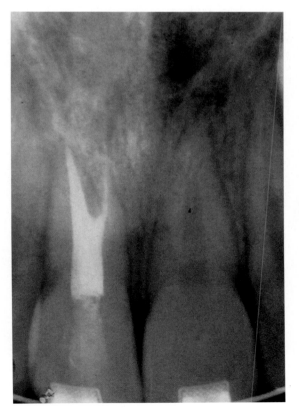

FIG. 24-37 A, Cleared tooth specimen of failed mesial root of mandibular molar. Note third mesial canal. B, Failed MB root of a maxillary molar. C, Failed maxillary first molar. Missed MB-2 canal.

FIG. 24-38 Bifurcated canal in a maxillary central incisor.

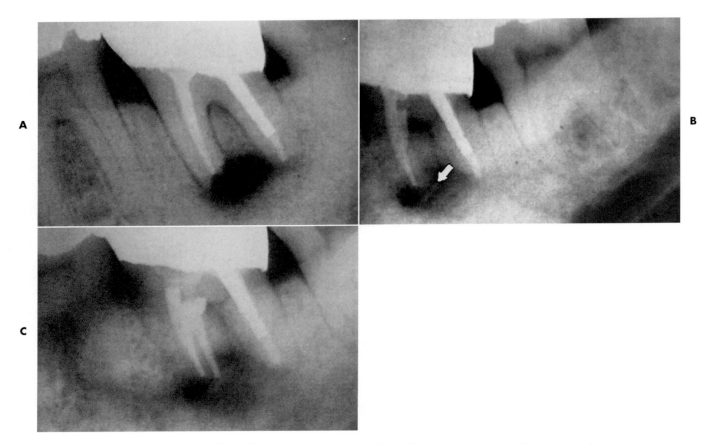

FIG. 24-39 A and **B,** Failing surgical treatment of mandibular second molar. Extreme mesially angled radiograph reveals outline of another canal. **C,** Retreatment completed.

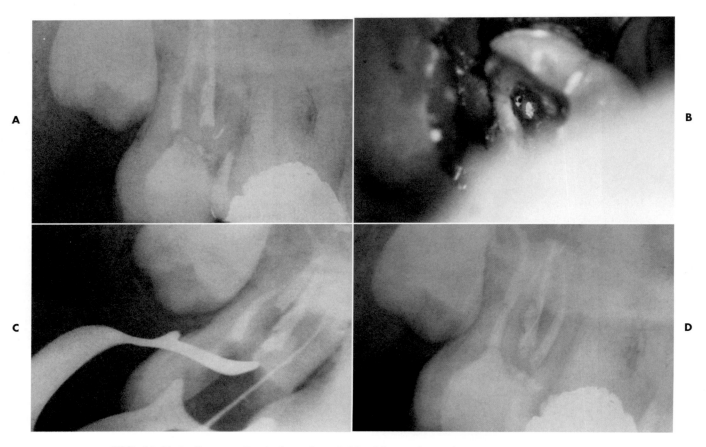

FIG. 24-40 A, Extreme distal view of tooth No. 15 reveals another canal mesial to MB-1.
B, Actual location of anomolous canal. **C,** File measurement. **D,** Retreatment completed.

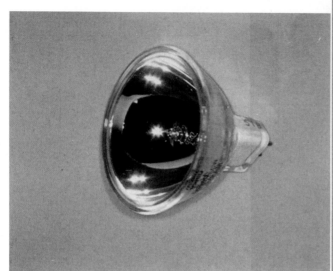

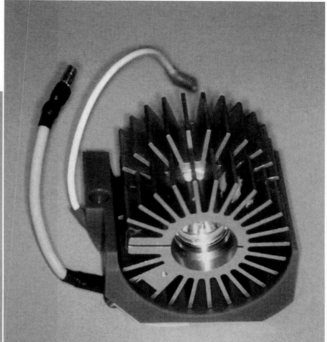

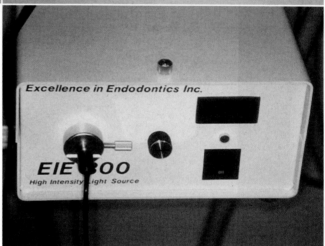

FIG. 24-41 A, Tungsten light bulb. **B,** Xenon light source. **C,** EIE/Analytic's metal halide light source.

Transillumination Methods

Transillumination with fiber-optic bundles can aid in the search for the difficult-to-locate canal. The illuminating light source should use either a xenon or metal halide bulb rather than the more standard tungsten bulbs (Fig. 24-41). Tungsten bulbs cannot provide enough lumens of light to penetrate soft tissue, bone, or dentin (Fig. 24-42, *A*). Standard tungsten light sources provide 3000 lumens, whereas metal halide and xenon sources supply twice that amount. The fiber optic cable must be composed of *glass* fibers because plastic fiber cables cannot withstand the significantly higher heat levels of the brighter light sources. Frequently, it is helpful to turn off the main microscope light while experimenting with various angulations of the fiber-optic wand to highlight the color and translucency differences that act as a road map in locating the hidden canal (Fig. 24-42, *B*). For dilacerated canals, transillumination can help locate the break-off canal and simplify its instrumenta-

tion by reducing blind guesswork and aimless probing with small-gauge files (Fig. 24-43). Finally, transillumination is extremely effective in locating fractures and following their apical extent into the canal (Fig. 24-44).

Troughing Methods: Using the "White Line Test"

The skillful use of the operating microscope has enabled the diligent clinician to search for missed canals much more successfully than in the past.[12,13] Fig. 24-45 and Plates 24-8 to 24-10 show how the CT-4 is used to create the initial troughing groove in the attempt to locate an MB-2 canal. The CT-4 is used in a dusting or etching, back-and-forth action with the water turned off while the assistant uses the Stropko irrigator to keep the operative site free from dentinal dust and pulpal debris. As the assistant applies a steady stream of air to the trough, any pulp tissue present becomes desiccated and turns white (Fig. 24-46, *A* and *B*, and Plates 24-11 and 24-12). This

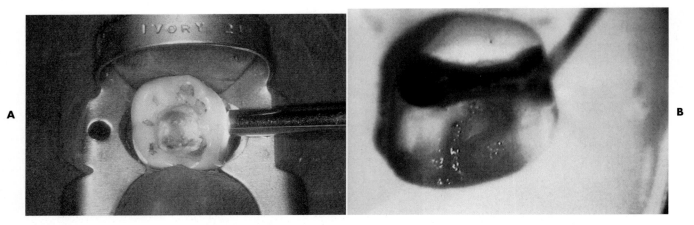

FIG. 24-42 A, Transillumination of pulpal floor reveals calcified pulp of mesiolingual canal. **B,** Removal of calcification reveals three mesial canals in same root.

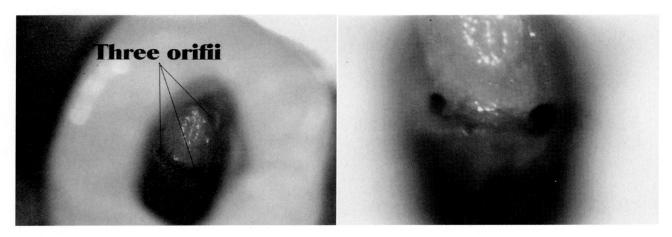

FIG. 24-43 All three orifices of this trifurcated root canal system can be seen.

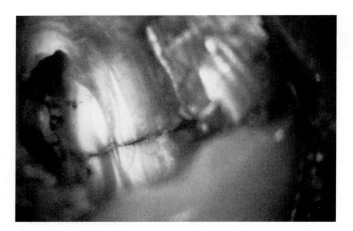

FIG. 24-44 Crown and root fractures can be examined to their end.

"white line" is a virtual road map to the missed canal; the microscope and ultrasonics provide the tools to locate the canal without endangering any adjacent structures or removing dentin unnecessarily. Figs. 24-47 and 24-48 demonstrate several retreatment cases using this technique.

Staining Methods

If a white line is not visible, the trough can be stained using a food dye or caries indicator (Ultradent caries indicator, South Jordan, Utah) (Fig. 24-49). After staining and flushing with water, difficult-to-see pulp can be identified (Fig. 24-50 and Plates 24-13 to 24-15).

Staining can be particularly helpful in looking for canals where there has been significant leakage around restorations and the pulpal floor is deeply discolored.

Bubble Tests

The action of sodium hypochlorite on vital or necrotic tissue produces oxygen bubbles. A single drop of sodium hypochlorite, carefully placed in a troughing groove, reacts with any pulp tissue and produces oxygen bubbles, which may be seen under high magnification (Fig. 24-51). The observant clinician must see where the *first* bubbles appear to be able to determine where the canal is located[12,13].

RETREATMENT OF COMPLETED BUT INADEQUATE THERAPY

Complete but inadequate treatment refers to cases that have had definitive and comprehensive treatment but fail to meet the standards of care needed to ensure long-term

Text continued on p. 815

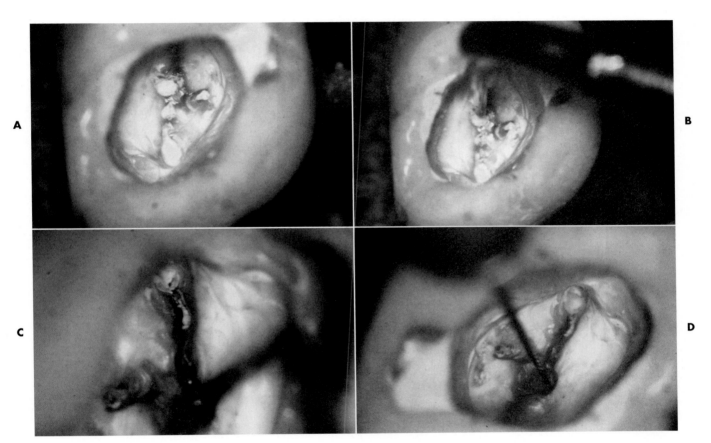

FIG. 24-45 A, Coronal view of access of completed case showing calcified pulp still remaining. **B,** CT-4 ultrasonic tip used to remove calcified pulp. Note unrestricted visual access possible. **C,** Examination of troughing groove; "white line" is visible after drying with Stropko air-water irrigator. **D,** Instrument placed in MB-2 canal.

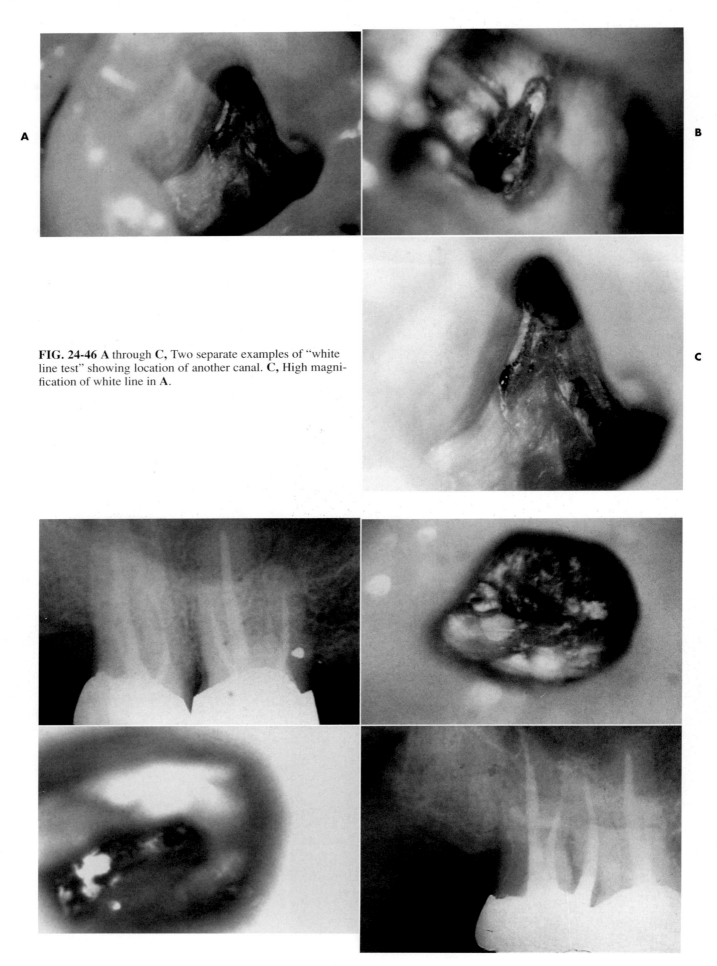

FIG. 24-46 A through **C,** Two separate examples of "white line test" showing location of another canal. **C,** High magnification of white line in **A.**

FIG. 24-47 Retreatment of maxillary second molar. Uncovered MB-2 was found. All four canals were retreated.

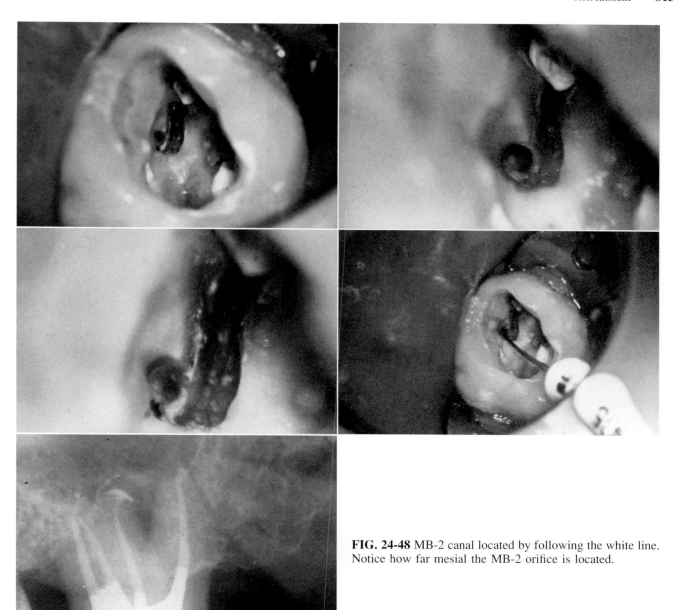

FIG. 24-48 MB-2 canal located by following the white line. Notice how far mesial the MB-2 orifice is located.

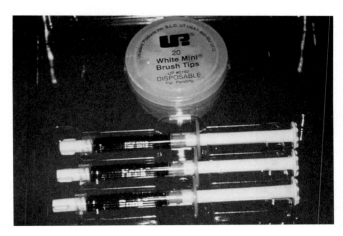

FIG. 24-49 Ultradent's caries indicator is used to find difficult-to-locate pulp.

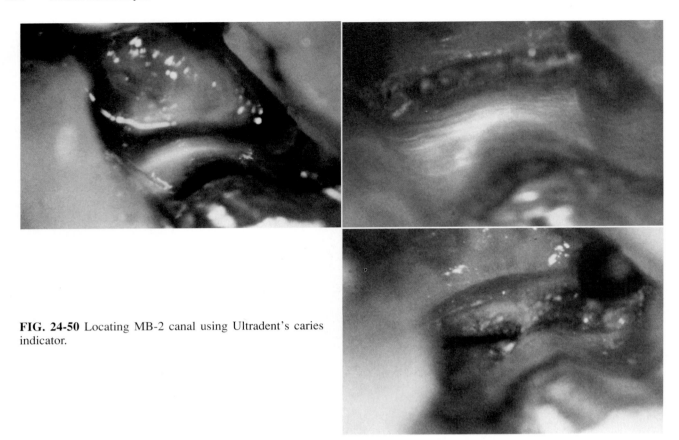

FIG. 24-50 Locating MB-2 canal using Ultradent's caries indicator.

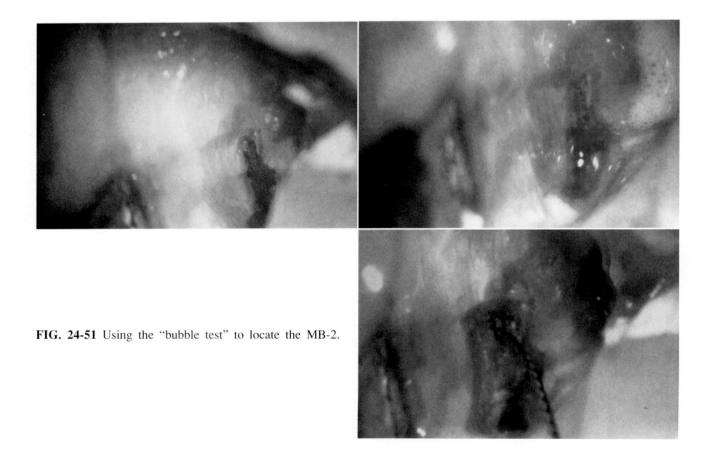

FIG. 24-51 Using the "bubble test" to locate the MB-2.

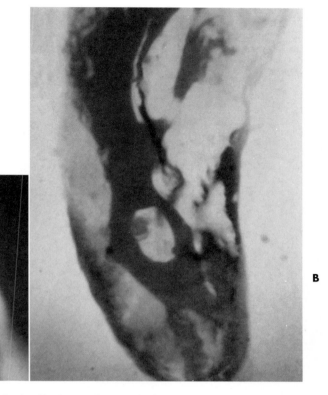

FIG. 24-52 A, Anatomic complexity. **B,** Anatomic complexity.

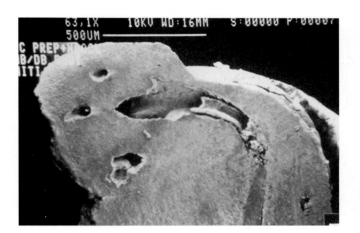

FIG. 24-53 Apex blocked by debris prevented apical instrumentation of final 2 mm.

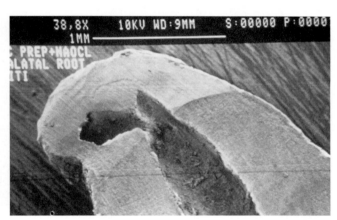

FIG. 24-54 Failure to instrument around abrupt curvatures with subsequent ledging.

success; this includes complete debridement of the root canal system and hermetic sealing of all apical *and* coronal orifices.

Underextended Fillings

In cases that are filled short and are failing, *it must be assumed that infected pulpal remnants are present apical to the obturation material.* Successful retreatment of these cases involves removal of the obturation material and thorough instrumentation and obturation of the canal to the radiographic terminus. Reasons for failure to obturate to the apex are as follows:

1. Anatomic complexity (Fig. 24-52)
2. Apical blockage caused by pulpal or dentinal debris (Fig. 24-53)

3. Ledge formation coronal to apex (Fig. 24-54)
4. Inadequate shape preventing apical seating of gutta-percha cone
5. Blockage by instrument (Fig. 24-55)

Abrupt demarcations of curvature are commonplace in the apical thirds of roots.[26,34,69,70] Failure to appreciate the subtleties of apical anatomy results in endodontic therapy that is neither well performed nor predictable in its success. The importance of early coronal enlargement in the instrumentation of the apical anatomy is discussed in Chapter 8. The tactile awareness gained by adequately removing restrictive coronal dentin is paramount. If coronal dentin is adequately removed, exploration of the delicate apical anatomy is simplified. Fig. 24-56

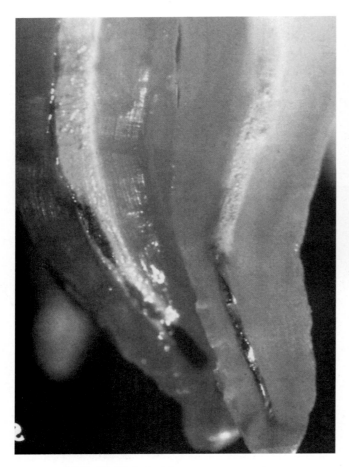

FIG. 24-55 Apical instrument separation.

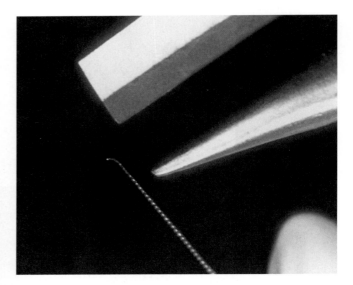

FIG. 24-56 Buchanan file bender.

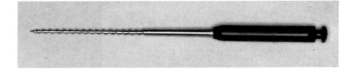

FIG. 24-57 GPX gutta-percha remover.

shows the file bender, which allows the clinician to place delicate and defined curvatures on file tips that greatly facilitate the gentle probing required to accomplish this task. Although a straight file can course around a gradual curve, it does not negotiate around an abrupt curvature. Forcing a straight stainless steel file apically seldom directs it *into* a curvature; rather, such action usually creates a ledge or divot into the dentin that complicates subsequent apical instrumentation (see Fig. 24-54). Bypassing a ledge created in apical dentin is very difficult.

Removal of gutta-percha–based obturation materials

Mechanical methods. Retreatment usually begins with the removal of the obturating material. In the case of gutta-percha, it is also helpful to identify the cementing medium used. Epoxy and resin-based sealers are more difficult to remove than zinc oxide–eugenol cements. If the gutta-percha is poorly condensed, or comprises only a single cone, it can be removed as one piece, using a small-gauge Hedström file to engage the cone and then applying coronal force on the Hedström file. If the gutta-percha is well compacted or condensed, a GPX instrument (Fig. 24-57) can be used in a slow-speed handpiece. This instrument is essentially a reverse McSpadden compactor, which melts the gutta-percha and directs it coronally. Care must be taken with the GPX to avoid fracturing the instrument inside the canal, thus further complicating the retreatment.

Ultrasonic Methods. Gutta-percha can be removed by thermal softening, either via heated pluggers or specialized ultrasonic tips. These tips are heated when activated by ultrasonic energy and are fine enough to work around curvatures. After the gutta-percha is heated, it can be removed with hand files.

Chemical Methods. Various solvents have been used to soften the gutta-percha and dissolve the cement.[27,31,74] Chloroform, eucalyptol, xylene, turpentine, halothane, and acetone, for example, are good solvents for isoprene rubber but are toxic to tissue; some are suspected carcinogens.[6,15,64] Postoperative periapical irritation should be expected whenever these solvents are used. They allow an advantageous passive instrumentation in removing the gutta-percha and sealer and decrease the likelihood of inadvertent alteration of the canal caused by mechanical removal methods. Taking advantage of the wicking effect of paper points to absorb the solvent also aids in the complete removal of the obturating material.

After removal of the gutta-percha, negotiation of the canal to the terminus begins with an evaluation of the access and coronal enlargement of the canal. Attempting delicate instrumentation of apical anatomy without adequate enlargement of the coronal two thirds of the canal makes a difficult task almost impossible. After the appropriate coronal canal shape is created with Gates-Glidden or shaping files, inspection of the apical one third of the canal using the operating microscope is undertaken. This inspection requires a clean canal, free of debris, and

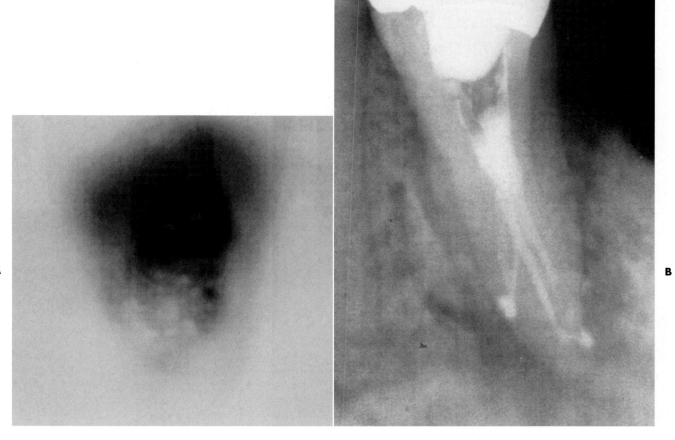

FIG. 24-58 A, Complex anatomy such as this can be inspected and deciphered with the aid of the microscope. **B,** Properly cleaned and filled canals. Trifurcation can be seen.

one that is absolutely dry. The technique for cleaning must address the need to clean *both* organic and inorganic material from the canal walls, down to the apical extent of the preparation. The technique for accomplishing this cleansing follows:

1. Flush with 5.25% sodium hypochlorite and activate with small-gauge ultrasonic files at the lowest possible power.
2. Rinse with sterile water to remove all sodium hypochlorite.
3. Irrigate with EDTA and activate with small-gauge ultrasonic files.
4. Rinse with sterile water to remove all EDTA.
5. Rinse with 100% ethyl alcohol.
6. Dry with paper points followed by air-only Stropko drying (Fig. 24-58, *A*).

This technique results in a clean, dry environment, where critical visual discernment is essential. This inspection demands the use of the highest powers of magnification and requires a trained eye, sensitive to minute differences in color. Frequently, information gathered during this critical inspection is sufficient to detect the reasons for the endodontic failure. Corrective measures can now be undertaken to address the problem. For example, if the main canal bifurcates apically and the bifurcation can be seen, the clinician places the appropriate bend in the file and directs the file purposely instead of by random picking (see Fig. 24-58).

Irrigation with sodium hypochlorite and EDTA[8,10,14], com-

bined with gentle probing with small curved files, results in complete instrumentation of many problematic apexes. After-confirming instrumentation to the radiographic terminus (by radiograph or apex locator), the canal should be shaped and sealed with gutta-percha.

Overextended Fillings

Overextension of gutta-percha fillings presents a unique problem for the retreating dentist. Not only must the dentist deal with a foreign body present in periapical tissue[75], but he or she also must establish the *reason why* the filling is overextended. Usually fillings are overextended because the natural apical constricture has been transported. Reestablishing a viable resistance form may not be possible if the apical transportation or zipping is extensive.

Often the presence of excess gutta-percha is *not* the cause of failure, but instead the cause of failure is actually the lack of a tight apical seal.[5,44,62,75] *Endodontists refer to such cases as overextended but undercompacted* (Fig. 24-59). Canals that are properly sealed and have slight excess filling material are generally successful.[22] However, if the excess filling material perforates through cortical bone and impinges on the mucoperiosteum, apical surgery is the only procedure that can resolve the problem (Fig. 24-60).[3]

In retreating teeth with overextended fills, success depends on disinfection of the canal and hermetic sealing of the entire

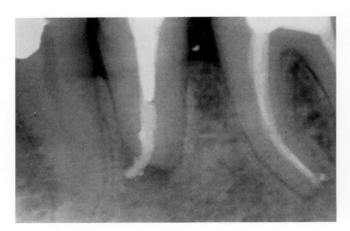

FIG. 24-59 Overextended but undercompacted gutta-percha resulting in a poor apical seal.

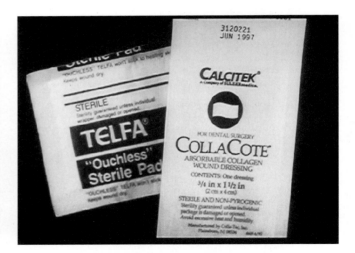

FIG. 24-61 CollaCote.

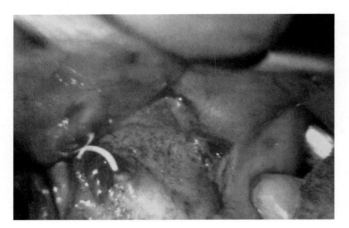

FIG. 24-60 Overextended gutta-percha impinging on the periosteum.

canal system from coronal access to apex. Removal of the filling material from the periapical tissue, although desirable, is not always necessary.

Methods for removal of gutta-percha are identical for both underextended and overextended fills. Occasionally, it *is* possible to remove gutta-percha cones from the periapical tissue through the canal by a fortuitous placement of Hedström files (aided by the microscope), which can engage the gutta-percha mass as one entity without shredding it.

After the gutta-percha has been removed, a tapered canal resistance form must be created if anatomically possible. If the apical foramen is badly transported and no resistance form is possible, the apex can be blocked mechanically by a bioabsorbable barrier such as CollaCote (bovine collagen, Fig. 24-61) or by calcium sulfate. One may also attempt to generate a physiologic barrier using calcium hydroxide. Because of its strong bacteriocidal properties, limited toxicity, and easy placement, interim calcium hydroxide therapy is recommended where inroot resorption is present. Many failing overextended canals exhibit resorption around the apex (Fig. 24-62), and

there is research to show that calcium hydroxide is a powerful inhibitor of inflammatory resorption.[23,33,55]

Whatever method is used to create an apical barrier, it is prudent to allow the highly bacteriocidal 5.25% sodium hypochlorite an opportunity to work longer for thorough disinfection.

Obturation methods for these cases are not different in any' fundamental way from those of standard obturation, other than perhaps the use of less vertical pressure because of the delicate nature of the apical barrier.

Poorly Compacted Fillings

Canal fillings extended to the radiographic terminus but undercompacted are the least vexing of retreatment cases, providing that the canal anatomy has not been irreversibly altered. Poorly compacted fillings are the result of either inadequate shape or careless technique. Sometimes the more carelessly a case is performed, the easier it is to retreat. This is especially true in retreating teeth that contain paste fillings. Because of minimal instrumentation, the paste can be removed and standard instrumentation and obturation can proceed (Fig. 24-63).

Role of Lateral and Furcal Canals: Retrograde Periodontitis

In only rare cases is the packing of the lateral canals important because the natural defenses of the body appear to be capable of containing a limited bacterial assault if the infective agent is not virulent[25,54]. Nevertheless, *it is important to fill these minuscule tributaries*. They gain tremendous importance if the coronal seal is not hermetic. Bacterial leakage occurring under and around well-fitting crowns is scientifically well established and commonplace.[47,56,65,66] Although the blood supply of the ligament is capable of containing a limited bacterial invasion, it is now faced with an unending bacterial assault. This process of reinfection is called *retrograde periodontitis*.[61] The pathogenesis of retrograde periodontitis demonstrates that the coronal seal is every bit as important as the apical seal. Dentin-bonded resins are now being used to complete the "coronal endodontics" to decrease the likelihood of retrograde infection.

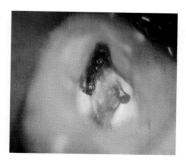

PLATE 24-1 Preliminary troughing groove created in maxillary molar. Notice the mesial extension of the preparation toward the wall of the mesial marginal ridge.

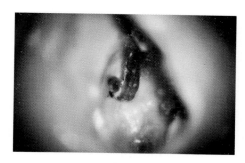

PLATE 24-2 High-magnification view of white line.

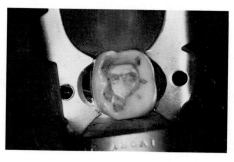

PLATE 24-3 Transgingival fiberoptic wand illumination of calcified pulp. Notice how the illumination easily distinguishes between calcified pulp and normal dentin.

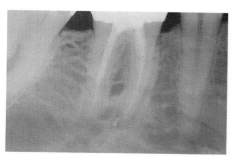

PLATE 24-4 Symptomatic mandibular first molar subsequent to retreatment therapy. Patient had delayed sensitivity to heat.

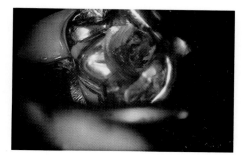

PLATE 24-5 Preliminary access to tooth in Plate 24-12. Calcified pulp has not been removed and is evident under distobuccal cusp.

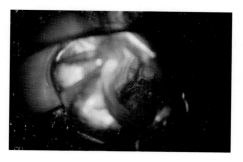

PLATE 24-6 Calcified pulp removed with UT-4 ultrasonic tip. A missed DB canal is visible.

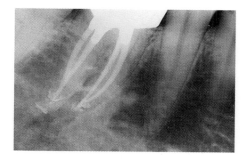

PLATE 24-7 Final radiograph of retreatment of all four canals.

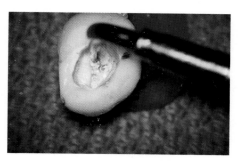

PLATE 24-8 Access view of failed endodontic therapy, with calcified pulp clearly evident as the darker material.

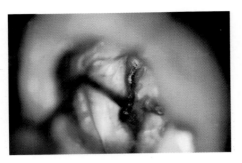

PLATE 24-9 High-magnification view of completed troughing, showing location of MB-2 canal at the termination of the white line.

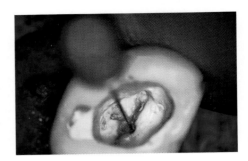

PLATE 24-10 No. 10 file entering into MB-2 canal.

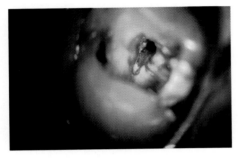

PLATE 24-11 White line clearly evident after drying with Stropko irrigator.

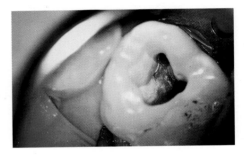

PLATE 24-12 Desiccated pulpal floor demonstrating white line connecting MB-1 and MB-2.

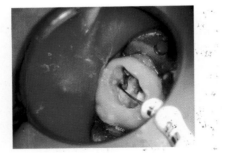

PLATE 24-13 Instrument placed in MB-2 canal from previous example. MB-2 canal is at the terminal end of the white line.

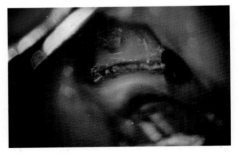

PLATE 24-14 High-magnification view of pulpal remnant after staining with caries indicator solution (Ultradent). Notice white line on axial wall of trough.

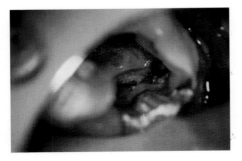

PLATE 24-15 No. 10 file placed in MB-2 canal of tooth in Plate 24-8.

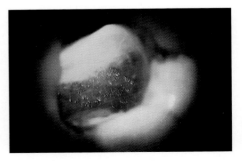

PLATE 24-16 High-magnification view of pulpal floor, demonstrating large pulp stones.

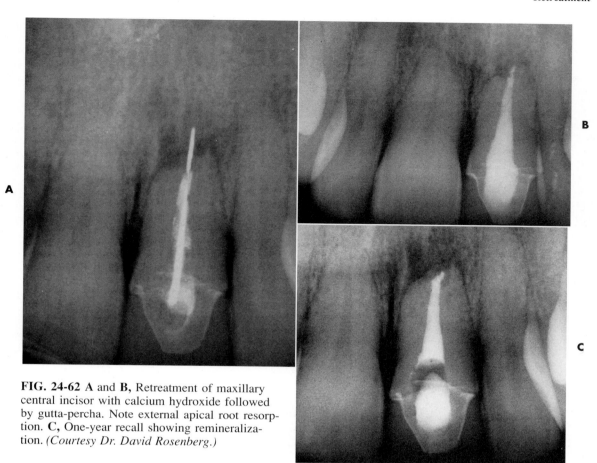

FIG. 24-62 **A** and **B,** Retreatment of maxillary central incisor with calcium hydroxide followed by gutta-percha. Note external apical root resorption. **C,** One-year recall showing remineralization. *(Courtesy Dr. David Rosenberg.)*

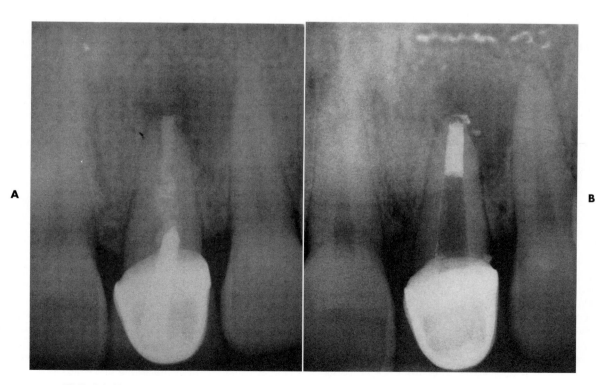

FIG. 24-63 **A,** Paste filling. **B,** Case retreated with gutta-percha. *(Case courtesy Dr. David Rosenberg.)*

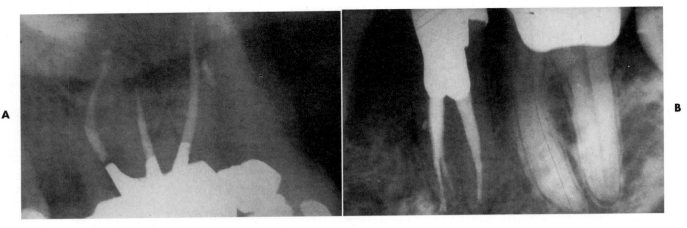

FIG. 24-64 **A,** Placement of amalgam cores into all three canal orifices. **B,** Placement of amalgam deep into canals.

Removal of Canal Obstructions

The introduction of the operating microscope has greatly simplified the removal of obstructions from any location within the canal. A list of the most common obstructions follows:
1. Resins, composites, restorative cements
2. Amalgam
3. Fractured posts
4. Sectional silver points
5. Separated instruments

Amalgam

At its minimal level the access preparation is completed by placing a restorative material, commonly amalgam or composite resin. The restorative material is placed or condensed on the furcal floor (or at the entry to the canal orifice in anterior teeth). Some clinicians advocate placing the material down into the canal to both aid in the retention of the material and to enhance the quality of the coronal seal (Fig. 24-64); however, this complicates retreatment if it should be necessary. Historically, the approach to the dilemma has been apical surgery or removal of the restorative material by excavation with small burs. This method is fraught with multiple pitfalls including furcal perforation, lateral root perforation, and hollowing out and weakening of the root.

Use of the microscope for removing metallic obstructions from the canal orifices has eliminated most of the guesswork and significantly reduced the procedural risks. Using specialized ultrasonic tips and high magnification, materials such as alloys, composite resins, cements, and glass-ionomers can be removed with little risk. Because the removal of the restorative material occurs under extreme scrutiny and with laserlike control, it is possible to remove the material and not endanger the adjacent dentin or enlarge the preparation (Fig. 24-65)

The technique is as follows:
1. Place the tooth access under high magnification (>12×).
2. Position the assistant so that the Stropko irrigator can be accurately placed.
3. If necessary, use supplemental fiberoptic illumination to distinguish the restorative material from dentin as outlined on p. 819. If the occluding material is tooth-colored resin instead of amalgam, this identification is accom-

plished by having the assistant desiccate the material using the air-only Stropko irrigator (Fig. 24-66).
4. After identifying the restorative material, activate the ultrasonic unit with the appropriate tip. With the assistant continually brushing away debris with the Stropko, the clinician brushes the tip back and forth or circumferentially around the restorative material, using a *very* light touch and keeping the tip *continuously* moving. All restorative materials can be removed in this way, even resins or silver amalgam condensed down into canals (Fig. 24-67).

Fractured posts

Posts fractured deep within the canal can be removed in a similar manner. Most posts that fracture subcrestally do so from metal fatigue failure, and the remaining segment in the root still possesses its original retentive capacity. Prior methods of removal used large trephine burs that frequently weakened the root from the overenlargement of the canals that is required to accommodate these burs. With the ultrasonic method, channels can be created down the facial and lingual sides of the post, where the dentin thickness is greatest. These channels are capable of reducing the retention sufficiently to loosen the post. This technique minimizes dentin removal and is performed without guesswork.

Sectional silver points

It is postulated that the pathogenesis of silver cone failure occurs when serum enzymes react with the silver ions to form silver salts, which are nonspecific cellular toxins.[60,71] Although macrophages and lymphocytes mount an attack against these toxins, the infinite supply of silver ions precludes their elimination. *Performing surgery on failing silver cone cases is futile because it will likely fail* (Fig. 24-68).[21] Indeed, one of the reasons for the unusually high failure rate of all endodontic cases reported in retrospective studies of surgeries performed may very well be due to the inclusion in those studies of large numbers of failing silver point cases.[18]

The microscopic approach to silver point removal has simplified this sometimes frustrating procedure. For cones that do not have significant retention, simply vibrating them lightly with a CT-4 or UT-4 and removing them with forceps is all

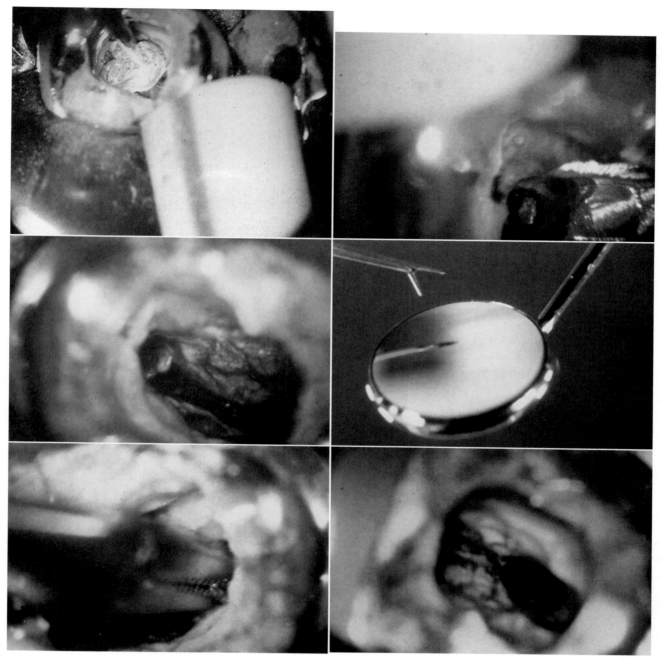

FIG. 24-65 Ultrasonic CT-4 tip used to remove amalgam from around silver point. After amalgam removal, silver point removed with microforceps.

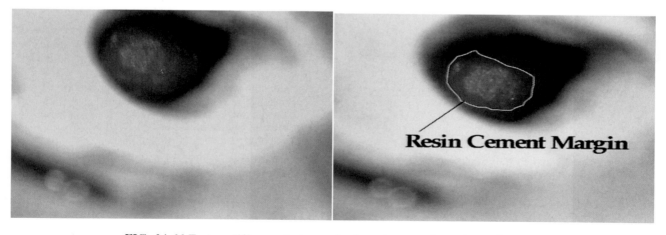

FIG. 24-66 Texture difference between dentin and composite resin can be seen.

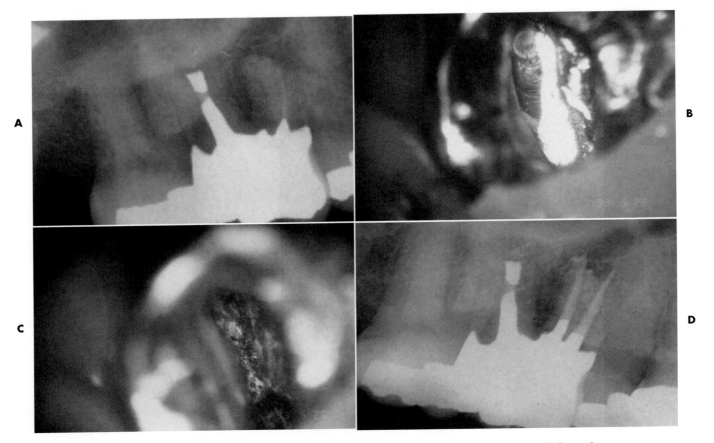

FIG. 24-67 Removal of deeply placed amalgam before locating missed calcified MB-2 canal. A, Amalgam core placed. B, Amalgam core to be removed with CT-4. C, "White line" leads to MB-2 canal. D, Retreatment completed.

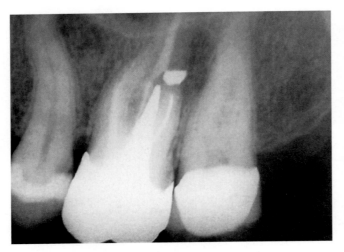

FIG. 24-68 Inappropriate surgical repair of failed silver point root canal therapy. Such attempts may lead to external root resorption and eventual failure.

that is required. If the cones are embedded in a cement (as was common practice years ago), ultrasonic vibration with a CT-4 under medium magnification differentially removes the cement without weakening or severing the silver cones coronally. Before ultrasonics and microscope-level magnification,

these cones were frequently amputated in the process of removing the cement with a bur, thereby complicating the case. If a purchase can be obtained on the silver cone, it is far easier to remove it with one of the many forceps available (see Fig. 24-65, *D*).

If the silver cone case has been well placed, the silver cone probably has a great deal of mechanical retention because of the parallel design of the preparation and the frictional engagement of the cone with the canal wall. These cases are managed as though they were fractured post cases. Under high magnification and with the assistant applying the air-only Stropko irrigator, a troughing groove is prepared around the cone with a Slim Jim 4, UT-4A or UT-4B ultrasonic tip (Fig. 24-69) (EIE/Analytic, Orange, Calif.). If a sectional cone has been used and the severed cone occurs in the midroot, the troughing may need to be restricted to the buccal and lingual sides of the cone to preserve the mesiodistal dentin (Fig. 24-70). Nearly all silver cones can be removed with this technique, even those with cones tightly wedged into the apical third.

Separated instruments

Instrument separation is a dentist's worst nightmare because in most cases it is a result of operator error and therefore avoidable. Although instrument breakage may be caused by a manufacturing defect; separation more commonly occurs because the dentist is using the instrument inappropriately, forcing the

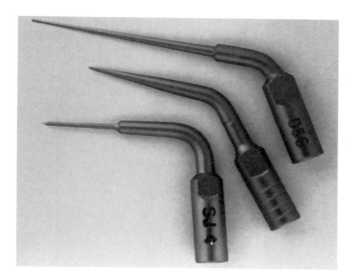

FIG. 24-69 Instruments used to remove files.

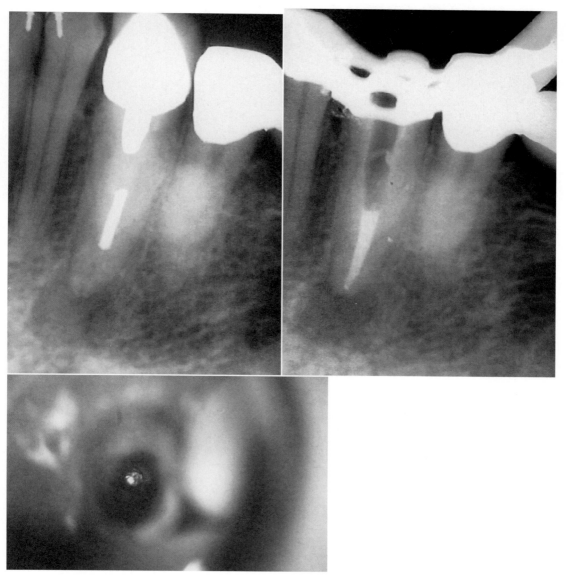

FIG. 24-70 Retreatment of silver point root canal therapy with coronal dentin bonding cement. The microscope enables very accurate removal of dentin, thereby eliminating the mechanical retention of the silver point.

instrument, or is using it past its useful life. These situations can usually be avoided by the careful clinician. However, automated instrumentation has led to a much higher incidence of instrument separation.

Instrument separations can be divided into two major categories:

I. Stainless steel and carbon steel instruments
   A. Gates-Glidden burs, Peeso burs, broaches
   B. Standard files, reamers, Hedström files, ultrasonic files
II. Hand- and machine-driven nickel-titanium instruments

Separated instrument removal techniques. Removal of instrument fragments is a microscopic procedure. The tech-

niques to be described cannot be performed with loupes except at the most coronal orifice level; deeper separations require magnifications and lighting levels far exceeding those obtainable with loupes and headlights (Chapter 5).

The basic techniques for instrument removal are similar for all the different kinds of instruments but differ in some critical details. The overall strategy involves creating a "staging platform" coronal to the separated fragment (Fig. 24-71, *A* and *B*). This staging platform provides the necessary working area from which all additional procedures take place. *Attempting instrument removal procedures without an adequate staging platform greatly complicates the procedure.* The staging platform creates a flat plateau that is easily cleaned of debris and greatly

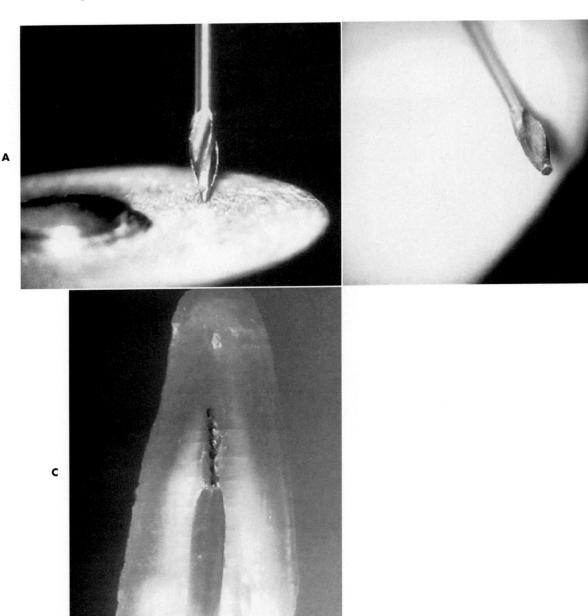

FIG. 24-71 A and **B,** Modification of Gates-Glidden bur with Carborundum disk. **C,** Creation of a flat staging platform using modified Gates-Glidden burs.

enhances the clinician's ability to discriminate fine detail. *It is important to realize that when an instrument fractures, it rarely remains in the center of the canal; to locate the instrument requires an ability to clearly inspect the lateral walls.* To create a staging platform, a series of Gates-Glidden burs is modified with a Carborundum disk as shown in Fig. 24-71, *A* and *B*. The working end of the bur is flattened to the midbud level, creating a true side-cutting bur. These burs are used in sequence to create a straight line path *from coronal access to the level of the fragment.* Straight-line access is critical. After the staging platform has been established, it must be cleaned and dried.

Since the debris is composed of both organic and inorganic material, a dual irrigation approach is recommended. Heated sodium hypochlorite is flooded into the chamber and canal. With a UT-4A or UT-4B ultrasonic tip, the solution is activated, as the lowest power setting with the lightest possible touch is used. The ultrasonic tip is rapidly moved over the staging platform and instrument head. The only goal here is to activate the sodium hypochlorite and potentiate the dissolving of the organic component of the debris. After flushing the canal with sterile saline, the same procedure is repeated with EDTA. The EDTA dissolves the inorganic component of the debris and essentially creates a platform free of smear layer. After activating the EDTA with ultrasonics, the canal is flushed with sterile saline again; 100% ethyl alcohol is used as a final rinse. Because visibility depends on dryness, any moisture compromises inspection. *The 100% ethyl alcohol rinse is essential to adequately dry the canal and platform area.* After removing the ethyl alcohol, the canal is gently dried with an air-only

Stropko side-venting needle for thorough detailed inspection. This entire procedure is summarized in Fig. 24-72.

Inspection of the staging platform occurs at high magnification (i.e., ×16 to ×22). *After inspection, an evaluation is made to determine how the fragment is lodged; then a strategy is designed for the removal of the fragment.* The fragment may require only simple circumferential troughing, or it may require troughing on only one side of the instrument. Frequently, it can be seen that the access requires additional refinement to establish straight-line access. Generally, the finer the ultrasonic tip, the less aggressive cutting action it possesses.

Most stainless and carbon steel instruments move coronally if a 1.5 to 2 mm trough is established around them and the fragment then activated with ultrasonic energy as demonstrated in Fig. 24-73.

If the fragment does not move coronally after troughing and vibration with ultrasonics, it can be removed with the Cancellier instruments. This technique requires 2 mm of exposed fragment. The Cancellier instruments are a graduated series of cannulas that can be attached to a threaded hand carrier, as depicted in Fig. 24-74. Estimate the approximate circumference of the exposed fragment and select the appropriately sized Cancellier cannula. Select a cannula that maximizes the contact area between the instrument and the cannula (Fig. 24-75) to apply cyanoacrylate glue onto the distal end of the Cancellier instrument with a hand file. The Cancellier instrument is then placed over the exposed instrument fragment and held in place while the assistant places one drop of methyl methacrylate monomer alongside the Cancellier instrument and directs

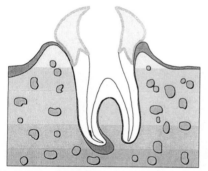

1. Problem: Separated instrument at the bottom of the root end canal.

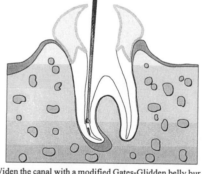

2. Widen the canal with a modified Gates-Glidden belly bur all the way down to the instrument.

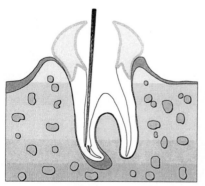

3. Use a Fine Spreader ultrasonic tip to create a trough around the broken file or instrument.

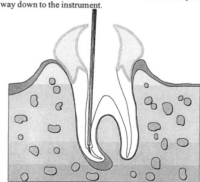

4. Put Superglue on the hollow end of the correct size Cancellier instrument. Place the Cancellier on top of the broken instrument and withdraw from canal. Use acetone to remove glue from instrument.

FIG. 24-72 Steps in preparing a staging platform for close examination.

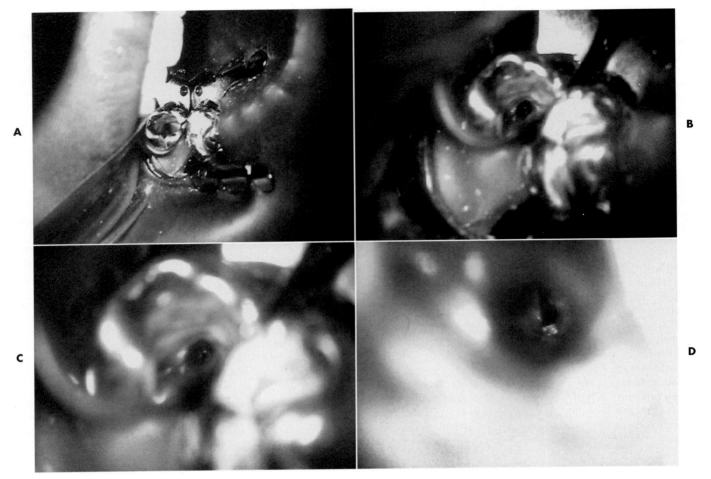

FIG. 24-73 A through D, Various microscopic magnifications showing troughing around separated instrument. C, Higher magnification of fractured instrument. D, Highest magnification shows a clear view of the fractured instrument.

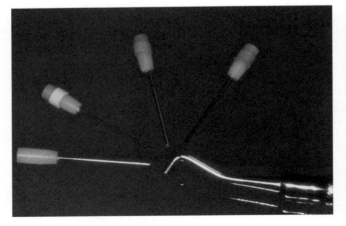

FIG. 24-74 Cancellier series of instruments.

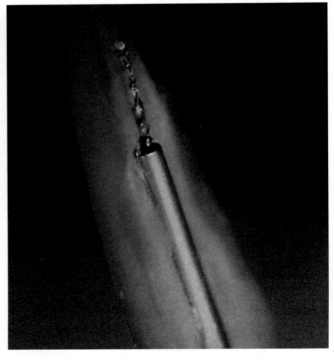

FIG. 24-75 Engagement of Cancellier instrument-extraction with separated instrument.

the monomer down the Cancellier instrument with a Stropko-syringe (Fig. 24-76). The monomer initiates a flash-set of the cyanoacrylate glue. After the glue sets, the hand carrier is un-threaded from the cannula, and gentle coronal pressure is used to deliver the fractured fragment (Fig. 24-77). The troughing, the sizing, and the placement of the Cancellier instruments are performed using high magnification. Once the clinician develops these sophisticated skills, even instruments in the apical third of roots can be removed (see Fig. 24-77).

Fractured nickel-titanium instruments present a unique chal-lenge to the dentist. Because of the thermodynamic properties of nickel-titanium, ultrasonic vibration of these instruments produces a rapid heating and spontaneous disintegration of the metal. For this reason the troughing procedure must be per-formed with great precision so as to avoid metal contact dur-ing creation of the trough. After the troughing is completed, the instrument fragment can be removed by either the Cancel-lier technique (recommended) or by reducing the ultrasonic power setting to its minimum and attempting to vibrate the ex-posed fragment coronally; this requires water to minimize heat buildup. Water irrigation during vibration obstructs visibility, making the removal of nickel-titanium instruments more diffi-cult than the removal of stainless steel instruments, which can be removed without water irrigation. The technique for removal of nickel-titanium ThermaFil carriers is identical to the removal of nickel-titanium files.

PERFORATION REPAIR

The ideal material for sealing perforations should be bio-compatible, seal hermetically, and support a healing response in the periodontal ligament. This material should chemically bond to dentin, should allow for easy placement, be able to withstand the compressive and tensile forces to which dentin is subjected, be radiopaque, have a similar modulus of elastic-

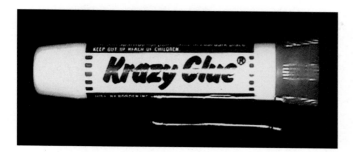

FIG. 24-76 Cyanoacrylate cement.

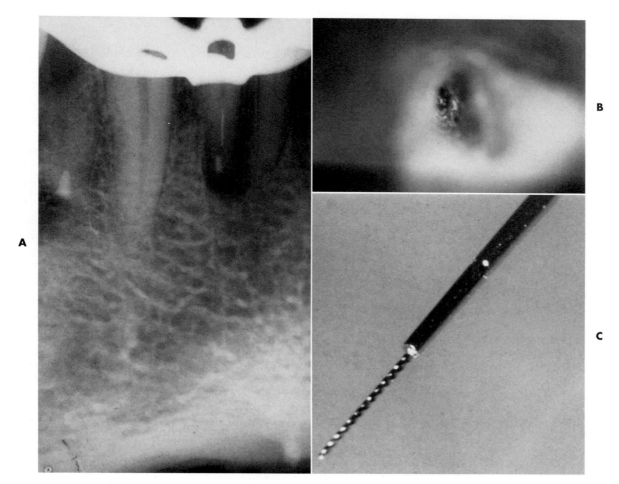

FIG. 24-77 A through **E,** Separated instrument cases showing use of the Cancellier instru-ments. **E,** Complete periapical remineralization. *Continued*

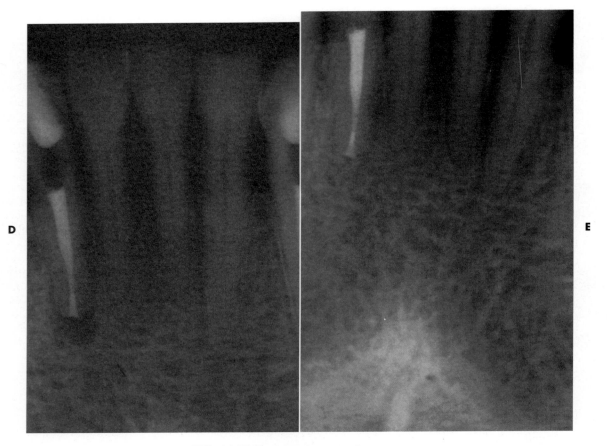

FIG. 24-77 For legend see previous page.

ity to dentin, and allow for the growth of cementoblasts on its surface. Such a dental material does not yet exist. Long-term retrospective studies evaluating perforation repair have yet to be undertaken[28,37,38.40].

Classification of perforations

A formal classification of perforations has not been established.[58] Perforations, however, can be classified by size (micro or macro), location (supracrestal or subcrestal), type (strip, zip, or furcal), length of time before repair (immediate or delayed), and degree of bone destruction. Each of these categories is significant and needs to be evaluated prior to treatment.

Size of perforation. Successful perforation repair depends on (1) hermetic sealing of the perforation and (2) reestablishment of a healthy periodontal ligament.[58] *The success of the hermetic seal decreases as the circumferential length of the perforation increases because the greater the perimeter, the higher the possibility of marginal leakage.*

The probability of successful reattachment of the periodontal ligament is dependent on the size of surface area that must be repaired; for that reason, larger perforations are less likely to be successfully repaired. For example, a large No. 8 round bur perforation through the furcal floor has a much lesser chance of successful repair than a No. 8 reamer perforation through the furcal floor.

Location of perforation. Perforations can be located anywhere within the root or pulp chamber. The significance of the location relates to whether the perforation is coronal (supracrestal) to the level of the alveolar bone or apical (subcrestal) to the level of the alveolar bone. Supracrestal perforations have a more guarded prognosis because they are exposed to the oral environment.[48] A long-term hermetic seal is unlikely to endure in this environment with the reparative materials we presently possess.

Subcrestal perforations have the theoretic advantage of being able to be sealed off from the oral environment but the disadvantage of being difficult to inspect because of their deeper location. Most subcrestal perforations are located on the lateral root surface and, as such, are difficult to view even with a microscope.

Type of perforation. The type of perforation (i.e., strip or furcal) will determine how easily the defect can be repaired. A strip perforation is typically an irregular, oval-shaped window located on the lateral root surface that can only be examined obliquely. A furcal perforation, however, can be inspected with direct vision and therefore, has a much higher likelihood of being sealed accurately.

Length of time before repair. Perforations repaired immediately after the occurence have the best prognosis.[37,38,60,63] Delayed repairs risk the development of inflammation and concentration of inflammatory mediators situated adjacent to the site of injury, with subsequent breakdown of the collagen fibrils of the periodontal ligament and eventual loss of supporting alveolar bone. Frequently, tissue from the gingival sulcus or peiodontal ligament invaginates through the perforation,

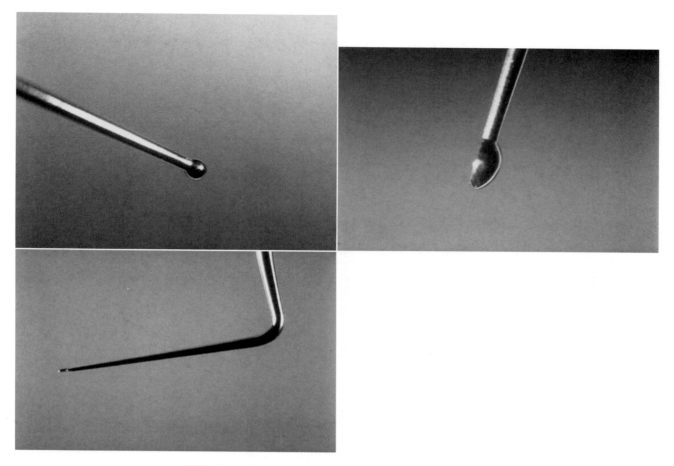

FIG. 24-78 Sharp series of perforation repair instruments.

creating a situation that is difficult to manage as this granulomatous tissue is hyperplastic and hypervascular. This tissue can be very difficult to remove and nearly always results in an operative site where hemostasis cannot be controlled. The use of nonspecific cellular intravascular clotting agents (e.g., ferric subsulfate) commonly used to control bleeding is contraindicated, as these chemicals can irreversibly damage delicate alveolar bone.[41,42]

Degree of bone destruction. The amount of bone destruction before repair also affects the prognosis. If little or no bone destruction is present, the perforation can remain a subcrestal defect and gain the advantage of not being exposed to the oral environment. If bone destruction is present, however, then contamination of the defect by oral microorganisms greatly compromises the prognosis.[58] Alveolar bone also provides the vascularity necessary to mount a competent reparative or regenerative response.

Techniques in perforation repair

Historically, perforation techniques have been directed to effecting a hermetic seal at the margins of the perforation. Before the introduction of microscopic techniques, these procedures were less predictable. *Perforation repair is most effective when performed under the microscope.* Fig. 24-78 illustrates the specialized armamentarium that has been developed to take advantage of the greater visual control possible using the microscope. These instruments are miniaturized restorative tools configured to operate within the limited confines of a root. Perforation repairs made with these instruments use the higher powers of magnification and refined tactile skills. Fig. 24-79 illustrates one such case using Super EBA as the reparative material. A discussion of the various reparative materials appears in Chapter 18.

It is not desirable to have the restorative material expressed into the ligament during its placement. Since all the currently used materials are either flowable or moldable at the time of placement, material expressed into the ligament is akin to leaving an overhang in restorative dentistry. However, in restorative dentistry, overhangs can be removed, whereas in perforation repairs, there is no access to subcrestal areas to allow trimming of the excess. For this reason, resorbable, biologic matrixes are used to pack the ligament space and provide a barrier that prevents the extraneous insertion of sealing material into the periodontal ligament space. Materials used for this barrier formation are bovine collagen (CollaCote), calcium sulfate, mineral trioxide, decalcified freeze-dried bone, or synthetic bone substitutes. Well-controlled long-term evaluation of these materials is ongoing.[59,63]

THE MICROSCOPE

The operating microscope has achieved a central position in the development of innovative techniques in all phases of endodontics. This section will review the uses of the operating microscope in endodontics.

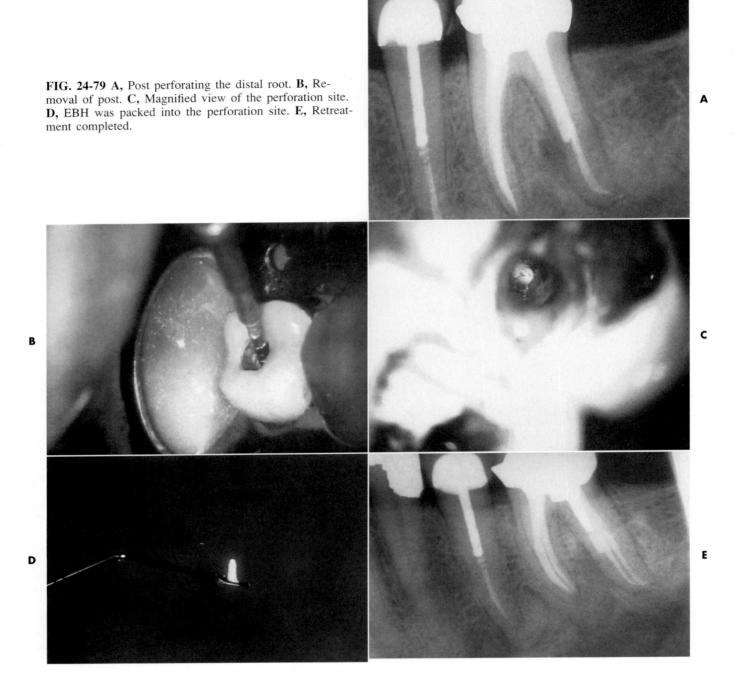

FIG. 24-79 A, Post perforating the distal root. **B,** Removal of post. **C,** Magnified view of the perforation site. **D,** EBH was packed into the perforation site. **E,** Retreatment completed.

Optical Principles

Operating microscopes used in endodontics are composed of a main section (body) that houses the objective lens and a binocular section that holds the eyepieces (Fig. 24-80).

Simple microscopes magnify at one fixed magnification, which is calculated by multiplying the focal length of the objective lens by the magnifying power of the eyepieces. More advanced microscopes contain a *magnification changer* (Fig. 24-81), which is a series of intermediate lenses placed between the objective lens and eyepieces that provides for a range of magnifications depending on the number of lenses (steps) placed in the changing turret.[26a,51a]

Microscopes used in endodontics require a three-step or five-step magnification changer. Useful magnification needed for endodontics are 2.5× to 40×.[29,12,13]

Operating microscopes are *Galilean* optical devices, meaning that the optical path is parallel rather than convergent. Gallilean optics are always focused at infinity and are referred to as infinity-corrected optics.[51a,53a] This means that the user is focused at infinity even though the object of observation is actually at the focal length of the objective lens (200 to 300 mm).

The advantage of Gallilean optics is that the parallel light beams may be "split" without sacrificing the stereopsis of the

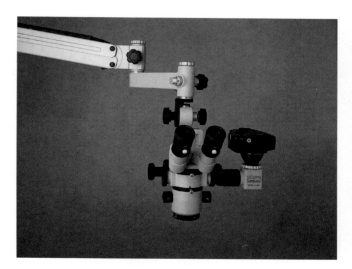

FIG. 24-80 The operating microscope.

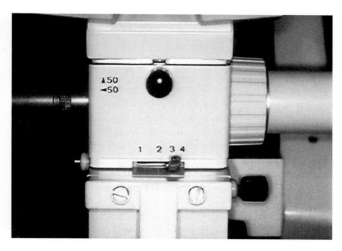

FIG. 24-82 35-mm camera and videocamera mounted to operating microscope.

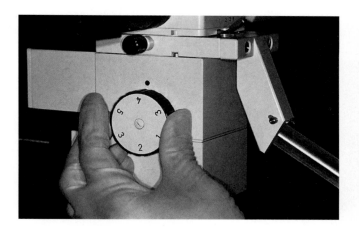

FIG. 24-81 The five-step magnification changer.

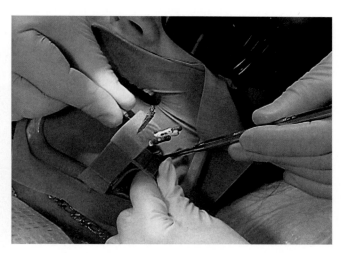

FIG. 24-83 Universal hand signal for a K-file.

viewer. The light is split by a *beam splitter* placed between the magnification changer and the binoculars. This division of the light allows accessory devices to be added to the microscope, such as assistants' viewports, videocameras (cine), and 35-mm cameras (Fig. 24-82).

Positioning

The correct positioning of the doctor, patient, assistant, and microscope is essential for the efficient utilization of microscopic techniques. Well-trained clinicians are capable of performing all endodontic procedures using the microscope with an efficiency far exceeding that of nonmicroscopic practitioners. The efficient use of the microscope depends upon positioning skills that result in a minimal need to reposition the microscope despite constantly changing fields of view and magnification ranges.

The patient is seated in the Trendelenberg position with the head and neck supported; many microscopic procedures require the hyperextension of the patient's head. The doctor then assumes an upright posture and positions the microscope

to conform to this upright posture. After comfortable positioning of the doctor and the microscope, the patient is raised or lowered to the appropriate height so that the patient's tooth is in focus. The assistant then positions the assistant's scope so the he or she is upright and comfortable as well.

Ergonomics

Endodontic procedures performed under the microscope require a disciplined and methodical approach. Well-trained clinicians understand the value of distinct, well-controlled hand movements and the importance of skilled dental assistants. A series of *universal hand signals* has been developed, which facilitate the passing of instruments under the microscope without having to look away from the oculars. One example is shown in Fig. 24-83.

Many of the microscopic techniques recently developed require very stable hand movements in a range where physiologic hand tremor becomes a significant issue. Proper hand, arm, and elbow placement is essential if these motions are to be minimized.[20a,50a,51b]

The Role of the Microscope in Nonsurgical Endodontics

Every aspect of conventional endodontics is enhanced by a microscopic approach, from diagnosis to final restoration. Examining caries, crown margins, subgingival defects, and fractures, and even detecting crown/root mobility, is more easily accomplished under the higher magnification and lighting levels of the operating microscope (Fig. 24-84).[12,13,57a,57b]

Access preparations inspected at 12× to 15× gain an added dimension of precision, eliminating much guesswork and unnecessary removal of tooth structure; minor errors in access openings are a significant factor in endodontic failure. Highly illuminated and magnified inspection of the pulpal floor and orifice openings results in far fewer iatrogenic injuries while simultaneously allowing for the discovery of aberrant canal anatomy or the uncovering and instrumentation of atypical canal morphology. Coronal or pulp chamber obstructions are easily distinguished from primary or secondary dentin.

The Role of the Microscope in Retreatment Endodontics

Calcified canals, complex anatomy, separated instruments, and abberant canal location are all clinical situations where the use of the microscope is paramount in producing a competent solution. Indeed, sophisticated skill development of microscopic techniques can reduce the need for a surgical approach considerably.

Use of the Microscope in Surgical Endodontics

The introduction of the operating microscope to endodontics has greatly enhanced the ability of the surgeon to inspect, prepare, and seal the apical ramifications. Before this technology was available, skillful surgery required the use of high-powered loupes and surgical headlights. Although these enhancements provided the surgeon increased visibility, the surgical assistant frequently struggled with limited visibility and access. Because the range of magnification needed for periapical procedures varies from 3 to 30 times, the surgeon is forced to change loupes frequently during the procedure. The operating microscope provides commanding visual control over the surgical site for both the doctor and the first surgical assistant, in addition to providing five times the illumination of surgical headlights.[12,13,14a,51c] This powerful instrument enables the surgeon to change powers rapidly and with ease throughout the surgery. Having the first surgical assistant at the microscope permits the addition of another pair of skilled hands into the surgical site and greatly facilitates the delicate procdures performed there. True surgical microscopes have the

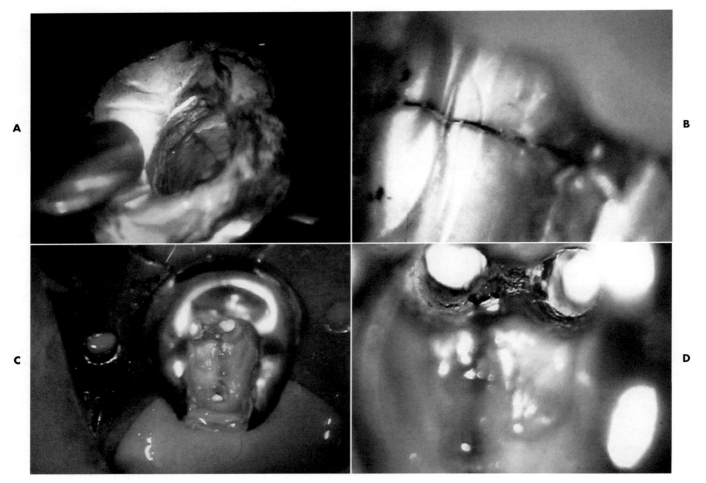

24-84 A, Low magnification of distal marginal ridge fracture. **B,** High magnification of same fracture. **C,** Medium magnification of furcal floor. **D,** High magnification of furcal floor. Note obturation of furcal canal.

capability of adding documentation modules that allow simultaneous video and 35-mm photography with virtually no interruption in the surgical routine. This comprehensive documentation capability has applications in patient, doctor, and assistant education. It also provides a permanent record for insurance and legal purposes.

Microscopic Armamentarium

The microsurgical approach to endodontic surgery has necessitated the development of a dedicated surgical armamentarium specifically designed for microsurgical procedures. The miniaturization of instruments to the appropriate scale allows the surgeon to take full advantage of the enhanced vision the microscope provides. Miniaturized optical grade retromirrors introduced into the surgical site allow examination in intimate detail of the apical anatomy of the beveled root system[2]. These mirrors also permit close inspection of furcal defects and lateral root surfaces that previously were hidden from view. Particularly invaluable is the ability to inspect at high magnification and high illumination the lingual aspects of beveled roots, second canal systems, isthmuses, and aberrant portals of exit: all can be clearly seen. Additionally, the surgeon may decrease the bevel placed on these roots and can now section them more perpendicular to the long axis of the root. A highly skilled surgeon can section the root perpendicular to the long axis and inspect, prepare, and seal the root end indirectly using a mirror.

Working with upside-down images using a micromirror in tandem with an operating microscope demands a series of progressive skills that are mastered more easily by a dentist than any other health professional. The development of microsurgical skills requires patience, practice, and an extraordinary amount of coordination among the surgical team. Achieving competence in this skill is well worth the effort and goes a long way toward reducing the stress level that surgeons typically experience while performing difficult posterior surgery.

The application of the operating microscope not only to surgical endodontics but also to nonsurgical endodontics points to the next era in endodontics, in which previously untreatable cases will be handled with great expertise by highly trained practitioners for the benefit of their patients. For the many benefits the operating microscope provides, it represents the evolving state of the art and science in endodontics.

REFERENCES

1. American Association of Endodontists: *Glossary of contemporary terminology for endodontics,* 1994.
2. Abdel-Fattah RA: Diagnosis and prevention of temporomandibular joint (TMJ) or odontostomatognathic (OSG) injury in dental practice, *Todays FDA* 2:1c, 6c-8c, 1990.
2a. Apotheker H: A microscope for use in dentistry, *J Microsurg* 3:7, 1981.
3. Alantar A, Tarragano H, Lefevre B: Extrusion of endodontic filling material into the insertions of the mylohyoid muscle: a case report, *Oral Surg Oral Med Oral Pathol* 78:646, 1994.
4. Allebring M, Haegerstam G: Invasive dental treatment, pain reports, and disease conviction in chronic facial pain patients: a retrospective study, *Acta Odontol Scand* 1:41, 1995.
5. Augsburger RA, Peters DD: Radiographic evaluation of extruded obturation materials, *J Endod* 16:492, 1990.
6. Barbasa S, Burkard DH, Larz S: Cytotoxic effects of gutta percha solvents, *J Endod* 20:6, 1994.
7. Barkhodar RN, Stewart GG: The potential of periodontal pocket formation associated with untreated accessory root canals, *Oral Surg Oral Med Oral Pathol* 70:769, 1990.
8. Baumgartner JC, Mader CI: A scanning electron microscopic evaluation of four root canal irrigation regimens, *J Endod* 13:147, 1987.
9. Berbert A, Filho MT, Ueno AH, Bramante CM: The influence of ultrasound in removing intraradicular posts, *Int Endodont J* 28:54, 1995.
10. Berutti E, Marini R: A scanning electron microscopic evaluation of the debridement capability of sodium hypochlorite at different temperatures, *J Endod* 22:467, 1996.
11. Borg E, Grendahl HG: Endodontic measurements in digital radiographs acquired by a photostimulable, storage phosphorsystem, *Endodont Dent Traumatol* 12:20, 1996.
12. Carr GB: Microscopes in endodontics, *J Calif Dent Assoc* 20:55, 1992.
13. Carr GB: Endodontics at the crossroads, *J Calif Dent Assoc* 24:20, 1996.
14. Cunningham W, Joseph E: Effect of temperature on the bactericidal action of sodium hypochlorite endodontic irrigant, *Oral Surg* 50:569, 1980.
14a. Daniel RK: Microsurgery: through the looking glass, *N Engl J Med* 300:1251, 1975.
15. Davidson IWF, Summer DD, Parker JC: Chloroform, a review of its metabolism, teratogenic, mutagenic and carcinogenic potential, *Drug Chem Toxicol* 5:1, 1982.
16. Engstrom B et al: Correlation of positive cultures with the prognosis for root canal therapy, *Odontol Revy* 15:257, 1964.
17. Friedman S, Moshonor J, Trope M: Resistance to vertical fracture of roots, previously fractured and bonded with glass ionomer cement, composite resin and cyanoacrylate cement, *Endodont Dent Traumatol* 9:40, 1993.
18. Frank AL, Glick DH, Patterson SS, Weine FS: Long-term evaluation of surgically placed amalgam fillings, *J Endod* 18:391, 1992.
19. Friedman S, Stabholz A: Endodontic retreatment retreatment: case selection and technique. I. Criteria for case selection, *J Endod* 12:28, 1986.
20. Gilles J, Reader A: An SEM investigation of the mesiolingual canal in human maxillary first and second molars, *Oral Surg* 70:638, 1990.
20a. Glenncross DJ: The control of skilled movements, *Psychol Bull,* 1977.
21. Goon WW, Lugassy AA: The periapical electrolytic corrosion in the failure of silver point endodontic restorations: report of two cases, *Quintessence Int* 26:629, 1995.
22. Halse A, Molven O: Overextended gutta percha and Kloropercha N-o root canal fillings: radiographic findings after 10-17 years, *Acta Odontol Scand* 20:171, 1987.
23. Hammerstrom LE, Blomloef LB, Feiglin B, Lindskog SF: Effect of calcium hydroxide treatment on periodontal repair and root resorption, *Endodonts Dent Traumatol* 2:184, 1986.
24. Harness DM, Donlon WC, Eversole LR: Comparison of clinical characteristics in myogenic TMJ internal derangement and atypical facial pain patients, *Clin J Pain* 8:4, 1990.
25. Hess JC, Culieras JM, Lamiable N: A scanning electron microscopic investigation of principal and accessory foramina on the root surfaces of human teeth: thoughts about endodontic pathology and therapeutics, *J Endod* 9:275, 1983.
26. Hess W: *Anatomy of the root canals of the teeth of permanent dentition, part I,* ed 3, New York, 1925, William Wood.
26a. Hoerenz P: The operating microscope. I. Optical principles, *J Microsurg* 1:364, 1980.
27. Hunter KR, Doblecki W, Pelleu GB: Halothane an eucalyptol as alternative to chloroform for softening gutta percha, *J Endod* 17:310, 1991.
28. Jew RC, Weine FS, Keene JJ, Smulson MH: A histological tissues adjacent to root perforations filled with Cavit, *Oral Surg* 54:124, 1982.
29. Kakehashi S, Stanley HR, Fitzgerald RJ: The effect of surgical exposure of dental pulps in germ-free and conventional laboratory rats, *Oral Surg* 20:340, 1965.
30. Kaplan SD, Tanzilli JP, Raphael D, Moodnick RM: A comparison of the marginal leakage of retrograde techniques, *Oral Surg* 54:583, 1982.
31. Kaplowitz GJ: Evaluation of gutta percha solvents, *J Endod* 16:539, 1990.

32. Kersten HW, Wesselink PR, Thoden van Velzen SK: The diagnostic reliability of the buccal radiograph after root canal filling, *Int Endodont J* 20:20, 1987.

33. Kontakiotis E, Nakou M: In vitro study of the indirect action of calcium hydroxide on the anaerobic flora of the root canal canal, *Int Endodont J* 28:285, 1995.

34. Kucukay IK: Root canal ramifications in mandibular incisors and efficacy of low temperatures injection thermoplasticized gutta percha filling, *Oral Surg* 20:236, 1994.

35. Kvinnsland I, Heyeraas KJ: Effect of traumatic occlusion on CGRP and SP immunoreactive nerve fibre morphology in rat pulp and periodontium, *Histochemistry* 97:111, 1992.

36. Langeland K, Block RM, Grossman LI: A histopathologic and histobacteriologic study of 35 periapical lesions specimens, *J Endod* 3:8, 1977.

37. Lantz B, Persson PA: Experimental root perforation in dogs' teeth: a roentgen study, *Odontol T* 16:238, 1965.

38. Lantz B, Persson PA: Periodontal tissue reactions after root perforations in dogs' teeth: a histological study, *Odontol T* 75:209, 1967.

39. Lavelle CL, Wu CJ: Digital radiographic images will benefit endodontic services, *Endodont Dent Traumatol* 11:253, 1995.

40. Lee SJ, Monsef M, Torabinejad M: Sealing ability of a mineral trioxide aggregate for repair of lateral root perforations, *J Endod* 19:541, 1993.

41. Lemon RR, Jeansonne BG, Boggs WS: Ferric sulfate hemostasis: effect on osseous wound healing. II. With curettage and irrigation, *J Endod* 19:174, 1993.

42. Lemon RR, Steele PJ, Jeansonne BG: Ferric sulfate hemostasis: effect on osseous wound healing. I. Left in situ for maximum exposure, *J Endod* 19:170, 1993.

43. Lin LM et al: Clinical, radiographic, and histologic study of endodontic treatment failures, *Oral Surg Oral Med Oral Pathol* 71:603, 1991.

44. Lin LM, Skribner JE, Gaengler P: Factors associated with endodontic treatment failures, *J Endod* 18:625, 1992.

45. Lin LM et al: Clinical and histological study of endodontic treatment failures, *Oral Surg* 11:603, 1991.

46. Machtou P, Sarfati P, Cohen AG: Postremoval prior to retreatment, *J Endod* 15:552, 1989.

47. Madison S, Swanson K, Chiles SA: An evaluation of coronal microleakage in endodontically treated teeth. II. Sealer types, *J Endod* 13:109, 1987.

48. Martin LR, Gilbert B, Dickerson AW: Management of endodontic perforations, *Oral Surg Oral Med Oral Pathol* 54:668, 1982.

49. Meister F, Lommel TJ, Gerstein H: Diagnosis and possible causes of vertical root fracture, *Oral Surg* 49:243, 1980.

50. Mellonig JT, Bowers GM, Cotton WR: Comparison of bone graft materials. II. New bone formation with autografts and allografts: a histological evaluation, *J Periodontol* 52:297, 1981.

50a. Murrell KFH: Ergonomics: *man in his working environment,* London, 1965, Chapman Hall.

51. Neff P: Trauma from occlusion: restorative concerns (review), *Dent Clin North Am* 39:335, 1995.

51a. Owen ER: Practical microsurgery. I. A choice of optical aids, *Med J Aust* 1:244, 1971.

51b. Patkin M: Ergonomics applied to microsurgery, *Austr NZ J Surg* 47:320, 1977.

51c. Pecora G, Andreana S: Use of dental operating microscope in endodontic surgery, *Oral Surg Oral Med Oral Path* 75:751, 1993.

52. Pineda F, Kuttler U: Mesiodistal and buccolingual roentgenographic investigations of 7275 root canals, *Oral Surg* 33:101, 1972.

53. Pitt DL, Natkin E: Diagnosis and treatment of vertical root fractures, *J Endod* 9:333, 1983.

53a. Rock JA, Berquist CA, et al: Comparison of the operating microscope and loupes, *Fertil Steril* 41:229, 1984.

54. Rubach WC, Mitchell DF: Periodontal disease, accessory canals and pulpal pathosis, *J Periodontol* 54:1, 1964.

55. Safavi KE, Nichols FC: Effect of $Ca(OH)_2$ on bacterial lipopolysaccharide, *J Endod* 19:76, 1993.

56. Saunders WP, Saunders EM: Coronal leakage as a cause of failure in root canal therapy: a review, *Endodont Dent Traumatol* 10:105, 1994.

57. Schilder H: Filling root canals in three dimensions, *Dent Clin North Am* 11:723, 1967.

57a. Selden HS: The role of the dental operating microscope in endodontics, *Pa Dent J* 53:36, 1986.

57b. Selden HS: The role of the dental operating microscope in improved nonsurgical trearment of "calcified" canals, *Oral Surg Oral Med Oral Pathol* 68:93, 1989.

58. Seltzer S, Sinai IH, August D: Periodontal effects of root perforations before and during endodontic procedures, *J Dent Res* 49:332, 1970.

59. Seltzer et al: Endodontic failures: an analysis based on clinical roentgenographic and histologic findings. I & II, *Oral Surg* 23:500, 1967.

60. Seltzer S et al: A scanning electron examination of silver cones removed from endodontically treated teeth, *Oral Surg* 33:589, 1972.

61. Simring M, Goldberg M: The pulpal periodontal approach: retrograde periodontitis, *J Periodontol* 35:22, 1964.

62. Sjogren U, Hagglund B, Sundqvist G, Wing K: Factors affecting the long-term results of endodontic treatment, *J Endod* 16:498, 1990.

63. Sonis ST et al: Healing of spontaneous periodontal defects in dogs treated with xerogenic demineralized bone, *J Periodontol* 52:297, 1985.

64. Squire RA: Ranking animal carcinogens: a proposed regularity approach, *Science* 214:877, 1981.

65. Swanson KS, Madison S: An evaluation of coronal microleakage in endodontically treated teeth. I. Time periods, *J Endod* 12:56, 1987.

66. Torabinejad M, Ung B, Kettering JD: In vitro bacterial penetration of coronally unsealed endodontically treated teeth, *J Endod* 16:566, 1990.

67. van Nieuwenhuysen JP, Aouar M, D'Hoore W: Retreatment or radiographic monotoring in endodontics, *Int Endodont J* 27:75, 1994.

68. Velvart P: Das Operationsmikroskop, neue Dimensionen in der Endodontie, *Schweiz Monatsschr Zahnmed* 106:357, 1996.

69. Vertucci FJ: Root canal morphology of mandibular premolars, *J Am Dent Assoc* 97:47, 1978.

70. Vertucci F, Seelig A, Gillis R: Root canal morphology of human maxillary second premolar, *Oral Surg* 38:456, 1974.

71. Weine FW, Rice RT: Handling previously treated silver points cases: removal, retreatment and tooth retention, *Compend Contin Educ Dent* 7:652, 1986.

72. Weine F et al: Canal configuration in the mesiobuccal root of the maxillary first molar and its endodontic significance, *Oral Surg* 28:419, 1969.

73. Weller RN, Niemczyk SP, Kim S: Incidence and position of the canal isthmus. I. Mesiobuccal root of the maxillary first molar, *J Endod* 21:380, 1995.

74. Wourms DJ et al: Alternative solvents to chloroform for gutta percha removal, *J Endod* 16:539, 1990.

75. Yusuf H: The significance of the presence of foreign material periapically as a cause of failure of root treatment, *Oral Surg Oral Med Oral Pathol* 54:566, 1982.

PART FOUR

ISSUES IN ENDODONTICS

Chapter **25**

The Future

Stephen Cohen

In the next decade the application of new knowledge and information will be the primary means by which the quality and effectiveness of endodontic therapy will be enhanced. The growth and preeminence of technologic advancement and the accelerating pace of discovery in the disciplines of basic science ensure an ever-expanding universe of new information, new devices, better materials, and sophisticated technologies. What is less certain is the context in which dentists will use this new knowledge and information for the benefit of their patients.

The appropriate application of this new knowledge and information will depend to some extent on each dentist's commitment to ongoing improvement of his or her clinical skills. However, the creation of the proper context for the application of these skills will depend on how willing each dentist is to work with the following new realities of health care:

- Need for full and effective communication with patients in explaining endodontic issues and treatment choices: Patient preferences must be honored and patients' autonomy must be respected in the formation of a dentist-patient partnership for decision making.
- Need to forge a closer connection between dental generalists and dental specialists and between dentists and physicians
- Need for a dramatic upgrading of each dentist's diagnostic skills: The increasingly complex care issues of an aging and multiethnic population require more accurate and timely disease identification.

These new realities of care for patients will be accompanied by new realities in care delivery systems and devices.

These will include the following:

- Widespread adoption of engine-driven instruments: Improved materials, better machining of canal enlarging instruments, and improvements in the dentist's tactile sense will lead to the use of engine-driven instruments as the norm in endodontic therapy.
- Agreement that hand-filing instruments should be regarded as disposable instruments
- Significant increase in the use of digital imaging devices: The possibility of smaller pixelation and lower cost will drive this change.
- Agreement that enhanced magnification and illumination should be the clinical standard
- Acceptance of new concepts such as scanning devices to detect pulp blood flow when they can be easily applied
- Increase in the understanding of the best methods for achieving profound local anesthesia for endodontic treatment: This development will allow more dentists to render pain-free endodontic therapy and will lead more patients to see endodontic treatment as a desirable method for relieving pain, swelling, and infection.

Meeting this rich future in endodontics means redefining the purpose of endodontic therapy according to these new realities. Endodontists must come to see themselves as valuable members of a health care team with no special status, but with a deep commitment to finding what is best for each patient. This must be the context in which new knowledge and information is evaluated, embraced, and applied. The result will be patient-centered, patient-sensitive, and effective endodontic care worthy of the challenges of the twenty-first century.

Challenge

Richard E. Walton
William T. Johnson
Lisa R. Wilcox

CHAPTER 1: DIAGNOSTIC PROCEDURES

1. Anesthetic testing is most effective in localizing pain
   a. to a specific tooth.
   b. to the mandible or maxilla.
   c. across the midline of the face.
   d. to a posterior tooth.

2. Areas of rarefaction are evident on radiographic examination when
   a. the tooth is responsive to cold.
   b. the tooth is responsive to percussion.
   c. a tooth fracture has been identified.
   d. the cortical layer of bone has been eroded.

3. Irreversible pulpitis is often defined by
   a. a moderate response to percussion.
   b. a painful response to cold that lingers.
   c. a short painful response to cold.
   d. a short painful response to heat.

4. The majority of patients with presenting symptoms of severe odontogenic pain have a diagnosis of
   a. periodontal abscess.
   b. irreversible pulpitis.
   c. acute apical periodontitis.
   d. acute apical abscess.

5. Medical history of coronary heart disease is significant
   a. and contraindicates endodontic treatment.
   b. because many medications impact dental treatment.
   c. and indicates the need for premedication with antibiotics.
   d. and contraindicates local anesthetic with epinephrine.

6. The best approach for diagnosis of odontogenic pain is
   a. radiographic examination.
   b. percussion.
   c. visual examination.
   d. a step-by-step, sequenced examination and testing approach.

7. Of the following, which is the most likely to have referred pain?
   a. irreversible pulpitis
   b. reversible pulpitis
   c. acute apical periodontitis
   d. phoenix abscess

8. A sinus tract that drains out on the face (through skin) is mostly likely from
   a. nonodontogenic pathosis.
   b. a periodontal abscess.
   c. periradicular (endodontic) pathosis.
   d. pericoronitis of a mandibular third molar.

9. A test cavity
   a. is the first test in diagnostic sequence.
   b. often results in a dull pain response.
   c. is employed when all other test findings are equivocal.
   d. should be performed with local anesthetic.

10. When the patient reports severe pain on biting, the percussion test should
    a. not be performed.
    b. be performed with only a blunt instrument.
    c. be performed only on the facial surface.
    d. be performed first with digital pressure.

11. When pulp stones are clearly evident on radiographs, this indicates
    a. a normal pulp.
    b. the patient is likely to experience pulpal pain in the future.
    c. root canal treatment is necessary (there is irreversible pulpitis).
    d. a pulp that has been injured in the past but has recovered.

12. Radiographically the acute apical abscess
    a. is generally of larger size than other lesions.
    b. has more diffuse margins than other lesions.
    c. often contains radiopacities (calcification).
    d. may not be evident.

13. A false-negative response to the pulp tester may occur
    a. primarily in anterior teeth.
    b. in a patient with a history of trauma.
    c. most often in teenagers.
    d. in the presence of periodontal disease.

14. The lateral periodontal abscess is best differentiated from the acute apical abscess by
    a. pulp testing.
    b. radiographic appearance.
    c. location of swelling.
    d. probing patterns.

15. The acute apical abscess is best differentiated from the acute apical periodontitis by
    a. pulp testing.
    b. radiographic appearance.
    c. presence of swelling.
    d. degree of mobility.
16. Chronic apical periodontitis is best differentiated from acute apical periodontitis by
    a. pulp testing and radiographic appearance.
    b. pulp testing and nature of symptoms.
    c. radiographic appearance and nature of symptoms.
    d. pulp testing, radiographic appearance, and nature of symptoms.

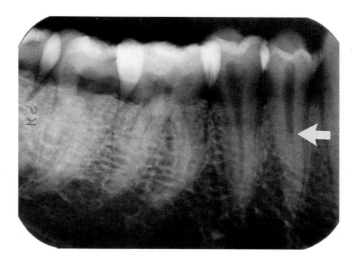

17. The abrupt change *(arrow)* in radiographic appearance in the illustration above likely indicates
    a. calcific metamorphosis.
    b. a dense accumulation of diffuse calcification.
    c. an increased density of overlying bone.
    d. a bifurcation into two canals.

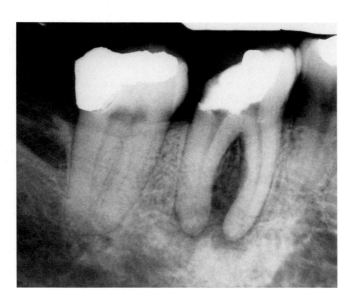

18. The patient in the preceding illustration reports severe, throbbing pain in the mandibular right molar region. The pain is exaggerated by cold. Which tooth and which tissue is *likely* the source of pain?
    a. first molar/pulp
    b. first molar/periapex
    c. second molar/pulp
    d. second molar/periapex

CHAPTER 2: OROFACIAL DENTAL PAIN EMERGENCIES: ENDODONTIC DIAGNOSIS AND MANAGEMENT

1. The degree of pulp pathosis
   a. can be determined by the level of pain a patient experiences.
   b. can be related to the level of response of the electrical pulp tester.
   c. can be correlated best when a diagnosis of irreversible pulpitis is established.
   d. does not correlate well with the level of pain a patient perceives.
2. When treating a patient in pain, all the following are considered key to the psychodynamic exchange between the patient and dentist *except* one. Which is this *exception?*
   a. The patient's symptoms and complaints should be given serious consideration.
   b. The dentist should display empathy and be nonjudgmental.
   c. The dentist should display confidence and professionalism.
   d. The patient should be informed that treatment may not result in relief of the symptoms.
   e. The patient should be made aware of the procedures and physical sensations that will be experienced in treatment.
3. In describing the sensory innervation of the dental pulp
   a. A delta fibers are high threshold myelinated fibers that transmit sharp momentary pain.
   b. C fibers are low threshold unmyelinated fibers that produce pain in response to inflammatory mediators.
   c. the domination of C fiber stimulation produces pain that is not well localized.
   d. the sharp well-localized pain to cold testing is conducted by both A delta and C fiber stimulation.
4. Which of the following induces hyperalgesia in local nerve fibers?
   a. prostaglandin and seratonin
   b. lysosomal enzymes
   c. calcitonin gene-related peptide
   d. substance P
5. Each of the following statements are correct regarding trigeminal neuralgia *except* one. Which is this *exception?*
   a. The onset occurs in midlife and is unilateral in location.
   b. The pain occurs unilaterally but often involves more than one division of the trigeminal nerve.
   c. The pain is characteristically sharp, lasts for several hours, and is induced by a trigger point.
   d. The pain mimics pain of pulpal origin in that thermal sensitivity and tingling is often encountered just before an attack.

6. A patient complains of pain of 3 days' duration on the left side of the face, which the patient relates is dull and constant. The patient notes the pain increases on positional changes such as bending over and when jogging. The most likely diagnosis is
   a. myocardial infarction.
   b. maxillary sinusitis.
   c. atypical facial pain.
   d. irreversible pulpitis.

7. Which of the following most likely indicates pain that is not of pulpal origin?
   a. unilateral pain that radiates over the face to the ear
   b. pain that has paresthesia as a component
   c. pain that is described as throbbing and intermittent
   d. pain that is increased during mastication

8. A complete medical history is essential when treating an emergency dental patient
   a. to identify patients with conditions that would contraindicate root canal treatment.
   b. to determine conditions that might require modifications in the approach to treatment.
   c. to protect the health care team from potential bloodborne pathogens and other infectious diseases the patient may have.
   d. for medical-legal protection and to determine if the medical status will impact the prognosis for root canal treatment.

9. When a patient complains of severe pain that cannot be localized,
   a. the pain is most likely periradicular in origin and likely to persist even when the necrotic pulp is removed.
   b. treatment procedures should be delayed and the condition managed with analgesic medications.
   c. the cause is most likely nonodontogenic in origin.
   d. selective administration of local anesthesia can lead to a definitive diagnosis.
   e. the pulp of more than one tooth will be involved and the pathosis produces a synergistic hyperalgesia response within the central nervous system.

10. A patient's chief complaint is severe pain from the mandibular right first molar, tooth No. 30, when eating ice cream and drinking ice tea. Clinical examination reveals MOD amalgam restorations in all posterior teeth. The margins appear intact and no cracks or caries is detected. Pulp testing indicates all teeth in the quadrant are responsive to electrical pulp testing. Application of cold fails to reproduce the symptoms. Which of the following actions should be taken?
    a. The patient should be dismissed and asked to return when the symptoms increase and the pain to cold becomes prolonged.
    b. Initiate root canal treatment by performing a pulpotomy/pulpectomy on tooth No. 30.
    c. Place a rubber dam on individual teeth and apply ice cold water.
    d. Remove the restoration in tooth No. 30, place a sedative restoration, and prescribe a nonsteroidal antiinflammatory agent.

11. A patient complains of pain to biting pressure and sensitivity to cold in the maxillary left posterior quadrant that subsides within seconds of removal of the stimulus. Clinical examination reveals teeth Nos. 2 and 3 exhibit occlusal amalgams. Which of the following test or actions is most appropriate based on the chief complaint?
    a. Obtain periapical radiographs of the posterior teeth.
    b. Examine with transillumination.
    c. Perform electrical pulp testing.
    d. Perform percussion/palpation testing.

12. A practitioner refers a patient for root canal treatment. The clinician should obtain a new preoperative radiograph
    a. when the film from the referring dentist is more than a month old.
    b. in cases when an emergency treatment procedure was performed.
    c. when the film from the referring dentist reveals a radiolucent area that has a "hanging drop" appearance.
    d. immediately before examining the patient.

13. Which of the following is true regarding the periodontal ligament injection when treating a tooth with a pulpal diagnosis of reversible pulpitis?
    a. There will be a decrease in pulpal blood flow when anesthetic agents with a vasoconstrictor are used.
    b. Damage to the supporting structures can cause continued symptoms.
    c. The periodontal ligament injection is contraindicated when block or infiltration injections are not effective.
    d. The periodontal ligament injection can be employed as primary anesthesia in teeth that exhibit single roots regardless of the number of canals.

14. A patient describes pain on chewing and sensitivity to cold that goes away immediately with removal of the stimulus. The mandibular left second molar, tooth No. 18, exhibits a mesial occlusal crack. The tooth is caries free, and no restorations are present. Periodontal probing depths are 3 mm or less. Which of the following statements is correct?
    a. The pulpal diagnosis is normal pulp, and the tooth should be prepared and restored with a mesial-occlusal bonded amalgam.
    b. The pulpal diagnosis is reversible pulpitis, and the tooth should be restored with a crown.
    c. The pulpal diagnosis is irreversible pulpitis, and root canal treatment should be performed, a bonded amalgam placed, and a crown fabricated.
    d. A radiograph will likely reveal a radiolucent area associated with the mesial root.
    e. The prognosis for the tooth is unfavorable.

15. Treatment of severe throbbing pain associated with the maxillary left first molar, tooth No. 14, is best managed by
    a. pulpotomy.
    b. partial pulpectomy.
    c. pulpectomy.
    d. analgesic agents.
    e. analgesic and antibiotic agents.

16. Leaving a tooth open for drainage in cases of an acute apical abscess
    a. is the recommended method of managing the emergency patient.
    b. may affect the outcome of treatment.
    c. is appropriate providing the patient is also placed on an antibiotic.
    d. should be considered in addition to soft tissue incision and drainage.
17. Administration of antibiotics in treatment of an acute apical abscess secondary to pulp necrosis
    a. is considered an aid to establishing drainage.
    b. will provide adequate levels of the drug at the site of tissue damage.
    c. is effective when the abscess is still primarily an immunologic reaction.
    d. should occur before the clinician initiates root canal treatment procedures.
18. A 21-year-old female model requires emergency treatment of a soft fluctuant swelling over the facial alveolar process of the maxillary left lateral incisor, tooth No. 10. The swelling is visible because of a high lip line. Which of the following statements is correct regarding performing incision and drainage?
    a. The incision should be placed vertically and go directly to bone.
    b. The incision should be horizontal in the attached gingiva at the base of the swelling.
    c. If drainage occurs with the initial incision, blunt dissection is not necessary.
    d. The placement of a drain is necessary for 24 to 48 hours.
19. Incision and drainage of an indurated swelling
    a. should be delayed until it becomes fluctuant.
    b. can reduce pain caused by tissue distention.
    c. provide a purulent exudate for culture and sensitivity testing.
    d. are not indicated, as antibiotic treatment will result in resolution of the lesion.
20. Flare-ups during root canal treatment
    a. are more common in teeth with vital pulp tissue when compared to teeth with pulp necrosis.
    b. are more common in teeth with apical radiolucent areas when compared to teeth with normal periapical tissues.
    c. are associated more frequently with single-visit endodontic procedures.
    d. are more common in symptomatic teeth exhibiting pulp necrosis.
    e. are more common in multirooted teeth.
21. Apical trephination through the faciobuccal cortical plate is advocated
    a. as a mechanism for releasing exudate.
    b. as a routine procedure for relief of pain when the offending tooth has been obturated.
    c. for treatment of severe recalcitrant pain.
    d. between multiple-visit endodontic procedures to prevent the occurrence of a flare-up.

22. A 22-year-old white man requires root canal treatment for pain and swelling in the mandibular anterior area. He notes that his dentist has been treating teeth Nos. 25 and 26 for several months and that swelling has occurred following each visit for cleaning and shaping. Clinical examination reveals swelling located on the alveolar process in the area of the incisor teeth. Teeth Nos. 25 and 26 are tender to palpation and percussion. The clinician should
    a. perform diagnostic tests on the other incisor.
    b. open teeth Nos. 25 and 26, debride these teeth, and place calcium hydroxide as an antimicrobial intracanal medicament.
    c. open teeth Nos. 25 and 26, debride these teeth, and perform incision and drainage.
    d. open teeth Nos. 25 and 26, debride these teeth, and leave the teeth open for drainage.
    e. perform incision and drainage and prescribe an antibiotic for supportive care.

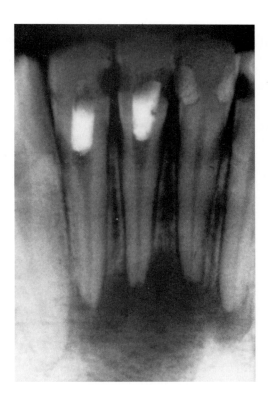

CHAPTER 3: NONODONTOGENIC FACIAL PAIN AND ENDODONTICS: PAIN SYNDROMES OF THE JAWS THAT SIMULATE ODONTALGIA

1. Pain in the absence of identifiable disease is recognized as
    a. acute pain.
    b. inflammation mediated.
    c. hypersensitivity.
    d. chronic pain.
2. Given time, diffuse pain of odontogenic origin will
    a. be referred.
    b. readily abate.
    c. tend to localize to a specific site.
    d. be controlled with analgesics.

3. Trigeminal neuralgia can be treated with
   a. analgesics.
   b. anesthesia to the trigger area.
   c. lysis of the terminal nerve endings.
   d. anticonvulsant drugs.

4. Cluster headache differs from migraine in being
   a. unilateral and involving the teeth.
   b. principally a female complaint.
   c. unilateral and involving the eye.
   d. bilateral.

5. Acute maxillary sinusitis often
   a. results in referred pain to a single tooth.
   b. results in referred pain to the orbit and maxillary posterior teeth.
   c. is exacerbated by cold testing.
   d. results in swelling in the maxillary posterior vestibule.

6. Degenerative joint disease often
   a. results in posterior displacement of the meniscus.
   b. results in malocclusion.
   c. allows for wide mouth opening.
   d. leads to adhesions and arthritic changes.

7. Of the facial pain syndromes, that which most often mimics odontogenic pain is
   a. trigeminal neuralgia.
   b. cluster headache.
   c. atypical facial pain.
   d. phantom tooth pain.

8. Atypical facial pain can be treated most effectively by
   a. microvascular decompression.
   b. radiofrequency gangliolysis.
   c. NSAIDs.
   d. tricyclic antidepressant drugs.

9. Phantom tooth (deafferentation) pain may
   a. occur briefly after tooth extraction.
   b. be simply a peripheral phenomenon.
   c. occur for an extended period after pulp extirpation.
   d. be managed by analgesics.

10. A definite diagnosis of facial causalgia can be made
    a. by lidocaine infiltration.
    b. by use of analgesics.
    c. by use of ipsilateral stellate ganglion block.
    d. by observation of symptoms.

11. Myalgic pain in the muscles of mastication may often be best diagnosed by
    a. identifying trigger point foci in the affected muscle.
    b. ruling out endodontic etiologies.
    c. determining if occlusal equilibration will relieve the pain.
    d. having the patient lie on his or her back; if the pain subsides, it likely is myalgia.

12. Pain syndromes that are not organically based generally are of what nature?
    a. short duration, sharp
    b. short duration, dull (aching)
    c. long duration, sharp
    d. long duration, dull (aching)

13. The atypical pain entity known as neuralgia-inducing cavitational osteonecrosis (NICO) has what treatment consideration?
    a. Most resolve spontaneously without treatment.
    b. The majority of patients demonstrate a favorable long-term outcome after treatment.
    c. Because the entity is inflammatory, it responds favorably to steroid therapy.
    d. Most patients have only temporary relief from treatment.

14. Proproceptive signals terminate in the
    a. caudate nucleus of V.
    b. mesencephalic nucleus.
    c. interpolaris nucleus of V.
    d. gasserian ganglion.

15. Each of the following is characteristic of chronic pain *except* one. Which is this *exception?*
    a. pain that shows no organic basis
    b. pain that becomes more intense as the day progresses
    c. pain that occurs in association with a motor deficit
    d. pain that is not localized

16. A 50-year-old male patient has a presenting chief complaint of severe, lancinating, shooting pain in the right mandibular anterior region that lasts for several seconds. Root canal treatment of the mandibular right central and lateral incisors has not provided relief. The most likely etiologic basis for the pain in this case is
    a. odontalgia.
    b. trigeminal neuralgia.
    c. cardiogenesis.
    d. cluster headaches.

17. Each of the following is characteristic of cluster headaches *except* one. Which is this *exception?*
    a. The disease generally affects females in the fifth and sixth decades and mimics pulpitis in the maxillary posterior teeth.
    b. The onset of pain is common after consumption of alcoholic beverages.
    c. The pain is unilateral in the maxilla, sinus, and retro-orbital area.
    d. The pain has an acute onset that lasts 30 to 45 minutes.
    e. Symptoms tend to occur at approximately the same time each day.

18. Neuralgia-inducing cavitational osteonecrosis is best managed with
    a. amitriptyline.
    b. prednisone.
    c. root canal treatment or extraction.
    d. surgical curettage.

19. Which of the following can occur with the administration of carbamazepine (Tegretol)?
    a. agranulocytosis
    b. electrolyte imbalance
    c. renal toxicity
    d. adrenal suppression
    e. increased intraocular pressure

20. A common feature of pain secondary to malignant disease is
    a. paresthesia.
    b. hyperalgesia.
    c. myalgia.
    d. referred pain.

CHAPTER 4: CASE SELECTION AND TREATMENT PLANNING

1. Electronic apex locators may be useful when
   a. the patient is physically impaired.
   b. anatomic structures overlay the root apex.
   c. a pregnant patient wishes to avoid x-ray exposure.
   d. all of the above.
2. Antibiotic premedication for patients with prosthetic joints is
   a. empiric and on the recommendation of the patient's orthopedist.
   b. scientifically valid and supported by numerous research studies.
   c. the same as for the American Heart Association regimen for infective endocarditis prophylaxis.
3. Elective endodontic treatment is contraindicated when the patient
   a. is a borderline diabetic.
   b. had a heart attack within the last 6 months.
   c. has had numerous opportunistic infections secondary to HIV infection.
   d. has an implanted pacemaker.
4. External resorptions
   a. are untreatable.
   b. can only be distinguished surgically from internal resorptions.
   c. appear to be superimposed over the root canal.
5. Referral of difficult cases is indicated when the dentist
   a. does not have the indicated equipment.
   b. does not have the indicated training and experience.
   c. is not sure what procedures are indicated.
   d. all of the above.
6. One-appointment root canal treatment
   a. is best performed in association with trephination or root end surgery.
   b. may predispose the patient to postoperative flare-ups.
   c. is equally successful as multiple-appointment root canal treatment.
   d. all of the above.
7. Multiple-appointment root canal treatment is indicated when
   a. the procedure will be lengthy and difficult for the patient.
   b. there is uncontrollable drainage from the canal.
   c. the dentist does not have time to complete the procedure.
   d. all of the above.
8. Root end surgery is indicated for endodontic failure when
   a. the dentist suspects a missed canal.
   b. there has been coronal leakage.
   c. a cast post and core and a well-fitting crown are present.
   d. all of the above.
9. Prognosis for root canal treatment is worse when the patient
   a. has pain as a presenting symptom.
   b. has an interappointment flare-up.
   c. has class III mobility and loss of bone support (probing defects).
   d. has a small periradicular radiolucent lesion.

10. Endodontic treatment is contraindicated when
    a. the patient has no motivation to maintain the tooth.
    b. the canal appears to be calcified.
    c. a large periapical lesion is present.
    d. the tooth needs periodontal crown lengthening before restoration.

CHAPTER 5: PREPARATION FOR TREATMENT

1. Transmission of HIV
   a. is more likely than the hepatitis B virus.
   b. could not occur from a stick of a file used in a canal with necrotic tissue.
   c. is unlikely from a patient without symptoms.
   d. can occur via either blood or saliva.
2. OSHA standards are established to protect the
   a. dental support personnel only.
   b. patient only.
   c. dentist and dental support personnel.
   d. dentist, dental support personnel, and patient.
3. Radiation exposure from a single full-mount survey
   a. is comparable to a single chest film.
   b. is comparable to a barium study of the intestines.
   c. is less with higher kilovoltages.
   d. would be sufficient to cause skin cancer if all exposures were at one site.
4. The recommended antibiotics for a patient with a total joint replacement who is allergic to penicillin or cephalosporin is
   a. amoxicillin.
   b. erythromycin.
   c. clindamycin.
   d. tetracycline.
5. The most effective method for controlling the pain that often occurs after cleaning and shaping is to administer
   a. an analgesic shortly before the procedure.
   b. equal amounts of the analgesic before and during the procedure.
   c. the analgesic at the conclusion of the procedure.
   d. the analgesic with instructions to the patient to take it if necessary.
6. The cone length/beam angulation that gives the most accurate tooth length is
   a. long cone, parallel.
   b. long cone, bisecting.
   c. short cone, parallel.
   d. short cone, bisecting.
7. The cone angulation in the following illustration on the next page is
   a. mesial.
   b. distal.
   c. parallel.
   d. bisecting.

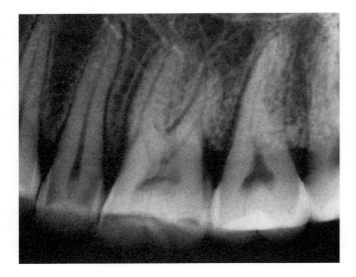

Questions 8 and 9 refer to the following illustration.

8. The radiopaque structure overlying the buccal roots is
   a. zygoma.
   b. floor of the maxillary sinus.
   c. coronoid process.
   d. eyeglass frame.

9. The best way to "move" this structure away from the buccal apexes of both molars is to reposition the cone
   a. inferiorly (decrease the vertical angle).
   b. superiorly (increase the vertical angle).
   c. mesially (the beam is directed more distally).
   d. distally (the beam is directed more mesially).

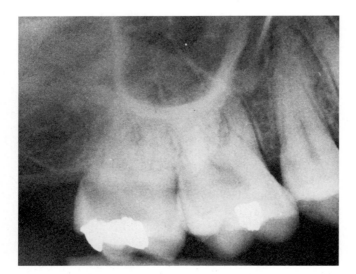

10. Why does the tooth in the following illustration appear elongated?
    a. There is excessive positive vertical angle to the cone.
    b. There is insufficient positive vertical angle to the cone.
    c. The film is not parallel to the tooth.
    d. The film is bent.

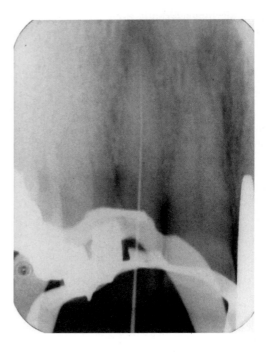

11. The radiopaque structure (arrow) in the following illustration is
    a. condensing osteitis.
    b. trabeculation.
    c. lamina dura.
    d. root surface.

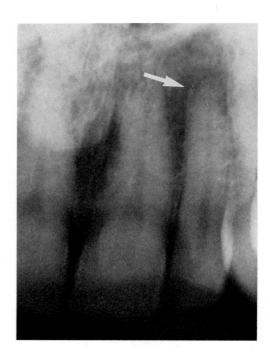

12. The view in the following illustration is a mesially angled (beam is directed distally) film. The unobturated root is the
    a. buccal root.
    b. lingual root.

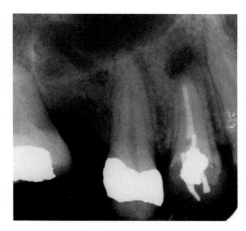

13. Of the following, the best way to identify the radiolucency *(arrow)* in the following illustration is to
    a. perform a pulp test.
    b. perform an incisional biopsy.
    c. perform an excisional biopsy.
    d. observe over time to evaluate for changes.

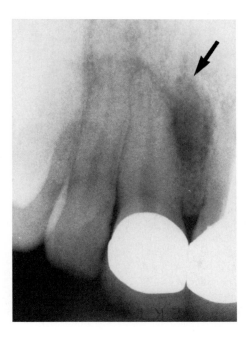

14. An advantage of digitized radiography in endodontic treatment is
    a. the image quality is better for working length radiographs.
    b. an x-ray generating source is not required.
    c. that one apparatus can be used for multiple applications, that is, occlusal, panographic, periapical, etc.
    d. there are no considerations as to infection control.

15. A situation in which a rubber dam need not be placed is
    a. when the clamp impinges on the gingiva, causing discomfort.
    b. when the chamber or canal may be difficult to locate on access.
    c. when the tooth is rotated, preventing placement of a clamp.
    d. none; there are no situations in which a rubber dam is not placed.

16. Endodontic files
    a. are best disposed of after one use.
    b. are considered reusable sharps.
    c. may be picked up by hand before decontamination.
    d. may be disposed of in "generic refuse."

17. Informed consent information for endodontic therapy excludes
    a. alternatives to recommended treatment.
    b. procedure and prognosis.
    c. a description of OSHA regulations.
    d. foreseeable and material risk.

18. X-ray units should be
    a. optimally capable of using 70 kVp.
    b. pointed in shape (cone).
    c. collimated to reduce exposure level, not to exceed 7 cm at the skin surface.
    d. collimated to reduce exposure level, not to exceed 9 cm at the skin surface.

19. Radiographic contrast can be directly affected by altering
    a. milliamperage.
    b. exposure time.
    c. kilovoltage.
    d. angulation.

20. With the cone moved to the distal and directed toward the mesial, the mesiobuccal root of the first molar
    a. is projected mesially on the film.
    b. is projected distally on the film.
    c. does not move.
    d. appears to move lingually.

21. To enhance crown preparation and retention when an infrabony defect exists, crown lengthening is completed by
    a. electrosurgery.
    b. conventional gingivectomy.
    c. laser surgery.
    d. apically positioned flap, reverse bevel.

CHAPTER 6: ARMAMENTARIUM AND STERILIZATION

1. The patient is exposed to the least amount of radiation when
    a. Radiovisiography is used.
    b. Ektaspeed film is used.
    c. Ultraspeed film is used.

2. Patients with a latex allergy
   a. can be treated safely without a rubber dam.
   b. can be treated with a rubber dam if there is no direct skin contact.
   c. can be treated with a nonlatex rubber dam.
3. The temporary restorative material, Cavit, is
   a. a zinc oxide–eugenol type of material.
   b. superior to other materials in in vitro resistance to bacterial leakage.
   c. prepared by mixing a powder and liquid.
   d. more durable than IRM or composite.
4. The best way to clean dental instruments before sterilization is by
   a. ultrasonic cleaning for 5 minutes in a perforated basket.
   b. hand scrubbing, using a brush and heavy rubber gloves.
   c. rinsing under a forceful water spray.
5. Steam sterilization is achieved when the load has
   a. reached 250° C for 15 minutes.
   b. reached 250° F for 15 minutes.
   c. reached 250° C for 30 minutes.
   d. reached 250° F for 30 minutes.
6. An advantage of rapid steam autoclave over traditional autoclave is
   a. rapid steam autoclave will not corrode steel instruments.
   b. rapid steam autoclave is safe for all types of materials.
   c. instruments do not have to be air dried at the end of the cycle.
   d. rapid steam autoclave has a shorter sterilization cycle than traditional autoclave.
7. The chemical vapor sterilizer
   a. uses a reusable chemical.
   b. requires adequate ventilation in the area where it is used.
   c. achieves sterilization when heated to 270° F at 20 psi for 10 minutes.
   d. does not destroy heat-sensitive materials.
8. Dental water line contamination can be reduced by
   a. discharging water lines without handpieces each week.
   b. running high-speed handpieces for 20 seconds between patients.
   c. properly sterilizing handpieces after patient care.
9. Gutta-percha is best sterilized by
   a. immersion in full-strength sodium hypochlorite.
   b. immersion in rubbing alcohol.
   c. dry heat.
   d. bead sterilizer.
10. The effect of sterilization on endodontic files is
    a. negative and proportional to the number of times sterilized.
    b. neutral; no effect is seen on physical properties.
    c. positive; it restores to the files flexibility lost over time.

CHAPTER 7: TOOTH MORPHOLOGY AND CAVITY PREPARATION

1. Studies of the apical root canal system have shown that
   a. accessory canals are capable of being cleaned mechanically at least 60% of the time.
   b. more than 60% of teeth examined showed accessory canals that were impossible to clean mechanically.
   c. apical foramina were located at the apex 80% of the time.
   d. canals terminate in the shape of a delta 45% of the time.
2. The fourth canal is often found in
   a. the mesiobuccal root of the maxillary first molar.
   b. the mesial root of the maxillary first premolar.
   c. the palatal root of the maxillary first molar.
   d. the distobuccal root of the maxillary first molar.
3. Entry into a maxillary central incisor is made
   a. below (apical to) the cingulum in the direction of the long axis of the tooth.
   b. just coronal to the cingulum in the direction of the long axis of the tooth.
   c. to include the marginal ridges.
   d. with a slow-speed bur.
4. A perforation during access preparation is more likely in which area?
   a. maxillary premolar on the mesial at the cementoenamel junction.
   b. mandibular molar on the distal.
   c. maxillary anterior on the lingual.
   d. mandibular anterior on the lingual.
5. It is desirable to remove as much of the existing restoration as possible as part of the access. Why?
   1. The restoration, or any part remaining, weakens the tooth.
   2. Visibility will be improved.
   3. Bits of restoration may later be shaved off and drop or be forced into canals.
   a. 1 and 2
   b. 1 and 3
   c. 2 and 3
   d. 1, 2, and 3
6. A round bur is used in preparation of anterior teeth to remove
   a. the lingual dentin shoulder.
   b. the incisal enamel triangle.
   c. the overhanging enamel rods.
   d. all of the above.
7. The outline form of the access opening in a maxillary central incisor is
   a. trapezoid.
   b. round.
   c. rectangular.
   d. triangular.
8. The dentin that must be removed to obtain straight-line access in the mesiobuccal canal of the mandibular molar is located where in the root?
   a. more mesially, toward the proximal.
   b. more distally, toward the furcation.
   c. more facially.
   d. more lingually.

9. A dens in dente is most common in the
   a. maxillary central incisor.
   b. maxillary lateral incisor.
   c. mandibular second premolar.
   d. mandibular central incisor.

10. If there are two canals in the distal of a mandibular first molar they usually
    a. each have their own apical foramen.
    b. begin as a single canal and bifurcate in the apical half.
    c. begin as two canals and join and exit as one.
    d. are smaller than the mesial canals.

11. In a mandibular incisor the most common surface for perforation is
    a. labial.
    b. lingual.
    c. mesial.
    d. distal.

12. Of the following, which is the most challenging aspect of treating a C-shaped mandibular molar?
    a. locating the chamber during access
    b. avoiding perforation into the furcation
    c. exceptionally long, small canals
    d. difficulty in debridement

13. Choose the letter below that corresponds to the correct access opening for a maxillary first premolar.

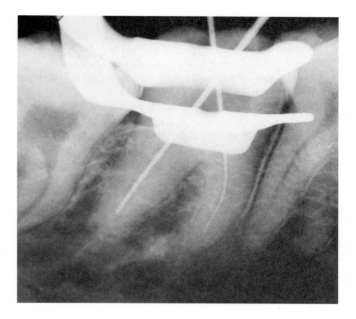

15. The solid line in the following illustration is the outline of the original canal. The dotted line indicates what the final shape (in cross section) of the enlarged canal should be. Select the drawing which demonstrates the preferred final shape of the preparation.

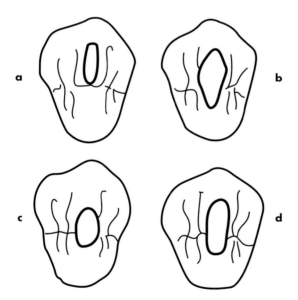

14. The instrument in the following illustration is in only one of two canals in the mesial root. The cone is directed from the mesial angle. From which dentin shoulder must tooth structure be removed to gain straight-line access in this canal?
    a. mesiobuccal
    b. mesiolingual
    c. distobuccal
    d. distolingual

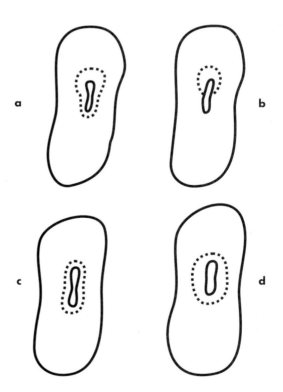

16. Most maxillary central incisors have
    a. a single canal with numerous irregularities.
    b. a single canal that is smooth and naturally tapered.
    c. a likelihood of exhibiting a distinct second canal.
17. If the chamber is obscured by a crown or is calcified, the recommended action is to
    a. obtain a vertically angled radiograph to visualize the chamber.
    b. make the initial opening with a low-speed handpiece to maximize the chances of finding the chamber.
    c. start the access without the rubber dam to use as many anatomic cues as possible.
18. The access outline form
    a. should be somewhat smaller than the form created by connecting the root canal orifices.
    b. reflects the shape of the crown of the tooth.
    c. should extend onto the tooth's marginal ridges.
    d. all of the above.
19. A root that seldom contains two canals is the
    a. distobuccal root of the maxillary molar.
    b. mandibular central incisor.
    c. maxillary second premolar.
    d. distal root of the mandibular molar.
20. Perforation of the maxillary anterior is usually
    a. to the facial of the root.
    b. to the lingual of the root.
    c. done with Gates-Glidden burs during straight-line access.
    d. done with a slow-speed handpiece while removing pulp horns.
21. The maxillary first premolar
    a. canal orifices lie beneath the central groove.
    b. is similar in length to the maxillary canine.
    c. may have one, two, or three canals.

CHAPTER 8: CLEANING AND SHAPING THE ROOT CANAL SYSTEM

1. All the following are objectives of shaping *except* one. Which is this *exception?*
   a. to provide a tapered space so that obturating instruments can fit freely in the root canal system
   b. to provide access for instruments and irrigants during treatment procedures
   c. to remove necrotic tissue and bacteria
   d. to remove dentin using a variety of instruments to enlarge the root canal space in three dimensions
2. Apical patency is maintained for each of the following reasons *except* one. Which is this *exception?*
   a. to preserve the apical anatomy
   b. to enhance the flushing action of the irrigant
   c. to loosen debris
   d. to maintain obturating materials within the root
3. Irrigation with sodium hypochlorite exhibits all the following properties *except* one. Which is this *exception?*
   a. mechanical flushing
   b. lubrication of instruments
   c. destruction of microbes
   d. dissolution of necrotic tissue
   e. hemostasis

4. Root canals should be cleaned, shaped, and obturated to the constricture for each of the following reasons *except* one. Which is this *exception?*
   a. The constriction is the narrowest diameter of the canal.
   b. Lateral and accessory canals are common in the apical 1 to 2 mm of the canal.
   c. The clinician can easily identify the constriction.
   d. Obturating materials are maintained within the root canal system.
5. Which of the following is true of apex locators?
   a. Resistance apex locators are preferred to frequency and impedance apex locators.
   b. Apex locators are helpful in initial placement of working length files.
   c. Repeated identical readings indicating the apical foramen are a reliable indication of the canal length.
   d. Readings indicating accessory canals are not possible because of the small size of the accessory canals.
6. The balanced force technique is best described by which of the following statements?
   a. The file is passively placed to the point of first binding and then rotated one to two turns in a counterclockwise direction.
   b. Dentin is engaged with the file rotating in a clockwise direction for a quarter turn followed by a counterclockwise rotation with inward pressure for at least one third of a revolution.
   c. The file is oscillated back and forth 30 to 60 degrees as it is positioned apically, followed by a clockwise rotation of 180 degrees before removal.
   d. A file is placed passively to a point of first binding and then rotated in a clockwise rotation of at least 180 degrees using apical pressure, followed by a counterclockwise rotation to evacuate debris.
7. Each of the following are components of recapitulation *except* one. Which is this *exception?*
   a. loosening of debris and tissue in the apical portion of the canal, which could produce blockage
   b. reintroduction of files previously used in cleaning and shaping procedures
   c. irrigation with sodium hypochlorite
   d. sterilization and disinfection of the radicular space
8. RC-Prep and Glyoxide
   a. have lubricating properties.
   b. are used during the later stages of shaping the canal to reduce ledge formation.
   c. digest collagenous components of the dental pulp.
   d. prevent the formation of the smear layer during canal preparation.
9. The most important factor(s) in removing debris from the root canal space during the preparation phase of treatment is(are)
   a. frequency and volume of the irrigant.
   b. the use of chelating agents.
   c. the use of a small patency file.
   d. sonic activation of files.
10. The ability to discern the apical foramen during working length determination is enhanced by which of the following?
    a. the use of small Nos. 8 to 10 files
    b. paper point placement
    c. coronal canal preparation
    d. canal curvature in the apical 1 to 2 mm

11. Which of the following is most responsible for short underfilled canals?
    a. severe curvatures
    b. packing debris
    c. canal ledging
    d. calcification of the canal
12. Preparing the curved canal in multiple planes
    a. permits preservation of the natural curvature.
    b. increases the risk of furcal perforation.
    c. requires Gates-Glidden drills.
    d. accomplishes the cleaning phase of canal preparation.
13. The apical control zone is
    a. defined by the apical constriction.
    b. established by three or more 0.5-mm step-backs.
    c. defined by parallel walls in the apical 2 to 3 mm.
    d. established by maintaining apical patency.
14. The crown-down technique has the following advantages *except* one. Which is this *exception?*
    a. enhances the action of the irrigant
    b. removes tissue and debris before they can be packed apically
    c. prevents changes in working length during canal preparation
    d. does *not* prevent changes in working length during canal preparation.
15. The Profile rotary instruments
    a. produce an accentuated smear layer.
    b. operate at low speeds and variable speeds.
    c. conform to ISO standards for instrument design.
    d. prepare the canal from the apex to the crown.

CHAPTER 9: OBTURATION OF THE CLEANED AND SHAPED ROOT CANAL SYSTEM

1. Paraformaldehyde-containing obturating materials
    a. eliminate bacteria that remain in the canals.
    b. mummify tissue remnant in canals.
    c. reduce posttreatment pain.
    d. are below standards of care for root canal treatment.
2. Gutta-percha in contact with connective tissue is
    a. relatively inert.
    b. immunogenic.
    c. unstable.
    d. carcinogenic.
3. It is preferable to not extrude sealer beyond the apex because the sealer
    a. usually does not resorb.
    b. often stains (tattoo) the tissue.
    c. is a tissue irritant and may delay healing.
    d. promotes bacterial growth.
4. Considering lateral versus vertical condensation, studies have shown
    a. lateral condensation results in a better seal.
    b. vertical condensation results in a better seal.
    c. either consistently fills lateral canals.
    d. sealability with either largely depends on the shape of the prepared canal.
5. A problem with nickel-titanium spreaders is
    a. a tendency to buckle under compaction pressure.
    b. a tendency to breakage during condensation.
    c. they create greater wedging force, leading to root fracture.
    d. they do not penetrate as deeply as stainless steel spreaders under equal forces.

6. Moderate extrusion of obturating materials beyond the apex is undesirable because
    1. there is more likelihood of postoperative discomfort.
    2. sealer is toxic to tissue.
    3. there is a poorer prognosis.
    a. 1 and 2
    b. 2 only
    c. 1 only
    d. 1, 2, and 3
7. One-visit root canal treatment is acceptable
    1. when the pulp is vital and symptomatic.
    2. when the pulp is necrotic and not symptomatic.
    3. when the pulp is necrotic and symptomatic.
    a. 1 only
    b. 1 and 2
    c. 2 only
    d. 2 and 3
8. A potentially beneficial application of heated (softened) injected gutta-percha is
    a. when there is an open apex.
    b. when there are aberrations or irregularities of the canal.
    c. when the clinician cannot master lateral condensation.
    d. when canals are curved and small, after preparation.
9. An advantage of thermocompaction over vertical compaction (gutta-percha heat-softening) techniques is
    a. thermocompaction is more rapid.
    b. thermocompaction adapts better to canal irregularities.
    c. thermocompaction is not technique sensitive.
    d. no special devices or instruments are required for thermocompaction.
10. The obturation of the incisor shown in the following illustration is inadequate because
    a. it appears short of the prepared length.
    b. there is variable radiodensity (incomplete condensation) throughout its length.
    c. there is a space between the temporary restoration and the gutta-percha.
    d. the diagnosis was pulp necrosis and chronic apical periodontitis; the canal should be filled to the apical foramen.

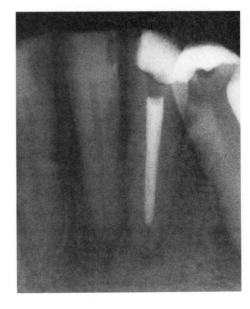

11. This dark tooth has a history of trauma and root canal treatment. It is likely that the discoloration is primarily due to (see illustration below)
    a. remnants of necrotic tissue.
    b. a leaking restoration.
    c. blood pigments in the dentinal tubules.
    d. obturating materials not removed from the chamber.

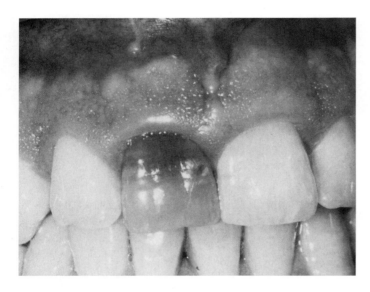

12. Of the following, what is the most likely cause of failure of root canal treatment on the lateral incisor? (see illustration below)
    a. The silver point corrodes.
    b. The canal is filled too close to the apex.
    c. There is coronal leakage.
    d. The silver point does not adapt to the prepared canal space.

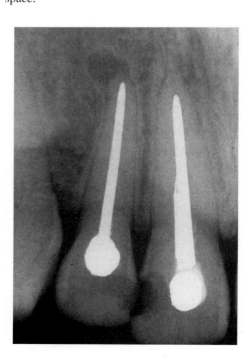

13. The most likely cause of a gross overfill (gutta-percha and sealer out the apex) is
    a. lack of an apical seat or stop.
    b. use of excessive amounts of sealer.
    c. use of excessive apical pressure on the spreader.
    d. use of a too-small master cone.
14. The master cone should
    a. never have "tug back" resistance.
    b. always be softened with solvent after a stop has been prepared.
    c. be the largest cone that will fit at or 0.5 mm short of the working length.
    d. fit 1.5 mm from the radiographic apex.

CHAPTER 10: RECORDS AND LEGAL RESPONSIBILITIES

1. As related to changes in a patients record,
   a. any changes are forbidden.
   b. alteration is permitted if dated.
   c. additions are forbidden.
   d. additions are permitted if dated.
2. Standard of care, as defined by courts,
   a. requires absolute perfection.
   b. describes what a reasonably careful and prudent clinician would do under similar circumstances.
   c. does not allow for individual variations of treatment.
   d. is equivalent to customary practice.
3. The doctrine of informed consent does *not* require that patients
   a. be advised of reasonably foreseeable risks of treatment.
   b. be advised of reasonable alternatives.
   c. forfeit their right to do as they see fit with their own body.
   d. be advised of the consequences of nontreatment.
4. A periodontal examination of a patient referred for endodontic treatment
   a. should be performed on the entire dentition.
   b. must be performed at least on the tooth to be treated.
   c. is necessary only if there is evidence of periodontal involvement.
   d. is necessary only if requested by the referring dentist.
5. A dentist may legally
   a. refuse to treat a new patient despite severe pain and infection.
   b. be bound to see a former patient on recall after treatment is completed.
   c. discharge a patient from his or her practice at any time.
   d. refuse to treat a patient who has an outstanding balance on his or her account.
6. If a patient who is HIV seropositive requests that the dentist not inform the staff of the condition, the dentist should
   a. refuse to treat the patient.
   b. tell the staff in private, then treat the patient using extra precautions.
   c. not tell the staff, but treat the patient with great caution.
   d. not tell the staff and require the patient to sign a private guarantee that the patient will be liable if someone contracts the virus.

7. As related to technologic or biologic advances,
   a. any clinician, including generalists, must remain current.
   b. only specialists must remain current.
   c. generalists must learn of new advances only if they have problems with existing technology.
   d. patients must be advised of all alternative, new techniques.

8. A specialist may be held liable who
   a. informs the patient that the general practitioner performed substandard care (the general practitioner may hold the specialist liable).
   b. fails to disclose to the patient or referring dentist evident pathosis other than the tooth the specialist is treating.
   c. fails to locate a very small canal that is not evident radiographically.
   d. mistakenly initiates treatment on the wrong tooth in a difficult diagnosis situation.

9. Of the following, the dentist's best approach to avoiding legal action by a patient is to
   a. tell patients that they have no malpractice insurance.
   b. attend continuing education courses frequently to remain informed of current techniques.
   c. refer all major patient complaints to peer review.
   d. demonstrate genuine interest in the welfare of each patient.

10. The illustration below is a radiograph of a patient who has been referred for treatment of the first premolar. Regarding problems with the second premolar, the endodontist
    a. need not inform the patient or the referring dentist unless there are symptoms.
    b. need not inform the patient or the referring dentist unless the patient asks for an opinion on other teeth on the radiograph.
    c. must inform both the patient and the referring dentist.
    d. need not inform the patient, only the referring dentist.

11. One month previous, a general dentist used the technique (pulpotomy with paraformaldehyde-containing paste) shown in the following illustration to treat a patient with an acute apical abscess and then placed a crown. The patient continues to have pain and swelling. As regarding malpractice, the generalist is
    a. liable because unacceptable treatment procedures were followed.
    b. liable because the patient should not have persistent symptoms regardless of the technique used.
    c. not liable if the patient is now referred to the appropriate specialist who can correctly treat the case.
    d. not liable if the general dentist performs additional treatment on the tooth for no fee.

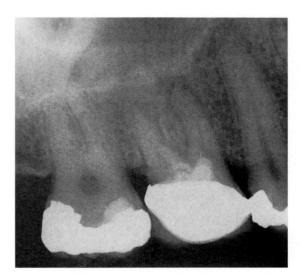

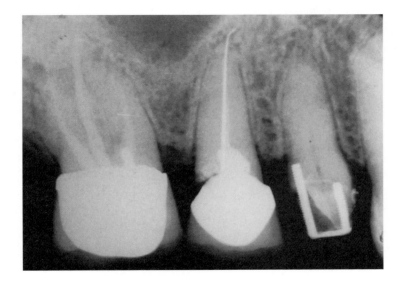

CHAPTER 11: PULP DEVELOPMENT, STRUCTURE, AND FUNCTION

1. The tissue fluid pressure of the pulp is such that through dentin
   a. there is an inward flow of fluid.
   b. there is an outward flow of fluid.
   c. there is no flow of fluid.
   d. direction of flow varies, depending on whether the pulp is inflamed.

Questions 2 and 3 refer to the following illustration.

2. In the above photomicrograph of the pulp, the structure indicated by the arrow
   a. transmits motor impulses.
   b. transmits sensory impulses.
   c. carries tissue fluids out of the pulp.
   d. is an artifact.

3. The morphology of the odontoblast layer indicates the above section is from
   a. a developing pulp.
   b. the coronal pulp.
   c. the midradicular pulp.
   d. the pulp in the apical third.

4. The ultrastructure of the cell body of the odontoblast demonstrates structures that indicate
   a. protein synthesis.
   b. protein degradation.
   c. phagocytosis.
   d. a relatively undifferentiated cell.

5. When odontoblasts die, they are replaced by differentiation of
   a. undifferentiated mesenchymal cells.
   b. fibroblasts.
   c. undifferentiated odontoblasts.
   d. preodontoblasts.

6. The major component of the pulp in the following illustration is (see illustration on following page)
   a. collagen.
   b. cells.
   c. support structures (vessels and nerves).
   d. water.

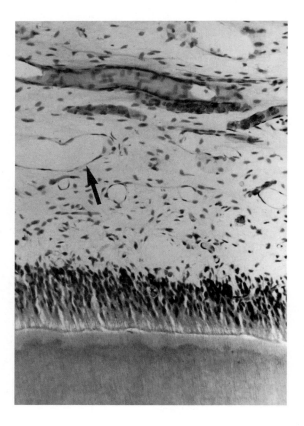

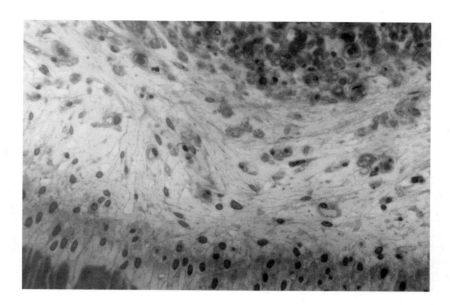

Questions 7 and 8 refer to the following illustration.

7. The pulpal structure shown by the large arrow transmits
    a. pain from dentin stimulation.
    b. pain from pulpal injury.
    c. impulses to vascular smooth muscle.
    d. proprioception.

8. The structures *(small arrows)*
    a. transmit pain from dentin stimulation.
    b. transmit pain from pulpal injury.
    c. synthesize and secrete collagen.
    d. phagocytose foreign substances.

9. The size, morphology, and location (adjacent to odonto-blasts) of the vessel *(arrow)* in the following illustration would indicate this is a
    a. venule.
    b. arteriole.
    c. arteriovenous anastomosis.
    d. capillary.

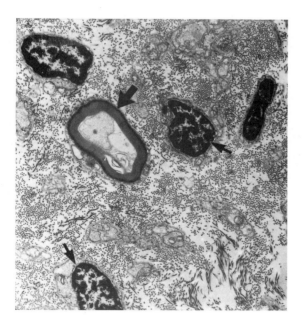

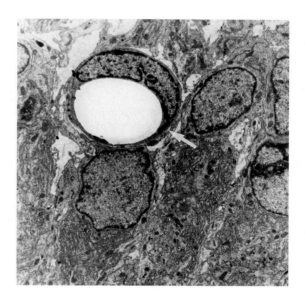

10. A histologic section at the level of the arrow in the tooth with calcific metamorphosis in the following illustration likely would show
    a. total calcification with normal-appearing (regular) dentin.
    b. total calcification with a very irregular dentin.
    c. total calcification with a cementum-like tissue.
    d. remnants of soft tissue surrounded by a cementum-like tissue.

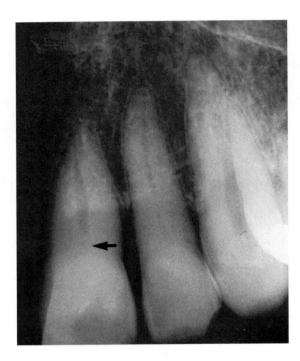

11. Lymphatics in the dental pulp
    a. transmit lymphocytes to inflamed regions.
    b. would not be necessary because of the extensive blood vessel network.
    c. cannot be demonstrated morphologically because they are identical to venules.
    d. participate in the removal of tissue fluids.
12. Growth factors are likely to be involved in tooth formation. What is at least one probable function of these factors?
    a. signaling epithelial mesenchymal interactions
    b. one of the eruptive forces located in the apical region
    c. disruption of Hertwig's epithelial root sheath
    d. collagen maturation in the dental papilla
13. The nerve fibers of the pulp are
    a. mainly myelinated fibers at the time of tooth eruption.
    b. easily damaged by inflammation.
    c. only sensory.
    d. unevenly distributed throughout the pulp.
14. Painful pulpitis associated with an inflamed or degenerating pulp
    a. is caused by a decrease of intrapulpal pressure.
    b. results from a reduction of nerve cell permeability.
    c. is associated with stimulation of A fibers.
    d. is most likely due to nociceptive fiber activity.

15. The cell-rich zone
    a. is more prominent in the radicular pulp than the coronal pulp.
    b. has increased mitotic activity following death of odontoblasts.
    c. is the result of the central migration of cells from the periphery following completion of dentin formation.
    d. contains mainly macrophages and endothelial cells and few fibroblasts.
16. Fibroblasts
    a. are the least numerous cells of the pulp.
    b. are capable of giving rise to cells that may differentiate into macrophages.
    c. increase in numbers as blood vessels and nerves decrease with age.
    d. undergo active differentiation in the pulp.
17. Secondary dentin formation is an appositional process occurring after eruption and
    1. in molars is greatest on the floor of the chamber.
    2. in premolars is greatest on the occlusal aspect of the chamber.
    3. is synonymous with reparative (irritation) dentin.
       a. 1 only
       b. 2 only
       c. 1 and 2
       d. 2 and 3
18. Pulpal calcifications
    a. may compromise the pulpal blood supply.
    b. are of no significance in root canal therapy.
    c. have an organic matrix of collagen.
    d. occur only after eruption.
19. The dendritic cell is most similar to which cell type?
    a. fibroblast
    b. T lymphocyte
    c. mesenchymal cell
    d. macrophage
20. The histodifferentiation stage of tooth development is characterized by
    a. initiation and proliferation of ameloblasts and odontoblasts.
    b. cellular elements acquiring their functional assignments.
    c. apposition of cementum.
    d. cell division, incremental apposition, and calcification of enamel.
21. The pathways of pulpal inflammation and infection are strongly influenced by
    a. the two structural proteins in the pulp: collagen and elastin.
    b. dental materials that depress pulpal metabolic activity.
    c. the state of polymerization of the ground substance components in the pulp.
    d. osmotic pressures as regulated by proteoglycans.
22. When the pulp is injured, it responds with inflammation. Why does it not have good capability for recovery if badly damaged?
    1. It has no collateral blood supply.
    2. It lacks lymph drainage.
    3. It is encased in a noncompliant environment.
       a. 1 and 2
       b. 1 and 3
       c. 2 and 3
       d. 1, 2, and 3

23. Dentin formation begins
    a. before the formation.
    b. during the bud stage.
    c. during the bell stage.
    d. during the cap stage.

CHAPTER 12: PERIAPICAL PATHOLOGY

1. In acute inflammation the first cells to pass through the blood vessel walls into the tissue are
    a. eosinophils.
    b. lymphocytes.
    c. monocytes.
    d. polymorphonuclear neutrophilic leukocytes.
2. In the inflammatory process, which of the following cell types function as phagocytes?
    a. macrophages and lymphocytes
    b. lymphocytes and neutrophils
    c. plasma cells and basophils
    d. neutrophils and macrophages
3. Which of the following results may be expected following surgery when both the buccal and lingual cortical plates have been lost?
    a. ankylosis
    b. scar tissue formation
    c. osteosclerosis
    d. persistent inflammation
4. A foreign body reaction is characterized by the presence of
    a. neutrophils.
    b. plasma cells.
    c. giant cells.
    d. fibroblasts.
5. The periapical lesion that would most likely contain bacteria within the lesion is
    a. an abscess.
    b. a cyst.
    c. a granuloma.
    d. a condensing osteitis.
6. Opsonization facilitates
    a. mitosis of lymphocytes.
    b. chemotaxis of neutrophils.
    c. vasodilation.
    d. phagocytosis.
7. A sinus tract associated with a suppurative apical periodontitis usually
    a. is lined with epithelium throughout its length.
    b. should be cauterized or removed surgically.
    c. does not heal unless the microorganisms are curetted from the apical area.
    d. requires no special treatment other than root canal treatment of the offending tooth.
8. What is the usual histologic picture of the pulp in a tooth with a chronic apical periodontitis (dental granuloma)?
    a. Pulpal abscess develops in the coronal pulp with chronic inflammation in the radicular pulp.
    b. There is necrotic pulp.
    c. The majority of the pulp exhibits chronic inflammation.
    d. Chronic inflammation in the coronal pulp and the radicular pulp appears normal.
9. Chronic apical periodontitis (granuloma) presents a histologic picture that is most consistent with
    a. infection.
    b. early cyst formation.
    c. healing.
    d. immune response.
10. Of the following periapical diagnoses, which would most likely contain bacteria within the lesion?
    a. suppurative apical periodontitis
    b. apical cyst
    c. chronic apical periodontitis
    d. acute apical periodontitis
11. When bacteria are recovered periapically, most studies show that there are
    a. anaerobes only.
    b. aerobes only.
    c. variable, mixed flora.
    d. only phagocytosed bacteria.
12. Studies have demonstrated a correlation between clinical and radiographic signs and symptoms of periapical pathosis and the presence of which specific microorganism?
    a. *Streptococcus mutans*
    b. *Prevotella melaninogenica*
    c. *Staphylococcus aureus*
    d. no specific microorganism(s)
13. The presence of C9 complement fragment in the inflamed periapex suggests that the complement system participates in
    a. opsonization.
    b. increasing vascular permeability.
    c. degranulation of mast cells.
    d. cell lysis.
14. Elevated levels of IgE have been identified in a periapical granuloma after canal instrumentation. This may represent which type of hypersensitivity reaction?
    a. type I (immediate hypersensitivity)
    b. type II (immediate cytotoxic hypersensitivity)
    c. type III (immune complex hypersensitivity)
    d. type IV (delayed hypersensitivity)
15. In the following periapical biopsy specimen, the arrows indicate (see illustration on following page)
    a. an immune response.
    b. a foreign body reaction.
    c. an actinomyces infection.
    d. an acute inflammatory response.

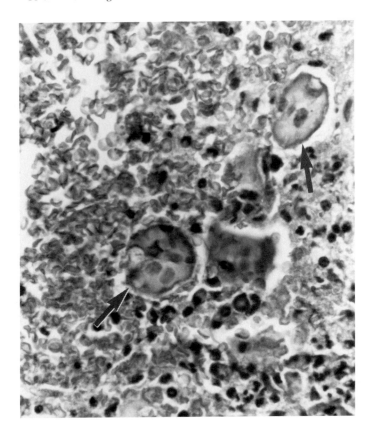

16. The predominant inflammatory cell type in the illustration below is
    a. lymphocytes.
    b. most cells.
    c. neutrophilic leukocytes.
    d. plasma cells.

CHAPTER 13: MICROBIOLOGY AND IMMUNOLOGY

1. Pulpal and periradicular pathosis results primarily from
   a. traumatic injury because of heat during cavity preparation.
   b. bacterial invasion.
   c. toxicity of dental materials.
   d. immunologic reactions.
2. Which of the following statements regarding the organisms producing pulpal pathosis is correct?
   a. The organisms are primarily facultative streptococci.
   b. Single isolates (monoinfection) produce the most severe reactions.
   c. Isolates tend to be polymicrobial and anaerobic.
   d. Organisms infecting the pulp tend to be aerobic when compared to organisms commonly found in periradicular tissues.
3. Which of the following statements is correct regarding the *Bacteroides* species?
   a. Pure isolates are common from infected root canals with periradicular pathosis.
   b. The organisms have been associated with periradicular pathosis that exhibits signs and symptoms.
   c. The organisms supply hemin and vitamin K to other bacteria in the polymicrobial ecologic mixture.
   d. The organisms are gram-positive anaerobic cocci and were previously classified as *Porphyromonas*.
4. Which of the following statements is correct regarding dentin?
   a. The tubules are wider at the pulp dentin border when compared to the dentinoenamel junction.
   b. Viable dentin is easily invaded by microorganisms when compared to dentin of nonvital teeth.
   c. Sound dentin beneath a carious lesion is free of microorganisms.
   d. Dentin permeability is uniform throughout the root.

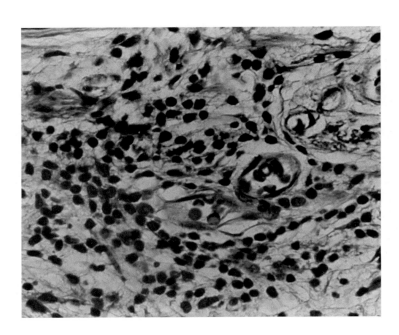

5. The smear layer produced during root canal treatment is best described as
   a. an amorphous layer of inorganic material.
   b. a partial barrier to bacterial penetration.
   c. an organic matrix composed of pulp tissue remnants.
   d. the condensation of calcium and phosphate ions that form within the tubules, forming plugs.

6. Cavitation that results from dental caries
   a. develops as acid-producing bacteria invade the tubules, causing demineralization and proteolytic species digesting the organic matrix.
   b. permits rapid infection of the pulp via the dentinal tubules.
   c. occurs slowly with proteolytic bacteria removing the organic matrix before demineralization.
   d. results in irreversible pulpal inflammation, since the bacteria within the tubules cannot be removed.

7. Which of the following statements best describes anachoresis?
   a. the attraction of blood-borne microorganisms to inflamed tissue during a bacteremia
   b. the process of carious invasion, cavitation, and exposure of the pulp from bacteria
   c. bacteria located in dentinal tubules and the pulp that are seeded to the systemic circulation, inducing disease in other areas of the body
   d. the process of anaerobic organisms causing disease

8. The initial cellular reaction of the dental pulp to microorganisms invading dentin is
   a. infiltration of polymorphonuclear neutrophil leukocytes.
   b. infiltration of plasma cells and lymphocytes.
   c. tubular sclerosis and deposition of secondary dentin.
   d. proliferation of fibroblasts that differentiate into new odontoblasts.

9. When the pulp is initially exposed by caries, the microorganisms
   a. are α-hemolytic streptococci and lactobacilli.
   b. are *Porphyromonas* and *Prevotella.*
   c. are facultative and obligate anaerobes.
   d. do not reflect the normal oral flora.

10. Organisms implicated in causing severe spreading abscesses include
    a. *Fusobacterium.*
    b. *Campylobacter.*
    c. *Enterococci.*
    d. *Bacteroides.*

11. Neuropeptides originate from
    a. somatosensory nerves.
    b. the cell wall of vascular channels.
    c. activation of the complement cascade.
    d. mast cells.

12. Nonsteroidal antiinflammatory agents produce a reduction in which of the following?
    a. Substance P
    b. Prostaglandins
    c. Calcitonin gene-related peptide
    d. Arachidonic acid

13. Abscess formation in the dental pulp is most likely to occur
    a. with activation of the cell-mediated immunologic response.
    b. when B lymphocytes are present.
    c. with release of lysosomal enzymes from leukocytes.
    d. with the formation of antigen-antibody complexes.

14. Which of the following statements is correct in relation to the periradicular lesion that has formed in response to dental caries and subsequent pulp necrosis?
    a. Bacteria are a common finding in the granuloma that develops.
    b. T-helper cells predominate over T-suppressor cells.
    c. Formation of the granuloma is mediated through a specific immunologic response.
    d. The release of interleukins can mediate bone resorption.

15. Which of the following is correct regarding tumor necrosis factor (TNF)?
    a. TNF is a potent stimulator of bone resorption.
    b. TNF enhances collagen formation.
    c. TNF-β (lymphotoxin) is produced primarily by activated macrophages.
    d. TNF-α produces bone resorption, whereas TNF-β induces osseous formation.

16. Disinfection of the root canal is
    a. mainly accomplished by mechanical means.
    b. the result of irrigants such as sodium hypochlorite.
    c. related to the use of intracanal medicaments from the phenolic and aldehyde groups.
    d. accomplished by placement of calcium hydroxide in multiple-visit endodontic treatment.

17. Each of the following statements regarding initial Gram staining is correct *except* one. Which is this *exception?*
    a. Microbial disease can be identified.
    b. Gram-negative species can be identified.
    c. No specific identification of genus or species is possible.
    d. Viable organisms can be distinguished from dead microbes.

18. The material of choice for temporization of teeth during multiple-appointment endodontic treatment is
    a. IRM.
    b. Cavit.
    c. TERM.
    d. zinc oxide–eugenol.

19. Following root canal treatment, a final restoration should be placed within
    a. 30 days.
    b. 3 months.
    c. 6 months.
    d. 1 year.

CHAPTER 14: INSTRUMENTS, MATERIALS, AND DEVICES

1. Pulp stimulation with cold
   a. is best accomplished with carbon dioxide snow (dry ice).
   b. is an accurate assessment of pulp vitality.
   c. directly stimulates nerve fibers in the pulp, producing the sensation of pain.
   d. is best determined with a stream of air from the air-water syringe.

2. With regard to electrical pulp testing, which of the following is correct?
   a. Positive responses can be used for differential diagnosis of pulp pathosis.
   b. The device employs a pulsating alternating current with a duration of 1 to 15 ms.
   c. The device employs a low current with a high potential difference in voltage.
   d. Gingival and periodontal tissues are more sensitive to testing when compared to the dental pulp.

3. Direct digital radiographic images
   a. are produced by a charged coupled device and do not require x-ray imaging.
   b. have the advantage of being manipulated, which facilitates interpretation.
   c. have greater resolution when compared to traditional film.
   d. captured by the sensor cover a greater area than traditional film.

4. Nickel-titanium instruments
   a. exhibit a high elastic modulus, which provides flexibility.
   b. on the application of stress exhibit a transformation from the austenitic crystalline phase a martensitic structure.
   c. cannot be strained to the same level as stainless steel without permanent deformation.
   d. are easier to prebend before placement in the canal than stainless steel.

5. A barbed broach is most useful for
   a. removal of cotton, paper points, and other objects in the radicular space.
   b. removal of vital pulp tissue from fine canals.
   c. initial planing of the canal walls.
   d. coronal orifice enlargement before establishing a corrected working length.

6. In comparing K-type files to reamers, the K-type file
   a. has more flutes per millimeter, which increases flexibility.
   b. differs, as the file is manufactured by twisting a tapered square (cross-sectional) steel wire.
   c. is more effective in removing debris.
   d. is the least flexible when comparing instruments of the same size.

7. Hedström files are
   a. manufactured by machining a round cross-sectional steel wire.
   b. effective when used in a reaming action.
   c. safer than K-type files, since external signs of stress are more visible as changes in flute design.
   d. aggressive because of a negative rake angle that is parallel to the canal wall.

8. The Profile rotary instruments
   a. are used at a range of 1500 to 2000 rpm.
   b. are nickel-titanium instruments manufactured in half sizes.
   c. exhibit ISO/ANSI standardized sizes.
   d. incorporate radial lands in the flute design.

9. LightSpeed rotary instruments
   a. prepare the canal from the orifice to the apex.
   b. provide a simple armamentarium for canal preparation.
   c. are available in standardized ISO/ANSI sizes of Nos. 8 through 140.
   d. exhibit a standardized taper of 0.04 mm/mm.
   e. have a long cylindric shaft.

10. Piezoelectric ultrasonic devices differ from magnetostrictive devices in that the piezoelectric unit
    a. transfers more energy to the file.
    b. produces heat that requires a coolant.
    c. uses RispiSonic, ShaperSonic, and TrioSonic files.
    d. vibrates at 2 to 3 kHz.

11. Ultrasonic root canal instrumentation produces
    a. acoustic microstreaming.
    b. cavitation.
    c. implosion.
    d. a bactericidal action.

12. Sodium hypochlorite used as a root canal irrigating solution
    a. is buffered to a pH of 12 to 13, which increases toxicity.
    b. exhibits a chelating action on dentin.
    c. should be used in higher concentrations because of the increased amount of free chlorine available.
    d. has a low surface tension that permits the solution to flow into irregularities.

13. When used as an endodontic irrigant, ethylenediaminetetraacetic acid (EDTA)
    a. must be completely removed following use to prevent continued action and destruction of dentin.
    b. is a rapid and efficient method of removing the smear layer.
    c. acts on organic and inorganic components of the smear layer.
    d. penetrates deep into dentin and enhances root canal preparation.

14. Calcium hydroxide is advocated as an interappointment medicament primarily because of
    a. its ability to dissolve necrotic tissue.
    b. its antimicrobial activity.
    c. its ability to stimulate hard tissue formation at the apical foramen.
    d. its ability to temporarily seal the canal space.

15. Heating of gutta-percha
    a. produces a transformation to the beta phase.
    b. followed by cooling results in crystallization in the alpha phase.
    c. with the Obtura system produces more shrinkage when compared to the Ultrafil system.
    d. with the Obtura system requires less heat when compared to the Ultrafil system.
    e. enhances adherence.

16. An advantage to AH26 as an endodontic sealer is
    a. the release of formaldehyde.
    b. low toxicity.
    c. solubility in chloroform.
    d. dentin adhesion.

17. N$_2$, Endomethasone, and Reibler's paste are sealers that
    a. produce liquefaction necrosis in the periradicular tissues.
    b. induce healing in the apical pulp wound following vital pulp extirpation.
    c. can cause periapical inflammation.
    d. do not produce a seal when used in combination with a core material.

18. When used as a temporary restoration in multivisit nonsurgical endodontic treatment, TERM
    a. seals better than Cavit.
    b. is the material of choice when strength of the restoration is a requirement.
    c. is a zinc oxide–reinforced material that can be light cured.
    d. has a eugenol component that functions as a bacterial barrier.

19. Based on instrument design and method of manufacturing, which of the following is most susceptible to fracture?
    a. K-type file fabricated from tapered square stainless steel wire
    b. K-flex file fabricated from rhomboidal stainless steel wire
    c. Hedström file fabricated from round stainless steel wire
    d. Reamer fabricated from triangular stainless steel wire

20. As noted in the following photomicrograph, the intracanal instrument is
    a. a specialized design (neither a reamer nor a file).
    b. altered to make it more flexible.
    c. untwisted, likely occurring during canal preparation.
    d. a noncutting canal explorer.

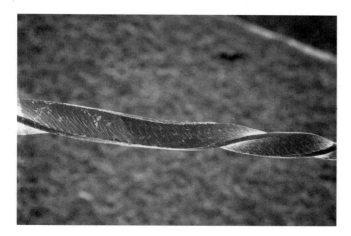

CHAPTER 15: PULPAL REACTION TO CARIES AND DENTAL PROCEDURES

1. The most common response in the dentin deep to caries is
   a. increased permeability.
   b. alteration of collagen.
   c. dissolution of peritubular dentin.
   d. dentinal sclerosis.

2. Relatively few bacteria are found in a pulp abscess because of the
   a. immune response of pulp tissue.
   b. high tissue pH in the adjacent inflammation.
   c. mechanical blockage of sclerotic dentin.
   d. antibacterial products of neutrophils.

3. A periodontal ligament injection of 2% lidocaine with 1:100,000 epinephrine causes the pulp circulation to
   a. cease for about 30 minutes.
   b. remain the same.
   c. increase markedly.
   d. decrease slightly.

4. Of the following, the highest incidence of pulp necrosis is associated with
   a. class V preparations on root surface.
   b. inlay preparations.
   c. partial veneer restorations.
   d. full crown preparations.

5. Acid etching of dentin before insertion of the restorative material
   a. protects the pulp from bacterial invasion.
   b. enhances bacterial penetration of the dentin.
   c. destroys odontoblastic processes in the tubules.
   d. decreases the pulp response to the restorative material.

6. The response of the pulp to a recently placed amalgam without a cavity lining is usually
   a. slight to moderate inflammation.
   b. moderate to severe inflammation.
   c. slight but increasingly severe with time.
   d. usually none.

7. The smear layer on dentin walls acts to prevent pulpal injury by
   a. reducing diffusion of toxic substance through the tubules.
   b. resisting the effects of acid etching of the dentin.
   c. eliminating the need for a cavity liner or base.
   d. its bactericidal activity against oral microorganisms.

8. A common histologic change in the pulp in response to moderately deep dentin caries is
   a. chronic inflammation.
   b. acute inflammation.
   c. vasoconstriction.
   d. increased numbers of odontoblasts.

9. Hypersensitivity is best relieved or controlled by
   a. opening the tubules to permit release of intrapulpal pressure.
   b. root planing to remove surface layers that are hypersensitive.
   c. applying antiinflammatory agents to exposed dentin.
   d. blocking exposed tubules on the dentin surface.

10. Deeper cavity preparations have more potential for pulpal damage because
    1. tubule diameter and density increases; therefore, there is increasing permeability.
    2. there is more vibration to pulp cells.
    3. odontoblastic processes are more likely to be severed.
       a. 1 only
       b. 3 only
       c. 1 and 3
       d. 2 and 3

11. Agents that clean, dry, or sterilize the cavity are
    a. best used in deep cavities.
    b. indicated when a patient reports symptoms.
    c. generally very damaging to the pulp.
    d. generally not useful.
12. Of the following, which is the best way to prevent pulp damage during cavity preparation?
    a. Retain the smear layer.
    b. Use sharp burs with a brush stroke.
    c. Use adequate air coolant.
    d. Use adequate water coolant.
13. Which is the major reason why class II restorations with composite are damaging to the pulp?
    a. Microleakage occurs at the occlusal surface
    b. Microleakage occurs at the gingival margin.
    c. Toxic chemicals are released from the composite and diffuse into the pulp.
    d. Polymerization shrinkage distorts cusps and opens gaps.
14. A pulp has been damaged and is inflamed because of deep caries and cavity preparation. What material placed on the floor of the cavity aids the pulp in resolving the inflammation?
    a. calcium hydroxide
    b. zinc oxide–eugenol
    c. steroid formulations
    d. none, there is no material that promotes healing.
15. A cusp fractures and exposes dentin but not the pulp. What is the probable response in the pulp?
    a. severe damage with irreversible inflammation
    b. mild to moderate inflammation
    c. pain but no inflammation
    d. no pulp response
16. The following illustration shows a section of pulp/dentin underlying an area of cavity preparation, which was done 1 day previous. The best description of the pulp reaction is
    a. there is no reaction; the pulp appears normal.
    b. the odontoblast layer is disrupted and there is mild inflammation.
    c. odontoblasts are aspirated into tubules and there is mild inflammation.
    d. odontoblasts are absent and there is extravasation of erythrocytes.

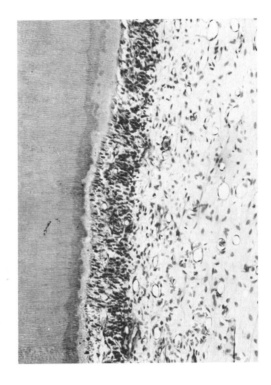

17. This is an area of pulp close to a carious exposure. The inflammatory response is primarily (see illustration below)
    a. acute.
    b. chronic.
    c. giant cell.
    d. vascular.

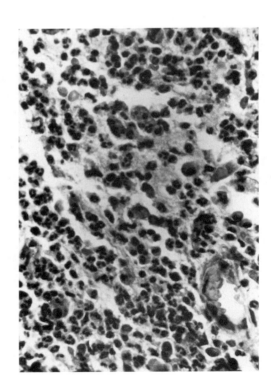

CHAPTER 16: TRAUMATIC INJURIES

1. If several teeth are out of alignment following trauma, the most reasonable explanation is
   a. luxation.
   b. subluxation.
   c. alveolar fracture.
   d. root fracture.

2. Initial vitality testing of traumatized teeth is most useful to
   a. establish a baseline for comparison with future testing.
   b. determine whether root canal treatment is indicated.
   c. determine if the blood supply to the pulp is compromised.
   d. predict the prognosis.

3. A normal periapical radiograph of a traumatized tooth is useful for
   a. visualizing most root fractures.
   b. visualizing concussion injuries.
   c. gathering baseline information.
   d. locating foreign objects.

4. Crown infraction
   a. may indicate luxation injury.
   b. is rarely seen on transillumination.
   c. seldom requires a follow-up examination.
   d. describes the process of necrosis in the coronal pulp.

5. Uncomplicated crown fracture
   a. is an indication for a dentin bonded restoration.
   b. requires baseline pulp testing.
   c. involves root canal treatment if the exposed dentin is sensitive to cold stimulus.
   d. has a questionable long-term prognosis.
   e. is managed differently in young versus older patients.

6. In a complicated crown fracture
   a. exposure to the oral cavity permits rapid bacterial penetration through the pulp.
   b. inflammation is limited to the coronal 2 mm of the exposed pulp for the first 24 hours.
   c. the tooth is normally managed by root canal treatment and restoration.

7. The success of vital pulp therapy in a trauma case is chiefly dependent on
   a. the age of the patient at the time of trauma.
   b. the size of the initial pulp exposure.
   c. the material used to cap the pulp.
   d. the placement of a bacteria-tight restoration.

8. Root fractures in which the coronal segment is slightly mobile, with no coronal dislocation and mild symptoms should be managed by
   a. rigid fixation for 2 to 4 months and periodic evaluation afterward.
   b. removal of the coronal segment and orthodontic extrusion and subsequent root canal treatment of the apical segment.
   c. nonrigid fixation for 7 to 10 days, initiation of root canal treatment, placement of calcium hydroxide, and permanent root canal filling after 4 to 6 months.
   d. none of the above; no treatment is necessary.

9. Replacement resorption
   a. results from direct contact between root dentin and bone.
   b. is managed by surgical exposure and repair with a biocompatible material.
   c. results when at least 75% of the root surface is damaged.
   d. can be avoided by timely endodontic intervention.

10. Pulp necrosis is most likely to occur after
    a. midroot fracture.
    b. intrusive luxation.
    c. concussion.
    d. complicated crown fracture.

11. Cervical root resorption
    a. is a common self-limiting result of luxation injury.
    b. causes significant pulpal symptoms.
    c. can be arrested by root canal treatment.
    d. may extend coronally to present as a pink spot on the crown.

12. Internal root resorption is
    a. more common in permanent than deciduous teeth.
    b. simple to differentiate from other types of resorption.
    c. characterized histologically by inflammatory tissue with multinucleated giant cells.
    d. ruled out when there is no response to pulp testing.

13. A luxated tooth should be splinted
    a. if the tooth is mobile after repositioning.
    b. until the root canal treatment is completed.
    c. with the composite as close to the gingiva as possible.
    d. if any of the above occur.

14. A pulpotomy (coronal pulp removal) is indicated when there is a crown fracture with pulp exposure and
    a. root formation is incomplete and the crown is fractured in the cervical third.
    b. the pulp has been exposed longer than 1 week.
    c. the pulp is hypersensitive to cold.
    d. any portion of the fracture extends to the root.

15. Which medium of storage for an avulsed tooth is best for prolonged extraoral periods?
    a. Hanks balanced salt solution
    b. Milk
    c. Distilled water
    d. Patient saliva

16. If a fully formed tooth has suffered an intrusive injury and the crown is partially exposed, what is the recommended treatment?
    a. Leave alone and allow to erupt spontaneously.
    b. Splint for 7 to 10 days, then observe.
    c. Orthodontically reposition into correct alignment within 3 to 4 weeks.
    d. Reposition with forceps.

17. The most important factor for managing avulsions is
    a. speed of replantation.
    b. decontamination of the root surface.
    c. timely initiation of root canal treatment.
    d. proper preparation of the socket.

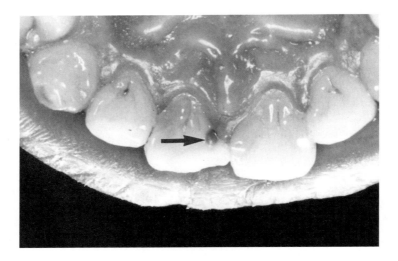

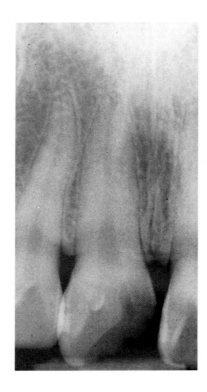

The following case study and questions refer to the illustrations (above): Three days ago, this 22-year-old patient fractured (complicated crown) the mesioincisal surface, exposing the pulp *(arrow)*. The pulp is sensitive to explorer contact.

18. The preferred treatment is
    a. one-visit root canal treatment.
    b. pulpotomy on the first visit and complete root canal treatment on the second visit.
    c. pulp extirpation, placement of calcium hydroxide for at least 6 months, and then root canal treatment.
    d. partial pulpotomy (Cvek technique).

19. The long-term prognosis (success) is affected primarily by
    a. how long the pulp has been exposed.
    b. microleakage of the restoration.
    c. the size of the exposure.
    d. the amount of root development (maturity).

CHAPTER 17: ENDODONTIC PHARMACOLOGY

1. Odontogenic pain is usually caused by
   a. noxious physical stimuli.
   b. the release of inflammatory mediators.
   c. stimulation of sympathetic fibers in the pulp.
   d. edema produced in a ridged noncompliant root canal system.

2. Which of the following best describes the neural innervation of the dental pulp?
   a. A delta fibers transmit pain to the trigeminal nucleus.
   b. C fibers transmit pain to the superior cervical ganglion.
   c. Sympathetic fibers are not blocked with application of local anesthetic agents.
   d. A delta fibers play the predominant role in encoding inflammatory pain.

3. Nociceptive signals are transmitted primarily to the
   a. nucleus caudalis.
   b. limbic system.
   c. reticular system.
   d. superior cervical ganglion.

4. Referred pain may be caused by neural convergence onto which of the following types of neurons?
   a. efferent neurons
   b. local circuit neurons
   c. projection fibers
   d. descending neurons

5. Which of the following statements is true regarding descending fibers?
   a. They inhibit transmission of nociceptive information.
   b. They are not affected by endogenous opioid peptides.
   c. They transmit information from the cerebral cortex to the thalamus.
   d. They are sympathetic fibers that modulate blood flow in the pulp after sensory stimulation.

6. Hyperalgesia is characterized by the following *except* one. Which is this *exception?*
   a. Hyperalgesia is primarily a central mechanism.
   b. Spontaneous pain is present.
   c. The pain threshold is reduced.
   d. Hyperalgesia produces an increased pain perception to a noxious stimuli.

7. Regarding etodolac (Lodine), which of the following statements is correct?
   a. The drug exhibits minimal gastrointestinal irritation when compared to ibuprofen.
   b. When compared to ibuprofen, etodolac has a more profound analgesic action.
   c. Studies indicate etodolac is unique, as the drug does not have a peripheral analgesic mechanism of action.
   d. This drug can be prescribed for adult patients with aspirin hypersensitivity.

8. Activation of the μ-opioid receptor
   a. blocks nociceptive signals from the trigeminal nucleus to higher brain centers.
   b. blocks transmission of signals from the thalamus to the cerebral cortex.
   c. induces the release of endorphins.
   d. blocks the release of dynorphins.

9. Opioids are frequently used in combination with other drugs because
   a. the nonsteroidal antiinflammatory drugs in combination with the opioid act synergistically on the μ-opioid receptor.
   b. the combination permits a lower dosage of the opioid, which can reduce side effects.
   c. opioids do not act peripherally.
   d. opioids are not antipyretic.

10. Which of the following is true for the use of codeine as an analgesic agent?
    a. Codeine prescribed in 60-mg doses is more effective than 650 mg of aspirin.
    b. Codeine prescribed in 30-mg doses is more effective than 600 mg of acetaminophen.
    c. Codeine prescribed in 30-mg doses is more effective than a placebo.
    d. Codeine prescribed in 60-mg doses is more effective than a placebo.

11. Management of pain of endodontic origin should focus on which of the following?
    a. removing the peripheral mechanism of hyperalgesia
    b. providing an adequate level of nonsteroidal antiinflammatory analgesic agent
    c. prescribing an appropriate antibiotic in cases where pain is the result of infection
    d. using long-acting local anesthetic agents to break the pain cycle

12. Which of the following best describes a "flexible plan" for prescribing analgesic agents?
    a. A maximal dose of an opioid is administered. If pain persists, the opioid is supplemented with a nonsteroidal antiinflammatory agent or acetaminophen. Dosages are then alternated.
    b. A maximal dose of a nonsteroidal antiinflammatory agent or acetaminophen is administered. If pain persists, the drug is supplemented with an opioid. Dosages are then alternated.
    c. Patients are advised to take the maximal dose of a nonsteroidal antiinflammatory agent a day before the appointment and then as necessary for postoperative pain.
    d. Patients are advised to take an opioid agent a day before the appointment and then as necessary for postoperative pain.

13. Nonsteroidal antiinflammatory agents administered in combination with cyclosporine may
    a. increase the risk of nephrotoxicity.
    b. induce bone marrow suppression.
    c. decrease the activity of the cyclosporine.
    d. result in increased concentrations of the nonsteroidal agent in the blood plasma.

14. Nonsteroidal antiinflammatory agents administered in combination with anticoagulants may
    a. increase the prothrombin time.
    b. result in a decreased bleeding time.
    c. increase the bioavailability of the anticoagulant.
    d. produce no adverse effect.

15. Indomethacin administered in combination with sympathomimetic agents results in
    a. a decreased blood pressure.
    b. an increased blood pressure.
    c. a decreased water retention.
    d. a decreased absorption of indomethacin, requiring a higher dosage.

16. Odontogenic pain is transmitted to the central nervous system via a three-neuron pathway. The second order neuron
    a. connects the pulpal C fibers with the medullary dorsal horn.
    b. connects the trigeminal ganglion to the thalamus.
    c. connects the nucleus caudalis to the thalamus.
    d. connects the thalamus to the cerebral cortex.

CHAPTER 18: SURGICAL ENDODONTICS

1. Each of the following is a primary concern when evaluating a patient for endodontic surgery *except* one. Which is this *exception?*
   a. blood dyscrasias
   b. "brittle diabetes"
   c. patients receiving renal dialysis
   d. positive test results for HIV infection

2. Patients reporting that they are receiving renal dialysis treatment may exhibit which of the following?
   a. Altered drug metabolism
   b. Normal wound healing (however, a greater susceptibility to infection)
   c. Hypertension
   d. Venous-venous shunts

3. During a presurgical workup the patient should be advised to
   a. begin taking nonsteroidal antiinflammatory analgesics 3 days before the surgical appointment.
   b. begin chlorhexidine rinses 2 days before the appointment.
   c. refrain from eating the day of the scheduled surgery.
   d. take an antibiotic for 7 to 10 days beginning on the day of surgery.

4. The dual entry technique for local anesthesia involves
   a. initial injection of a long-acting local anesthetic agent followed by 2% lidocaine 1:50,000 epinephrine for hemostasis.
   b. initial injection of 2% lidocaine 1:100,000 epinephrine followed by a long-acting local anesthetic following the procedure for pain control.
   c. block anesthesia followed by local infiltration in the gingival tissues for hemostasis.
   d. block anesthesia followed by injection of lidocaine 1:50,000 directly into the periradicular lesion.

5. Hemostasis is enhanced during endodontic surgery by
   a. depositing the anesthetic agent in the alveolar mucosa.
   b. injecting into the attached gingival tissue.
   c. injecting into tissues that have a high concentration of β_2-adrenergic receptors.
   d. injecting into the periodontal ligament of the involved tooth.

6. A mucogingival flap is contraindicated when there is
   a. 8 to 10 mm of attached gingiva.
   b. the patient exhibits a low lip line.
   c. there is a large periradicular lesion.
   d. a porcelain-fused-to-metal restoration is present in the area where flap reflection is required.

7. Postoperative swelling and ecchymosis is most often the result of
   a. employing a mucogingival flap.
   b. crushing the reflected tissue with the retractor.
   c. the failure to use a local anesthetic agent with a vasoconstrictor.
   d. central bleeding in the osseous defect that is not controlled before flap closure.

8. Tissue removed during apical surgery
   a. is almost always inflammatory and therefore does not require microscopic examination.
   b. should be placed in formalin, stored, and submitted for microscopic examination if healing fails to occur.
   c. is nonodontogenic in approximately 10% of the cases.
   d. should be submitted only when root resorption is evident on the radiograph or during the surgical procedure.

9. Apical root resection
   a. is more difficult in cases where the root exhibits a lingual inclination.
   b. should be oblique to expose all apical ramifications.
   c. projects the canal toward the buccal in an oblique resection.
   d. made perpendicular to the canal to expose the largest number of dentinal tubules.

10. Methylene blue dye is used in root end surgery to
    a. provide hemostasis in the osseous crypt.
    b. distinguish the periodontal membrane from tooth structure.
    c. evaluate the sealing ability of the core filling material following root end resection.
    d. promote coagulation and initiate healing following closure of the flap.

11. When used in root end surgery, ferric sulfate
    a. induces hemostasis by collagen activation of platelet aggregation.
    b. is a necrosing agent that causes intravascular coagulation.
    c. is nontoxic and preferred over CollaCote as an intraosseous hemostatic agent.
    d. should be applied in a dry aseptic field.

12. In preparing the root end to receive a root end filling material
    a. the microhandpiece with a quarter round bur is the preferred device to prepare down the long axis of the root.
    b. roots with more than one canal require two separate and distinct preparations to ensure the seal.
    c. the ideal depth is at least 3 mm.
    d. retention is required only when silver amalgam is the restorative material.

13. During endodontic surgery a "tracking groove" is
    a. established 0.5 to 1 mm deep.
    b. placed in the root end with an ultrasonic handpiece using the lowest power setting.
    c. required to guide bur in the microhandpiece.
    d. placed in the cortical plate of bone to hold the retractor and prevent crushing of the reflected tissues.

14. Ultrasonic root end preparation
    a. permits the clinician to include irregularities of the canal in the preparation.
    b. permits the clinician to use acute bevels during root end surgery.
    c. requires a larger osseous window when compared to the microhandpiece.
    d. is performed dry to permit visualization and accurate preparation.

15. In comparing IRM, Super EBA, and amalgam as root end filling materials, which of the following is true?
    a. Super EBA exhibits less eugenol than IRM.
    b. IRM is less toxic than Super EBA.
    c. Super EBA exhibits polymethyl methacrylate.
    d. There is little difference in the sealing ability of the materials; however, over time they are inferior to amalgam.

16. Postsurgical compression of the wound site
    a. permits suturing from the attached to the unattached mucosa.
    b. may produce local areas of ischemia and delay healing.
    c. permits complete closure of the vertical releasing incision and permits healing by primary intention.
    d. decreases the thickness of the coagulum.

17. Pain management following root end surgery should include
    a. opiate narcotic agents, as they do not interfere with hemostasis.
    b. preoperative administration of aspirin.
    c. antibiotics to prevent infection and subsequent pain.
    d. application of an ice pack intermittently for 24 to 48 hours.

18. In performing root end surgery of a maxillary lateral incisor that does not exhibit a periradicular lesion, the clinician can locate the root end by employing each of the following techniques *except* one. Which is this *exception?*
    a. Obtain a parallel preoperative radiograph for measurement.
    b. Note color differences between root and bone.
    c. Place a radiopaque object in the entry point and expose a film.
    d. Prepare a conservative osseous window at the measured length of the root.

19. The 40-year-old woman in the following illustration requires treatment for a sinus tract associated with tooth No. 21. She relates a history of previous root canal treatment followed several years later by root end surgery. Records from the endodontist who performed the surgery indicate Super EBA was used as the root end filling material. The clinical examination reveals a sinus tract, normal mobility, and no tenderness to percussion; probing depths are 3 mm. The most likely cause for failure in this case is
   a. coronal microleakage.
   b. vertical root fracture.
   c. failure to include the isthmus in the preparation.
   d. post perforation.
   e. periodontal abscess.

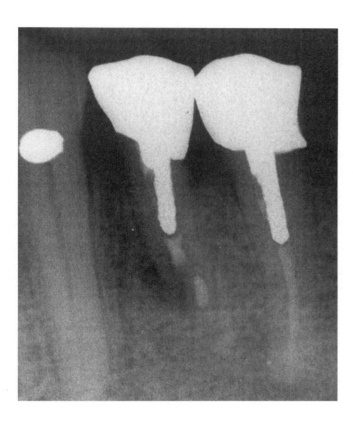

CHAPTER 19: MANAGEMENT OF PAIN AND ANXIETY

1. The majority of life-threatening systemic complications arise
   a. during or immediately following injection of local anesthetic agents.
   b. in conjunction with surgical procedures such as tooth extraction.
   c. during the pulp extirpation phase of root canal treatment.
   d. as a result of bleeding from patients with known blood dyscrasias.

2. Which of the following tooth groups is the most difficult to anesthetize?
   a. maxillary premolars
   b. maxillary molars
   c. mandibular premolars
   d. mandibular molars

3. Each of the following is a factor that affects onset of local anesthesia *except* one. Which is this *exception?*
   a. diffusion of the local anesthetic through the lipid-rich nerve sheath
   b. the pK_a for the anesthetic agent
   c. the pH of the tissue
   d. the protein-binding ability of the local anesthetic agent

4. A decrease in the tissue pH
   a. increases the free base of the local anesthetic agent.
   b. results in fewer anesthetic molecules entering the nerve sheath.
   c. changes the pK_a value for a given local anesthetic agent.
   d. decreases protein binding of the local anesthetic agent.

5. Failure to obtain adequate anesthesia after an appropriately administered nerve block is most likely the result of
   a. pH changes in the pulp tissue caused by inflammation.
   b. morphologic neurodegenerative changes and inflammatory mediators.
   c. insufficient volume of the local anesthetic injected.
   d. tolerance to the anesthetic agent.

6. Each of the following can influence the duration of action of a local anesthetic agent *except* one. Which is this *exception?*
   a. variation in the individual patient's response to the drug
   b. anatomic variations
   c. the type of injection
   d. larger than recommended doses

7. When comparing amide and ester local anesthetic agents, which of the following statements is true?
   a. Esters are more likely to produce systemic toxicity when compared to amides.
   b. Amides are more allergenic when compared to esters.
   c. Amides are more effective than ester anesthetic agents.
   d. Esters and amides are equally effective; however, esters are more likely to produce adverse reactions.

8. A patient is anesthetized using a posterior superior alveolar nerve block to perform endodontic treatment on the maxillary right first molar. Adequate anesthesia is not obtained. In this situation the clinician should consider
   a. anesthetizing the anterior superior nerve.
   b. anesthetizing the middle superior alveolar nerve.
   c. performing a palatal subperiosteal injection.
   d. repeating the posterior superior alveolar nerve block.

9. An infiltration injection is given to a patient for endodontic treatment of a maxillary second premolar. Adequate anesthesia is not obtained. Which of the following injections should be considered?
   a. anterior superior alveolar block
   b. posterior superior alveolar block
   c. palatal infiltration
   d. maxillary second division nerve block
   e. greater palatine nerve block

10. Infiltration in the mandible may be an effective technique treating
    a. the mandibular central incisor.
    b. the mandibular canine.
    c. the mandibular first premolar.
    d. the mandibular second molar.

11. Advantages to using the Gow-Gates technique include
    a. the increased vascularity of the tissue at the site of injection.
    b. the injection can be employed when the patient cannot open the mouth wide.
    c. anesthesia of the buccal and mylohyoid nerves.
    d. a rapid onset of anesthesia with a shorter duration of action.

12. In performing the Akinosi technique
    a. the needle is inserted at the height of the mucogingival junction of the most posterior maxillary tooth.
    b. the needle is passed lingual to the mandibular ramus until osseous tissue is contacted.
    c. injection at the neck of the mandibular condyle is critical.
    d. an incision in the soft tissue overlying the alveolar process, trephination of the cortical bone, and injection into the medullary bone are required.

13. The Stabident local anesthesia system is employed
    a. as a true intraosseous injection.
    b. as a modified periodontal ligament injection.
    c. to limit the adverse reactions to vasopressor components of local anesthetic cartridges.
    d. as a method of administering intrapulpal anesthesia when other injection techniques have proven to be inadequate.

14. Prescriptions for analgesic agents should
    a. include instructions for administration at regular time intervals.
    b. indicate the patient only needs the medication when they experience pain.
    c. be provided to patients in pain 1 day before initiating root canal treatment to establish effective blood levels.
    d. include immediate preoperative administration of opioids when pulp pathosis is the cause.

15. For emergency treatment of patients with pulp pathosis, oral sedation
    a. is indicated when deep sedation of the fearful patient is desired.
    b. with barbiturates should be considered.
    c. with midazolam may provide an amnesia effect.
    d. with a short-acting agent permits the patient to leave the dental office without an escort.

16. The use of nitrous oxide inhalation sedation
    a. produces a significant analgesic effect when used in conjunction with local anesthetic agents.
    b. is difficult in managing endodontic patients because of the application of the rubber dam.
    c. should be considered if oral sedation cannot be employed.
    d. should be used only when an auxiliary of the same sex as the patient is present to assist.

CHAPTER 20: BLEACHING OF NONVITAL AND VITAL DISCOLORED TEETH

1. Discoloration caused by pulp necrosis or intrapulpal hemorrhage is
   a. primarily in dentin.
   b. related to the length of time the tooth has been discolored.
   c. due to tissue by-products or iron sulfides, or both.
   d. is related to all of the above.

2. Excessive fluoride ingested during tooth development may result in
   a. teeth that are discolored when they erupt.
   b. gray-blue discoloration.
   c. enamel hypoplasia.

3. The pulp horn area of anterior teeth should be cleaned to
   a. facilitate straight-line access.
   b. to remove necrotic tissue.
   c. to enhance the area for retention of the acid-etched composite.

4. Single-tooth discoloration is most frequently caused by
   a. necrotic pulp associated with trauma.
   b. tetracycline staining.
   c. obturation materials remaining in the chamber.

5. Of available intracoronal bleaching agents,
   a. sodium perborate is recommended for intracoronal bleaching.
   b. 5.25% hydrogen peroxide is the most common concentration.
   c. carbamide peroxide–based agents are the safest.
   d. the most common are reducing agents.

6. When bleaching a tooth, one must
   a. verify pulp horns are exposed and clean.
   b. remove existing restorations within the chamber.
   c. remove obturating materials below the gingival margins.
   d. perform all of the above.

7. Sodium perborate as a bleaching agent
   a. may be placed as dry granules within the chamber.
   b. should be mixed with 30% hydrogen peroxide and placed in the chamber.
   c. should have the consistency of wet sand when placed.
   d. need not actually contact dentin to be effective.

8. Thermocatalytic technique for bleaching
   a. is associated with external cervical root resorption.
   b. involves using a heat source of 95 to 110° F.
   c. gives better long-term success than walking bleach.

9. Safer nonvital bleaching is accomplished by
   a. evaluation of periodontal tissues before and after treatment.
   b. avoidance of heat, acid-etching agents, and strong concentrations of bleaching agents.
   c. use of internal barriers at the level of the cementoenamel junction.
   d. use of rubber dam.
   e. all of the above.

10. The optimal post bleaching restoration is
    a. fill the chamber with calcium hydroxide powder and place a composite restoration.
    b. fill the chamber with white zinc phosphate cement and place a bonded composite restoration.
    c. etch the chamber and fill with a dentin bonded composite.

11. Mouthguard vital bleaching
    a. is best with mild discolorations.
    b. has a good long-term prognosis for color stability.
    c. is effective for the yellow/brown form of tetracycline stains.
    d. is associated with development of irreversible pulpal damage.

CHAPTER 21: RESTORATION OF THE ENDODONTICALLY TREATED TOOTH

1. Following restoration with a crown, pulp degeneration
    a. may not be evident for many years.
    b. is signaled by acute symptoms.
    c. occurs soon after cementation.
    d. is usually identified by radiographic changes.
2. A principal advantage of a ferrule is
    a. the incidence of root fracture is reduced.
    b. the incidence of recurrent caries is reduced.
    c. a shorter post may be used.
    d. occlusal forces are distributed through the root.
3. The incidence of fractures of teeth when not restored with a crown is lowest in
    a. anterior teeth.
    b. premolars.
    c. molars.
    d. no tooth group; there is no difference.
4. From the following, the greatest loss of coronal strength is
    a. an access preparation in an unrestored, noncarious maxillary incisor.
    b. an access preparation in an unrestored, noncarious maxillary molar.
    c. an access preparation in an unrestored, noncarious mandibular molar.
    d. a MOD preparation in a noncarious premolar with no access preparation.
5. Endodontic access through existing crowns
    a. usually has no effect on porcelain strength.
    b. does not cause separation of the porcelain veneer from the metal substructure.
    c. often leads to excessive removal of coronal tooth structure.
    d. should not be performed.
6. The primary function of a dowel is to
    a. retain the core materials.
    b. strengthen the tooth.
    c. transmit forces apically.
    d. decrease the risk of root fracture.
7. An axiom for restoring an endodontically treated tooth is that
    a. all teeth should be restored with a crown.
    b. all posterior teeth should be restored with cuspal protection.
    c. if a crown is placed, there should be a dowel.
    d. anterior teeth are less likely than posterior teeth to require a crown.

8. Guidelines for dowel length in a tooth with normal periodontal support include
    a. half the length of the canal.
    b. the coronal length of the tooth.
    c. two thirds the bone-supported length of the tooth.
    d. the same length as the core height.
9. Dowel features that contribute the greatest retention include
    a. parallel sides and moderate diameter.
    b. tapered and serrated surface.
    c. parallel sides and serrated surface.
    d. tapered and smooth surface.
10. Compared to nickel-chrome dowels, titanium dowels are
    a. stronger.
    b. less radiopaque.
    c. more allergenic.
    d. more economical.
11. Which is more prone to cause root fracture?
    a. a parallel as compared to a tapered post
    b. a passive as compared to a snug post
    c. a very short as compared to a long post
    d. an antirotational as compared to a round post
12. The microleakage phenomenon is potentially greatest with
    a. composite resin core.
    b. amalgam core.
    c. glass-ionomer core.
    d. cast post and core.
13. Which material should be avoided in teeth with high aesthetic value?
    a. composite resin
    b. amalgam
    c. glass-ionomer
    d. cast post and core
14. Composite cores
    a. are anticarcinogenic.
    b. should be used only in teeth with significant remaining structure.
    c. are dimensionally stable.
    d. are all of the above.
15. Tapered dowels are indicated in roots
    a. with small diameter.
    b. with a significantly tapered canal system.
    c. of short length.
    d. that require no additional preparation following root canal treatment.
16. The major cause of failure of endodontically treated posterior teeth that are periodontally compromised is
    a. recurrent periodontal disease.
    b. root fracture.
    c. endodontic failure.
    d. caries.

17. In the example in the following illustration, what is the error as regarding the post?
    a. It is too long.
    b. It is too small in diameter.
    c. It should be tapered.
    d. It likely is unnecessary.

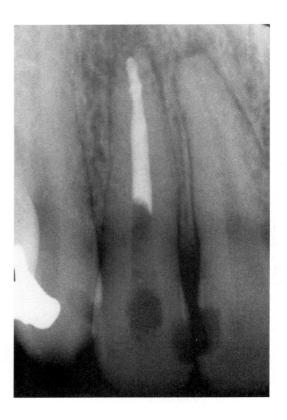

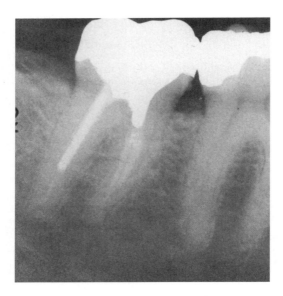

18. The root canal treatment in the following illustration has just been completed. When and how should this tooth be restored?
    a. Restore soon, with an acid-etched composite.
    b. Restore soon, with a full crown and post and core.
    c. Delay until there is evidence of healing. Then restore with a post and core and full crown.
    d. Restore soon. Place a post and acid-etched composite. Do not place a crown.

CHAPTER 22: PEDIATRIC ENDODONTIC TREATMENT

1. The basic morphologic difference between primary and permanent teeth is
   a. the thickness of dentin between the pulp and enamel is greater in primary teeth.
   b. the enamel is thick on primary teeth.
   c. the pulp chamber is comparatively smaller in primary teeth than in permanent teeth.
   d. the pulp horns are higher in primary molars than in permanent molars.

2. Radiographically in primary teeth
   a. pathologic changes in the periradicular tissues are most often apparent at the apexes rather than the furcation in molars.
   b. the presence of calcified masses within the pulp is indicative of acute pulpal disease.
   c. by the time internal resorption is visible the only treatment is extraction.
   d. pathologic bone and root resorption is always indicative of nonvital pulp.

3. Which of the following diagnostic tests are usually reliable for determining pulpal status in primary teeth?
   a. thermal pulp tests
   b. electrical pulp tests
   c. percussion test
   d. none of the above

4. Indirect pulp therapy
   a. is indicated only in the treatment of teeth with deep carious lesions in which there is no clinical evidence of pulpal degeneration of periapical pathosis.
   b. removes much of the bacteria present in the dentin.
   c. includes placing calcium hydroxide or zinc oxide–eugenol over the remaining caries and permanently restoring the tooth with amalgam.
   d. involves all of the above.

5. Direct pulp capping is recommended for primary teeth with
   a. carious exposures.
   b. mechanical exposures.
   c. calcification in the pulp chamber.
   d. all of the above.

6. A calcium hydroxide pulpotomy performed on a young permanent tooth is judged to be successful when
   a. the patient is asymptomatic.
   b. the tooth responds to pulp testing.
   c. normal root development continues.
   d. all of the above occur.

7. Formocresol pulpotomy on a primary tooth is indicated when
   a. there is a history of spontaneous toothache.
   b. the inflammation or infection is confined to the coronal pulp.
   c. the pulp does not hemorrhage.
   d. there is only apical pathosis.

8. An increasingly popular technique for pulpotomy in primary teeth is
   a. formocresol.
   b. calcium hydroxide.
   c. electrosurgery.
   d. laser surgery.

9. Glutaraldehyde may be preferred to formocresol for primary pulpotomy because it
   a. has less systemic distribution beyond the pulp.
   b. has a better prognosis.
   c. is not antigenic.
   d. is less readily metabolized.

10. Each of the following statements regarding primary tooth anatomy is correct *except* one. Which is this exception?
    a. The root-crown ratio is smaller than that of permanent teeth.
    b. The roots are narrower than those of permanent teeth.
    c. The molar roots are more divergent than those of permanent molars.
    d. The roots are shorter than those of permanent teeth.

11. Which of the following is an indication for root canal treatment of primary teeth?
    a. radiographic evidence of internal resorption in the roots
    b. periapical lesion
    c. presence of a dentigerous or follicular cyst
    d. mechanical or carious perforation of the chamber floor

12. Access openings on primary incisors
    a. are from the facial surface.
    b. are from the lingual surface.
    c. are through the incisal edge.
    d. are different for maxillary and mandibular teeth.

13. Which of the following is true in placing zinc oxide–eugenol in a primary tooth?
    a. The technique is not important.
    b. The overfill has a poorer prognosis than a flush fill.
    c. The paste should be a thick mix.
    d. All of the above are true.

CHAPTER 23: GERIATRIC ENDODONTICS

1. As related to dental visits by the older patient,
   a. older patients have fewer visits per year than younger patients.
   b. the number of visits by older patients should decrease in the future.
   c. most visits are for comprehensive procedures.
   d. dental visits of older patients are for less complicated procedures as compared to younger patients.

2. Secondary dentin formation in the radicular pulp in an older patient
   a. is less likely to occur in response to abrasion than in younger patients.
   b. may result in complete pulp obliteration.
   c. may compromise the blood supply and cause pulp necrosis.
   d. does not require an irritant.

3. In the older patient, as compared to a younger patient, pulpal inflammation from caries
   a. is less likely to be as painful as in a younger patient.
   b. usually progresses more slowly.
   c. is less likely to occur.
   d. is more likely to be acute than chronic.

4. The nerve supply in the pulps of older patients
   a. make thermal testing more accurate than electrical testing.
   b. is more dense than in younger pulp.
   c. makes a test cavity a better diagnostic test than in younger patients.
   d. shows fewer peripheral branches coronally than in younger pulps.

5. An abrupt midroot radiographic disappearance of a canal usually indicates
   a. a bifurcation in the canal.
   b. secondary dentin formation apically.
   c. concentrations of dystrophic calcifications apically.
   d. a diminished (often unnegotiable) sized canal.

6. In the older patient, as compared to the younger patient, the exit of the canal (apical foramen) is
   a. closer to the radiographic apex.
   b. closer to the true apex.
   c. easier to detect tactily.
   d. more variable because of cementum formation.

7. Single-visit root canal treatment in an older patient
   a. should be avoided because there is more likely to be an increase in postappointment pain.
   b. should be avoided because it decreases successful prognosis.
   c. is acceptable if it is more convenient for the patient.
   d. should be avoided to place an intracanal medicament.

8. In the older patient, as compared to the younger patient, a general statement on healing of periapical pathosis is that healing
   a. is less predictable.
   b. occurs more slowly.
   c. patterns are similar but possibly with less mineralization.
   d. is more likely to occur by scarring.

9. In the elderly patient, as compared to extraction, root canal treatment is
   a. usually more emotionally traumatic.
   b. usually more tissue traumatic.
   c. often less expensive in the long run.
   d. more likely to result in postappointment complication.

10. A postsurgical problem that tends to be more common in the older patient (compared to the younger patient) is
    a. ecchymosis (discoloration).
    b. increased swelling.
    c. increased pain.
    d. slower healing of incision margins.

11. Periapical radiographs should be prescribed
    a. before discussion of the chief complaint.
    b. after discussing the chief complaint with the patient.
    c. just before the clinical examination.
    d. after completing the clinical examination.

12. With aging
    a. lateral canals enlarge and become more clinically significant.
    b. gingival recession exposes cementum and dentin, which is less resistant to caries.
    c. the cementodentinal junction locates progressively more coronally.
    d. all of the above occur.

13. In geriatric patients
    a. there is a direct correlation between the nature of response to electrical pulp testing and the degree of inflammation.
    b. there is a reduced volume and increased neural component of the pulp.
    c. tooth discoloration usually is not indicative of pulpal death.
    d. diffuse pain of vague origin is unlikely to be odontogenic.

14. In evaluating success and failure of endodontic treatment in aged patients, a consideration is that
    a. the bone of the aged patient is more mineralized than that of a younger patient.
    b. overlooked canals are seldom a problem because they are usually calcified.
    c. there may be failure even though the patient has no symptoms.
    d. cold sensitivity is the usual symptom that indicates a missed canal.

15. Endodontic surgery in elderly patients
    a. requires more anesthetic and vasoconstrictor than in younger patients.
    b. may be somewhat easier because the vestibule is deeper.
    c. is risky because inadequate blood supply may result in postsurgical osteomyelitis.
    d. has been demonstrated to be much less successful than in younger patients.

16. The radiolucent structure at the periapex of the premolar in the following illustration is likely
    a. a maxillary sinus.
    b. an endodontic apical pathosis.
    c. a fibroosseous lesion.
    d. a bony trabecular pattern.

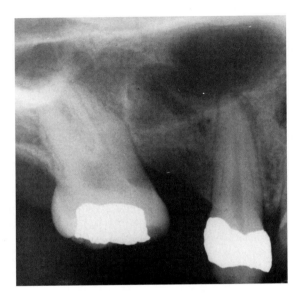

17. The elevated structure facial to the crowned first molar in the following illustration is likely
    a. an acute apical abscess.
    b. a periodontal abscess.
    c. a fibroma.
    d. exostoses.

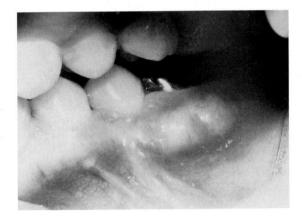

CHAPTER 24: RETREATMENT

1. Canals may be missed during treatment because of
   a. calcification.
   b. anomalous location.
   c. inadequate access.
   d. all of the above.

2. Canals that appear calcified radiographically
   a. are seldom able to be instrumented.
   b. have a different appearance than the surrounding dentin.
   c. should be opened up with rotary rather than ultrasonic instruments.

3. The bubble test is used to
   a. determine the presence of a lateral canal after obturation.
   b. locate a difficult-to-find canal.
   c. verify an oral/antral communication with the canal.

4. Presence of excess gutta-percha beyond the apex is usually caused by
   a. use of too small a master cone.
   b. excessive heating and compaction during warm vertical condensation.
   c. destruction of the natural apical constriction.

5. Lateral or furcal canals are
   a. commonplace.
   b. not able to be mechanically cleaned.
   c. not routinely obturated.
   d. seldom the sole cause of endodontic failure.
   e. all of the above.

6. Retreatment has the most favorable prognosis when
   a. the cause of failure is identified and is correctable.
   b. the patient is asymptomatic.
   c. gutta-percha was used instead of paste.
   d. a surgical microscope is used.

7. Crowns should be removed before retreatment
   a. in most cases to facilitate visibility.
   b. to permit better radiographic interpretation.
   c. when recurrent caries is present, causing coronal leakage.

8. Clinically successful cases with radiographically unsatisfactory obturation
   a. should always be retreated.
   b. should usually be retreated if a new prosthetic restoration is planned.
   c. should be retreated if a post is to be placed.

9. An apical barrier can be created
   a. mechanically with hand instruments.
   b. by placing calcium hydroxide and waiting for apexification.
   c. by placing a mechanical blockage such as CollaCote.
   d. all of the above.

10. Removal of objects can be facilitated by
    a. straight-line access.
    b. a good light source.
    c. magnification.
    d. all of the above.

TEST YOUR KNOWLEDGE

Questions 1 to 3 relate to the radiograph above right.

The patient does not have symptoms. All teeth shown in the radiograph respond to pulp testing, except the canine.

1. The radiolucent structure *(arrow)* at the apex of the canine is likely
   a. maxillary fracture.
   b. apical pathosis.
   c. nasopalatine duct.
   d. nutrient canal.

2. The radiographic appearance internally indicates
   a. there likely are two canals superimposed.
   b. dentinogenesis imperfecta.
   c. dense accumulations of linear calcifications.
   d. calcific metamorphosis.

3. The recommended treatment/reason for the treatment is
   a. root canal treatment; there is pulp pathosis.
   b. root end resection and root end filling; there is pathosis, but the pulp space is too small to attempt root canal treatment.
   c. no treatment; there is no pathosis.
   d. extraction.

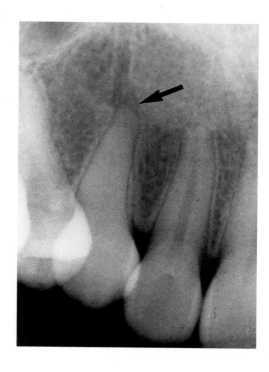

Questions 4 to 8 relate to the photograph on the following page.

Tooth No. 30 (first molar) causes the patient prolonged pain to cold and episodes of spontaneous pain. The tooth responds to probing with an explorer into the carious lesion. There is no pain to percussion or palpation and no swelling. Periodontal probing is within normal limits.

4. What is the pulpal diagnosis?
   a. reversible pulpitis
   b. irreversible pulpitis
   c. necrosis
   d. unknown, pending further information

5. What is the periapical diagnosis?
   a. normal
   b. acute apical periodontitis
   c. chronic apical periodontitis
   d. acute apical abscess

6. What is the likely appearance of the pulp histologically?
   a. Coronal pulp is necrotic; radicular pulp is inflamed.
   b. Coronal pulp is inflamed; radicular pulp is normal.
   c. The entire pulp is inflamed.
   d. The entire pulp is necrotic.

7. What is the likely appearance of the periapex histologically?
   a. normal structures
   b. acute inflammation, no bone resorption
   c. acute inflammation, bone resorption
   d. chronic inflammation, bone resorption
8. What *minimal* immediate treatment is indicated?
   a. None. Schedule the patient for future evaluation.
   b. Complete canal preparation at this visit.
   c. Remove the caries and place a sedative temporarily.
   d. Pulpotomy or partial pulpectomy

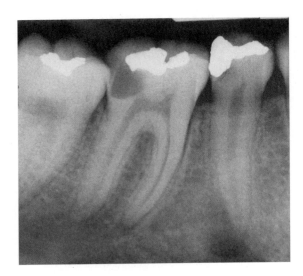

Questions 9 to 13 relate to this radiograph and photograph. (See illustrations below and on next page.)

A 50-year-old woman comes to the clinic complaining of sharp sensitivity with chewing on the lower left second molar. She reports a period of cold sensitivity 6 months prior but has not had any cold tenderness for several months. The third and first molars respond to pulp testing; the second molar does not respond. There is no pain to palpation, but the tooth is tender to percussion on the cusps and tender to biting on a bite stick. There is an isolated 6-mm probing defect on distal. *Photograph:* The shallow occlusal alloy has been removed.

9. What is the pulpal diagnosis for tooth No. 18?
   a. normal
   b. hypersensitive
   c. irreversible pulpitis
   d. necrosis
10. What type of bacteria would likely be found in the pulp?
    a. gram-positive aerobes
    b. gram-negative anaerobes
    c. mixed flora
    d. none
11. What is the likely cause of the patient's pain?
    a. inflamed pulp
    b. apical abscess
    c. cracked tooth
    d. periodontal abscess
12. What additional tests are indicated?
    a. cold test
    b. heat test
    c. test cavity
    d. transillumination
13. What type of permanent restoration is indicated?
    a. occlusal amalgam
    b. occlusal bonded composite
    c. pin-retained amalgam
    d. full cast crown

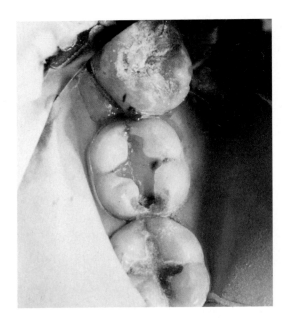

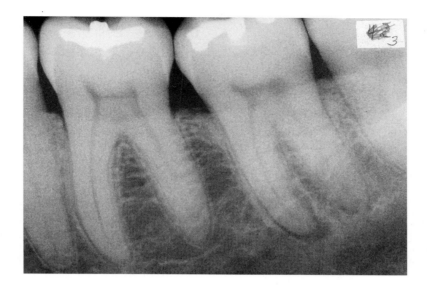

Questions 14 to 20 relate to this radiograph and photograph. (See illustration below.)

   The patient reports "a bad toothache for 2 days. I can't bite on these lower right front teeth." There is pain on pressure and palpation in the region of the lateral incisor and canine. The premolar (small amalgam) is asymptomatic. The lateral and premolar respond to pulp testing; the canine does not respond. There is no swelling. There is an aphthous ulcer on the facial attached gingiva of the lateral. All probings are normal. The lateral and canine have moderate mobility.

14. Which tooth and tissue are the probable source of pain?
    1. lateral
    2. canine
    3. pulp
    4. periapical tissue
       a. 1 and 3
       b. 2 and 3
       c. 2 and 4
       d. 1, 2, and 4

15. What is the likely pulpal/periapical diagnosis for the lateral incisor?
    a. irreversible/phoenix abscess
    b. normal/chronic apical periodontitis
    c. necrosis/phoenix abscess
    d. reversible/normal

16. What is the likely pulpal/periapical diagnosis for the canine?
    a. irreversible pulpitis/phoenix abscess
    b. normal/chronic apical periodontitis
    c. necrosis/phoenix abscess
    d. necrosis/suppurative apical periodontitis

17. Which teeth (tooth) require(s) endodontic treatment?
    a. lateral incisor only
    b. canine only
    c. both the lateral incisor and canine
    d. neither at present observation

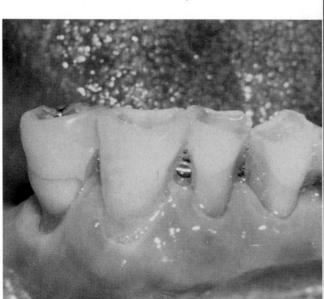

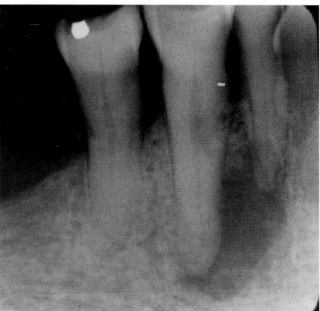

18. Which bacteria have been related to this pathosis?
    a. gram-negative rods, anaerobic
    b. gram-positive rods, anaerobic
    c. gram-negative cocci, aerobic
    d. gram-positive cocci, aerobic
19. Of the following inflammatory cells, which would likely predominate periapically?
    a. lymphocytes
    b. polymorphonuclear neutrophilic leukocytes
    c. plasma cells
    d. macrophages
20. Looking at the radiograph and clinical photograph, what is the likely cause of the pulpal and periapical pathosis?
    a. incisal attrition
    b. cervical erosion
    c. caries
    d. impact trauma

Questions 21 to 25 relate to this radiograph. (See illustration below.)

The patient reports severe, continuous pain in the mandibular right quadrant. She states that the pain began when she was drinking iced tea last evening and the pain has not subsided. She slept poorly last night. Medical history is noncontributory.

Amalgams were placed a few months ago after removal of deep caries on both molars. She has increased pain on lying down. The pain is not relieved with analgesics. She cannot localize the pain to an individual tooth. Pulp testing shows response on the premolar and second molar. The first molar does not respond. Cold water application causes intense, diffuse pain in the region. Percussion and palpation are not painful. Probings are normal.

21. Which tooth (teeth) is (are) the most likely cause of her pain?
    a. premolar
    b. first molar
    c. second molar
    d. b and c

22. What is the pulpal/periapical diagnosis for the first molar?
    a. necrosis/chronic apical periodontitis
    b. necrosis/phoenix abscess
    c. irreversible pulpitis/chronic apical periodontitis
    d. irreversible pulpitis/acute apical periodontitis
23. What is the pulpal/periapical diagnosis for the second molar?
    a. irreversible pulpitis/normal
    b. irreversible pulpitis/acute apical periodontitis
    c. irreversible pulpitis/acute apical abscess
    d. normal/normal
24. What should be the minimal emergency treatment on the offending tooth (teeth)?
    a. Remove the amalgam and place a sedative dressing. Prescribe analgesics and antibiotics.
    b. Do a complete canal preparation. Place a cotton pellet of formocresol.
    c. Reduce the occlusion and prescribe antibiotics.
    d. Perform a pulpotomy and place a dry cotton pellet.
25. Inferior alveolar injection is indicated. If the offending tooth (teeth) is (are) not anesthetized, what is the likely reason?
    a. There is a decreased pH in the region favoring formation of cations.
    b. The anesthetic solution is diluted by the inflammatory fluids.
    c. There may be morphologic changes in the nerves that originate in the inflamed areas; these nerves becomes more excitable.
    d. Because of inflammation, there is increased circulation in the area; this carries away the anesthetic very rapidly.

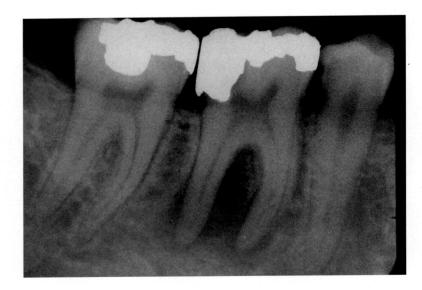

Questions 26 to 28 relate to this radiograph. (See illustration below.)

The patient has no adverse signs or symptoms. Surgery was several years ago. There are no probing defects. The canine responds to pulp testing.

26. What diagnosis is likely?
    a. chronic apical periodontitis
    b. foreign body reaction
    c. apical radicular cyst
    d. scar tissue
27. What is the likely cause?
    a. continued irritation from an undebrided, unsealed canal
    b. adverse reaction to corrosion of the amalgam
    c. coronal leakage
    d. perforation of both cortical plates
28. What should the treatment plan be?
    a. Replace the crown; retreat the canal.
    b. Perform another surgery and place another root end material.
    c. Place the patient on antibiotics to resolve the lesion.
    d. No treatment is needed.

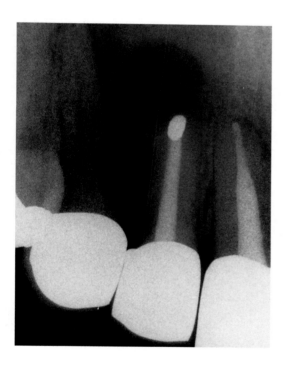

Questions 29 to 35 relate to the radiograph and clinical photograph. (See illustration below and on next page.)

A 58-year-old woman has swelling in the maxillary anterior area that has steadily increased for two days. She denies thermal sensitivity and tenderness to biting pressure. The swelling is between teeth Nos. 9 (central incisor) and 10 (lateral incisor). There is normal mobility, and probing depths are 4 to 5 mm with the distofacial surface of tooth No. 9 probing 8 mm. There is no tenderness to percussion, but there is tenderness to palpation. Pulp tests reveal that teeth Nos. 8, 9, 10, and 11 are responsive to electrical pulp testing and to thermal stimulation with carbon dioxide snow (dry ice).

29. Based on the above information, the clinical photograph, and the radiograph, what is the pulpal diagnosis for tooth No. 9?
    a. normal
    b. reversible pulpitis
    c. irreversible pulpitis
    d. necrotic
30. Based on the above information, the clinical photograph, and the radiograph, what is the pulpal diagnosis for tooth No. 10?
    a. normal
    b. reversible pulpitis
    c. irreversible pulpitis
    d. necrotic
31. What is the periradicular diagnosis for tooth No. 9?
    a. normal
    b. chronic apical periodontitis
    c. chronic suppurative apical periodontitis
    d. acute apical periodontitis
    e. acute periodontal abscess
32. Which of the following is the most likely the cause of swelling associated with teeth Nos. 9 and 10?
    a. pulp necrosis
    b. periodontal disease
    c. a developmental groove defect
    d. vertical root fracture
    e. peripheral giant cell granuloma

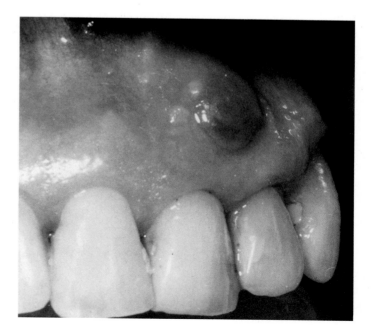

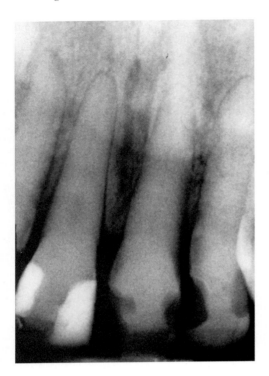

33. Which of the following is most important in determining if this lesion is of periodontal origin or of pulpal origin?
    a. percussion
    b. a periapical radiograph
    c. periodontal mobility and mobility assessment
    d. pulp testing
    e. periodontal probing

34. Treatment of this case requires
    a. periodontal scaling, root planing of the area, and drainage.
    b. root canal debridement of tooth No. 9 followed by incision and drainage.
    c. analgesic and antibiotic treatment until the involved tooth can be localized.
    d. flap reflection to inspect the root for a vertical root fracture or lateral canal.
    e. Surgical excision and biopsy.

35. Which of the following statements is true regarding the effects of periodontal treatment procedures on the dental pulp?
    a. Scaling and root planing procedures remove cementum, expose dentinal tubules, which are invaded and result in pulp inflammation.
    b. Citric acid application appears to produce pulpal inflammation when used in conjunction with reattachment procedures.
    c. Hypersensitivity may result from scaling but is a sign of pulpal pathosis/inflammation.
    d. Scaling and root planing procedures may produce deposition of reparative dentin.

ANSWER KEY

Chapter 1

1. b	7. a	13. b
2. d	8. c	14. a
3. b	9. c	15. c
4. b	10. d	16. c
5. b	11. a	17. d
6. d	12. d	18. c

Chapter 2

1. d	9. b	16. b
2. d	10. c	17. a
3. c	11. b	18. a
4. a	12. b	19. b
5. b	13. a	20. d
6. b	14. b	21. c
7. b	15. c	22. a
8. b		

Chapter 3

1. d	8. d	15. c
2. c	9. c	16. b
3. d	10. c	17. a
4. c	11. a	18. d
5. b	12. d	19. a
6. d	13. b	20. a
7. c	14. b	

Chapter 4

1. d	5. d	8. c
2. a	6. c	9. c
3. b	7. d	10. a
4. c		

Chapter 5

1. d	8. a	15. b
2. c	9. a	16. b
3. c	10. d	17. c
4. c	11. c	18. c
5. a	12. b	19. c
6. a	13. a	20. a
7. c	14. a	21. d

Chapter 6

1. a	5. b	8. b
2. c	6. d	9. a
3. b	7. b	10. b
4. a		

Chapter 7

1. b	8. a	15. c
2. a	9. b	16. a
3. b	10. c	17. c
4. a	11. a	18. b
5. c	12. d	19. a
6. a	13. d	20. a
7. d	14. c	21. c

Chapter 8

1. c	6. b	11. c
2. d	7. d	12. a
3. e	8. a	13. b
4. c	9. a	14. d
5. b	10. c	15. a

Chapter 9

1. d	6. d	11. d
2. a	7. b	12. d
3. c	8. b	13. a
4. d	9. a	14. c
5. a	10. a	

Chapter 10

1. d	5. b	9. d
2. b	6. a	10. c
3. c	7. a	11. a
4. b	8. b	

Chapter 11

1. b	9. d	17. a
2. c	10. d	18. c
3. b	11. d	19. d
4. a	12. a	20. b
5. b	13. d	21. c
6. d	14. d	22. b
7. a	15. b	23. c
8. c	16. d	

Chapter 12

1. d	7. d	12. b
2. d	8. b	13. d
3. b	9. d	14. a
4. c	10. a	15. b
5. a	11. c	16. a
6. d		

Chapter 13

1. b	8. b	14. d
2. c	9. a	15. a
3. b	10. d	16. a
4. a	11. a	17. d
5. b	12. b	18. a
6. a	13. c	19. a
7. a		

Chapter 14

1. a	8. d	15. e
2. c	9. e	16. b
3. b	10. a	17. c
4. b	11. a	18. b
5. a	12. a	19. c
6. a	13. b	20. c
7. a	14. b	

Chapter 15

1. d	7. a	13. b
2. d	8. a	14. d
3. a	9. d	15. b
4. d	10. c	16. b
5. b	11. d	17. a
6. a	12. d	

Chapter 16

1. c	8. a	14. a
2. a	9. a	15. a
3. c	10. b	16. c
4. a	11. d	17. a
5. b	12. c	18. d
6. b	13. a	19. b
7. d		

Chapter 17

1. a	7. a	12. b
2. a	8. a	13. a
3. a	9. b	14. a
4. c	10. d	15. b
5. a	11. a	16. c
6. a		

Chapter 18

1. d	8. c	14. a
2. a	9. a	15. a
3. b	10. b	16. d
4. a	11. b	17. d
5. a	12. c	18. d
6. d	13. a	19. c
7. b		

Chapter 19

1. a	7. c	12. a
2. d	8. b	13. a
3. d	9. a	14. a
4. b	10. d	15. c
5. c	11. c	16. d
6. d		

Chapter 20

1. d	5. a	9. e
2. c	6. d	10. b
3. b	7. c	11. a
4. c	8. a	

Chapter 21

1. a	7. d	13. b
2. a	8. b	14. b
3. a	9. c	15. b
4. d	10. a	16. a
5. c	11. c	17. d
6. a	12. c	18. a

Chapter 22

1. d	6. c	10. a
2. c	7. b	11. b
3. d	8. c	12. d
4. d	9. a	13. d
5. b		

Chapter 23

1. c	7. c	13. c
2. d	8. c	14. c
3. a	9. c	15. b
4. d	10. a	16. a
5. a	11. d	17. d
6. d	12. b	

Chapter 24

1. d	5. e	8. c
2. b	6. a	9. d
3. b	7. c	10. d
4. c		

Test Your Knowledge

1. d	13. d	25. c
2. d	14. c	26. d
3. c	15. d	27. d
4. b	16. c	28. d
5. a	17. b	29. a
6. b	18. a	30. a
7. a	19. b	31. e
8. d	20. a	32. b
9. d	21. c	33. d
10. c	22. a	34. a
11. c	23. a	35. d
12. d	24. d	

Index